The Essential Guide to Prescription Drugs

The Essential Guide to Prescription Drugs

1990 EDITION

James W. Long, M.D.

Harper & Row, Publishers, New York
Grand Rapids, Philadelphia, St. Louis, San Francisco
London, Singapore, Sydney, Tokyo, Toronto

THE ESSENTIAL GUIDE TO PRESCRIPTION DRUGS 1990. Copyright © 1977, 1980, 1982, 1985, 1987, 1988, 1989 by James W. Long. All rights reserved. Printed in the United States of America. No part of this book may be used or reproduced in any manner whatsoever without written permission except in the case of brief quotations embodied in critical articles and reviews. For information address Harper & Row, Publishers, Inc., 10 East 53rd Street, New York, N.Y. 10022.

Designed by C. Linda Dingler

Library of Congress Catalog Card Number 87-657561
ISSN 0894-7058
ISBN 0-06-055171-2   89 90 91 92 93 HC 10 9 8 7 6 5 4 3 2 1
ISBN 0-06-096394-8 (pbk.)   90 91 92 93 HC 10 9 8 7 6 5 4

Contents

SECTION SIX:
Tables of Drug Information

Author's Note for the 1990 Edition

Upon reflection on significant changes in health care services and public awareness that have occurred during the last decade, it seems prudent to rethink the mission of this book and the nature of the information it should provide. Several forces signal the need for change: the rapid increase in the introduction of new and more powerful drugs that require greater knowledge and vigilance by both physician and patient; the expanding emphasis on multiple-drug regimens for treating serious disorders; and the growing tendency of more informed individuals to assume an active role (some would say "take charge") in the management of their drug therapy. Changes of progress always require appropriate adjustments.

This new edition of the Guide will enhance its character as a responsible "bridge text" that can better facilitate the exchange of information between health care providers (physicians, dentists, nurses, pharmacists) and consumers. The drugs included for presentation (always limited by the size of the book) will be confined to those of major importance. They will be selected primarily on the basis of the seriousness of the disorder being treated and the complexity of the drug's actions and usage. The scope of information presented for each drug will provide the breadth and depth of detail required to achieve optimal therapeutic benefit with minimal risk and harm—in language suitable for the reading public. Drugs of minor and fading importance (though used widely) will be omitted to allow the inclusion of the major drugs in current use. Information regarding drug advantage and choice will attempt to reflect medical consensus at the time of writing.

While some readers may be disappointed that "their drug" is not presented in a given edition, it is the author's opinion that the overriding need is for information in depth that relates to those drugs and disorders that impact most significantly on the health and well-being of the public at large.

Newly added features of this edition include: (1) a separate information category in each Drug Profile detailing the drug's effect on sexual function; (2) ten new Drug Profiles of major drugs, eight of them introduced (or soon to be introduced) for use in the United States since publication of the last edition; (3) expansion of the information categories dealing with *New Drugs in Development, Current Controversies in Drug Management, Possible Advantages of This Drug,* and *Drug of Choice* designations; (4) the provision of names, addresses and telephone numbers of national organizations that provide helpful information and guidance to those with the major disorders presented in Section Two.

As noted in each previous edition, no claim is made that all known actions, side-effects, adverse effects, precautions, interactions, etc., for a drug are included in the information provided in the six sections that comprise this book. While diligent care was taken to ensure the accuracy of the information provided during the preparation of this revision, the continued accuracy and currentness are ever subject to change relative to the dissemination of new information derived from drug research, development and general usage.

1
HOW TO USE THIS BOOK

2
GUIDELINES FOR SAFE
AND EFFECTIVE DRUG USE

1

How to Use This Book

Your physician has advised you to take a drug (or drugs), or you have been directed to administer a drug (or drugs) to someone under your care. The kind and amount of information you have been given about how to use these drugs, and what to expect from them, will vary tremendously. In many instances it will not be practical or possible for the physician to provide you with *all* the information that could be considered appropriate and useful, or it will be difficult for you to remember it. From time to time you will find it desirable—even necessary—to seek clarification and guidance about some aspect of drug action or drug use. The aim of this book is to give you the kind of information you may need to supplement the direction and guidance you receive from your physician.

The book consists of six sections. The first section will give you the orientation and insight necessary to appreciate the complexities of modern drug therapy and help you to make the best use of the information contained in Sections Two through Six.

Section Two presents useful information regarding the role of drugs in treating 25 common chronic disorders that require long-term drug therapy. A synopsis of each disorder is followed by information categories that cover drug selection, the goals of drug treatment and an overview of drug management during the period of therapy. A list of the disorders reviewed is found in the introduction to the section.

Section Three is a compilation of Drug Profiles covering 220 prescription (and several nonprescription) drugs used widely in the United States and Canada. The selection of each drug was based upon three considerations: the extent of its use; the urgency of the

3

conditions for which it is prescribed; the volume and complexity of the information essential to its proper utilization. The Drug Profiles are arranged alphabetically by generic name. (Some generic names have spellings similar to other generic names; be careful not to confuse one with another.)

The Profile of each drug is presented in a uniform sequence of information categories. (When you become familiar with the format, you will be able to find quickly specific items of information on any drug, without having to read the entire Profile.) Each Drug Profile contains 42 (or more) separate categories of information. The principal categories include the following.

Year Introduced

This tells you how long the drug has been in general use. The older the drug, the more likely its full spectrum of actions is known and the less likely its continued use will produce new surprises. The date given represents the year the drug was introduced for human use anywhere in the world.

Drug Class

This identifies the principal therapeutic class(es) to which the drug belongs. When appropriate, the chemical and/or pharmacological class designations are also given. You will find it helpful to recognize the class of the drug you are taking because many actions, reactions and interactions with other drugs are often shared by drugs of the same class. Throughout this book (and in most literature on drug information) you will find reference to drugs by their class designation. (Section Four provides alphabetically arranged listings of the classes of drugs referred to in this guide.)

Prescription Required

This indicates whether a drug is a prescription or a nonprescription (over-the-counter) purchase. Because there are significant differences in prescription requirements between the United States and Canada, the designation for each country is given when appropriate.

Controlled Drug

Drugs subject to regulation under the Controlled Substances Act of 1970 (those with potential for abuse) are so designated by the particular schedule that governs their dispensing in the United States. A corresponding schedule is also given for Canada when applicable.

A description of the Schedules of Controlled Drugs is found inside the back cover of this guide.

Available for Purchase by Generic Name

Increasing interest in the availability of prescription drugs for purchase by their generic names has been prompted by two issues of major significance. The first is concerned with the cost of prescription drugs. The comparison shopper realizes that in general the cost of prescription medication is significantly less when a generic equivalent of a brand name product is purchased. The second issue relates to what is termed "bioavailability and bioequivalence"—the comparative composition, quality and effectiveness of the generic versus the brand name drug product. Further discussion of bioavailability and bioequivalence of drug products will be found in the Glossary, Section Five.

Brand Names

These are provided to confirm that you are consulting the correct Drug Profile. They may also help you to recognize a brand name that identifies this drug as one that produced in you an unfavorable reaction on previous use. Brand names are listed for the United States and for Canada (♦). A combination drug (a drug product with more than one active ingredient) is identified by [CD] following the brand name.

In a few instances a particular brand name in current use in both the United States and Canada will represent entirely different generic drugs (in a single drug product), or a significantly different mixture of generic ingredients (in a combination drug product). The generic composition of such brand name products is identified by country in the index. Travelers between the two countries who obtain their medications by brand name in either country are advised to ascertain that they are being provided the intended generic drug(s) in every instance.

Benefits versus Risks

A deliberate attempt is made here to crystallize the "pros" and "cons" for each drug. The format adopted for this category utilizes capital letters to give weight (emphasis) to the drug's principal benefits and risks, and lower case letters are used for benefits and risks of lesser significance. A glance reveals the comparative "weights" of the two columns and provides an initial and tentative impression as to whether a drug's benefits exceed its risks, or vice versa, or whether its benefits and risks seem to be roughly equivalent.

This presentation is not intended to be the principal basis for decision on whether or not to use the drug. Its purpose is to enjoin the reader to be more circumspect and discriminating in his or her use of drugs. The failure to give adequate attention to the individualization of drug selection and dosage is perhaps the greatest weakness seen in the current management of drug therapy.

Principal Uses

A drug may be available as a single drug product or in combination with other drugs. In this section of the Profile under the designation As a Single Drug Product, you will find the primary use(s) of the drug when used alone. Under the designation As a Combination Drug Product [CD], you will find the primary use(s) when combined with other active drugs within the same tablet, capsule, etc. The uses stated are those determined by consensus within the medical community and substantiated by current scientific study. Combination drugs have been developed because some conditions that warrant drug therapy have more than one cause, are characterized by a variety of symptoms or may be treated in more than one way. Where appropriate, in this guide, the logic for combining certain drugs to enhance their therapeutic value is explained. When you find the designation for Combination Drugs [CD] in the Brand Name list at the beginning of the Drug Profile, read under the Principal Uses section to learn more about the drug's use in combination products.

How This Drug Works

This simplified explanation is limited to consideration of how the drug acts to produce its principal (intended) therapeutic effect(s). If a specific method of action has not been established, the currently held theory is given.

Available Dosage Forms and Strengths

This represents a composite of available manufacturers' dosage forms (tablets, capsules, elixirs, etc.) and strengths, without company identification. Included are those dosage forms appropriate for use by outpatients and in extended care facilities and nursing homes. Dosage forms limited to hospital use are not included. Refer to Dosage Forms and Strengths in the Glossary for an explanation of those few abbreviations used to designate the strengths of each dosage form.

Usual Adult Dosage Range

The dosage information given represents a carefully derived consensus by appropriate authorities and is the currently recommended standard. It is provided as a guide that indicates the amount of the drug that is reasonably expected to be both effective and safe when properly used for its intended purpose. Under certain circumstances, your physician may elect to modify this "standard" dosage scheme. Adhere strictly to his or her prescribed dosages and schedules.

Dosing Instructions

Specific guidance is given here regarding the timing of oral medication with regard to food intake. In addition, there are occasions when an individual finds it difficult or impossible to swallow a tablet or a capsule, and the drug to be taken is not available in a liquid dosage form. On those occasions when the patient's condition urgently requires the medication, one may wish to crush the tablet or open the capsule and mix the contents with a palatable food or beverage for administration. Many of today's drugs are available in a bewildering array of solid dosage forms, some of which should *not* be altered to accommodate administration. This information category identifies those dosage forms of each drug that may be and those that should not be altered for administration. In addition, your pharmacist can provide appropriate guidance if you should need it.

Usual Duration of Use

Many factors influence the period of time required for any drug to exert beneficial effects. Among them are the nature and severity of the symptoms being treated, the formulation and strength of the drug, the presence or absence of food in the stomach, the ability of the patient to respond and the concurrent use of other drugs. The information in this category is helpful in preventing premature termination of medication in treatment situations where improvement may seem to you to be unreasonably delayed. Where appropriate, limitations in the duration of use are given.

This Drug Should Not Be Taken If

This category consists of the *absolute* contraindications to the use of the drug (see Contraindications in Glossary). It is most important that you alert your physician or dentist if any information in this category applies to you.

Inform Your Physician Before Taking This Drug If

This category lists the *relative* contraindications to the use of the drug. Here again, it is important that you communicate all relevant information to your physician or dentist.

Possible Side-Effects

This category describes the natural, expected and usually unavoidable actions of the drug—the normal and anticipated consequences of taking it. It is important that you maintain a realistic perspective that balances properly the occurrence of side-effects and the goals of treatment. Consult your physician for guidance whenever side-effects are troublesome or distressing, so that appropriate adjustments of your treatment program can be made.

Possible Adverse Effects

This category includes those unusual, unexpected and infrequent drug effects that are commonly referred to as adverse drug reactions. For the sake of evaluation, adverse effects are classified as mild or serious in nature. It is always wise to inform your physician as soon as you have reason to suspect you may be experiencing an adverse drug effect. Serious adverse reactions usually announce their development initially in the form of mild, unthreatening symptoms. It is important that you remain alert to significant changes in your well-being when you are taking a drug that is known to be capable of producing a serious adverse effect. It is also possible to experience an adverse reaction that has not yet been reported. Do not discount the possibility of an adverse effect just because it is not listed in this category. Following standard practice, some adverse reactions (and interactions) of certain drugs are listed, as a precaution, because these reactions are associated with the use of a particular class of drugs. Although the literature may not document such reactions in connection with the use of an individual drug within that class, the possibility of their occurrence must be considered.

A word of caution is appropriate here. You have consulted your physician for medical evaluation and management. He or she has advised you to take a drug (or administer it to someone else). It is important that you recognize and understand that *in the vast majority of instances a properly selected drug has a comparatively small chance of producing serious harm.* Most of the drugs included in this book produce serious adverse effects rarely. Knowledge that a drug is capable of causing a serious adverse reaction should not deter you from using it when it has been properly selected and its use will be carefully supervised.

Possible Effects on Sexual Function

The growing interest and concern of the medical community and the general public regarding the potential effects of many drugs on sexual function justify this designated category for the provision of relevant information. This aspect of drug performance has not received the professional scrutiny or public disclosure commensurate with its importance. Currently available information (often inadequate and vague) from all reliable sources is presented for consideration. In the interest of compliance and effective management, both physician and patient are well advised to discuss frankly the full significance of any potential effect that proposed drug therapy could have on all aspects of sexual expression.

Adverse Effects That May Appear Similar to Natural Diseases or Disorders

The failure to recognize that a given symptom or disorder is actually drug induced occurs with surprising frequency. Quite often this inadvertent error is compounded by the administration of yet another drug to relieve the "symptoms" (unrecognized manifestations) of a drug being taken on a regular basis. For milder symptoms (*e.g.*, the nasal congestion and diarrhea caused by reserpine), the oversight may not be too serious. But in the case of parkinsonlike effects of some drugs, the mistake can be devastating. This category can alert you to this common flaw in the management of drug therapy.

Natural Diseases or Disorders That May Be Activated by This Drug

Similar to the situation described in the previous category, many drugs in common use are capable of "activating" latent disorders that may not be recognized as drug induced. The development of a new and seemingly unrelated disorder during the course of any treatment program should arouse suspicion that it may be drug related.

Caution

This category provides information on certain aspects of drug action and/or drug use that require special emphasis. Occasionally these warnings may relate to information provided in other categories.

When included here, such entries are of sufficient importance to warrant repetition.

Precautions for Use by Infants and Children

In addition to mandatory adjustments of drug dosage for infants and children under twelve years of age, some drugs and/or treatment situations call for special precautions. This category provides such information for selected drugs. When administering *any* drug (whether prescription or over-the-counter drug), it is advisable to ask the attending physician about precautions to observe or procedures to follow.

Precautions for Use by Those over 60 Years of Age

Changes in body composition and function occur naturally as part of normal aging. As would be expected, there is enormous individual variation in the speed with which such changes occur and the degree of these changes. With regard to medical management—and to drug therapy in particular—the assessment of one's "age" must be based upon the individual's mental and physical condition and never upon years alone. In general, however, it should be recognized that changes that accompany aging may affect the actions of the body on the drug, as well as the actions of the drug on the body. Appropriate precautions are outlined in this category.

Advisability of Use During Pregnancy: Pregnancy Category

Information regarding the safe use of a particular drug during pregnancy was one of the most forceful concerns that led to the formal petitioning of the Food and Drug Administration in 1975 for the provision of such guidance to the public. Most category designations are labeled "tentative" at this time in recognition of the fact that data not readily available now may be advanced by pharmaceutical manufacturers as they negotiate with the FDA to eventually determine final category assignments. The FDA definitions of the five Pregnancy Categories are listed inside the back cover of the book. It should be noted that the FDA does not make the initial category assignment; this is the responsibility of the manufacturer that markets the drug. The initial designation is then subject to review and modification by the FDA as deemed appropriate. The Pregnancy Category designations presented in each Profile were determined by the author after thorough review of pertinent literature and consultation with appropriate authorities. They are offered at this time for initial guidance only. They are in no sense "official" and do not have the endorsement of either the manufacturer or the FDA.

Advisability of Use If Breast-Feeding

Information presented here includes what could be ascertained regarding the effects of the drug on milk production, the presence of the drug in human milk and the possible effects of the drug on the nursing infant. Prudent recommendations are given where appropriate.

Suggested Periodic Examinations While Taking This Drug

This category lists those examinations your physician may recommend you undergo while taking the drug(s) he or she has prescribed, in order to monitor your reaction to them and the course of your condition. You should remember that the advisability of performing such examinations varies greatly from one situation to another, and is best left to the judgment of your physician. The selection and timing of examinations are based on many variables, including your past and present medical history, the nature of the condition under treatment, the dosage and anticipated duration of drug use and your physician's observations of your response to treatment. There may be many occasions when he or she will feel no examinations are necessary.

To assure optimal results from drug treatment, it is important that you keep your physician informed of all developments you think may be drug related.

While Taking This Drug, Observe the Following: Marijuana Smoking

The widespread "social" use of marijuana by virtually all age groups has led to inquiries regarding the possibility of interactions between the pharmacologically active chemicals in marijuana smoke and medicinal drugs in common use. Currently available literature on the health aspects of marijuana use contains very little practical information concerning the potential for drug interactions. The limited information presented in this category of selected Drug Profiles represents those *possible interactions* that are considered likely to occur in view of the known pharmacological effects of the principal components of marijuana and of the medicinal drug reviewed in the Profile. In most instances, the interaction statements are not based on documented evidence since very little is available. However, the conclusions stated—derived by logical inductive reasoning—represent the concurrence of authorities with expertise in this field.

While Taking This Drug, Observe the Following: Other Drugs

For clarification of this confusing and often controversial area of drug information, this category is divided into five subcategories of possible interactions between drugs. Observe carefully the wording of each subcategory heading (see also Interaction in Glossary). Some of the drugs listed as possible interactants do not have a representative Profile in Section Three. If you are using one of these drugs, consult your physician or pharmacist for guidance regarding potential interactions. A brand name (or names) that follows the generic name of an interacting drug is given for purposes of illustration only. It is not intended to mean that the particular brand(s) named have interactions that are different from other brands of the same generic drug. If you are taking the generic drug, *all* brand names under which it is marketed are to be considered as possible interactants.

Driving, Hazardous Activities

In addition to driving motor vehicles, the information in this category applies to any activity of a dangerous nature such as operating machinery, working on ladders, using power tools and handling weapons.

Aviation Note

Until the publication of Dr. Stanley Mohler's *Medication and Flying: A Pilot's Drug Guide* in 1982, there was no authoritative source of current drug information written specifically to serve the needs of civil aviation. The military airman enjoys the expert guidance and surveillance provided by the flight surgeon, but no tightly structured control system exists for his civilian counterpart. However, the need for practical information regarding the possible effects of medicinal drugs on flight performance is the same for pilots in all settings. This category is designed to inform the civilian pilot how a particular drug may affect his or her eligibility to fly and when it is advisable or necessary to consult a designated Aviation Medical Examiner or an FAA medical officer.

Occurrence of Unrelated Illness

This category relates to those drugs that require careful regulation of daily doses to maintain a constant drug effect within critical limits. Anticoagulants, antidiabetic medication and digitalis are examples of such drugs. Emphasis is given to those interim illnesses, separate from the condition for which the drug has been prescribed, that might affect the established schedule of drug use.

Discontinuation

This aspect of drug use is often overlooked when a plan of drug therapy is first discussed. However, for some drugs it is mandatory that the patient be fully informed on *when* to discontinue, when *not* to discontinue and precisely *how* to discontinue use of the drug.

Another consideration in discontinuation is the need to adjust the dosage schedules of other drugs being taken concurrently. The physician who is primarily responsible for your overall management must be kept informed of *all* the drugs you are taking at a given time.

The remaining information categories in the Drug Profile are self-explanatory.

Section Four is a presentation of Drug Classes arranged alphabetically according to their chemical or therapeutic class designation. The drugs within each class are listed alphabetically by their generic names. Because of their chemical composition and biological activities, some drugs will appear in two or more classes. For example, the drug product with the brand name Diuril will be represented by its generic name, chlorothiazide, in three drug classes: the Thiazide Diuretics (a chemical classification), the Diuretics (a drug action classification) and the Antihypertensives (a disease-oriented classification).

Frequently in the Drug Profiles in Section Three you are advised to "See (a particular) Drug Class." This alerts you to a possible contraindication for drug use, or to possible interactions with certain foods, alcohol or other drugs. In each case, you can determine the more readily recognized brand names for each drug listed generically within a drug class by consulting the appropriate Drug Profile. Timely use of these references will enable you to avoid many possible hazards of medication.

Section Five is a glossary of drug-related terms used throughout the book. The preferred use of each term is explained. Frequent references to the Glossary are made in the Drug Profiles. Use of the Glossary will increase your understanding of how to recognize and interpret significant drug effects.

Section Six consists of tables of drug information. The title and introductory material explain the content and purpose of each table. The information in the tables is drawn from certain information categories in the Profiles and is rearranged to emphasize pertinent aspects of drug behavior. The tables are intended to provide another source of ready reference.

The index of Brand and Generic Names in the back of the book is a single alphabetical listing that provides page references to the appropriate Drug Profile(s) for all drugs found in this book. Its usefulness will be enhanced if you read first the introductory explanation of the special features of this combined index.

2

Guidelines for Safe and Effective Drug Use

DO NOT

- pressure your physician to prescribe drugs that, in his or her judgment, you do not need.
- take prescription drugs on your own or on the advice of friends and neighbors because your symptoms are "just like theirs."
- offer drugs prescribed for you to anyone else without a physician's guidance.
- change the dose or timing of any drug without the advice of your physician (except when the drug appears to be causing adverse effects).
- continue to take a drug that you feel is causing adverse effects, until you are able to reach your physician for clarification.
- take *any* drug (prescription or nonprescription) while pregnant or nursing an infant until you are assured by your physician that no harmful effects will occur to either mother or child.
- take any more medicines than are absolutely necessary. (The greater the number of drugs taken simultaneously, the greater the likelihood of adverse effects.)
- withhold from your physician important information about previous drug experiences. He or she will want to know both beneficial and undesirable drug effects you have experienced in the past.
- take any drug in the dark. Identify every dose of medicine carefully in adequate light to be certain you are taking the drug intended.

- keep drugs on a bedside table. Drugs for emergency use, such as nitroglycerin, are an exception. It is advisable to have only one such drug at the bedside for use during the night.

DO

- know the name (and correct spelling) of the drug(s) you are taking. It is advisable to know both the brand name and the generic name.
- read the package labels of all nonprescription drugs to become familiar with the contents of the product.
- follow your physician's instructions regarding dosage schedules as closely as possible. Notify him or her if it becomes necessary to make major changes in your treatment routine.
- thoroughly shake all liquid suspensions of drugs to ensure uniform distribution of ingredients.
- use a standardized measuring device for giving liquid medications by mouth. The household "teaspoon" varies greatly in size.
- follow your physician's instruction on dietary and other treatment measures designed to augment the actions of the drugs prescribed. This makes it possible to achieve desired drug effects with smaller doses. (A familiar example is the reduction of salt intake during drug treatment for high blood pressure.)
- keep your personal physician informed of all drugs prescribed for you by someone else. Consult him or her regarding nonprescription drugs you intend to take on your own initiative at the same time that you are taking drugs prescribed by him or her.
- inform your anesthesiologist, surgeon and dentist of *all* drugs you are taking, prior to any surgery.
- inform your physician if you become pregnant while you are taking any drugs from any source.
- keep a written record of *all* drugs (and vaccines) you take during your entire pregnancy—name, dose, dates taken and reasons for use.
- keep a written record of *all* drugs (and vaccines) to which you become allergic or experience an adverse reaction. This should be done for each member of the family, especially the elderly and infirm.
- keep a written record of *all* drugs (and vaccines) to which *your children* become allergic or experience an adverse reaction.
- inform your physician of all known or suspected allergies, especially allergies to drugs. Be certain that this information is included in your medical record. (Allergic individuals are four times more prone to drug reactions than those who are free of allergy).

- inform your physician promptly if you think you are experiencing an overdose, a side-effect or an adverse effect from a drug.
- determine if it is safe to drive a car, operate machinery or engage in other hazardous activities while taking the drug(s) prescribed.
- determine if it is safe to drink alcoholic beverages while taking the drug(s) prescribed.
- determine if any particular foods, beverages or other drugs should be avoided while taking the drug(s) prescribed.
- keep all appointments for follow-up examinations to determine the effects of the drugs and the course of your illness.
- ask for clarification of any point that is confusing or difficult to understand, at the time the drug(s) are prescribed or later if you have forgotten. Request information in writing if circumstances justify it.
- discard all outdated prescription drugs. This will prevent the use of drugs that have deteriorated with time.
- store all drugs to be retained for intermittent use out of the reach of children to prevent accidental poisoning.

PREVENTING ADVERSE DRUG REACTIONS

Our knowledge of the mechanisms of adverse reactions is very limited. For the most part, we cannot identify with certainty the person who is at greater risk of experiencing a true adverse effect. Available tests for the early detection of toxicity are of definite value, but they do not provide as full a measure of protection as we could wish.

As our understanding of drug actions and reactions expands, it becomes more apparent that there *is* a sizable proportion of adverse effects that are, to some extent, predictable and preventable. The exact percentage of preventable reactions is yet to be determined, but several contributing factors are now well recognized, and specific recommendations are available to guide both physican and patient. These fall into eleven categories of consideration.

Previous Adverse Reaction to a Drug

There is evidence to indicate that an individual who has experienced an adverse drug reaction in the past is more likely to have adverse reactions to other drugs, even though the drugs are unrelated. This suggests that some individuals may have a genetic (inborn) predisposition to unusual and abnormal drug responses. *The patient should inform the physician of any history of prior adverse drug experiences.*

Allergies

Individuals who are allergic by nature (hayfever, asthma, eczema, hives) are more likely to develop allergies to drugs than are non-allergic individuals. The allergic patient must be observed very closely for the earliest indication of a developing hypersensitivity to any drug. Known drug allergies must be noted in the medical record. The patient must inform every physician and dentist consulted that he or she is allergic by nature and is allergic to specific drugs by name. *The patient should provide this information without waiting to be asked.* The physician will then be able to avoid those drugs that could provoke an allergic reaction, as well as those related drugs to which the patient may have developed a cross-sensitivity.

Contraindications

Both patient and physician must strictly observe all known contraindications to any drug under consideration. *Absolute contraindications* include those conditions and situations that prohibit the use of the drug for any reason. *Relative contraindications* include those conditions that, in the judgment of the physician, do not preclude the use of the drug altogether, but make it essential that special considerations be given to its use to prevent the intensification of preexisting disease or the development of new disease. Such conditions and situations usually require adjustment of dosage, additional supportive measures and close supervision.

Precautions in Use

The patient should know about any special precautions to observe while taking the drug. This includes the advisability of use during pregnancy or while nursing an infant; precautions regarding exposure to the sun (or ultraviolet lamps); the avoidance of extreme heat or cold, heavy physical exertion, etc.

Dosage

The patient must adhere to the prescribed dosage schedule as closely as possible. *This is most important with those drugs that have narrow margins of safety.* Circumstances that interfere with taking the drug as prescribed (nausea, vomiting, diarrhea) must be reported to the physician so that appropriate adjustments can be made.

Interactions

Much is known today about how some drugs can interact unfavorably with certain foods, alcohol and other drugs to produce serious adverse effects. *The patient must be informed regarding all likely interactants* that could alter the action of the drug he or she is using. If, during the course of treatment, the patient has reason to feel he or she has discovered a new interaction of importance, the physician should be informed so that its full significance can be determined. (It is through such observations that much of our understanding of drug interactions has come.)

Warning Symptoms

Experience has shown that many drugs will produce symptoms that are actually early indications of a developing adverse effect. Examples include the appearance of severe headaches and visual disturbances *before* the onset of a stroke in a woman taking oral contraceptives; the development of acid indigestion and stomach distress *before* the activation of a bleeding peptic ulcer in a man taking phenylbutazone (Butazolidin) for shoulder bursitis. *It is imperative that the patient be familar with those symptoms and signs that could be early indicators of impending adverse reactions.* With this knowledge he or she can act in his or her own behalf by discontinuing the drug and consulting the physician for additional guidance.

Examinations to Monitor Drug Effects

Certain drugs (less than half of those in common use) are capable of damaging vital body tissues (bone marrow, liver, kidney, eye structures, etc.)—especially when these drugs are used over an extended period. Such adverse effects are relatively rare, and many of them are not discovered until the drug has been in wide use for a long time. As our knowledge of such effects accumulates, we learn which kinds of drugs (that is, which chemical structures) are most likely to produce such tissue reactions. Hence, we know those drugs that should be monitored periodically to detect as early as possible any evidence of tissue injury resulting from their use. *The patient should cooperate fully with the physician in the performance of periodic examinations for evidence of adverse drug effects.*

Advanced Age and Debility

The altered functional capacity of vital organs that accompanies advancing age and debilitating disease can greatly influence the body's response to drugs. Such patients tend not to tolerate drugs with inherent toxic potential well; it is usually necessary for them to use smaller doses at longer intervals. *The effects of drugs on the elderly and severely ill are often unpredictable.* The frequent need for dosage adjustments or change in drug selection requires continuous observation of these patients if adverse effects are to be prevented or minimized.

Appropriate Drug Choice

The drug(s) selected to treat any condition should be the most appropriate of those available. Many adverse reactions can be prevented if both physician and patient exercise good judgment and restraint. *The wise patient will not demand overtreatment.* He or she will cooperate with the physician's attempt to balance properly the seriousness of the illness and the hazard of the drug.

Polypharmacy

This term refers to the concurrent use by an individual of several drugs prescribed separately by two (or more) physicians for different disorders—often without appropriate communication between patient and prescriber. This frequent practice is conducive to potentially serious drug/drug interactions. *The patient should routinely inform each physican (and dentist) consulted of all the drugs— prescription and nonprescription—that he or she may be taking at the time.* It is mandatory that each physician have this information before prescribing additional drugs.

DRUGS AND THE ELDERLY

Advancing age brings changes in body structure and function that may alter significantly the action of drugs. An impaired digestive system may interfere with drug absorption. Reduced capacity of the liver and kidneys to metabolize and eliminate drugs may result in the accumulation of drugs in the body to toxic levels. By impairing the body's ability to maintain a "steady state" (homeostasis), the aging process may increase the sensitivity of many tissues to the actions of drugs, thereby altering greatly the responsiveness of the nervous and circulatory systems to standard drug doses. If aging should cause deterioration of understanding, memory, vision or physical coordination, people with such impairments may not always use drugs safely and effectively.

Adverse reactions to drugs occur three times more frequently in the older population. An unwanted drug response can render a functioning and independent older person whose health and reserves are at marginal levels, confused, incompetent or helpless. For these reasons, drug treatment in the elderly must always be accompanied by the most careful consideration of the individual's health and tolerances, the selection of drugs and dosage schedules and the possible need for assistance in treatment routines.

Guidelines for the Use of Drugs by the Elderly

- Be certain that drug treatment is necessary. Many health problems of the elderly can be managed without the use of drugs.
- Avoid if possible the use of many drugs at one time. It is advisable to use not more than three drugs concurrently.
- Dosage schedules should be as uncomplicated as possible. When feasible, a single daily dose of each drug is preferable.
- In order to establish individual tolerance, treatment with most drugs is usually best begun by using smaller than standard doses. Maintenance doses should also be determined carefully. A maintenance dose is often smaller for persons over 60 years of age than for younger persons.
- Avoid large tablets and capsules if other dosage forms are available. Liquid preparations are easier for the elderly or debilitated to swallow.
- Have all drug containers labeled with the drug name and directions for use in large, easy-to-read letters.
- Ask the pharmacist to package drugs in easy-to-open containers. Avoid "child-proof" caps and stoppers.
- Do not take any drug in the dark. Identify each dose of medicine carefully in adequate light to be certain you are taking the drug intended.
- To avoid taking the wrong drug or an extra dose, do not keep drugs on a bedside table. Drugs for emergency use, such as nitroglycerin, are an exception. It is advisable to have only one such drug at the bedside for use during the night.
- Drug use by older persons may require supervision. Observe drug effects continuously to ensure safe and effective use.
- Remember the adage: "Start low, go slow and (when appropriate) learn to say no."

Drugs Best Avoided by the Elderly Because of Increased Possibility of Adverse Reactions

antacids (high sodium)*   cyclophosphamide
barbiturates*   diethylstilbestrol

*See Drug Class, Section Four.

estrogens
indomethacin
monoamine oxidase inhibitors
   (MAOI's)* type A

oxyphenbutazone
phenacetin
phenylbutazone
tetracyclines*

Drugs That Should Be Used by the Elderly in Reduced Dosages Until Full Effect Has Been Determined

anticoagulants (oral)*
antidepressants*
antidiabetic drugs*
antihistamines*
antihypertensives*
anti-inflammatory drugs*
barbiturates*
beta-blockers*
colchicine
cortisonelike drugs*
digitalis preparations*
diuretics* (all types)

ephedrine
epinephrine
haloperidol
isoetharine
nalidixic acid
narcotic drugs
prazosin
pseudoephedrine
quinidine
sleep inducers (hypnotics)*
terbutaline
thyroid preparations

Drugs That May Cause Confusion and Behavioral Disturbances in the Elderly

amantadine
antidepressants*
antidiabetic drugs*
antihistamines*
anti-inflammatory drugs*
atropine* (and drugs containing
   belladonna)
barbiturates*
benzodiazepines*
carbamazepine
cimetidine
digitalis preparations*
diuretics*
ergoloid mesylates

levodopa
meprobamate
methocarbamol
methyldopa
narcotic drugs
pentazocine
phenytoin
primidone
reserpine
sedatives
sleep inducers (hypnotics)*
thiothixene
tranquilizers (mild)*
trihexyphenidyl

Drugs That May Cause Orthostatic Hypotension in the Elderly

antidepressants*
antihypertensives*
diuretics* (all types)
phenothiazines*

sedatives
tranquilizers (mild)*
vasodilators*

*See Drug Class, Section Four.

Drugs That May Cause Constipation and/or Retention of Urine in the Elderly

amantadine
androgens
antidepressants*
antiparkinsonism drugs*
atropinelike drugs*
epinephrine

ergoloid mesylates
isoetharine
narcotic drugs
phenothiazines*
terbutaline

Drugs That May Cause Loss of Bladder Control (Urinary Incontinence) in the Elderly

diuretics* (all types)
sedatives
sleep inducers (hypnotics)*

tranquilizers (mild)*

THERAPEUTIC DRUG MONITORING
(Measuring Drug Levels in Blood)

The routine use of measuring drug levels in blood as an aid in managing drug therapy has evolved gradually over the past 20 years. Because individuals vary so greatly in the nature and degree of their responses to drugs, it became apparent that greater precision in determining optimal dosage for the individual was needed. For many drugs, the responses observed by the physician (clinical changes) clearly indicate that the drug is working as intended and that the dosage scheme is satisfactory. However, for some drugs—especially those with narrow safety margins—the toxic reactions closely resemble the symptoms of the disorder for which the drugs are prescribed. In many instances the patient's response is not in keeping with his or her clinical condition or program of drug therapy. By measuring the blood levels of certain drugs at appropriate times, the physician can adjust dosage schedules more accurately, predict drug response more precisely, reduce the risk of toxicity and achieve greater benefit.

The timing of the blood samples is an important consideration. As a general rule, the best time for sampling is just before the next scheduled dose of the drug to be measured (the "trough" level). Sampling should be avoided during the two hours following oral administration; during this absorption period, blood levels do not represent tissue levels of the drug.

*See Drug Class, Section Four.

The following drugs are those most suitable for therapeutic drug monitoring. If you are using any of these on a regular basis, consult your physician regarding the advisability or need for periodic measurement of drug levels in your blood.

Generic Name	Brand Name(s)
acetaminophen	Datril, Tylenol, etc.
amikacin	Amikin
amitriptyline	Amitril, Elavil, Endep, etc.
aspirin (other salicylates)	Bufferin, Ecotrin, etc.
carbamazepine	Tegretol
chloramphenicol	Chloromycetin
chlorpromazine	Thorazine
ciprofloxacin	Cipro
clonazepam	Clonopin
desipramine	Norpramin, Pertofrane
digitoxin	Crystodigin
digoxin	Lanoxin
disopyramide	Norpace
doxepin	Adapin, Sinequan
dyphylline	Brophylline, Neothylline, etc.
ethosuximide	Zarontin
ethotoin	Peganone
gentamicin	Garamycin
gold salts	Auranofin, Myochrisine, etc.
imipramine	Imavate, Tofranil, etc.
isoniazid	INH, Niconyl, etc.
kanamycin	Kantrex
lidocaine	Xylocaine, etc.
lithium	Lithobid, Lithotabs, etc.
mephenytoin	Mesantoin
mephobarbital	Mebaral
methotrexate	Mexate
methsuximide	Celontin
nortriptyline	Aventyl, Pamelor
paramethadione	Paradione
phenobarbital	Luminal, etc.
phensuximide	Milontin
phenytoin	Dilantin
primidone	Mysoline
procainamide	Pronestyl
propranolol	Inderal
protriptyline	Vivactil
quinidine	Cardioquin, Quinaglute, etc.

theophylline   Aminophylline, Theo-Dur, et
thioridazine   Mellaril
tobramycin   Nebcin
trimethadione   Tridione
valproic acid   Depakene

THE USE
OF DRUGS IN TREATING
CHRONIC DISORDERS

Chronic Disorders Reviewed in This Section

Acne
Alzheimer's Disease
Angina Pectoris
Asthma
Cholesterol Disorders
Congestive Heart Failure
Crohn's Disease
Depression
Diabetes
Epilepsy
Glaucoma
Gout
Hypertension (High Blood Pressure)
Hypothyroidism
Menopause
Migraine Headache
Myasthenia Gravis
Osteoarthritis
Osteoporosis
Parkinson's Disease
Peptic Ulcer
Psoriasis
Rheumatoid Arthritis
Schizophrenia
Ulcerative Colitis

INTRODUCTION

Of the 200 drugs prescribed most frequently by physicians in the United States in 1988, 130 (65%) are used in the treatment of chronic disorders. This section provides an overview of the management of some of the more common disorders that require drug therapy for long periods of time, some of them for life. As you read this section, you will become familiar with important principles in the use of selected drugs and will gain perspectives that can help you to understand what your physician is attempting to accomplish with the therapy recommended. Since the lack of reasonable compliance by the patient is one of the major causes of failure in today's use of drugs, your greater understanding will encourage you to cooperate fully with your physician's instructions so that together you can achieve the greatest benefit with the least risk from the drugs prescribed.

Although drugs are essential to the rational treatment of most chronic disorders, proper attention must also be given to other treatment procedures, of equal importance. Examples include adherence to the appropriate diet in the management of diabetes, cessation of smoking in the treatment of angina (coronary artery disease), weight control in the treatment of high blood pressure (hypertension) and the use of "allergy shots" (immunotherapy) in the management of asthma. The intelligent use of drugs can make a significant contribution, but it must be recognized that drugs have their limitations and should be looked upon as but one part of a comprehensive and integrated treatment program.

WARNING: Each physician develops his or her own favored approach to the use of drugs. This is based upon knowledge of the drug's characteristics plus personal experience and observation of drug performance. The treatment program recommended by your physician may vary somewhat from the guidelines provided in this book. It is important that you follow your physician's instructions precisely as given—that you comply fully. If you question any aspect of drug selection, dosage schedule, drug effects, etc., consult your physician before attempting any modification of your drug treatment program on your own. *Under no circumstances should you attempt to initiate prescription drug therapy for yourself or others without the full knowledge and guidance of a qualified physician.*

ACNE

Other Name: Acne vulgaris

Prevalence in USA: Approximately 4.6 million cases: 2.4% of the population under 18 years of age; 3% of the population 18 to 44 years of age.

Age Group: Most common in adolescents and young adults. Usually begins at puberty (9 to 12 years of age) and subsides at 18 to 20 years of age. A small percentage of cases will persist into the twenties and thirties.

Male to Female Ratio: Slightly more common in women.

Principal Features: Common acne is a disorder of the hair follicles and sebaceous (oil-producing) glands of the skin. It is characterized by the formation of open comedones (blackheads), closed comedones (whiteheads), inflammed papules (pimples) and pustules in the superficial layers of the skin. The deep form of acne includes the formation of inflammed nodules and pus-filled cysts. These skin changes occur most commonly on the face, but are also found on the neck, chest, shoulders and upper back. The degree of inflammation will vary from mild to severe throughout the course of the disorder. It is often worse in the winter and better during the summer, probably due to the beneficial effects of sun exposure.

Causes: Acne is primarily due to overactivity of the oil-producing sebaceous glands. This usually begins with the changes of puberty when the associated increase in sex hormones (principally androgens) stimulates the growth and production of the glands. The opening of the gland becomes plugged with a mixture of dead skin cells, oils and bacteria, resulting in a comedo; this progresses to the formation of fatty acids within the gland that causes inflammation, swelling and eventual rupture into the skin. Contributing causes include familial predisposition, excessive heat and humidity, poor personal hygiene, the use of oil-based cosmetics and exposure to industrial oils and tars.

Drugs That Can Cause This Disorder: The following drugs can initiate acne or aggravate existing acne:
androgens (male hormonelike drugs)
cortisonelike drugs
cytotoxic drugs (those used to treat various types of cancer)
methotrexate
oral contraceptives that contain norethindrone or norgestrel (Brevicon, Loestrin, Lo/Ovral, Micronor, Modicon, Norinyl, Norlestrin, Norlutin, Nor-Qd, Ortho-Novum, Ovcon, Ovral, Ovrette)
progesterone
The following drugs can cause acnelike eruptions but do not cause true comedo formation:
bromides
disulfiram
iodides
isoniazid
lithium
phenobarbital
phenytoin
quinine
thiouracil
trimethadione
vitamin B-12

Drugs Used to Treat This Disorder
Locally (Topically)
- benzoyl peroxide (Benoxyl, Clearasil, Epi-Clear, Topex, etc.).
- tretinoin (retinoic acid preparations, Retin-A).
- antibiotic lotions.
- metronidazole gel (MetroGel).

Internally (Systemically)
- tetracycline (see Drug Profile).
- erythromycin (see Drug Profile).
- isotretinoin (see Drug Profile).
- prednisone (see Drug Profile).
- ibuprofen (see Drug Profile).

Goals of Drug Treatment
Improvement and control are the primary objectives; cure is not possible.
Prevention of new blemishes.
Prevention of scarring.
Note: Appropriate treatment, conscientiously followed, is beneficial in 95% of all cases.

Drug Management
Local (Topical) Drug Treatment
Often sufficient to control superficial acne with mild to moderate inflammation.

May be used concurrently with internal (systemic) treatment for control of deep acne with severe inflammation, nodule and cyst formation.

Start treatment slowly; determine tolerance by applying small amounts of low-concentration products to small areas of skin.

Limit applications to once or twice daily.

Apply to *dry* skin, one-half hour after washing.

Use soap and water to remove skin oils; wash skin no more than twice daily.

Avoid abrasive preparations.

Irritation from topical drugs is common; true allergy is uncommon.

Use of Benzoyl Peroxide
1. This is the single most effective drug for the topical treatment of acne. Many preparations are available without prescription.
2. Its principal action is anti-infective; its primary use is treating superficial, inflammatory, papulo-pustular acne.
3. Start with a 5% preparation; apply once daily—in the morning.
4. This drug inactivates tretinoin (retinoic acid); do not apply these two drugs at the same time.

Use of Tretinoin (Retinoic Acid)
1. This is the only practical drug available for the topical management of comedones. It does require a prescription.
2. It is used in all forms of acne to facilitate the removal of existing comedones and to prevent the formation of new ones.
3. Start with the 0.01% gel; increase the strength of the preparation as needed and tolerated.
4. Apply once daily—in the evening or at bedtime.
5. This drug may require continual use for up to 12 weeks to obtain initial benefit; continued control will require maintenance treatment for months or years.
6. Drying and irritation of the skin are common. However, deliberate irritation and peeling are not necessary for benefit.
7. This drug may increase skin sensitivity to sunlight; use sun screen preparations if necessary, but avoid them if possible.

Use of Topical Antibiotics
1. Erythromycin is the drug of choice; tetracycline and clindamycin preparations are also used.
2. These anti-infective drugs are used primarily to treat inflammatory acne; they do not clear existing lesions but do prevent the development of new ones.
3. May be used concurrently with benzoyl peroxide or tretinoin.
4. Apply twice daily—morning and evening.
5. These drugs may require continual use for 3 to 4 weeks to obtain significant improvement.

Internal (Systemic) Drug Treatment

Required for control of moderate to severe deep acne (inflammatory nodules, cysts, abscesses) and to reduce permanent scarring.

A firm commitment to conscientious treatment for many months or years is often required to accomplish desired results.

Use of Tetracycline
1. Generally considered to be the drug of choice for long-term use. (See Drug Profile for complete description.)
2. May be used alone or concurrently with benzoyl peroxide or tretinoin.
3. Begin treatment with 500 mg to 1000 mg daily for 4 weeks or until a satisfactory result is obtained. Then reduce gradually to the smallest effective dose for long-term maintenance; this may be as low as 250 mg every 1 to 3 days.
4. This is best taken on an empty stomach, 1 hour before or 2 hours after eating.
5. Continual use for 3 months may be required to obtain optimal benefit.
6. If tetracycline is not effective or cannot be tolerated, erythromycin is the next drug of choice.

Use of Isotretinoin
1. This drug is reserved for the treatment of severe acne that has not responded to conventional management. (See Drug Profile for complete description.)
2. Its primary action is to inhibit the production of sebum (a mix of sebaceous oils and skin cell debris). This reduces the source of fatty acids that cause inflammatory reaction.
3. ***Do not use this drug during pregnancy. Use effective birth control measures while taking it.***
4. Continual use for 20 or more weeks is usually required to produce significant benefit.
5. Monitor triglyceride blood levels during use; if level exceeds 400 mg, reduce the dose; if level exceeds 600 mg, discontinue this drug.
6. Use this drug with caution in those with type I diabetes or inflammatory bowel disease (Crohn's disease, ulcerative colitis).

Use of Prednisone
1. Cortisonelike drugs may induce acne in some individuals. However, it may be useful for some with extensive, severe inflammatory acne that is unresponsive to other treatments.
2. Initiate treatment with 30 mg to 45 mg of prednisone daily, gradually reducing this dose within 1 month. Low-dose maintenance using 2.5 mg each evening may extend control. (See Drug Profile for complete description.)

Use of Ibuprofen
1. This anti-inflammatory drug may enhance the beneficial effects of systemic tetracyline. (See Drug Profile of Ibuprofen for complete description.)
2. A trial of 600 mg 4 times per day is warranted for those with severe inflammatory acne that has shown limited benefit from standard drug therapy.

Use of Oral Contraceptives
1. High-estrogen birth control pills that contain a nonandrogenic progestin (ethynodrel, norethisterone, norethynodrel) are sometimes used to treat severe acne.
2. The beneficial action of these preparations is the reduction of sebum formation.
3. Because of the inherent risks, this use of oral contraceptives is generally not recommended. (See Drug Profile for complete description.)

Ancillary Drug Treatment (as required)

Condition	*Drug Treatment*
For candidiasis (yeast infection of genital or anal region, a complication of long-term antibiotic or oral contraceptive use):	clotrimazole (Lotrimin) nystatin (Mycostatin)

Note: Drug selection, dosage and administration schedule must be determined by the physician for each patient individually.

Resource for Additional Information and Services

Acne Research Institute
1587 Monrovia Avenue
Newport Beach, CA 92663
Phone: (714) 722-1805

Telecommunications services: 1-800-235-2263 (outside CA); 1-800-225-2263 (inside CA)
Publications available.

ALZHEIMER'S DISEASE

Other Names: Alzheimer's presenile and senile dementia, senile dementia (Alzheimer type)

Prevalence in USA: Approximately 2.5 million; more than 7% of the American population aged over 65 years; the cause of 50% of all progressive dementias.

Age Group: Occurs occasionally under 50 years of age; uncommon before 65 years; the majority occurs over 65 years: mild dementia in 5% and moderate to severe in 10–20%. Moderate to severe dementia occurs in 20% of all over 80.

Male to Female Ratio: More common in women.

Principal Features

Insidious onset leading to progressive and permanent decline of all intellectual functions.

Mood changes: apathy, depression, irritability, anxiety, paranoia.

Loss of recent memory, inability to recall facts of common knowledge, disorientation, confusion, all worse at night.

Impaired attention, understanding, judgment. Loss of ability to think abstractly, to use language correctly, to calculate.

Eventual gait disturbances, incoordination of movements.

Social skills may be retained until late in course of disease.

Course is from 3 to 20 years, with mean duration of 7 years.

Causes: Degeneration of nerve cells in the areas of the brain that control intellectual functions. Actual cause of degeneration is unknown. Genetic predisposition appears probable; Alzheimer type dementia is four times more frequent among family members than in the general population. There is a history of previous head injury in 15% to 20% of cases. One common feature is a marked deficiency of the nerve transmitter acetylcholine.

Drugs That Can Cause This Disorder: No drugs cause true Alzheimer's dementia. However, 3% of all dementias are drug induced. The following drugs can cause symptoms in the elderly that resemble Alzheimer's disease (see Drug Classes, Section Four):

antidepressants	butyrophenones
atropinelike drugs	cortisonelike drugs
barbiturates	digitalis preparations
benzodiazepines	MAO inhibitors

Drugs Used to Treat This Disorder

No specific or truly effective drug treatment is available at this time.

Ergoloid mesylates (Deapril-ST, Hydergine) are tried during the early stages to relieve symptoms; benefits are infrequent, negligible and fleeting. (See Drug Profile, Section Three.)

Experimental drugs: choline, lecithin, physostigmine (none are curative or significantly beneficial).

Goals of Drug Treatment

Temporary improvement of alertness and memory.

Relief of confusion, depression and behavioral disturbances.

Drug Management

Keep all medications to a minimum.

If any drug is used, start treatment with small doses, increase the dosage cautiously and monitor the response very closely.

Avoid drugs with strong atropinelike effects and strong sedative effects.

Ergoloid mesylates may act as a mild antidepressant and may improve mood. If it is tolerated well, a trial of 6 months is justified.

Lecithin may increase the acetylcholine content of brain tissue and temporarily improve memory in some individuals. It is available in health food stores without prescription. It is safe to try. Ask your physician for guidance.

Use antipsychotics (Haldol, Mellaril, etc.) and sedatives (chloral hydrate, Benadryl, etc.) only when clearly needed. Use the smallest dose that proves to be effective.

Ancillary Drug Treatment (as required)

Condition	*Drug Treatment*
For agitation, confusion:	haloperidol (Haldol)
	thioridazine (Mellaril)
	thiothixene (Navane)
For insomnia:	chloral hydrate (Noctec, Somnos, etc.)
	diphenhydramine (Benadryl)
For depression:	trazodone (Desyrel)
For constipation:	docusate (Colace, Doxinate, Surfak, etc.)

Note: Drug selection, dosage and administration schedule must be determined by the physician for each patient individually.

Resource for Additional Information and Services

Alzheimer's Disease and Related Disorders Association
70 East Lake Street, Suite 600
Chicago, IL 60601
Phone: 1-800-621-0379; (312) 853-3060

Available 24 hours a day, 7 days a week.
Sends packet of information; offers information by phone.
National network of 180 chapters and 1200 support groups.

ANGINA PECTORIS

Other Names: Coronary artery insufficiency, coronary artery disease, coronary heart disease, ischemic heart disease

Prevalence in USA: Approximately 6 million; coronary artery disease is the leading cause of death in the USA.

Age Group: Under 45 years—0.2% of population; 45 to 64 years—6.5% of population; over 65 years—11% of population.

Male to Female Ratio: Under 45 years—1.5 to 1; 45 to 64 years—3 to 1; 65 to 74 years—1.8 to 1; over 75 years—1 to 1.

Principal Features
Classical Angina-of-Effort (Exertional Angina): A moderate to severe discomfort (pain, pressure, tightness, fullness, squeezing or burning sensation) usually located deeply behind the breastbone (but may be felt in the jaw, neck, shoulder, arms, upper back or pit of the stomach). It is characteristically brought on by physical exertion, a large meal, emotional stress or exposure to cold; it usually lasts 1 to 3 minutes and disappears with rest.
Variant (Prinzmetal's) Angina: Usually occurs at rest, and is unpredictable and unrelated to the situations that provoke effort angina. It often occurs between midnight and 8 a.m. The two types of angina can coexist. Acute anginal pain may be accompanied by weakness, sweating, shortness of breath or nausea.

Causes
Exertional Angina: Due to atherosclerosis (thickening and hardening) of segments of coronary arteries. Contributory causes of these arterial changes include heredity (genetic susceptibility), hypertension, high blood cholesterol, diabetes and smoking.
Variant (Prinzmetal's) Angina: Due to spontaneous spasm of segments of coronary arteries; the cause of the spasm is not known. Anemia, hyperthyroidism, aortic valve disease and heart rhythm disorders predispose to angina.

Drugs That Can Cause This Disorder: The following drugs do not cause coronary artery disease per se, but they can affect heart function adversely and induce or intensify angina in susceptible individuals:

amphetamines
beta blocker drugs (abrupt
　withdrawal)
bromocriptine
cocaine
epinephrine
ergot preparations
5-fluouracil
hydralazine
indomethacin
isoetharine
isoproterenol
metaproterenol
methysergide
nifedipine (first dose)
nylidrin
oral contraceptives
phenylpropanolamine
prazosin
terbutaline
thyroid

Drugs Used to Treat This Disorder
Nitrate Preparations
  • nitroglycerin lingual aerosol (Nitrolingual Spray).
  • nitroglycerin sublingual tablets (Nitrostat).
  • nitroglycerin buccal tablets (Susadrin).
  • nitroglycerin prolonged-action forms (Nitro-Bid, etc.).
  • nitroglycerin ointment (Nitrol, etc.).
  • nitroglycerin patches (Nitrodisc, Nitro-Dur, etc.).
  • isosorbide dinitrate (Isordil, Sorbitrate).

- erythrityl tetranitrate (Cardilate).
- pentaerythritol tetranitrate (Peritrate).

Beta Blocker Drugs
- atenolol (Tenormin).
- labetalol (Normodyne, Trandate).
- metoprolol (Lopressor).
- nadolol (Corgard).
- propranolol (Inderal).

Other beta blockers are used but have not yet been approved by the FDA for specific use in the management of angina.

Calcium Blocker Drugs
- nicardipine (Cardene).
- nifedipine (Adalat, Procardia).
- diltiazem (Cardizem).
- verapamil (Calan, Isoptin).

Others
- aspirin (for its antiplatelet action).
- dipyridamole (Persantine). Antianginal effect is questionable and under review.

Goals of Drug Treatment

Prompt relief of acute anginal attack.

Prevention of anticipated angina by use of nitroglyerin just before physical activity.

Long-term prevention of angina; reduced frequency, severity and duration of recurrent anginal episodes.

Prevention of heart rhythm disturbances.

Prevention of heart attack (myocardial infarction).

Drug Management

For Stable Exertional Angina

Frequency and severity of angina-of-effort remain at a constant level.

Nitroglycerin spray or sublingual tablet for relief of acute attacks.

Long-acting nitrates and/or a beta blocker.

If control is not adequate, add a calcium blocker.

For Unstable Angina

Frequency and severity of angina increase over time; angina occurs with exertion and at rest, is less responsive to treatment.

Hospitalization in coronary care unit.

Mild sedation with benzodiazepines (Valium, etc.).

Combined use of nitrates, beta blocker and calcium blocker.

Aspirin, for antiplatelet effect.

For Variant (Prinzmetal's) Angina

Anginal attacks primarily at rest.

Nitroglycerin spray or sublingual tablets.

Long-acting nitrates.

Calcium blocker.

Avoid beta blockers (unless it is established that both types of angina are present).

Use of Nitroglycerin

1. Nitroglycerin is the mainstay of managing angina. Always have a supply of fresh, active tablets available. Keep them in the original dark glass bottle, tightly closed, no cotton added. Do not transfer them to a metal or plastic container.
2. The sublingual tablet will produce a mild stinging sensation under the tongue, flushing of the face and throbbing in the head. These reactions are normal and indicate that the drug is active and you are having a good response.
3. Use nitrolycerin promptly and as often as necessary, no matter how often. Unless instructed otherwise, do not consciously keep count of the tablets used.
4. If the lingual spray or sublingual tablet causes weakness, dizziness or faintness, sit down or lie down until the sensation passes.
5. Use the spray or tablet to prevent an attack by taking it just before starting a specific physical activity that is known to induce angina.
6. If anginal pain persists after taking 3 successive sublingual tablets (1 tablet at 3-to-5-minute intervals for 3 doses), consult your physician immediately or seek assistance at the nearest hospital emergency room.
7. Nitroglycerin ointment may be used at bedtime to prevent angina during sleep. Follow the instructions for application carefully. Do not use your fingers. Do not rub the ointment into the skin.
8. Nitroglycerin patches (discs) may induce tolerance to the drug and cause it to be less effective with continuous use. The intermittent use of oral dosage forms may be more effective for long-term treatment. Ask your physician for guidance.
9. If you have glaucoma, consult your physician regarding the periodic measurement of your internal eye pressures while using long-term nitrates for angina.
10. Following long-term use, nitrates should be discontinued gradually to prevent symptoms of withdrawal.

Use of Beta Blocker Drugs

1. Do not use this type of drug without your physician's knowledge and guidance.
2. Beta blockers are not recommended for mild angina that is well controlled by nitrates. Their use is generally reserved for severe and unstable angina.
3. Beta blockers are not recommended for variant (Prinzmetal's) vasospastic angina.
4. If your angina worsens with the use of a beta blocker drug, notify your physician promptly.
5. Atenolol (Tenormin) and metoprolol (Lopressor) are preferred for individuals with asthma, emphysema, diabetes or peripheral circulatory disorders.
6. Atenolol (Tenormin) and nadolol (Corgard) are effective with once-daily dosage and tend to cause less depression and insomnia.

7. Beta blocker drugs must not be discontinued suddenly. Abrupt withdrawal can cause severe angina and increase the risk of heart attack (myocardial infarction).

Use of Calcium Blocker Drugs

1. A calcium blocker is the drug of choice for treating variant (Prinzmetal's) angina.
2. Nifedipine (Adalat, Procardia) is the most potent antianginal calcium blocker. However, angina may worsen if the heart rate increases excessively.
3. Verapamil (Calan, Isoptin) can delay the excretion of digoxin and increase the risk of digoxin toxicity. Dosage adjustments may be necessary.
4. These drugs can be used initially by individuals who should not use beta blockers.

Current Controversies in Drug Management

The nitrate drugs are well established as effective therapeutic agents for the management of angina and congestive heart failure, two conditions that require long-term drug therapy. Recent studies have shown that the "standard" practice of continuous administration of nitrates can lead to the development of tolerance (see Glossary) and loss of effectiveness. Tolerance is most likely to occur with frequent dosing and the use of prolonged-action capsules or tablets and the use of transdermal nitroglycerin patches. Continuous treatment with nitrates produces tolerance within 24 hours of the first dose and complete loss of effect when continued for one week or more. The intermittent use of nitrates ("pulse" dosing) causes only partial tolerance and is more effective for long-term protection. Intermittent rather than continuous nitrate dosing is now recommended for treating angina and congestive heart failure.

Comments: Current guidelines for the optimal use of nitrates include the following recommendations.

- Take isosorbide dinitrate (Isordil, short-acting form) 2 or 3 (but not 4) times daily; take at 8:00 a.m. and 1:00 or 3:00 p.m., or at 8:00 a.m., 1:00 p.m. and 5:00 p.m.; no dosing again until the following 8:00 a.m.
- Take the prolonged-action dosage forms of isosorbide dinitrate at 8:00 a.m., only once daily.
- Use the nitroglycerin patch for only 12 hours daily, from 8:00 a.m. to 8:00 p.m.; leave it off during the night.
- Long nitrate-free intervals appear to preserve responsiveness to the drug.

Ancillary Drug Treatment (as required)

Condition	*Drug Treatment*
For anxiety:	benzodiazepines (Valium, etc.) (See Drug Class, Section Four.)
For hypertension:	see Profile of Hypertension in this section
For congestive heart failure:	see Profile of Congestive Heart Failure in this section
For hyperthyroidism:	methimazole (Tapazole) propylthiouracil propranolol (Inderal)
For anemia:	iron preparations

Note: Drug selection, dosage and administration schedule must be determined by the physician for each patient individually.

Resource for Additional Information and Services

Heartlife (Heart Disease Heart Line)
P.O. Box 54305
Atlanta, GA 30308
Phone: 1-800-241-6993; (404) 523-0826

Available 9:00 a.m.–4:00 p.m. EST, M–F; Spanish-speaking counselor available.
Publications available.

ASTHMA

Other Names: Bronchial asthma, reversible airway disease, reversible obstructive airway disease

Prevalence in USA: Approximately 7 million, 3% of population (includes 1.5 million school-age children).

Age Group: Under 18 years—2.5 million; 18 to 44 years—2.7 million; 45 to 64 years—1.6 million; 65 to 74 years—726,000; 75 years and over—308,000.

Male to Female Ratio: About equal.

Principal Features: Recurring acute attacks of shortness of breath, wheezing (labored breathing), a sensation of tightness in the chest and cough, with symptom-free intervals between attacks. Episodes of active asthma may last an hour to several days. The acute attack begins with tightening of muscles in the walls of bronchial tubes (airways), which causes constriction and reduced air flow. This is followed by swelling of the lining of bronchial tubes and the excessive production of mucus, both of which cause additional narrowing of the airways, forced breathing and coughing. Severe asthma may be accompanied by sweating, insomnia and bluish discoloration of the face and extremities (cyanosis). Asthma that begins in infancy (under 2 years of age) may persist into adulthood. With onset after 2 years, 50% of asthma cases will "outgrow" the disorder by 16 years. Asthma with onset in adulthood is often severe and persistent.

Causes

Extrinsic (Allergic) Asthma: Due to a true allergy (allergen-antibody reaction); hereditary susceptibility to the development of allergies. Common allergens are house dust (and mites in house dust), pollens, animal danders, feathers, wool, molds.

Intrinsic (Idiosyncratic) Asthma: Due to an unusual individual sensitivity (not a true allergy). Onset usually 35 to 45 years of age; 10% to 15% are sensitive to aspirin and have nasal polyps.

Exercise-induced Asthma: Usually in children and young adults; occurs alone or with other types of asthma; often worse 15 minutes after exercise.

Asthma "Triggers": Cold air, smoke, cooking odors, respiratory infections, emotional stress.

Drugs That Can Cause This Disorder

acetaminophen
aspirin (and substitutes)
beta blocker drugs
erythromycin
griseofulvin
hydralazine
ibuprofen
indomethacin
ketoprofen
mefenamic acid
monoamine oxidase inhibitors
naproxen
nitrofurantoin
oral contraceptives
penicillin
pentazocine
phenothiazines
phenylbutazone
procainamide
propoxyphene
reserpine
tartrazine dye

Drugs Used to Treat This Disorder

Xanthine Preparations
- aminophylline (Aminophyllin, Aminodur, etc.).
- oxtriphylline (Brondecon, Choledyl).
- theophylline (Bronkodyl, Slo-bid, Theo-Dur, etc.).

Beta-Adrenergic Drugs
- albuterol (Proventil, Ventolin).
- terbutaline (Brethine, Bricanyl).
- metaproterenol (Alupent, Metaprel).
- isoetharine (Bronkometer, Bronkosol).
- isoproterenol (Isuprel, Medihaler-Iso, etc.).

Cortisonelike Steroids
- beclomethasone aerosol (Beclovent, Vanceril).
- prednisolone (Delta-Cortef, Sterane, etc.).
- prednisone (Deltasone, Meticorten, etc.).

Others
- cromolyn (Intal).
- ipratropium (Atrovent).
- oxygen.

Goals of Drug Treatment

Prompt relief of acute asthmatic attacks.

Prevention of recurrent acute attacks.

Stabilization of lung function: freedom from asthma to the greatest degree possible, with a minimal use of drugs.

Prevention of later complications: bronchiectasis, emphysema, heart disease (cor pulmonale).

Drug Management

For Extrinsic (Allergic) Asthma

For occasional and predictable acute attacks, start treatment with beta-adrenergic inhalers.

For attacks of increasing frequency and duration, add albuterol or terbutaline tablets or a long-acting oral theophylline preparation.

For severe acute attacks or aggravation of chronic asthma, add beclomethasone aerosol inhaler.

If control is not adequate, use albuterol (or terbutaline) tablets and a theophylline preparation concurrently.

If control is still inadequate, add cromolyn on a regular basis.

If an adequate trial of all of the above fails to produce satisfactory relief and control, add cortisonelike steroids (tablets by mouth).

For Intrinsic (Idiosyncratic, Late-Onset) Asthma

Attacks may be less responsive to the use of the bronchodilators (beta-adrenergics and theophylline) as outlined above.

Earlier control may require the use of cromolyn and steroid preparations on a regular schedule.

For Exercise-induced Asthma

Try cromolyn on a regular schedule for prevention of attacks that follow exercise.

Use albuterol or terbutaline inhalation 5 to 10 minutes before exercise and following exercise for prevention.

Long-acting theophylline preparations may be effective in children for prevention.

Use of Theophylline Preparations

1. Theophylline elixir and uncoated tablets are used for prompt relief of acute asthma.
2. Theophylline sustained-release forms (Slo-bid, Slo-phyllin, Theo-Dur) are used for smooth maintenance therapy of chronic asthma. Theophylline blood levels are helpful in determining optimal dosage schedules.

3. Theophylline potentiates beta-adrenergic bronchodilators and increases their effectiveness.
4. See the Drug Profile of Theophylline in Section Three for important drug interactions.

Use of Beta-Adrenergic Bronchodilators
1. These presssurized inhalers are potent drugs that must be used cautiously. Avoid excessive use; follow dosage schedules precisely.
2. They are most effective at the beginning of an asthmatic attack and before exercise that induces asthma.
3. For the most effective use of aerosol bronchodilators, learn the correct procedure: exhale through the mouth to empty lungs; squirt and inhale the first dose at the same time; hold your breath and count to 10, then exhale. If necessary, use a second inhalation in 10 to 15 minutes.
4. Limit inhalations to 1 or 2 at a time, and at least 3 to 4 hours apart.
5. Do not use isoproterenol (Isuprel) aerosol and epinephrine (Adrenalin) aerosol concurrently.

Use of Cortisonelike Steroids
1. Steroids are not bronchodilators; they will not relieve acute asthma. This includes beclomethasone.
2. Their use should be restricted to the treatment of severe acute and chronic asthma that is not controlled by conventional drugs.
3. Steroids should never be used as the sole drug for managing asthma.
4. For short-term use: when an acute attack is prolonged and fails to respond to bronchodilators; steroids are very effective when used for 7 to 10 days of a "burst and taper" schedule—high initial dose followed by gradual dose reduction and withdrawal.
5. For long-term use: when asthma becomes severe and continuous and cannot be controlled by other drugs; a trial period of 2 to 4 weeks of steroids will determine effectiveness. The optimal long-term use consists of a relatively large single dose of prednisone (or prednisolone) every other morning (alternate-day schedule). This provides adequate asthma control with minimal adverse effects of long-term steroid use.
6. The steroid beclomethasone, inhaled in aerosol form, is used to control asthma as steroid tablets are withdrawn.

Use of Cromolyn
1. Cromolyn is not a bronchodilator; it will not relieve acute asthma.
2. It is used only by inhalation; powder and liquid aerosol forms are available.
3. A trial of cromolyn (as an asthma preventive) should begin while you are free of asthma, before acute attacks occur.
4. When used on a regular schedule, cromolyn is 70% to 75% effective in preventing recurrences of acute asthma.

5. It is most effective in preventing extrinsic (allergic) asthma, and least effective in preventing intrinsic (idiosyncratic) asthma. It may or may not prevent exercise-induced asthma but is worth a trial.
6. Cromolyn should be used on a regular basis for 8 to 10 weeks to evaluate its protective benefit.
7. For best results, a beta-adrenergic aerosol should be used 10 minutes before inhaling cromolyn.

Ancillary Drug Treatment (as required)

Condition	*Drug Treatment*
For anxiety:	promethazine (Phenergan). Note: Avoid *all* sedatives in active asthma.
For pain, mild to moderate:	acetaminophen (Tylenol, etc.)
For pain, severe:	methotrimeprazine (Levoprome). This does not depress respiration.
For bacterial infection of respiratory tract (complicating asthma):	ampicillin amoxicillin trimethoprim and sulfamethoxazole tetracycline (avoid during pregnancy and under 8 years of age)
For viral infection of respiratory tract (triggering asthma):	steroids: prednisone and methylprednisolone

Note: Drug selection, dosage and administration schedule must be determined by the physician for each patient individually.

Resources for Additional Information and Services

Asthma and Allergy Foundation of America
1717 Massachusetts Avenue, N.W., Suite 305
Washington, DC 20036
Phone: (202) 265-0265

Publications available.

National Asthma Center
3800 East Colfax Avenue
Denver, CO 80206
Phone: 1-800-222-5864

Available 8:00 a.m.–5:00 p.m. MST, M–F
Publications available.

National Foundation for Asthma
P.O. Box 30069
Tucson, AZ 85751
Phone: (602) 323-6046
Publications available.

CHOLESTEROL DISORDERS

Other Names: Dyslipidemia, hypercholesterolemia, hyperlipidemia, hyperlipoproteinemia, hypertriglyceridemia, lipid transport disorder, lipoprotein disorder

Prevalence in USA: An estimated 25% of adults are thought to have a total cholesterol level in the "too high" range: 200 to 240 mg (current standard). 0.1% of the population has congenital (familial) hypercholesterolemia. 1.0% of the population has congenital (familial) hypertriglyceridemia.

Age Group: In the USA, the low-density lipoprotein (LDL) cholesterol begins to rise after adolescence and continues to rise for 30 years. Significant elevations of LDL cholesterol levels are found in the 20-to-50-year age group.

Male to Female Ratio: 25 to 54 years of age: men show moderately higher levels of total cholesterol and LDL cholesterol; 55 years and older: women show moderately higher levels of total cholesterol and LDL cholesterol.

Principal Features
The principal blood fats (lipids)—notably cholesterol and triglycerides—are combined in the liver with proteins (to form lipoproteins) that facilitate their transport to body tissues. There are normally 3 major classes of lipoproteins: very low-density lipoproteins (VLDL), low-density lipoproteins (LDL) and high-density lipoproteins (HDL). Each class contains differing proportions of fat and protein. VLDL consists of five-sixths triglycerides and one-sixth cholesterol. While circulating in the blood, VLDL is transformed first to intermediate-density lipoprotein (IDL), which is 30% cholesterol and 40% triglyceride, and then to low-density lipoprotein (LDL), which carries from 60% to 75% of the total blood cholesterol. High levels of LDL cholesterol are associated *statistically* with an increased risk of coronary heart disease—the higher the level, the higher the risk. HDL carries less than 25% of the total blood cholesterol. It is thought to assist with the removal of LDL cholesterol from the blood and body tissues. High levels of HDL cholesterol appear to be protective against coronary heart disease—the higher the HDL level, the lower the risk.

The principal cholesterol disorders are classified into 5 major types according to the nature of the lipoprotein abnormality and associated clinical features. Types I and V are not associated with the development of atherosclerosis. Types II, III and IV are associated with the atherosclerotic process that causes coronary heart disease and peripheral vascular disorders. The lipoprotein features of these classes are as follows:

Type IIa: increased total cholesterol and LDL cholesterol; normal triglycerides.

Type IIb: increased total cholesterol, LDL cholesterol and VLDL; moderately increased triglycerides.

Type III: increased IDL cholesterol (abnormal form); increased triglycerides.

Type IV: normal total cholesterol, increased VLDL, decreased HDL cholesterol; increased triglycerides.

Causes: The major cholesterol disorders are primarily hereditary (familial) and therefore genetically determined. Secondary causes can contribute to congenital lipid disorders or can independently account for abnormalities of blood lipid metabolism. Among the secondary causes are the following conditions: Hypothyroidism, biliary cirrhosis, nephrosis, anorexia nervosa and acute intermittent porphyria can cause significant increases in blood cholesterol levels. Diabetes, chronic alcoholism, chronic kidney failure and acute hepatitis can cause significant increases in blood triglyceride levels. However, the most apparent secondary cause of lipid disorders is the high dietary cholesterol and fat content consumed by the American public.

Drugs That Can Cause This Disorder: The following drugs have been reported to cause abnormal increases in cholesterol blood levels: anabolic (male-hormonelike) steroids, chenodiol, disopyramide, thiazide diuretics (see Drug Class, Section Four), trimeprazine. The following drugs have been reported to cause abnormal increases in triglyceride blood levels: cortisonelike drugs (see Drug Class, Section Four), estrogens, isotretinoin, oral contraceptives, thiazide diuretics (see Drug Class, Section Four), timolol.

Drugs Used to Treat This Disorder

Drugs that inhibit synthesis of cholesterol and lipoprotein: lovastatin (Mevacor), niacin (nicotinic acid, Nicobid, Nicotinex, etc.).

Drugs that hasten the clearance of lipoproteins in the bloodstream: clofibrate (Atromid-S), gemfibrozil (Lopid).

Drugs that accelerate breakdown and elimination of lipoproteins: cholestyramine (Questran), colestipol (Colestid), probucol (Lorelco).

Other drugs used less often: dextrothyroxine (Choloxin), neomycin.

New Drugs in Development for Treating This Disorder

Drugs of the lovastatin class: mevastatin (Compactin), pravastatin (Eptastatin), simvastatin (Synvinolin). These drugs, for the most part,

significantly reduce total and LDL cholesterol and raise HDL cholesterol. They may prove to be effective in lower dosage and therefore
less likely to cause adverse effects.

Drugs of the fibric acid class: fenofibrate. This drug (in use in Europe
for several years) effectively reduces LDL cholesterol and triglycerides, raises HDL cholesterol and is well tolerated.

Goals of Drug Treatment

Normalization of blood lipid levels to currently accepted standards:
total cholesterol of less than 200 mg; LDL cholesterol of less than 130
mg; triglycerides of less than 250 mg (in the absence of other significant lipid abnormalities).

Avoidance or reduction of adverse drug effects.

Prevention, retardation or reversal of atherosclerotic arterial changes
throughout the body to reduce the risk of coronary heart disease,
peripheral vascular disease and stroke.

Note: The following values reflect the evolving opinion regarding the
"normalcy" of blood lipids over the past 15 years:

Normal Upper Limit	1975	1980	1989
Total cholesterol	300	280	200
LDL cholesterol		180	130
Triglycerides	200	165	150

A "normal" HDL cholesterol range is 40 to 80.

Drug Management

Introduction

Our present understanding of how cholesterol disorders are causally
related to the development of atherosclerosis (coronary and peripheral vascular disease) is incomplete and controversial. While large
population studies have demonstrated that high cholesterol blood levels are associated statistically with an increased incidence of atherosclerosis, cholesterol values alone have low predictability for the actual development of coronary heart disease on an individual basis.
The somewhat exaggerated emphasis on "statistical significance" has
resulted in the creation of unrealistic risk ratios based on minor
changes in blood lipid levels that are meaningless in the light of wide
individual variability and the unreproducibility of laboratory test results as currently obtained. Determination of isolated blood lipid levels provides at best an incomplete appraisal of an individual's status
regarding an inclination to develop atherosclerosis. They represent
only one aspect of a disease process in which many other causative
factors are involved. An understanding of the complex interactions of
the numerous cholesterol-triglyceride-apoprotein linkages (lipoprotein fractions) is the key to learning which components and what
concentrations can be relied upon to predicate an increased risk for
the consequent development of atherosclerosis. For example, high levels of apolipoproteins (a), AI and B are much stronger predictors than

cholesterol values for identifying those at high risk for atherosclerotic heart disease. Anyone who has reason to be concerned about a possible cholesterol disorder is well advised to reduce dietary fat and cholesterol intake. The majority of individuals with elevated blood lipid values do not require drug therapy to manage their disorder. Before starting a long-term, expensive and somewhat risky program of drug treatment, the concerned individual should first seek a detailed evaluation at a reputable lipid research center, either in person or by submission of appropriate blood samples and medical information.

Determining the Need for Treatment

Observe the following procedures for the measurement of blood lipid values:

1. Do not alter your regular diet in preparation for testing. You should not be on a reducing diet.
2. You should be free of any kind of infection.
3. Avoid all alcoholic beverages for 24 hours prior to testing.
4. Fast for 12 to 16 hours prior to testing.
5. Your blood samples should be examined by a reliable laboratory that has established a record for providing accurate, precise and reproducible test results.
6. For proper evaluation, a blood lipid profile should include values for total cholesterol, LDL and HDL cholesterol fractions and triglycerides.
7. Obtain blood lipid measurements on at least 2 separate occasions (3 if in doubt) and use the average of the test results.

When to Treat

Current recommendations regarding initiation of treatment are based on the following guidelines. Either diet therapy alone or diet plus drug therapy is recommended when the blood lipid values exceed those stated in the table.

	DIET ALONE		DIET AND DRUGS	
Age Group	*Cholesterol*	*LDL*	*Cholesterol*	*LDL*
20–29	200	140	220	160
30–39	220	155	240	175
Over 40	240	160	260	185

How to Treat

1. Diet modification is the primary treatment for all individuals with elevated blood lipid levels. The total caloric intake should be designed to achieve ideal body weight. The initial diet should restrict saturated fats to 10% of the total calories and restrict cholesterol to less than 300 mg daily. This low-fat, low-cholesterol diet should be adhered to for 4 to 6 months to fully evaluate its effectiveness. Individuals with severe blood lipid disorders may require the guidance of a registered dietitian.

2. If an adequate trial of dietary therapy fails to lower blood lipid values to acceptable levels, consideration may be given to adding a trial of drug therapy while dietary modification continues. No single drug is appropriate for treating all blood lipid disorders. The choice of the initial drug depends upon the specific nature of the lipoprotein abnormality. Begin with an adequate trial of a single drug. If the response is insufficient, substitute another drug or add a second drug as appropriate. Measure blood lipid levels 4 to 6 weeks after starting drug treatment and at 3-month intervals until a stable response is obtained.

3. To reduce LDL cholesterol (the most common form of cholesterol disorder in the USA):

   weight reduction if necessary

   diet low in saturated fats and cholesterol

   effective drugs:

       cholestyramine (Questran)

       colestipol (Colestid)

       lovastatin (Mevicor)

       niacin (nicotinic acid)

4. To reduce VLDL triglycerides:

   weight reduction

   diet low in saturated fats and cholesterol

   alcohol restriction

   effective drugs:

       niacin (nicotinic acid)

       gemfibrozil (Lopid)

5. To reduce IDL (abnormal lipoprotein):

   weight reduction

   diet low in saturated fats and cholesterol

   effective drugs:

       niacin (nicotinic acid)

       gemfibrozil (Lopid)

       clofibrate (Atromid-S), not recommended due to serious adverse drug effects

6. To raise HDL cholesterol:

   weight reduction

   smoking cessation

   regular exercise

   modest use of alcohol (no more than 1 to 2 drinks daily)

   avoidance of progestin-containing contraceptives

   no specific drug recommended currently

Notes on Specific Lipid-Lowering Drugs

(See the respective Drug Profiles in Section Three for a complete discussion.)

Lovastatin (Mevacor)

The prototype of a new and most promising class of drugs

Recent studies show it to be more effective and better tolerated than cholestyramine.

Can reduce total cholesterol 22% to 33%

Can reduce LDL cholesterol 32% to 42%

Can reduce triglycerides 8% to 27%

Can raise HDL cholesterol slightly

More effective in women than in men

Most effective when used in combination with cholestyramine or colestipol

Infrequent adverse drug effects: indigestion, localized muscle pain

Cholestyramine (Questran) and colestipol (Colestid)

Have demonstrated effectiveness in reducing the development of coronary heart disease

Currently the drugs of choice for treating Type IIa hyperlipidemia

Can reduce total cholesterol 20%

Can reduce LDL cholesterol 23% to 27%

Can raise HDL cholesterol slightly

Triglycerides unchanged or increased

Cause severe constipation in 20% of users

Cause decreased absorption of many other drugs (due to binding)

Large doses cause deficiencies of vitamins A, D, E and K; calcium; iron

Niacin (nicotinic acid)

Used to treat Types IIa, IIb, III and IV hyperlipidemia

Can reduce total cholesterol 25%

Can reduce LDL cholesterol 35%

Can reduce triglycerides 26%

Can raise HDL cholesterol 20%

Not well tolerated by many users

Advise use of timed-release dosage form; increase dose slowly over 2 to 3 months; take with meals; take one adult aspirin tablet 30 minutes before each dose to reduce skin flushing

Significant adverse effects: liver toxicity, reduced sugar tolerance, increased blood uric acid levels, stomach irritation

Gemfibrozil (Lopid)

Used primarily to treat Types IIb, III, IV and V hyperlipidemia

Can reduce total cholesterol 10%

Can reduce LDL cholesterol 11%

Can reduce triglycerides 35%

Can raise HDL cholesterol 11%

Significant adverse effects: reduced sugar tolerance, decreased white blood cell counts, doubled risk for gall stone formation, reduced libido in 12% of men

Should be discontinued if not beneficial after 3 months of treatment

Probucol (Lorelco)

Used primarily to treat Type IIa hyperlipidemia

Can reduce total cholesterol 10% to 15%

Can reduce LDL cholesterol 8%

Can reduce HDL cholesterol 23% (possibly undesirable)

Triglycerides unchanged or raised

Significant adverse effects: anemia, diarrhea
Of limited usefulness due to reduction of HDL cholesterol
May be used in combination with more effective drugs

Current Controversies in Drug Management

1. Should individuals with "moderate" elevations of cholesterol be treated initially with diet modification alone or with combined dietary and drug treatment?

   Comments

   Dietary reduction of saturated fats and cholesterol usually reduces blood cholesterol levels by no more than 10% to 20%; no significant benefit in morbidity or mortality has been demonstrated.

   Cholestyramine drug therapy reduces blood cholesterol levels by 25% with an associated 50% reduction in the risk of developing coronary heart disease.

   Generalizations are not always appropriate or applicable in therapeutic decisions. *Individual* assessment of benefit versus risk (and cost) must be made jointly by patient and physician. The early introduction of drug therapy is justified when there is a family history of premature coronary heart disease (before age 60), recent coronary bypass surgery or other risk factors, such as obesity, high blood pressure, diabetes or heavy use of tobacco.

2. Should individuals with "moderate" elevations of triglycerides (primarily) be treated with diet modification only or with combined dietary and drug treatment?

   Comments

   Not all forms of triglycerides are associated with increased risk for atherosclerosis. A detailed lipoprotein profile is necessary for specific recommendations. The triglycerides found primarily in chylomicrons (Types I and V disorders) are not atherogenic and drug therapy is not indicated. The triglycerides associated with IDL (Type III disorder) are atherogenic and require drug treatment.

Ancillary Drug Treatment (as required)

Condition	*Drug Treatment*
For constipation (due to cholestyramine or colestipol):	docusate (Colace, Dialose, Doxidan, Surfak, etc.)
	Citrucel
	Metamucil
For diarrhea (due to probucol):	diphenoxylate (Lomotil)
	loperamide (Imodium)
For associated diabetes mellitus:	see Profile of Diabetes in this section
For associated hypertension:	see Profile of Hypertension in this section

For associated hypothyroidism: see Profile of Hypothyroidism in
this section

Note: Drug selection, dosage and administration schedule must be determined
by the physician for each patient individually.

Resource for Additional Information and Services

Council on Arteriosclerosis of the American Heart Association
c/o The American Heart Association
7320 Greenville Avenue
Dallas, TX 75231
Phone: (214) 750-5431

Publications available.

CONGESTIVE HEART FAILURE

Other Names: Chronic heart failure, cardiac decompensation, myocardial
decompensation

Prevalence in USA: 2.3 million; 400,000 new cases annually.

Age Group: 45 to 54 years—2.6/1000 population; 55 to 64 years—7/1000
population; 65 to 74 years—15/1000 population.

Male to Female Ratio: 1.5 to 1.

Principal Features: The designation "congestive heart failure" refers to a
condition in which the heart is unable to pump enough blood to satisfy the needs of the body. Diseased heart muscle loses its contracting
power, allowing increased filling pressures inside the heart chambers
(ventricles); further stretching and weakening of muscle tissue leads
to muscle exhaustion and reduced pumping capacity; the forward
flow of blood is impaired and excessive volumes of blood accumulate
in vital areas throughout the body, producing congestion. Resulting
symptoms include shortness of breath (dyspnea), first with exertion
and later at rest; inability to breathe comfortably while lying down
(orthopnea); fatigue and weakness, especially in the legs; a dry cough;
night urination; swelling of the feet and ankles at the end of the day;
and vague discomfort in the chest and abdomen.

Causes: Primary causes of heart disease that ultimately lead to congestive
heart failure:

hypertension (75%)   myocarditis
coronary heart disease (10%)   diabetes (16%)
valvular heart disease (10%)   emphysema
congenital heart disease

Precipitating causes in predisposed individuals: reduction of therapy (most common), heart rhythm disorders, severe infections, obesity, pregnancy, anemia, hyperthyroidism, excessive heat and humidity.

Drugs That Can Cause This Disorder: In individuals with borderline heart function, the following drugs can precipitate congestive heart failure:
amantadine (Symmetrel)
beta-adrenergic-blocking drugs (see Drug Class, Section Four)
cortisonelike steroids (see Drug Class, Section Four)
disopyramide (Norpace)
nonsteroidal anti-inflammatory drugs (see Drug Class, Section Four)

Drugs Used to Treat This Disorder
- digitalis preparations: digitoxin, digoxin.
- diuretics (see Drug Class, Section Four).
- vasodilators: arterial dilators—hydralazine, prazosin; venous dilators—isosorbide dinitrate, nitroglycerin.
- calcium channel-blocking drugs: ditiazem, nifedipine, verapamil.
- ACE inhibitors: captopril, enalapril, lisinopril.
- milrinone (investigational only).
- oxygen.

New Drugs in Development for Treating This Disorder: Xamoterol (Carwin), a new heart muscle stimulant under study in Europe and in the US, has been shown to be significantly better than digoxin in treating chronic heart failure. This drug is not yet available for general use.

Goals of Drug Treatment
Improvement of the heart's pumping performance by the use of digitalis.
Reduction of the heart's workload by the use of arterial and venous vasodilators.
Removal of excess salt and water from the body by the use of diuretics.
Relief of symptoms—fatigue, shortness of breath, ankle swelling, etc.—by means of the above procedures.

Drug Management
For Early, Mild Congestive Heart Failure
Two variations of initial treatment are used widely:
1. Treatment is started with digitalis (digoxin or digitoxin). This may be the only drug used if response is satisfactory. If necessary, a thiazide diuretic (or equivalent) is added.
2. Treatment is started with a thiazide diuretic (or equivalent), given alone. This may give a very adequate response, especially in the elderly. If necessary, digoxin (or digitoxin) is added.
For Moderate to Severe Congestive Heart Failure
Digoxin (or digitoxin) and thiazide diuretics are used in maximal tolerated dosage.
As necessary, a stronger diuretic, such as furosemide or ethacrynic acid, is added.

If the response is inadequate, vasodilators are started: isosorbide dinitrate or nitroglycerin patches for venous dilation; hydralazine for arterial dilation.

If additional improvement is sought, captopril (or enalapril) may be tried as a replacement for the nitrates (isosorbide dinitrate or nitroglycerin).

For long-term maintenance, a combination of hydralazine and nitrates or hydralazine and captropril may be tried.

For congestive heart failure with angina and/or hypertension, a trial of nifedipine is justified.

Use of Digitalis

1. Should be started only when there is a firm diagnosis of heart failure. Periodic reassessment is necessary to determine continued need. Maintenance digitalis may not be necessary for life. Following correction of congestive heart failure, stable heart function may be achieved by using only diuretics and vasodilators.
2. Digoxin is the form of digitalis most frequently used. Because digoxin products vary in their absorbability, refill your prescriptions with the same brand to ensure uniform drug effects.
3. Take the exact dose at the same time each day.
4. Learn to count your pulse and check its regularity. Notify your physician if your pulse rate is below 60 beats/minute or your pulse rhythm changes significantly.
5. The elderly and individuals with hypothyroidism often have a reduced tolerance for digitalis; smaller doses are advisable.
6. Digitalis toxicity (overdosage) occurs in 20% of users; it is more common in the elderly. The earliest indications of toxicity are usually loss of appetite, nausea and vomiting; other indications include headache, facial pains, blurred vision, seeing "snowflakes" or yellowish-green halos, fatigue, weakness and disturbances of heart rhythm. The elderly may show confusion; rarely, seizures may occur.
7. Periodic blood levels can help to determine optimal dosage, especially if kidney function is impaired. The blood sample should be taken no less than 6 hours after the last dose.
8. See the Drug Profile of Digoxin in Section Three for important drug interactions.

Use of Diuretics ("Water Pills")

1. Thiazide (or equivalent) diuretics may suffice as the only drug treatment for mild heart failure in many elderly patients.
2. When possible, diuretics should be taken in the morning to minimize nighttime urination.
3. If your diuretic is one that increases the excretion of potassium in the urine, it is important that your blood level of potassium be checked periodically. An abnormally low potassium level can increase the risk of digitalis toxicity. Consult your physician regarding the advisability of omitting your diuretic every third day to minimize the loss of potassium.

4. If your diuretic is one that does not increase the excretion of potassium (amiloride, spironolactone, triamterene), you should not take a potassium supplement or eat excessive amounts of high-potassium foods.
5. If you use diuretics on a regular basis, consult your physician regarding the degree of salt restriction he or she recommends for you.
6. Many salt substitutes have a high potassium content. Ask your physician for guidance regarding the selection and use of commercially available salt substitutes.
7. In advanced congestive heart failure, you may be advised to use a thiazide diuretic concurrently with furosemide (or ethacrynic acid) and a potassium-saving diuretic; the combined actions of the three types of drugs give a maximal diuretic effect.

Use of Vasodilators
1. These are generally used when heart failure does not respond adequately to digitalis and diuretics.
2. These may be used earlier for those who cannot tolerate digitalis, and for those who need a vasodilator to treat hypertension (hydralazine) or angina (nifedipine).
3. Nitrate vasodilators (primarily venous dilators) contribute to the relief of shortness of breath.
4. Hydralazine (primarily an arterial dilator) contributes to the relief of fatigue and weakness.
5. Isosorbide dinitrate (venous) and hydralazine (arterial) vasodilators can be used concurrently to advantage; they are quite effective in the majority of cases of chronic congestive failure.
6. Prazosin (both an arterial and a venous dilator) is an alternative choice. However it causes fluid retention and requires increasing doses and additional diuretics with continued use.

Use of Oxygen
1. Oxygen must be properly humidified to prevent drying of tissues of the respiratory tract.
2. Administer by nasal prongs; avoid a mask.

Current Controversies in Drug Management
With the advent of new drugs and improved understanding of the altered physiology associated with congestive heart failure, controversy regarding drug selection for its treatment has increased. A consensus has emerged indicating that diuretics should now be considered the first-line drugs of choice, replacing digoxin.

Controversy continues, however, as to which drug should be added next if diuretics are inadequate. Some authorities favor digoxin as the second drug; others favor vasodilators (see above). Current evidence seems to favor vasodilators as the second drug, with digoxin added as a third drug when required. New studies show that angiotensin-converting enzyme (ACE) inhibitors (see above) can enhance treatment and prolong survival. Further experience and detailed analysis of drug performance are required to resolve current controversies.

Drug choices at this time will remain a matter of individual physician preference.

Ancillary Drug Treatment (as required)

Condition	*Drug Treatment*
For anxiety:	diazepam (only as needed)
For insomnia:	chloral hydrate (Noctec, Somnos)
For anemia:	iron preparations
For hypertension:	see Profile of Hypertension in this section

Note: Drug selection, dosage and administration schedule must be determined by the physician for each patient individually.

Resources for Additional Information and Services

Heartlife (Heart Disease Heart Line)
P.O. Box 54305
Atlanta, GA 30308
Phone: 1-800-241-6993; (404) 523-0826

Available 9:00 a.m.–4:00 p.m. EST, M–F; Spanish-speaking counselor available.
Publications available.

American Heart Association
7320 Greenville Avenue
Dallas, TX 75231
Phone: (214) 373-6300

Publications available.

CROHN'S DISEASE

Other Names: Regional enteritis, regional ileitis, granulomatous colitis, inflammatory bowel disease

Prevalence in USA: 1 million (includes 100,000 children); 15,000 new cases annually.

Age Group: Onset from infancy to 25 years of age; 15% to 30% have onset before puberty. Peak incidence is from 10 to 25 years of age.

Male to Female Ratio: Slightly more common in females.

Principal Features: An intermittent to chronic disorder of the small intestine and colon; one third of cases occur in the lower segment of the small intestine (the ileum), one third in the colon and one third in both. Less than 50% of cases involve the rectum. The onset is usually insidious, but may be rapid and resemble acute appendicitis. Symptoms include loss of appetite, fatigue, fever, loss of weight, abdominal cramps and pain after eating, nausea, vomiting, diarrhea (occasionally bloody), anal sores and retarded growth in children. There may also be inflammatory disorders in the skin, eyes, mouth and large joints. Children may experience fever and joint pains before any indications of disease in the intestine or colon. Adults may have a higher incidence of gallstones or kidney stones. This disorder often recurs throughout life.

Caution: The early manifestations of Crohn's disease may vary. Loss of appetite and weight may lead to the mistaken diagnosis of anorexia nervosa.

Causes: The primary cause is unknown. There is a familial clustering in 15% to 20% of cases. It is thought that an inherited susceptibility may predispose to unknown environmental factors capable of inducing the disorder.

Drugs That Can Cause This Disorder: By altering the normal balance of bacteria in the intestine, several antibiotics can cause a form of enteritis that might resemble Crohn's disease. These include some of the tetracyclines, penicillin and chloramphenicol. Antibiotic-induced enteritis is transient and easily corrected; no permanent damage occurs. The vitamin A derivative etretinate (Tegison) has been reported to cause Crohn's disease.

Drugs Used to Treat This Disorder
- sulfasalazine (Azulfidine).
- cortisonelike steroids, principally prednisone.
- azathioprine (Imuran); 6-mercaptopurine (Purinethol).
- metronidazole (Flagyl).
- antidiarrheals: diphenoxylate (Lomotil), loperamide (Imodium).
- antispasmodics: belladonna (Donnatal), dicyclomine (Bentyl).
- antibiotics: ampicillin (Amcill, etc.), tetracycline (Achromycin, etc.); used when appropriate for bacterial infections of intestine.

Goals of Drug Treatment
Induction of a remission (return to normal) during the active phase of the disease.
Relief of symptoms.
Protection of bowel, avoidance of complications.
Maintenance of general nutrition.

Drug Management
General Principles
For initial treatment of mild disease: sulfasalazine.
For moderate to severe disease: prednisone, used concurrently with sulfasalazine.
For acute recurrences: prednisone.

For long-term maintenance: sulfasalazine; avoid use of cortisonelike steroids (prednisone).

For active disease that fails to respond to combined use of sulfasalazine and prednisone: (1) a trial of metronidazole as replacement for sulfasalazine; (2) a trial of azathioprine or 6-mercaptopurine added to sulfasalazine and prednisone programs.

Use of Sulfasalazine

1. Used to initiate treatment in active disease.
2. About 50% effective when used with prednisone.
3. Most beneficial in treating Crohn's disease of the colon.
4. Usually not effective in preventing recurrences; however, it may be tried for long-term maintenance until a better treatment is developed.
5. Common adverse effects are headache, nausea and vomiting; take with or immediately following food.

Use of Cortisonelike Steroids (Prednisone, etc.)

1. Usually 60% to 70% effective during first 6 months of treatment; if use is extended to 12 months, only 20% to 30% remain in remission.
2. Good initial response in treating Crohn's disease of the colon, but the majority relapse within 1 year.
3. Long-term use for mild disease or to prevent recurrences is usually ineffective and is not advised.
4. Use primarily to control worsening symptoms and to suppress acute flare-ups. Continue use until a sustained improvement is established. Try to use the lowest effective dose.
5. When possible, an alternate-day dosing schedule is recommended: a single morning dose every 48 hours.
6. When appropriate, taper dose very slowly over a period of 4 to 12 months.
7. Repeated intermittent short courses are preferable to continual long-term use.
8. Crohn's disease of the rectum should be treated with steroid suppositories and retention enemas.

Use of Antidiarrheals

1. Use very cautiously and as sparingly as possible.
2. Excessive use can induce two complications: (1) paralytic (adynamic) ileus, a paralysis of the small intestine that results in a functional obstruction; (2) toxic megacolon, a marked distention of the colon with air, and a danger of perforation.

Use of Adsorbents

1. Cholestyramine (Questran) and aluminum hydroxide (Amphojel) can adsorb bile in the intestine and reduce bile-induced diarrhea.
2. These adsorbents can also adsorb other drugs being used concurrently. Schedule all dosages to ensure maximal effectiveness—adequate spacing between adsorbents and other active drugs.

Use of Immunosuppressants

1. Azathioprine (Imuran) and 6-mercaptopurine (Purinethol) may be tried when sulfasalazine and prednisone have failed to control the disease after an adequate trial.
2. Either one may be tried as an adjunct to the established treatment program.
3. A trial of 4 to 6 months of treatment is often necessary to determine effectiveness.
4. These drugs make it possible to reduce the dose of steroids or withdraw them completely in some individuals.

Use of Antibiotics

1. Appropriately selected antibiotics may be used to treat a diarrhea due to specific bacterial overgrowth (superinfection).
2. Antibiotics should not be taken concurrently with sulfasalazine.

Ancillary Drug Treatment (as required)

Condition	Drug Treatment
For anemia (common):	iron preparations, vitamin B-12, folic acid (as required)
For malnutrition:	multiple vitamins and the minerals calcium, magnesium, zinc
For depression:	see Profile of Depression in this section

Note: Drug selection, dosage and administration schedule must be determined by the physician for each patient individually.

Resource for Additional Information and Services

American Digestive Disease Society
7720 Wisconsin Avenue
Bethesda, MD 20814
Phone: (301) 652-9293

Telecommunications services: Gutline, available to the public every Tuesday evening from 7:30 to 9:00 p.m.
Publications available.

DEPRESSION

Other Names: Depressive reaction (reactive depression, secondary depression), depressive illness (biologic depression, major depressive disorder), affective disorder: depressive phase of manic-depressive disorder

Prevalence in USA: Approximately 30 million; 5% to 8% of general population. One third of all depressions are severe enough to require medical treatment.

Age Group: Can occur at any age. Peak occurrence is between 25 and 44 years of age.

Male to Female Ratio: 1 male to 2 females; 25% of women and 10% of men will experience depression during their lifetime.

Principal Features

Depressive Reaction: A situational (exogenous) reactive depression that represents an understandable adaptive response to a significant loss or stressful life situation; a sense of despondency and distress, comparatively mild to moderate, usually self-limiting with a duration of 2 weeks to 6 months.

Depressive Illness: A spontaneous (endogenous) unexplained and seemingly unprovoked depression of moderate to severe degree; characterized by (1) a depressed mood—sadness, dejection, hopelessness, despair; (2) reduced energy level—loss of interest, fatigue, inability to function effectively; (3) negative self-image—sense of inferiority, incompetence, exaggerated guilt. Common features include loss of appetite, broken sleep, early morning awakening, constipation. Often clears spontaneously in 6 to 12 months, even without treatment.

Causes: Depressive reactions are normal mood responses to the stresses and strains of daily life. The primary cause of major depressive illness is unknown. Research indicates that in many cases there appears to be a genetic (constitutional) predisposition to depression. The actual onset of depressive illness is attributed to a deficiency of certain brain chemicals—the neurotransmitters norepinephrine, dopamine and/or serotonin. What initiates the deficiency is not known.

Drugs That Can Cause This Disorder: Drug-induced depressions are more likely to occur in those who are genetically susceptible to depression. The following drugs are known to cause depression:

benzodiazepines (in excess)	levodopa
certain beta-blocking drugs	methyldopa
clonidine	oral contraceptives
cortisonelike steroids	some phenothiazines
digitalis (toxicity)	reserpine (and related drugs)
indomethacin	

Drugs Used to Treat This Disorder

Bicyclic Antidepressant
- fluoxetine (Prozac).

Tricyclic Antidepressants (TCA's)
- amitriptyline (Elavil, Endep).
- amoxapine (Asendin).
- desipramine (Norpramin, Pertofrane).
- doxepin (Adapin, Sinequan).
- imipramine (Imavate, Presamine, Tofranil).

- nortriptyline (Aventyl, Pamelor).
- protriptyline (Vivactil).

Tetracyclic Antidepressant
- maprotiline (Ludiomil).

Monoamine Oxidase Inhibitors (MAOI's) Type A
- phenelzine (Nardil).
- tranylcypromine (Parnate).

Other Drugs
- alprazolam (Xanax)
- lithium (Eskalith, Lithane, Lithobid, Lithotab)
- methylphenidate (Ritalin)
- trazodone (Desyrel)

Goals of Drug Treatment
Alleviation of symptoms.
Termination of depression, restoration of normal mood.
Prevention of recurrence.
Prevention of swing from depression to manic psychosis (in manic-depressive disorder).

Drug Management
For Depressive Reactions: Reactive depressions are often mild and self-limiting; they usually respond well to supportive psychotherapy. Drug treatment is not necessary for everyone who is depressed. If this type of depression becomes severe or is unreasonably prolonged, a tricyclic antidepressant (or a new generation equivalent) may be tried for 1 month to determine its effectiveness.

For Depressive Illness: Major endogenous depressions are usually very responsive to an appropriate and adequate trial of antidepressant drug therapy. Spontaneous remissions often occur within 6 to 12 months, but recovery can be initiated earlier and greatly accelerated by proper medication. Adequate dosage and a sufficient period of treatment are essential to a successful outcome.

Treatment is usually started with a tricyclic antidepressant or one of the newer equivalents. If response is inadequate after a reasonable trial, another tricyclic or similar antidepressant should be tried. If this fails, a monoamine oxidase inhibitor may be considered. Some cyclic depressions respond better to lithium than to tricyclic antidepressants.

Not all depressions are recurrent. For a first episode, the antidepressant drug may be gradually reduced and discontinued after 3 to 6 months of a stable mood, free of depression.

For the 50% of depressions that are recurrent, the optimal maintenance dose of the most effective drug should be determined and continued indefinitely.

Use of Tricyclic Antidepressants (TCA's)
1. These are the drugs of choice when drug treatment is deemed necessary.

2. They are 60% to 75% effective in treating major endogenous depressive illness. They may also be effective in treating severe reactive depressions.

3. Continual use on a regular schedule for 2 to 5 weeks is necessary to determine a drug's effectiveness in relieving depression.

4. Treatment with all antidepressants is necessarily empirical; a period of trial and error is unavoidable for both the selection of the best drug and the determination of optimal dosage.

5. If one TCA (or equivalent) shows no significant benefit after 3 weeks of adequate dosage, it is advisable to try another drug of the same or similar class.

6. During drug trials, and during maintenance treatment later, stay with the same brand (manufacturer) to ensure uniform results.

7. Periodic measurement of blood levels of the drug can be helpful in determining optimal dosage. (See Therapeutic Drug Monitoring in Section One.)

8. Most drugs of this class cause drowsiness, especially during the first several weeks of use. Avoid alcoholic beverages and use extreme caution in driving and engaging in all hazardous activities.

9. When the correct total daily dose has been determined, it can usually be taken as a single dose at bedtime.

10. Use these drugs cautiously if you have glaucoma, prostatism or a heart rhythm disorder.

11. Avoid rapid withdrawal of TCA's; abrupt discontinuation may cause restlessness, headache, anxiety, insomnia, muscle aches, nausea. Withdraw gradually over a period of 10 to 14 days.

12. See the Drug Profiles of respective TCA's in Section Three for important drug interactions.

Use of Newer ("Second Generation") Antidepressants

1. Maprotiline (Ludiomil) may act more rapidly than TCA's; it is quite sedating. Avoid if you have a seizure disorder.

2. Alprazolam (Xanax) is sedating. After long-term use, withdraw gradually to avoid possible seizures.

3. Amoxapine (Asendin) is less sedating. It can cause parkinsonlike symptoms, restlessness and tardive dyskinesia (rarely). Do not use longer than 3 to 4 months.

4. Trazodone (Desyrel) is also sedating, but it has little or no atropinelike effects. It is very useful in the elderly and for those with glaucoma or prostatism.

Use of Monoamine Oxidase Inhibitors (MAOI's) Type A

1. Used to treat biologic endogenous depressions that do not respond to TCA's.

2. Also useful for treating "atypical" and neurotic depressions that are characterized by marked anxiety, phobias, hypochondriasis, excessive eating and excessive sleeping.

3. Continual use on a regular schedule for 2 to 5 weeks is necessary to determine effectiveness in relieving depression.

4. Avoid concurrent use of over-the-counter diet pills, nose drops and cold and allergy preparations.
5. Avoid foods and beverages that contain tyramine and similar compounds. (See Tyramine in Glossary.)
6. If switching from a TCA to a MAOI, allow a "washout" period of 7 to 10 days before starting the MAOI. If switching from a MAOI to a TCA, allow a "washout" period of 14 days before starting the TCA.
7. MAOI's can cause low blood pressure, overstimulation, insomnia, confusion, nausea, vomiting, diarrhea and fluid retention.
8. MAOI's can provoke an abrupt swing from depression to manic psychosis in manic-depressive disorder.
9. MAOI's can activate psychosis in those with schizophrenia.
10. Do not discontinue these drugs suddenly. A rebound depression can follow abrupt withdrawal.
11. See the Drug Profiles of respective MAOI's in Section Three for important drug interactions.

Use of Lithium
1. Can be 70% effective in stabilizing mood, especially in bipolar manic-depressive illness; reduces the frequency and severity of attacks of both mania and depression.
2. Often effective in preventing recurrences of depression in unipolar (depression only) disorders.
3. Must be taken in divided doses to avoid stomach irritation and excessively high (toxic) blood levels.
4. When lithium proves to be effective in preventing recurrence of depression, it is very important to continue maintenance treatment when feeling well and free of depression.
5. Periodic measurements of blood levels are mandatory to maintain effective concentrations and to prevent toxicity. Blood samples should be taken 12 hours after the last dose.
6. Mild side-effects (not toxicity) include loss of appetite, metallic taste, indigestion, nausea, thirst, fatigue, tremor, fluid retention, acne.
7. Early toxic effects include vomiting, dizziness, unsteadiness, weakness, slurred speech, muscle twitching, confusion.
8. While taking lithium, maintain a high liquid intake, but avoid excessive coffee, tea and cola drinks.
9. Do not restrict your salt intake.
10. Use lithium cautiously if you have heart disease, kidney disease or a thyroid disorder.
11. Check thyroid and kidney functions before and during lithium therapy.

Use of Other Antidepressant Drugs
1. Methylphenidate (Ritalin) may be tried for long-term treatment of selected elderly persons with depression.
2. Alprazolam (Xanax), a benzodiazepine tranquilizer, may be useful for short-term treatment of minor depression.

Ancillary Drug Treatment (as required)

Condition	*Drug Treatment*
For mild anxiety:	alprazolam (Xanax)
For severe anxiety and agitation:	thioridazine (Mellaril) thiothixene (Navane)
For psychosis:	amitriptyline and perphenazine (Etrafon, Triavil)
For constipation:	docusate (Colace, Doxinate, etc.)

Note: Drug selection, dosage and administration schedule must be determined by the physician for each patient individually.

Resources for Additional Information and Services

Depressives Anonymous: Recovery From Depression
329 East 62nd Street
New York, NY 10021
Phone: (212) 689-2600

Publications available.

Emotions Anonymous
P.O. Box 4245
St. Paul, MN 55104
Phone: (612) 647-9712

Telecommunications services: Telephone referrals to local chapters.
Publications available.

National Depressive and Manic Depressive Association
222 South Riverside Plaza
Chicago, IL 60606
Phone: (312) 993-0066

Telecommunications services: Offers information, one-to-one support, referrals.
Publications available.

DIABETES

Other Names: Diabetes mellitus; insulin-dependent diabetes mellitus (IDDM), type I; non-insulin-dependent diabetes mellitus (NIDDM), type II

Prevalence in USA: Approximately 10 million: 6 million known, 4 million undiagnosed; 2% to 4% of the population, with a 6% increase (new cases) annually.

Age Group: Under 18 years—90,000; 18 to 44 years—880,000; 45 to 64 years—2.6 million; 65 to 74 years—1.6 million; 75 years and over—800,000.

Male to Female Ratio: Type I—same incidence in men and women. Type II—greater incidence in women.

Principal Features: A disorder of carbohydrate, protein and fat metabolism that renders the body unable to convert foods properly into energy for vital functions.

Type I (10% to 15% of All Diabetes): Occurs most commonly in children and adolescents, with peak onset from 11 to 14 years; can begin at any age. Individuals are usually thin or normal weight (nonobese). Requires lifelong insulin for control of blood sugar and prevention of acidosis.

Type II (85% to 90% of All Diabetes): Most common after 40 years of age, with peak onset from 45 to 64 years. Up to 90% of individuals are obese. Does not require lifelong insulin for control; not prone to development of acidosis.

Characteristic symptoms include excessive hunger and thirst, excessive urination, unexplained weight loss, blurred vision, fatigue, itching of skin, anal and vaginal yeast infections and delayed healing of wounds.

Causes: Primary causes are unknown, but a genetic (hereditary) predisposition appears certain for both types of diabetes. In addition, some individuals who develop type I diabetes may have a genetic susceptibility to viral infection of the pancreas that initiates destruction of the tissue cells that produce insulin. In type I diabetes the pancreas produces very little or no insulin. In type II diabetes insulin production may be normal or partially reduced, but not absent; the diabetes is due to insulin resistance in body tissues.

Drugs That Can Cause This Disorder: In susceptible individuals and those with latent diabetes, the following drugs may induce diabetic manifestations; these are usually mild in nature and reversible:

cortisonelike steroids	phenothiazines
ethacrynic acid	phenytoin
furosemide	propranolol
indomethacin	thiazide diuretics
lithium	tricyclic antidepressants
oral contraceptives	

Drugs Used to Treat This Disorder

The Insulins: See Drug Profile of Insulin in Section Three.

The Sulfonylureas (Oral Hypoglycemic Drugs)
- acetohexamide (Dymelor).
- chlorpropamide (Diabinese).
- glipizide (Glucotrol).
- glyburide (Diabeta, Micronase).

- tolazamide (Tolinase).
- tolbutamide (Orinase).

New Drugs in Development for Treating This Disorder: Nazlin, a nasal insulin product, is now in clinical trials to evaluate its effectiveness and determine proper dosage. This dosage form will be absorbed through the nose, providing rapid absorption that more closely resembles the body's natural release of insulin.

Goals of Drug Treatment

Normalization of carbohydrate, protein and fat metabolism insofar as possible; control of blood sugar; elimination of acidosis.

Elimination of symptoms; restoration of well-being.

Prevention of hypoglycemia (insulin "shock").

Prevention of recurrent acidosis.

Promotion of normal growth and development in diabetic children.

Prevention or minimization of late complications.

Achievement of normal life expectancy.

Drug Management

General Principles

"Good control" consists of the optimal balance of properly selected foods, exercise and drugs—either insulin or a sulfonylurea in correct dosage. The degree of control is estimated by periodic measurement of blood-sugar levels or urine sugar content.

"Tight control" consists of maintaining a fasting blood sugar between 100 and 140 mg, and a 2-hour (after eating) blood sugar betweeen 100 and 200 mg. Consideration must be given to the possible benefits of "tight control" versus the possible risks of inducing hypoglycemia.

"Tight control" is appropriate for the young diabetic who is otherwise healthy, free of coronary artery and cerebral circulatory disease, capable of excellent self-care and not living alone. It is not appropriate for the elderly, those with circulatory disorders of the brain or heart, those with established complications of long-standing diabetes and those with other serious disorders.

Although more expensive and inconvenient, the home monitoring of blood-sugar levels is the method of choice for managing diabetic control. The blood-sugar strips Chemstrip bG and Visidex II are recommended for this purpose.

The use of urine-testing strips for the detection of urine sugar and ketones is a useful and practical alternative to the use of blood-sugar strips. Regular testing of urine before meals and at bedtime provides adequate information for the proper adjustment of insulin dosage schedules and the prevention of hypoglycemia and acidosis. Accuracy is improved when the bladder is first emptied and the urine for testing is collected 30 minutes later; the sugar content of this second voiding is more representative of the current blood-sugar level.

If urine testing reveals the repeated presence of ketones, consult your physician promptly.

The following drugs can cause a *false positive* test result for urine sugar when using Clinitest: aspirin (with doses larger than 2400 mg/day), ascorbic acid (vitamin C), cephalosporins, chloral hydrate, chloramphenicol, isoniazid, levodopa, methyldopa, nalidixic acid, penicillin G, probenecid, streptomycin.

The following drugs can cause a *false negative* test result for urine sugar when using Diastix or Testape: aspirin (with doses larger than 2400 mg/day), ascorbic acid (vitamin C), levodopa, methyldopa.

The following drugs can cause a *false positive* test result for urine ketones when using Acetest or Ketostix: aspirin (in moderate to high doses), levodopa, phenazopyridine (Ketostix only).

Learn to recognize the early indications of hypoglycemia and what to do to correct it. Signs that warn of a developing insulin reaction include hunger, sweating, headache, dizziness, nervousness, trembling, blurred vision, drowsiness, confusion, inability to think, sense of inebriation. At the first indication of impending hypoglycemia, take sugar immediately: 5 small sugar cubes; or 2 teaspoonsful or 2 packets of granulated sugar; or ½ to 1 cup of fruit juice; or 1 candy bar. An alternative treatment is the injection of 1 mg of glucagon, repeated in 5 to 10 minutes if necessary. Glucagon is a pancreatic hormone that increases the level of blood sugar.

Learn to recognize the early indications of acidosis. These include the slow development of increasing thirst, excessive urination, drowsiness, fatigue, nausea, vomiting, stomach pain.

The use of beta-blocking drugs (especially in high doses) may predispose to hypoglycemia and mask its symptoms.

For Type I, IDDM

Insulin is a lifelong requirement for control. Sulfonylureas (oral hypoglycemics) are not effective and should not be used.

Insulin requirements will vary continually throughout a lifetime. Therefore, you must learn how to manage your diabetes on a day-by-day basis, modifying insulin types and dosage schedules as necessary, according to the results of regular blood- or urine sugar testing.

For the newly diagnosed diabetic who is not acutely ill and is without complications, the usual American procedure for initiating treatment is to give a single morning dose of 15 to 30 units of an intermediate-acting insulin (NPH or Lente) before breakfast; the dose is then increased by 5 units every 48 hours as required to achieve normal blood-sugar levels. The British method is to start with 6 to 10 units of an intermediate-acting insulin given twice daily, before the morning and evening meals. Either method will relieve most symptoms in 90% of cases within 4 days.

The optimal schedule of insulin injections for regulating the disordered metabolism is determined by periodic monitoring of blood-sugar levels at appropriate times during the 24-hour day. In this way individual patterns of blood-sugar fluctuation and response to insulin can be studied so that the most appropriate types and doses of insulin are given in proper relationship to eating.

A most effective and practical method of providing adequate insulin for the average diabetic is to give a mixture (1 injection) of a rapid-acting insulin (Regular) and an intermediate-acting insulin (NPH or Lente) 20 to 30 minutes before the morning and evening meals, just 2 injections daily. This scheme provides for easy modification of doses of each type of insulin as necessary to obtain smooth control throughout 24 hours.

During periods of stress—infections, injuries, surgery—insulin requirements will increase. Consult your physician for guidance if you have difficulty in making the necessary adjustments of insulin dosage, food intake, etc.

Even during periods of fasting, small amounts of insulin are necessary to control blood sugar and prevent acidosis.

For Type II, NIDDM

Diet is of primary importance and should be tried diligently before starting drugs. Dietary goals are reduction of blood sugar and correction of obesity. Seventy-five percent of cases of Type II diabetes can be controlled by diet alone.

If an adequate trial of dietary management fails, either sulfonylurea drugs (oral hypoglycemics) or insulin may be added to the treatment program. If the blood sugar is only moderately above normal, a sulfonylurea may be tried. If the blood sugar is quite high and the individual is thin, it is best to initiate drug treatment with insulin. After the blood sugar has been stabilized for 3 to 4 weeks, the insulin may be withdrawn and a sulfonylurea may be started to determine its effectiveness.

The major reaction to sulfonylureas is hypoglycemia. It is most likely to occur in the elderly, in alcoholics and in those with significant impairment of liver or kidney function. Hypoglycemic reactions occur most frequently with the use of chlorpropamide (Diabinese), the longest acting sulfonylurea.

If you experience a primary failure (on initial trial) or a secondary failure (after a temporary period of effectiveness) on attempting control with a sulfonylurea, you may need insulin to manage your diabetes successfully.

Insulin is used primarily to control the levels of blood sugar. It is not required to prevent acidosis except under stressful conditions, such as infections, trauma or surgery.

Type II diabetes is often well controlled with a single daily dose of an intermediate-acting insulin. Some individuals with a high degree of insulin resistance may require unusually high doses of insulin to achieve satisfactory control.

Use of Insulins

1. Twenty percent of all diabetics require insulin for satisfactory control.
2. Available insulins differ in their times of peak action and duration of action. An understanding of these differences is necessary for planning an insulin schedule and adjusting it to control your in-

Type of insulin	Peak action (hours)	Duration (hours)	Hypoglycemia most likely to occur
Short-acting			
Regular	2–4	5–7	Before lunch
Semilente	2–8	12–16	Before lunch
Actrapid	2.5–5	8	Before lunch
Semitard	7	9	Early afternoon
Velosulin	2–5	8	Before lunch
Humulin R	2–5	6–8	Before lunch
Intermediate-acting			
Lente	8–12	18–28	Late afternoon
NPH	6–12	18–28	Late afternoon
Monotard	7–15	18–24	Late afternoon
Lentard	8–12	16–24	Late afternoon
Insulatard	4–12	16–24	Mid-afternoon
Humulin N	6–12	14–24	Late afternoon
Novolin N	4–12	18–24	Mid-afternoon
Long-acting			
Protamine Zinc	14–24	24–36	During night–early morning
Ultralente	18–24	32–36	During night–early morning
Ultratard	10–28	24–36	During night–early morning

dividual pattern of blood-sugar fluctuations during each 24-hour day. The accompanying table illustrates the characteristics of the three principal types of insulin.

3. The peak action times and the duration of action vary greatly from person to person. Each individual will show variations of absorption from one injection site to another and from day to day. Insulin programs must be tailored to each person individually based on response to trials. All insulin schedules need adjustment from time to time.

4. Most insulin-dependent diabetics require from 20 to 60 units of insulin daily. If the requirement reaches 200 units/day, a marked degree of insulin resistance has developed. This is best treated with highly purified pork insulin or human insulin.

5. Most of the time satisfactory control can be achieved with an intermediate-acting insulin, or with the addition of a short-acting insulin. Regular insulin can be mixed with either Lente or NPH in the same syringe and given as a single injection. The mixture retains the short and intermediate characteristics of action.

6. Long-acting insulins are rarely necessary and are seldom used.

7. Hypoglycemia that occurs during the night (excessive insulin effect) causes a "rebound" hyperglycemia that is detected by blood- or urine sugar testing the next morning. This is known as the Somogyi effect. The proper adjustment is to reduce the dose of the long-

acting insulin taken in the morning or the dose of the intermediate-acting insulin taken before the evening meal; this will prevent the nocturnal hypoglycemia that causes the confusing high blood or urine sugar on arising.

8. If a true allergy to insulin develops, or if the fatty tissue under the skin at the sites of insulin injection should disappear (lipoatrophy), change to highly purified pork or human insulin.

9. If insulin use is to be intermittent (as in some cases of type II diabetes), it is best to use human insulin to reduce the possibility of developing insulin antibodies that cause insulin resistance.

10. Insulin pumps using either Regular or Ultralente insulin have been developed for use in selected individuals. While they are capable of providing excellent control, their use is quite complex and demanding. They are suitable only for the highly motivated and educated individual who needs and is dedicated to achieving "tight control."

Use of Sulfonylureas (Oral Hypoglycemic Drugs)

1. These drugs are used only for the treatment of type II, NIDDM, in those whose diabetes is not adequately controlled by diet and exercise and who cannot or will not take insulin.

2. The best candidates for a trial of sulfonylureas
   - are over 50 years old.
   - are otherwise healthy.
   - are not allergic to "sulfa" drugs.
   - have no tendency to develop acidosis.
   - have an insulin requirement of less than 30 units/day.
   - prefer tablets by mouth to injections.

3. Sulfonylureas are not suitable for treating
   - type I, insulin-dependent diabetes.
   - the acutely ill diabetic with acidosis.
   - the diabetic with infection or with injury, or undergoing surgery.
   - the diabetic using long-term cortisonelike steroids.
   - the pregnant diabetic.
   - the diabetic whose blood sugar is over 300 mg.

4. Sulfonylureas should be used with caution in treating
   - the very old.
   - alcoholics.
   - those taking multiple drugs.
   - those with significantly impaired liver or kidney function.
   - those who comply poorly with recommendations.

5. Recommended dosage schedules:

Short-acting	**Duration**	**Doses/day**
tolbutamide	6–12 hrs.	2–3

Intermediate-acting

acetohexamide	12–24 hrs.	1–2
glipizide	18–30 hrs.	1–2
glyburide	10–30 hrs.	1–2
tolazamide	10–18 hrs.	1–2

Long-acting

chlorpropamide	60 hrs.	1

6. All sulfonylureas can cause hypoglycemia. Because of its accumulative effects and long period of action, chlorpropamide requires the greatest caution in use; any hypoglycemic reaction is apt to be quite prolonged.

7. Sulfonylureas as a group have a high rate of primary failure (40%). A primary failure is an inability to control hyperglycemia after 3 months of continual treatment with adequate dosage. Secondary failures (25% to 30%) occur when a sulfonylurea drug loses its effectiveness after an initial period of demonstrated ability to control hyperglycemia.

8. During apparently successful long-term use of a sulfonylurea, it is prudent to periodically reduce the dosage and gradually withdraw the drug to determine if its continued use is justified. The success rate of adequate control by long-term use of sulfonylureas is no more than 20% to 30%.

9. There appears to be no general support for the concurrent use of sulfonylureas and insulin. If it is found that insulin is necessary for adequate control, the customary practice is to discontinue the sulfonylurea.

Ancillary Drug Treatment (as required)

Condition	*Drug Treatment*
For yeast infections of skin:	ciclopirox (Loprox) clotrimazole (Lotrimin) haloprogin (Halotex) miconazole (Micatin) nystatin (Mycostatin)
For yeast infections of the vagina:	clotrimazole (Gyne-Lotrimin, Mycelex-G) miconazole (Monistat)
For diabetic diarrhea:	diphenoxylate (Lomotil) loperamide (Imodium)
For peripheral neuritis:	carbamazepine (Tegretol) and amitriptyline (Elavil) concurrently
For neurogenic bladder:	bethanechol (Urecholine)
For high blood pressure:	see Profile of Hypertension in this section

Note: Drug selection, dosage and administration schedule must be determined by the physician for each patient individually.

Resources for Additional Information and Services

American Diabetes Association
National Service Center
P.O. Box 25757
1660 Duke Street
Alexandria, VA 22313
Phone: 1-800-232-3472; (703) 549-1500

Publications available.

Joslin Diabetes Center
One Joslin Place
Boston, MA 02215
Phone: 1-800-223-1138; (617) 732-2400

Available 9:00 a.m.–5:00 p.m. EST, M–F. Spanish-speaking counselors available. Offers public information on specific diabetic needs.
Publications available.

Juvenile Diabetes Foundation
432 Park Avenue South, 16th Floor
New York, NY 10016
Phone: 1-800-223-1138; (212) 889-7575

Publications, films, tapes available.

EPILEPSY

Other Names: Seizure disorders, convulsive disorders

Prevalence in USA: Approximately 2 million, 1% of the population.

Age Group: 24% of epileptics are under 18 years of age; 53% are 18 to 44 years; 18% are 45 to 64 years; 4% are 65 to 74 years; 1% is 75 years and older.

Male to Female Ratio: About equal.

Principal Features: True epilepsy is a chronic disorder characterized by recurring seizures lasting from a few seconds to several minutes and requiring specific medication for prevention and control. Sixty-six percent of epileptic patients require lifelong drug therapy. The principal types of epilepsy include:

Tonic-Clonic Seizures (Grand Mal): Sudden attacks that begin with an involuntary cry, followed by a loss of consciousness and falling, violent convulsive movements of the head, trunk and extremities, excessive salivation and sometimes loss of bladder and/or rectal control. The seizure lasts from 1 to 3 minutes. The individual awakens spontaneously, is dazed, confused and exhausted, and usually falls into a deep sleep that lasts several hours. The subject cannot remember the episode.

Absence Seizures (Petit Mal): These begin between 2 and 12 years of age; 90% cease by 20 years; 50% go on to develop tonic-clonic seizures by 20 years. The seizure consists of a sudden, momentary lapse of consciousness lasting several seconds (30 at the most), during which the subject has a blank stare and is oblivious of surroundings; there is no actual loss of consciousness, no fall and no convulsion; there may be a minor twitching of an eyelid or facial muscle, chewing movements or a jerk of a hand or arm. Such episodes may recur more than 100 times a day. Following each seizure, the subject resumes normal functioning as though nothing had happened; the attack is not remembered.

Complex Partial Seizures (Psychomotor or Temporal Lobe Epilepsy): This type comprises 40% of all epilepsies. It consists of sudden alterations of behavior that involve speech, hearing, memory and emotional response. Some episodes begin with an "aura" that may take the form of distorted vision, unpleasant odors, visual and auditory hallucinations and bizarre illusions; the subject may walk about aimlessly, talk irrationally, laugh, engage in purposeless and inappropriate actions, such as striking at walls in anger or fear. When the seizure ends, the subject is confused and does not recall what has happened.

Causes: The actual epileptic seizure is due to a sudden, abnormal and excessive electrical discharge within the brain. Normal electrical impulses of 80/second are suddenly increased to 500/second. In primary epilepsy the basic cause is unknown; there is usually a familial (genetic) predisposition. Secondary epilepsy can be a complication following head injuries, bacterial meningitis and malaria; it is often associated with cerebral palsy, mental retardation, brain tumors and cysts and hydrocephalus.

Drugs That Can Cause This Disorder: The following drugs have been reported to cause seizures or to aggravate existing epileptic disorders:

amphetamines
antihistamines
chloroquine
cimetidine (with large doses in the elderly)
cycloserine
isoniazid
metronidazole

monoamine oxidase inhibitors (MAOI's)
nalidixic acid
oral contraceptives
phenothiazines
tricyclic antidepressants
vincristine

Drugs Used to Treat This Disorder (in order of preference)
Generalized Tonic-Clonic Seizures (Grand Mal)
- phenytoin (Dilantin).
- phenobarbital (Luminal).
- carbamazepine (Tegretol).
- primidone (Mysoline).

Absence Seizures (Petit Mal)
- ethosuximide (Zarontin).
- valproic acid (Depakene).
- trimethadione (Tridione).
- clonazepam (Clonopin).

Complex Partial Seizures (Psychomotor, Temporal Lobe)
- carbamazepine (Tegretol).
- phenytoin (Dilantin).
- primidone (Mysoline).
- clonazepam (Clonopin).
- valproic acid (Depakene).

Goals of Drug Treatment

Complete prevention of seizures if possible (or marked reduction in frequency), with no (or minimal) adverse drug effects.

Restoration of ability to function independently.

Promotion of participation in school, employment and societal activities.

Drug Management

General Principles

Each individual who is subject to epilepsy experiences a pattern of seizures that is unique; the onset, frequency, severity and specific type (or types) of seizures are never exactly the same as those experienced by someone else.

The drugs used to control epilepsy are selected according to the specific type(s) of seizures the patient experiences.

Antiepileptic drugs are not curative; they are used to control seizures—to reduce their frequency and severity. Seizures should be prevented whenever possible; repeated, uncontrolled convulsions can cause significant brain damage.

When the drug of choice is used in adequate dosage to manage a correctly diagnosed type of epilepsy, seizures can be controlled completely in 60% of patients and substantially reduced in another 20%.

In every case a period of trial and error is necessary to find the most effective drug, the optimal dose and the correct timing of use.

Complete control of seizures with one drug is the ideal; this is possible in 85% of cases. If one drug does not give adequate control, a second drug may be added. The first drug may be continued or gradually withdrawn, depending upon individual response.

Dosage schedules are adjusted gradually to achieve the maximum of seizure control with the minimum of drug side-effects.

Because of the wide variation in drug absorption and elimination from person to person, the periodic measurement of drug levels in blood is necessary to determine the optimal dosage for each drug. An attempt is made to establish for each individual that drug level which will ensure freedom from seizures without toxic drug effects. Blood samples for measurement are usually taken just before the morning dose. (See Therapeutic Drug Monitoring in Section One.)

All antiepileptic drugs have toxic effects when taken in large doses; dosage adjustments are often necessary to prevent toxicity. However, the controllable risks of proper use do not justify withholding treatment in view of the much greater risks resulting from uncontrolled repeated seizures.

Birth defects are two to three times higher in children whose parents (father or mother) are using antiepileptic drugs, especially phenytoin, trimethadione and valproic acid. Consult your physician regarding the best course of action for you in managing your epilepsy during pregnancy.

Do not discontinue any antiepileptic drug suddenly unless advised to do so by your physician. Normally the dosage should be reduced gradually over a period of several weeks. Abrupt withdrawal can cause status epilepticus—a prolonged period of continual seizures without interruption.

Any consideration of discontinuing antiepileptic medications permanently should be made jointly with your physician. Such consideration can be made for absence seizures (petit mal) after a period of 2 to 3 years without a seizure. For other types of epilepsy, a period of 3 to 5 years is advisable. Seizures tend to return in 20% to 50% of cases after stopping medication. Any attempt to withdraw medication must be done very gradually over a period of several months.

Use of Phenytoin

1. Used to control all types of epilepsy except absence seizures.
2. A drug blood level within the therapeutic range correlates well with a decrease in seizure frequency and relative freedom from toxic effects.
3. Due to variation of absorbability among available products, it is advisable to stay with the same brand to gain and maintain control.
4. When the daily maintenance requirement has been established, it may be taken in a single dose.
5. Possible adverse effects include a measleslike rash within the first 2 weeks, excessive growth of hair (5%) and enlargement of the gums (30%).
6. Indications of early toxicity include rapid involuntary eye movements (nystagmus), dizziness, unsteadiness, lethargy and slurred speech.
7. If another drug is added for concurrent use, any significant interaction will occur within 6 weeks.

Use of Phenobarbital

1. Used to control all types of epilepsy except absence seizures.
2. Use with caution if liver or kidney function is impaired.
3. Should be taken twice a day with the largest dose at bedtime.
4. More sedative than phenytoin and carbamazepine, but relatively free of long-term adverse effects.
5. Indications of early toxicity include drowsiness, unsteadiness and impaired thinking.

Use of Primidone
1. Closely related to phenobarbital. Used to control all types of epilepsy except absence seizures.
2. Must be taken in divided doses because of its sedative effect.
3. Indications of early toxicity are the same of those for phenobarbital.

Use of Ethosuximide
1. Used to control absence seizures and some myoclonic seizures. About 75% effective in reducing the frequency of absence seizures when used in adequate dosage.
2. Indications of early toxicity include headache, drowsiness and dizziness.

Use of Valproic Acid
1. Used primarily to control both simple and complex absence seizures. Also used adjunctively to control all other types of epilepsy. It may control both absence and tonic-clonic seizures in the same individual.
2. Multiple doses are necessary to maintain 24-hour control.
3. Avoid use in presence of liver disease.
4. A possible side-effect is weight gain.
5. Monitor for indications of liver toxicity.
6. If used concurrently with other antiepileptic drugs, the periodic measurement of blood levels of all drugs being used is necessary to ensure adequate dosage and prevent toxicity.

Use of Carbamazepine
1. Used to control both tonic-clonic seizures and partial complex seizures (psychomotor epilepsy).
2. Should be taken with food to improve absorption.
3. Avoid use in presence of liver disease or impaired function.
4. Indications of early toxicity include double vision, blurred vision, dizziness, unsteadiness and tremor.
5. Routine, periodic, complete blood counts are mandatory to detect early bone marrow toxicity.

Ancillary Drug Treatment (as required)

Condition	*Drug Treatment*
For increased seizures before or after menstruation:	acetazolamide (Diamox)
For anxiety:	benzodiazepines (Tranxene, Valium, etc.)
For depression:	see Profile of Depression in this section

Note: Drug selection, dosage and administration schedule must be determined by the physician for each patient individually.

Resources for Additional Information and Services

American Epilepsy Society
179 Allyn Street, #304

Hartford, CT 06103
Phone: (203) 246-6566

Publications available.

Epilepsy Concern Service Group
1282 Wynnewood Drive
West Palm Beach, FL 33409
Phone: (305) 586-4804

Promotes formation of self-help groups.
Publications and telephone referrals available.

Epilepsy Foundation of America
4351 Garden City Drive, Suite 406
Landover, MD 20785
Phone: 1-800-EFA-1000 (outside MD); (301) 459-3700

Provides a low-cost pharmacy program for members.
Publications and audiovisual materials available.

GLAUCOMA

Other Names: Primary glaucoma, secondary glaucoma

Prevalence in USA: 1.7 million known, an estimated 1 million undiagnosed; 2% of the population over 40 years of age.

Age Group: Under 18 years—13,000; 18 to 44 years—124,000; 45 to 64 years—513,000; 65 to 74 years—534,000; 75 years and over—527,000.

Male to Female Ratio: Under 45 years—same incidence in men and women; 45 to 64 years—more common in men; 65 years and over—more common in women.

Principal Features: A chronic disorder characterized by abnormally high internal eye pressure that destroys the optic nerve and causes partial to complete loss of vision. Principal types include

Chronic Open-Angle (Simple, Wide-Angle) Glaucoma: The most common type, a primary glaucoma that is rare in children and young adults; usually begins after 30. The rise in intraocular pressure is gradual; the loss of vision is insidious and slowly progressive. Usually both eyes are affected. Characteristic symptoms include blurring of vision, frequent need for change of glasses, occasional headache, colored halos seen around electric lights and impaired visual adaptation to the dark.

Acute/Chronic Angle-Closure (Narrow-Angle, Closed-Angle) Glaucoma: A primary glaucoma that usually occurs after 60. The acute glaucoma attack begins in one eye; the rise in intraocular pressure is sudden and dramatic. Within a few hours the patient experiences severe headache, throbbing eye pain, blurred vision, halos around lights, tearing, swollen eyelids, nausea and vomiting. Initially the episode may be misdiagnosed as an acute abdominal disorder, such as gallbladder disease. Attacks of lesser severity can recur in chronic fashion.

Secondary Glaucoma: The rise in intraocular pressure is a consequence of a preexistent condition, such as infection (uveitis), eye tumor, enlarged cataract or long-term treatment with cortisonelike drugs. Headache, halos and blurred vision occur in proportion to the degree and duration of increased pressure.

Causes: Increased intraocular pressure is due to an imbalance between production and drainage of the liquid (aqueous humor) in the front portion of the eye; obstruction to normal drainage is the main mechanism. The primary types of glaucoma occur in individuals with hereditary predisposition, but specific initiating causes responsible for the rise in pressure are not known. Secondary types of glaucoma are associated with other eye disorders: uveitis, tumors, cataracts, hemorrhage, injury. "Steroid responders" develop increased pressure after 1 to 8 weeks of using cortisonelike steroids.

Drugs That Can Cause This Disorder: The following drugs do not cause true, permanent glaucoma, but they can increase intraocular pressure and thereby precipitate an attack of acute angle-closure glaucoma or aggravate chronic open-angle glaucoma:

amyl nitrite	nitroglycerin
atropine and atropinelike drugs	phenylephrine
cortisonelike drugs	tolazoline
epinephrine	tricyclic antidepressants
isosorbide dinitrate	

Drugs Used to Treat This Disorder

Eye Drops/Inserts (for Local Effects)
- carbachol (Carbacel, Isopto Carbachol).
- demecarium (Humorsol).
- dipivefrin (DPE, Propine).
- echothiopate (Phospholine).
- epinephrine (Epifrin, Epitrate, Glaucon, Lyophrin).
- phenylephrine (Neo-Synephrine, Ocusol).
- pilocarpine solution (Almocarpine, Isoptocarpine, etc.).
- pilocarpine inserts (Ocuserts Pilo-20, Pilo-40).
- timolol (Timoptic).

Internal Medications (for Systemic Effects)
- acetazolamide (Diamox).
- glycerine (Glyrol, Osmoglyn).

Goals of Drug Treatment

Prompt reduction of intraocular pressure in acute angle-closure glaucoma; stabilization of eye status in preparation for corrective eye surgery.

Gradual reduction and long-term normalization of intraocular pressure in chronic, simple, open-angle glaucoma.

Prevention of optic nerve damage; preservation of vision.

Drug Management

General Principles

Drug treatment cannot cure but can control glaucoma.

Factors that can increase intraocular pressure and reduce the effectiveness of drugs include emotional stress (anger, fear, worry); heavy physical exertion; straining with defecation; tight collars, belts and girdles; upper respiratory infections.

Periodic measurement of intraocular pressure is most advisable during long-term use of cortisonelike steroid drugs, especially eye drops and ointments.

Soft contact lens can act as a drug reservoir for pilocarpine (when administered in eye-drop solutions).

Some individuals cannot use pilocarpine Ocuserts successfully; some cannot retain them in the eye, and the loss may be unnoticed; some cannot tolerate the foreign-body sensation.

Pilocarpine is the pupil-constricting (miotic) drug of choice for use in the elderly. The stinging sensation felt on initial use usually disappears with continued application. Some blurring of distant vision is unavoidable.

Timolol (a beta blocker) is as effective as pilocarpine in treating open-angle and secondary glaucoma; twice daily dosage (every 12 hours) is usually sufficient; it should be used very cautiously in those with asthma, slow heart rates or borderline congestive heart failure.

Epinephrine may be used concurrently with pilocarpine (or other miotic drugs) for greater effectiveness in reducing intraocular pressure; it is important that the pilocarpine be used first and be allowed to act for 5 minutes before using epinephrine. Avoid use in presence of high blood pressure (hypertension). Do not use discolored solutions of epinephrine.

Acetazolamide is usually reserved for glaucoma that is unresponsive to eye drops alone. Effectiveness is improved when both are used concurrently.

For Chronic Open-Angle Glaucoma

Eye drops: pilocarpine, timolol, carbachol, epinephrine, dipivefrin, demecarium.

Internal medications: acetazolamide.

Most cases are controlled by eye drops alone.

Treatment is started with the weakest strength; the most effective strength and dosage schedule are determined by trial and error.

Acetazolamide is not used routinely; it is added after an adequate trial of eye drops fails to maintain normal intraocular pressure.

For Acute Angle-Closure Glaucoma (Acute Attack)

Eye drops: pilocarpine, timolol.

Internal medications: glycerine and water mixture, acetazolamide.

The initial treatment is designed to lower intraocular pressure as rapidly as possible to prevent irreversible damage to the optic nerve. Eye drops and internal medications are used concurrently. The combination can reduce the pressure rapidly and abort the acute attack. The ultimate treatment for this condition is surgical.

For Chronic, Recurrent Episodes of Subacute Angle-Closure Glaucoma
Eye drops: pilocarpine and timolol concurrently.
Internal medications: glycerine and water; acetazolamide is used only during the acute phase, not long-term.
The ultimate treatment is surgical.

For Secondary Glaucoma
Eye drops: atropine, cortisonelike steroids.
Internal medications: cortisonelike steroids, acetazolamide.
When appropriate, corrective treatment is directed at the primary eye disorder that is causing increased intraocular pressure.

For Cortisone-Induced Glaucoma
Discontinue all cortisonelike steroids if possible.
Eye drops: pilocarpine, timolol, demecarium.
Internal medications: acetazolamide.

Ancillary Drug Treatment (as required)

Condition	*Drug Treatment*
For itching, burning, redness of eyes:	naphazoline (Naphcon, Privine, Vasoclear) tetrahydralazine (Visine)

Note: Drug selection, dosage and administration schedule must be determined by the physician for each patient individually.

Resources for Additional Information and Services

Foundation for Glaucoma Research
490 Post Street, Suite 1042
San Francisco, CA 94102
Phone: (415) 986-3162

Publications available.

National Society to Prevent Blindness
National Center for Sight
500 East Remington Road
Schaumburg, IL 60173
Phone: 1-800-221-3004; (312) 843-2020

Available 9:00 a.m.–4:00 p.m. CST, M–F.
Answers questions about vision problems.
Provides publications and films on specific problems and conditions.

GOUT

Other Names: Gouty arthritis, podagra (gouty arthritis of the big toe), hyperuricemia (abnormally high blood uric acid)

Prevalence in USA: Approximately 2.3 million, 2.8% of males in middle age. Hyperuricemia occurs in 5% to 10% of the population; 1% to 2% will have gout manifestations during a lifetime.

Age Group: Under 18 years—12,000; 18 to 44 years—316,000; 45 to 64 years—1.01 million; 65 to 74 years—494,000; 75 years and over—396,000.

Male to Female Ratio: Approximately 95% in men, 5% in women.

Principal Features: Gout consists of a group of related disorders having a single underlying feature—abnormally high blood levels of uric acid; this is referred to as hyperuricemia and implies a blood level of more than 7.0 mg of uric acid per 100 ml of blood. (The normal ranges generally recognized are 2.5 to 8.0 mg for men and 1.5 to 7.0 mg for women.) During the early years of primary (genetic) gout, hyperuricemia may exist without any symptoms to indicate its presence. During a lifetime, a small minority of these individuals will experience recurrent acute attacks of severe joint pain with tender swelling (usually one joint in an upper or lower limb), episodes of kidney stones, serious impairment of kidney function or the development of tophi—localized deposits of uric acid salts in the skin, on earlobes, on tendons and bones in and around joints (tophaceous gout).

Causes: Primary gout is due to an inherited defect in the metabolism of purines—end products of protein digestion. In approximately 10% of cases the defect results in an overproduction of uric acid; in 90% the defect is responsible for decreased excretion of uric acid by the kidneys. Either defect causes hyperuricemia. When tissue fluids cannot dissolve excessive levels of uric acid (due to saturation), uric acid crystals are deposited in joints (acute arthritis), kidneys (kidney damage and stone formation) and in soft tissue (tophi).

Drugs That Can Cause This Disorder: The following drugs can raise the blood level of uric acid and precipitate acute gouty arthritis in susceptible individuals:

acetazolamide	furosemide
alcohol	levodopa
antineoplastic drugs	nicotinic acid
aspirin (less than 2 grams/day)	pyrazinamide
ethacrynic acid	thiazide diuretics
ethambutol	triamterene

Drugs Used to Treat This Disorder

For Reducing Blood and Tissue Levels of Uric Acid
- allopurinol (Lopurin, Zyloprim).
- probenecid (Benemid).
- sulfinpyrazone (Anturane).

For Treating and Preventing Acute Attacks of Arthritis
- colchicine.
- fenoprofen (Nalfon).
- ibuprofen (Advil, Motrin, Nuprin, Rufen).
- indomethacin (Indocin).
- naproxen (Naprosyn).
- oxyphenbutazone (Oxalid).
- phenylbutazone (Azolid, Butazolidin).
- piroxicam (Feldene).
- prednisone (Deltasone, Meticorten, Orasone, etc.).
- sulindac (Clinoril).
- tolmetin (Tolectin).

Goals of Drug Treatment

Prompt relief of symptoms of acute attack of gouty arthritis.

Maintenance of blood uric acid level below 6 mg/100 ml. (Prevention of recurrent attacks of acute arthritis, kidney stone formation, kidney damage and tophi formation.)

Dissolution of existing tophi.

Drug Management

General Principles

Only 20% of individuals with hyperuricemia will develop manifestations of gout during their lifetime. At present there is no way of identifying those who will.

Gouty arthritis is the most responsive to treatment and the most easily controlled of all types of arthritis.

The patient and physician together should determine by trial and error which drug is most effective and acceptable for treating acute attacks of gouty arthritis.

After the acute attack of arthritis has subsided, minor symptoms may persist for 2 to 3 months. If maintenance treatment with antigout drugs is started, it is advisable to use low-dose colchicine concurrently to prevent recurrent flare-ups.

Measurement of the amount of uric acid in a 24-hour collection of urine can identify the overproducer of uric acid (greater than 800 mg) and the underexcretor (less than 800 mg). The overproducer is best treated with allopurinol; the underexcretor is best treated with probenecid or sulfinpyrazone.

Authorities differ on whether and when to initiate long-term treatment for hyperuricemia. Conservative opinion: initiate drug therapy only after 2 or more episodes of gouty arthritis or kidney stone within a year. Many first attacks are not followed by recurrent episodes. Withholding long-term treatment avoids the risks of adverse drug reactions. Aggressive opinion: initiate drug therapy after the first episode of gouty arthritis or kidney stone to prevent recurrent attacks and reduce the risks of kidney damage and tophi formation. Hyperuricemia is often present for 20 years or more before the first attack; bone, cartilage and kidney damage may already have occured. The risks of untreated hyperuricemia are thought to exceed the risks of long-term drug therapy. The prudent physician will consider the pros and cons of each case individually and make the decision jointly with the patient.

Once long-term treatment is started with allopurinol and/or probenecid or sulfinpyrazone, it should be maintained for life. Start-stop treatment has no lasting benefit and may precipitate acute attacks. Low-dose colchicine should be taken preventively until the uric acid blood level is stabilized below 6.0 mg/100ml and there have been no acute attacks for 6 to 12 months.

Acute attacks of gouty arthritis can be precipitated by injury, surgery, systemic infections and severe medical illnesses. Colchicine may be used preventively to minimize acute episodes of arthritis when such events occur.

Patients with kidney stones should use allopurinol to treat hyperuricemia; probenecid and sulfinpyrazone should be avoided because they increase the uric acid content of urine.

Do not take aspirin (or other salicylates) in doses of less than 2 grams while taking probenecid or sulfinpyrazone. It abolishes the effectiveness of these drugs and raises the blood level of uric acid.

Avoid fasting to lose weight; fasting can raise the blood level of uric acid. Treat obesity by long-term reduction of food intake and gradual loss of weight.

While taking antigout drugs on a regular basis, drink 2 to 3 quarts of liquids daily to ensure a copious flow of dilute urine.

Use of Allopurinol
1. Used to lower the blood level of uric acid by reducing its formation. Of no value in treating the acute attack, and should not be started until all symptoms of acute arthritis have subsided.
2. The drug of choice for individuals who
   - are overproducers of uric acid (more than 800 mg/24-hour urine excretion).
   - are over 60 years of age.
   - have impaired kidney function.
   - are subject to kidney stones.
   - have tophi formations.
   - are allergic or overly sensitive to probenecid or sulfinpyrazone.
3. The total daily requirement may be taken in a single dose.
4. Once started, a commitment should be made to a lifetime of continual use.
5. May be combined with all other antigout drugs as appropriate for increased effectiveness.

6. Recommended for use prior to and during chemotherapy or irradiation therapy for selected cancers to counteract resulting hyperuricemia.
7. Serious toxicity is extremely rare.

Use of Colchicine

1. Used to treat acute attacks of gouty arthritis. It does not lower the blood level of uric acid.
2. For the quickest response and best results, treatment should be started as soon as possible after the onset of symptoms. If started within the first 12 hours, colchicine gives effective relief of acute arthritis in 90% of cases.
3. The long-term use of low-dose colchicine is very effective in preventing recurrent acute attacks of gouty arthritis.
4. Its use is recommended during the early months of maintenance therapy with allopurinol and/or probenecid or sulfinpyrazone to prevent flare-ups of acute arthritis.
5. Use with caution and reduce the dose in the presence of liver disease or impaired liver function.
6. Colchicine is destroyed by exposure to light. Be sure your supply is fresh and fully effective.

Use of Indomethacin (and Other Nonsteroidal Anti-inflammatory Drugs)

1. Now considered by many authorities to be the drug(s) of choice for treating acute attacks of gouty arthritis. They relieve pain and inflammation, but do not lower the blood level of uric acid.
2. When given promptly and in adequate dosage, these drugs usually provide relief within 6 to 12 hours and complete recovery in 3 days.
3. Take with food to prevent stomach irritation and indigestion.
4. Avoid in the presence of active peptic ulcer disease. Use with caution in hypertension and congestive heart failure.

Use of Phenylbutazone or Oxyphenbutazone

1. Used to provide prompt relief of acute gouty arthritis. It reduces pain and inflammation effectively, but does not lower the blood level of uric acid.
2. Because of its rare but very serious potential for causing bone marrow depression, this drug should never be used for long-term treatment. Treatment courses of no more than 5 to 7 days are advised.
3. This drug should not be used by the elderly (over 60 years of age).

Use of Prednisone (or Similar Cortisonelike Steroids)

1. Used to abort acute attacks of gouty arthritis. Relieves inflammation, swelling and pain, but does not lower the blood level of uric acid.
2. Should be used only after adequate trials of all other appropriate drugs have failed to relieve the acute attack.
3. "Rebound" attacks are common following withdrawal of steroid medications.
4. Not recommended for frequently repeated or long-term use.

Use of Probenecid or Sulfinpyrazone

1. Used to lower the blood level of uric acid by increasing its excretion in the urine. Of no value in treating the acute attack, and should not be started until acute arthritis has subsided.
2. Best suited for individuals who
   - are underexcretors of uric acid (less than 800 mg/24-hour urine excretion).
   - are under 60 years of age.
   - have good kidney function.
   - have no history of kidney stones.
3. Should not be used by those who
   - are overproducers of uric acid (more than 800 mg/24-hour urine excretion).
   - have impaired kidney function and low urine volume.
   - are subject to kidney stones.
4. Begin treatment with small doses to avoid precipitating an acute attack of arthritis.
5. Must be taken in 2 to 4 doses/day.
6. If the tolerance of either drug is limited, the two drugs can be taken concurrently in reduced dosage.
7. Ensure a high intake of liquids (up to 3 quarts daily). Effectiveness is improved by the concurrent use of sodium bicarbonate or potassium citrate.

Ancillary Drug Treatment (as required)

Condition	Drug Treatment
For mild pain:	acetaminophen (Tylenol, etc.). Do not use aspirin or other salicylates.
For severe pain:	codeine or meperidine (Demerol)
For diarrhea due to colchicine:	paregoric or loperimide (Imodium)
For high blood pressure:	see Profile of Hypertension in this section
For "secondary" gout due to chemotherapy for leukemia, lymphoma, multiple myeloma, polycythemia:	allopurinol (Zyloprim)

Note: Drug selection, dosage and administration schedule must be determined by the physician for each patient individually.

Resources for Additional Information and Services

Arthritis Foundation
1314 Spring Street, N.W.

Atlanta, GA 30309
Phone: (404) 872-7100

Publications available.

Association for People With Arthritis
P.O. Box 954
6 Commercial Street
Hicksville, NY 11802
Phone: 1-800-323-2243

Publications available.

HYPERTENSION

Other Names: Arterial hypertension, essential hypertension, primary hypertension, secondary hypertension high blood pressure

Prevalence in USA: 26.5 million—15% of adult white population; 25% of adult black population.

Age Group: Under 18 years—184,000; 18 to 44 years—5.6 million; 45 to 64 years—10.8 million; 65 to 74 years—6 million; 75 years and over—3.8 million.

Male to Female Ratio: Under 45 years—same incidence in men and women; 45 to 64 years—slightly more common in women; 65 years and over—more common in women (2 to 1).

Principal Features: During the early years of high blood pressure there are usually no symptoms. Brief periods of sudden elevation of blood pressure above usual levels may cause throbbing headaches and/or dizziness. After years of untreated high blood pressure, manifestations of "target organ" disease include stroke (blood clot or hemorrhage in the brain), impaired vision (retinal hemorrhage and deterioration), heart attack (myocardial infarction), congestive heart failure and kidney failure (uremia).

Causes: In primary (essential) hypertension (95% of all hypertension), no specific cause is apparent. There is a definite hereditary predisposition; 80% of hypertensive individuals have a close relative with high blood pressure. In those who are genetically susceptible, obesity and high salt intake contribute significantly to the development of hypertension. Secondary hypertension (5% of all hypertension) is due to a demonstrable (and sometimes curable) cause: narrowing of the main artery to one or both kidneys, chronic kidney disease, adrenalin or renin producing tumors, coarctation of the aorta.

Drugs That Can Cause This Disorder: The following drugs (or drug combinations) can cause significant elevations of blood pressure:

amphetamines and related drugs
carbenoxolone
ephedrine
ergot preparations
licorice
oral contraceptives
phenylephrine
phenylpropanolamine
pseudoephedrine
tricyclic antidepressants taken
   concurrently with appetite
   suppressants, decongestants
   or antihistamines

Drugs Used to Treat This Disorder
Diuretics
- thiazides (see Drug Class, Section Four).
- chlorthalidone (Hygroton).
- quinethazone (Hydromox).
- metolazone (Diulo, Zaroxolyn).
- indapamide (Lozol).
- bumetanide (Bumex).
- furosemide (Lasix).
- *potassium-saving diuretics:* amiloride (Midamor); spironolactone (Aldactone); triamterene (Dyrenium).

Drugs Acting on the Sympathetic Nervous System
Beta-Adrenergic-Blocking Drugs
- acebutolol (Sectral).
- atenolol (Tenormin).
- labetalol (Normodyne, Trandate).
- metoprolol (Lopressor).
- nadolol (Corgard).
- penbutolol (Levatol).
- pindolol (Visken).
- propranolol (Inderal).
- timolol (Blocadren).

Alpha-Adrenergic-Blocking Drugs
- prazosin (Minipres).
- terazosin (Hytrin).

Centrally Acting Drugs (in the Brain)
- clonidine (Catapres).
- guanabenz (Wytensin).
- guanfacine (Tenex).
- methyldopa (Aldomet).

Peripherally Acting Drugs (in Peripheral Blood Vessels)
- guanadrel (Hylorel).
- guanethidine (Ismelin).
- reserpine (Serpasil).

Direct Vasodilators
- hydralazine (Apresoline).
- minoxidil (Loniten).

Calcium Channel-Blocking Drugs
- diltiazem (Cardizem).
- nicardipine (Cardene).
- nifedipine (Procardia).
- verapamil (Calan, Isoptin).

Angiotensin Converting Enzyme (ACE) Inhibitors
- captopril (Capoten).
- enalapril (Vasotec).
- lisinopril (Prinivil, Zestril).

Goals of Drug Treatment

Maintenance of blood pressure below 140/90, or as close as possible to this level with an acceptable program of drug therapy (minimal drug side-effects and expense).

Prevention or postponement of "target organ" disease in the brain, retina (eye), heart, major blood vessels and kidneys.

Drug Management

General Principles

Although hypertension is difficult to define precisely, blood pressure is considered to be abnormally high if the systolic level is 140 or above or the diastolic level is 90 or above.

Hypertension may be classified as follows:
Diastolic pressure less than 85—normal
Diastolic pressure of 85 to 89—high normal
Diastolic pressure of 90 to 104—mild hypertension
Diastolic pressure of 105 to 114—moderate hypertension
Diastolic pressure of 115 or above—severe hypertension
Systolic pressure less than 140—normal
Systolic pressure of 140 to 159—borderline systolic hypertension
Systolic pressure of 160 or above—systolic hypertension

Most men who develop primary hypertension will have a diastolic pressure of 90 or above by age 35, most women by age 40 to 45.

An adequate program of drug therapy for hypertension will postpone serious disability and death for most hypertensive individuals.

The selection of antihypertensive drugs for initial treatment is based upon the range of the abnormally high pressures recorded on repeated measurements *and* the status of the "target organs" (brain, heart, kidneys and blood vessels) at the time hypertension is discovered.

One practical and effective approach to drug therapy for hypertension initiates treatment with a single drug and adds stronger drugs in stepwise fashion as needed to control blood pressure:

Step 1 begin treatment with	either a diuretic or a beta blocker drug.
Step 2 if necessary, add	clonidine, methyldopa or prazosin (or a diuretic or a beta blocker if not used in Step 1)

| Step 3 if necessary, add | hydralazine, a calcium channel blocker or an ACE inhibitor |
| Step 4 if necessary, add | guanethidine or minoxidil |

For most individuals, the initial drug treatment will normalize blood pressure within the first 2 months. Up to 60% of cases are controlled with a diuretic alone; 50% can be controlled with a beta blocker alone. From 70% to 80% of all hypertensive individuals will achieve satisfactory blood pressure control by compliance with Step 1 or Step 2 drug therapy. The majority of the remainder can be controlled by Steps 3 and 4.

Tranquilizers and sedatives are not effective for lowering elevated blood pressure and should not be relied upon as primary treatment for hypertension.

Obtain a blood pressure measuring instrument (preferably an aneroid manometer, arm cuff and stethoscope) and ask your physician to teach you how to take your own blood pressure. Measurements of blood pressure made at home (or at work) are far more representative of your actual day-by-day pressures than are readings made in the physician's office. By taking your own blood pressure at home, at work and at varying times and under different circumstances, you can create a record that clearly reflects your response to the antihypertensive drugs prescribed for you.

Read the Drug Profiles (Section Three) of the drugs you are taking. If you think you may be experiencing any of the side-effects or adverse effects listed in the Profile, discuss this with your physician so appropriate adjustments can be made. It is to your benefit to work along with your physician until a satisfactory selection of drugs is reached.

Avoid isometric exercises—body building, weight lifting, push-ups; these raise the blood pressure significantly. Consult your physician regarding the advisability of isotonic exercises—walking, bicycling, swimming.

Consumption of more than 2 ounces of alcohol daily can raise the blood pressure. One ounce of alcohol is present in 2 ounces of 100-proof whiskey, in 8 ounces of wine, or in 24 ounces of beer.

Five percent of oral contraceptive users will develop a diastolic blood pressure of over 90. If this occurs, the contraceptive pill should be discontinued for 6 months and the blood pressure monitored. Women with this sensitivity should use an alternative method of contraception.

The elderly individual with hypertension must approach antihypertensive drug therapy very cautiously. Goals of drug treatment are more liberal; reduction of pressures to 140–160/95–100 are usually adequate. This can usually be achieved with small doses of a diuretic. If a Step 2 drug is needed, methyldopa is better tolerated than the other choices. However, the response to all drugs must be observed closely. Drugs that cause emotional depression in the young individual can cause symptoms in the elderly that closely resemble senile dementia.

In type I diabetes, thiazides are well tolerated, but beta blockers may mask the symptoms of hypoglycemia. In type II diabetes, thiazides are best avoided; small doses of furosemide or spironolactone are preferable. Beta blockers can impair insulin release.

After blood pressure has been well controlled for a year, consideration may be given to a "step-down" reduction of both drug dosage and the number of drugs used. The blood pressure response to the gradual withdrawal of drugs must be monitored very carefully. A recent study showed that 28% of the group of hypertensives studied had normal blood pressure one year after discontinuing all antihypertensive medication. Your physician can determine if and when you meet the criteria for attempting to discontinue your program of drug treatment.

Treatment of Hypertension According to Severity

For Borderline Hypertension (120–160/90–94)

- Reduce excessive weight.
- Reduce salt intake moderately.
- Reduce stress in daily living.
- Avoid excessive consumption of alcohol.
- Stop smoking.
- Avoid isometric exercise.
- Increase isotonic exercise.
- Defer drug treatment for 3 to 6 months to determine effectiveness of above measures.

For Mild Hypertension (140–160/95–104) (80% of All Hypertensives)

- Urge all of the above measures.
- Begin Step 1 drug treatment: Use a single drug—currently a thiazide diuretic or a beta blocker. Some authorities are now advocating a trial of a calcium channel blocker or an ACE inhibitor for initiating treatment.

For Moderate Hypertension (140–180/105–114)

- Begin with Step 2 drug treatment; it is not likely that a single drug will control this degree of hypertension.
- A diuretic will enhance the effectiveness of a beta blocker, a calcium channel blocker, or a centrally acting drug.

For Severe Hypertension (160+/115+)

- Adequate control may require Step 3 or Step 4 drug treatment. When multiple drugs are used, smaller doses of individual drugs are often effective and better tolerated. A trial-and-error approach is often necessary to determine the most effective and acceptable combination of drugs.

For Isolated Systolic Hypertension (160+/85–90)

- This is usually found in the elderly. Cautious and conservative drug treatment is recommended for those under age 70.
- Calcium channel-blocking drugs may be very effective for this type of hypertension.
- If a diuretic is used, avoid dehydration and potassium loss.
- If methyldopa is used, monitor for any tendency to depression or dementia.

Use of Diuretics
1. Used as Step 1 or Step 2 drugs, diuretics are most appropriate for treating hypertensives who are black or elderly, those with congestive heart failure or kidney failure and those who cannot use a beta blocker drug.
2. A thiazide diuretic is the initial drug tried in the majority of cases. It is effective in a single dose taken in the morning.
3. While using thiazide diuretics, observe for loss of potassium (10% of users), increased blood level of uric acid (66% of users) and increased blood-sugar level.
4. Spironolactone and triamterene are as effective as thiazides in reducing blood pressure; they are used to prevent potassium loss.
5. The more potent diuretics furosemide and ethacrynic acid are no more effective than the thiazides for reducing blood pressure.
6. The most practical and reliable way to prevent a significant decline in the potassium blood level is to use a potassium-saving diuretic— amiloride, spironolactone or triamterene. The use of high-potassium foods is often unreliable. Compliance with the long-term use of oral potassium supplements is very poor.
7. It is advisable to discontinue the use of diuretics gradually to prevent fluid retention (edema) after withdrawal.

Use of Beta-Adrenergic-Blocking Drugs
1. Used as Step 1 or Step 2 drugs, beta blockers are most appropriate for treating hypertensives who are young, those who have an overactive heart (fast rate, palpitation, premature beats) and those with gout, migraine headaches and angina (coronary artery disease).
2. Avoid beta blockers if you have asthma, emphysema or a history of heart block or congestive heart failure.
3. These drugs characteristically cause fatigue and lethargy. Propranolol and metoprolol can cause emotional depression.
4. When propranolol is used alone, 10% of users can experience an increase in blood pressure. It is advisable to use a diuretic prior to starting propranolol in sensitive individuals.
5. Avoid sudden discontinuation of beta blockers, especially in the presence of coronary artery disease. Abrupt withdrawal can cause rapid heart rate, palpitation and intensification of angina; myocardial infarction has been reported.

Use of Labetalol (an Alpha- and Beta-Adrenergic Blocker)
1. This drug may be effective when the beta blockers have failed to control blood pressure.
2. Functions primarily as a vasodilator in the elderly, with no significant alteration of heart function.
3. Avoid in presence of asthma, emphysema, heart block and congestive heart failure.

Use of Clonidine
1. Characteristically causes drowsiness, fatigue and dry mouth. Is capable of causing depression.

2. Do not discontinue this drug abruptly; sudden withdrawal can cause a severe rebound hypertension with higher blood pressure than prior to treatment. Withdraw over 2 to 4 days.
3. After discontinuation of clonidine, delay the start of a beta blocker drug for 48 hours.

Use of Methyldopa

1. Usually causes lethargy and fatigue at beginning of treatment; these often subside with continued use. Is also capable of causing depression.
2. This drug causes salt and water retention; a diuretic should be taken concurrently.
3. Discontinue this drug if any of the following develop: emotional depression, drug fever, breast enlargement, milk production, indications of liver toxicity (loss of appetite, nausea, jaundice).
4. Sudden discontinuation of this drug can cause agitation, insomnia, rapid heart rate and intensification of angina.

Use of Prazosin

1. In 10% of users, this drug can provoke an idiosyncratic reaction that results in a sudden extreme drop in blood pressure following the first dose. It is advisable to begin treatment with a bedtime dose and a warning to arise cautiously the next morning in anticipation of possible orthostatic hypotension (see Glossary).
2. This drug can cause fluid retention and can aggravate angina. It is best used in conjunction with a diuretic and a beta blocker.
3. Do not use this drug concurrently with hydralazine or guanethidine because of the potential for additive postural hypotension.
4. A rapid loss of effectiveness can limit this drug's long-term usefulness.

Use of Hydralazine

1. This drug is rarely used alone. It can cause fluid retention and should be used concurrently with a diuretic.
2. This drug characteristically increases heart activity, which can be counteracted by the concurrent use of a beta blocker drug.
3. Use cautiously in the presence of angina (coronary artery disease).
4. Monitor for possible development of a lupuslike drug reaction.

Use of Reserpine

1. Limit the daily dose to 0.25 mg or less.
2. Avoid completely if you have a history of depression.
3. This drug can cause salt and water retention; a diuretic should be used concurrently.
4. Do not use this drug concurrently with methyldopa; the combination can cause marked sedation, excessive dreaming and sexual impotence.
5. Observe for the following possible adverse effects: drowsiness, lethargy, depression (can be very insidious), nightmares, nasal congestion, acid indigestion (possible ulcer), diarrhea, impotence, parkinsonlike syndrome.

Use of Guanethidine

1. This is the most potent antihypertensive drug in general use. It is usually reserved to treat the most severe cases of hypertension and those that have been difficult to control.
2. It causes marked orthostatic hypotension. Users should avoid prolonged sitting (without moving the legs) and prolonged standing (without walking around); these are conducive to excessive drops in blood pressure and resultant fainting. Users should also arise cautiously in the morning to avoid fainting shortly after getting out of bed.
3. This drug causes salt and water retention and should be taken concurrently with a diuretic.
4. Tricyclic antidepressants can reduce this drug's antihypertensive effectiveness.

Use of Minoxidil

1. This drug is a potent, long-acting vasodilator. Its use is usually restricted to treating those whose blood pressure cannot be controlled by conventional treatment with other drugs.
2. It is generally used concurrently with a diuretic and a beta blocker drug.
3. Observe for excessive growth of hair.

Use of Calcium Channel-Blocking Drugs

1. These drugs are approved by the U.S. Food and Drug Administration only for use in the management of angina (coronary artery disease). However, they are effective antihypertensives and are being used as such by many physicians.
2. They may be used as Step 1, 2, or 3 drugs in the management of hypertension.
3. They are especially useful in treating the elderly individual with isolated systolic hypertension.
4. Use these drugs with caution if a beta blocker drug is being used concurrently.
5. A dosage of 3 to 4 times daily is required.
6. Observe for fluid retention. Effectiveness is improved if a thiazide diuretic is taken concurrently.

Use of Angiotensin Converting Enzyme (ACE) Inhibitors

1. These may be used as Step 1, 2, 3, or 4 drugs in the management of hypertension.
2. To prevent an excessive drop in blood pressure, any diuretic in use should be discontinued 5 to 7 days before starting an ACE inhibitor. After the dose is stabilized, a diuretic may be resumed if necessary.
3. Captopril should be taken 1 hour before eating, 2 to 3 times daily, for maximal effectiveness. Enalapril may be taken once or twice daily without regard to eating.
4. Full effectiveness of these drugs may not be apparent until after several weeks of continual use.

5. These drugs may increase the blood potassium level. Do not use any commercial salt substitute (most of which contain potassium) without first consulting your physician.

Current Controversies in Drug Management

The standard "stepped-care" approach to treating hypertension usually recommends the use of a thiazide diuretic as the drug of choice to initiate therapy. If an adequate trial with thiazide therapy fails to lower the blood pressure sufficiently, other drugs of the various classes listed above are *added* in a somewhat arbitrary and rigid fashion. While the guidelines provided by a standardized approach were beneficial in promoting rational therapy, new information about the older drugs and the availability of many new and more effective drugs call for a reappraisal of drug selection for managing hypertension.

Recent review of thiazide drug performance discloses that (1) while they are effective in mild hypertension, they have not decreased the incidence of heart attacks; (2) they can cause loss of potassium and/or magnesium and thereby contribute to the development of dangerous heart rhythm disorders; and (3) they cause a 10% increase in LDL cholesterol blood levels and may increase the risk of coronary artery disease. Some authorities no longer consider thiazides to be the drugs of choice for initiating treatment; they also recommend that thiazides be used in the lowest effective dose to reduce the potential risks of long-term therapy.

Current recommendations call for a greater emphasis on individualization of drug management; this includes wider flexibility in selecting drugs for starting treatment and in substituting and deleting drugs as individual monitoring dictates. Several drug classes are admirably suited for initiating treatment and provide a broad spectrum of features that permit tailoring the drug to the individual characteristics of the patient.

Ancillary Drug Treatment (as required)

Condition	*Drug Treatment*
For thiazide-induced gout:	allopurinol (Zyloprim)
	probenecid (Benemid)
For drug-induced fluid retention:	bumetanide (Bumex)
For guanethidine-induced diarrhea:	diphenoxylate (Lomotil)
For tension headache:	acetaminophen (Tylenol, etc.)
For migraine headache (short-term use):	ibuprofen (Motrin, Advil, Nuprin)
	oxycodone (Percodan)
	Avoid ergotamine preparations.

For musculo-skeletal
pain, arthritis (long-
term use):   sulindac (Clinoril)

Note: Drug selection, dosage and administration schedule must be determined
by the physician for each patient individually.

Resources for Additional Information and Services

Citizens for the Treatment of High Blood Pressure
888 17th Street, N.W., Suite 904
Washington, DC 20006
Phone: (202) 466-4553

Publications available.

The Joint National Committee on Detection, Evaluation and Treat-
ment of High Blood Pressure
National Heart, Lung and Blood Institute
National Institutes of Health
Box 120/80
Bethesda, MD 20892
Phone: (301) 496-4000

Publication: *The 1988 Report of the Joint National Committee.*

National Institute of Hypertension Studies
13217 Livernois
Detroit, MI 48238
Phone: (313) 931-3427

Publications available.

HYPOTHYROIDISM

Other Names: Hypometabolism, myxedema, primary hypothyroidism,
secondary hypothyroidism

Prevalence in USA: 1.9 million—0.8% of the general population; 1 in 5000
newborn infants has hypothyroidism (cretinism).

Age Group: Juvenile hypothyroidism: under 18 years—2% of total incidence. Adult hypothyroidism: percentage of total incidence by age:
18 to 44 years—34%; 45 to 64 years—40%; 65 years and over—24%.

Male to Female Ratio: More common in women—8 to 1.

Principal Features: Hypothyroidism spans a wide spectrum from very
mild thyroid hormone deficiency (hypometabolism) with few nonspecific symptoms to severe deficiency (myxedema) that can be fatal

if not treated adequately. The most common form of hypothyroidism is the mild to moderate hormone deficiency seen primarily in women age 20 to 65. The onset is usually insidious and the early symptoms are so vague that medical attention is rarely sought. With progression of the deficiency, the subject gradually becomes aware of lethargy, fatigability, intolerance of cold, weight gain (with no increased food intake), loss of hair, vague muscle and joint pains, and irregular menstruation. The skin may become dry and scaly, the face may appear puffy (fluid retention), the speech slows, the voice becomes hoarse and the pattern of activity becomes sluggish. Hypothyroidism in the elderly can cause mental changes, confusion, paranoia, depression and dementia.

Causes: Primary hypothyroidism can be due to (1) a congenital defect in thyroid gland development or function; (2) an "autoimmune" impairment of thyroid hormone production (45% of cases); (3) a lack of iodine in the food or water supply; or (4) intentional thyroid gland suppression by the administration of radioactive iodine or by surgical removal of thyroid tissue (35% of cases). Secondary hypothyroidism is due to inadequate stimulation of thyroid gland function from the hypothalamus (in the brain) or from the pituitary gland (the "master" gland that regulates most hormone-producing glands).

Drugs That Can Cause This Disorder: The following drugs can impair the normal production of thyroid hormones and induce varying degrees of hypothyroidism (see Drug Classes, Section Four):

amiodarone	methimazole
cyclophosphamide	pentazocine
disulfiram (?)	phenylbutazone
ethionamide	propylthiouracil
iodine compounds (iodides)	sulfonylurea antidiabetic drugs
lithium	

Drugs Used to Treat This Disorder
- synthetic thyroxine (T-4) (Synthroid, Levothroid).
- synthetic liothyronine (T-3) (Cytomel).
- synthetic liotrix (combinations of T-4 and T-3) (Euthroid, Thyrolar).
- thyroid extract (animal origin) (Dessicated thyroid Armour).
- thyroglobulin (animal origin) (Proloid).

Goals of Drug Treatment
Adequate replacement of thyroxine; restoration of normal blood levels of T-4, T-3 and the Thyroid Stimulating Hormone (TSH).
Relief of symptoms associated with deficiency of thyroid hormones (hypothyroidism, cretinism, myxedema).

Drug Management
General Principles
Primary hypothyroidism is diagnosed by finding the blood level of the principal thyroid hormone—thyroxine (T-4)—below the normal

range and the blood level of the pituitary hormone—Thyroid Stimulating Hormone (TSH)—above the normal range.

Once the diagnosis of true primary hypothyroidism is established, treatment for life is generally thought to be necessary. However, periodic evaluation is advisable to determine the need for continual thyroid hormone replacement.

Individuals taking replacement thyroid hormones should be monitored every 6 to 12 months by measurements of T-4 and TSH along with evaluation of general well-being.

Until thyroid deficiency is adequately corrected, the subject may be overly sensitive to drugs that depress brain function—sedatives, tranquilizers, hypnotics, narcotic analgesics.

In treating hypothyroidism of infancy, avoid formula feedings that contain soybean extract; they can prevent the absorption of thyroxine and perpetuate cretinism.

Anxious, thin individuals usually require smaller doses of maintenance thyroxine than lethargic, obese individuals require. Significant reduction in weight (correction of obesity) is usually followed by a reduction in the daily requirement of maintenance thyroxine.

The use of thyroid hormones for weight reduction in the presence of normal thyroid function (no hormone deficiency) is unjustified and dangerous.

Hypothyroidism causes an increase in bone mass. Thyroid replacement therapy can result in a significant loss of bone (osteoporosis) in the lumbar vertebrae (spine). Consult your physician regarding the advisability of taking supplements of calcium and vitamin D during thyroid hormone replacement. (See Profile of Osteoporosis in this section.)

Use of Thyroxine

1. Hypothyroidism is best treated with a synthetic preparation of thyroxine (see Drug Profile, Section Three). This provides replacement that approximates most closely the normal status of thyroid hormones in circulating blood.

2. Young, basically healthy individuals with hypothyroidism may take thyroxine in full dosage—1 microgram per pound of body weight daily. This usually achieves normal blood levels of T-4 and TSH.

3. Older individuals, with incipient or established heart disease, should initiate thyroxine treatment with small doses that can be increased gradually over 2 to 3 months. This reduces the risk of precipitating disturbances of heart function, such as angina and abnormal rhythm.

4. Thyroxine should be taken in the morning on an empty stomach to ensure maximal absorption and uniform effectiveness.

5. Cholestyramine and colestipol can prevent absorption of thyroxine and liothyronine; for best results, take thyroxine (and/or liothyronine) first (preferably in the morning, fasting), 2 to 3 hours before the first daily dose of either cholestyramine or colestipol.

6. Observe for possible seasonal variation in your response to thyroxine replacement therapy. Some individuals may need less in warm months and more in cold months. If the winter dose of thyroxine is somewhat excessive for summer requirements, you may develop nervousness, insomnia, headaches, intolerance of heat and loss of weight. Consult your physician if you think dosage adjustment is necessary.
7. Long-term thyroxine therapy may lead to premature bone loss in the upper femur (thigh bone) in women. Periodic monitoring of thyroxine blood levels is advised to detect excessive dosage.
8. Do not purchase thyroxine tablets in large quantities (such as 500 to 1000). Thyroxine products can lose up to 6% of their potency per year. It is advisable to obtain a 3 to 6 months' supply (100 to 200 tablets) to ensure full-strength medication.

Ancillary Drug Treatment (as required)

Condition	*Drug Treatment*
For anemia:	iron preparations
	vitamin B-12 (if appropriate for type of anemia)
For constipation:	docusate (Colace, Doxinate, etc.)
	docusate with casanthranol (Peri-Colace, etc.)
For muscle or joint ache/ pain:	aspirin
	acetaminophen (Tylenol, Panadol, etc.)
	ibuprofen (Advil, Nuprin, etc.)

Note: Drug selection, dosage and administration schedule must be determined by the physician for each patient individually.

Resource for Additional Information and Services

American Thyroid Association
Mayo Clinic
200 First Street, S.W.
Rochester, MN 55905
Phone: (507) 284-4738

Maintains professional membership directory for geographical referrals.

MENOPAUSE

Other Names: Menopausal syndrome, estrogen withdrawal syndrome, female climacteric, change of life

Prevalence in USA: 12.8 million women (candidates for menopause).

Age Group: 45 to 55 years; the mean age of natural menopause is 50 years.

Principal Features: The term "menopause" refers to the permanent cessation of menstruation. This occurs naturally in most women between 45 and 55 years of age. The characteristic indication of the "change"—altered menstrual pattern with eventual cessation of menstrual periods—usually lasts from 6 to 18 months. The majority of women (85%) experience some physical effects of progressive estrogen withdrawal: recurring hot flushes, episodic sweating, shrinkage of breast tissue, reduction of vaginal secretions and a variety of nervous and emotional symptoms—anxiety, depression, insomnia, headaches, dizziness, nausea. For approximately 25%, the symptoms are of sufficient intensity to warrant a trial of estrogen replacement therapy. Up to 35% of menopausal women experience hot flushes for 5 or more years.

Causes: Natural menopause occurs spontaneously to terminate reproductive capability. Therapeutic menopause follows surgical removal of the uterus or ovaries and irradiation or removal of the pituitary gland.

Drugs That Can Cause This Disorder: The following drugs can cause cessation of menstruation for varying periods of time, sometimes permanently: busulfan, chlorambucil, cyclophosphamide, mechlorethamine, oral contraceptives and vincristine. The antiestrogen drug tamoxifen, used for the treatment of breast cancer, can cause hot flushes, dizziness and menstrual irregularities typical of the menopausal syndrome.

Drugs Used to Treat This Disorder
"Natural-type" estrogens are preferred:
- conjugated estrogens (Genisis, Premarin).
- esterified estrogens (Evex, Menest).
- estradiol cypionate (Depo-Estradiol, injection).
- estradiol valerate (Delestrogen, injection).
- estriol (Hormonin, a mixture of estriol, estradiol, and estrone).
- piperazine estrone sulfate (Ogen).
- micronized 17-B estradiol (Estrace).
- transdermal estradiol skin patch (Estraderm-50 and 100).

Goals of Drug Treatment
Reduction in the frequency and severity of hot flushes and night sweats with attendant insomnia.

Relief of nervous and emotional symptoms.

Prevention or relief of atrophic changes of the vulva, vagina and urethra.

Prevention of thinning of the skin.

Prevention of osteoporosis (long-term treatment).

Drug Management

General Principles

It is now generally held that for the well-informed menopausal woman who has obvious symptoms of estrogen deficiency and does not have any contraindications to its use, the benefits of estrogen replacement therapy outweigh the possible risks. The use of estrogen is considered effective and safe when prescribed appropriately and monitored properly.

As each women reaches the menopausal years (45 to 55), she should assess her own status and perceived needs. Next she should familiarize herself with the benefits and possible risks of estrogen replacement therapy. (See the Drug Profile of Estrogen, Section Three.) If she thinks she needs medical guidance and/or treatment, she should discuss all aspects of her situation with her physician and share in the decision regarding the use of hormones.

A clear indication for the use of estrogen should exist. It should not be given routinely to the menopausal woman, but should be reserved to treat those with symptoms of estrogen deficiency. Estrogen does not retard the natural progression of general aging; it should not be used for the sole purpose of "preserving femininity."

Before estrogen therapy is started, appropriate examinations should be performed and due consideration given to the following possible contraindications to the use of estrogen:

1. Pregnancy
2. History of deep venous thrombosis or pulmonary embolism
3. Present or previous cancer of the breast
4. Cancer of the uterus
5. Strong family history of breast or uterine cancer
6. Current liver disease or previous drug-induced jaundice
7. Chronic gallbladder disease, with or without stones
8. Abnormal elevation of blood fats (cholesterol, triglycerides, etc.)
9. History of porphyria
10. Large uterine fibroid tumors
11. Any estrogen-dependent tumor
12. Combination of obesity, varicose veins and cigarette smooking
13. Diabetes mellitus
14. Severe hypertension

In the young woman experiencing premature menopause (destruction or removal of both ovaries), the *long-term* use of estrogen replacement is justified, provided appropriate precautions are observed (see Guidelines below).

In the menopausal woman experiencing hot flushes and/or atrophic vaginitis, the *short-term* use of estrogen therapy is generally felt to be acceptable with appropriate supervision and guidance. Estrogen replacement therapy provides symptomatic relief; it is not a permanent cure for hot flushes. *Long-term* estrogen therapy for *all* women after the menopause cannot be justified. Treatment must be carefully individualized (see Guidelines below).

It is generally recommended that estrogens be taken cyclically. The customary schedule is from the 1st through the 25th day of each month, with no estrogen during the remaining days of the month. After 6 to 12 months of continuous use, the estrogen dose should be gradually reduced over a period of 2 to 3 months and then discontinued to assess the individual's need for resumption of use.

The lowest effective daily dose of estrogen should be determined and maintained for the duration of the treatment.

Vaginal cream preparations of estrogen may be considered instead of orally administered estrogen if the only indication is atrophic vaginitis. However, it should be noted that these preparations allow rapid absorption of estrogen into the systemic circulation, and do not permit accurate control of dosage. They should be used intermittently and only as needed to correct the symptoms of atrophic vaginitis. (Note: The estrogen in vaginal creams can be absorbed through the skin of the penis and cause tenderness of the breast in men.)

The unnecessary prolongation of estrogen therapy should be avoided. It is advisable to use estrogens in the lowest effective dose and for only as long as necessary to relieve symptoms.

Guidelines for the Use of Estrogens in Specific Deficiency States

I. The young woman (under 45 years of age) with both ovaries and uterus removed:
    1. Choice of estrogen: a conjugated "natural" estrogen (see list of estrogen preparations).
        The lowest effective dose should be used.*
    2. Dosage schedule: once daily from the 1st through the 25th day of each month.
        Note: If the uterus is present, it is advisable to add a progestin (medroxyprogesterone), 4 to 10 mg daily during the last 7 to 10 days of the estrogen course.**
    3. Duration of use: if well tolerated, until 50 years of age, when assessment of continued need is made individually.
    4. Periodic examinations:
        Base-line mammogram (low-radiation-dose xeroradiography); mammogram should be repeated only as necessary to evaluate possible breast tumor (American Cancer Society guideline).
        Self-examination of breasts monthly.
        Physician examination of breasts (and uterus if present) every 6 to 12 months.
        Measurement of blood pressure.

---

*The lowest effective dose is determined by keeping a daily "flush count" to ascertain the lowest daily dose that will reduce the frequency and severity of flushes to an acceptable level.
**The use of a supplemental progestin during the last 7 to 10 days of estrogen administration is still controversial. A possible benefit is the reduced potential for uterine cancer; a possible risk is the increased potential for coronary artery disease; a possible inconvenience is withdrawal bleeding (induced menstruation). The risks of this form of long-term progestin therapy are not known.

II. The woman experiencing the "menopausal syndrome" of hot flushes
and sweating (usually 45 to 55 years of age):
  A. Uterus not removed
   1. Choice of hormones and recommended dosage range:
Estrogen: conjugated equine estrogens—0.3 to 0.625 mg daily.
(See list of alternative estrogen preparations.)
Progestin: medroxyprogesterone—5 to 10 mg daily.
The lowest effective dose of estrogen should be used.*
   2. Dosage schedule:
Estrogen: once daily from the 1st through the 25th day of each
month.
Progestin: once daily during the last 7 to 10 days of the estrogen
course.**
   3. Duration of use: 6 to 12 months, followed by gradual reduction
of dose over a period of 2 to 3 months, and then discontinuation
to assess the need for continued use. Treatment should be resumed only if symptoms require it. An attempt should be made
to discontinue all hormones after 2 to 3 years of continual use,
unless a clear need for continuation is apparent.
   4. Periodic examinations:
Base-line mammogram (low-radiation-dose xeroradiography).
Low-dose mammogram annually (over 50 years of age) during
  continuous use of estrogen (American Cancer Society guideline).
Self-examination of breasts monthly.
Physician examination of breasts every 6 to 12 months.
Cervical cytology and endometrial biopsy (aspiration curettage)
  annually.
Blood pressure measurement every 3 to 6 months.
Two-hour blood sugar assay annually.
  B. Uterus removed
   1. Choice of estrogen and dose: conjugated equine estrogens—0.3
to 0.625 mg daily.
The lowest effective dose should be used.*
   2. Dosage schedule: once daily from the 1st through the 25th day
of each month.

*The lowest effective dose is determined by keeping a daily "flush count" to ascertain
the lowest daily dose that will reduce the frequency and severity of flushes to an
acceptable level.
**The use of a supplemental progestin during the last 7 to 10 days of estrogen admin-
istration is still controversial. A possible benefit is the reduced potential for uterine
cancer; a possible risk is the increased potential for coronary artery disease; a possible inconvenience is withdrawal bleeding (induced menstruation). The risks of this
form of long-term progestin therapy are not known.

3. Duration of use: 6 to 12 months, followed by gradual reduction of dose over a period of 2 to 3 months, and then discontinuation to assess the need for continued use. Treatment should be resumed only if symptoms require it. An attempt should be made to discontinue all hormones after 2 to 3 years of continual use.

4. Periodic examinations:

   Base-line mammogram (low-radiation-dose xeroradiography).

   Low-dose mammogram annually (over 50 years of age) during continuous use of estrogen (American Cancer Society guideline).

   Self-examination of breasts monthly.

   Physician examination of breasts every 6 to 12 months.

   Blood pressure measurement every 3 to 6 months.

   Two-hour blood sugar assay annually.

III. The woman in the "post-menopausal" period (usually over 55 years of age): treatment should be individualized as follows:

1. If there are no specific symptoms of estrogen deficiency (hot flushes or atrophic vaginitis), estrogen should not be given.

2. If specific symptoms of estrogen deficiency persist to a degree requiring subjective relief, the recommendations in category II apply. However, in addition to limiting courses of estrogen to 6 to 12 months followed by gradual withdrawal, dosage might be limited to 3 times weekly on a trial basis. Estrogen should be discontinued altogether as soon as possible. If only flushes persist beyond 60 years of age, all estrogen should be discontinued. Nonhormonal drugs such as clonidine, ergot preparations and certain sedatives may be substituted for the relief of hot flushes.

3. Although we do not yet have accurate and reliable predictive indicators, an attempt should be made to identify the woman who may be at high risk for the development of osteoporosis. The following features suggest the possibility of increased risk:

   (1) slender build, light-boned, white or Oriental race

   (2) a sedentary life style or restricted physical activity

   (3) a family history (mother or sister) of osteoporosis (reported by some investigators)

   (4) a low-sodium diet (also likely to be a low-calcium diet)

   (5) heavy smoking

   (6) excessive use of antacids that contain aluminum

   (7) long-term use of cortisone-related drugs

   (8) habitual use of carbonated beverages (reported by some investigators)

   (9) excessive consumption of alcohol

   (10) increased urinary excretion of calcium

For the woman thought to be at increased risk for the development of osteoporosis, estrogen treatment should be started within 3 years after menstruation ceases. The following schedule of estrogen therapy may be recommended for prevention: conjugated equine estrogens— 0.625 mg daily or 3 times weekly, for the first 3 weeks of each month.

Periodic examinations as outlined in category II above should be performed. Estrogen replacement therapy may continue indefinitely, always with appropriate supervision.

In addition to the prudent use of estrogen, regular exercise and a daily intake of 1500 mg of calcium and 400 units of vitamin D are generally thought to be beneficial in slowing the development of osteoporosis.

Ancillary Drug Treatment (as required)

Condition	Drug Treatment
For anxiety and/or depression:	alprazolam (Xanax), for intermittent, short-term use
For insomnia:	doxylamine (Unisom), available OTC diphenhydramine (Benadryl)
For headache:	aspirin acetaminophen (Tylenol, Panadol, etc.) ibuprofen (Advil, Nuprin, etc.)
For atrophic vaginitis and painful intercourse:	estrogen creams (Dienestrol, Estrace, Premarin)

Note: Drug selection, dosage and administration schedule must be determined by the physician for each patient individually.

Resource for Additional Information and Services

WARM (Women's Association for Research in Menopause)
128 East 56th Street
New York, NY 10022
Phone: (212) 418-0610

Operates support groups; gathers and disseminates information on menopause.

MIGRAINE HEADACHE

Other Names: Classic migraine, common migraine

Prevalence in USA: Approximately 30 million cases, 15% of the general population under 40 years of age.

Age Group: Under 18 years—0.8% of population; 18 to 44 years—4.7% of population; 45 to 64 years—5% of population; over 65 years—1.9% of population.

Male to Female Ratio

With onset at puberty, boys and girls are affected equally.
By age 40 there is a 3 to 2 predominance in women.

Principal Features

Migraine headaches may first appear in childhood but usually begin in the late teens or early twenties; they often cease after menopause. The migraine attack occurs in one of two patterns:

(1) Classic migraine (15% of the total) begins with an "aura" of symptoms that may precede the onset of headache by 15 to 20 minutes; these usually consist of visual manifestations described as blind spots, zig-zag effects or flashing lights. The attack may begin at any time of the day or night; the headache is usually (70% of attacks) located on one side of the head, but may spread to both sides before terminating. The pain is usually pulsating or throbbing in nature and varies in intensity from mild to severe. The migraine attack commonly (90% of attacks) includes nausea, vomiting and increased sensitivity to light and noise. Other associated features are scalp tenderness, dizziness, dry mouth, tremors, sweating and chilliness.

(2) Common migraine (85% of the total) begins as a headache without a warning "aura." Otherwise the pattern is essentially the same. Attacks may occur rarely (1 or 2 a year) or every few days; the average frequency is 2 to 4 per month. Individual episodes usually last from 12 to 48 hours.

Causes: The exact complex of mechanisms responsible for the migraine attack is not known. It is basically a disturbance in the autonomic nervous system that causes instability in the control of cerebral arteries. There is a positive family history in 70% of those who experience migraine attacks. The majority of women who experience migraine find frequent association of the episode with menstruation. Other factors that are reported to trigger migraine attacks include emotional stress, excessive fatigue, erratic patterns of eating and sleeping, bright sunlight, loud noises, and the use of alcohol. The following foods are thought to be responsible for migraine attacks in sensitive individuals: aged cheese, bananas, chicken livers, chocolate, citrus fruits, monosodium glutamate, onions, pickled herring, pork, red wine, excessive salt, shell fish, sodium nitrite, vinegar, yogurt.

Drugs That Can Cause This Disorder: The following drugs may induce migrainelike headaches or aggravate existing migraine syndromes:
aminophylline
analgesics (chronic use of acetaminophen or aspirin)
antihypertensive drugs that cause vasodilation
caffeine (chronic use may cause vascular headache)
estrogens (can worsen migraine in 50% of women)
hydralazine
indomethacin
nifedipine

nitrates
oral contraceptives
prazosin
reserpine

Drugs Used to Treat This Disorder

For Prevention of Migraine Attacks

Beta-Adrenergic-Blocking Drugs (Beta Blockers)
- propranolol (Inderal).
- nadolol (Corgard).
- atenolol (Tenormin).
- timolol (Blocadren).
- metoprolol (Lopressor).

Calcium Channel-Blocking Drugs (Calcium Blockers)
- nifedipine (Procardia).
- verapamil (Calan, Isoptin).

Anti-inflammatory Drugs (Aspirin Substitutes)
- naproxen (Naprosyn).
- ibuprofen (Motrin, Rufen, Advil, etc.).
- fenoprofen (Nalfon).

Antidepressants
- amitriptyline (Elavil, Endep).
- doxepin (Sinequan, Adapin).

methysergide (Sansert)
lithium (Lithane, Lithobid, etc.)

For Abortion and Relief of Migraine Attacks

Vasoconstrictor Drugs
- ergotamine: oral (Cafergot, Wigraine); rectal (Cafergot, Wigraine suppositories); sublingual (Ergostat, Ergomar, Wigrettes); inhalant (Medihaler ergotamine).
- isometheptene (Midrin).

Anti-inflammatory Drugs
- aspirin.
- meclofenamate (Meclomen).
- ibuprofen (Motrin, Rufen, Advil, etc.).
- naproxen (Naprosyn).
- diflunisal (Dolobid).

Opioid Analgesics
- codeine.
- meperidine (Demerol).

Goals of Drug Treatment

Prompt abortion and relief of the acute migraine attack.
Reduction in the frequency and severity of recurrent migraine attacks.
A permanent cure is not available.

Drug Management

Important note: Not every drug is effective with every patient. Trial and experimentation may be necessary to determine the most effective treatment for each individual.

For fewer than 3 attacks per month of mild to moderate migraine, use abortive medications at the onset of symptoms. Ergotamine and anti-inflammatory drugs are the medications of choice.

For 3 or more attacks per month and for severe, prolonged migraine, use preventive medications on a continual basis. Beta blockers are the drugs of choice to reduce the frequency and severity of recurrent migraine attacks.

Always try to take your medication as soon as possible after the first indications of a developing migraine attack.

Isometheptene (Midrin) is a mild, well-tolerated and safer drug than ergotamine; use it first to determine its effectiveness. Go to stronger drugs only as needed.

Metoclopramide (Reglan) is an effective addition to the treatment of migraine attacks; it often controls nausea and vomiting, and it enhances the effectiveness of other oral migraine drugs.

Antidepressants may be used concurrently with other preventive drugs. They may be very effective *even in the absence of depression*.

For best results, start the preventive treatment of menstrual migraine 3 days before the onset of menstruation and continue it until all spotting has ceased.

Use of Beta Blockers

1. These are the drugs of choice for long-term prevention of migraine attacks. Propranolol (Inderal) is the most widely used; nadolol (Corgard) is a good second choice.
2. The preventive dose varies greatly and must be determined by individual trial. Effective dosage ranges from 80 mg to 320 mg daily.
3. After a period of 6 to 12 months of good headache control, the dose may be reduced gradually and the drug eventually discontinued.

Use of Calcium Blockers

1. The preventive use of this class of drugs is still experimental in this country; they have been highly effective in Europe.
2. Verapamil (Calan, Isoptin) is the most effective of this class currently available in the USA. Nifedipine (Procardia) has been found to intensify migraine attacks in some individuals. Its use is not recommended.
3. A trial of 6 to 8 weeks is usually required to determine the preventive effectiveness of these drugs.
4. Observe for the development of fluid retention and constipation.

Use of Anti-inflammatory Drugs

1. These drugs are useful in both preventing and relieving migraine attacks. They are usually well tolerated and are not habit-forming.
2. Meclofenamate (Meclomen) is the fastest acting of the class and is very effective in aborting acute migraine.
3. Naproxen (Naprosyn) and fenoprofen (Nalfon) are also effective and widely used for intermittent prevention (as in menstrual migraine).
4. The prolonged-action forms of these drugs should be used cautiously, especially in the elderly, because of their potential for reducing kidney blood flow.

Use of Antidepressants
1. The long-term use of amitriptyline (Elavil, Endep, etc.) is effective in preventing all types of chronic headaches: tension headaches, migraine attacks and mixed forms.
2. Effectiveness is not dependent upon the drug's antidepressant action; the dose required for headache control is less than the antidepressant dose.
3. For migraine patients with sleep problems, the antidepressants of choice are amitriptyline, doxepin and trazodone because of their sedative effects. The total daily requirement is best given as a single dose at bedtime.
4. Desipramine (Norpramin, Pertofrane) is usually considered to have the fewest side-effects.

Use of Methysergide
1. While very effective as a migraine preventive, this drug is inherently dangerous. It can cause serious and life-threatening adverse effects with long-term use: formation of scar tissue (fibrosis) involving the heart, lungs, blood vessels and kidneys.
2. It is usually reserved to treat severe migraine that has not responded to safer drugs.
3. Its use should be limited to courses of no more than 4 to 6 months followed by drug-free intervals of 4 to 6 weeks.
4. This drug should not be used in the presence of valvular heart disease or serious blood vessel disorders.
5. The smallest effective dose should be determined; the total daily dosage should not exceed 8 mg.

Use of Ergotamine
1. This is the most effective abortive drug if taken early in the migraine attack; it can relieve the headache in 1 to 2 hours. It tends to be less effective if taken later.
2. It may be taken orally or sublingually in tablet form, rectally in the form of suppositories, by inhalation or by injection.
3. Dosage should be limited to no more than 6 mg/24 hours or 10 mg/week to prevent serious adverse effects. (See Drug Profile.)
4. Avoid concurrent use with dopamine, erythromycins, troleandomycin and beta blockers.
5. Avoid frequent and regular use; this drug can cause dependence (see Glossary). Long-term use on a daily basis can *cause* chronic migrainelike headaches.
6. Ergotamine "rebound" (return and intensification of headache) can be prevented by allowing 48 hours between courses.

Ancillary Drug Treatment (as required)

Condition	*Drug Treatment*
For nausea and vomiting:	metoclopramide (Reglan)

For preheadache visual
    disturbances: nitroglycerin, sublingual
                               isoproterenol (Isuprel), inhalation

Note: Drug selection, dosage and administration schedule must be determined by the physician for each patient individually.

Resource for Additional Information and Services

National Headache Foundation
5252 North Western Avenue
Chicago, IL 60625
Phone: 1-800-843-2256 (outside IL); 1-800-523-8858 (inside IL); (312) 878-5558

Publications available.

MYASTHENIA GRAVIS

Other Names: MG, autoimmune myasthenia gravis, myasthenia gravis pseudoparalytica

Prevalence in USA: Estimated to be 1 in 25,000. Approximately 24,000 documented cases. (Because many mild forms of this disorder are not recognized or reported, it is estimated that the prevalence may approach 100,000.)

Age Group: The autoimmune form of myasthenia gravis (over 90% of all forms of MG) can have its onset at any age from birth to 90 years. Thirty percent of all cases begin in women between puberty and 40 years of age, with the highest incidence in the twenties. Thirty percent of all cases begin in men after the age of 40, with the highest incidence in the fifties.

Male to Female Ratio
    Age of onset under 40 years—1 to 3
    Age of onset 30–50 years—1 to 1
    Age of onset over 40 years—3 to 1

Principal Features: Myasthenia gravis is a chronic disorder of neuromuscular function attributed to the presence of antibodies in the blood that impair the transmission of nerve impulses across the junction of nerve and muscle tissue. The characteristic symptoms are periods of fluctuating fatigue and early exhaustion of affected muscles. Involvement may be restricted to a single muscle group or may gradually expand to affect major muscle groups throughout the body. The first muscles to show abnormal fatigability in 50% of all cases are those of the eye, resulting in drooping eyelids and blurred or double vision; 25% of cases first become aware of weakness while speaking, chewing or swallowing; 20% first notice unusual weakness and fatigue in the arms or legs. The course of the disorder varies greatly from one person to another, but the point of maximal involvement is usually reached within 3 years. Stage 1, the "active" stage, is characterized by increasing disability and fluctuation of symptoms; it may last from 5 to 10 years. Stage 2, the "inactive" stage, is marked by less variation and greater stability. Stage 3, the "burned out" stage, is usually reached 14 to 20 years after the initial onset of symptoms; it generally represents the residual pattern of the disorder that must be managed for the remaining life of the individual. Spontaneous remissions occur in fewer than 10% of cases, and these may last only 2 to 3 years.

Causes: The current belief is that myasthenia gravis is an autoimmune disorder characterized by the formation of antibodies that impair acetylcholine receptors of the nerve-muscle junctions in affected voluntary muscles. Such antibodies are present in 80% to 90% of all MG patients. Their presence implies damage or destruction of receptors by autoimmune complexes. The resulting reduction of available receptors for nerve impulse transmission is responsible for the muscle weakness and easy fatigability that characterize this disorder. The mechanisms responsible for the formation of destructive antibodies are not understood. There is no clear pattern of heredity to account for the development of MG.

Drugs That Can Cause This Disorder

The drug penicillamine (Cuprimine, Depen), used to treat rheumatoid arthritis and Wilson's disease, can cause true myasthenia gravis in about 1% of users.

The following drugs may impair neuromuscular impulse transmission and should be avoided or used with great caution in patients with myasthenia gravis:

antihistamines	morphine
barbiturates	neomycin
beta blocker drugs	opioid analgesics
calcium channel blocker drugs	phenytoin
clindamycin	polymyxin A and B
colistimethate	procainamide
colistin	quinidine
gentamycin	quinine
kanamycin	streptomycin
lidocaine	tranquilizers
lithium	trimethadione
magnesium sulfate	tubocurarine

Drugs Used to Treat This Disorder

Cholinesterase Inhibitors
- ambenonium (Mytelase).
- neostigmine (Prostigmin).
- pyridostigmine (Mestinon).

Cortisonelike Drug (Corticosteroid)
- prednisone

azathioprine (Imuran)

Goals of Drug Treatment

The primary aim is to minimize disability; cure is not possible.

Prompt determination of the optimal drug regimen for each patient individually.

Smooth control of fluctuating muscle weakness and fatigability; restoration of sustained strength and endurance.

Prevention of both myasthenic crisis and cholinergic crisis.

Achievement of remission of the disease process.

Drug Management

Dosage requirements may vary from day to day, according to the course of the disorder, the physical demands of daily routines, the emotional state of the patient, etc. Doses should be adjusted according to need, larger doses being taken at times of greatest fatigue—as just before meals, to facilitate eating.

Restoration of muscle strength and endurance beyond 80% of normal status (before MG) is usually not possible. Learn by experience the limit of your response to the drugs that work best for you and do not exceed the optimal dose.

Cholinesterase inhibitors provide only transient symptomatic relief and are of limited usefulness in most cases of moderate to severe MG. They are most useful for nonprogressive eye muscle weakness and mild limb muscle weakness.

Use caution when taking drugs concurrently that can cause low blood potassium levels (hypokalemia). Many diuretics in wide use can cause potassium loss and thereby increase muscle weakness and fatigue.

Use of Cholinesterase Inhibitors

1. These drugs are generally used first to treat the newly diagnosed case of MG. A trial of 1 to 3 months is usually sufficient to determine their effectiveness.

2. The drug of choice must be determined for each patient individually by trial and error, as must the optimal dose and administration schedule.

3. Pyridostigmine (Mestinon) is usually preferred by most patients with ocular or mild nonprogressive MG.

4. These drugs are prone to irregular absorption and consequent variation in therapeutic effect. They are best taken with food to reduce stomach upset.

5. Careful dosage adjustment is mandatory. Underdosage can result in myasthenic crisis. Overdosage can result in cholinergic crisis. Both reactions can cause sudden muscle weakness and be life-threatening if respiration is seriously impaired. Sudden weakness occurring 1 hour after taking medication usually indicates overdosage (cholinergic crisis).

6. After prolonged use, these drugs may lose their effectiveness. Your ability to respond to them can be restored by reducing the dose or withdrawing them for several days. *However, this must be done under the supervision of your physician.*

7. Long-term treatment with high doses of these drugs may itself cause permanent changes in the motor end-plates and adversely affect neuromuscular transmission.

Use of Cortisonelike Drugs (Corticosteroids)

1. These drugs have become more widely used within the past 5 years for treating MG. Some physicians initiate treatment with prednisone if there are no contraindications. The usual course of treatment is 2 years, to minimize the possibility of relapse.

2. Prednisone is given initially in high doses daily until improvement begins, then changed to an alternate-day schedule. With sustained improvement and stabilization of function, the dose is gradually reduced to the smallest effective maintenance level.

3. A trial period of 60 days is usually necessary to determine the effectiveness of prednisone therapy for MG. For those who respond favorably, marked improvement occurs within 3 months and maximal improvement is usually attained within 9 months. Favorable results are reported in 80% of patients, with remissions in 25% to 35%.

4. Significant worsening of symptoms can occur in 48% of patients during the early phase of high-dose prednisone treatment. For this reason a trial of prednisone is best initiated in the hospital.

5. Approximately 90% of patients remain dependent upon long-term prednisone treatment for sustained improvement. Only 10% can withdraw successfully and remain in remission.

6. Observe carefully for the possible development of adverse effects that often accompany long-term use of cortisonelike drugs. See the Drug Profile of Prednisone in Section Three.

7. Some experts now recommend that thymectomy be done in serious cases *before* corticosteroids are used. A consensus is emerging that long-term corticosteroid therapy should be avoided if possible.

Use of Azathioprine (Imuran)

1. It is now felt that azathioprine is significantly less toxic than long-term steroid therapy. It is useful in reducing steroid requirement, and can produce improvement or remission when used alone.

2. It may be used alone or in conjunction with cortisonelike drugs to treat advanced stages of MG with severe disability.

3. For those who respond favorably, improvement usually begins within 3 to 12 months; maximal improvement may require continual treatment for 12 to 36 months. Approximately 53% of patients show some improvement using azathioprine alone, with 40% achieving temporary remission. However, continued improvement usually requires high doses.

4. Only 10% of patients show sustained improvement following discontinuation of this drug.

5. Observe carefully for the development of serious adverse effects. See the Drug Profile of Azathioprine in Section Three.

Ancillary Drug Treatment (as required)

Condition	Drug Treatment
For apathy, lethargy:	ephedrine
For hypokalemia:	potassium supplements (see Drug Profile)
For diarrhea:	diphenoxylate (Imodium)

Note: Drug selection, dosage and administration schedule must be determined by the physician for each patient individually.

Resource for Additional Information and Services

Myasthenia Gravis Foundation
53 West Jackson Boulevard, Suite 909
Chicago, IL 60604
Phone: (312) 427-6252

Sponsors 52 state groups and low-cost pharmacy service.
Publications: physicians' and nurses' manuals, patient handbooks, brochures, pamphlets.

OSTEOARTHRITIS

Other Names: Osteoarthrosis, degenerative arthritis, degenerative joint disease, hypertrophic arthritis

Prevalence in USA: 16 million—8.7% of the adult population; 10% of the elderly population.

Age Group: 55 years and over.

Male to Female Ratio: Same incidence in men and women.

Principal Features: Osteoarthritis is the most common joint disease and the major cause of disability of our older population. It is an insidious, slowly progressive deterioration of the surface cartilage on the ends of bones where they come together to form joints. During the early phases of change, there are no symptoms. With progressive destruction of protective cartilage, bone surface becomes exposed and irritated; this results in pain, stiffness and muscle spasm. As the central area of cartilage is destroyed, new bone and cartilage begin to form on the edges of the joint (spur formation). These degenerative changes can start as early as the fourth decade of life; they usually begin to cause symptoms in sixth and seventh decades; by age 75, all individuals have some degree of osteoarthritis in one or more joints.

The most commonly involved joints are: fingers, thumb, shoulders, hips, knees, base of the first toe, neck and lower (lumbar) spine. Progressive changes in the weight-bearing joints, principally the lower spine, hips and knees, eventually give rise to pain, deep ache and muscle spasm. Discomfort grows worse after prolonged activity that involves diseased joints.

Causes: There is no apparent initiating cause for primary osteoarthritis. The disorder does have a familial pattern, and it is thought that genetic biochemical defects in cartilage structure predispose some individuals to excessive "wear and tear" deterioration of vulnerable joints. Secondary osteoarthritis is due to congenital joint malformations, joint injuries and infections and other infrequent causes of bone and cartilage deterioration.

Drugs That Can Cause This Disorder: Although some drugs are capable of causing joint aches and pains (e.g., barbiturates, "sulfa" drugs, oral contraceptives, isoniazid, pyrazinamide), no drugs cause the bone and cartilage destruction characteristic of osteoarthritis. Rarely the systemic (internal) use of cortisonelike steroid drugs can cause aseptic necrosis of bone (destruction without infection); this can initiate a secondary form of osteoarthritis.

Drugs Used to Treat This Disorder

There are no drugs that can prevent, halt the progression of or reverse the degenerative changes of osteoarthritis. The following drugs are used to relieve pain, stiffness and muscle spasm.

Nonsteroidal Anti-inflammatory Drugs (NSAIDs)

Salicylates

- aspirin (Bufferin, Ascriptin, Cama, etc.).
- aspirin, enteric-coated (Easprin, Ecotrin, etc.).
- aspirin, zero-order-release (Zorpin).
- magnesium salicylate (Magan, Mobidin).
- choline magnesium salicylate (Trisilate).
- salsalate (Disalcid).
- diflunisal (Dolobid).
- sodium salicylate.

Indole Derivatives

- indomethacin (Indocin).
- sulindac (Clinoril).
- tolmetin (Tolectin).

Propionic Acid Derivatives

- fenoprofen (Nalfon).
- flurbiprofen (Ansaid).
- ibuprofen (Motrin, Rufen, Advil, etc.).
- ketoprofen (Orudis).
- naproxen (Naprosyn).
- suprofen (Suprol).

Fenamic Acid Derivatives

- meclofenamate (Meclomen).

- mefenamic acid (Ponstel).

Oxicam Derivative
- piroxicam (Feldene).

Phenylacetic Acid Derivative
- diclofenac (Voltaren).

Simple Analgesics
- acetaminophen (Tylenol, Panadol, etc.).
- propoxyphene (Darvon, etc.).
- codeine (Tylenol with codeine, etc.).
- hydrocodone (Vicodin, etc.).
- oxycodone (Percodan, Percocet, Tylox).

Muscle Relaxants
- carisoprodol (Soma).
- cyclobenzaprine (Flexeril).
- diazepam (Valium).
- methocarbamol (Robaxin).
- orphenadrine (Norflex).

Goals of Drug Treatment

Relief of pain and stiffness sufficient to permit continued activity, therapeutic exercise and physiotherapy.

Relief of associated anxiety and/or depression.

Drug Management

General Principles

Osteoarthritis is a chronic but slowly progressive disorder; although there is no curative treatment available, the symptoms are generally mild for long periods of time and can usually be relieved satisfactorily with available drugs.

Nonsteroidal anti-inflammatory drugs (NSAIDs) are the primary drugs of choice for managing osteoarthritis. Their principal actions are within the tissues of the diseased joint.

Simple analgesics, such as propoxyphene, codeine, oxycodone, etc., suppress pain perception in the brain; they are used to supplement the analgesic effects of NSAIDs.

Cortisonelike steroids by mouth should not be used in the management of osteoarthritis. They may be helpful when injected directly into osteoarthritis joints, sometimes providing prompt and lasting relief of pain and swelling. If effective, steroid injections may be repeated at intervals of 4 to 6 months for a limited number of times.

Symptomatic drug treatment will be more effective if it is supplemented by appropriate physiotherapy and the use of physical aids, such as canes, crutches, walkers, railings, etc.

Avoid prolonged and repeated overuse of diseased joints to (1) slow the progression of joint destruction and (2) minimize requirements for analgesic drugs.

Excessive body weight (obesity) can accelerate deterioration of weight-bearing joints. Prudent weight reduction programs are a most important part of treatment for osteoarthritis of the lower spine, hips and knees.

Use of Nonsteroidal Anti-inflammatory Drugs (NSAIDs)

1. These drugs are not thought to be able to favorably influence the natural course of osteoarthritis, but they can relieve pain and inflammation and thereby improve joint function and mobility.

2. Treatment is usually initiated with aspirin (lowest cost). Unfortunately, large doses (2 to 4 tablets of 325 mg each, 3 to 4 times daily) are often necessary to achieve satisfactory relief. The high blood levels required can cause ringing in the ears (tinnitus) and loss of hearing, especially in the elderly. Measurements of salicylate blood levels can be most helpful in establishing correct dosage. (See Therapeutic Drug Monitoring in Section One.)

3. Soluble aspirin preparations (regular aspirin, Bufferin, Ascriptin, etc.) often cause stomach ulceration and bleeding; they should be taken with food to minimize this effect.

4. The preferred forms of aspirin for continual use in large doses include (1) enteric-coated preparations and (2) zero-order-release tablets. (See list above.)

5. Salicylates other than aspirin can also be used. (See list above.) These cause significantly less stomach irritation; some are effective with twice daily dosage.

6. All NSAID aspirin substitutes are better tolerated than aspirin. However, they may share a cross-sensitivity in individuals who are allergic to aspirin and may induce asthmatic reactions.

7. An NSAID should be used on a regular schedule for a trial period of 3 to 4 weeks; if it is not effective, another one should be tried in sequence (selecting one from a different chemical group). An attempt is made to find the NSAID that provides the best relief with the fewest side-effects.

8. Authorities do not recommend the use of NSAIDs in combination with each other. A small dose of aspirin taken along with an NSAID may provide additional relief of pain.

9. NSAIDs have a potential for injuring the kidney and impairing kidney function. They should be used with caution in individuals over 50 years old, in those with hypertension, diabetes, congestive heart failure and especially in those taking diuretics.

10. NSAIDs can increase the effects of oral antidiabetic drugs (sulfonylureas) and anticoagulants. Dosage adjustments may be necessary.

Use of Narcoticlike Analgesics

1. In advanced cases of osteoarthritis, mild analgesics such as acetaminophen or propoxyphene may not provide adequate pain relief. Codeine, hydrocodone and oxycodone may be tried cautiously on an intermittent schedule to avoid tolerance and dependence.

2. The use of stronger narcotic (opioid) analgesics (morphine, meperidine, etc.) should be avoided completely. Their potential for causing dependence (addiction) precludes repetitious, long-term use in chronically painful disorders like osteoarthritis.

Use of Muscle Relaxants
1. Muscle spasm prevents exercise and use of affected joints. The cautious use of muscle relaxants in conjunction with physiotherapy may be beneficial in preserving joint mobility and muscle strength.
2. Muscle relaxants are most useful in managing osteoarthritis of the lower spine with associated lumbo-sacral muscle spasm.

Ancillary Drug Treatment (as required)

Condition	Drug Treatment
For anxiety and/or mild depression:	alprazolam (Xanax), for intermittent, short-term use
For moderate or severe depression:	trazodone (Desyrel) (see Profile of Depression in this section)
For drug-induced constipation:	docusate with casanthranol (Peri-Colace)

Note: Drug selection, dosage and administration schedule must be determined by the physician for each patient individually.

Resources for Additional Information and Services

Arthritis Foundation
1314 Spring Street, N.W.
Atlanta, GA 30309
Phone: (404) 872-7100
Publications available.

Association for People With Arthritis
P.O. Box 954
6 Commercial Street
Hicksville, NY 11802
Phone: 1-800-323-2243
Publications available.

OSTEOPOROSIS

Other Names: Osteopenia, type I postmenopausal or spinal osteoporosis (95% of all cases), type II senile osteoporosis

Prevalence in USA: 24 million—approximately 25% of white women over 60 years of age have osteoporosis; 1.3 million fractures due to osteoporosis occur annually.

Age Group: Type I osteoporosis—50 to 65 years. Type II osteoporosis—65 years and over.

Male to Female Ratio: Much higher incidence in women: 8 to 1.

Principal Features: Osteoporosis is a major disorder of bone in the elderly, occurring most often in postmenopausal women. As ovarian function declines and estrogen is withdrawn, the natural loss of bone mass is accelerated. This eventually weakens bone structure and predisposes to fractures that can result from minimal trauma. Osteoporosis can be localized in a single bone (a leg immobilized in a cast), but it is usually more widely distributed, with most fractures occurring in the spine, wrist and hip. The basic defect is a relative increase in the rate of bone destruction without a compensating increase in the reformation of new bone. There are usually no symptoms prior to the occurrence of a spontaneous or traumatic fracture. A sudden compression fracture of a vertebra in the middle or lower section of the spine can result from such minor strains as bending, lifting or sneezing; it causes immediate pain and disability lasting several weeks. Gradual compression of the vertebrae (usually painless) causes loss of height and the development of a stooped, rounded back ("dowager's hump"). A spontaneous fracture of a hip (femur) can occur on arising from a chair or while walking. Untreated osteoporosis can cause a loss of 30% to 60% of bone mass.

Causes: Primary osteoporosis is a normal consequence of aging. A woman loses approximately 50% of bone mass, and a man approximately 25%, during a normal life span. Type I primary osteoporosis refers to the estrogen withdrawal syndrome following menopause. Type II primary osteoporosis occurs later as a feature of senility. Secondary osteoporosis refers to the bone loss that is associated with other diseases and disorders: hyperthyroidism, hyperparathyroidism, adrenal cortical hormone excess (Cushing's syndrome or drug-induced), multiple myeloma, diabetes, and alcoholism.

Drugs That Can Cause This Disorder
- Cortisonelike steroids, especially in immobilized women over 50 years of age receiving large doses.
- Heparin, when used in long-term therapy.
- Methotrexate, when used in prepubertal children for long-term therapy.

Drugs Used to Treat This Disorder
Estrogens ("Natural-type" Estrogens Are Preferred)
- conjugated estrogens (Genisis, Premarin).
- esterified estrogens (Evex, Menest).
- estradiol cypionate (Depo-Estradiol, injection).
- estradiol valerate (Delestrogen, injection).
- estriol (Hormonin, a mixture of estriol, estradiol and estrone).
- piperazine estrone sulfate (Ogen).

- micronized 17-B estadiol (Estrace).
- transdermal estradiol skin patch (Estraderm-50 and 100).

Calcium Preparations
- calcium carbonate (40% calcium) (generic tablets, Alka-2, Biocal, Caltrate, OsCal-500, Tums).
- calcium gluconate (9% calcium) (generic tablets).
- calcium lactate (13% calcium) (generic tablets).
- dibasic calcium phosphate (31% calcium) (generic tablets).

Vitamin D Analogs
- calcifediol (Calderol).
- calcitriol (Rocaltrol).

Other Drugs
- calcitonin (Calcimar).
- fluorides (investigational).

Goals of Drug Treatment

Primary prevention: early initiation of estrogen therapy—during or immediately after menopause—to prevent acceleration of natural bone loss.

Secondary prevention: initiation of estrogen therapy 3 or more years following menopause (after some degree of osteoporosis is present) to arrest or retard progressive bone loss.

Prevention of osteoporosis-related fractures.

Relief of pain and muscle spasm associated with fracture of osteoporotic bone.

Drug Management

General Principles

It is now firmly established that excessive bone loss (osteoporosis) following menopause can be prevented or significantly reduced by the timely administration of low-dose estrogen.

Accurate assessment of bone mass for the detection of osteoporosis can be made by quantitative CAT scan of vertebrae and by photon absorptiometry of wrist bones. However, these procedures are expensive and not generally available.

Currently it is not feasible to screen all postmenopausal women for osteoporosis. To identify those who may benefit from estrogen used preventively, the following "risk factors" characterize the candidates for postmenopausal osteoporosis:

1. slender build, light-boned, white or Oriental race
2. a sedentary life style or restricted physical activity
3. a family history of osteoporosis (grandmother, mother, aunt or sister)
4. a high-protein diet
5. a low-sodium diet (also likely to be a low-calcium diet)
6. lifelong avoidance of dairy products
7. heavy smoking
8. excessive use of antacids that contain aluminum
9. long-term use of cortisonelike steroid drugs

   10. habitual use of carbonated beverages
   11. excessive consumption of alcohol
   12. increased urinary excretion of calcium
  Thyroid replacement therapy (in appropriate dosage) may increase bone loss and predispose to the development of osteoporosis in the vertebrae of the lower spine. If you are taking a thyroid preparation to correct hypothyroidism, consult your physician regarding a possible need for calcium and vitamin D supplements to prevent potential bone loss.

Use of Estrogens

1. Estrogen increases the absorption of dietary calcium and reduces the rate of calcium loss from bone. Recent studies have shown that estrogen can reduce the risk of hip fractures by as much as 66%.
2. Estrogen does not substantially increase bone mass; it does not enhance restoration of bone following loss.
3. To be effective in preventing significant osteoporosis, estrogen therapy must begin within 3 years after menopause. Available evidence seems to indicate that continued protection against the development of osteoporosis requires ongoing use of estrogen—probably for life by those at risk.
4. Fifty percent of women are protected by 0.3 mg of conjugated estrogens daily; close to 100% are protected by 0.625 mg daily. Your physician can advise the dose most appropriate for you.
5. For detailed information regarding the use of estrogen, see the Profile of Menopause in this section and the Drug Profile of Estrogen in Section Three.

Use of Calcium Preparations

1. Calcium supplementation of the diet is appropriate for preventing or treating osteoporosis because the calcium content of the diet is usually less than the ongoing requirement for the maintenance of normal bone density. The average dietary intake of calcium by women is 500 to 600 mg daily. The daily requirement for the postmenopausal woman is 1500 to 2000 mg (all sources).
2. There is some evidence that calcium supplements (taken alone) may reduce the rate of bone loss and the incidence of fracture, but further proof is needed. Calcium is most effective when taken in conjunction with vitamin D and estrogen.
3. Supplemental calcium must not be taken in excessive doses. The recommended daily intake of calcium is approximately 1000 mg if taking estrogen and 1500 mg if not taking estrogen.
4. Excessive intake of supplemental calcium (more than 2000 mg daily) can cause abnormal increases in the blood and urine levels of calcium and predispose to kidney stone formation.
5. The most appropriate calcium preparations to use for supplementation are listed above.
6. Calcium supplements made from bone meal or mineral clay (dolomite, montmorillomite) may contain lead or other toxic metals and should be avoided.

7. Calcium supplements may be more effective if taken as a single late-evening dose to suppress the normal nocturnal rise in parathyroid hormone that increases bone loss.

8. Calcium may decrease the effects of aspirin (and other salicylates), calcium channel-blocking drugs, iron and tetracyclines. Do not take calcium preparations within 2 hours of taking other drugs.

Use of Vitamin D Analogs

1. Elderly individuals with osteoporosis who have a normal life style are not likely to a have a vitamin D deficiency; they usually have an adequate supply from their diet and exposure to sunlight.

2. Shut-ins (those confined to home, nursing home or hospital) probably need a supplement of vitamin D. Currently recommended sources include Calderol and Rocaltrol.

3. When vitamin D is used, limit calcium intake to 600 to 700 mg daily to prevent excessive absorption and abnormally high calcium levels in blood and urine.

Use of Calcitonin (a Thyroid Hormone That Reduces Bone Loss)

1. Studies to date show that calcitonin in doses of 100 units daily can produce an increase in total body calcium (99% in bone) after 2 years of treatment. A favorable response was achieved in 70% of users.

2. Calcitonin is given by injection and is used in conjunction with calcium and vitamin D.

3. Studies using other dosage forms of calcitonin—oral, buccal (cheek), intranasal—are under way.

Use of Fluoride

1. The use of fluoride in the prevention and treatment of osteoporosis is still investigational. Directions for its optimal use have not been established.

2. A dose of 40 to 65 mg/day is required to stimulate bone formation. Adverse effects occur in over 30% of users; these include nausea, stomach pain, gastrointestinal bleeding, bone and joint pain and severe foot discomfort, often intense enought to preclude compliance with treatment.

3. Calcium must always be used concurrently with fluoride to avoid the development of osteomalacia (abnormal mineral composition of bone).

Ancillary Drug Treatment (as required)

Condition	*Drug Treatment*
For calcium-induced constipation:	docusate (Colace, etc.)
	docusate with casanthranol (Peri-Colace, etc.)

For fracture pain:	acetaminaphen with codeine (Tylenol with codeine)
	acetaminophen with propoxyphene (Darvocet-N 100)
	Avoid opiate analgesics stronger than codeine.
For muscle spasm:	diazepam (Valium)
For mild depression:	alprazolam (Xanax), for intermittent, short-term use
For marked depression:	trazodone (Desyrel)

Note: Drug selection, dosage and administration schedule must be determined by the physician for each patient individually.

Resources for Additional Information and Services

National Institute of Arthritis and Musculoskeletal and Skin Diseases
Information Office: Building 31, Room 4C32B
9000 Rockville Pike
Bethesda, MD 20892
Phone: Information Specialist, (301) 496-8188

Handles inquiries on arthritis, bone diseases (including osteoporosis), and skin diseases.

National Osteoporosis Foundation
1625 Eye Street, N.W., Suite 822
Washington, DC 20006
Phone: (202) 223-2226

Publications available.

WARM (Women's Association for Research in Menopause)
128 East 56th Street
New York, NY 10022
Phone: (212) 418-0610

Gathers and disseminates information on menopause-related subjects.

PARKINSON'S DISEASE

Other Names: Paralysis agitans, parkinsonism, parkinsonian syndrome

Prevalence in USA: Approximately 1.5 million—50,000 new cases annually; 1% of the population over 50 years old.

Age Group: 10% of cases under 40 years old; 20% of cases 40 to 50 years old; 70% of cases 50 years old and over. The mean age at onset is 58 to 62 years.

Male to Female Ratio: More common in men, 3 to 2.

Principal Features: Parkinson's disease is a slowly progressive, debilitating disorder of certain brain centers that contribute to the control and regulation of body movement. The earliest symptoms begin very insidiously; one arm or one leg (or the arm and leg on one side) will gradually develop a sense of weakness, retarded movement and stiffness. A fine tremor in a hand or foot will appear in 70% of cases; this occurs at rest and disappears with intentional use of the affected limb and while asleep. Symptoms may remain mild for years or they may progress steadily. Eventually the principal features of the disorder become generalized; the tremor spreads, most of the body musculature becomes rigid, the posture is stooped, movement is slow and jerky, the gait is shuffling and unsteady. Facial expression is lost; the voice grows weak and speech indistinct. Withdrawal and depression may occur as disability advances. Loss of mental acuity occurs in 30% of cases within 7 to 10 years. Currently available drug therapy can slow the progress of the disorder significantly for many, and life expectancy has been extended to equal the norms.

Causes: Primary Parkinson's disease is due to degeneration of the nerve cells in the brain that produce dopamine, one of the major nerve impulse transmitters. In most instances, the initiating cause of the cellular degeneration is unknown. Infrequently a virus infection of the brain (encephalitis) can initiate the degenerative process. Secondary parkinsonism can be caused by hardening of brain arteries, strokes, brain tumors, trauma, carbon monoxide or manganese poisoning and a few rare degenerative disorders of brain tissue.

Drugs That Can Cause This Disorder: The following drugs can block the action of dopamine and cause a form of secondary parkinsonism with features that are indistinguishable from primary Parkinson's disease: phenothiazines, droperidol, haloperidol, reserpine, chlorprothixene, thiothixene, methyldopa, metoclopramide, lithium. (See respective Drug Profiles in Section Three or Drug Classes in Section Four.)

Drugs Used to Treat This Disorder
- levodopa (Dopar, Larodopa).
- levodopa + carbidopa (Sinemet).
- levodopa + bensarazide (Prolopa in Canada).
- amantadine (Symmetrel).
- anticholinergics (atropinelike drugs): benztropine (Cogentin), diphenhydramine (Benadryl), trihexyphenidyl (Artane).
- bromocriptine (Parlodel).
- pergolide (Permax).
- selegiline (Eldepryl).

New Drugs in Development for Treating This Disorder: Sinemet CR-4, a new slow-release formulation of Sinemet, is now being tested in clinical trials. It is designed to reduce or eliminate the wearing-off phenomenon or end-of-dose failure that some individuals experience with standard Sinemet. Dosing frequency can be reduced by 25% to 50% and fluctuations in drug response minimized or eliminated throughout the day.

Goals of Drug Treatment

Improvement of overall function and mobility.
Reduction of muscular rigidity and tremor.
Reversal of slowed movement.
Improvement of posture, balance, gait, speech and writing.

Drug Management

General Principles

The symptoms of Parkinson's disease are due to a relative increase in the effects of acetylcholine in the brain centers that regulate body movement. The exaggerated acetylcholine effects are the result of a reduced supply of dopamine (primary Parkinson's disease) or to a blocking of dopamine action (drug-induced parkinsonism).

Drugs used to manage parkinsonism utilize three distinct mechanisms of action: (1) anticholinergic drugs reduce the excessive effects of acetylcholine; (2) levodopa is converted to dopamine in the brain, increasing its supply to restore a balance closer to normal; (3) bromocriptine serves as a substitute for dopamine by stimulating its receptor cells directly. Amantadine is thought to have both anticholinergic and direct-stimulating effects.

Appropriate drugs, properly used, can improve function and mobility for significant periods of time; up to 50% of those treated have no major disabilities after 10 years of disease.

The optimal drug program—either one drug used alone or two or more used in combination—is that which provides satisfactory relief of symptoms or the most acceptable compromise between symptom relief and drug side-effects. (Complete relief of symptoms may not be possible.)

Drug selection and dosage schedules *must be carefully individualized;* adjustments will be necessary throughout the course of this disorder. Daily fluctuations in symptoms and drug responses occur in almost every individual and vary greatly from person to person. A "trial-and-error" process is unavoidable in determining the best drug(s) and the best dosage schedule. For the best treatment results, keep your physician informed regarding all aspects of your response to the drugs prescribed.

Combinations of several drugs taken in small doses are often more beneficial than a single drug taken in large doses.

Use of Levodopa

1. Only 25% of levodopa taken alone by mouth enters the brain. The large doses required to be effective often cause unacceptable side-effects. To prevent this, levodopa is combined with carbidopa; the combination (marketed as Sinemet) permits a 75% dosage reduction of levodopa.

2. Levodopa is the most effective drug available in the USA and has been the drug of choice for managing primary parkinsonism for the past 15 years. Approximately 80% of users achieve 80% improvement in muscular rigidity and retarded movement.

3. Levodopa may be tried at any time during the course of this disorder. It is most effective during the first 2 to 5 years of use. However, authorities differ in their opinions as to the best time to use levodopa. Some advise early use—within the first year of symptoms—to obtain the fullest benefit possible. Others advise later use to delay the onset of side-effects and adverse effects that develop with long-term use of levodopa.

4. Levodopa is more completely absorbed when taken on an empty stomach. However, it may be necessary to take it following food to prevent nausea. If so, avoid meat when possible; proteins can interfere with absorption of levodopa.

5. After a year or more of continual use of levodopa, 80% of users will develop abnormal involuntary movements (dyskinesias) of various muscle groups—jerks and twitches of the head and face or semi-purposeful movement of the extremities. In 30% of the users these may be severe enough to interfere with normal functioning. They last for a few minutes to several hours and seem to coincide with the times of both high and low blood levels of levodopa.

6. Another 20% of users will experience "on-off" episodes—changes from relatively good function and mobility (drug effects "on") to marked loss of function and mobility (drug effects "off"). To minimize these periods of fluctuating effectiveness, levodopa may be taken in small doses every 1 to 3 hours throughout the day to maintain a more constant blood level.

7. Levodopa can cause a variety of mental disturbances: euphoria, hypomania, depression, confusion, nightmares, vivid hallucinations.

8. Levodopa should not be used concurrently with those antipsychotic drugs that block the action of dopamine; or with monoamine oxidase (MAO) inhibitors that increase the risk of a hypertensive crisis.

9. Some authorities advocate the use of "drug holidays" to reduce the toxic manifestations of levodopa. The very gradual withdrawal and reintroduction of the drug are essential to success.

Use of Amantadine

1. This drug probably releases dopamine from nerve cells and increases its availability. It may also seve as a dopamine substitute and stimulate receptor cells directly. It has anticholinergic effects that contribute to its effectiveness.

2. Amantadine may be tried first in all patients. It can produce a 15% to 25% improvement in 60% of users. A trial period of 1 week is usually adequate; if not beneficial or if mentality is adversely affected, discontinue use.

3. Amantadine may also be used in conjunction with anticholinergics and levodopa. It is usually well tolerated by the elderly.

4. This drug has a low incidence of side-effects. Ankle swelling and a reddish-blue mottling of the arms or legs may occur after 1 month to 1 year of use. These are not serious and are reversible.
5. Doses over 200 mg can cause excitement, increased tremor, jerkiness, insomnia and nightmares in sensitive individuals.
6. Amantadine may lose some of its effectiveness after 6 to 12 weeks of continual use.
7. In very rare cases the long-term use of this drug is associated with the unexpected development of congestive heart failure. If shortness of breath appears during exertion or while lying down or rouses you from sleep, report this promptly.
8. Recent reports indicate that this drug should not be stopped abruptly in the elderly patient (over 70 years of age). Sudden withdrawal can result in the prompt return of parkinsonian features and rapid deterioration.

Use of Anticholinergic Drugs
1. These atropinelike drugs are often used to initiate treatment when symptoms are mild. They can produce a 20% to 30% improvement by suppressing effects due to overactivity of acetylcholine: tremor, excessive salivation, rigidity and slow movement.
2. They may be used alone as long as symptoms remain mild. They may be combined with any of the other drugs used and at any stage of the disorder.
3. These drugs are not well tolerated by individuals over 70 years old. They can provoke latent glaucoma and can aggravate urinary retention in men with prostatism (see Glossary).
4. Unavoidable side-effects include blurring of near vision, dry mouth, constipation and urinary hesitancy. High doses may cause drowsiness, confusion, impaired memory, hallucinations and nightmares.
5. Following long-term use, these drugs must be discontinued very gradually to avoid a dangerous withdrawal syndrome.

Use of Bromocriptine
1. This drug may be used alone but is usually added to the treatment program at a later stage. It is the drug of choice for alleviating the abnormal involuntary movements associated with long-term levodopa use. It can also have a stabilizing effect when the "on-off" effects of levodopa therapy become apparent.
2. Bromocriptine is initiated with very small doses, and the dose is increased very slowly. Some individuals develop extreme hypotension (low blood pressure) with the first doses. It is advisable to try a test dose at bedtime for several days to determine individual blood pressure response.
3. This drug may not be effective in severe Parkinson's disease or in those with a poor response to levodopa.
4. High doses can cause acute personality changes, mood swings and other intolerable adverse effects; 40% of users discontinue this drug because of undesirable reactions.

5. This drug is an ergot derivative; it should be used with caution in the presence of angina, hypertension or any form of peripheral vascular disease.

Current Controversies in Drug Management

The difference of opinion among authorities regarding the best time to begin treatment with levodopa (Sinemet) has not been resolved to date. Those advocating early use—when symptoms are causing only mild disability—argue that the individual's quality of life is significantly improved and that his or her period of productive functioning is prolonged. Those advocating late introduction of levodopa—when symptoms are causing moderate to severe disability—argue that the early use of levodopa hastens the onset of adverse levodopa effects (abnormal involuntary movements, "wearing-off" effects, "on-off" effects). They propose the use of amantadine and/or anticholinergic drugs to manage the early period of mild disability and the later use of levodopa only if and when progression of symptoms requires greater relief. Studies to date have not been sufficiently conclusive to resolve the controversy.

One recently published study, however, does show that levodopa treatment started early (1 to 3 years after the onset of symptoms) significantly reduces mortality rates, especially those related to the disease itself.

Comment: The decision as to when levodopa therapy is to be started must be made jointly by the patient and the physician on an individual, case-by-case basis. The patient should be informed of the issues involved in making the decision and should share the resposibility for making the best decision for all concerned.

Ancillary Drug Treatment (as required)

Condition	Drug Treatment
For levodopa-induced drowsiness:	methylphenidate (Ritalin)
For levodopa-induced nausea:	diphenidol (Vontrol)
For action tremor:	propranolol (Inderal)
For muscle spasm and rigidity:	diazepam (Valium)
For nocturnal leg cramps:	quinine (Quinamm) at bedtime
For constipation:	docusate (Colace)
	docusate with casanthranol (Peri-Colace)
For insomnia:	chloral hydrate (Noctec, Somnos)
For ankle swelling:	hydrochlorothiazide (generic)
For depression:	amitriptyline (Elavil)
	desipramine (Norpramin)
	imipramine (Tofranil)

                                    trazodone (Desyrel)
                                    fluoxetine (Prozac)
For action tremor (that
    accompanies resting
    tremor):   propranolol (Inderal)

Note: Drug selection, dosage and administration schedule must be determined
by the physician for each patient individually.

Resources for Additional Information and Services

American Parkinson Disease Association
116 John Street, Suite 417
New York, NY 10038
Phone: 1-800-223-2732; (212) 732-9550

Available 8:30 a.m.–5:00 p.m. EST, M–F.
Provides publications, referrals, references and answers to inquiries regarding research and treatment.

Parkinson's Disease Foundation
Columbia Presbyterian Medical Center
640 West 168th Street
New York, NY 10032
Phone: (212) 923-4700

Serves as a source of information to patients and physicians on all aspects of Parkinson's disease.

United Parkinson Foundation
220 South State Street
Chicago, IL 60604
Phone: (312) 922-9734

Serves 28,000 members (patients, family members, medical personnel);
publishes reliable information on all aspects of Parkinson's disease.

PEPTIC ULCER

Other Names: Peptic ulcer disease, duodenal ulcer, gastric ulcer

Prevalence in USA: Approximately 20 million; 10% of the general population will have a symptomatic peptic ulcer sometime during life;
25% of men and 16% of women have scars of peptic ulcer disease on
autopsy examination.

Age Group: Duodenal ulcer occurs most commonly between 25 and 40
years. Gastric ulcer occurs most commonly between 40 and 55 years.
Of all ulcers, 1.9% occur under 18 years; 43% occur between 18 and

44 years; 36% occur between 45 and 64 years; 12.8% occur between 65 and 74 years; 6.3% occur at 75 years and over.

Male to Female Ratio: Duodenal ulcer: higher incidence in men—2 to 1. Gastric ulcer: same incidence in men and women.

Principal Features: Peptic ulcer disease refers to an intermittent disorder of the stomach and first portion of the small intestine (duodenum) that is characterized by the formation of ulcers in the lining of these organs. The tissues subject to ulceration are constantly bathed in digestive juices produced in the stomach; the principal components of these juices include hydrochloric acid and the digestive enzyme pepsin (hence "peptic" ulcer). Most individuals with peptic ulcer disease produce excessive amounts of acid and pepsin, which overwhelm the normal protection of the lining tissues and cause erosion (ulceration). The singular feature of an active duodenal ulcer is a gnawing or burning pain in the upper mid-abdomen that usually occurs between meals and in the early morning hours—when acid secretion is high. The pain is characteristically relieved by food or antacids. The pattern of pain-food-relief typifies active duodenal ulcer. Episodes of ulcer activation occur unpredictably, but are often more frequent and troublesome in the spring and fall of the year. By nature, peptic ulcer disease is a chronically recurrent disorder. The recurrence rate of duodenal ulcer is approximately 70% within 1 year and 90% within 2 years. Frequent recurrence predisposes to serious complications in 30% of ulcer patients, 10% to 15% will experience bleeding, 5% to 10% will suffer perforation of the duodenal wall and 5% will develop obstruction at the stomach outlet (pylorus) due to the extensive scarring that follows ulcer healing.

Causes: A predisposition to develop peptic ulcer disease appears to be hereditary. The primary initiating cause of ulceration is not known. Those individuals who produce excessive amounts of stomach acid and pepsin are often prone to the development of duodenal ulcer. Others with normal amounts of acid and pepsin develop ulceration because the protective mechanisms in the lining tissues are defective and inadequate. Certain states of physical stress (burns, trauma, surgery) can increase the incidence of peptic ulcer.

Drugs That Can Cause This Disorder: The following drugs can initiate ulceration of the stomach or duodenum in susceptible individuals or aggravate existing ulcers:

alcohol	cortisonelike steroids
aminophylline	phenylbutazone
aspirin and other nonsteroidal	reserpine (?)
anti-inflammatory drugs	

Drugs Used to Treat This Disorder
- antacids (Delcid, Maalox TC, Mylanta II, etc.).
- cimetidine (Tagamet).

- famotidine (Pepcid).
- misoprostol (Cytotec). Used for prevention and treatment.
- nizatidine (Axid).
- ranitidine (Zantac).
- sucralfate (Carafate).
- anticholinergic drugs (Darbid, Pro-Banthine, Robinul) for adjunctive use.

New Drugs in Development for Treating This Disorder: Current studies in 13 countries are showing that a new antiulcer drug, omeprazole (Losec), relieves symptoms and promotes ulcer healing more rapidly than other treatments in general use. Approval for marketing is expected within the next year.

Goals of Drug Treatment

Short-term control of stomach acidity sufficient to relieve pain and promote ulcer healing.

Long-term control of stomach acidity to prevent ulcer recurrence.

Prevention of complications.

Drug Management

General Principles

Most cases of peptic ulcer disease can be managed successfully by appropriate drug therapy. A treatment program of 4 to 6 weeks will heal up to 90% of duodenal ulcers. Surgery is needed only for the management of ulcer complications: uncontrolled bleeding, perforation, obstruction, persistent pain.

The four principal drugs used to promote healing of duodenal ulcer are all equally effective when taken in adequate dosage for 4 to 6 weeks. However, some individuals may respond more favorably to 2 (or more) drugs used concurrently. In the treatment of gastric ulcer, antacids are less effective than cimetidine, ranitidine, or sucralfate.

Anticholinergic (atropinelike) drugs are used only when ulcer symptoms are not adequately controlled by antacids and/or cimetidine or ranitidine.

Tranquilizers and sedatives should not be used routinely but only as necessary to relieve significant anxiety and nervous tension that could possibly contribute to hyperacidity.

If possible, it is advisable to avoid cortisonelike steroid therapy in the presence of active peptic ulcer or in those individuals who are subject to recurrently active peptic ulcer disease. If steroid treatment is necessary, antacids and/or cimetidine (or ranitidine) should be used protectively.

The chronic use of aspirin (and substitute nonsteroidal anti-inflammatory drugs) increases the chance of developing active peptic ulcer.

Cigarette smoking doubles the chance of developing peptic ulcer disease; it also delays healing significantly.

Caffeine-containing beverages (coffee, tea, cola) can stimulate stomach acid production and aggravate an existing ulcer.

Alcohol (in excess) can aggravate gastric ulcer and increase the risk of bleeding.

Use of Antacids

1. These drugs are used to neutralize stomach acids and thereby (1) relieve pain, heartburn and acid indigestion; and (2) correct hyperacidity and promote ulcer healing.
2. The antacids of choice are composed of magnesium aluminum hydroxide (Delcid, Maalox TC, Mylanta II). The optimal treatment schedule is 1 ounce taken 1 hour and 3 hours after meals and at bedtime until free of pain for 2 weeks; then 1 hour after meals and at bedtime for an additional 4 weeks.
3. Avoid long-term use of aluminum hydroxide and magnesium trisilicate preparations; they may cause depletion of phosphate and increase the risk of osteomalacia (softening of bones).
4. Avoid calcium-containing antacids (Alka-2, Titralac, Tums); these stimulate secretion of gastrin, a stomach hormone that in turn stimulates production of hydrochloric acid and pepsin, referred to as rebound hyperacidity.
5. When practical, antacid liquids (suspensions) are more effective than tablets.
6. Antacids can interfere with the absorption of cimetidine (but not ranitidine), digoxin, iron, isoniazid and tetracyclines.

Use of Histamine (H-2)-Blocking Drugs

1. These drugs reduce the production of hydrochloric acid by blocking the stomach's response to stimulation by histamine. They promote healing of peptic ulcer in 70% to 80% of cases when taken for 4 to 6 weeks.
2. Treatment with one of these drugs alone is a reasonable alternative to high-dose antacid therapy.
3. Cimetidine may cause confusion and unsteadiness in the elderly, especially those with impaired kidney function; infrequently it can cause breast enlargement and impotence in men; it increases the effects of warfarin when taken concurrently.
4. Ranitidine taken in a single dose at bedtime is as effective as other multidose drug regimens for healing peptic ulcer.
5. Ranitidine is less likely to cause confusion, unsteadiness, breast changes or altered sexual functions; in addition, it does not appear to be involved in any significant drug-drug interactions.
6. In the presence of liver disease or impaired liver function, avoid the concurrent use of ranitidine and acetaminophen to reduce the risk of liver toxicity.
7. Drugs of this class taken once daily at bedtime, can reduce the recurrence rate (in 1 year) for duodenal ulcer from 70% to 10%, and for gastric ulcer from 56% to 20%.

Use of Sucralfate

1. This drug is used for short-term (8 weeks') treatment of active duodenal ulcer. It promotes ulcer healing by forming a dense coating over the ulcer that protects it from the erosive action of hydro-

chloric acid. Its effectiveness is comparable to antacids and histamine blockers (cimetidine and ranitidine) when used alone.

2. Sucralfate should not be used in conjunction with antacids or histamine blockers.
3. Food may impair the effectiveness of sucralfate. The recommended
schedule is as follows:
  (1) If other drugs are being used concurrently, take these 1 hour
  before sucralfate.
  (2) Take sucralfate on an empty stomach, 1 hour before meals and
  at bedtime.
  (3) Food may be taken 1 hour after sucralfate.
4. This drug is very safe; it has no contraindications and minimal side-
effects—constipation (2%).
5. It can interfere with the absorption of tetracyclines and phenytoin.

Current Controversies in Drug Management

Should histamine (H-2)-blocking drugs (see above) be used intermittently or continuously in treating peptic ulcer disease?

Recently completed studies (219 patients followed for 5 years) have
shown that continuous treatment with cimetidine (Tagamet) is significantly more effective than intermittent treatment in preventing
recurrence of ulcer activity. Current recommendations call for continuous treatment (daily bedtime maintenance dosing) of anyone who
has two or more relapses within two years.

Comments: Such long-term treatment must be individualized; consult
your physician regarding its advisability for you. The optimal duration of such treatment and the long-term effects of chronic histamine
(H-2)-blocking drug use have not been determined.

Ancillary Drug Treatment (as required)

Condition	Drug Treatment
For persistant nocturnal ulcer pain:	isopropamide (Combid, Darbid) taken at bedtime
For constipation:	docusate (Colace, etc.) docusate with casanthranol (Peri-Colace, etc.)
For anxiety or nervous tension:	buspirone (Buspar) diazepam (Valium)
For headache, minor aches and pains:	acetaminophen (Tylenol, etc.) propoxyphene (Darvon) Avoid aspirin.

Note: Drug selection, dosage and administration schedule must be determined
by the physician for each patient individually.

Resources for Additional Information and Services

American Digestive Disease Society
7720 Wisconsin Avenue
Bethesda, MD 20814
Phone: (301) 652-9293

Telecommunications services: Gutline, available to the public every Tuesday evening from 7:30 to 9:00 p.m., EST.
Publications available.

National Ulcer Foundation
675 Main Street
Melrose, MA 02176
Phone: (617) 665-6210

Publication: newsletter concerning peptic ulcer disease.

PSORIASIS

Other Name: Psoriasis vulgaris

Prevalence in USA: 2% to 4% of the white population; less than 1% of the black population. 6% to 7% of individuals with psoriasis have associated arthritis (psoriatic arthritis).

Age Group: The usual onset is between 10 and 40 years of age. However, psoriasis may begin at any age.

Male to Female Ratio: Slightly more common in men in all age groups.

Principal Features

Psoriasis is the most common type of chronic, recurrent scaling dermatitis. It begins gradually, often with one or two small patches, and follows a course of irregular and unpredictable remissions and recurrences throughout life. The characteristic skin change consists of a well-demarcated pink to reddish patch (plaque), one to three inches in size, which is covered almost completely by dry, silvery scales. Removal of the scales exposes numerous small, red bleeding points. Itching, if present at all, is usually mild. The size, number and distribution of the patches varies greatly. They may remain localized to a few small areas or they may spread to involve the entire body surface. The areas most commonly involved include the scalp, back of the neck and the outer surfaces of the arms and legs, especially the elbows, knees and shins. Less commonly psoriasis may involve the eyebrows, armpits, palms of the hands, soles of the feet, finger nails, umbilicus and the anal and genital areas. A rare form may involve the back, hips and thighs. Very rarely patches may occur in the mouth or on the tongue. During remission the patches fade and clear, the skin heals without scarring and there is no alteration of hair in involved areas. Permanent remission is rare. Currently there is no curative treatment, but most cases can be controlled satisfactorily.

Usually the general health is not affected. Infrequently a more serious and extensive form of psoriasis may develop. An acute, generalized, pustular form with fever, weakness and systemic debility can occur. Another unusual type causes extensive inflammation and peeling of the skin. Approximately 7% of cases will develop a form of arthritis that resembles rheumatoid arthritis; this varies in severity from relatively mild to permanently disabling.

Causes: The primary, fundamental cause is unknown. Psoriasis is a genetically determined, hereditary defect of the factors that regulate skin growth. The characteristic scaly patch is caused by a ten-fold increase in the turnover rate of the surface cells of the skin. Precipitating factors that can "trigger" the development of psoriasis plaques include excessive sunburn, acute respiratory infections (such as "strep" throat), local injury to the skin, surgical incisions and vaccination.

Drugs That Can Cause This Disorder: Drugs cannot cause or initiate psoriasis in an individual with normal skin (hereditary defect absent). However, a few drugs can exacerbate existing psoriasis. These include beta blockers, chloroquine, hydroxychloroquine, lithium, quinidine and the withdrawal of cortisonelike drugs.

Drugs Used to Treat This Disorder
Lubricants: lotions, creams, ointments; used to reduce water loss from psoriasis plaques. Examples: Lac-Hydrin, Moisturel lotion, Eucerin Creme, Aquaphor Creme, Vaseline Petroleum Jelly.

Keratolytic agents: used to remove scale. Examples: 6% salicylic acid (Keralyt Gel), 10% to 20% urea in petrolatum.

Coal tar preparations: used with and without ultraviolet light. Examples: Aquatar, Estar, Fototar, psoriGel, P&S Plus.

Anthralin preparations: used with and without ultraviolet light. Examples: Dithroceme, Lasan.

Cortisonelike preparations: topical creams, gels and ointments for local use. Examples: Aristocort, Cyclocort, Diprolene, Kenalog, Lidex, Topicort, Valisone, others.

Psoralen preparations: used with ultraviolet light. Example: methoxsalen, topical and oral forms.

Methotrexate: see Drug Profile, Section Three.

Etretinate: see Drug Profile, Section Three.

Fish oil containing eicosapentanoic acid (EPA): for relief of itching and inflammation.

New Drugs in Development for Treating This Disorder
Vitamin A derivatives similar to etretinate and isotretinoin are currently under investigation.

Cyclosporine, a drug in current use to prevent rejection in organ transplant surgery, appears to be effective for psoriasis when used in small doses; this use is currently under investigation. It can cause dramatic clearing of generalized psoriasis, but its long-term adverse effects preclude its use except in very severe and resistant cases.

Goals of Drug Treatment

Acceleration of clearing of active plaques; this can usually be achieved in close to 90% of cases.

Prevention of recurrence of plaques; while remissions of several months can be achieved, permanent remission is not possible with currently available drugs.

Drug Management

Topical Use of Drugs

1. Coal tar preparations: method of action is not fully known. Available in solutions, bath oils, shampoos, lotions and ointments.

   When used in conjunction with ultraviolet light (UVL), they can produce remissions lasting 6 to 12 months.

   Can cause burning, stinging reactions ("tar smarts") in skin on exposure to sun or large doses of UVL.

2. Anthralin preparations: interfere with DNA synthesis and skin cell reproduction.

   Available in creams, ointments and paste.

   Apply only to psoriasis plaques; can irritate normal skin and stain it brown.

   More effective when used in conjunction with UVL.

3. Cortisonelike preparations for local use: reduce inflammation, swelling and itching of psoriasis plaques.

   These are the drugs most commonly used in the current management of mild to moderate psoriasis.

   Available in lotions, creams and ointments. Lotions are preferred for treating the scalp; creams are preferred for treating the armpits and groin; ointments are preferred for remaining skin areas. The ointment is more effective when used under occlusive dressings.

   These drugs are used primarily when (1) the skin is "sore" and vulnerable to the irritant effects of other drugs; (2) other drugs are unacceptable for cosmetic reasons; (3) results with coal tar or anthralin preparations alone are unsatisfactory.

   Prolonged use without interruption can cause skin atrophy and loss of drug effectiveness.

   Possible side-effects: rosacealike skin changes, excessive hair growth (at point of application), lowered resistance to infection, systemic absorption, glaucoma (when applied around eyes).

Systemic Use of Drugs

1. Psoralens: inhibit DNA synthesis and suppress skin cell reproduction.

Available as methoxsalen and trioxsalen for both local and systemic use.

These are photosensitizing drugs and are used in conjunction with ultraviolet light in the A range; the combined treatment program is referred to as PUVA. The drug is taken orally 2 hours before UVL exposure; food impairs absorption and should be avoided. Treatments are given 2 to 4 times per week until the skin is clear. Maintenance treatment is given every 1 to 3 weeks to prevent recurrence. Protective glasses should be worn during treatment and for 8 hours following treatment to prevent cataracts.

Side-effects include itching, nausea and accelerated aging of the skin.

When properly used, this form of treatment produces improvement in 2 to 3 weeks and clearance of plaques within 1 to 3 months in 75% to 80% of cases.

2. Methotrexate: reduces the turnover rate of superficial skin cells.

This drug is reserved for use in treating severe, resistant cases of psoriasis, especially the generalized pustular forms and those with chronic extensive plaque formation that have not responded to safer treatment measures. It may also be beneficial in cases of psoriatic arthritis.

This drug can be highly effective. However, it has very serious potential toxicity. It can depress bone marrow function, damage liver tissue and impair kidney function.

Avoid alcohol, aspirin and aspirin substitutes while taking this drug.

See the Drug Profile in Section Three for a complete discussion.

3. Etretinate:

This vitamin A derivative may be used alone or in conjunction with other appropriate treatments, especially PUVA. It provides excellent relief in severe pustular psoriasis and when there is involvement of the palms and soles.

This drug should be used only to treat severe, resistant forms of psoriasis that have failed to respond to standard treatments. It can cause major birth defects, significant elevations of blood triglycerides and toxic effects on bone marrow, liver and kidney tissue.

See the Drug Profile in Section Three for a complete discussion.

Current Controversies in Drug Management

Should doses of psoralen and ultraviolet light (PUVA) and the duration of treatment be reduced to lessen the long-term risk of developing skin cancer?

Comments: PUVA treatment is an established, highly effective therapy for severe psoriasis. The best results are obtained when relatively high doses and extended treatment periods are used. Two recently published research reports demonstrate a significantly increased risk of developing two types of skin cancer five years after initial treatment with PUVA. The risk for squamous cell skin cancer was 12 times greater for those who received over 260 PUVA treatments than for those who received 160 or fewer treatments. The risk for basal cell skin cancer was moderately increased and also dose-related. It is recommended that PUVA treatment dosage be reduced by alternating it with other treatment methods, even if this means less than complete clearing of the skin.

Ancillary Drug Treatment (as required)

Condition	*Drug Treatment*
For itching:	hydroxyzine (Atarax, Vistaril)

Note: Drug selection, dosage and administration schedule must be determined by the physician for each patient individually.

Resources for Additional Information and Services

National Institute of Arthritis and Musculoskeletal and Skin Diseases
Information Office: Building 31, Room 4C32B
9000 Rockville Pike
Bethesda, MD 20892
Phone: Information Specialist, (301) 496-8188

Handles inquiries on arthritis, bone diseases, and skin diseases (including psoriasis).

Psoriasis Research Association
107 Vista del Grande
San Carlos, CA 94070
Phone: (415) 593-1394

Publications available.

RHEUMATOID ARTHRITIS

Other Names: Atrophic arthritis, chronic inflammatory arthritis, proliferative arthritis

Prevalence in USA: Approximately 7 million—2% to 3% of the general population.

Age Group: Affects all ages—infancy to senescence. Usual onset is between 20 and 50 years. Mean age at onset is 30 to 40 years.

Male to Female Ratio: In 20-to-50-year age group—more common in women, 3 to 1. Over 50 years—same incidence in men and women.

Principal Features: Rheumatoid arthritis is a highly complex inflammatory disorder that can affect several systems of the body simultaneously. It is quite variable in its manifestations: it may last a few days or up to 50 years; it may affect a single joint or up to 60 joints; it may involve the skin, the eyes, the nervous system, the lungs, the heart and blood vessels and the spleen; it can be mild, moderately severe or life-threatening in its most virulent forms. It usually begins with fatigue, poor appetite, loss of weight, morning stiffness and joint pains. Initially the small joints of the hands, wrists and feet are affected; larger joints may be affected later. The painful and destructive disease of the joints is the major feature of this disorder. The disease process begins with a severe inflammation of the joint lining (synovial membrane). This is followed by the formation of thick granulation tissue that ultimately destroys joint cartilage, bone and adjacent ligaments. The affected joints are swollen, warm, tender, stiff and painful to use; after a sustained period of active disease, joint destruction results in irreversible deformity. All of the joints that are affected will show evidence of disease within the first 2 years. Ten percent of cases will have a spontaneous complete remission (recovery) within 6 to 24 months after the onset of symptoms.

Causes: A specific definitive cause for rheumatoid arthritis has not been established. However, there is evidence to support the theory that the disease process is initiated by a virus that infects the joints of individuals who are genetically susceptible because of a defective immune system.

Drugs That Can Cause This Disorder: There are no drugs that induce true rheumatoid arthritis. The following drugs may aggravate an active or latent arthritis: iron dextran, isoniazid and pyrazinamide (in combination), oral contraceptives (?).

Drugs Used to Treat This Disorder: There are no drugs that can cure rheumatoid arthritis. The drugs currently available for use in managing this form of arthritis fall into 2 groups: (1) those that relieve symptoms but do not alter the basic disease process—do not produce remission; (2) those that may retard or arrest the disease and initiate remission.

Drugs Used to Relieve Symptoms
  Salicylates
* aspirin (Bufferin, Ascriptin, Cama, etc.).
* aspirin, enteric-coated (Easprin, Ecotrin, etc.).
* aspirin, zero-order-release (Zorprin).
* magnesium salicylate (Magan, Mobidin).
* choline magnesium salicylate (Trisilate).
* salsalate (Disalcid).
* diflunisal (Dolobid).
* sodium salicylate (Pabalate).

Other Nonsteroidal Anti-inflammatory Drugs (NSAIDs)
Indole derivatives:
- indomethacin (Indocin).
- sulindac (Clinoril).
- tolmetin (Tolectin).

Propionic acid derivatives:
- fenoprofen (Nalfon).
- flurbiprofen (Ansaid).
- ibuprofen (Motrin, Rufen, etc.).
- ketoprofen (Orudis).
- naproxen (Naprosyn).
- suprofen (Suprol).

Fenamic acid derivative: meclofenamate (Meclomen).
Oxicam derivative: piroxicam (Feldene).
Phenylacetic acid derivative: diclofenac (Voltaren).

Cortisonelike Steroid Drugs
- prednisone.
- triamcinolone (Aristocort).
- dexamethasone (Decadron).
- methylprednisolone (Medrol).

Immunosuppressive Drugs
- azathioprine (Imuran).
- chlorambucil (Leukeran).
- cyclophosphamide (Cytoxan).
- methotrexate (Mexate).

Drugs Used to Produce Remission
Gold Preparations
- auranofin (Ridaura).
- aurothioglucose (Solganal).
- gold sodium thiomalate (Myochrysine).

hydroxychloroquine (Plaquenil)
penicillamine (Cuprimine, Depen)

Goals of Drug Treatment

Relief of pain, tenderness and stiffness.
Control of inflammation in joint tissues.
Production of remission; arrest of active disease.
Prevention of joint destruction; preservation of joint function.

Drug Management

General Principles

Rheumatoid arthritis can be the most difficult of all arthritic disorders
to control; in its more severe forms, it is the most damaging to joint
tissues. Its course is usually intermittent to chronic. No cure is
known. If adequate treatment is started early, severe crippling can
often be prevented or minimized.

Every case of rheumatoid arthritis is a unique, individual problem; successful management depends upon a treatment program that is carefully individualized.

Many drugs are available to treat rheumatoid arthritis. None is curative, and none is effective in all cases. Drugs that control inflammation can provide symptomatic relief but do not modify the underlying disease process; they cannot induce a remission. Disease-altering drugs are used in an attempt to modify the actual disease process and thereby initiate a remission. If successful, maintenance drug treatment may be continued for months or years.

Treatment is usually started with the safest and best tolerated drugs. There is marked individual variation in response to most drugs; this is very apparent with the use of the nonsteroidal anti-inflammatory drugs (aspirin substitutes). Trial-and-error experimentation is necessary to find the most effective and acceptable anti-inflammatory drug for each person.

Drug treatment of rheumatoid arthritis often requires a combination of drugs. The more severe forms of this arthritis respond more favorably when a disease-modifying drug is added to an established program of salicylates or NSAIDs. (See drugs listed above.)

Use of Salicylates

1. Aspirin is often the first drug used to provide adequate anti-inflammatory effects; it must be taken in large doses. A trial of salicylates is indicated in all cases of rheumatoid arthritis. (Avoid if there is a history of aspirin allergy, peptic ulcer disease, gastritis or gastrointestinal bleeding.)
2. Aspirin preparations that are designed for absorption in the small intestine (instead of in the stomach) are preferred: Disalcid, Easprin, Ecotrin, Zorprin.
3. The measurement of salicylate blood levels is advisable to determine the optimal dose of the salicylate used and to avoid serious toxicity.
4. Warning symptoms of early salicylate toxicity are ringing in the ears (tinnitus) and loss of hearing. However, these may not occur in the very young or in the elderly.
5. Approximately 50% of patients cannot tolerate the large doses of aspirin required to achieve adequate anti-inflammatory effects. Other salicylates may be tried or a nonsteroidal anti-inflammatory drug may be substituted.

Use of Other Nonsteroidal Anti-inflammatory Drugs (NSAIDs)

1. These may be used as substitutes for aspirin by those who cannot tolerate (or should not take) salicylates; or they may be used to initiate treatment at the outset.
2. As a group, the NSAIDs are not superior to salicylates in anti-inflammatory effect, but they are generally better tolerated.
3. These drugs produce significant decrease in morning stiffness, improve comfort and function and may be more effective than aspirin for some.
4. Fenoprofen and naproxen are among the more active NSAIDs; a trial of 2 weeks will identify those who can respond favorably.

5. Response to NSAIDs is highly variable from person to person. If an NSAID from one chemical class proves to be ineffective or unacceptable, a drug from another class within the NSAID group should be tried. A trial of 2 weeks is usually adequate to determine effectiveness and tolerance. (See drugs listed above.)

Use of Cortisonelike Steroid Drugs

1. Steroids are used infrequently and for short periods of time in both acute and chronic stages of rheumatoid arthritis. They are always added to existing drug programs as needed. Their use is justified, in small doses, to control acute "flares" of inflammation that prevent any degree of mobility in severely diseased joints.

2. Steroids provide a powerful anti-inflammatory effect, but they do not alter the underlying disease process or induce remission. They should be used to provide short-term comfort as necessary but not to abolish all symptoms.

3. Long-term maintenance use of steroids—even in small doses—must be avoided. Risks of excessive use include cataracts, osteoporosis, muscle wasting, atherosclerosis.

Use of Immunosuppressive Drugs

1. These highly toxic and hazardous drugs are used only when arthritis activity persists in spite of combined treatment with NSAIDs and disease-modifying agents. They are used in an attempt to prevent further joint destruction, deformity and disability.

2. Cyclophosphamide is the most effective drug of this group. Its use is reserved for patients with disabling systemic complications of rheumatoid arthritis.

3. Methotrexate is often the first choice of this group to try in the treatment of severe rheumatoid arthritis that has not responded to conventional therapy. In low dosage it can be very effective in approximately 50% of patients. Potential risks include severe depression of the bone marrow, liver damage, ulceration of the mouth and intestine and birth defects. Avoid alcohol and salicylates during methotrexate therapy.

Use of Gold Preparations

1. Based upon long experience with its use, gold is the standard disease-modifying drug for treating rheumatoid arthritis. It is often the first choice to add to an established program of NSAID therapy.

2. Gold is used only when arthritis cannot be controlled with safer drugs. A trial of 6 months or longer is necessary to determine its ability to induce remission. Approximately 50% of patients respond favorably.

3. Risks of gold therapy include dermatitis, kidney damage and blood cell and bone marrow toxicity. Treatment should be stopped immediately if any of the following develop: skin rash, mouth ulcers, fever, sore throat, abnormal bleeding or bruising.

Use of Hydroxychloroquine
1. This drug is used to treat mild or moderately severe rheumatoid arthritis. It can be very effective in some cases, relieving symptoms and retarding disease activity.
2. A trial of 6 months is necessary to determine this drug's ability to induce remission.
3. After 1 year of continual use, this drug can (rarely) damage eye structures and impair vision. Corneal deposits, retinal pigmentation and optic neuritis have been reported. The estimated incidence is 1 in 1000 to 1 in 2000 patients.
4. Other possible adverse drug effects include skin rash, abnormally low white blood cell count and peripheral neuritis (see Glossary).
5. This drug can aggravate existing psoriasis.

Use of Penicillamine
1. This drug is an effective substitute for gold therapy when a disease-modifying drug is needed.
2. A trial of 6 to 12 months is necessary to determine its ability to induce remission.
3. For maximal effectiveness, this drug should be taken on an empty stomach.
4. This is a potent drug; it can cause the following adverse effects: dermatitis, kidney damage, blood cell and bone marrow toxicity, bronchiolitis (dry cough and shortness of breath) and a pattern of muscular weakness similar to myasthenia gravis.

Ancillary Drug Treatment (as required)

Condition	*Drug Treatment*
For additional analgesia:	propoxyphene (Darvon)
	hydrocodone (Vicodin) (for short-term, intermittent use only)
For night pain:	indomethacin (Indocin) (taken with food at bedtime)
For anemia:	iron preparations
	folic acid (if appropriate for type of anemia)
For anxiety and tension:	diazepam (Valium)
For depression:	tricyclic antidepressants (see Profile of Depression in this section)
For drug-induced peptic ulcer:	cimetidine (Tagamet)
	famotidine (Pepcid)
	nizatidine (Axid)
	ranitidine (Zantac) (see Profile of Peptic Ulcer in this section)

Note: Drug selection, dosage and administration schedule must be determined by the physician for each patient individually.

Resources for Additional Information and Services

American Juvenile Arthritis Organization
1314 Spring Street
Atlanta, GA 30309
Phone: (404) 872-7100

Publications available.

Arthritis Foundation (parent organization)
1314 Spring Street
Atlanta, GA 30309
Phone: (404) 872-7100

Publications available.

Association for People With Arthritis
P.O. Box 954
6 Commercial Street
Hicksville, NY 11802
Phone: 1-800-323-2243

Publications available.

SCHIZOPHRENIA

Other Name: Dementia praecox

Prevalence in USA: Approximately 2.4 million—1% of the general population; 100,000 new cases annually.

Age Group: Onset most common between 16 and 25 years of age. Onset uncommon after 30 and rare after 40 years of age.

Male to Female Ratio: Equal incidence in men and women.

Principal Features: Schizophrenia refers to a group of disorders of the brain manifested by severe disturbances of the mind and personality. Cardinal features are abnormal thinking, behavior and mood; the schizophrenic pattern is characterized by misinterpretation of reality, withdrawal, delusions, hallucinations (usually auditory), bizarre or regressive behavior. It usually begins early in life, may be mild and transient in nature or may develop into a psychosis of major dimension that is intermittent or chronic for life. The first group—referred to as schizophreniform—experiences one episode of varying severity (often in response to stress), responds well to treatment and has no relapse after treatment is stopped. The second group—classical chronic schizophrenia—experiences recurrent episodes of disabling symptoms that require long-term antipsychotic drug therapy for control. Most of this group will relapse if maintenance treatment is stopped. A variety of subtypes are identified according to their dominant features: delusions of persecution and grandeur (paranoid type); primitive mentality, markedly disorganized thought and behavior (hebephrenic type); withdrawn, negativistic, uncommunicative, apathetic behavior pattern (catatonic); disorganized thinking, delusions, hallucinations accompanied by either mania or depression (schizoaffective); insidious loss of motivation and ambition, avoidance of interpersonal relationships (simple type); mixed or indefinite symptom complex (undifferentiated type). Though the presentations may vary according to type, the same group of antipsychotic drugs is used to treat all types without distinction.

Causes: The fundamental cause of schizophrenia is unknown. No anatomical or biochemical abnormality of the brain has been identified. Studies suggest that a genetic predisposition is necessary for the development of schizophrenia, rendering the subject vulnerable to disturbances of neurochemical transmission of nerve impulses or to alterations of brain circuitry. Effective antipsychotic drugs block dopamine receptors in certain brain cells; this suggests that increased dopamine activity is somehow responsible for the schizophrenic syndrome.

Drugs That Can Cause This Disorder: The following drugs may aggravate existing schizophrenia or produce schizophrenialike symptoms in normal individuals:

albuterol

alcohol (intoxication)

amantadine

amphetamines (abuse)

anticonvulsants

apomorphine

atropinelike drugs

bromides

bromocriptine

cimetidine

cocaine

cortisonelike steroids

digitalis

disopyramide

disulfiram (toxicity)

indomethacin

isoniazid

levodopa

methyldopa

propranolol

tocainide

triazolam

Drugs Used to Treat This Disorder
Phenothiazines
Aliphatic type:
  • chlorpromazine (Thorazine)
Piperidine type:
  • thioridazine (Mellaril)
  • mesoridazine (Serentil)
Piperazine type:
  • perphenazine (Trilafon)
  • trifluoperazine (Stelazine)
  • fluphenazine (Prolixin, Permitil)

Thioxanthenes
- thiothixene (Navane).

Butyrophenones
- haloperidol (Haldol).

Dibenzoxazepines
- loxapine (Loxitane).

Dihydroindolones
- molindone (Moban).

Goals of Drug Treatment

Good control of symptoms with the lowest possible dose of antipsychotic drug.

Determination of the most effective drug and dosage schedule for each individual: intermittent dosage (as needed) versus continual long-term dosage.

Prevention of relapse (recurrent psychotic episode).

Improvement of capacity to function in society as normally as possible.

Drug Management

General Principles

The primary management of schizophrenia is based upon the rational use of antipsychotic drugs. Psychotherapy and drug therapy are considered to be complementary; psychotherapy can improve the patient's social adjustment; drug therapy can control disabling symptoms and make the situation somewhat manageable. Drug therapy is not curative.

If appropriate drug treatment is started early, 30% to 50% of patients will have a satisfactory remission; another 30% will improve sufficiently to live outside of a hospital. Drug therapy can abolish delusions, hallucinations, hyperactivity and combative behavior. Approximately 10% to 20% of patients do not respond to any drugs currently available.

The initial treatment of an acute psychotic episode consists of a course of carefully selected antipsychotic drugs taken for 6 to 12 months. Many individuals will respond favorably to one drug and not at all to another. History of previous drug use and response can be very helpful in selecting a drug for the management of recurrent episodes.

Current practice is to attempt withdrawal of antipsychotic drugs from all patients who have had a good response to drug treatment during their first episode of schizophrenia. This allows identification of those who will have a self-limited type of schizophrenia (schizophreniform disorder) and will do well without maintenance drug therapy. From 15% to 30% of patients will recover spontaneously following the initial episode and drug withdrawal. Antipsychotic drugs should be discontinued gradually over a period of 1 to 2 weeks.

The majority of schizophrenic patients will require continual drug therapy for long periods of time—possibly for life. Many will relapse rapidly and severely after drugs are discontinued. The nature of the drug maintenance program is determined by the type and frequency of continuing psychotic symptoms and the pattern of relapses experienced by each individual. When the patient complies well, maintenance drug therapy is successful in 85% of cases.

The principal action of antipsychotic drugs is to block dopamine receptors in the brain. By blocking dopamine action in the mesolimbic system, the drugs control the abnormal manifestations of schizophrenia; by blocking dopamine action in the nigrostriatal system, the drugs cause parkinsonism (and related adverse effects). Thus parkinsonism is now recognized as an *unavoidable* side-effect of most antipsychotic drugs. It is usually very responsive to the anticholinergic drugs used to treat Parkinson's disease, but not to levodopa. (See Profile of Parkinson's Disease in this section.)

It is generally recommended that antiparkinsonism drugs *not* be used routinely while taking antipsychotic drugs. Reasons given are:

(1) antiparkinsonism drugs can produce toxic brain syndromes

(2) they can interfere with the effectiveness of antipsychotic drugs

(3) they may increase the risk of developing tardive dyskinesia

Tardive dyskinesia (see Glossary) is one of the most serious adverse effects of long-term antipsychotic drug use. The reported incidence ranges from 3% after 1 year of medication to 21% after 7 years of medication. It appears to occur more frequently in elderly women.

"Drug holidays" of 4 to 6 weeks without medication are being used by some physicians treating chronic schizophrenia to reduce the risk of developing tardive dyskinesia. Among those who have been on maintenance therapy for 1 year without relapsing, 66% will not relapse within 6 months after stopping medication. For this group of patients, a "drug holiday" is feasible and possibly beneficial.

Antipsychotic drugs usually improve behavior. However, excessively high doses can cause a toxic state that worsens behavior. Drug response and tolerance vary greatly from person to person and must be monitored carefully in each individual.

Patients with schizo-affective disorders will probably require an antipsychotic drug and an additional drug for the affective component; this could be either lithium or an antidepressant.

Lithium may aggravate the neurological complications of antipsychotic drug therapy. The concurrent use of these two drugs requires caution and careful monitoring.

Use of Phenothiazines

1. Because of its numerous side-effects, chlorpromazine (the first phenothiazine) is used less frequently.

2. Because of its relatively greater sedative effects, thioridazine is favored for treatment of acute psychotic episodes. It causes parkinsonism (and possibly tardive dyskinesia) less frequently.

3. Fluphenazine is less sedating but is thought to have a higher risk for causing parkinsonism and tardive dyskinesia.

4. Trifluoperazine is thought to be preferable for the elderly schizophrenic because it has less sedative and atropinelike side-effects.

Use of Thiothixene
1. This antipsychotic drug is thought to be more effective for the retarded and regressed schizophrenic.
2. Because of its mild antidepressant effect, this drug is preferred for the schizo-affective patient who has features of depression.
3. This drug has less sedative and atropinelike side-effects, but a higher risk for causing parkinsonism.

Use of Haloperidol
1. This drug is reported to be effective in patients who are not responsive to chlorpromazine.
2. It can control aggressive behavior without causing significant sedation.
3. Although it has a relatively high potential for causing parkinsonism (and related effects), it is useful in the elderly because it is less sedating and has fewer atropinelike side-effects.

Use of Loxapine
1. This drug is especially useful in treating the paranoid schizophrenic.
2. It is less sedating than chlorpromazine and equal to haloperidol in effectiveness.

Use of Molindone
1. This is the only antipsychotic drug that appears to contribute to weight loss; many antipsychotic drugs tend to promote weight gain.
2. This drug is as effective as other major antipsychotics and is less sedating than many.

Current Controversies in Drug Management

Is "low-dose" antipsychotic drug therapy feasible for maintenance following release from the hospital?

The vast majority of schizophrenic individuals will experience a return of symptoms shortly after discontinuing a stabilizing maintenance dose of effective medication. Conventional practice has not favored reduction of dosage that proved effective for long-term maintenance. Recent studies have shown that many responsive and stabilized schizophrenic patients can be maintained satisfactorily at home (following hospital discharge) with one-fifth of the usually prescribed dose of injectable, long-acting fluphenazine: 5 mg every 2 weeks instead of the standard 25 mg dose. Patients on low-dose maintenane therapy adjusted better to family and work situations, were less apathetic and experienced fewer adverse drug effects. The lower dosage may also reduce the potential for the development of tardive dyskinesia (see Glossary).

Ancillary Drug Treatment (as required)

Condition	*Drug Treatment*
For anxiety:	buspirone (Buspar)
For depression:	see Profile of Depression in this section

For insomnia: chloral hydrate (Noctec, etc.)
                           temazepam (Restoril)
                           triazolam (Halcion)
For constipation: docusate (Colace, etc.)
                           docusate with casanthranol (Peri-Colace)
For parkinsonism: benztropine (Cogentin)
                           trihexyphenidyl (Artane)
For akathisia (marked
  restlessness):   propranolol (Inderal)
                           diphenhydramine (Benadryl)

Note: Drug selection, dosage and administration schedule must be determined
  by the physician for each patient individually.

Resources for Additional Information and Services

American Schizophrenia Association
900 North Federal Highway
Boca Raton, FL 33432
Phone: 1-800-847-3802

National Mental Health Association
1021 Prince Street
Alexandria, VA 22314
Phone: (703) 684-7722

Publications: *FOCUS*; also provides pamphlets and films.

National Mental Health Consumers' Association
311 South Juniper Street, Room 902
Philadelphia, PA 19107
Phone: (215) 735-2465

Publications available.

Schizophrenics Anonymous
1209 California Road
Eastchester, NY 10709
Phone: (914) 337-2252

Twenty-five local groups. A self-help organization sponsored by the
American Schizophrenia Association. Conduct meetings for discussion of all aspects of managing and coping with schizophrenia.

ULCERATIVE COLITIS

Other Names: Idiopathic proctocolitis, inflammatory bowel disease

Prevalence in USA: 1 million (includes 100,000 children); 15,000 new cases
  annually.

Age Group: Peak incidence occurs between 19 and 49 years of age; 75% of cases develop before the age of 40.

Male to Female Ratio: Same incidence in men and women.

Principal Features: Ulcerative colitis is a chronically recurrent disorder of the colon (large intestine) and rectum characterized by inflammation and ulceration. Its course follows a pattern of frequent spontaneous remissions and recurrences without apparent cause. It may be associated with disease in other organs of the body, notably the skin, joints, eye, liver and blood vessels, making it a multiple system disorder. The principle symptoms of the diseased colon are abdominal cramping and bloody diarrhea; associated symptoms include fatigue, weakness, occasional low-grade fever, weight loss, anemia and dehydration. The more severe forms of ulcerative colitis can be very difficult to control.

Causes: The basic cause of ulcerative colitis is not known. Theories of possible causes include infection, environmental toxins, psychological stress, sensitivities to foods and "autoimmunity"—a disorder of the immune system that results in the selective destruction of body tissues. There is some evidence that indicates a familial pattern, suggesting a hereditary susceptibility to a causative agent.

Drugs That Can Cause This Disorder: No drugs initiate true ulcerative colitis. However, the following anti-infective drugs can cause pseudomembranous colitis, a disorder that closely resembles an acute attack of ulcerative colitis:

amoxicillin	penicillin
ampicillin	tetracycline
cephalosporins	trimethoprim and
chloramphenicol	sulfamethoxsazole in
clindamycin	combination
lincomycin	

Drugs Used to Treat This Disorder
Anti-inflammatory Drugs
- 5-aminosalicylic acid (5-ASA)
- mesalamine (Rowasa) rectal suspension
- sulfasalazine (Azulfidine)

Cortisonelike Steroids
- prednisone, prednisolone (generic).
- hydrocortisone enemas (Cortenema).
- methylprednisolone enema (Medrol Enpak).

Antidiarrheals
- diphenoxylate (Lomotil).
- loperamide (Imodium).

Antispasmodics
- dicyclomine (Bentyl).
- propantheline (Pro-Banthine).

Immunosuppressive Drugs
- azathioprine (Imuran).
- 6-mercatopurine (Purinethol).

Goals of Drug Treatment
Control of pain and diarrhea.

Prompt control of acute attacks; surppression of inflammation and ulceration.

Induction of a remission.

Prevention of recurrence of acute attacks.

Drug Management
General Principles

The majority (up to 90%) of cases of active ulcerative colitis respond well to medical treatment or have a spontaneous remission. Approximately 20% have a prolonged remission after the first acute attack.

Studies indicate that 55% of individuals who experience ulcerative colitis remain in remission at any given time during the course of the disorder. To minimize the risks of long-term drug use, the smallest dose of maintenance drugs (azulfidine and steroids) that prevents recurrence should be determined.

It is essential that every recurrence of acute colitis (relapse) be treated promptly and vigorously. Chronically active ulcerative colitis predisposes to a higher than normal incidence of cancer of the colon and rectum. Estimates are 3% after the first 10 years of disease, increasing to 20% per decade thereafter. Everyone subject to ulcerative colitis should have a thorough examination of the colon and rectum annually regardless of the status of the disorder.

Antidiarrheal drugs should be used with extreme caution. Excessive use can induce a paralysis of colon activity and increase the risk of developing toxic megacolon—a massive distention of the colon with air; perforation constitutes a surgical emergency.

Iron preparations for anemia should not be taken during a period of acute inflammation or active ulceration. Withhold iron therapy until a remission is established.

Use of Sulfasalazine
1. This effective and reliable drug is used to treat acute attacks of active colitis and to prevent relapse during periods of remission.
2. It is used concurrently with cortisonelike steroids during acute attacks to control inflammation and ulceration and to induce remission.
3. During the quiescent phase of colitis, it is used in small doses (up to 2 grams/day) for the long-term maintenance of remission. It may be taken indefinitely.
4. This drug is best taken with or following food to reduce stomach irritation.
5. The long-term use of this drug can impair folic acid absorption and may cause a folic acid deficiency. Consult your physician regarding the need for a supplement.

6. During long-term use, it is advisable to monitor blood cell counts to detect the development of anemia or abnormally low white blood cells.

7. Mesalamine, the active derivative of sulfasalazine, is used in the form of a rectal suspension (retention enema), taken at bedtime for night-long action. The initial course of treatment is from 3 to 6 weeks. Carefully read and follow the printed instructions that are provided with this drug.

Use of Cortisonelike Steroids

1. These drugs are the mainstay of treatment for acute, active ulcerative colitis. They can induce remission in 70% to 80% of cases.

2. Steroids should be used when there are obvious symptoms of disease activity: diarrhea, bloody stools, nocturnal bowel movements, anemia, weight loss, etc. They are also of value in treating the systemic manifestations of this disorder: dermatitis, arthritis, iritis, etc.

3. To ensure prompt and adequate control of acute inflammation, initial dosage should be high. Response usually occurs within 10 to 14 days.

4. After a remission has been induced, steroid dosage is reduced to a minimum that will stabilize the colon and prevent relapse. The long-term maintenance use of steroids is controversial. If individual circumstances warrant the continual use of low-dose steroids, it is preferable to use alternate-day dosage—a single morning dose every 48 hours. This is effective in preventing recurrence for some patients and it carries a lower risk of causing adverse effects.

5. When the inflammation and ulceration are limited to the rectum, steroids can be administered in the form of enemas, foams and suppositories for local application. This minimizes systemic effects.

6. The long-term use of steroids (even in small doses) can cause significant adverse effects:
   • susceptibility to infection.
   • mineral and water imbalance.
   • reduced tolerance for sugar, potential for diabetes.
   • cataracts.
   • hypertension.
   • acne, excessive hair growth.
   • muscle wasting.
   • mental disturbances.
   • osteoporosis.
   • peptic ulcer activation.
   • retarded growth in children.

Ancillary Drug Treatment (as required)

Condition	*Drug Treatment*
For abdominal cramps:	dicyclomine (Bentyl)
	propantheline (Pro-Banthine)
	Use these sparingly.
For diarrhea:	diphenoxylate (Lomotil)
	loperamide (Imodium)
	Use these sparingly.
For anxiety:	buspirone (Buspar), nonsedating
	diazepam (Valium), sedating
For depression:	see Profile of Depression in this section
For anemia:	iron preparations (not during acute stage of colitis)
	folic acid (if appropriate for type of anemia)

Note: Drug selection, dosage and administration schedule must be determined by the physician for each patient individually.

Resource for Additional Information and Services

American Digestive Disease Society
7720 Wisconsin Avenue
Bethesda, MD 20814
Phone: (301) 652-9293

Telecommunications services: Gutline, available to the public every Tuesday evening from 7:30 to 9:00 p.m.
Publications available.

DRUG PROFILES

NOTE

The designation [CD] following the brand name of any drug in these Profiles indicates a combination drug (a drug product with more than one active ingredient).

ACEBUTOLOL
(a se BYU toh lohl)

Introduced: 1973

Class: Antihypertensive, heart rhythm regulator, beta-adrenergic blocker

Prescription: USA: Yes

Controlled Drug: USA: No

Available as Generic: No

Brand Name: Sectral

BENEFITS versus RISKS

Possible Benefits	*Possible Risks*
EFFECTIVE ANTIHYPERTENSIVE in mild to moderate high blood pressure	CONGESTIVE HEART FAILURE in advanced heart disease Worsening of angina in coronary heart disease (abrupt withdrawal) Masking of low blood sugar (hypoglycemia) in drug-treated diabetes

---

▷ **Principal Uses**

As a Single Drug Product: The treatment of mild to moderately severe high blood pressure. May be used alone or concurrently with other antihypertensive drugs, such as diuretics. Also used to prevent premature ventricular heartbeats.

How This Drug Works: By blocking certain actions of the sympathetic nervous system, this drug
- reduces the rate and contraction force of the heart, thus lowering the ejection pressure of the blood leaving the heart.
- reduces the degree of contraction of blood vessel walls, resulting in their relaxation and expansion and consequent lowering of the blood pressure.
- prolongs the conduction time of nerve impulses through the heart, of benefit in the management of certain heart rhythm disorders.

Available Dosage Forms and Strengths
Capsules — 200 mg, 400 mg

▷ **Usual Adult Dosage Range:** Initially 400 mg daily, either as a single dose in the morning or as 200 mg taken morning and evening (12 hours apart). The usual maintenance dose is 400 to 800 mg/24 hours. The total dose should not exceed 1200 mg/24 hours, given as 600 mg twice daily. **Note: Actual dosage and administration schedule must be determined by the physician for each patient individually.**

▷ **Dosing Instructions:**   May be taken without regard to eating. Capsule may be opened for administration. Do not discontinue this drug abruptly.

Usual Duration of Use: Continual use on a regular schedule for 10 to 14 days is usually necessary to determine this drug's effectiveness in lowering the blood pressure or abolishing premature heartbeats. The long-term use of this drug will be determined by the course of your blood pressure over time and your response to the overall treatment program (weight reduction, salt restriction, smoking cessation, etc.). Consult your physician on a regular basis.

Possible Advantages of This Drug
Causes less slowing of the heart rate than most other beta blocker drugs. Less likely to cause asthma (in susceptible individuals) when used in low doses.

Currently a "Drug of Choice" for initiating treatment of hypertension with a single drug, especially for those subject to bronchial asthma or diabetes.

▷ **This Drug Should Not Be Taken If**
- you have had an allergic reaction to it previously.
- you have congestive heart failure.
- you have an abnormally slow heart rate or a serious form of heart block.
- you are taking, or have taken within the past 14 days, any monoamine oxidase (MAO) type A inhibitor drug (see Drug Class, Section Four).

▷ **Inform Your Physician Before Taking This Drug If**
- you have had an adverse reaction to any beta blocker drug in the past (see Drug Class, Section Four).
- you have a history of serious heart disease, with or without episodes of heart failure.
- you have a history of hay fever (allergic rhinitis), asthma, chronic bronchitis or emphysema.
- you have a history of overactive thyroid function (hyperthyroidism).
- you have a history of low blood sugar (hypoglycemia).
- you have impaired liver or kidney function.
- you have diabetes or myasthenia gravis.
- you are currently taking any form of digitalis, quinidine or reserpine, or any calcium blocker drug (see Drug Class, Section Four).
- you plan to have surgery under general anesthesia in the near future.

Possible Side-Effects (natural, expected and unavoidable drug actions)
Lethargy and fatigability (11%), cold extremities (0.2%), slow heart rate, light-headedness in upright position (see Orthostatic Hypotension in Glossary).

▷ **Possible Adverse Effects** (unusual, unexpected and infrequent reactions)
If any of the following develop, consult your physician promptly for guidance.

Mild Adverse Effects
   Allergic Reactions: Skin rash, itching.
   Headache, dizziness, insomnia, abnormal dreams.
   Indigestion, nausea, constipation, diarrhea.
   Joint and muscle discomfort, fluid retention (edema).
Serious Adverse Effects
   Mental depression (2%), anxiety.
   Chest pain, shortness of breath, precipitation of congestive heart failure.
   Induction of bronchial asthma (in asthmatic individuals).

▷ **Possible Effects on Sexual Function:** Impotence (2%), decreased libido, Peyronie's disease (see Glossary).

CAUTION
   1. **Do not discontinue this drug suddenly** without the knowledge and guidance of your physician. Carry a notation on your person that you are taking this drug.
   2. Consult your physician or pharmacist before using nasal decongestants usually present in over-the-counter cold preparations and nose drops. These can cause sudden increases in blood pressure when taken concurrently with beta blocker drugs.
   3. Report the development of any tendency to emotional depression.

Precautions for Use
   By Infants and Children: Safety and effectiveness for use by those under 12 years of age have not been established. However, if this drug is used, observe for the development of low blood sugar (hypoglycemia) during periods of reduced food intake.
   By Those over 60 Years of Age: Proceed **cautiously** with all antihypertensive drugs. Unacceptably high blood pressure should be reduced without creating the risks associated with excessively low blood pressure. Start treatment with small doses, and monitor the blood pressure response frequently. Sudden, rapid and excessive reduction of blood pressure can predispose to stroke or heart attack. Total daily dosage should not exceed 800 mg. Observe for dizziness, unsteadiness, tendency to fall, confusion, hallucinations, depression or urinary frequency.

▷ **Advisability of Use During Pregnancy**
   Pregnancy Category: B (tentative). See Pregnancy Code inside back cover.
   Animal studies: No significant increase in birth defects found in rats or rabbits.
   Human studies: Information from adequate studies of pregnant women is not available.
   Use this drug only if clearly needed. Ask physician for guidance.

Advisability of Use if Breast-Feeding
   Presence of this drug in breast milk: Yes.
   Avoid drug or refrain from nursing.

Habit-Forming Potential: None.

Effects of Overdosage: Weakness, slow pulse, low blood pressure, fainting, cold and sweaty skin, congestive heart failure, possible coma and convulsions.

Possible Effects of Long-Term Use: Reduced heart reserve and eventual heart failure in susceptible individuals with advanced heart disease.

Suggested Periodic Examinations While Taking This Drug (at physician's discretion)
Measurements of blood pressure, evaluation of heart function.

▷ **While Taking This Drug, Observe the Following**
  Foods: No restrictions. Avoid excessive salt intake.
  Beverages: No restrictions. May be taken with milk.
▷ *Alcohol:* Use with caution until the combined effect has been determined. Alcohol may exaggerate this drug's ability to lower the blood pressure and may increase its mild sedative effect.
  Tobacco Smoking: Nicotine may reduce this drug's effectiveness in treating high blood pressure. In addition, high doses of this drug may potentiate the constriction of the bronchial tubes caused by regular smoking.
▷ *Other Drugs*
  Acebutolol may ***increase*** the effects of
  • other antihypertensive drugs and cause excessive lowering of the blood pressure. Dosage adjustments may be necessary.
  • reserpine (Ser-Ap-Es, etc.) and cause sedation, depression, slowing of the heart rate and lowering of the blood pressure.
  Acebutolol ***taken concurrently*** with
  • clonidine (Catapres) requires close monitoring for rebound high blood pressure if clonidine is withdrawn while acebutolol is still being taken.
  • insulin requires close monitoring to avoid undetected hypoglycemia (see Glossary).
  The following drugs may ***decrease*** the effects of acebutolol
  • indomethacin (Indocin), and possibly other "aspirin substitutes," may impair acebutolol's antihypertensive effect.
▷ *Driving, Hazardous Activities:* Use caution until the full extent of drowsiness, lethargy and blood pressure change has been determined.
  Aviation Note: The use of this drug ***is a disqualification*** for piloting. Consult a designated Aviation Medical Examiner.
  Exposure to Sun: No restrictions.
  Exposure to Heat: Caution advised. Hot environments can lower the blood pressure and exaggerate the effects of this drug.
  Exposure to Cold: Caution advised. Cold environments can enhance the circulatory deficiency in the extremities that may occur with this drug. The elderly should take precautions to prevent hypothermia (see Glossary).

Heavy Exercise or Exertion: It is advisable to avoid exertion that produces light-headedness, excessive fatigue or muscle cramping. The use of this drug may intensify the hypertensive response to isometric exercise.

Occurrence of Unrelated Illness: The fever that accompanies systemic infections can lower the blood pressure and require adjustment of dosage. Illnesses that cause nausea or vomiting may interrupt the regular dosage schedule. Ask your physician for guidance.

Discontinuation: It is advisable to avoid sudden discontinuation of this drug in all situations. If possible, gradual reduction of dose over a period of 2 to 3 weeks is recommended. Ask your physician for specific guidance.

ACETAMINOPHEN
(a set a MEE noh fen)

Other Names: APAP, paracetamol

Introduced: 1893

Class: Mild analgesic and antipyretic

Prescription: No

Controlled Drug: No

Available as Generic: Yes

Brand Names: Actifed-A [CD], Anacin-3, Anexsia [CD], Anexsia 7.5 [CD], ◆Apo-Acetaminophen, ◆Atasol, ◆Atasol Forte, Bromo-Seltzer [CD], Children's Fevernol, Contac Severe Cold Formula Caplets [CD], CoTylenol Children's Liquid Cold Formula [CD], CoTylenol Tablets [CD], Darvocet-N 50/100 [CD], Datril Extra Strength, Demerol-APAP [CD], Dimetapp-A Preparations [CD], Dolene AP-65 [CD], Drixoral Plus [CD], ◆Empracet-30, -60 [CD], Empracet w/Codeine No. 3, 4 [CD], ◆Emtec-30 [CD], Excedrin [CD], Excedrin P.M. [CD], ◆Exdol, ◆Exdol Strong, ◆Exdol-8, -15, -30 [CD], Fioricet [CD], Hycomine Compound [CD], ◆Lenoltec w/Codeine No. 1, 2, 3, 4 [CD], Lorcet Plus [CD], Lortab [CD], Ornex [CD], ◆Oxycocet [CD], Panadol, Parafon Forte [CD], Percocet [CD], ◆Percocet-Demi [CD], Percogesic [CD], Phenaphen, Phenaphen w/Codeine No. 2, 3, 4 [CD], ◆Robaxacet [CD], ◆Robigesic, ◆Rounox, ◆Rounox w/Codeine [CD], Sine-Aid [CD], Sine-Off Extra Strength Capsules [CD], Singlet [CD], Sinubid [CD], Sinutab Maximum Strength [CD], Sinutab No Drowsiness Tablets [CD], Sinutab Tablets [CD], St. Joseph Aspirin-Free, Sudafed Sinus Maximum Strength [CD], Talacen [CD], Tapar, Tempra, Triaminicin [CD], Trigesic [CD], Tycolet [CD], Tylenol, Tylenol w/Codeine No. 1, 2, 3, 4 [CD], ◆Tylenol Sinus Medication [CD], Tylox [CD], Valadol, Vanquish [CD], Vicodin [CD], Vicodin ES [CD], Wygesic [CD], Zydone [CD]

```
┌─────────────────────────────────────────────────────────────┐
│                    BENEFITS versus RISKS                     │
├─────────────────────────────────────────────────────────────┤
│      Possible Benefits              Possible Risks           │
│  EFFECTIVE RELIEF OF MILD       Rare anemia, liver or kidney │
│     TO MODERATE PAIN              damage (with prolonged or  │
│  REDUCTION OF FEVER               excessive use)             │
└─────────────────────────────────────────────────────────────┘
```

▷ **Principal Uses**

As a Single Drug Product: To relieve mild to moderate pain from any cause, and to reduce high fever. It is often used instead of aspirin for these purposes.

As a Combination Drug Product [CD]: Often combined with other analgesics to enhance pain relief. Also combined with antihistamines and decongestants to relieve the discomfort of respiratory tract infections; and with muscle relaxants to augment the relief of discomfort associated with muscle spasm.

How This Drug Works: The mechanism of its analgesic action is not completely known. It may reduce the tissue concentrations of prostaglandins (chemicals involved in the production of pain) more effectively in the brain than in peripheral tissues. This could explain its reasonably good analgesic effect and its weak anti-inflammatory effect.

Available Dosage Forms and Strengths

Capsules —	325 mg, 500 mg
Effervescent granules —	325 mg (buffered)
Elixir —	120 mg, 160 mg, 325 mg per 5-ml teaspoonful
Liquid —	160 mg per 5-ml teaspoonful, 500 mg per 15-ml tablespoonful
Solution —	100 mg per ml, 120 mg per 2.5 ml
Suppositories —	120 mg, 125 mg, 325 mg, 600 mg, 650 mg
Tablets —	160 mg, 325 mg, 500 mg, 650 mg
Tablets, chewable —	80 mg, 160 mg
Wafers —	120 mg

▷ **Usual Adult Dosage Range:**   325 to 650 mg/4 hours as needed, or 1000 mg (1 gram)/4 to 6 hours (not to exceed 4 times/24 hours). **Note: For long-term use, actual dosage and administration schedule must be determined by the physician for each patient individually.**

▷ **Dosing Instructions:**   May be taken on empty stomach or with food or milk. Capsule may be opened for administration.

Usual Duration of Use: Continual use (at above dosage) should not exceed 10 days at a time. For long-term use under physician supervision, the daily dosage should not exceed 2600 mg/24 hours. Recently published studies reveal that uninterrupted long-term use can cause significant kidney damage. Ask your physician for guidance.

▷ **This Drug Should Not Be Taken If**
  • you have had an allergic reaction to any dosage form of it previously.

▷ **Inform Your Physician Before Taking This Drug If**
  • you have impaired liver or kidney function.
  • you are currently taking any anticoagulant drug ("blood thinner").

Possible Side-Effects (natural, expected and unavoidable drug actions)
  Drowsiness (in sensitive individuals).

▷ **Possible Adverse Effects** (unusual, unexpected and infrequent reactions)
  If any of the following develop, consult your physician promptly for guidance.
  Mild Adverse Effects
  Allergic Reactions: Skin rash, hives (rare).
  Impaired thinking and concentration.
  Serious Adverse Effects
  Allergic Reactions: Swelling of the vocal cords, difficult breathing, anaphylactic reaction (see Glossary). Hemolytic anemia (see Glossary).
  Fever, sore throat (abnormally low white blood cell count).
  Abnormal bleeding or bruising (reduced blood platelet count, see Glossary).
  Decreased urine volume, bloody urine (kidney damage).
  Jaundice (liver damage).

▷ **Possible Effects on Sexual Function:**   None reported.

  CAUTION
  1. If you have bronchial asthma and you are also allergic to aspirin, use this drug with caution until your sensitivity to it has been determined.
  2. If you are taking an oral anticoagulant drug ("blood thinner"), high-dose acetaminophen may alter your response to it and increase the risk of abnormal bleeding. Ask physician for guidance.
  3. Avoid the long-term use of this drug concurrently with aspirin or aspirin substitutes. This combination, especially in high doses, can increase the risk of kidney damage.

Precautions for Use
  By Infants and Children: Dosage is based upon age; ask physician for guidance if in doubt. Do not exceed 5 doses/24 hours. Continual use should not exceed 5 days at a time without physician guidance.
  By Those over 60 Years of Age: Do not exceed a total dose of 2600 mg/24 hours. Prolonged use in excessive doses can cause anemia, liver damage with jaundice and kidney damage.

▷ **Advisability of Use During Pregnancy**
  Pregnancy Category: B (tentative). See Pregnancy Code inside back cover. Animal studies: No birth defects due to this drug have been demonstrated.

Human studies: Is used in all stages of pregnancy. No evidence of adverse effects on mother or fetus has been documented when used in recommended doses for short periods of time.

Advisability of Use if Breast-Feeding
Presence of this drug in breast milk: Yes.
No adverse effects on nursing infants reported.

Habit-Forming Potential: None.

Effects of Overdosage: Nausea, vomiting, stomach pain, drowsiness, stupor, convulsions, coma, jaundice (in 2 to 5 days after large overdose).

Possible Effects of Long-Term Use: Formation of abnormal hemoglobin (methemoglobin). Development of anemia.

Suggested Periodic Examinations While Taking This Drug (at physician's discretion)
None required for short-term use.
During long-term use, examination for abnormal hemoglobin, anemia, reduced white blood cell or platelet counts, liver and kidney function.

▷ **While Taking This Drug, Observe the Following**
Foods: No restrictions.
Beverages: No restrictions. May be taken with milk or juices.
▷   *Alcohol:* No interactions expected.
Tobacco Smoking: No interactions expected.
▷   *Other Drugs*
Acetaminophen may ***increase*** the effects of
• oral anticoagulants if the acetaminophen is taken continually in daily doses of 2000 mg or more.
The following drug may ***increase*** the effects of acetaminophen
• diflunisal (Dolobid) may increase the risk of acetaminophen toxicity.
▷   *Driving, Hazardous Activities:* Usually no restrictions. Be alert to the rare occurrence of drowsiness and/or impaired thinking, and restrict activities accordingly.
Aviation Note: Usually no restrictions. However, it is advisable to observe for the possible occurrence of drowsiness or impaired thinking and to restrict activities accordingly.
Exposure to Sun: No restrictions.

ACETAZOLAMIDE
(a set a ZOHL a mide)

Introduced: 1953

Class: Anticonvulsant, antiglaucoma, diuretic, sulfonamides

Prescription: USA: Yes
Canada: Yes

Controlled Drug: USA: No
Canada: No

Available as Generic: USA: Yes
Canada: No

Brand Names: ✦Acetazolam, Ak-Zol, ✦Apo-Acetazolamide, Dazamide, Diamox, Diamox Sequles

---

BENEFITS versus RISKS

Possible Benefits	*Possible Risks*
REDUCTION OF INTERNAL EYE PRESSURE in selected cases of glaucoma	Acidosis with long-term use
	Increased risk of kidney stone
	Rare bone marrow, liver or kidney injury
CONTROL OF ABSENCE (PETIT MAL) SEIZURES	
TREATMENT OF PERIODIC PARALYSIS	

▷ **Principal Uses**
As a Single Drug Product: Primarily to treat certain types of glaucoma. Also used with other anticonvulsant drugs to manage petit mal epilepsy. Used less frequently to treat familial periodic paralysis and to prevent altitude sickness.

How This Drug Works: By inhibiting the action of the enzyme carbonic anhydrase, it decreases the formation of fluid (the aqueous humor) in the eye and increases the volume of urine.

Available Dosage Forms and Strengths
Capsules, prolonged-action — 500 mg
Injections — 500 mg per vial
Tablets — 125 mg, 250 mg

▷ **Usual Adult Dosage Range:** For glaucoma: 250 to 1000 mg/24 hours, in 2 or 3 doses. For epilepsy: 250 to 1000 mg/24 hours. As a diuretic: 250 to 375 mg/24 hours, in one morning dose. **Note: Actual dosage and administration schedule must be determined by the physician for each patient individually.**

▷ **Dosing Instructions:** Best taken with food or milk to prevent stomach irritation. Tablet may be crushed. Diamox Sequels may be opened, but do not chew or crush contents for administration.

Usual Duration of Use: Treatment of glaucoma and epilepsy require long-term use. If taken to control seizures, do not stop this drug abruptly. Consult your physician on a regular basis.

▷ **This Drug Should Not Be Taken If**
- you have had an allergic reaction to any dosage form of it previously.
- you have serious liver or kidney disease.
- you have Addison's disease.

▷ **Inform Your Physician Before Taking This Drug If**
- you have had an allergic reaction to any "sulfa" drug in the past.
- you have gout or lupus erythematosus.

Possible Side-Effects (natural, expected and unavoidable drug actions)
Drowsiness, temporary nearsightedness.

▷ **Possible Adverse Effects** (unusual, unexpected and infrequent reactions)
If any of the following develop, consult your physician promptly for guidance.
Mild Adverse Effects
Allergic Reactions: Skin rash, hives, drug fever.
Reduced appetite, indigestion, nausea.
Fatigue; weakness; dizziness; tingling of face, arms or legs.
Serious Adverse Effects
Allergic Reactions: Hemolytic anemia (see Glossary), spontaneous bruising (reduced blood platelet count, see Glossary).
Bone marrow depression (see Glossary)—fatigue, weakness, fever, sore throat, abnormal bleeding or bruising.
Hepatitis with jaundice (see Glossary)—yellow eyes and skin, dark-colored urine, light-colored stools.

▷ **Possible Effects on Sexual Function:**   Decreased libido (male and female), impotence (both infrequent). Effects may begin after 2 weeks of use and subside when drug is discontinued.

▷ **Adverse Effects That May Mimic Natural Diseases or Disorders**
Toxic liver reaction may suggest viral hepatitis.
Lupus erythematosus–like syndrome.

Natural Diseases or Disorders That May Be Activated by This Drug
Gout, acidosis secondary to chronic obstructive lung disease—asthma, bronchitis, emphysema.

CAUTION
1. Observe for possible loss of drug effectiveness when used as a diuretic or to control seizures.
2. Emotional depression may occur and not be recognized as an adverse effect of this drug.
3. This drug may cause an excessive loss of potassium from the body. Consult your physician regarding the need for a high-potassium diet or potassium supplements.

Precautions for Use
By Infants and Children: Excessive dosage may cause drowsiness and numbness of the face and extremities. Not recommended for use as a diuretic in children.
By Those over 60 Years of Age: Do not exceed recommended doses. Increased dosage may cause excessive loss of sodium and potassium, with resultant weakness, confusion, numbness in the extremities and

nausea. If taking a digitalis preparation (digitoxin, digoxin), consult your physician regarding the need for a high-potassium diet or potassium supplements.

▷ **Advisability of Use During Pregnancy**

Pregnancy Category: C (tentative). See Pregnancy Code inside back cover.

Animal studies: Limb and skeletal defects reported in mice and rats.

Human studies: Information from adequate studies of pregnant women is not available.

Avoid completely during the first 3 months and during labor and delivery.

Advisability of Use if Breast-Feeding

Presence of this drug in breast milk: Yes.

Diuretic effect of drug may temporarily impair milk production.

Monitor nursing infant closely and discontinue drug or nursing if adverse effects develop.

Habit-Forming Potential: None.

Effects of Overdosage: Drowsiness, numbness and tingling, thirst, nausea, vomiting, confusion, excitement, convulsions, coma.

Possible Effects of Long-Term Use: The development of low blood potassium and/or acidosis.

Suggested Periodic Examinations While Taking This Drug (at physician's discretion)

Complete blood cell counts, measurements of blood sodium, potassium and uric acid levels, liver and kidney function tests.

▷ **While Taking This Drug, Observe the Following**

Foods: Consult your physician regarding the advisability of eating a high-potassium diet. See Section Six for the Table of High Potassium Foods.

Beverages: No restrictions. May be taken with milk.

▷ *Alcohol:* Use with caution until the combined effect has been determined. Alcohol may impair the anticonvulsant effect of this drug and reduce its control of seizures.

Tobacco Smoking: No interactions expected.

▷ *Other Drugs*

Acetazolamide may *increase* the effects of

• quinidine.

Acetazolamide may *decrease* the effects of

• lithium.

▷ *Driving, Hazardous Activities:* Usually no restrictions. Be alert to the possible occurrence of drowsiness or dizziness.

Aviation Note: The use of this drug *may be a disqualification* for piloting. Consult a designated Aviation Medical Examiner.

Exposure to Sun: No restrictions.

ACYCLOVIR
(ay SI kloh ver)

Introduced: 1979

Class: Antiviral

Prescription: USA: Yes
    Canada: Yes

Controlled Drug: USA: No
    Canada: No

Available as Generic: No

Brand Name: Zovirax

BENEFITS versus RISKS

Possible Benefits	*Possible Risks*
HASTENED RECOVERY FROM INITIAL EPISODE OF GENITAL HERPES PREVENTION OF RECURRENCE OF GENITAL HERPES	Nausea, vomiting, diarrhea (8% in long-term use) Nervousness, depression (less than 3%) Joint and muscle pain (3%)

▷ **Principal Uses**

As a Single Drug Product: Treatment of initial episodes and prevention of recurrent episodes of genital herpes in selected individuals.

How This Drug Works: By inhibiting DNA replication of the herpes simplex virus, this drug arrests the multiplication and spread of the infecting virus and thus reduces the severity and duration of the herpes infection.

Available Dosage Forms and Strengths
    Capsules — 200 mg
    Ointment — 5%

▷ **Usual Adult Dosage Range:** For initial episode of genital herpes—200 mg/4 hours for a total of 5 capsules daily for 10 consecutive days (total dose of 50 capsules). For intermittent recurrence—200 mg/4 hours for a total of 5 capsules daily for 5 consecutive days (total dose of 25 capsules). Begin treatment at the earliest indication of recurrence. For prevention of frequent recurrence—200 mg taken 3 to 5 times daily for up to 6 months. For the ointment form—cover all infected areas every 3 hours for a total of 6 times daily for 7 consecutive days. Begin treatment at the earliest indication of infection. **Note: Actual dosage and administration schedule must be determined by the physician for each patient individually.**

▷ **Dosing Instructions:** May be taken without regard to eating. Capsule may be opened for administration. Take the full course of the exact dose prescribed. Use a finger cot or rubber glove to apply the ointment.

Usual Duration of Use: Continual use on a regular schedule for 10 days is usually necessary to determine this drug's effectiveness in reducing the severity and duration of the initial infection. Continual use for 4 to 6 months may be necessary to prevent frequent recurrence of herpes eruptions.

▷ **This Drug Should Not Be Taken If**
- you have had an allergic reaction to any dosage form of it previously.

▷ **Inform Your Physician Before Taking This Drug If**
- you have impaired liver or kidney function.
- you are taking any other drugs at this time.

Possible Side-Effects (natural, expected and unavoidable drug actions)
With use of capsules—none.
With use of ointment—mild pain, burning or stinging at site of application (28%).

▷ **Possible Adverse Effects** (unusual, unexpected and infrequent reactions)
If any of the following develop, consult your physician promptly for guidance.
Mild Adverse Effects
Allergic Reaction: Skin rash.
Headache, dizziness, nervousness, insomnia, depression, fatigue.
Nausea, vomiting, diarrhea.
Joint pains, muscle cramps.
Acne, hair loss.
Serious Adverse Effects
Superficial thrombophlebitis, enlarged lymph glands.

▷ **Possible Effects on Sexual Function:**   Altered timing and pattern of menstruation.

CAUTION
1. This drug does not eliminate all herpes virus and is not a permanent cure. Observe for possible recurrence and resume treatment at the earliest indication of active infection.
2. Avoid sexual intercourse while herpes blisters and inflammation are visible.
3. Do not exceed the prescribed dosage.
4. Inform physician if the frequency and severity of recurrent infections do not improve.

Precautions for Use
By Infants and Children: Safety and effectiveness for use by those under 12 years of age have not been established.
By Those over 60 Years of Age: Avoid dehydration. Drink 2 to 3 quarts of liquids daily.

▷ **Advisability of Use During Pregnancy**
Pregnancy Category: C (tentative). See Pregnancy Code inside back cover.
Animal studies: No birth defects found in mouse, rat or rabbit studies.

Human studies: Information from adequate studies of pregnant women is not available.
Avoid use if possible. Use only if clearly needed.

Advisability of Use if Breast-Feeding
Presence of this drug in breast milk: Unknown.
Avoid drug or refrain from nursing.

Habit-Forming Potential: None.

Effects of Overdosage: Possible impairment of kidney function.

Possible Effects of Long-Term Use: Development of strains of herpes virus that are resistant to this drug.

Suggested Periodic Examinations While Taking This Drug (at physician's discretion)
Kidney function tests.

▷ **While Taking This Drug, Observe the Following**
Foods: No restrictions.
Beverages: No restrictions. May be taken with milk. Drink 2 to 3 quarts of liquids daily.
▷ *Alcohol:* Use caution until the combined effects have been determined. Dizziness or fatigue may be accentuated.
Tobacco Smoking: No interactions expected.
▷ *Other Drugs*
The following drugs may *increase* the effects of acyclovir
• probenecid (Benemid) may delay its elimination.
▷ *Driving, Hazardous Activities:* Use caution if dizziness or fatigue occurs.
Aviation Note: The use of this drug **may be a disqualification** for piloting. Consult a designated Aviation Medical Examiner.
Exposure to Sun: No restrictions.

ALBUTEROL
(al BYU ter ohl)

Other Name: Salbutamol

Introduced: 1968

Class: Antiasthmatic, bronchodilator

Prescription: USA: Yes
    Canada: Yes

Controlled Drug: USA: No
    Canada: No

Available as Generic: No

Brand Names: ✦Novosalmol, Proventil Inhaler, Proventil Repetabs, Proventil Tablets, Ventolin Inhaler, Ventolin Rotacaps, Ventolin Tablets

```
┌─────────────────────────────────────────────────────────────────┐
│                    BENEFITS versus RISKS                          │
│                                                                   │
│       Possible Benefits              Possible Risks               │
│    VERY EFFECTIVE RELIEF OF       Increased blood pressure        │
│       BRONCHOSPASM                Fine hand tremor                 │
│                                   Irregular heart rhythm (with    │
│                                     excessive use)                │
└─────────────────────────────────────────────────────────────────┘
```

▷ **Principal Uses**

As a Single Drug Product: To relieve acute bronchial asthma and to reduce the frequency and severity of chronic, recurrent asthmatic attacks.

How This Drug Works: It is thought that by increasing the production of cyclic AMP, this drug relaxes constricted bronchial muscles to relieve asthmatic wheezing.

Available Dosage Forms and Strengths

Aerosol — 90 mcg per actuation
Capsules for inhalation — 200 mcg
Solution for inhalation — 0.83 mg per ml, 5 mg per ml
Syrup — 2 mg per 5-ml teaspoonful
Tablets — 2 mg, 4 mg
Tablets, prolonged-action — 4 mg

▷ **Usual Adult Dosage Range:**   Inhaler—1 to 2 inhalations (90 to 180 mcg) up to 4 times daily, every 4 to 6 hours. Tablets—2 to 4 mg 3 to 4 times daily, every 4 to 6 hours. **Do not exceed** 8 inhalations (720 mcg)/ 24 hours, or 32 mg (tablet form)/24 hours. **Note: Actual dosage and administration schedule must be determined by the physician for each patient individually.**

▷ **Dosing Instructions:**   May be taken on empty stomach or with food or milk. Tablet may be crushed. For inhaler, follow the written instructions carefully. Do not overuse.

Usual Duration of Use: According to individual requirements. Do not use beyond the time necessary to terminate episodes of asthma.

▷ **This Drug Should Not Be Taken If**
  • you have had an allergic reaction to any dosage form of it previously.
  • you currently have an irregular heart rhythm.
  • you are taking, or have taken within the past 2 weeks, any mono-amine oxidase (MAO) type A inhibitor drug (see Drug Class, Section Four).

▷ **Inform Your Physician Before Taking This Drug If**
  • you have any type of heart or circulatory disorder, especially high blood pressure or coronary heart disease.
  • you have diabetes.
  • you are taking any form of digitalis or any stimulant drug.

Possible Side-Effects (natural, expected and unavoidable drug actions)
Aerosol—dryness or irritation of mouth or throat, altered taste.
Tablet—nervousness, palpitation.

▷ **Possible Adverse Effects** (unusual, unexpected and infrequent reactions)
If any of the following develop, consult your physician promptly for guidance.
Mild Adverse Effects
Headache (7%), dizziness (2%), restlessness, insomnia, fine tremor of hands (20%).
Nausea (2%), heartburn, vomiting.
Leg cramps (3%), flushing of skin.
Serious Adverse Effects
Rapid or irregular heart rhythm, increased blood pressure, difficult urination.

▷ **Possible Effects on Sexual Function:**   None reported.

Natural Diseases or Disorders That May Be Activated By This Drug
Latent coronary artery disease, diabetes or high blood pressure.

CAUTION
1. Concurrent use of this drug by inhalation with beclomethasone aerosol (Beclovent, Vanceril) may increase the risk of toxicity due to fluorocarbon propellants. It is advisable to use albuterol aerosol 20 to 30 minutes *before* beclomethasone aerosol. This will reduce the risk of toxicity and will enhance the penetration of beclomethasone.
2. The excessive or prolonged use of this drug by inhalation can reduce its effectiveness and cause serious heart rhythm disturbances, including cardiac arrest.

Precautions for Use
By Infants and Children: Safety and effectiveness of use in children under 12 years of age have not been established.
By Those over 60 Years of Age: Avoid excessive and continual use. If acute asthma is not relieved promptly, other drugs will have to be tried. Observe for the development of nervousness, palpitations, irregular heart rhythm and muscle tremors.

▷ **Advisability of Use During Pregnancy**
Pregnancy Category: C (tentative). See Pregnancy Code inside back cover.
Animal studies: Cleft palate reported in mice.
Human studies: Information from adequate studies of pregnant women is not available.
Avoid use during first 3 months if possible.

Advisability of Use if Breast-Feeding
Presence of this drug in breast milk: Unknown.
Avoid drug or refrain from nursing.

Habit-Forming Potential: None.

Effects of Overdosage: Nervousness, palpitation, rapid heart rate, sweating, headache, tremor, vomiting, chest pain.

Possible Effects of Long-Term Use: Loss of effectiveness.

Suggested Periodic Examinations While Taking This Drug (at physician's discretion)
Blood pressure measurements, evaluation of heart status.

▷ **While Taking This Drug, Observe the Following**
Foods: No restrictions.
Beverages: Avoid excessive use of caffeine-containing beverages—coffee, tea, cola, chocolate.
▷ *Alcohol:* No interactions expected.
Tobacco Smoking: No interactions expected.
▷ *Other Drugs*
Albuterol *taken concurrently* with
  • monoamine oxidase (MAO) type A inhibitor drugs may cause excessive increase in blood pressure and undesirable heart stimulation.
▷ *Driving, Hazardous Activities:* Use caution if excessive nervousness or dizziness occurs.
Aviation Note: The use of this drug *is a disqualification* for piloting. Consult a designated Aviation Medical Examiner.
Exposure to Sun: No restrictions.
Heavy Exercise or Exertion: Use caution. Excessive exercise can induce asthma in sensitive individuals.

ALLOPURINOL
(al oh PURE i nohl)

Introduced: 1963

Class: Antigout

Prescription: USA: Yes
Canada: Yes

Controlled Drug: USA: No
Canada: No

Available as Generic: USA: Yes
Canada: No

Brand Names: ◆Alloprin, ◆Apo-Allopurinol, Lopurin, ◆Novopurol, ◆Purinol, Zurinol, Zyloprim

BENEFITS versus RISKS	
Possible Benefits	*Possible Risks*
EFFECTIVE CONTROL OF GOUT CONTROL OF HIGH BLOOD URIC ACID due to polycythemia, leukemia, cancer and chemotherapy	Increased frequency of acute gout initially Peripheral neuritis Allergic reactions in skin, blood vessels and liver Bone marrow depression (questionable)

▷ **Principal Uses**

As a Single Drug Product: Used primarily in the long-term management of gout to *prevent* episodes of acute gout. (It does not relieve the symptoms of acute gout attacks.) Also used to prevent abnormally high blood levels of uric acid in individuals who have recurrent uric acid kidney stones, and in those receiving chemotherapy or radiation therapy for cancer.

How This Drug Works: By inhibiting the action of the tissue enzyme xanthine oxidase, this drug decreases the conversion of purines (protein nutrients) to uric acid.

Available Dosage Forms and Strengths

Tablets — 100 mg, 300 mg (and 200 mg in Canada)

▷ **Usual Adult Dosage Range:**   Initially 100 mg/24 hours. Increase by 100 mg/24 hours at intervals of 1 week until uric acid blood level is 6 mg/dl or less. Usual dose is 200 to 300 mg/24 hours for mild gout, and 400 to 600 mg/24 hours for moderate to severe gout. Daily doses of 300 mg or less may be taken as a single dose. Doses exceeding 300 mg daily should be divided into 2 or 3 equal portions; for the high uric acid levels associated with cancer, 600 to 800 mg/24 hours, divided into 3 equal portions. **Note: Actual dosage and administration schedule must be determined by the physician for each patient individually.**

▷ **Dosing Instructions:**   Best taken with food or milk to reduce stomach irritation. Tablet may be crushed. Drink 2 to 3 quarts of liquids daily.

Usual Duration of Use: According to individual requirements. Blood uric acid levels usually begin to decrease in 48 to 72 hours and may reach a normal range in 1 to 3 weeks. Regular use for several months may be required to prevent attacks of acute gout. Continual use for many years may be necessary for adequate control. Consult your physician on a regular basis.

▷ **This Drug Should Not Be Taken If**
- you have had an allergic reaction to any dosage form of it previously.
- you are experiencing an acute attack of gout at the present time.

▷ **Inform Your Physician Before Taking This Drug If**
- you have a personal or family history of hemochromatosis.
- you have a history of liver or kidney disease.
- you have had a blood cell or bone marrow disorder.
- you have any type of convulsive disorder (epilepsy).

Possible Side-Effects (natural, expected and unavoidable drug actions)

An increase in the frequency and severity of episodes of acute gout may occur during the first several weeks of drug use. Consult your physician regarding the need for other drugs during this period.

▷ **Possible Adverse Effects** (unusual, unexpected and infrequent reactions)
If any of the following develop, consult your physician promptly for guidance.

Mild Adverse Effects

Allergic Reactions: Skin rash, hives, itching, drug fever.

Headache, dizziness, drowsiness.

Nausea, vomiting, diarrhea, stomach cramps.

Loss of scalp hair.

Serious Adverse Effects

Allergic Reactions: Severe skin reactions, high fever, chills, joint pains, swollen glands, kidney damage.

Hepatitis with or without jaundice (see Glossary)—yellow eyes and skin, dark-colored urine, light-colored stools.

Bone marrow depression (see Glossary)—questionable.

Seizures, peripheral neuritis.

Macular eye damage, cataract formation—questionable.

▷ **Possible Effects on Sexual Function:**   Less than 1% and causal relationship not established: male infertility, male breast enlargement, impotence.

▷ **Adverse Effects That May Mimic Natural Diseases or Disorders**

Toxic liver reaction may suggest viral hepatitis.

Severe skin reactions may resemble the Stevens-Johnson syndrome (erythema multiforme).

CAUTION

1. During the early weeks of treatment, the frequency of acute attacks of gout may increase. These subside with continuation of treatment.
2. This drug will not relieve the symptoms of acute gout. It should not be started during the presence of acute gout symptoms.
3. Vitamin C in doses of 2 grams or more daily may acidify the urine and increase the risk of kidney stone formation during the use of allopurinol.
4. The concurrent use of thiazide diuretics (see Drug Class, Section Four) is reported to cause a possible allergic-type kidney damage. Avoid this drug combination.

Precautions for Use

By Infants and Children: Monitor closely for allergic skin reactions and blood cell disorders. This drug may increase the toxicity of azathioprine (Imuran) or mercaptopurine (Purinethol) in children receiving chemotherapy for cancer.

By Those over 60 Years of Age: The natural decline in kidney function makes it advisable to use smaller initial and maintenance doses of this drug.

▷ **Advisability of Use During Pregnancy**

Pregnancy Category: C (tentative). See Pregnancy Code inside back cover.

Animal studies: Results are conflicting and inconclusive.

Human studies: Information from adequate studies of pregnant women is not available.

Avoid use of drug during the first 3 months. Use during the last 6 months only if clearly needed.

Advisability of Use if Breast-Feeding
Presence of this drug in breast milk: Yes.
Avoid drug or refrain from nursing.

Habit-Forming Potential: None.

Effects of Overdosage: Nausea, vomiting or diarrhea may occur as a result of individual sensitivity. No serious toxic effects expected.

Possible Effects of Long-Term Use: None identified.

Suggested Periodic Examinations While Taking This Drug (at physician's discretion)
Blood uric acid levels, complete blood cell counts, liver and kidney function tests. If appropriate, eye examinations for possible cataract formation or macular damage. A cause-and-effect relationship (see Glossary) between this drug and eye changes has not been established.

▷ **While Taking This Drug, Observe the Following**
Foods: Follow physician's advice regarding the need for a low-purine diet.
Beverages: No restrictions. May be taken with milk.
▷ *Alcohol:* No interactions expected.
Tobacco Smoking: No interactions expected.
▷ *Other Drugs*
Allopurinol may *increase* the effects of
- azathioprine (Imuran) and mercaptopurine (Purinethol), making it necessary to reduce their dosages.
- oral anticoagulants (see Drug Class, Section Four) in *some* individuals.
- theophylline (aminophylline, Elixophyllin, Theo-Dur, etc.)
Allopurinol *taken concurrently* with
- ampicillin may increase the incidence of skin rash.
▷ *Driving, Hazardous Activities:* Drowsiness may occur in some individuals. Determine sensitivity before engaging in hazardous activities.
Aviation Note: The use of this drug *may be a disqualification* for piloting. Consult a designated Aviation Medical Examiner.
Exposure to Sun: No restrictions.

ALPRAZOLAM
(al PRAY zoh lam)

Introduced: 1973

Class: Mild tranquilizer, benzodiazepines

Prescription: USA: Yes
Canada: Yes

Controlled Drug: USA: C-IV*
Canada: No

Available as Generic: No

Brand Name: Xanax

BENEFITS versus RISKS

Possible Benefits	*Possible Risks*
RELIEF OF ANXIETY AND NERVOUS TENSION in 75% of users	Habit-forming potential with prolonged use
Wide margin of safety with therapeutic doses	Minor impairment of mental functions with therapeutic doses

---

▷ **Principal Uses**

As a Single Drug Product: Used primarily as a mild tranquilizer for the short-term relief of mild to moderate anxiety and nervous tension. It is also used to relieve anxiety associated with depression and to prevent or relieve panic attacks.

How This Drug Works: It is thought that this drug produces a calming effect by enhancing the action of the nerve transmitter gamma-aminobutyric acid (GABA), which in turn blocks the arousal of higher brain centers.

Available Dosage Forms and Strengths
Tablets — 0.25 mg, 0.5 mg, 1 mg

▷ **Usual Adult Dosage Range:** 0.25 mg to 0.5 mg 3 times daily. The maximal dose is 4 mg/24 hours, taken in divided doses. **Note: Actual dosage and administration schedule must be determined by the physician for each patient individually.**

▷ **Dosing Instructions:** May be taken on empty stomach or with food or milk. Tablet may be crushed for administration. Do not discontinue this drug abruptly if taken for more than 4 weeks.

Usual Duration of Use: Several days to several weeks. Avoid prolonged and uninterrupted use. Continual use should not exceed 8 weeks without evaluation by your physician.

*See Schedules of Controlled Drugs inside back cover.

▷ **This Drug Should Not Be Taken If**
- you have had an allergic reaction to it previously.
- you are pregnant (first 3 months).
- you have acute narrow-angle glaucoma.
- you have myasthenia gravis.

▷ **Inform Your Physician Before Taking This Drug If**
- you are allergic to other benzodiazepine drugs (see Drug Class, Section Four).
- you are pregnant (last 6 months) or planning pregnancy.
- you are breast-feeding.
- you have a history of depression or serious mental illness (psychosis).
- you have a history of alcoholism or drug abuse.
- you have impaired liver or kidney function.
- you have open-angle glaucoma.
- you have a seizure disorder (epilepsy).
- you have severe chronic lung disease.

Possible Side-Effects (natural, expected and unavoidable drug actions)
Drowsiness, light-headedness.

▷ **Possible Adverse Effects** (unusual, unexpected and infrequent reactions)
If any of the following develop, consult your physician promptly for guidance.
Mild Adverse Effects
Allergic Reactions: Skin rash, hives.
Headache, dizziness, fatigue, blurred vision, dry mouth.
Nausea, vomiting, constipation.
Serious Adverse Effects
Confusion, hallucinations, depression, unexpected excitement, agitation (paradoxical reaction).

▷ **Possible Effects on Sexual Function:**   Rare but documented: inhibited female orgasm (5 mg/day); impaired ejaculation (3.5 mg/day); decreased libido, impaired erection (4.5 mg/day); altered timing and pattern of menstruation (0.75 to 4 mg/day).

CAUTION
1. This drug should not be discontinued abruptly if it has been taken continually for more than 4 weeks.
2. The concurrent use of some over-the-counter drug products that contain antihistamines (allergy and cold preparations, sleep aids) can cause excessive sedation in sensitive individuals.

Precautions for Use
By Infants and Children: Safety and effectiveness for use by those under 18 years of age have not been established.
By Those over 60 Years of Age: The starting dose should be 0.25 mg 2 or 3 times daily. Monitor for excessive drowsiness, dizziness, unsteadiness and incoordination (possible low blood pressure).

▷ **Advisability of Use During Pregnancy**

Pregnancy Category: D (tentative). See Pregnancy Code inside back cover.

Animal studies: Diazepam (a closely related benzodiazepine) can cause cleft palate in mice and skeletal defects in rats. No information available for alprazolam.

Human studies: Some studies suggest a possible association between the use of diazepam and defects such as cleft lip and heart deformities. Information from adequate studies on the use of alprazolam by pregnant women is not available.

Avoid use during entire pregnancy if possible.

Advisability of Use if Breast-Feeding

Presence of this drug in breast milk: Probably yes.

Avoid drug or refrain from nursing.

Habit-Forming Potential: This drug can produce psychological and/or physical dependence (see Glossary) if used in large doses for an extended period of time.

Effects of Overdosage: Marked drowsiness, weakness, feeling of drunkenness, staggering gait, tremor, stupor progressing to deep sleep or coma.

Possible Effects of Long-Term Use: Psychological and/or physical dependence.

Suggested Periodic Examinations While Taking This Drug (at physician's discretion)

None required for short-term use.

▷ **While Taking This Drug, Observe the Following**

Foods: No restrictions.

Beverages: Avoid excessive intake of caffeine-containing beverages: coffee, tea, cola. This drug may be taken with milk.

▷ *Alcohol:* Use with extreme caution and in very small amounts until the combined effect is determined. Alcohol may increase the sedative effects of alprazolam. Alprazolam may increase the intoxicating effects of alcohol. Avoid alcohol completely—throughout the day and night— if you find it necessary to drive or to engage in *any* hazardous activity.

Tobacco Smoking: Heavy smoking may reduce the calming action of alprazolam.

Marijuana Smoking

Occasional (once or twice weekly): Mild increase in the sedative effect of this drug.

Daily: Marked increase in the sedative effect of this drug.

▷ *Other Drugs*

Alprazolam may *increase* the effects of

• digoxin (Lanoxin), and cause digoxin toxicity.

Alprazolam may *decrease* the effects of
- levodopa (Sinemet, etc.), and reduce its effectiveness in treating Parkinson's disease.

The following drugs may *increase* the effects of alprazolam
- cimetidine (Tagamet).
- disulfiram (Antabuse).
- isoniazid (INH, Rifamate, etc.).
- oral contraceptives.
- valproic acid (Depakene).

The following drugs may *decrease* the effects of alprazolam
- rifampin (Rimactane, etc.).
- theophylline (aminophylline, Theo-Dur, etc.).

▷ *Driving, Hazardous Activities:* This drug can impair mental alertness, judgment, physical coordination and reaction time. Avoid hazardous activities accordingly.

Aviation Note: The use of this drug *is a disqualification* for piloting. Consult a designated Aviation Medical Examiner.

Exposure to Sun: No restrictions.

Discontinuation: If it has been necessary to use this drug for an extended period of time, do not discontinue it abruptly. Reduce dose gradually at the rate of 1 mg every 3 days.

AMANTADINE
(a MAN ta deen)

Introduced: 1966

Class: Antiparkinsonism, antiviral

Prescription: USA: Yes
Canada: Yes

Controlled Drug: USA: No
Canada: No

Available as Generic: USA: Yes
Canada: No

Brand Names: Symadine, Symmetrel

BENEFITS versus RISKS	
Possible Benefits	*Possible Risks*
PARTIAL RELIEF OF RIGIDITY, TREMOR AND IMPAIRED MOTION in all forms of parkinsonism (in 60% of users) PREVENTION AND TREATMENT OF REPIRATORY TRACT INFECTIONS CAUSED BY INFLUENZA TYPE A VIRUSES*	Skin rashes, mild to severe Confusion, hallucinations Congestive heart failure Increased prostatism (see Glossary) Abnormally low white blood cell counts

*This drug is not effective for the prevention or treatment of viral infections other than those caused by influenza type A viruses.

▷ **Principal Uses**

As a Single Drug Product: This drug has two primary uses: (1) to treat all forms of parkinsonism, and (2) to prevent and treat respiratory tract infections caused by strains of influenza type A virus.

How This Drug Works: Not completely known. It is thought that by increasing the availability of the nerve impulse transmitter known as dopamine in certain nerve centers, this drug reduces the muscular rigidity, tremor and impaired movement associated with all forms of parkinsonism. By blocking the penetration of infectious material from virus particles into tissue cells, this drug prevents the development of influenza type A.

Available Dosage Forms and Strengths
Capsules — 100 mg
Syrup — 50 mg per 5-ml teaspoonful

▷ **Usual Adult Dosage Range:** Antiparkinsonism: 100 mg once or twice daily. The total daily dose should not exceed 400 mg. Antiviral: 200 mg once daily; or 100 mg/12 hours. **Note: Actual dosage and administration schedule must be determined by the physician for each patient individually.**

▷ **Dosing Instructions:** May be taken with or following meals. The capsule may be opened for administration.

Usual Duration of Use: Continual use on a regular schedule for up to 2 weeks is usually necessary to determine this drug's effectiveness in relieving the symptoms of parkinsonism. Long-term use (months to years) requires periodic evaluation of response and dosage adjustment. Consult your physician on a regular basis. Following exposure to influenza type A, maximal protection requires continual daily dosage for at least 10 days. During influenza epidemics, this drug may be given for 6 to 8 weeks.

Currently a "Drug of Choice" for prevention of influenza Type A infection (70% to 90% effective), and for treatment of such infections (50% reduction of severity and length of illness).

▷ **This Drug Should Not Be Taken If**
• you have had an allergic reaction to it previously.

▷ **Inform Your Physician Before Taking This Drug If**
• you have any type of seizure disorder.
• you have a history of serious emotional or mental disorder.
• you have a history of heart disease, especially previous heart failure.
• you have impaired liver or kidney function.
• you have a history of peptic ulcer disease.
• you have eczema or recurring eczemalike skin rashes.
• you are taking any drugs for emotional or mental disorders.

Possible Side-Effects (natural, expected and unavoidable drug actions)
Light-headedness, dizziness, weakness, feeling of impending faint in up-right position (see Orthostatic Hypotension in Glossary). Dry mouth, constipation. Reddish-blue network pattern or patchy discoloration of the skin of the legs and feet (livedo reticularis); this is transient and unimportant.

▷ **Possible Adverse Effects** (unusual, unexpected and infrequent reactions)
If any of the following develop, consult your physician promptly for guidance.
Mild Adverse Effects
Allergic Reaction: Skin rash.
Headache, nervousness, irritability, inability to concentrate, insomnia, nightmares.
Unsteadiness, visual disturbances, slurred speech.
Loss of appetite, nausea, vomiting.
Serious Adverse Effects
Allergic Reaction: Severe eczemalike skin rashes.
Idiosyncratic Reactions: Confusion, depression, hallucinations.
Swelling (fluid retention) of the arms, feet or ankles.
Development of congestive heart failure (rare).
Aggravation of prostatism (see Glossary).
Abnormally low white blood cell counts: fever, sore throat, infections.

▷ **Possible Effects on Sexual Function:**   None reported.

▷ **Adverse Effects That May Mimic Natural Diseases or Disorders**
Mood or mental changes, confusion or hallucinations may suggest a psychotic disorder.
Swelling of the legs and feet may suggest (but not necessarily be in-dicative of) heart, liver or kidney disorder.

Natural Diseases or Disorders That May Be Activated by This Drug
Latent epilepsy, incipient congestive heart failure.

CAUTION
1. This drug has a narrow margin of safety. Do not exceed a total dose of 400 mg/24 hours. Observe closely for indications of adverse ef-fects with doses over 200 mg/24 hours.
2. After an initial period of benefit lasting 3 to 6 months, this drug may lose its effectiveness in the treatment of parkinsonism. If this occurs, consult your physician regarding dosage adjustment or drug replacement.
3. This drug is reported to increase susceptibility to German measles. Avoid exposure to anyone with active German measles infection.
4. Observe for early indications of congestive heart failure: shortness of breath on exertion or during the night while sleeping, mild cough, swelling of the feet and ankles. Report these developments promptly to your physician.

Precautions for Use
By Infants and Children: Safety and effectiveness for use by those under 1 year of age have not been established.
By Those over 60 Years of Age: Observe for the possible development of confusion, delirium, hallucinations and disorderly conduct. Prostatism may be aggravated by this drug.

▷ **Advisability of Use During Pregnancy**
Pregnancy Category: C (tentative). See Pregnancy Code inside back cover.
Animal studies: Birth defects reported in rat studies; no defects reported in rabbit studies.
Human studies: Information from adequate studies of pregnant women is not available. Avoid this drug during the first 3 months if possible. Ask your physician for guidance.

Advisability of Use if Breast-Feeding
Presence of this drug in breast milk: Yes.
The nursing infant may develop skin rash, vomiting or retention of urine. Avoid drug or refrain from nursing.

Habit-Forming Potential: While not habituating, this drug does have a potential for abuse because of its ability to cause euphoria, hallucinations and feelings of detachment.

Effects of Overdosage: Hyperactivity, disorientation, confusion, visual hallucinations, aggressive behavior, severe toxic psychosis, seizures, heart rhythm disturbances, drop in blood pressure.

Possible Effects of Long-Term Use: Livedo reticularis (see Possible Side-Effects above). Congestive heart failure in predisposed individuals.

Suggested Periodic Examinations While Taking This Drug (at physician's discretion)
White blood cell counts, liver and kidney function tests.
Evaluation of heart function.

▷ **While Taking This Drug, Observe the Following**
Foods: No restrictions.
Beverages: No restrictions. May be taken with milk.
▷ *Alcohol:* Use caution until combined effects have been determined. This combination may impair mental function and lower blood pressure excessively.
Tobacco Smoking: No interactions expected.
Marijuana Smoking: No interactions expected.
▷ *Other Drugs*
Amantadine may ***increase*** the effects of
• those atropinelike drugs that are used to treat parkinsonism, especially benztropine (Cogentin), orphenadrine (Disipal) and trihexyphenidyl (Artane). Amantadine can increase their therapeutic effectiveness. However, if doses are too large, these drugs taken

concurrently with amantadine may cause mental confusion, delirium, hallucinations and nightmares.

- levodopa (Dopar, Larodopa, Sinemet, etc.), and enhance its therapeutic effectiveness. However, this combination may cause acute mental disturbances.

The following drugs may *increase* the effects of amantadine

- amphetamine and amphetaminelike stimulant drugs may cause excessive stimulation and adverse behavioral effects.

▷ *Driving, Hazardous Activities:* This drug may cause drowsiness, dizziness, blurred vision or confusion. If these drug effects occur, avoid all hazardous activities.

Aviation Note: The use of this drug *may be a disqualification* for piloting. Consult a designated Aviation Medical Examiner.

Exposure to Sun: No restrictions.

Exposure to Heat: No restrictions.

Exposure to Cold: Use caution. Excessive chilling may enhance the development of livedo reticularis (see Possible Side-Effects above).

Discontinuation: When used to treat parkinsonism, this drug should not be stopped abruptly. Sudden discontinuation may cause an acute parkinsonian crisis. When used to treat influenza A infections, this drug should be continued for 48 hours after the disappearance of all symptoms.

AMBENONIUM
(am bee NOH ni um)

Introduced: 1956

Class: Antimyasthenic

Prescription: USA: Yes
Canada: No

Controlled Drug: USA: No
Canada: No

Available as Generic: USA: No
Canada: No

Brand Name: Mytelase Caplets

BENEFITS versus RISKS	
Possible Benefits	*Possible Risks*
MODERATELY EFFECTIVE TREATMENT OF OCULAR AND MILD FORMS OF MYASTHENIA GRAVIS (symptomatic relief of muscle weakness)	Cholinergic crisis (overdose): excessive salivation, nausea, vomiting, stomach cramps, diarrhea, shortness of breath (asthmalike wheezing), excessive weakness

▷ **Principal Uses**

As a Single Drug Product: Used primarily to treat the ocular and milder forms of myasthenia gravis by providing temporary relief of muscle weakness and fatigability. Because of its potential for serious adverse effects, its use is generally reserved for treating those individuals who cannot use neostigmine (Prostigmin) or pyridostigmine (Mestinon).

How This Drug Works: This drug inhibits cholinesterase, the enzyme that destroys acetylcholine. This results in higher levels of acetylcholine, the nerve transmitter that facilitates the stimulation of muscular activity. The net effects are increased muscle strength and endurance.

Available Dosage Forms and Strengths
Tablets — 10 mg

▷ **Usual Adult Dosage Range:**   Initially: 2.5 to 5 mg 3 or 4 times daily; adjust dosage as needed and tolerated at intervals of 48 hours. Maintenance: up to 300 mg/24 hours; the average dose is 15 to 100 mg/24 hours. It is advisable to try to determine the smallest dose that will provide the greatest strength. **Note: Actual dosage and administration schedule must be determined by the physician for each patient individually.**

▷ **Dosing Instructions:**   Take with food or milk to reduce the intensity of side-effects. Larger portions of the daily maintenance dosage should be timed according to the pattern of fatigue and weakness. The tablet may be crushed for administration.

Usual Duration of Use: Continual use on a regular schedule (with dosage adjustment) for 10 to 14 days is usually necessary to determine this drug's effectiveness in relieving the symptoms of myasthenia gravis. Long-term use (months to years) requires periodic evaluation of response and dosage adjustment. Consult your physician on a regular basis.

▷ **This Drug Should Not Be Taken If**
- you have had an allergic reaction to it previously.

▷ **Inform Your Physician Before Taking This Drug If**
- you have any type of seizure disorder.
- you are subject to heart rhythm disorders or bronchial asthma.
- you have recurrent urinary tract infections.
- you have prostatism (see Glossary).
- you plan to have surgery under general anesthesia in the near future.

Possible Side-Effects (natural, expected and unavoidable drug actions)
Small pupils, watering of eyes, slow pulse, low blood pressure, excessive salivation, nausea, vomiting, stomach cramps, diarrhea, urge to urinate, increased sweating.

▷ **Possible Adverse Effects** (unusual, unexpected and infrequent reactions)
If any of the following develop, consult your physician promptly for guidance.
Mild Adverse Effects
Allergic Reaction: Skin rash.
Nervousness, anxiety, unsteadiness, muscle cramps or twitching.
Serious Adverse Effects
Confusion, slurred speech, seizures, difficult breathing (asthmatic wheezing).
Increased muscle weakness or paralysis.
Excessive vomiting or diarrhea may induce abnormally low blood potassium levels (hypokalemia). This will accentuate muscle weakness.

▷ **Possible Effects on Sexual Function:**   None reported.

▷ **Adverse Effects That May Mimic Natural Diseases or Disorders**
Seizures may suggest the possibility of epilepsy.

Natural Diseases or Disorders That May Be Activated by This Drug
Latent bronchial asthma.

CAUTION
1. Certain drugs can block the action of this drug and reduce its effectiveness in treating myasthenia gravis. (See *Other Drugs* below.) Consult your physician before starting any new drug, prescription or over-the-counter.
2. The dosage schedule of this drug must be carefully individualized for each patient. Variations in response may occur from time to time. Because generalized muscle weakness is a major symptom of both myasthenia crisis (underdosage) and cholinergic crisis (overdosage), it may be difficult to recognize the correct cause. As a rule, weakness that begins within 1 hour after taking this drug probably represents overdosage; weakness that begins 3 or more hours after taking this drug is probably due to underdosage. Observe these time relationships and inform your physician.
3. During long-term use of this drug, observe for the possible development of resistance to the drug's therapeutic action (loss of effectiveness). Consult your physician regarding the advisability of discontinuing this drug for a few days to see if responsiveness can be restored.

Precautions for Use
By Infants and Children: Dosage and administration schedule should be determined by a qualified pediatric neurologist.
By Those over 60 Years of Age: Avoid high doses that are more likely to cause serious adverse effects.

▷ **Advisability of Use During Pregnancy**
Pregnancy Category: C (tentative). See Pregnancy Code inside back cover.
Animal studies: No information available.

Human studies: Information from adequate studies of pregnant women is not available.

There are no reports of birth defects due to the use of this drug during pregnancy. However, there are reports of significant muscular weakness in 10% to 20% of newborn infants whose mothers had taken this class of drugs during pregnancy. Ask your physician for guidance.

Advisability of Use if Breast-Feeding

Presence of this drug in breast milk: Probably not.

Monitor nursing infant closely and discontinue drug or nursing if adverse effects develop.

Habit-Forming Potential: None.

Effects of Overdosage: Generalized muscular weakness, blurred vision, very small pupils, slow heart rate, difficult breathing (wheezing), excessive salivation, nausea, vomiting, stomach cramps, diarrhea, muscle cramps or twitching. This syndrome constitutes the cholinergic crisis.

Possible Effects of Long-Term Use: Development of tolerance (see Glossary) with loss of therapeutic effectiveness.

Suggested Periodic Examinations While Taking This Drug (at physician's discretion)

Assessment of drug effectiveness and dosage schedule for optimal therapeutic results.

▷ **While Taking This Drug, Observe the Following**

Foods: No restrictions.

Beverages: No restrictions. May be taken with milk.

▷ *Alcohol:* Use caution until the combined effects are determined. Weakness and unsteadiness may be accentuated.

Tobacco Smoking: No interactions expected.

▷ *Other Drugs*

The following drugs may *decrease* the effects of ambenonium

- atropine (belladonna).
- clindamycin (Cleocin).
- guanadrel (Hylorel).
- guanethidine (Esimil, Ismelin).
- procainamide (Procan SR, Pronestyl).
- quinidine (Cardioquin, Duraquin, etc.).
- quinine (Quinamm).

▷ *Driving, Hazardous Activities:* This drug may cause blurred vision, confusion or generalized weakness. Restrict activities as necessary.

Aviation Note: The use of this drug *is a disqualification* for piloting. Consult a designated Aviation Medical Examiner.

Exposure to Sun: No restrictions.

Exposure to Heat: Use caution. This may cause excessive sweating and increased weakness.

Exposure to Environmental Chemicals: Avoid excessive exposure (inhalation, skin contamination) to the insecticides Baygon, Diazinon and Sevin. These can accentuate the potential toxicity of this drug.

Discontinuation: Do not discontinue this drug abruptly without your physician's knowledge and guidance.

AMILORIDE
(a MIL oh ride)

Introduced: 1967

Class: Diuretic

Prescription: USA: Yes
    Canada: Yes

Controlled Drug: USA: No
    Canada: No

Available as Generic: Yes

Brand Names: Midamor, ✦Moduret [CD], Moduretic [CD]

BENEFITS versus RISKS	
Possible Benefits	*Possible Risks*
EFFECTIVE DIURETIC WITHOUT LOSS OF POTASSIUM	ABNORMALLY HIGH BLOOD POTASSIUM with excessive use Rare bone marrow depression

▷ **Principal Uses**

As a Single Drug Product: To eliminate excessive fluid retention (edema).

As a Combination Drug Product [CD]: It is combined with other diuretics of the thiazide class primarily to prevent the loss of potassium from the body.

How This Drug Works: It is thought that this drug promotes the loss of sodium and water from the body and the retention of potassium by altering the enzyme systems of the kidney that control the formation of urine.

Available Dosage Forms and Strengths

Tablets — 5 mg

▷ **Usual Adult Dosage Range:** Initially 5 mg once daily, preferably in the morning. May increase up to 15 mg daily as needed and tolerated. Should not exceed 20 mg/24 hours. **Note: Actual dosage and administration schedule must be determined by the physician for each patient individually.**

▷ **Dosing Instructions:** Preferably taken on arising, with the stomach empty. For best results, withhold food for 4 hours. May be taken with food if necessary to reduce stomach irritation. Tablet may be crushed for administration.

Usual Duration of Use: As needed for elimination of edema or maintenance of normal blood pressure. Intermittent or alternate-day use is recommended to minimize imbalance of sodium and potassium. Consult your physician on a regular basis.

▷ **This Drug Should Not Be Taken If**
   • you have had an allergic reaction to any dosage form of it previously.
   • your blood potassium level is above the normal range.
   • your kidneys are not producing urine.

▷ **Inform Your Physician Before Taking This Drug If**
   • you have diabetes or glaucoma.
   • you have a history of kidney disease or impaired kidney function.
   • you are taking any other diuretic, blood pressure drug, any form of digitalis or lithium.

Possible Side-Effects (natural, expected and unavoidable drug actions)
   Abnormally high blood potassium level (10% of users), abnormally low blood sodium level, dehydration, constipation.

▷ **Possible Adverse Effects** (unusual, unexpected and infrequent reactions)
   If any of the following develop, consult your physician promptly for guidance.
   Mild Adverse Effects
   Allergic Reactions: Skin rash, itching.
   Headache, dizziness, weakness, fatigue, numbness and tingling.
   Dry mouth, nausea, vomiting, stomach pains, diarrhea.
   Loss of scalp hair.
   Serious Adverse Effects
   Idiosyncratic Reactions: Joint and muscle pains.
   Excessively high blood potassium level—marked fatigue and weakness, confusion, numbness and tingling of lips and extremities, slow and irregular heartbeats.
   Increased internal eye pressure (of concern in glaucoma).
   Mental depression, visual disturbances, ringing in ears, tremors.
   Aplastic anemia (see Glossary)—unusual fatigue or weakness, fever, sore throat, abnormal bleeding or bruising.

▷ **Possible Effects on Sexual Function:** More than 1%: decreased libido and impotence (5 to 10 mg/day).

▷ **Adverse Effects That May Mimic Natural Diseases or Disorders**
   Nervousness, confusion and/or depression may resemble spontaneous mental disorder.

Natural Diseases or Disorders That May Be Activated by This Drug
   Preexisting peptic ulcer, latent glaucoma.

CAUTION
1. Do not take potassium supplements, and do not increase your intake of high-potassium foods.
2. If taking any form of digitalis, report as directed for periodic measurements of your blood potassium level.
3. Do not discontinue this drug abruptly unless directed to do so by your physician.

Precautions for Use
By Infants and Children: Safety and effectiveness for use by those under 12 years of age have not been established.

By Those over 60 Years of Age: The natural decline in kidney function may predispose to excessive retention of potassium in the body. It is advisable to limit use of this drug to periods of 2 to 3 weeks if possible. Overdosage and extended use can cause excessive loss of body water, increased viscosity of the blood and an increased tendency to abnormal blood clotting (thrombosis, heart attack, stroke).

▷ **Advisability of Use During Pregnancy**
Pregnancy Category: B (tentative). See Pregnancy Code inside back cover.
Animal studies: No birth defects reported.
Human studies: Information from adequate studies of pregnant women is not available.
Use only if clearly needed.

Advisability of Use if Breast-Feeding
Presence of this drug in breast milk: Unknown, but probably present.
This drug may suppress milk production.
Avoid drug if possible. If use is necessary, monitor nursing infant closely and discontinue drug or nursing if adverse effects develop.

Habit-Forming Potential: None.

Effects of Overdosage: Thirst, drowsiness, fatigue, weakness, nausea, vomiting, confusion, numbness and tingling of face and extremities, irregular heart rhythm, shortness of breath.

Suggested Periodic Examinations While Taking This Drug (at physician's discretion)
Complete blood cell counts; measurements of blood levels of sodium, potassium and chloride; kidney function tests; and assessment of water balance (state of hydration).

▷ **While Taking This Drug, Observe the Following**
Foods: No restrictions. Avoid excessive restriction of salt. Avoid excessive amounts of high-potassium foods.
Beverages: No restrictions. May be taken with milk.
▷ *Alcohol:* Use with caution until the combined effect has been determined. Alcohol can exaggerate the blood-pressure-lowering effect of this drug and cause orthostatic hypotension (see Glossary).

Tobacco Smoking: No interactions expected.
▷ *Other Drugs*
  Amiloride may ***increase*** the effects of
  • other blood-pressure-lowering drugs. Dosage adjustments may be necessary.
  Amiloride may ***decrease*** the effects of
  • digoxin (Lanoxin, etc.), and reduce its effectiveness in treating heart failure.
  Amiloride ***taken concurrently*** with
  • spironolactone (Aldactone, Aldactazide) or triamterene (Dyrenium, Dyazide) may cause excessive (dangerous) increase in blood potassium levels. Avoid the concurrent use of these drugs.
  • lithium may cause lithium accumulation to toxic levels.
▷ *Driving, Hazardous Activities:* This drug may cause drowsiness, dizziness and orthostatic hypotension in sensitive individuals. If these drug effects occur, avoid hazardous activities.
Aviation Note: The use of this drug ***may be a disqualification*** for piloting. Consult a designated Aviation Medical Examiner.
Exposure to Sun: No restrictions.
Exposure to Heat: Caution advised. Excessive perspiration can cause water, sodium and potassium imbalance. Hot environments can cause lowering of blood pressure.
Occurrence of Unrelated Illness: Consult your physician if you contract an illness that causes vomiting or diarrhea.
Discontinuation: With high dosage or prolonged use, withdraw this drug gradually. Sudden withdrawal can cause excessive loss of potassium from the body.

AMITRIPTYLINE
(a mee TRIP ti leen)

Introduced: 1961   **Class:** Antidepressant

Prescription: USA: Yes   **Controlled Drug:** USA: No
  Canada: Yes   Canada: No

Available as Generic: Yes

Brand Names: Amitril, ✦Apo-Amitriptyline, Elavil, ✦Elavil Plus [CD], Emitrip, Endep, Etrafon [CD], Etrafon-A [CD], Etrafon-Forte [CD], ✦Levate, Limbitrol [CD], ✦Novotriptyn, Triavil [CD]

BENEFITS versus RISKS

Possible Benefits	*Possible Risks*
EFFECTIVE RELIEF OF ENDOGENOUS DEPRESSION in 60% to 75% of users	ADVERSE BEHAVIORAL EFFECTS: Confusion, disorientation, hallucinations
	CONVERSION OF DEPRESSION TO MANIA in manic-depressive disorders
	Irregular heart rhythms
	Rare blood cell abnormalities

▷ **Principal Uses**

As a Single Drug Product: To relieve the symptoms associated with spontaneous (endogenous) depression, and to initiate the restoration of normal mood. This drug should be used only when a diagnosis of a true, primary depression of significant degree has been established. It should not be used to treat the symptoms of mild and transient (reactive) depression that may be associated with many life situations in the absence of a bona fide affective illness.

As a Combination Drug Product [CD]: This drug is available in combination with chlordiazepoxide, a mild tranquilizer of the benzodiazepine class. This combination is used to relieve anxiety that may accompany depression. This drug is also available in combination with perphenazine, a strong tranquilizer of the phenothiazine class. This combination is used to relieve severe agitation that may accompany depression.

How This Drug Works: It is thought that this drug relieves depression by slowly restoring to normal levels certain constituents of brain tissue (norepinephrine and serotonin) that transmit nerve impulses.

Available Dosage Forms and Strengths
Tablets — 10 mg, 25 mg, 50 mg, 75 mg, 100 mg, 150 mg

▷ **Usual Adult Dosage Range:**   Initially 25 mg 2 to 4 times daily. Dose may be increased cautiously as needed and tolerated by 10 to 25 mg daily at intervals of 1 week. Usual maintenance dose is 50 to 100 mg/24 hours. Total dose should not exceed 150 mg/24 hours. When the optimal requirement is determined, it may be taken at bedtime as one dose. **Note: Actual dosage and administration schedule must be determined by the physician for each patient individually.**

▷ **Dosing Instructions:**   May be taken without regard to meals. Tablet may be crushed for administration.

Usual Duration of Use: Some benefit may be apparent within 1 to 2 weeks, but adequate response may require continual use for 4 to 6 weeks or longer. Long-term use should not exceed 6 months without evaluation regarding the need for continuation of the drug. Consult your physician on a regular basis.

▷ **This Drug Should Not Be Taken If**
- you are allergic to any of the drugs bearing the brand names listed above.
- you are taking or have taken within the past 14 days any monoamine oxidase (MAO) type A inhibitor drug (see Drug Class, Section Four).
- you are recovering from a recent heart attack.
- you have narrow-angle glaucoma.

▷ **Inform Your Physician Before Taking This Drug If**
- you are allergic or sensitive to any other tricyclic antidepressant (see Drug Class, Section Four).
- you have a history of any of the following: diabetes, epilepsy, glaucoma, heart disease, prostate gland enlargement or overactive thyroid function.
- you plan to have surgery under general anesthesia in the near future.

Possible Side-Effects (natural, expected and unavoidable drug actions)
Drowsiness, blurred vision, dry mouth, constipation, impaired urination.

▷ **Possible Adverse Effects** (unusual, unexpected and infrequent reactions)
If any of the following develop, consult your physician promptly for guidance.
Mild Adverse Effects
Allergic Reactions: Skin rash, hives, swelling of face or tongue, drug fever (see Glossary).
Headache, dizziness, weakness, fainting, unsteady gait, tremors.
Peculiar taste, irritation of tongue or mouth, nausea, indigestion.
Fluctuation of blood sugar levels.
Serious Adverse Effects
Allergic Reactions: Hepatitis, with or without jaundice (see Glossary).
Confusion, hallucinations, agitation, restlessness, nightmares.
Heart palpitation and irregular rhythm.
Bone marrow depression (see Glossary)—fatigue, weakness, fever, sore throat, abnormal bleeding or bruising.
Peripheral neuritis (see Glossary)—numbness, tingling, pain, loss of strength in arms and legs.
Parkinson-like disorders (see Glossary)—usually mild and infrequent; more likely to occur in the elderly.

▷ **Possible Effects on Sexual Function:** Decreased libido (8%), increased libido (antidepressant effect), impotence (19%), inhibited female orgasm, inhibited ejaculation, male and female breast enlargement, milk production, swelling of testicles. These effects usually disappear within 2 to 10 days after discontinuation of the drug.

▷ **Adverse Effects That May Mimic Natural Diseases or Disorders**
Liver toxicity may suggest viral hepatitis.

Natural Diseases or Disorders That May Be Activated by This Drug

Latent diabetes, epilepsy, glaucoma, impaired urination due to prostate gland enlargement.

CAUTION

1. Dosage must be adjusted for each person individually. Report for follow-up evaluation and laboratory tests as directed by your physician.
2. It is advisable to withhold this drug if electroconvulsive therapy (ECT, "shock" treatment) is to be used to treat your depression.

Precautions for Use

By Infants and Children: Safety and effectiveness for use by those under 12 years of age have not been established.

By Those over 60 Years of Age: During the first 2 weeks of treatment, observe for the development of confusion, agitation, forgetfulness, disorientation, delusions and hallucinations. Reduction of dosage or discontinuation may be necessary. Unsteadiness may predispose to falling and injury. This drug can increase the degree of impaired urination associated with prostate gland enlargement (prostatism).

▷ Advisability of Use During Pregnancy

Pregnancy Category: C (tentative). See Pregnancy Code inside back cover.

Animal studies: Skull deformities reported in rabbits.

Human studies: No defects reported in 21 exposures. Information from adequate studies of pregnant women is not available.

Avoid use of drug during first 3 months. Use during last 6 months only if clearly needed.

Advisability of Use if Breast-Feeding

Presence of this drug in breast milk: Yes, in small amounts.

Monitor nursing infant closely and discontinue drug or nursing if adverse effects develop.

Habit-Forming Potential: Psychological or physical dependence is rare and unexpected.

Effects of Overdosage: Confusion, hallucinations, marked drowsiness, heart palpitations, dilated pupils, tremors, stupor, deep sleep, coma, convulsions.

Suggested Periodic Examinations While Taking This Drug (at physician's discretion)

Complete blood cell counts, liver function tests, serial blood pressure readings and electrocardiograms.

▷ While Taking This Drug, Observe the Following

Foods: No restrictions. This drug may increase the appetite and cause excessive weight gain.

Beverages: No restrictions. May be taken with milk.

▷ *Alcohol:* Avoid completely. This drug can markedly increase the intoxicating effects of alcohol and accentuate its depressant action on brain function.

Tobacco Smoking: May hasten the elimination of this drug. Higher doses may be necessary.

▷ *Other Drugs*

Amitriptyline may *increase* the effects of
- atropinelike drugs (see Drug Class, Section Four).

Amitriptyline may *decrease* the effects of
- clonidine (Catapres).
- guanethidine (Ismelin).

Amitriptyline *taken concurrently* with
- monoamine oxidase (MAO) type A inhibitor drugs may cause high fever, delirium and convulsions (see Drug Class, Section Four).
- thyroid preparations may impair heart rhythm and function. Ask physician for guidance regarding adjustment of thyroid dose.

▷ *Driving, Hazardous Activities:* This drug may impair mental alertness, judgment, physical coordination and reaction time. Avoid hazardous activities.

Aviation Note: The use of this drug *is a disqualification* for piloting. Consult a designated Aviation Medical Examiner.

Exposure to Sun: Use caution until sensitivity to sun has been determined. This drug may cause photosensitivity (see Glossary).

Exposure to Heat: This drug can inhibit sweating and impair the body's adaptation to hot environments, increasing the risk of heat stroke. Avoid saunas.

Exposure to Cold: The elderly should use caution and avoid conditions conducive to hypothermia (see Glossary).

Discontinuation: It is advisable to discontinue this drug gradually. Abrupt withdrawal after long-term use can cause headache, malaise and nausea.

AMOXAPINE
(a MOX a peen)

Introduced: 1970

Class: Antidepressant

Prescription: USA: Yes
Canada: Yes

Controlled Drug: USA: No
Canada: No

Available as Generic: No

Brand Name: Asendin

```
┌─────────────────────────────────────────────────────────────────┐
│                    BENEFITS versus RISKS                          │
│                                                                   │
│      Possible Benefits              Possible Risks                │
│   EFFECTIVE RELIEF OF          ADVERSE BEHAVIORAL                  │
│     PRIMARY DEPRESSIONS:         EFFECTS: Confusion, delusions,    │
│     Endogenous, neurotic, reactive   disorientation, hallucinations│
│   Well tolerated by most persons  CONVERSION OF DEPRESSION        │
│                                    TO MANIA in manic-depressive    │
│                                    disorders                       │
│                                  Rare blood cell abnormalities     │
└─────────────────────────────────────────────────────────────────┘
```

▷ **Principal Uses**

> *As a Single Drug Product:* To provide symptomatic relief in all types of depression, and to initiate the restoration of normal mood.

How This Drug Works: It is thought that by increasing the availability of certain nerve impulse transmitters (norepinephrine and serotonin) in brain tissue, this drug relieves the symptoms associated with depression.

Available Dosage Forms and Strengths

> Tablets — 25 mg, 50 mg, 100 mg, 150 mg

▷ **Usual Adult Dosage Range:**   Initially 50 mg 3 times daily. Dose may be increased cautiously on the third day as needed and tolerated to 100 mg 3 times daily. Usual maintenance dose is 200 to 300 mg/24 hours. Total dosage should not exceed 400 mg/24 hours. When determined, the optimal requirement may be taken at bedtime as one dose, not to exceed 300 mg. **Note: Actual dosage and administration schedule must be determined by the physician for each patient individually.**

▷ **Dosing Instructions:**   May be taken without regard to meals. Tablet may be crushed for administration.

Usual Duration of Use: Benefit may be apparent within 4 to 7 days in some individuals, but continual use on a regular schedule for 2 to 3 weeks is usually necessary to determine this drug's effectiveness. Long-term use should not exceed 6 months without evaluation regarding the need for continuation. Consult your physician on a regular basis.

▷ **This Drug Should Not Be Taken If**
- you have had an allergic reaction to it previously.
- you are taking or have taken within the past 14 days any monoamine oxidase (MAO) type A inhibitor drug (see Drug Class, Section Four).
- you are recovering from a recent heart attack.

▷ **Inform Your Physician Before Taking This Drug If**
- you are allergic or overly sensitive to other antidepressant drugs.
- you have a history of any of the following: diabetes, epilepsy, glaucoma, heart disease, paranoia, prostate gland enlargement, schizophrenia or overactive thyroid function.
- you plan to have surgery under general anesthesia in the near future.

Possible Side-Effects (natural, expected and unavoidable drug actions)
Drowsiness, blurred vision, dry mouth, constipation, impaired urination.

▷ **Possible Adverse Effects** (unusual, unexpected and infrequent reactions)
If any of the following develop, consult your physician promptly for guidance.

Mild Adverse Effects
Allergic Reactions: Skin rash, hives, swellings, drug fever (see Glossary).
Insomnia, nervousness, palpitations, dizziness, unsteadiness, tremors, fainting.
Peculiar taste, indigestion, nausea, vomiting.

Serious Adverse Effects
Behavioral effects: anxiety, confusion, excitement, disorientation, hallucinations, delusions.
Aggravation of paranoid psychosis and schizophrenia.
Aggravation of epilepsy (seizures).
Parkinson-like disorders (see Glossary).
Peripheral neuritis (see Glossary)—numbness, tingling, pain, loss of strength in arms and legs.
Reduced white blood cell count—fever, sore throat.

▷ **Possible Effects on Sexual Function:** Decreased libido (150 mg/day), increased libido (antidepressant effect), inhibited ejaculation (75 to 150 mg/day), painful ejaculation (75 mg/day), inhibited female orgasm (100 mg/day), female breast enlargement/milk production (300 mg/day), altered menstrual timing and pattern (300 mg/day), swelling of testicles. These effects usually disappear within 2 to 10 days after discontinuation of the drug.

Natural Diseases or Disorders That May Be Activated by This Drug
Latent epilepsy, glaucoma, prostatism.

CAUTION
1. The dosage of this drug must be adjusted carefully for each person individually. This requires observation of symptom improvement and, in some instances, the measurement of drug levels in the blood.
2. Observe for early indications of toxicity: confusion, agitation, rapid heartbeat.
3. It is advisable to withhold this drug if electroconvulsive therapy (ECT, "shock" treatment) is to be used.

Precautions for Use
By Infants and Children: Safety and effectiveness for use by those under 16 years of age have not been established.
By Those over 60 Years of Age: During the first 2 weeks of treatment, observe for the development of confusion, restlessness, agitation, forgetfulness, disorientation, delusions and hallucinations. Reduction of dosage or discontinuation may be necessary. Observe for unsteadiness that may predispose to falling and injury. This drug can increase the

degree of impaired urination associated with prostate gland enlargement (prostatism). It is advisable to take the total dose at bedtime to reduce the risk of postural hypotension (see Glossary).

▷ **Advisability of Use During Pregnancy**
Pregnancy Category: C (tentative). See Pregnancy Code inside back cover.
   Animal studies: Reveal toxic effects on the embryo in rats and rabbits but no birth defects in the newborn.
   Human studies: Information from adequate studies of pregnant women is not available.
   Avoid drug during first 3 months. Use during the last 6 months only if clearly needed.

Advisability of Use if Breast-Feeding
Presence of this drug in breast milk: Yes, in small amounts.
Monitor nursing infant closely and discontinue drug or nursing if adverse effects develop.

Habit-Forming Potential: None.

Effects of Overdosage: Confusion, hallucinations, marked drowsiness, tremors, dilated pupils, cold skin, stupor, coma, convulsions, rapid heartbeat, low blood pressure.

Suggested Periodic Examinations While Taking This Drug (at physician's discretion)
   Complete blood cell counts, serial blood pressure readings and electrocardiograms.

▷ **While Taking This Drug, Observe the Following**
Foods: No restrictions. Drug may increase appetite and cause excessive weight gain.
Beverages: No restrictions. May be taken with milk.
▷ *Alcohol:* Avoid completely. This drug can markedly increase the intoxicating effects of alcohol and accentuate its depressant action on brain function.
Tobacco Smoking: May hasten the elimination of this drug. Higher doses may be necessary.
▷ *Other Drugs*
   Amoxapine may *increase* the effects of
   • atropinelike drugs (see Drug Class, Section Four).
   Amoxapine may *decrease* the effects of
   • clonidine (Catapres).
   • guanethidine (Ismelin).
   Amoxapine *taken concurrently* with
   • monoamine oxidase (MAO) type A inhibitor drugs may cause high fever, delirium and convulsions (see Drug Class, Section Four).
   • thyroid preparations may impair heart rhythm and function. Ask physician for guidance regarding adjustment of thyroid dose.

▷ *Driving, Hazardous Activities:* This drug may impair mental alertness, judgment, physical coordination and reaction time. Avoid hazardous activities.

Aviation Note: The use of this drug *is a disqualification* for piloting. Consult a designated Aviation Medical Examiner.

Exposure to Sun: Use caution until sensitivity to sun has been determined. This drug may cause photosensitivity (see Glossary).

Exposure to Heat: This drug can inhibit sweating and impair the body's adaptation to hot environments, increasing the risk of heat stroke. Avoid saunas.

Exposure to Cold: The elderly should use caution and avoid conditions conducive to hypothermia (see Glossary).

Discontinuation: It is advisable to discontinue this drug gradually. Abrupt withdrawal after long-term use can cause headache, malaise and nausea.

AMOXICILLIN
(a mox i SIL in)

Introduced: 1969

Class: Antibiotic, penicillins

Prescription: USA: Yes
Canada: Yes

Controlled Drug: USA: No
Canada: No

Available as Generic: USA: Yes
Canada: No

Brand Names: Amoxil, ✦Apo-Amoxi, Augmentin [CD], ✦Clavulin [CD], Larotid, ✦Novamoxin, Polymox, Trimox, Utimox, Wymox

---

BENEFITS versus RISKS

Possible Benefits	*Possible Risks*
EFFECTIVE TREATMENT OF INFECTIONS due to susceptible microorganisms	ALLERGIC REACTIONS, mild to severe, in 3% of the general population and 15% of allergic individuals
	Superinfections (yeast)
	Drug-induced colitis

▷ **Principal Uses**

As a Single Drug Product: To treat certain infections of the skin and soft tissues; of the ear, nose and throat; and of the genitourinary tract, including gonorrhea.

How This Drug Works: This drug destroys susceptible infecting bacteria by interfering with their ability to produce new protective cell walls as they multiply and grow.

Available Dosage Forms and Strengths
>   Capsules — 150 mg, 500 mg
>   Chewable tablets — 125 mg, 250 mg
>   Oral suspension — 125 mg, 250 mg per 5-ml teaspoonful
>   Pediatric drops — 50 mg per ml

▷ **Usual Adult Dosage Range:** 250 to 500 mg/8 hours. The usual maximal dose is 4500 mg/24 hours. **Note: Actual dosage and administration schedule must be determined by the physician for each patient individually.**

▷ **Dosing Instructions:** May be taken on an empty stomach or with food, milk, fruit juice, ginger ale or other cold drinks. Capsule may be opened for administration.

Usual Duration of Use: For all streptococcal infections—not less than 10 consecutive days (without interruption) to reduce the possibility of developing rheumatic fever or glomerulonephritis. For all other infections—as long as necessary to eradicate the infection.

▷ **This Drug Should Not Be Taken If**
- you have had an allergic reaction to any dosage form of it previously.
- you are certain you are allergic to *any* form of penicillin.

▷ **Inform Your Physician Before Taking This Drug If**
- you suspect you may be allergic to penicillin or you have a history of a previous "reaction" to penicillin.
- you are allergic to cephalosporin antibiotics (Ancef, Ceporan, Ceporex, Kafocin, Keflex, Keflin, Kefzol, Loridine).
- you are allergic by nature (hay fever, asthma, hives, eczema).

Possible Side-Effects (natural, expected and unavoidable drug actions)
Superinfections (see Glossary), often due to yeast organisms.

▷ **Possible Adverse Effects** (unusual, unexpected and infrequent reactions)
If any of the following develop, consult your physician promptly for guidance.
Mild Adverse Effects
Allergic Reactions: Skin rashes, hives, itching.
Irritations of mouth and tongue, "black tongue," nausea, vomiting, mild diarrhea, dizziness (rare).
Serious Adverse Effects
Allergic Reactions: Anaphylactic reaction (see Glossary), severe skin reactions, drug fever, swollen painful joints, sore throat, abnormal bleeding or bruising.

▷ **Possible Effects on Sexual Function:** None reported.

CAUTION
1. Take the exact dose and the full course prescribed.
2. This drug should not be used concurrently with antibiotics like erythromycin or tetracycline.

Precautions for Use
By Infants and Children: A generalized rash occurs in approximately 90% of individuals who take this drug during an episode of infectious mononucleosis. This drug may cause diarrhea, which sometimes necessitates discontinuation.

By Those over 60 Years of Age: Natural changes in the skin may predispose to prolonged itching reactions in the genital and anal regions. Report such reactions promptly.

▷ Advisability of Use During Pregnancy
Pregnancy Category: B (tentative). See Pregnancy Code inside back cover.
Animal studies: No information available.
Human studies: Information from adequate studies of pregnant women indicates no increased risk of birth defects in 3546 pregnancies exposed to penicillin derivatives.
Ask physician for guidance.

Advisability of Use if Breast-Feeding
Presence of this drug in breast milk: Yes.
The nursing infant may be sensitized to penicillin and may be at risk for developing diarrhea or yeast infections.
Avoid drug if possible or refrain from nursing.

Habit-Forming Potential: None.

Effects of Overdosage: Possible nausea, vomiting and/or diarrhea.

Possible Effects of Long-Term Use: Superinfections, often due to yeast organisms.

Suggested Periodic Examinations While Taking This Drug (at physician's discretion)
Complete blood cell counts.

▷ While Taking This Drug, Observe the Following
Foods: No restrictions.
Beverages: No restrictions. May be taken with milk, fruit juices or carbonated drinks.
▷ *Alcohol:* No interactions expected.
Tobacco Smoking: No interactions expected.
▷ *Other Drugs*
Amoxicillin may *decrease* the effects of
- oral contraceptives in some women, and impair their effectiveness in preventing pregnancy.

The following drugs may *decrease* the effects of amoxicillin
- antacids reduce the absorption of amoxicillin.
- chloramphenicol (Chloromycetin).
- erythromycin (Erythrocin, E-Mycin, etc.).
- tetracyclines (Achromycin, Declomycin, Minocin, etc.). (See Drug Class, Section Four.)

▷ *Driving, Hazardous Activities:* Usually no restrictions. Be alert to the rare occurrence of dizziness and/or nausea, and restrict activities accordingly.

Aviation Note: The use of this drug *may be a disqualification* for piloting. Consult a designated Aviation Medical Examiner.

Exposure to Sun: No restrictions.

Special Storage Instructions: Oral suspension and pediatric drops should be refrigerated.

Observe the Following Expiration Times: Do not take the oral suspension or drops of this drug if older than 7 days when kept at room temperature or 14 days when kept refrigerated.

AMPICILLIN
(am pi SIL in)

Introduced: 1961

Class: Antibiotic, penicillins

Prescription: USA: Yes
Canada: Yes

Controlled Drug: USA: No
Canada: No

Available as Generic: Yes

Brand Names: Amcill, ✦Ampicin, ✦Ampicin PRB [CD], ✦Ampilean, ✦Apo-Ampi, 500 Kit [CD], ✦Novo-Ampicillin, Omnipen, Omnipen Pediatric Drops, ✦Penbritin, Polycillin, Polycillin Pediatric Drops, Polycillin-PRB [CD], Principen, Probampacin [CD], ✦Pro-Biosan, Totacillin

---

BENEFITS versus RISKS

Possible Benefits	*Possible Risks*
EFFECTIVE TREATMENT OF INFECTIONS due to susceptible microorganisms	ALLERGIC REACTIONS, mild to severe, in 3% of the general population and 15% of allergic individuals
	Superinfections (yeast)
	Drug-induced colitis

▷ **Principal Uses**

As a Single Drug Product: To treat certain infections of the skin and soft tissues, of the respiratory tract, of the gastrointestinal tract, and of the genitourinary tract (including gonorrhea in females). Also used to treat certain types of septicemia and meningitis.

As a Combination Drug Product [CD]: May be combined with probenecid (Benemid) to delay the elimination of ampicillin by the kidney and thereby increase its level in the blood. This combination drug is designed primarily for the treatment of gonorrhea in males and females.

How This Drug Works: This drug destroys susceptible infecting bacteria by interfering with their ability to produce new protective cell walls as they multiply and grow.

Available Dosage Forms and Strengths

Capsules — 250 mg, 500 mg

Oral suspension — 100 mg per ml, 125 mg, 250 mg, 500 mg per 5-ml teaspoonful

Pediatric drops — 100 mg per ml

▷ **Usual Adult Dosage Range:** 250 to 500 mg/6 hours. The usual maximal dose is 6000 mg/24 hours. **Note: Actual dosage and administration schedule must be determined by the physician for each patient individually.**

▷ **Dosing Instructions:** Best taken on an empty stomach, 1 hour before or 2 hours after eating. Capsule may be opened for administration.

Usual Duration of Use: For all streptococcal infections—not less than 10 consecutive days (without interruption) to reduce the possibility of developing rheumatic fever or glomerulonephritis. For all other infections—as long as necessary to eradicate the infection.

▷ **This Drug Should Not Be Taken If**
- you have had an allergic reaction to any dosage form of it previously.
- you are certain you are allergic to *any* form of penicillin.

▷ **Inform Your Physician Before Taking This Drug If**
- you suspect you may be allergic to penicillin or you have a history of a previous "reaction" to penicillin.
- you are allergic to cephalosporin antibiotics (Ancef, Ceporan, Ceporex, Kafocin, Keflex, Keflin, Kefzol, Loridine).
- you are allergic by nature (hay fever, asthma, hives, eczema).

Possible Side-Effects (natural, expected and unavoidable drug actions)

Superinfections (see Glossary), often due to yeast organisms.

▷ **Possible Adverse Effects** (unusual, unexpected and infrequent reactions) **If any of the following develop, consult your physician promptly for guidance.**

Mild Adverse Effects

Allergic Reactions: Skin rashes, hives, itching.

Irritations of mouth and tongue, "black tongue," nausea, vomiting, mild diarrhea, dizziness (rare).

Serious Adverse Effects

Allergic Reactions: Anaphylactic reaction (see Glossary), severe skin reactions, drug fever, swollen painful joints, sore throat, abnormal bleeding or bruising.

▷ **Possible Effects on Sexual Function:**   None reported.

CAUTION

1. Take the exact dose and the full course prescribed.
2. This drug should not be used concurrently with antibiotics like erythromycin or tetracycline.

Precautions for Use

By Infants and Children: A generalized rash occurs in approximately 90% of individuals who take this drug during an episode of infectious mononucleosis. This drug may cause diarrhea, which sometimes necessitates discontinuation.

By Those over 60 Years of Age: Natural changes in the skin may predispose to prolonged itching reactions in the genital and anal regions. Report such reactions promptly.

▷ **Advisability of Use During Pregnancy**

Pregnancy Category: B (tentative). See Pregnancy Code inside back cover.

Animal studies: No birth defects due to this drug found in mice or rats.

Human studies: Information from adequate studies of pregnant women indicates no increased risk of birth defects in 3546 pregnancies exposed to penicillin derivatives.

Ask physician for guidance.

Advisability of Use if Breast-Feeding

Presence of this drug in breast milk: Yes, in small amounts.

The nursing infant may be sensitized to penicillin and may be at risk for developing diarrhea or yeast infections.

Avoid drug if possible or refrain from nursing.

Habit-Forming Potential: None.

Effects of Overdosage: Possible nausea, vomiting and/or diarrhea.

Possible Effects of Long-Term Use: Superinfections, often due to yeast organisms.

Suggested Periodic Examinations While Taking This Drug (at physician's discretion)

Complete blood cell counts.

▷ **While Taking This Drug, Observe the Following**

Foods: No restrictions.

Beverages: No restrictions. May be taken with milk.

▷ *Alcohol:* No interactions expected.

Tobacco Smoking: No interactions expected.

▷ *Other Drugs*
  Ampicillin may *decrease* the effects of
  • oral contraceptives in some women, and impair their effectiveness in preventing pregnancy.
  The following drugs may *decrease* the effects of ampicillin
  • antacids reduce the absorption of amoxicillin.
  • chloramphenicol (Chloromycetin).
  • erythromycin (Erythrocin, E-Mycin, etc.).
  • tetracyclines (Achromycin, Declomycin, Minocin, etc.). (See Drug Class, Section Four.)
▷ *Driving, Hazardous Activities:* Usually no restrictions. Be alert to the rare occurrence of dizziness and/or nausea, and restrict activities accordingly.
  Aviation Note: The use of this drug *may be a disqualification* for piloting. Consult a designated Aviation Medical Examiner.
  Exposure to Sun: No restrictions.
  Special Storage Instructions: Oral suspension and pediatric drops should be refrigerated.
  Observe the Following Expiration Times: Do not take the oral suspension or drops of this drug if older than 7 days when kept at room temperature or 14 days when kept refrigerated.

ASPIRIN*
(AS pir in)

Other Names: ASA, acetylsalicylic acid

Introduced: 1899

Class: Mild analgesic, anti-inflammatory, antipyretic, salicylates

Prescription: USA: No
  Canada: No

Controlled Drug: USA: No
  Canada: No

Available as Generic: Yes

*In the United States *aspirin* is an official generic designation. In Canada *Aspirin* is the Registered Trade Mark of the Bayer Company Division of Sterling Drug Limited.

Brand Names: Alka-Seltzer Effervescent Pain Reliever & Antacid [CD], Alka-Seltzer Plus [CD], Anacin [CD], Anacin Maximum Strength [CD], ◆Anacin w/Codeine [CD], ◆Ancasal, A.S.A. Enseals, ◆Asasantine [CD], Ascriptin [CD], Ascriptin A/D [CD], Aspergum, ◆Aspirin*, ◆Astrin, Axotal [CD], Azdone [CD], Bayer Aspirin, Bayer Children's Chewable Aspirin, Bufferin [CD], Bufferin Arthritis Strength [CD], Bufferin Extra Strength [CD], Bufferin w/Codeine [CD], Cama Arthritis Pain Reliever [CD], Cope [CD], ◆Coryphen, ◆Coryphen-Codeine [CD], Darvon Compound [CD], Darvon Compound-65 [CD], Darvon w/ASA [CD], ◆Darvon-N Compound [CD], Darvon-N w/ASA [CD], Dolene Compound-65 [CD], Easprin, Ecotrin Preparations, 8-Hour Bayer, Empirin, Empirin w/Codeine No. 2, 4 [CD], ◆Entrophen, Excedrin [CD], Fiorinal [CD], Fiorinal w/Codeine [CD], ◆Fiorinal-C 1/4, -C 1/2 [CD], 4-Way Cold Tablets [CD], Lortab ASA [CD], Maximum Bayer Aspirin, Measurin, Midol Caplets [CD], Norgesic [CD], Norgesic Forte [CD], ◆Novasen, ◆Novopropoxyn Compound [CD], ◆Oxycodan [CD], Percodan [CD], Percodan-Demi [CD], ◆Phenaphen [CD], ◆Phenaphen No. 2, 3, 4 [CD], ◆Riphen-10, Robaxisal [CD], ◆Robaxisal-C [CD], ◆Sal-Adult, ◆Sal-Infant, Sine-Off Tablets [CD], St. Joseph Children's Aspirin, ◆Supasa, Synalgos [CD], Synalgos-DC [CD], Talwin Compound [CD], Talwin Compound-50 [CD], ◆Triaphen-10, Trigesic [CD]

BENEFITS versus RISKS

Possible Benefits	*Possible Risks*
EFFECTIVE RELIEF OF MILD TO MODERATE PAIN and INFLAMMATION	Stomach irritation, bleeding, and/or ulceration
REDUCTION OF FEVER	Hearing loss
PREVENTION OF BLOOD CLOTS (as in heart attack, phlebitis and stroke)	Decreased numbers of white blood cells and platelets
	Hemolytic anemia

▷ **Principal Uses**

As a Single Drug Product: To relieve mild to moderate pain from any cause, to provide symptomatic relief in conditions characterized by inflammation and to reduce high fever. A major use is to treat musculoskeletal disorders, especially acute and chronic arthritis. It is also used selectively in low dosage to prevent platelet embolism to the brain (in men) and to reduce the risk of thromboembolism in patients recovering from a recent heart attack, in those with artificial heart valves and in those undergoing hip surgery. (See Blood Platelets in the Glossary.)

---

*In the United States *aspirin* is an official generic designation. In Canada *Aspirin* is the Registered Trade Mark of the Bayer Company Division of Sterling Drug Limited.

As a Combination Drug Product [CD]: Frequently combined with other mild or strong analgesic drugs to enhance pain relief. Also combined with antihistamines and decongestants in many cold preparations to relieve the headache and general discomfort that often accompany respiratory infections.

How This Drug Works: Aspirin reduces the tissue concentrations of prostaglandins, chemicals involved in the production of inflammation and pain. By modifying the temperature-regulating center in the brain, dilating blood vessels in the skin, and increasing sweating, aspirin hastens the loss of body heat and reduces fever. By preventing the production of thromboxane in blood platelets, aspirin inhibits the aggregation of platelets and the initiation of blood clots.

Available Dosage Forms and Strengths

Capsules, enteric-coated — 500 mg

Capsules, enteric-coated granules — 325 mg

Gum tablets — 227.5 mg

Suppositories — 60 mg, 120 mg, 125 mg, 130 mg, 195 mg, 200 mg, 300 mg, 325 mg, 600 mg, 650 mg, 1.2 grams

Tablets — 65 mg, 81 mg, 325 mg, 500 mg

Tablets, chewable — 81 mg

Tablets, enteric-coated — 325 mg, 500 mg, 650 mg, 975 mg

Tablets, prolonged-action — 650 mg, 800 mg

▷ **Usual Adult Dosage Range:**   For pain or fever—325 to 650 mg/4 hours as needed. For arthritis (and related conditions)—3600 to 5400 mg daily in divided doses. For the prevention of blood clots—80 to 150 mg/24 to 48 hours. **Note: For long-term use, actual dosage and administration schedule must be determined by the physician for each patient individually.**

▷ **Dosing Instructions:**   Take with food, milk, or a full glass of water to reduce stomach irritation. Regular tablets may be crushed and capsules opened for administration. Enteric-coated tablets, prolonged-action tablets, A.S.A. Enseals, Cama tablets and Ecotrin tablets should not be crushed.

Usual Duration of Use: Short-term use is recommended—3 to 5 days. Daily use should not exceed 10 days without physician supervision. Continual use on a regular schedule for 1 week is usually necessary to determine this drug's effectiveness in relieving the symptoms of chronic arthritis. Long-term use requires periodic evaluation of response and dosage adjustment. Consult your physician on a regular basis.

▷ **This Drug Should Not Be Taken If**
- you have had an allergic reaction or unfavorable response to any form of aspirin previously.

- you have any type of bleeding disorder (such as hemophilia).
- you have active peptic ulcer disease.
- it has an odor resembling vinegar. This is due to the presence of acetic acid and indicates the decomposition of aspirin.

▷ **Inform Your Physician Before Taking This Drug If**
- you are taking any anticoagulant drug.
- you are taking oral antidiabetic drugs.
- you have a history of peptic ulcer disease or gout.
- you have lupus erythematosus.
- you are pregnant or planning pregnancy.
- you plan to have surgery of any kind in the near future.

Possible Side-Effects (natural, expected and unavoidable drug actions)
Mild drowsiness in sensitive individuals.

▷ **Possible Adverse Effects** (unusual, unexpected and infrequent reactions)
If any of the following develop, consult your physician promptly for guidance.
Mild Adverse Effects
Allergic Reactions: Skin rash, hives, nasal discharge (resembling hay fever), nasal polyps.
Stomach irritation, heartburn, nausea, vomiting, constipation.
Serious Adverse Effects
Allergic Reactions: Acute anaphylactic reaction (see Glossary), asthma, unusual bruising due to allergic destruction of blood platelets (see Glossary).
Idiosyncratic Reactions: Hemolytic anemia (see Glossary).
Erosion of stomach lining, with silent bleeding.
Activation of peptic ulcer, with or without hemorrhage.
Bone marrow depression (see Glossary)—fatigue, weakness, fever, sore throat, abnormal bleeding or bruising.
Hepatitis with jaundice (see Glossary)—yellow skin and eyes, dark-colored urine, light-colored stool (very rare).
Kidney damage, if used in large doses or for a prolonged period of time.

▷ **Possible Effects on Sexual Function:**   None reported.

▷ **Adverse Effects That May Mimic Natural Diseases or Disorders**
Liver damage may suggest viral hepatitis.

CAUTION
1. It is most important to understand that aspirin is a drug. While it is one of our most useful drugs, we have an unrealistic sense of safety and unconcern regarding its action within the body and its potential for adverse effects.
2. In order to know if you are taking aspirin, make it a point to learn the contents of all drugs you take—those prescribed by your physician and those you purchase over-the-counter (OTC) without prescription.

3. Limit the dose of aspirin to no more than 3 tablets (975 mg) at one time, allow at least 4 hours between doses and take no more than 10 tablets (3250 mg) in 24 hours without physician supervision.
4. Remember that aspirin can
   • cause new illnesses.
   • complicate existing illnesses.
   • complicate pregnancy.
   • complicate surgery.
   • interact unfavorably with other drugs.
5. When your physician asks "Are you taking any drugs?" the answer is yes if you are taking aspirin. This also applies to *any* nonprescription drug you may be taking. (See OTC Drugs in the Glossary.)

Precautions for Use

By Infants and Children: Reye syndrome (brain and liver damage in children, often fatal) can follow flu or chicken pox in children and teenagers. While the exact cause and nature of the syndrome are not known, some reports suggest that the use of aspirin by children with flu or chicken pox can increase the risk of developing this complication. Consult your physician before giving aspirin to a child or teenager with chicken pox, flu or similar infection.

Usual dosage schedule for children:

Up to 2 years of age—consult physician.

2 to 4 years of age—160 mg/4 hours, up to 5 doses/24 hours.

4 to 6 years of age—240 mg/4 hours, up to 5 doses/24 hours.

6 to 9 years of age—320 mg/4 hours, up to 5 doses/24 hours.

9 to 11 years of age—400 mg/4 hours, up to 5 doses/24 hours.

11 to 12 years of age—480 mg/4 hours, up to 5 doses/24 hours.

Do not exceed 5 days of continual use without consulting your physician.

Give all doses with food, milk or a full glass of water.

By Those over 60 Years of Age: The natural decline in kidney function can reduce your tolerance for aspirin. Observe for indications of excessive dosage: nervous irritabilty, confusion, ringing in the ears, deafness, loss of appetite, nausea and stomach irritation. Aspirin can cause excessive bleeding from the stomach in sensitive individuals. This can occur as "silent" bleeding of small amounts over an extended period of time, resulting in anemia. In addition, sudden hemorrhage can occur, even without a history of stomach ulcer. Observe stools for gray to black discoloration—an indication of stomach bleeding.

▷ **Advisability of Use During Pregnancy**

Pregnancy Category: D (tentative). See Pregnancy Code inside back cover.

Animal studies: Significant birth defects due to this drug have been reported.

Human studies: Information from studies of pregnant women indicates no increased risk of birth defects in 32,164 pregnancies exposed to aspirin. However, studies show that the regular use of salicylates during pregnancy is often detrimental to the health of the mother and to the welfare of the fetus. Excessive use of salicylate drugs can cause anemia, hemorrhage before and after delivery and an increased incidence of stillbirths and newborn deaths. It is advisable to limit the use of aspirin during pregnancy to small doses and for brief periods of time, and to avoid aspirin altogether during the last 3 months.

Advisability of Use if Breast-Feeding
Presence of this drug in breast milk: Yes.
Avoid drug or refrain from nursing.

Habit-Forming Potential: Use of this drug in large doses for a prolonged period of time may cause a form of psychological dependence (see Glossary).

Effects of Overdosage: Stomach distress, nausea, vomiting, ringing in the ears, dizziness, impaired hearing, sweating, stupor, fever, deep and rapid breathing, muscular twitching, delirium, hallucinations, convulsions.

Possible Effects of Long-Term Use
A form of psychological dependence (see Glossary).
Anemia due to chronic blood loss from erosion of stomach lining.
The development of stomach ulcer.
The development of "aspirin allergy"—nasal discharge, nasal polyps, asthma.
Kidney damage.
Excessive prolongation of bleeding time, of major importance in the event of injury or surgery.

Suggested Periodic Examinations While Taking This Drug (at physician's discretion)
Complete blood cell counts.
Kidney function tests and urine analyses.
Liver function tests.

▷ **While Taking This Drug, Observe the Following**
Foods: No restrictions.
Nutritional Support: If supplementing the diet with vitamin C, take no more than the recommended daily allowance. Do not take large doses of vitamin C while taking aspirin on a regular basis.
Beverages: No restrictions. May be taken with milk.
▷ *Alcohol:* No interactions expected. However, the concurrent use of alcohol and aspirin may significantly increase the possibility of erosion and ulceration of the stomach lining and may result in bleeding.
Tobacco Smoking: No interactions expected.
▷ *Other Drugs*
Aspirin may *increase* the effects of
• oral anticoagulants, and cause abnormal bleeding. Dosage adjustment is often necessary.

- oral antidiabetic drugs and insulin, and cause hypoglycemia (see Glossary). Dosage adjustment is often necessary.
- heparin, and cause abnormal bleeding.
- methotrexate, and increase its toxic effects.
- valproic acid (Depakene).

Aspirin may *decrease* the effects of
- beta-adrenergic-blocking drugs (see Drug Class, Section Four).
- captopril (Capoten).
- probenecid (Benemid), and reduce its effectiveness in the treatment of gout—with aspirin doses of less than 2 grams/24 hours.
- spironolactone (Aldactone), and reduce its diuretic effect.
- sulfinpyrazone (Anturane), and reduce its effectiveness in the treatment of gout—with aspirin doses of less than 2 grams/24 hours.

The following drugs may *increase* the effects of aspirin
- acetazolamide (Diamox).
- para-aminobenzoic acid (Pabalate).
- vitamin C, taken as ascorbic acid and in large doses, may acidify the urine in some individuals and cause aspirin accumulation and toxicity.

The following drugs may *decrease* the effects of aspirin
- antacids, in regular continual use.
- cortisonelike drugs (see Drug Class, Section Four).
- urinary alkalizers (sodium bicarbonate, sodium citrate).

▷ *Driving, Hazardous Activities:* No restrictions or precautions.

Aviation Note: Usually no restrictions. However, it is advisable to observe for the possible occurrence of mild drowsiness and to restrict activities accordingly.

Exposure to Sun: No restrictions.

Discontinuation: The use of aspirin should be discontinued completely at least 1 week before surgery of any kind.

ATENOLOL
(a TEN oh lohl)

Introduced: 1973

Class: Antianginal, antihypertensive, beta-adrenergic blocker

Prescription: USA: Yes
Canada: Yes

Controlled Drug: USA: No
Canada: No

Available as Generic: No

Brand Names: Tenoretic [CD], Tenormin

BENEFITS versus RISKS

Possible Benefits	*Possible Risks*
EFFECTIVE ANTIANGINAL DRUG in the management of effort-induced angina EFFECTIVE, WELL-TOLERATED ANTIHYPERTENSIVE in mild to moderate high blood pressure	CONGESTIVE HEART FAILURE in advanced heart disease Worsening of angina in coronary heart disease (abrupt withdrawal) Masking of low blood sugar (hypoglycemia) in drug-treated diabetes Provocation of bronchial asthma (with high doses)

▷ **Principal Uses**

As a Single Drug Product: Used primarily to treat (1) classical, effort-induced angina pectoris; (2) mild to moderately severe high blood pressure. May be used alone or concurrently with other antihypertensive drugs, such as diuretics.

How This Drug Works: By blocking certain actions of the sympathetic nervous system, this drug
- reduces the rate and contraction force of the heart, thus lowering the ejection pressure of the blood leaving the heart and reducing the oxygen requirement for heart function.
- reduces the degree of contraction of blood vessel walls, resulting in their relaxation and expansion and consequent lowering of blood pressure.

Available Dosage Forms and Strengths
Tablets — 50 mg, 100 mg

▷ **Usual Adult Dosage Range:** Initially 50 mg once daily. Dose may be increased gradually at intervals of 7 to 10 days as needed and tolerated up to 100 mg/24 hours. The usual maintenance dose is 50 to 100 mg/24 hours. The total dose should not exceed 100 mg/24 hours. **Note: Actual dosage and administration schedule must be determined by the physician for each patient individually.**

▷ **Dosing Instructions:** May be taken without regard to eating. Tablet may be crushed for administration. Do not discontinue this drug abruptly.

Usual Duration of Use: Continual use on a regular schedule for 10 to 14 days is usually necessary to determine this drug's effectiveness in lowering blood pressure. The long-term use of this drug will be determined by the course of your blood pressure over time and your response to the overall treatment program (weight reduction, salt restriction, smoking cessation, etc.). Consult your physician on a regular basis.

Possible Advantages of This Drug: The least likely of all beta blocker drugs to cause central nervous system adverse effects: confusion, halluci- nations, nervousness, nightmares.

Currently a "Drug of Choice" for initiating treatment of hypertension with a single drug, especially for those subject to bronchial asthma or di- abetes.

▷ **This Drug Should Not Be Taken If**
- you have had an allergic reaction to it previously.
- you have congestive heart failure.
- you have an abnormally slow heart rate or a serious form of heart block.
- you are taking, or have taken within the past 14 days, any monoamine oxidase (MAO) type A inhibitor drug (see Drug Class, Section Four).

▷ **Inform Your Physician Before Taking This Drug If**
- you have had an adverse reaction to any beta blocker drug in the past (see Drug Class, Section Four).
- you have a history of serious heart disease, with or without episodes of heart failure.
- you have a history of hay fever (allergic rhinitis), asthma, chronic bronchitis or emphysema.
- you have a history of overactive thyroid function (hyperthyroidism).
- you have a history of low blood sugar (hypoglycemia).
- you have impaired liver or kidney function.
- you have diabetes or myasthenia gravis.
- you are currently taking any form of digitalis, quinidine or reserpine, or any calcium blocker drug (see Drug Class, Section Four).
- you plan to have surgery under general anesthesia in the near future.

Possible Side-Effects (natural, expected and unavoidable drug actions)
Lethargy, fatigability, cold extremities, slow heart rate, light-headed- ness in upright position (see Orthostatic Hypotension in Glossary).

▷ **Possible Adverse Effects** (unusual, unexpected and infrequent reactions)
If any of the following develop, consult your physician promptly for guidance.
Mild Adverse Effects
Allergic Reactions: Skin rash, itching.
Headache, dizziness, drowsiness, abnormal dreams.
Indigestion, nausea, diarrhea.
Joint and muscle discomfort, fluid retention (edema).
Serious Adverse Effects
Mental depression, anxiety.
Chest pain, shortness of breath, precipitation of congestive heart failure.
Induction of bronchial asthma (in asthmatic individuals).

▷ **Possible Effects on Sexual Function:** Decreased libido and impaired po- tency (50 to 100 mg/day). This beta blocker is less likely to cause reduced erectile capacity than most other drugs of this class.

CAUTION
1. **Do not discontinue this drug suddenly** without the knowledge and guidance of your physician. Carry a notation on your person that you are taking this drug.
2. Consult your physician or pharmacist before using nasal decongestants usually present in over-the-counter cold preparations and nose drops. These can cause sudden increases in blood pressure when taken concurrently with beta blocker drugs.
3. Report the development of any tendency to emotional depression.

Precautions for Use

By Infants and Children: Safety and effectiveness for use by those under 12 years of age have not been established. However, if this drug is used, observe for the development of low blood sugar (hypoglycemia) during periods of reduced food intake.

By Those over 60 Years of Age: Proceed **cautiously** with all antihypertensive drugs. Unacceptably high blood pressure should be reduced without creating the risks associated with excessively low blood pressure. Start treatment with small doses, and monitor the blood pressure response frequently. Sudden, rapid and excessive reduction of blood pressure can predispose to stroke or heart attack. Total daily dosage should not exceed 100 mg. Observe for dizziness, unsteadiness, tendency to fall, confusion, hallucinations, depression or urinary frequency.

▷ Advisability of Use During Pregnancy

Pregnancy Category: C (tentative). See Pregnancy Code inside back cover.
Animal studies: Increased resorptions of embryo and fetus reported in rats, but no birth defects.
Human studies: Information from adequate studies of pregnant women is not available.
Avoid use of drug during the first 3 months if possible. Avoid use during labor and delivery because of the possible effects on the newborn infant.

Advisability of Use if Breast-Feeding

Presence of this drug in breast milk: Yes.
Avoid drug if possible. If drug is necessary, observe nursing infant for slow heart rate and indications of low blood sugar.

Habit-Forming Potential: None.

Effects of Overdosage: Weakness, slow pulse, low blood pressure, fainting, cold and sweaty skin, congestive heart failure, possible coma and convulsions.

Possible Effects of Long-Term Use: Reduced heart reserve and eventual heart failure in susceptible individuals with advanced heart disease.

Suggested Periodic Examinations While Taking This Drug (at physician's discretion)

Measurements of blood pressure, evaluation of heart function.

▷ **While Taking This Drug, Observe the Following**

Foods: No restrictions. Avoid excessive salt intake.

Beverages: No restrictions. May be taken with milk.

▷ *Alcohol:* Use with caution until the combined effect has been determined. Alcohol may exaggerate this drug's ability to lower blood pressure and may increase its mild sedative effect.

Tobacco Smoking: Nicotine may reduce this drug's effectiveness in treating high blood pressure. In addition, high doses of this drug may potentiate the constriction of the bronchial tubes caused by regular smoking.

▷ *Other Drugs*

Atenolol may *increase* the effects of

- other antihypertensive drugs and cause excessive lowering of blood pressure. Dosage adjustments may be necessary.
- reserpine (Ser-Ap-Es, etc.) and cause sedation, depression, slowing of heart rate and lowering of blood pressure.

Atenolol *taken concurrently* with

- clonidine (Catapres) requires close monitoring for rebound high blood pressure if clonidine is withdrawn while atenolol is still being taken.
- insulin requires close monitoring to avoid undetected hypoglycemia (see Glossary).

The following drugs may *decrease* the effects of atenolol

- indomethacin (Indocin), and possibly other "aspirin substitutes," may impair atenolol's antihypertensive effect.

▷ *Driving, Hazardous Activities:* Use caution until the full extent of drowsiness, lethargy, and blood pressure change has been determined.

Aviation Note: The use of this drug *is a disqualification* for piloting. Consult a designated Aviation Medical Examiner.

Exposure to Sun: No restrictions.

Exposure to Heat: Caution advised. Hot environments can lower blood pressure and exaggerate the effects of this drug.

Exposure to Cold: Caution advised. Cold environments can enhance the circulatory deficiency in the extremities that may occur with this drug. The elderly should take precautions to prevent hypothermia (see Glossary).

Heavy Exercise or Exertion: It is advisable to avoid exertion that produces light-headedness, excessive fatigue, or muscle cramping. The use of this drug may intensify the hypertensive response to isometric exercise.

Occurrence of Unrelated Illness: The fever that accompanies systemic infections can lower blood pressure and require adjustment of dosage. Illnesses that cause nausea or vomiting may interrupt the regular dosage schedule. Ask your physician for guidance.

Discontinuation: It is advisable to avoid sudden discontinuation of this drug in all situations. If possible, gradual reduction of dose over a period of 2 to 3 weeks is recommended. Ask your physician for specific guidance.

ATROPINE*
(A troh peen)

Other Names: Belladonna alkaloids, hyoscyamine, scopolamine

Introduced: 1831

Class: Antispasmodic, atropinelike drugs, anticholinergics

Prescription: USA: Yes
Canada: No

Controlled Drug: USA: No
Canada: No

Available as Generic: Yes

Brand Names: Barbidonna [CD], Barbidonna Elixir [CD], Belladenal [CD], Belladenal-S [CD], ♦Belladenal Spacetabs [CD], ♦Bellergal [CD], Bellergal-S [CD], ♦Bellergal Spacetabs [CD], Butibel [CD], Cafergot P-B [CD], Chardonna-2 [CD], Donnagel [CD], ♦Donnagel w/Neomycin [CD], Kinesed [CD], Lomotil [CD], Pyridium Plus [CD], Urised [CD], ♦Wigraine [CD]

BENEFITS versus RISKS

Possible Benefits	*Possible Risks*
EFFECTIVE ANTISPASMODIC ACTION in spastic disorders of the stomach and intestine	Increased internal eye pressure (important in glaucoma)
	Constipation (may be quite marked)
	Urinary retention (in predisposed persons)

▷ **Principal Uses**

As a Single Drug Product: Used primarily for its antispasmodic effect in the treatment of spastic disorders of the digestive tract and lower urinary tract.

As a Combination Drug Product [CD]: Frequently combined with mild sedatives (especially barbiturates) to utilize their calming effects in the management of functional disorders associated with anxiety and nervous tension. The combination of a mild tranquilizer and an antispasmodic medication is more effective than either drug used alone.

---

*Atropine, hyoscyamine and scopolamine are the principal belladonna alkaloids. The characteristics of atropine are representative of the group.

How This Drug Works: By blocking the action of the chemical (acetylcholine) that transmits impulses at parasympathetic nerve endings, this drug prevents stimulation of muscular contraction and glandular secrection within the organs involved. This results in reduced overall activity, including the prevention or relief of muscle spasm.

Available Dosage Forms and Strengths

Injection — 0.05 mg, 0.1 mg, 0.3 mg, 0.4 mg, 0.5 mg, 0.8 mg, 1 mg, 1.2 mg, all per ml

Tablets — 0.4 mg

Tablets, soluble — 0.3 mg, 0.4 mg, 0.6 mg

▷ **Usual Adult Dosage Range:**   0.3 to 1.2 mg/4 to 6 hours. **Note: Actual dosage and administration schedule must be determined by the physician for each patient individually.**

▷ **Dosing Instructions:**   For maximal absorption and effect, this drug should be taken 30 to 60 minutes before eating. Regular tablets may be crushed and regular capsules may be opened for administration. Prolonged-action and sustained-release dosage forms should be taken whole (neither crushed nor opened).

Usual Duration of Use: Continual use on a regular schedule for 2 to 5 days is usually necessary to determine this drug's effectiveness in relieving the symptoms of spastic disorders of the digestive system. Limit use to the relief of symptoms as necessary. Ask physician for guidance regarding long-term use.

▷ **This Drug Should Not Be Taken If**
* you have had an allergic reaction or unfavorable response to any atropine or belladonna preparation in the past.
* your stomach cannot empty properly into the intestine (pyloric obstruction).
* you are unable to empty the urinary bladder completely.
* you have glaucoma (narrow-angle type).
* you have severe ulcerative colitis.

▷ **Inform Your Physician Before Taking This Drug If**
* you have glaucoma (open-angle type).
* you have angina or coronary heart disease.
* you have chronic bronchitis.
* you have a hiatal hernia or peptic ulcer disease.
* you have enlargement of the prostate gland.
* you have myasthenia gravis.
* you plan to have surgery under general anesthesia in the near future.

Possible Side-Effects (natural, expected and unavoidable drug actions)

Blurring of near vision (impairment of focus), dryness of mouth and throat, constipation, hesitancy in urination.

▷ **Possible Adverse Effects** (unusual, unexpected and infrequent reactions)
If any of the following develop, consult your physician promptly for guidance.
Mild Adverse Effects
Allergic Reactions: Skin rash, hives.
Light-headedness, dizziness, unsteadiness.
Dilation of pupils, causing sensitivity to light.
Flushing and dryness of skin, reduced sweating.
Serious Adverse Effects
Allergic Reactions: Severe skin reactions—exfoliative dermatitis.
Idiosyncratic Reactions: Paradoxical excitement, nervousness, confusion, delirium.
Increased internal eye pressure, development of glaucoma in susceptible individuals.

▷ **Possible Effects on Sexual Function:** Inhibited female orgasm, reduced male fertility (0.4 to 0.6 mg/dose).

Natural Diseases or Disorders That May Be Activated by This Drug
Latent glaucoma (narrow-angle type), latent myasthenia gravis.

CAUTION
1. Use cautiously in the presence of asthma and chronic bronchitis. This drug can thicken bronchial secretions and promote retention of mucous plugs.
2. Many over-the-counter medications (see OTC Drugs in the Glossary) for allergies, colds and coughs contain antihistamines that can augment this drug's drying effects. Ask your physician or pharmacist for guidance before using such preparations.

Precautions for Use
By Infants and Children: Children are particularly vulnerable to atropine toxicity. Start with low doses and increase cautiously as needed and tolerated. Observe for idiosyncratic reactions consisting of flushing, high fever, agitation, rapid pulse and breathing. Children with Down's syndrome or brain damage are more susceptible to this type of reaction.
By Those over 60 Years of Age: Observe for agitation, confusion, loss of short-term memory, disorientation, visual and auditory hallucinations, delirium. This drug can increase the degree of impaired urination associated with prostate gland enlargement (prostatism).

▷ **Advisability of Use During Pregnancy**
Pregnancy Category: C (tentative). See Pregnancy Code inside back cover.
Animal studies: Birth defects reported in mouse studies.
Human studies: No increase in birth defects reported in 1198 exposures to this drug. Information from adequate studies of pregnant women is not available.
Avoid drug completely during first 3 months.

Advisability of Use if Breast-Feeding
Presence of this drug in breast milk: Yes, in very small amounts.
Monitor nursing infant closely and discontinue drug or nursing if adverse effects develop.

Habit-Forming Potential: None.

Effects of Overdosage: Dilated pupils, blurring of near vision, dryness of mouth and throat, heart palpitation, impaired urination, high fever, hot skin, excitement, confusion, hallucinations, delirium, convulsions, coma.

Possible Effects of Long-Term Use: Chronic constipation, severe enough to result in fecal impaction. (Constipation should be treated promptly with effective laxatives.)

Suggested Periodic Examinations While Taking This Drug (at physician's discretion)
Measurement of internal eye pressure to detect any significant increase that could indicate developing glaucoma.

▷ **While Taking This Drug, Observe the Following**
Foods: Avoid constipating foods, such as cheeses. Follow the diet prescribed by your physician.
Beverages: Avoid large amounts of tea (may be constipating).
▷   *Alcohol:* No interactions expected.
Tobacco Smoking: No interactions expected.
▷   *Other Drugs*
Atropine may ***increase*** the effects of
• all other drugs having atropinelike actions (see Drug Class, Section Four).
Atropine may ***decrease*** the effects of
• haloperidol (Haldol), and reduce its effectiveness.
• phenothiazines (Thorazine, etc.), and reduce their effectiveness.
• pilocarpine eye drops, and reduce their effectiveness in lowering internal eye pressure in the treatment of glaucoma.
▷   *Driving, Hazardous Activities:* This drug may cause drowsiness, dizziness or blurred vision. Avoid hazardous activities if these drug effects occur.
Aviation Note: The use of this drug ***is a disqualification*** for piloting. Consult a designated Aviation Medical Examiner.
Exposure to Sun: No restrictions.
Exposure to Heat: Use extreme caution. The use of this drug in hot environments may significantly increase the risk of heat stroke.
Heavy Exercise or Exertion: Use caution in warm or hot environments. This drug may impair normal perspiration (heat loss) and interfere with the regulation of body temperature.
Discontinuation: Avoid prolonged and unnecessary use of this drug. When symptoms have been controlled for an adequate period of time, and

discontinuation appears possible, reduce the dose gradually over a period of several days.

AURANOFIN
(aw RAY noh fin)

Introduced: 1976

Class: Antiarthritic, gold compounds

Prescription: USA: Yes
Canada: Yes

Controlled Drug: USA: No
Canada: No

Available as Generic: No

Brand Name: Ridaura

BENEFITS versus RISKS

Possible Benefits	*Possible Risks*
REDUCTION OF JOINT PAIN, TENDERNESS AND SWELLING in active, severe RHEUMATOID ARTHRITIS Medication effective when taken by mouth	SIGNIFICANTLY REDUCED LEVELS OF RED AND WHITE BLOOD CELLS AND BLOOD PLATELETS (1% to 3%) LIVER DAMAGE WITH JAUNDICE (less than 0.1%) Diarrhea (47%), ulcerative colitis (less than 0.1%) Skin rash (24%) Mouth sores (13%)

▷ **Principal Uses**

As a Single Drug Product: Used *only* for the treatment of adults with active, severe rheumatoid arthritis who have had an inadequate and disappointing response to aspirin, aspirin substitutes and other antiarthritic drugs and treatment programs. It is usually added to a well-established program of antiarthritic drugs of the aspirin-substitute class.

How This Drug Works: Its method of action is unknown. It suppresses but does not cure arthritis and associated synovitis.

Available Dosage Forms and Strengths

Capsules — 3 mg

▷ **Usual Adult Dosage Range:** 6 mg daily, taken either as one dose every 24 hours or as two doses of 3 mg each every 12 hours. If response is inadequate after 6 months of regular continual use, the dose may be increased to 9 mg daily, taken as 3 doses of 3 mg each. If response remains inadequate after 3 months of 9 mg daily, this drug should be discontinued. **Note: Actual dosage and administration schedule must be determined by the physician for each patient individually.**

▷ **Dosing Instructions:** Take with or following food to reduce stomach irritation. Take the capsule whole with milk or a full glass of water.

Usual Duration of Use: Continual use on a regular schedule for 3 to 4 months is usually necessary to determine this drug's effectiveness in reducing the joint pain, tenderness and swelling associated with rheumatoid arthritis. The extent of long-term use will be determined by the degree of benefit and the pattern of adverse effects experienced by the individual patient. Consult your physician on a regular basis.

▷ **This Drug Should Not Be Taken If**
- you have had an allergic reaction or serious adverse effect from previous use of gold.
- you have active ulcerative colitis.
- you have a current blood cell or bone marrow disorder.
- you have active liver or kidney disease.
- you are pregnant or breast-feeding.
- you are taking penicillamine or antimalarial drugs for your arthritis.

▷ **Inform Your Physician Before Taking This Drug If**
- you are allergic by nature, or have a history of allergic reactions to drugs.
- you have diabetes.
- you have a history of heart disease, high blood pressure, circulatory disorders, liver or kidney disease, or ulcerative colitis.
- you are taking any other drugs at this time.
- you are planning pregnancy in the near future.

Possible Side-Effects (natural, expected and unavoidable drug actions)
Metallic taste.

▷ **Possible Adverse Effects** (unusual, unexpected and infrequent reactions)
If any of the following develop, consult your physician promptly for guidance.
Mild Adverse Effects
Allergic Reactions: Itching, skin rash.
Sores in mouth and throat and on tongue, loss of appetite, nausea, vomiting, stomach cramps, diarrhea.
Headache, partial or complete hair loss.
Serious Adverse Effects
Allergic Reactions: Severe skin reactions, exfoliative dermatitis.
Fever, cough, shortness of breath, drug-induced pneumonia and lung damage.
Liver damage with jaundice, ulcerative colitis.
Kidney damage.

Blood cell and bone marrow toxicity—fatigue, weakness, sore throat, abnormal bleeding or bruising.

Peripheral neuritis—pain, numbness, weakness of arms and legs.

▷ **Possible Effects on Sexual Function:**   None reported.

Possible Delayed Adverse Effects: Adverse effects from gold may occur many months after treatment has been discontinued. This is due to accumulation of gold in body tissues and its slow elimination. Report any indications of possible toxicity to your physician promptly.

▷ **Adverse Effects That May Mimic Natural Diseases or Disorders**
Fever, cough and chest discomfort may suggest respiratory tract infections such as bronchitis or pneumonia.

Liver damage may suggest viral hepatitis.

CAUTION
1. Periodic examinations (blood and urine tests) are mandatory during the use of this drug. Keep all appointments as directed by your physician.
2. Inform your physician promptly of any indications of possible toxic reactions. If there is a delay in reaching your physician, discontinue this drug until you obtain medical guidance.

Precautions for Use
By Infants and Children: Safety and effectiveness for use by those under 12 years of age have not been established.

By Those over 60 Years of Age: Tolerance to gold usually decreases with advancing age. Use small doses initially and observe closely for indications of adverse effects.

▷ **Advisability of Use During Pregnancy**
Pregnancy Category: C (tentative). See Pregnancy Code inside back cover.

Animal studies: Rabbit studies revealed an increase in resorptions, abortions and birth defects.

Human studies: Information from adequate studies of pregnant women is not available.

The manufacturer does not recommend the use of this drug during pregnancy.

Advisability of Use if Breast-Feeding
Presence of this drug in breast milk: Yes.

Avoid drug or refrain from nursing.

Habit-Forming Potential: None.

Effects of Overdosage: Nausea, vomiting, diarrhea, confusion, delirium, peripheral neuritis.

Suggested Periodic Examinations While Taking This Drug (at physician's discretion)
Complete blood cell counts, urine analyses, liver and kidney function tests.

▷ **While Taking This Drug, Observe the Following**
Foods: No restrictions.
Beverages: No restrictions. May be taken with milk.
▷ *Alcohol:* Use caution until the combined effects have been determined.
Alcohol may intensify the irritant effect of this drug on the gastrointestinal tract.
Tobacco Smoking: No interactions expected.
▷ *Other Drugs*
Auranofin may *increase* the effects of
• phenytoin (Dilantin), by increasing its blood level. Monitor closely for indications of phenytoin toxicity.
▷ *Driving, Hazardous Activities:* Usually no restrictions.
Aviation Note: The use of this drug *may be a disqualification* for piloting. Consult a designated Aviation Medical Examiner.
Exposure to Sun: Use caution. This drug may cause photosensitivity (see Glossary). Avoid sun and sun lamps if a drug-induced rash occurs.

AZATADINE
(a ZA ta deen)

Introduced: 1977   **Class:** Antihistamines

Prescription: USA: Yes   **Controlled Drug:** USA: No
　　　　　　Canada: Yes   Canada: No

Available as Generic: No

Brand Names: Optimine, Trinalin Repetabs [CD]

BENEFITS versus RISKS	
Possible Benefits	*Possible Risks*
EFFECTIVE RELIEF OF ALLERGIC RHINITIS AND ALLERGIC SKIN DISORDERS	Mild sedation Atropinelike effects Rare blood cell disorders: hemolytic anemia, abnormally low white blood cell and platelet counts

▷ **Principal Uses**
As a Single Drug Product: Used primarily to provide symptomatic relief in allergic and related disorders: seasonal and perennial allergic rhinitis (hay fever), allergic conjunctivitis, and vasomotor rhinitis; also in hives and localized swellings (angioedema) of allergic origin.

As a Combination Drug Product [CD]: This drug is combined with a decongestant drug to enhance its ability to reduce tissue swelling and
secretions in allergic and infectious disorders of the upper respiratory
tract—hay fever, head colds and sinusitis.

How This Drug Works: Antihistamines reduce the intensity of the allergic
response by blocking the action of histamine after it has been released
from sensitized tissue cells in the eyes, nose and skin.

Available Dosage Forms and Strengths
Tablets — 1 mg

▷ **Usual Adult Dosage Range:**   1 to 2 mg/12 hours as needed (twice daily).
**Note: Actual dosage and administration schedule must be determined
by the physician for each patient individually.**

▷ **Dosing Instructions:**   Take with food or milk to prevent stomach irritation.
The prolonged-action (combination) tablet should be swallowed
whole (not crushed or chewed).

Usual Duration of Use: Continual use on a regular schedule for 2 to 3 days
is usually necessary to determine this drug's effectiveness in relieving
the symptoms of allergic rhinitis and dermatosis. It may be necessary
to take this drug throughout the entire pollen season, depending upon
individual sensitivity. However, antihistamines should not be taken
continually (without interruption) for long-term use. Limit their use
to periods that require symptomatic relief.

▷ **This Drug Should Not Be Taken If**
   • you have had an allergic reaction to any dosage form of it previously.
   • you are currently undergoing allergy skin tests.
   • you are taking, or have taken within the past 14 days, any monoamine
     oxidase (MAO) type A inhibitor drug (see Drug Class, Section Four).

▷ **Inform Your Physician Before Taking This Drug If**
   • you have had any allergic reactions or unfavorable responses to the
     previous use of antihistamines.
   • you have glaucoma (narrow-angle type) or asthma.
   • you have difficulty emptying the urinary bladder, especially if due to
     prostate gland enlargement.
   • you are taking an anticoagulant at this time.
   • you plan to have surgery under general anesthesia in the near future.

Possible Side-Effects (natural, expected and unavoidable drug actions)
Drowsiness; sense of weakness; blurred vision; dryness of the nose,
mouth and throat; impaired urination.

▷ **Possible Adverse Effects** (unusual, unexpected and infrequent reactions)
**If any of the following develop, consult your physician promptly for
guidance.**

Mild Adverse Effects
Allergic Reaction: Skin rash.
Headache, nervous agitation, dizziness, confusion.
Reduced tolerance for contact lenses.
Thickening of bronchial secretions in asthma or bronchitis.
Indigestion, nausea, vomiting.

Serious Adverse Effects
Hemolytic anemia (see Glossary).
Abnormally low white blood cell count—fever, sore throat, infections.
Abnormally low blood platelet count—abnormal bleeding or bruising.

▷ **Possible Effects on Sexual Function:** Shortened menstrual cycle (early arrival of expected menstrual onset).

CAUTION
1. Discontinue this drug 4 days before diagnostic skin testing procedures in order to prevent false negative test results.
2. Do not use this drug if you have active bronchial asthma, bronchitis or pneumonia. It can thicken bronchial mucus and make it more difficult to remove (by absorption or coughing).

Precautions for Use
By Infants and Children: Safety and effectiveness for use by those under 12 years of age have not been established.
By Those over 60 Years of Age: You may be more susceptible to the development of drowsiness, dizziness, and unsteadiness, and to impairment of thinking, judgment and memory. This drug can increase the degree of impaired urination associated with prostate gland enlargement (prostatism).

▷ **Advisability of Use During Pregnancy**
Pregnancy Category: B (tentative). See Pregnancy Code inside back cover.
Animal studies: Reproduction studies of rats and rabbits revealed no increase in birth defects.
Human studies: Information from adequate studies of pregnant women is not available.
Avoid this drug during the last 3 months because of the potential risk for serious adverse effects on the newborn infant.

Advisability of Use if Breast-Feeding
Presence of this drug in breast milk: Unknown.
Avoid drug or refrain from nursing.

Habit-Forming Potential: None.

Effects of Overdosage: Drowsiness; unsteadiness; faintness; marked dryness of mouth, nose and throat; flushing of face; shortness of breath; hallucinations; convulsions.

Possible Effects of Long-Term Use: Tardive dyskinesia (see Glossary) has been reported in association with the long-term use of several widely used antihistamines. It is advisable to avoid the prolonged, continual use of antihistamines without interruption.

Suggested Periodic Examinations While Taking This Drug (at physician's discretion)
Complete blood cell counts.

▷ **While Taking This Drug, Observe the Following**
Foods: No restrictions.
Beverages: No restrictions. May be taken with milk.
▷ *Alcohol:* Use with extreme caution until the combined effects have been determined. The combination of antihistamine and alcohol can produce rapid and marked sedation.
Tobacco Smoking: No interactions expected.
▷ *Other Drugs*
Azatadine may *increase* the effects of
• all sedatives, sleep-inducing drugs, tranquilizers, analgesics, and narcotic drugs, and produce oversedation.
Azatadine may *decrease* the effects of
• oral anticoagulants (Warfarin, etc.), by hastening their elimination from the body. Consult physician regarding prothrombin time testing and dosage adjustment.
The following drugs may *increase* the effects of azatadine
• monoamine oxidase (MAO) type A inhibitor drugs (see Drug Class, Section Four) may prolong the action of antihistamines.
▷ *Driving, Hazardous Activities:* This drug can impair mental alertness, judgment, coordination and reaction time. Avoid hazardous activities until the full sedative effects have been determined.
Aviation Note: The use of this drug *may be a disqualification* for piloting. Consult a designated Aviation Medical Examiner.
Exposure to Sun: Use caution. This drug may cause photosensitivity in some individuals (see Glossary).

AZATHIOPRINE
(ay za THI oh preen)

Introduced: 1965

Class: Antiarthritic, immunosuppressive

Prescription: USA: Yes
Canada: Yes

Controlled Drug: USA: No
Canada: No

Available as Generic: No

Brand Name: Imuran

BENEFITS versus RISKS	
Possible Benefits	*Possible Risks*
REDUCTION OF JOINT PAIN, TENDERNESS AND SWELLING in active, severe RHEUMATOID ARTHRITIS (66% of users) PREVENTION OF REJECTION IN ORGAN TRANSPLANTATION	UNACCEPTABLE ADVERSE EFFECTS IN 15% OF USERS REDUCED LEVELS OF WHITE BLOOD CELLS (28% in rheumatoid arthritis, 50% in kidney transplants) REDUCED LEVELS OF RED BLOOD CELLS AND PLATELETS LIVER DAMAGE WITH JAUNDICE (less than 1%) POSSIBLE INCREASED RISK OF MALIGNANCY (3%)

▷ **Principal Uses**

As a Single Drug Product: Used primarily as an immunosuppressant to prevent rejection in organ transplantation (mainly kidney transplants). Also used to manage active, severe rheumatoid arthritis (in adults) that has failed to respond adequately to conventional treatment. Progression of the arthritic process may be slowed or even stopped. Lesser uses include treatment of lupus erythematosus, ulcerative colitis, chronic active hepatitis and other "autoimmune" disorders.

How This Drug Works: Not fully known. It is thought that by impairing purine metabolism, blocking production of DNA and RNA, and inhibiting cell multiplication, this drug suppresses the immune reaction that is responsible for such "autoimmune" disorders as rheumatoid arthritis, lupus erythematosus, etc.

Available Dosage Forms and Strengths

Injection — 100 mg per 20-ml vial

Tablets — 50 mg

▷ **Usual Adult Dosage Range:** As immunosuppressant—3 to 5 mg/kilogram of body weight daily, 1 to 3 days before transplantation surgery; for postoperative maintenance—1 to 2 mg/kilogram of body weight daily. As antiarthritic—1 mg/kilogram of body weight daily for 6 to 8 weeks; increase dose by 0.5 mg/kilogram of body weight every 4 weeks as needed and tolerated. Maximal daily dose is 2.5 mg/kilogram of body weight. Total dose may be taken once daily or divided into 2 equal doses taken 12 hours apart. **Note: Actual dosage and administration schedule must be determined by the physician for each patient individually.**

▷ **Dosing Instructions:** Take with or following food to reduce stomach irritation. Tablet may be crushed for administration.

Usual Duration of Use: Continual use on a regular schedule for 12 weeks is usually necessary to determine this drug's effectiveness in favorably modifying the course of rheumatoid arthritis. This drug has been used successfully for periods of up to 11 years. Consult your physician on a regular basis.

▷ **This Drug Should Not Be Taken If**
  • you have had an allergic reaction to it previously.
  • you are pregnant, and this drug is prescribed to treat rheumatoid arthritis.
  • you have an active blood cell or bone marrow disorder.
  • you are taking, or have recently taken, any form of chlorambucil (Leukeran), cyclophosphamide (Cytoxan) or melphalan (Alkeran).

▷ **Inform Your Physician Before Taking This Drug If**
  • you have any kind of active infection.
  • you have any form of cancer.
  • you have gout or are taking allopurinol (Zyloprim).
  • you have a history of blood cell or bone marrow disorders.
  • you have impaired liver or kidney function.
  • you are taking any form of gold, penicillamine or an antimalarial drug for arthritis.
  • you plan pregnancy in the near future.

Possible Side-Effects (natural, expected and unavoidable drug actions)
  Development of infection (2.4%).

▷ **Possible Adverse Effects** (unusual, unexpected and infrequent reactions)
  If any of the following develop, consult your physician promptly for guidance.
  Mild Adverse Effects
  Allergic Reaction: Skin rash (2%).
  Loss of appetite, nausea, vomiting, diarrhea (19%).
  Sores on lips and in mouth.
  Serious Adverse Effects
  Allergic Reactions: Drug fever (see Glossary), joint and muscle pain.
  Pancreatitis—severe stomach pain with nausea and vomiting (0.18%).
  Bone marrow depression (see Glossary)—fatigue, weakness, fever, sore throat, abnormal bleeding or bruising.
  Liver damage—yellow eyes and skin, dark-colored urine, light-colored stools (0.37%). (See Hepatitis and Jaundice in Glossary.)
  Drug-induced pneumonia—cough, shortness of breath.
  Development of cancer—skin cancer, reticulum-cell sarcoma, lymphoma, leukemia (3.3%).

▷ **Possible Effects on Sexual Function:** Reversal of male infertility that is due to the body's production of autoantibodies to sperm; this drug suppresses the formation of autoantibodies and permits the normal accumulation of sperm as they are produced.

Possible Delayed Adverse Effects: Bone marrow depression may become apparent many weeks after discontinuing this drug.

▷ **Adverse Effects That May Mimic Natural Diseases or Disorders**
Liver damage may suggest viral hepatitis.

CAUTION
1. Report promptly any indications of a developing infection—fever, chills, lip or mouth sores, etc.
2. Inform your physician promptly if you become pregnant.
3. Periodic blood counts are mandatory for the safe use of this drug. Report for examinations as directed.

Precautions for Use
By Infants and Children: Safety and effectiveness for use by those under 12 years of age have not been established.
By Those over 60 Years of Age: To reduce the risk of possible toxic reactions, the minimal effective dose should be determined and maintained.

▷ **Advisability of Use During Pregnancy**
Pregnancy Category: D (tentative). See Pregnancy Code inside back cover.
Animal studies: Birth defects reported in rodent studies.
Human studies: Two incidents of birth defects reported.
Information from adequate studies of pregnant women is not available.
Avoid completely during entire pregnancy if possible.

Advisability of Use if Breast-Feeding
Presence of this drug in breast milk: Unknown.
Avoid drug or refrain from nursing.

Habit-Forming Potential: None.

Effects of Overdosage: Immediate—nausea, vomiting, diarrhea. Delayed—lowered white blood cell and platelet counts.

Possible Effects of Long-Term Use: Susceptibility to infection, bone marrow depression, development of malignancies.

Suggested Periodic Examinations While Taking This Drug (at physician's discretion)
Complete blood cell counts, liver function tests.

▷ **While Taking This Drug, Observe the Following**
Foods: No restrictions.
Beverages: No restrictions. May be taken with milk.
▷ *Alcohol:* No interactions expected.
Tobacco Smoking: No interactions expected.

▷ *Other Drugs*

Azathioprine may **decrease** the effects of
- oral anticoagulants (warfarin, etc.), and make it necessary to increase their dosage.
- certain muscle relaxants (gallamine, pancuronium, tubocurarine), and make it necessary to increase their dosage.

The following drugs may **increase** the effects of azathioprine
- allopurinol (Zyloprim) may increase its activity and toxicity and make it necessary to reduce its dosage.

▷ *Driving, Hazardous Activities:* No restrictions.

Aviation Note: The use of this drug **may be a disqualification** for piloting. Consult a designated Aviation Medical Examiner.

Exposure to Sun: No restrictions.

Discontinuation: If possible, do not discontinue this drug suddenly. A gradual reduction in dosage is preferable. Consult your physician for a withdrawal schedule.

BACAMPICILLIN
(bak am pi SIL in)

Introduced: 1979

Class: Antibiotic, penicillins

Prescription: USA: Yes
    Canada: Yes

Controlled Drug: USA: No
    Canada: No

Available as Generic: No

Brand Names: ✦Penglobe, Spectrobid

BENEFITS versus RISKS

Possible Benefits	*Possible Risks*
EFFECTIVE TREATMENT OF INFECTIONS due to susceptible microorganisms	ALLERGIC REACTIONS, mild to severe, in 3% of the general population and 15% of allergic individuals Superinfections (yeast) Drug-induced colitis

---

▷ **Principal Uses**

As a Single Drug Product: To treat certain infections of the skin and skin structures, of the upper and lower respiratory tract, and of the genitourinary tract, including gonorrhea.

How This Drug Works: During its absorption from the gastrointestinal tract, bacampicillin is converted to ampicillin. The unique chemical modification that characterizes bacampicillin permits its more rapid and complete absorption than ampicillin. When given in equivalent doses, bacampicillin provides peak blood levels that are 3 times higher than the levels provided by unmodified ampicillin. Thus bacampicillin can be effective when given every 12 hours; ampicillin requires a dosage schedule of every 6 hours. (See the Drug Profile of ampicillin.)

Available Dosage Forms and Strengths
Oral suspension — 125 mg per 5-ml teaspoonful
Tablets — 400 mg

▷ **Usual Adult Dosage Range:**   400 to 800 mg/12 hours. **Note: Actual dosage and administration schedule must be determined by the physician for each patient individually.**

▷ **Dosing Instructions:**   Tablets may be taken without regard to eating. The oral suspension should be taken on an empty stomach, 1 hour before or 2 hours after eating. The tablet may be crushed for administration.

Usual Duration of Use: Continual use on a regular schedule for 5 to 7 days is usually necessary to determine this drug's effectiveness in eradicating the infection. Treatment is usually continued for 2 to 3 days after all indications of infection are gone. Treatment for all streptococcal infections should be for no less than 10 consecutive days (without interruption) to reduce the possibility of developing rheumatic fever or glomerulonephritis.

▷ **While Taking This Drug, Observe the Following**
▷ *Other Drugs*
Bacampicillin *taken concurrently* with
- allopurinol (Zyloprim) substantially increases the incidence of skin rash.
- disulfiram (Antabuse) can cause a disulfiramlike reaction (see Glossary). Avoid the concurrent use of these 2 drugs.

The following drugs may *decrease* the effects of bacampicillin
- chloramphenicol (Chloromycetin).
- erythromycins (E-Mycin, Erythrocin, etc.).
- sulfonamides ("Sulfa" drugs, see Drug Class, Section Four).
- tetracyclines (see Drug Class, Section Four).

Note: The information categories provided in this Profile are appropriate for bacampicillin. For specific information that is normally found in those categories that have been omitted from this Profile, the reader is referred to the Drug Profile of ampicillin.

BECLOMETHASONE
(be kloh METH a sohn)

Introduced: 1976

Class: Antiallergic, antiasthmatic, cortisonelike drugs

Prescription: USA: Yes
Canada: Yes

Controlled Drug: USA: No
Canada: No

Available as Generic: No

Brand Names: Beclovent, ✦Beclovent Rotacaps, ✦Beclovent Rotahaler, Beconase AQ Nasal Spray, Beconase Nasal Inhaler, ✦Propaderm, Vancenase AQ Nasal Spray, Vancenase Nasal Inhaler, Vanceril

BENEFITS versus RISKS	
Possible Benefits	*Possible Risks*
EFFECTIVE RELIEF OF ALLERGIC RHINITIS EFFECTIVE CONTROL OF SEVERE, CHRONIC ASTHMA	FUNGUS INFECTIONS OF THE MOUTH AND THROAT Localized areas of "allergic" pneumonia

▷ **Principal Uses**

As a Single Drug Product: Used primarily to treat bronchial asthma in those individuals who do not respond to bronchodilators and who require cortisonelike drugs for asthma control. This inhalation dosage form is significantly more advantageous than cortisone taken by mouth (swallowed) or by injection in that it works locally on the tissues of the respiratory tract and does not require absorption and systemic distribution. This prevents the more serious adverse effects that usually result from the long-term use of cortisone taken for systemic effects.

How This Drug Works: Not established. One possibility is that by increasing the amount of cyclic AMP in appropriate tissues, this drug may thereby increase the concentration of epinephrine, which is an effective bronchodilator and antiasthmatic. Additional benefit may be due to the drug's ability to reduce local inflammation in the lining tissues of the respiratory tract.

Available Dosage Forms and Strengths

Nasal inhaler — 16.8 grams (200 doses of 42 mcg each)
Nasal spray — 0.042%
Oral inhaler — 16.8 grams (200 doses of 42 mcg each)

▷ **Usual Adult Dosage Range:**   Nasal inhaler—1 inhalation (42 mcg) 2 to 4 times daily. Oral inhaler—2 inhalations (84 mcg) 3 or 4 times daily. For severe asthma—12 to 16 inhalations daily. The maximal daily dose should not exceed 20 inhalations. **Note: Actual dosage and administration schedule must be determined by the physician for each patient individually.**

▷ **Dosing Instructions:**   May be used as needed without regard to eating. Rinse the mouth and throat (gargle) with water thoroughly after each inhalation.

Usual Duration of Use: Continual use on a regular schedule for 1 to 4 weeks is usually necessary to determine this drug's effectiveness in

relieving severe, chronic allergic rhinitis and in controlling severe, chronic asthma. Long-term use requires the supervision and guidance of the physician. Consult your physician on a regular basis.

▷ **This Drug Should Not Be Taken If**
- you have had an allergic reaction to any of the drugs bearing the brand names listed above.
- you are experiencing severe acute asthma or status asthmaticus that requires more intense treatment for prompt relief.
- your asthma can be controlled by bronchodilators and other antiasthmatic drugs that are not related to cortisone.
- your asthma requires cortisonelike drugs infrequently for control.
- you have a form of nonallergic bronchitis with asthmatic features.

▷ **Inform Your Physician Before Taking This Drug If**
- you are now taking or have recently taken any cortisone-related drug (including ACTH by injection) for any reason (see Drug Class, Section Four).
- you have a history of tuberculosis of the lungs.
- you have chronic bronchitis or bronchiectasis.
- you think you may have an active infection of any kind, especially a respiratory infection.

Possible Side-Effects (natural, expected and unavoidable drug actions)
Fungus infections (thrush) of the mouth and throat.

▷ **Possible Adverse Effects** (unusual, unexpected and infrequent reactions)
If any of the following develop, consult your physician promptly for guidance.
Mild Adverse Effects
Allergic Reaction: Skin rash (rare).
Dryness of mouth, hoarseness, sore throat.
Serious Adverse Effects
Allergic Reaction: Localized areas of "allergic" pneumonitis (lung inflammation).
Bronchospasm, asthmatic wheezing (rare).

▷ **Possible Effects on Sexual Function:** None reported.

Natural Diseases or Disorders That May Be Activated by This Drug
Cortisone-related drugs that have systemic effects can impair immunity and lead to reactivation of "healed" or quiescent tuberculosis of the lungs. Individuals with a history of tuberculosis must be observed closely during use of this drug by inhalation.

CAUTION
1. This drug does not act primarily as a brochodilator and should not be relied upon for the immediate relief of acute asthma.
2. If you were using any cortisone-related drugs for treatment of your asthma *before* transferring to this inhaler drug, it may be necessary

to resume the former cortisone-related drug if you experience injury or infection of any kind, or if you require surgery. Be sure to notify your attending physician of your prior use of cortisone-related drugs taken either by mouth or by injection.

3. If you experience a return of severe asthma while using this drug, notify your physician immediately so that additional supportive treatment with cortisone-related drugs by mouth or injection can be provided as needed.

4. It is advisable to carry a card of personal identification with a notation (if applicable) that you have used cortisone-related drugs within the past year. During periods of stress it may be necessary to resume cortisone treatment in adequate dosage.

5. An interval of approximately 5 to 10 minutes should separate the inhalation of bronchodilators such as epinephrine, isotharine, or isoproterenol (which should be used first) and the inhalation of this drug. This sequence will permit greater penetration of beclomethasone into the bronchial tubes. The delay between inhalations will also reduce the possibility of adverse effects from the propellants used in the two inhalers.

Precautions for Use

By Infants and Children: Safety and effectiveness for use of the nasal inhaler by those under 12 years of age have not been established. Safety and effectiveness for use of the oral inhaler by those under 6 years of age have not been established. The maximal daily dose in children 6 to 12 years of age should not exceed 10 inhalations.

By Those over 60 Years of Age: Individuals with bronchiectasis should be observed closely for the development of lung infections.

▷ Advisability of Use During Pregnancy

Pregnancy Category: C (tentative). See Pregnancy Code inside back cover.

Animal studies: Mouse, rat and rabbit studies reveal significant birth defects due to this drug.

Human studies: Information from adequate studies of pregnant women is not available.

Avoid drug during the first 3 months. Use infrequently and only as clearly needed during the last 6 months.

Advisability of Use if Breast-Feeding

Presence of this drug in breast milk: Probably yes.

Avoid drug or refrain from nursing.

Habit-Forming Potential:

With recommended dosage, a state of functional dependence (see Glossary) is not likely to develop.

Effects of Overdosage:

Indications of cortisone excess (due to systemic absorption)—fluid retention, flushing of the face, stomach irritation, nervousness.

Suggested Periodic Examinations While Taking This Drug (at physician's discretion)

Inspection of nose, mouth and throat for evidence of fungus infection.

Assessment of the status of adrenal function in individuals who have used cortisone-related drugs over an extended period of time prior to using this drug.

X-ray examination of the lungs of individuals with a prior history of tuberculosis.

▷ **While Taking This Drug, Observe the Following**

Foods: No specific restrictions beyond those advised by your physician.

Beverages: No specific restrictions.

▷ *Alcohol:* No interactions expected.

Tobacco Smoking: No interactions expected. However, smoking can affect the condition under treatment and reduce the effectiveness of this drug. Follow your physician's advice.

▷ *Other Drugs*

The following drugs may *increase* the effects of beclomethasone

* inhalant bronchodilators—epinephrine, isoetharine, isoproterenol.
* oral bronchodilators—aminophylline, ephedrine, terbutaline, theophylline, etc.

▷ *Driving, Hazardous Activities:* No restrictions.

Aviation Note: The use of this drug and the disorder for which this drug is prescribed *may be disqualifications* for piloting. Consult a designated Aviation Medical Examiner.

Exposure to Sun: No restrictions.

Occurrence of Unrelated Illness: Acute infections, serious injuries, and surgical procedures can create an urgent need for the administration of additional supportive cortisone-related drugs given by mouth and/or injection. Notify your physician immediately in the event of new illness or injury of any kind.

Discontinuation: If the regular use of this drug has made it possible to reduce or discontinue maintenance doses of cortisonelike drugs by mouth, *do not* discontinue this drug abruptly. If you find it necessary to discontinue this drug for any reason, consult your physician promptly. It may be necessary to resume cortisone preparations and to institute other measures for satisfactory management.

Special Storage Instructions : Store at room temperature. Avoid exposure to temperatures above 120 degrees F (49 degrees C). Do not store or use this inhaler near heat or open flame. Protect from light.

BENZTROPINE
(BENZ troh peen)

Introduced: 1954

Class: Antiparkinsonism, atropine-like drugs

Prescription: USA: Yes
Canada: No

Controlled Drug: USA: No
Canada: No

Available as Generic: USA: No
Canada: Yes

Brand Names: ◆Apo-Benztropine, ◆Bensylate, Cogentin, ◆PMS Benztropine

---

BENEFITS versus RISKS

Possible Benefits	*Possible Risks*
PARTIAL RELIEF OF SYMPTOMS OF PARKINSON'S DISEASE	Atropinelike side-effects: blurred vision, dry mouth, constipation, impaired urination

---

▷ **Principal Uses**

As a Single Drug Product: Used adjunctively in the management of all types of parkinsonism to relieve the characteristic rigidity, tremor and sluggish movement. Should it fail to provide adequate relief, it may be supplemented with more potent drugs such as levodopa and bromocriptine. This drug is also used to control the parkinsonian reactions that can result from the use of certain antipsychotic drugs, such as the phenothiazines and related compounds.

How This Drug Works: By restoring a more normal balance of the chemical activities responsible for the transmission of nerve impulses within the basal ganglia of the brain, this drug relieves the symptoms of parkinsonism.

Available Dosage Forms and Strengths
Injection — 1 mg per ml
Tablets — 0.5 mg, 1 mg, 2 mg

▷ **Usual Adult Dosage Range:**   For Parkinson's disease—0.5 to 2 mg daily, taken in a single dose at bedtime. For drug-induced parkinsonian reactions—1 to 4 mg daily, either in a single dose or in 2 to 3 divided doses. The total daily dose should not exceed 6 mg. **Note: Actual dosage and administration schedule must be determined by the physician for each patient individually.**

▷ **Dosing Instructions:**   May be taken with or following food to reduce stomach irritation. Tablet may be crushed for administration.

Usual Duration of Use: Continual use on a regular schedule for 2 to 4 weeks is usually necessary to determine this drug's effectiveness in relieving the symptoms of parkinsonism and to determine the optimal dosage schedule. Long-term use (months to years) requires physician supervision and guidance. Consult your physician on a regular basis.

▷ **This Drug Should Not Be Taken If**
   • you have had an allergic reaction to any dosage form of it previously.
   • it is prescribed for a child under 3 years of age.

▷ **Inform Your Physician Before Taking This Drug If**
- you have experienced an unfavorable reaction to atropine or atropinelike drugs in the past.
- you have glaucoma or myasthenia gravis.
- you have heart disease or high blood pressure.
- you have a history of liver or kidney disease.
- you have difficulty emptying the urinary bladder, especially if due to an enlarged prostate gland.
- you are taking, or have taken within the past 2 weeks, any monoamine oxidase (MAO) type A inhibitor drug (see Drug Class, Section Four).

Possible Side-Effects (natural, expected and unavoidable drug actions)
Nervousness, blurring of vision, dryness of mouth, constipation, impaired urination. (These often subside as drug use continues.)

▷ **Possible Adverse Effects** (unusual, unexpected and infrequent reactions)
If any of the following develop, consult your physician promptly for guidance.
Mild Adverse Effects
Allergic Reaction: Skin rashes.
Headache, dizziness, drowsiness, muscle cramps.
Indigestion, nausea, vomiting.
Serious Adverse Effects
Idiosyncratic Reactions: Abnormal behavior, confusion, delusions, hallucinations, agitation.

▷ **Possible Effects on Sexual Function**
Reversal of male impotence due to the use of fluphenazine (a phenothiazine antipsychotic drug).
Male infertility (0.5 to 6 mg/day).

Natural Diseases or Disorders That May Be Activated by This Drug
Latent glaucoma, latent myasthenia gravis.

CAUTION
1. Many over-the-counter (OTC) medications for allergies, colds and coughs contain drugs that can interact unfavorably with this drug. Ask your physician or pharmacist for guidance before using such preparations.
2. This drug may aggravate tardive dyskinesia (see Glossary). Ask physician for guidance.

Precautions for Use
By Infants and Children: Safety and effectiveness for use by those under 3 years of age have not been established. Children are especially susceptible to the atropinelike effects of this drug.
By Those over 60 Years of Age: Small doses are advisable until your response has been determined. You may be more susceptible to the development of impaired thinking, confusion, nightmares, hallucina-

tions, increased internal eye pressure (glaucoma) and impaired urination associated with prostate gland enlargement (prostatism).

▷ **Advisability of Use During Pregnancy**
Pregnancy Category: C (tentative). See Pregnancy Code inside back cover.
Animal studies: No data available.
Human studies: Information from adequate studies of pregnant women is not available.
Avoid use if possible, especially close to delivery. This drug can impair the proper functioning of the infant's intestinal tract following birth.

Advisability of Use if Breast-Feeding
Presence of this drug in breast milk: Unknown.
Avoid drug or refrain from nursing.

Habit-Forming Potential: None with recommended doses. At higher doses it may cause euphoria and hallucinations, creating a potential for abuse.

Effects of Overdosage: Weakness; drowsiness; stupor; impaired vision; rapid pulse; excitement; confusion; hallucinations; dry, hot skin; skin rash; dilated pupils.

Possible Effects of Long-Term Use: Increased internal eye pressure—possible glaucoma, especially in the elderly.

Suggested Periodic Examinations While Taking This Drug (at physician's discretion)
Measurement of internal eye pressure at regular intervals.

▷ **While Taking This Drug, Observe the Following**
Foods: No restrictions.
Beverages: No restrictions.
▷   *Alcohol:* Use caution until the combined effects have been determined. Alcohol may increase the sedative effects of this drug.
Tobacco Smoking: No interactions expected.
▷   *Other Drugs*
Benztropine may **decrease** the effects of
• haloperidol (Haldol), and reduce its effectiveness.
• phenothiazines (Thorazine, etc.), and reduce their effectiveness.
The following drugs may **increase** the effects of benztropine
• antihistamines may add to the dryness of mouth and throat.
• tricyclic antidepressants (Elavil, etc.) may add to the effects on the eye and further increase internal eye pressure (dangerous in glaucoma).
• monoamine oxidase (MAO) type A inhibitor drugs may intensify all effects of this drug (see Drug Class, Section Four).
▷   *Driving, Hazardous Activities:* Drowsiness and dizziness may occur in sensitive individuals. Avoid hazardous activities until full effects and tolerance have been determined.

Aviation Note: The use of this drug *is a disqualification* for piloting. Consult a designated Aviation Medical Examiner.

Exposure to Sun: No restrictions.

Exposure to Heat: Use caution. This drug may reduce sweating, cause an increase in body temperature, and contribute to the development of heat stroke.

Heavy Exercise or Exertion: Use caution. Avoid in hot environments.

Discontinuation: Do not discontinue this drug abruptly. Ask physician for guidance in reducing the dose gradually.

BITOLTEROL
(bi TOHL ter ohl)

Introduced: 1985

Class: Antiasthmatic, bronchodilator

Prescription: Yes

Controlled Drug: No

Available as Generic: No

Brand Name: Tornalate

BENEFITS versus RISKS	
Possible Benefits	*Possible Risks*
EFFECTIVE PREVENTION AND RELIEF OF ASTHMA for 5 to 8 hours	Fine hand tremor (14%)
	Nervousness (5%)
	Throat irritation (5%)
	Irregular heart rhythm (with excessive use)

▷ **Principal Uses**

As a Single Drug Product: To relieve acute bronchial asthma and to reduce the frequency and severity of chronic, recurrent asthmatic attacks.

How This Drug Works: It is thought that by increasing the production of cyclic AMP, this drug relaxes constricted bronchial muscles to relieve asthmatic wheezing.

Available Dosage Forms and Strengths

Aerosol inhaler — 15 ml (300 inhalations of 0.37 mg each)

▷ **Usual Adult Dosage Range:** For acute bronchospasm—2 inhalations at intervals of 1 to 3 minutes, followed by a third inhalation in 3 to 4 minutes if needed. For prevention of bronchospasm—2 inhalations/8 hours. **Note: Actual dosage and administration schedule must be determined by the physician for each patient individually.**

▷ **Dosing Instructions:** May be used without regard to eating. Follow the written directions for use carefully. Do not overuse.

Usual Duration of Use: According to individual requirements. Do not use beyond the time necessary to terminate episodes of acute asthma. Ask physician for guidance regarding duration of use for prevention of asthma attacks.

▷ **This Drug Should Not Be Taken If**
- you have had an allergic reaction to it previously.
- you currently have an irregular heart rhythm.
- you are taking, or have taken within the past 2 weeks, any mono-amine oxidase (MAO) type A inhibitor drug (see Drug Class, Section Four).

▷ **Inform Your Physician Before Taking This Drug If**
- you have any type of heart or circulatory disorder, especially high blood pressure or coronary heart disease.
- you have diabetes, epilepsy or an overactive thyroid gland.
- you are taking any form of digitalis or any stimulant drug.

Possible Side-Effects (natural, expected and unavoidable drug actions)
Dryness or irritation of mouth or throat (5%).

▷ **Possible Adverse Effects** (unusual, unexpected and infrequent reactions)
If any of the following develop, consult your physician promptly for guidance.
Mild Adverse Effects
Headache (4%), dizziness (3%), nervousness (5%), insomnia (less than 1%), fine tremor of hands (14%).
Nausea (3%), indigestion.
Serious Adverse Effects
Rapid or irregular heart rhythm or increased blood pressure can occur with excessive use.

▷ **Possible Effects on Sexual Function:** None reported.

Natural Diseases or Disorders That May Be Activated by This Drug
Latent coronary artery disease, diabetes or high blood pressure.

CAUTION
1. Concurrent use of this drug by inhalation with beclomethasone aerosol (Beclovent, Vanceril) may increase the risk of toxicity due to fluorocarbon propellants. It is advisable to use bitolterol aerosol 20 to 30 minutes *before* beclomethasone aerosol. This will reduce the risk of toxicity and will enhance the penetration of beclomethasone.
2. The excessive or prolonged use of this drug by inhalation can reduce its effectiveness and cause serious heart rhythm disturbances.

Precautions for Use
By Infants and Children: Safety and effectiveness for use by children under 12 years of age have not been established.

By Those over 60 Years of Age: Avoid excessive and continual use. If acute asthma is not relieved promptly, other drugs will have to be tried. Observe for the development of nervousness, palpitations, irregular heart rhythm and muscle tremors.

▷ **Advisability of Use During Pregnancy**
Pregnancy Category: C (tentative). See Pregnancy Code inside back cover.
Animal studies: Cleft palate reported in mice.
Human studies: Information from adequate studies of pregnant women is not available.
Avoid use during first 3 months if possible.

Advisability of Use if Breast-Feeding
Presence of this drug in breast milk: Unknown.
Avoid drug or refrain from nursing.

Habit-Forming Potential: None.

Effects of Overdosage: Nervousness, palpitation, rapid heart rate, sweating, headache, tremor, vomiting, chest pain.

Possible Effects of Long-Term Use: Loss of effectiveness.

Suggested Periodic Examinations While Taking This Drug (at physician's discretion)
Blood pressure measurements, evaluation of heart status.

▷ **While Taking This Drug, Observe the Following**
Foods: No restrictions.
Beverages: Avoid excessive use of caffeine-containing beverages—coffee, tea, cola, chocolate.
▷ *Alcohol:* No interactions expected.
Tobacco Smoking: No interactions expected.
▷ *Other Drugs*
Bitolterol *taken concurrently* with
• monoamine oxidase (MAO) type A inhibitor drugs (see Drug Class, Section Four) may cause excessive increase in blood pressure and undesirable heart stimulation.
▷ *Driving, Hazardous Activities:* Use caution if excessive nervousness or dizziness occurs.
Aviation Note: The use of this drug *is a disqualification* for piloting. Consult a designated Aviation Medical Examiner.
Exposure to Sun: No restrictions.
Heavy Exercise or Exertion: Use caution. Excessive exercise can induce asthma in sensitive individuals.

BROMOCRIPTINE
(broh moh KRIP teen)

Introduced: 1975

Class: Antiparkinsonism, dopamine agonist, ergot derivative

Prescription: USA: Yes
Canada: Yes

Controlled Drug: USA: No
Canada: No

Available as Generic: No

Brand Name: Parlodel

BENEFITS versus RISKS

Possible Benefits	*Possible Risks*
PARTIAL RELIEF OF SYMPTOMS OF PARKINSON'S DISEASE	ABNORMAL INVOLUNTARY MOVEMENTS AND ALTERED BEHAVIOR in 20% to 35% of users taking high doses
PREVENTION OF LACTATION following childbirth	Raynaud's phenomenon (see Glossary) in 30% to 60% of users taking high doses
CORRECTION OF INFERTILITY AND ABSENT MENSTRUATION in women with high prolactin levels	

▷ **Principal Uses**

As a Single Drug Product: This drug is used primarily to
1. Treat the manifestations of Parkinson's disease. It may be used as the initial drug in treating those with early-stage symptoms. More often it is used in conjunction with levodopa when it is found that levodopa is losing its effectiveness, or the patient cannot tolerate the adverse effects of levodopa and dosage adjustment or withdrawal is necessary.
2. Suppress the production of milk and thereby prevent the breast congestion and engorgement that normally follow childbirth.
3. Treat those disorders that are due to excessive production of prolactin by the pituitary gland: absence of menstruation, infertility, and inappropriate production of milk.

How This Drug Works: By directly stimulating the dopamine receptor sites in the corpus striatum of the brain, this drug helps to offset the deficiency of dopamine that is responsible for the rigidity, tremor, and sluggish movement characteristic of Parkinson's disease. By inhibiting the production of the hormone prolactin by the anterior pituitary gland, this drug
• reduces the amount of prolactin in the blood to below the level required to stimulate the breast glands to produce milk.

Parlodel

- reduces abnormally high levels of prolactin in the blood, restoring it to normal levels that permit menstrual regularity and fertility.

Available Dosage Forms and Strengths
Capsules — 5 mg
Tablets — 2.5 mg

▷ **Usual Adult Dosage Range:**   For Parkinson's disease—initially 1.25 to 2.5 mg once daily; for maintenance, 2.5 to 100 mg daily in divided doses. Increase dose by no more than 2.5 to 5 mg on alternate days. The usual dosage range is 10 to 40 mg daily. Do not exceed 300 mg daily. For suppression of lactation—2.5 mg 2 times a day for 14 days; may extend to 21 days if needed. For absent menstruation and infertility— initially 1.25 to 2.5 mg daily; for maintenance, 2.5 mg 2 or 3 times a day. **Note: Actual dosage and administration schedule must be determined by the physician for each patient individually.**

▷ **Dosing Instructions:**   Take with food or milk to reduce stomach irritation. Capsule may be opened and tablet may be crushed for administration.

Usual Duration of Use: Continual use on a regular schedule for 3 to 4 months is usually necessary to determine this drug's effectiveness in controlling the symptoms of Parkinson's disease. Treatment for 4 to 12 weeks restores fertility and normal menstruation in most women; however, treatment may be necessary for 6 to 12 months. Long-term use (up to 3 years or more) must be under physician supervision and guidance. Consult your physician on a regular basis.

▷ **This Drug Should Not Be Taken If**
- you have had an allergic reaction to it previously.
- you have had a serious adverse effect from any ergot preparation in the past.
- you have severe coronary artery disease or peripheral vascular disease.
- you are pregnant.

▷ **Inform Your Physician Before Taking This Drug If**
- you have constitutionally low blood pressure.
- you are taking any antihypertensive drugs or phenothiazines (see Drug Classes, Section Four).
- you have any degree of coronary artery disease, especially with a history of a "heart attack" (myocardial infarction).
- you have a history of heart rhythm abnormalities.
- you have impaired liver function.
- you have a seizure disorder (epilepsy).

Possible Side-Effects (natural, expected and unavoidable drug actions)
Fatigue, lethargy, light-headedness in upright position (see Orthostatic Hypotension in Glossary).

▷ **Possible Adverse Effects** (unusual, unexpected and infrequent reactions)
If any of the following develop, consult your physician promptly for guidance.
Mild Adverse Effects
Allergic Reaction: Skin rash.
Headache, drowsiness, dizziness, fainting, nervousness, nightmares.
Nasal congestion, dry mouth, loss of appetite, nausea, vomiting, stomach cramps, constipation, diarrhea.
Serious Adverse Effects
Abnormal involuntary movements, confusion, hallucinations, incoordination, visual disturbances, depression, seizures.
Swelling of feet and ankles (edema).
Loss of urinary bladder control, inability to empty bladder.
Indications of "ergotism": numbness and tingling of fingers, cold hands and feet, muscle cramps of legs and feet.
Vomiting blood, bloody or black stools (gastrointestinal bleeding).

▷ **Possible Effects on Sexual Function:**   Rare occurrence of impotence. However, this drug can correct impotence and reduced libido when these conditions are due to increased blood levels of prolactin (a pituitary hormone).

▷ **Adverse Effects That May Mimic Natural Diseases or Disorders**
Effects on mental function and behavior may resemble psychotic disorders.

Natural Diseases or Disorders That May Be Activated by This Drug
Coronary artery disease with anginal syndrome, Raynaud's syndrome.

CAUTION
1. During treatment of parkinsonism, avoid excessive and hurried activity as improvement occurs; this will reduce the risk of falls and injury.
2. The neurological and psychiatric disturbances due to this drug may last for 2 to 6 weeks after stopping it.
3. During treatment to reduce the blood level of prolactin and restore normal menstruation and fertility, it is mandatory that you use a barrier method of contraception to prevent pregnancy. Oral contraceptives should not be used while taking bromocriptine.
4. If pregnancy occurs, notify your physician immediately.

Precautions for Use
By Infants and Children: Safety and effectiveness for use by those under 15 years of age have not been established.
By Those over 60 Years of Age: Your initial test dose should be 1.25 mg. Observe closely for any tendency to light-headedness or faintness on attempting to stand after this first dose. You may be more susceptible to the development of impaired thinking, confusion, agitation, nightmares, hallucinations, nausea or vomiting. Close monitoring and careful dosage adjustments are mandatory.

▷ **Advisability of Use During Pregnancy**
　　Pregnancy Category: X (tentative). See Pregnancy Code inside back cover.
　　Animal studies: Rabbit studies reveal an increase in cleft lip.
　　Human studies: Serious birth defects have been reported in infants
　　　whose mothers took this drug during early pregnancy. Because the
　　　incidence of these defects (3.3%) does not exceed that reported for the
　　　general population, a cause-and-effect relationship is uncertain. In-
　　　formation from adequate studies of pregnant women is not available.
　　Pending further studies, it is recommended that this drug not be taken
　　　during the entire pregnancy.

Advisability of Use if Breast-Feeding
　　This drug prevents the production of milk and makes nursing impos-
　　　sible.

Habit-Forming Potential:　None.

Effects of Overdosage:　Weakness, low blood pressure, nausea, vomiting,
　　diarrhea, confusion, agitation, hallucinations, loss of consciousness.

Possible Effects of Long-Term Use:　Drug-induced changes in the lung tis-
　　sue, thickening of the pleura and pleural effusion (fluid formation
　　within the chest cage). These effects appear to be reversible after dis-
　　continuation of the drug. Fibrosis (scar tissue formation) in the back
　　wall of the abdominal cavity and contractures of the extremities have
　　also been reported.

Suggested Periodic Examinations While Taking This Drug (at physician's
　　discretion)
　　Blood pressure measurements; CAT scan of the pituitary gland for en-
　　largement due to tumor; pregnancy test; blood tests for anemia; eval-
　　uation of heart, lung and liver functions.

▷ **While Taking This Drug, Observe the Following**
　　Foods: No restrictions.
　　Beverages: No restrictions. May be taken with milk.
▷　*Alcohol:* Use caution until the combined effects have been determined.
　　　Alcohol can exaggerate the blood-pressure-lowering effects and sed-
　　　ative effects of this drug.
▷　*Other Drugs*
　　Bromocriptine *taken concurrently* with
　　• antihypertensive drugs (and other drugs that can lower blood pres-
　　　sure) requires careful monitoring for excessive drops in pressure. Dos-
　　　age adjustments may be necessary.
　　The following drugs may *decrease* the effects of bromocriptine
　　• phenothiazines (see Drug Class, Section Four). Theoretically, brom-
　　　ocriptine and phenothiazines have opposite effects on the utilization
　　　of dopamine in the brain. It is probably best to avoid the concurrent
　　　use of these drugs until the results of further studies are available.

Driving, Hazardous Activities: Be alert to the possible occurrence of orthostatic hypotension, dizziness, drowsiness or impaired coordination.
Aviation Note: Parkinsonism *is a disqualification* for piloting. The use of
this drug otherwise *may be a disqualification* for piloting. Consult a
designated Aviation Medical Examiner.
Exposure to Sun: No restrictions.

BROMPHENIRAMINE
(brohm fen IR a meen)

Introduced: 1957   **Class:** Antihistamines

Prescription: USA: Varies   **Controlled Drug:** USA: No
Canada: No   Canada: No

Available as Generic: USA: Yes
Canada: No

Brand Names: ✦Dimedrine [CD], Dimetane, Dimetane Cough Syrup-DC
[CD], Dimetane-DC [CD], Dimetane Decongestant Elixir [CD], Di-
metane Decongestant Tablets [CD], Dimetane-DX [CD], ✦Dimetane
Expectorant [CD], ✦Dimetane Expectorant-C [CD], ✦Dimetane Ex-
pectorant-DC [CD], Dimetane Extentabs, Dimetane-Ten, Dimetapp
Preparations [CD], ✦Dimetapp-A Preparations [CD], ✦Dimetapp-C
[CD], ✦Dimetapp w/Codeine [CD], ✦Dimetapp-DM [CD], ✦Dimetapp
Infant Drops [CD], Disophrol [CD], Drixoral Plus [CD], Drixoral
Syrup [CD], Drixoral Tablets [CD], ✦Drixtab, Veltane

BENEFITS versus RISKS

Possible Benefits	*Possible Risks*
EFFECTIVE RELIEF OF	Mild sedation (23%)
ALLERGIC RHINITIS AND	Atropinelike effects
ALLERGIC SKIN DISORDERS	Rare blood cell disorders:
	abnormally low white blood
	cell and platelet counts

▷ **Principal Uses**
   As a Single Drug Product: Used primarily to provide symptomatic relief
   in allergic and related disorders: seasonal and perennial allergic rhinitis (hay fever), allergic conjunctivitis and vasomotor rhinitis; also in
   hives and localized swellings (angioedema) of allergic origin.

As a Combination Drug Product [CD]: This drug is combined with a decongestant drug to enhance its ability to reduce tissue swelling and secretions in allergic and infectious disorders of the upper respiratory tract—hay fever, head colds and sinusitis. It is also combined with decongestants, expectorants and codeine to increase their effectiveness in the symptomatic treatment of allergic and infectious disorders of the lower respiratory tract, often with associated coughing.

How This Drug Works: Antihistamines reduce the intensity of the allergic response by blocking the action of histamine after it has been released from sensitized tissue cells in the eyes, nose, respiratory passages and skin.

Available Dosage Forms and Strengths

Elixir — 2 mg per 5-ml teaspoonful
Injection — 10 mg per ml, 100 mg per ml
Tablets — 4 mg
Tablets, prolonged-action — 8 mg, 12 mg

▷ **Usual Adult Dosage Range:** 4 mg/4 to 6 hours, or 8 to 12 mg (prolonged-action form)/12 hours. Total daily dosage should not exceed 24 mg. **Note: Actual dosage and administration schedule must be determined by the physician for each patient individually.**

▷ **Dosing Instructions:** Take with food or milk to prevent stomach irritation. The prolonged-action forms should be swallowed whole (not crushed or chewed).

Usual Duration of Use: Continual use on a regular schedule for 2 to 3 days is usually necessary to determine this drug's effectiveness in relieving the symptoms of allergic rhinitis and dermatosis. It may be necessary to take this drug throughout the entire pollen season, depending upon individual sensitivity. However, antihistamines should not be taken continually (without interruption) for long-term use. Limit their use to periods that require symptomatic relief.

▷ **This Drug Should Not Be Taken If**
- you have had an allergic reaction to any dosage form of it previously.
- you are currently undergoing allergy skin tests.
- you are taking, or have taken within the past 14 days, any monoamine oxidase (MAO) type A inhibitor drug (see Drug Class, Section Four).

▷ **Inform Your Physician Before Taking This Drug If**
- you have had any allergic reactions or unfavorable responses to the previous use of antihistamines.
- you have glaucoma (narrow-angle type) or asthma.
- you have epilepsy or a seizure disorder.
- you have difficulty emptying the urinary bladder, especially if due to prostate gland enlargement.
- you plan to have surgery under general anesthesia in the near future.

Possible Side-Effects (natural, expected and unavoidable drug actions)

Drowsiness; sense of weakness; blurred vision; dryness of the nose, mouth and throat; impaired urination.

▷ **Possible Adverse Effects** (unusual, unexpected and infrequent reactions)

If any of the following develop, consult your physician promptly for guidance.

Mild Adverse Effects

Allergic Reaction: Skin rash.

Headache, nervous agitation, dizziness, confusion, tremor, blurred or double vision, ringing in ears.

Reduced tolerance for contact lenses.

Thickening of bronchial secretions in asthma or bronchitis.

Indigestion, nausea, vomiting, diarrhea.

Serious Adverse Effects

Hemolytic anemia (see Glossary).

Abnormally low white blood cell count—fever, sore throat, infections.

Abnormally low blood platelet count—abnormal bleeding or bruising.

▷ **Possible Effects on Sexual Function**

No adverse effects reported.

This drug has been used successfully to correct retrograde (backward) ejaculation, a condition that occurs occasionally in some men with diabetes.

Natural Diseases or Disorders That May Be Activated by This Drug

Latent epilepsy, glaucoma, prostatism (see Glossary).

CAUTION

1. Discontinue this drug 4 days before diagnostic skin testing procedures in order to prevent false negative test results.
2. Do not use this drug if you have active bronchial asthma, bronchitis or pneumonia. It can thicken bronchial mucus and make it more difficult to remove (by absorption or coughing).

Precautions for Use

By Infants and Children: This drug should not be used in premature or full-term newborn infants. Doses for children should be small. The young child is especially sensitive to the effects of antihistamines on the brain and nervous system.

By Those over 60 Years of Age: You may be more susceptible to the development of drowsiness, dizziness, and unsteadiness, and to impairment of thinking, judgment and memory. This drug can increase the degree of impaired urination associated with prostate gland enlargement (prostatism). The sedative effects of antihistamines in the elderly can cause a syndrome of underactivity that may be misinterpreted as senility or emotional depression.

▷ **Advisability of Use During Pregnancy**

Pregnancy Category: B (tentative). See Pregnancy Code inside back cover.

Animal studies: No information available.

Human studies: Information from adequate studies of pregnant women is not available. Birth defects have been reported in 10 infants whose mothers used this drug during the first 3 months of pregnancy.

Avoid this drug during the first 3 months, and the last 3 months because of the potential risk for serious adverse effects on the newborn infant.

Advisability of Use if Breast-Feeding
Presence of this drug in breast milk: Yes, in small amounts.
Avoid drug or refrain from nursing.

Habit-Forming Potential: None.

Effects of Overdosage: Drowsiness; unsteadiness; faintness; marked dryness of mouth, nose and throat; flushing of face; shortness of breath; hallucinations; convulsions; stupor progressing to coma.

Possible Effects of Long-Term Use: Tardive dyskinesia (see Glossary) has been reported in association with the long-term use of several widely used antihistamines. It is advisable to avoid the prolonged, continual use of antihistamines without interruption.

Suggested Periodic Examinations While Taking This Drug (at physician's discretion)
Complete blood cell counts.

▷ **While Taking This Drug, Observe the Following**
Foods: No restrictions.
Beverages: No restrictions. May be taken with milk.
▷ *Alcohol:* Use with extreme caution until the combined effects have been determined. The combination of antihistamine and alcohol can produce rapid and marked sedation.
Tobacco Smoking: No interactions expected.
▷ *Other Drugs*
Brompheniramine may *increase* the effects of
• all sedatives, sleep-inducing drugs, tranquilizers, analgesics and narcotic drugs, and produce oversedation.
The following drugs may *increase* the effects of brompheniramine
• monoamine oxidase (MAO) type A inhibitor drugs (see Drug Class, Section Four) may prolong the action of antihistamines.
▷ *Driving, Hazardous Activities:* This drug can impair mental alertness, judgment, coordination and reaction time. Avoid hazardous activities until the full sedative effects have been determined.
Aviation Note: The use of this drug *is a disqualification* for piloting. Consult a designated Aviation Medical Examiner.
Exposure to Sun: Use caution. Some drugs of this class can cause photosensitivity (see Glossary).

BUMETANIDE
(byu MET a nide)

Introduced: 1983   **Class:** Diuretic

Prescription: USA: Yes   **Controlled Drug:** USA: No

Available as Generic: No

Brand Name: Bumex

BENEFITS versus RISKS

Possible Benefits	*Possible Risks*
POTENT, EFFECTIVE DIURETIC BY MOUTH OR INJECTION	ABNORMALLY LOW BLOOD POTASSIUM with excessive use Impaired sexual function

▷ **Principal Uses**

As a Single Drug Product: To relieve edema (fluid retention) associated with congestive heart failure, liver disease or kidney disease.

How This Drug Works: By increasing the elimination of salt and water from the body (through increased urine production), this drug reduces the volume of fluid in the blood and body tissues and lowers the sodium content throughout the body.

Available Dosage Forms and Strengths

Injection — 0.25 mg per ml (2-ml ampules)

Tablets — 0.5 mg, 1 mg, 2 mg

▷ **Usual Adult Dosage Range:** 0.5 to 2 mg daily, usually taken in the morning as a single dose. If needed, an additional second or third dose may be taken later in the day at 4- to 5-hour intervals. The total daily dose should not exceed 10 mg. Alternate-day dosage (taken every other day) may be adequate for some individuals. **Note: Actual dosage and administration schedule must be determined by the physician for each patient individually.**

▷ **Dosing Instructions:** May be taken with or following food to reduce stomach irritation. Tablet may be crushed for administration.

Usual Duration of Use: Continual use on a regular schedule for 2 to 3 days is usually necessary to determine this drug's effectiveness in relieving edema. After maximal benefit has been achieved, intermittent use will reduce the risk of sodium, potassium and water imbalance. Long-term use requires the supervision and guidance of the physician. Consult your physician on a regular basis.

▷ **This Drug Should Not Be Taken If**

• you have had an allergic reaction to either dosage form previously.

• your kidneys are unable to produce urine.

▷ **Inform Your Physician Before Taking This Drug If**
- you are allergic to any form of "sulfa" drug.
- you are pregnant or planning pregnancy.
- you have impaired liver or kidney function.
- you have diabetes or a tendency to diabetes.
- you have a history of gout.
- you have impaired hearing.
- you are taking any form of cortisone, digitalis, oral antidiabetic drugs, insulin, probenecid (Benemid), indomethacin (Indocin), lithium or drugs for high blood pressure.
- you plan to have surgery under general anesthesia in the near future.

Possible Side-Effects (natural, expected and unavoidable drug actions)
Light-headedness on arising from sitting or lying position (see Orthostatic Hypotension in Glossary).
Increase in level of blood sugar, affecting control of diabetes.
Increase in level of blood uric acid, affecting control of gout.
Decrease in levels of blood potassium and sodium, resulting in muscle weakness and cramping.

▷ **Possible Adverse Effects** (unusual, unexpected and infrequent reactions)
If any of the following develop, consult your physician promptly for guidance.
Mild Adverse Effects
Allergic Reactions: Skin rashes, hives, itching.
Headache, dizziness, vertigo, fatigue, weakness, sweating, earache.
Nausea, vomiting, stomach pain, diarrhea.
Breast nipple tenderness, joint and muscle pains.
Serious Adverse Effects
Impaired hearing, precipitation of liver coma (in preexisting liver disease).

▷ **Possible Effects on Sexual Function:** Difficulty maintaining an erection; premature ejaculation (0.5 to 2 mg/day).

Natural Diseases or Disorders That May Be Activated by This Drug
Latent diabetes, gout.

CAUTION
1. Do not exceed recommended doses. Increased dosage can cause excessive excretion of water, sodium and potassium, with resultant loss of appetite, nausea, weakness, confusion and profound drop in blood pressure (circulatory collapse).
2. If you are also taking a digitalis preparation (digitoxin, digoxin), ensure an adequate intake of high-potassium foods to prevent potassium deficiency—a potential cause of digitalis toxicity.
3. If you are being treated for cirrhosis of the liver, do not increase your dose without consulting your physician. Excessive dosage can alter blood chemistry significantly and induce liver coma.

Precautions for Use

By Infants and Children: Safety and effectiveness for use by those under 18 years of age have not been established.

By Those over 60 Years of Age: Small doses are advisable until your individual response has been determined. You may be more susceptible to the development of impaired thinking, orthostatic hypotension, potassium loss and elevation of blood sugar. Overdosage and prolonged use of this drug can cause excessive loss of body water, thickening of the blood, and an increased tendency of the blood to clot, predisposing to stroke, heart attack or thrombophlebitis.

▷ **Advisability of Use During Pregnancy**

Pregnancy Category: C (tentative). See Pregnancy Code inside back cover.

Animal studies: High-dose studies of rats and rabbits reveal defects in bone development.

Human studies: Information from adequate studies of pregnant women is not available.

This drug should not be used during pregnancy unless a very serious complication of pregnancy occurs for which this drug is significantly beneficial.

Advisability of Use if Breast-Feeding

Presence of this drug in breast milk: Unknown.

Avoid drug or refrain from nursing.

Habit-Forming Potential: None.

Effects of Overdosage: Weakness, lethargy, dizziness, confusion, nausea, vomiting, muscle cramps, thirst, drowsiness progressing to deep sleep or coma, weak and rapid pulse.

Possible Effects of Long-Term Use: Impaired balance of water, salt, and potassium in blood and body tissues. Dehydration with resultant increase in blood viscosity and potential for abnormal clotting. Development of diabetes in predisposed individuals.

Suggested Periodic Examinations While Taking This Drug (at physician's discretion)

Complete blood cell counts; measurements of blood levels of sodium, potassium, chloride, sugar, uric acid; liver and kidney function tests.

▷ **While Taking This Drug, Observe the Following**

Foods: Consult your physician regarding the advisability of eating a high-potassium diet. See Section Six for the Table of High Potassium Foods. Follow your physician's instructions regarding the use of salt.

Beverages: No restrictions unless directed by your physician. May be taken with milk.

▷ *Alcohol:* Use with caution until the combined effect has been determined. Alcohol can exaggerate the blood-pressure-lowering effect of this drug and cause orthostatic hypotension (see Glossary).

Tobacco Smoking: No interactions expected. Follow your physician's advice regarding smoking.

▷ *Other Drugs*

Bumetanide may *increase* the effects of
- antihypertensive drugs. Careful adjustment of dosages is necessary to prevent excessive lowering of the blood pressure.

Bumetanide *taken concurrently* with
- aminoglycoside antibiotics (amikacin, gentamicin, kanamycin, neomycin, streptomycin, tobramycin, viomycin) may increase the risk of hearing loss.
- cortisone-related drugs may cause excessive loss of potassium from the body.
- digitalis-related drugs requires very careful monitoring and dosage adjustments to prevent serious disturbances of heart rhythm.
- lithium may increase the risk of lithium toxicity.

The following drugs may *decrease* the effects of bumetanide
- indomethacin (Indocin) may reduce its diuretic effect.

▷ *Driving, Hazardous Activities:* Use caution until the possible occurrence of dizziness, weakness or orthostatic hypotension (see Glossary) has been determined.

Aviation Note: The use of this drug *may be a disqualification* for piloting. Consult a designated Aviation Medical Examiner.

Exposure to Sun: No restrictions.

Occurrence of Unrelated Illness: Illnesses that cause vomiting or diarrhea can produce a serious imbalance of important body chemistry. Report such illnesses promptly.

Discontinuation: It may be advisable to discontinue this drug 5 to 7 days before major surgery. Consult your physician, surgeon, or anesthesiologist for guidance regarding dosage reduction or withdrawal.

BUSPIRONE
(byu SPI rohn)

Introduced: 1979   **Class:** Mild tranquilizer

Prescription: USA: Yes   **Controlled Drug:** USA: No

Available as Generic: No

Brand Name: Buspar

BENEFITS versus RISKS	
Possible Benefits	*Possible Risks*
EFFECTIVE RELIEF OF MILD TO MODERATE ANXIETY without significant sedation or risk of dependence	Mild dizziness, faintness or headache (uncommon) Rare restlessness, tremor and rigidity (with high doses)

▷ **Principal Uses**

As a Single Drug Product: Used to relieve anxiety and nervous tension states of mild to moderate severity. Because of its lack of significant sedative effects and of abuse potential, it is particularly useful in the elderly, the alcoholic and the addiction-prone individual.

How This Drug Works: Not completely established. This drug is thought to be a "mid-brain modulator" with effects on dopamine, norepinephrine and serotonin transmission activities. Its exact method of action is not understood.

Available Dosage Forms and Strengths
Tablets — 5 mg, 10 mg

▷ **Usual Adult Dosage Range:**   20 to 30 mg/day, in divided doses. Initially, 5 mg 3 times/day; if needed, increase dose by 5 to 10 mg/day every 3 to 4 days, with individual doses every 6 to 8 hours. The total daily dose should not exceed 60 mg. **Note: Actual dosage and administration schedule must be determined by the physician for each patient individually.**

▷ **Dosing Instructions:**   May be taken without regard to food. The tablet may be crushed for administration.

Usual Duration of Use: Continual use on a regular schedule for 7 to 10 days is usually necessary to determine this drug's effectiveness in relieving anxiety and nervous tension. Use intermittently and only as necessary; avoid prolonged and uninterrupted use.

Possible Advantages of This Drug
Relieves anxiety and nervous tension without causing significant sedation.
Does not cause withdrawal symptoms upon discontinuation.

▷ **This Drug Should Not Be Taken If**
• you have had an allergic reaction to it previously.

▷ **Inform Your Physician Before Taking This Drug If**
• you are taking other drugs that affect the function of the brain and nervous system: tranquilizers, sedatives, hypnotics, analgesics, narcotics, antidepressants, antipsychotic drugs, anticonvulsants or drugs for parkinsonism.
• you have impaired liver or kidney function.

Possible Side-Effects (natural, expected and unavoidable drug actions)
Infrequent and mild drowsiness (less than with benzodiazepines), lethargy, fatigue.

▷ **Possible Adverse Effects** (unusual, unexpected and infrequent reactions)
If any of the following develop, consult your physician promptly for guidance.

Mild Adverse Effects
Headache, dizziness, faintness, excitement, nausea.
Serious Adverse Effects
Depression (3%).
With high doses: restlessness, rigidity, tremors.

▷ **Possible Effects on Sexual Function:** Increased or decreased libido, inhibited ejaculation, impotence, breast milk production, altered timing and pattern of menstruation (10 to 40 mg/day).

CAUTION
Although this drug is reported to have no significant (or very mild) sedative effects and no potential for causing dependence, it should be used with caution and only when clearly needed. It has not been used by large numbers of people for long periods of time; some unexpected side-effects or adverse effects may become apparent after general use for several years.

Precautions for Use
By Infants and Children: Safety and effectiveness for use by those under 18 years of age have not been established.
By Those over 60 Years of Age: This drug should be tolerated much better than benzodiazepines and barbiturates when used by this age group. Observe for some possible increase in dizziness and/or weakness; use caution to avoid falls.

▷ **Advisability of Use During Pregnancy**
Pregnancy Category: B (tentative). See Pregnancy Code inside back cover.
Animal studies: No birth defects found in rat and rabbit studies.
Human studies: Information from adequate studies of pregnant women is not available.
Use this drug during pregnancy only when clearly needed. Until more experience has been gained from wider use, it is advisable to avoid this drug during the first 3 months of pregnancy.

Advisability of Use if Breast-Feeding
Presence of this drug in breast milk: Unknown; probably yes.
Avoid drug or refrain from nursing.

Habit-Forming Potential: None demonstrated in premarketing trials.

Effects of Overdosage: No experience reported. Probable effects would be increased dizziness, weakness and lethargy.

Possible Effects of Long-Term Use: None reported.

Suggested Periodic Examinations While Taking This Drug (at physician's discretion)
None required or recommended at the time of this writing.

▷ **While Taking This Drug, Observe the Following**
    Foods: No restrictions.
    Beverages: No restrictions.
▷ *Alcohol:* No interactions expected.
    Tobacco Smoking: No interactions expected.
▷ *Other Drugs:* No significant drug interactions have been reported at the time of this writing.
▷ *Driving, Hazardous Activities:* This drug may cause dizziness, faintness or fatigue. Restrict activities as necessary.
    Aviation Note: The use of this drug *may be a disqualification* for piloting. Consult a designated Aviation Medical Examiner.
    Exposure to Sun: No restrictions.

BUTALBITAL
(byu TAL bi tal)

Introduced: 1954

Class: Mild sedative, hypnotic, barbiturates

Prescription: USA: Yes
Canada: Yes

Controlled Drug: USA: C-III*
Canada: C

Available as Generic: No

Brand Names: Axotal [CD], Fioricet [CD], Fiorinal [CD], ✦Fiorinal-C1/4, C1/2 [CD], Fiorinal w/Codeine No. 1, 2, 3 [CD]

BENEFITS versus RISKS

Possible Benefits	*Possible Risks*
RELIEF OF ANXIETY AND NERVOUS TENSION	HABIT-FORMING POTENTIAL WITH EXCESSIVE USE Minor impairment of mental functions with usual doses Allergic skin rashes and hepatitis Rare blood cell changes: abnormally low white blood cell and blood platelet counts

---

▷ **Principal Uses**
    As a Single Drug Product: This barbiturate, with short to intermediate duration of action, is a mild sedative that is infrequently used alone to relieve anxiety and nervous tension.

*See Schedules of Controlled Drugs inside back cover.

As a Combination Drug Product [CD]: This drug is used primarily in combination with aspirin, caffeine and codeine to treat headaches associated with nervous tension. Because of the significant emotional component in the perception of pain, the addition of a mild sedative to a mixture of analgesics renders the combination more effective in relieving pain.

How This Drug Works: Not completely established. It is thought that this drug relieves nervous tension by reducing the amount of available norepinephrine, one of the chemicals responsible for nerve impulse transmission in the brain.

Available Dosage Forms and Strengths
   Capsules — 50 mg (in combination)
   Tablets — 50 mg (in combination)

▷ **Usual Adult Dosage Range:**   50 mg (in combination capsule or tablet)/4 hours as needed. Total daily dose should not exceed 6 capsules or tablets. **Note: Actual dosage and administration schedule must be determined by the physician for each patient individually.**

▷ **Dosing Instructions:**   Take with food or milk to prevent stomach irritation. The tablet may be crushed or the capsule opened for administration.

Usual Duration of Use: For short-term use only. Take only as needed to abort or relieve tension headaches. Avoid prolonged and uninterrupted use.

▷ **This Drug Should Not Be Taken If**
   • you have had an allergic reaction to any dosage form of it previously.
   • you have a history of porphyria.

▷ **Inform Your Physician Before Taking This Drug If**
   • you are allergic or overly sensitive to any barbiturate drug.
   • you are taking any other sedative drugs, tranquilizers, antihistamines or pain relievers.
   • you have epilepsy.
   • you have a history of liver or kidney disease.
   • you plan to have surgery under general anesthesia in the near future.

Possible Side-Effects (natural, expected and unavoidable drug actions)
   Drowsiness, lethargy and sense of mental and physical sluggishness as "hangover" effect.

▷ **Possible Adverse Effects** (unusual, unexpected and infrequent reactions)
   If any of the following develop, consult your physician promptly for guidance.
   Mild Adverse Effects
   Allergic Reactions: Skin rash; hives; localized swellings of eyelids, face or lips; drug fever (see Glossary).

Headache, dizziness.

Nausea, vomiting, diarrhea.

Serious Adverse Effects

Allergic Reactions: Drug-induced hepatitis, with or without jaundice (see Glossary).

Idiosyncratic Reactions: Paradoxical excitement and delirium (rather than sedation). This is more likely to occur in the presence of pain and in the elderly.

Abnormally low white blood cell count—infection, fever, sore throat.

Abnormally low blood platelet count—abnormal bleeding or bruising.

▷ **Possible Effects on Sexual Function:**   None reported.

▷ **Adverse Effects That May Mimic Natural Diseases or Disorders**
Drug-induced jaundice may suggest viral hepatitis.

Natural Diseases or Disorders That May Be Activated by This Drug
Acute intermittent porphyria.

CAUTION

This drug is most commonly used in combination with caffeine and/or aspirin. For complete information, be sure to read the Profiles of these two drugs.

Precautions for Use

By Infants and Children: Observe for possible paradoxical excitement and hyperactivity. Barbiturates should not be given to the hyperkinetic child.

By Those over 60 Years of Age: Small doses are advisable until tolerance has been determined. The elderly or debilitated may experience agitation, excitement, confusion and delirium with standard doses. This drug may also cause excessive lowering of body temperature (hypothermia). Keep dosage to a minimum during cold weather; dress warmly.

▷ **Advisability of Use During Pregnancy**

Pregnancy Category: D (tentative). See Pregnancy Code inside back cover.

Animal studies: No information available.

Human studies: Information from adequate studies of pregnant women is not available. However, some studies suggest that barbiturates taken during pregnancy are associated with a higher incidence of fetal abnormalities. This drug should be avoided during entire pregnancy.

Advisability of Use if Breast-Feeding

Presence of this drug in breast milk: Probably yes.

Avoid drug or refrain from nursing.

Habit-Forming Potential: If used for an extended period of time, this drug can cause both psychological and physical dependence (see Glossary).

Effects of Overdosage: Behavior similar to alcoholic intoxication: confusion, slurred speech, incoordination, staggering gait, drowsiness, deepening sleep, coma.

Possible Effects of Long-Term Use: Psychological and/or physical dependence. If dose is excessive, a form of chronic intoxication can occur: headache, impaired vision, slurred speech and depression.

Suggested Periodic Examinations While Taking This Drug (at physician's discretion)
With frequent or continual use, complete blood cell counts and liver function tests are desirable.

▷ **While Taking This Drug, Observe the Following**
Foods: No restrictions.
Beverages: No restrictions.
▷ *Alcohol:* Avoid completely. Alcohol can increase greatly the sedative and depressant actions of this drug on brain function.
Tobacco Smoking: No interactions expected.
▷ *Other Drugs*
Butalbital may *increase* the effects of
- other sedatives, hypnotics, tranquilizers, antihistamines and pain relievers, and cause oversedation. Ask your physician for guidance regarding dosage adjustments.

Butalbital may *decrease* the effects of
- oral anticoagulants of the coumarin drug class. Ask physician for guidance regarding prothrombin time testing and adjustment of the anticoagulant dose.
- beta blocker drugs (see Drug Class, Section Four).
- oral contraceptives (see Drug Profile, Section Three).
- cortisonelike drugs (see Drug Class, Section Four).
- doxycycline (Vibramycin, etc.).
- griseofulvin (Fulvicin, Grisactin, etc.).
- phenmetrazine (Preludin).
- quinidine (Quinaglute, Quinidex, etc.).
- theophylline (Bronkotabs, Quibron, Theo-Dur, etc.).

Butalbital *taken concurrently* with
- anticonvulsants may cause a change in the pattern of epileptic seizures. Dosage adjustments may be necessary to achieve a balance of drug actions that will give the best protection from seizures.
▷ *Driving, Hazardous Activities:* This drug can cause drowsiness and can impair mental alertness, judgment, physical coordination and reaction time. Avoid hazardous activities until its full sedative effects have been determined.
Aviation Note: The use of this drug *is a disqualification* for piloting. Consult a designated Aviation Medical Examiner.
Exposure to Sun: Use caution until sensitivity has been determined. Some barbiturates can cause photosensitivity (see Glossary).

Discontinuation: If it has been necessary to use this drug for an extended period of time, do not discontinue it abruptly. Ask physician for guidance during gradual withdrawal. It may also be necessary to adjust the doses of other drugs taken concurrently with it.

CAFFEINE
(KAF een)

Introduced: 4700 B.C. (tea)   **Class:** Stimulant, xanthines

Prescription: USA: No   **Controlled Drug:** USA: No
        Canada: No   Canada: No

Available as Generic: USA: Yes
        Canada: No

Brand Names: Anacin [CD], Anacin Maximum Strength [CD], ✦Anacin w/ Codeine [CD], Cafergot [CD], Cafergot-PB [CD], Cope [CD], Darvon Compound [CD], Darvon Compound-65 [CD], Darvon-N Compound [CD], Dolene Compound-65 [CD], Ercaf [CD], ✦Ergodryl [CD], Excedrin [CD], ✦Exdol-8, -15, -30 [CD], Fioricet [CD], Fiorinal [CD], ✦Fiorinal-C 1/4, -C 1/2 [CD], Fiorinal w/Codeine No. 1, 2, 3 [CD], Hycomine Compound [CD], ✦Lenoltec No. 1, 2, 3 [CD], Midol Caplets [CD], NoDoz, Norgesic [CD], Norgesic Forte [CD], ✦Novopropoxyn Compound [CD], Synalgos [CD], Synalgos-DC [CD], ✦Talwin Compound-50 [CD], Trigesic [CD], ✦Tylenol No. 1 [CD], ✦Tylenol No. 1 Forte [CD], ✦Tylenol w/Codeine No. 2, 3 [CD], Vivarin, Wigraine [CD], ✦Wigraine [CD]

BENEFITS versus RISKS

Possible Benefits	*Possible Risks*
RELIEF OF DROWSINESS AND FATIGUE	Nervousness, insomnia
	Irritability
RELIEF OF MIGRAINE AND RELATED HEADACHES (in combination drugs)	Impaired thinking
	Stomach irritation, heartburn, ulcer

▷ **Principal Uses**

As a Single Drug Product: This stimulant of brain activity is used primarily to prolong wakefulness and delay the onset of sleep.

As a Combination Drug Product [CD]: This drug is used most commonly in combination with ergotamine to treat vascular headaches, such as migraine and cluster headaches. Caffeine increases the absorption of ergotamine and renders it more effective.

How This Drug Works: By increasing the energy level of the chemical systems responsible for nerve tissue activity, this drug induces wakefulness and improves alertness and mental acuity. By constricting the walls of blood vessels, this drug corrects the excessive expansion (dilation) responsible for the pain of vascular headache.

Available Dosage Forms and Strengths
Capsules, prolonged-action — 200 mg, 250 mg
Tablets — 65 mg, 100 mg, 150 mg, 200 mg

▷ **Usual Adult Dosage Range:** 100 to 200 mg/4 hours, as needed. Prolonged-action forms: 200 to 250 mg/6 hours, as needed. **Note: For frequent or long-term use, actual dosage and administration schedule must be determined by the physician for each patient individually.**

▷ **Dosing Instructions:** If necessary, take with food or milk to prevent stomach irritation. The prolonged-action forms should be taken whole (not crushed or chewed). Do not take within 6 hours of retiring.

Usual Duration of Use: Short-term use advised. Avoid frequent or prolonged use without physician supervision.

▷ **This Drug Should Not Be Taken If**
  • you have had an allergic reaction to any dosage form of it previously.
  • you have severe heart disease.
  • you have an active peptic ulcer.

▷ **Inform Your Physician Before Taking This Drug If**
  • you have serious disturbances of heart rhythm.
  • you have a history of peptic ulcer disease.
  • you are subject to hypoglycemia.
  • you have epilepsy.

Possible Side-Effects (natural, expected and unavoidable drug actions)
Nervousness, insomnia, increased urine output. (Nature and degree of side-effects depend upon the size of the dose and the susceptibility of the individual.)

▷ **Possible Adverse Effects** (unusual, unexpected and infrequent reactions)
If any of the following develop, consult your physician promptly for guidance.
Mild Adverse Effects
Headache, irritability, light-headedness, feeling of drunkenness, impaired thinking and concentration.
Rapid, forceful heart action; palpitation.
Indigestion, stomach irritation, heartburn, nausea.
Serious Adverse Effects
Development of peptic ulcer (in susceptible individuals).

▷ **Possible Effects on Sexual Function:** None reported.

CAUTION
1. Do not exceed 250 mg/dose or 500 mg/24 hours.
2. Caffeine in excessive amounts can provoke migraine headache in susceptible individuals.

Precautions for Use

By Infants and Children: Use not recommended.

By Those over 60 Years of Age: Tolerance for caffeine often decreases after 60. You may be more susceptible to caffeine-induced nervousness, irritability, impaired thinking, tremor, insomnia, disturbed heart rhythm and acid indigestion.

▷ **Advisability of Use During Pregnancy**

Pregnancy Category: C (tentative). See Pregnancy Code inside back cover.
Animal studies: Significant birth defects are attributed to this drug.
Human studies: Information from studies of pregnant women indicates no increased birth defects in 12,696 exposures to this drug.
Avoid completely during first 3 months. Because caffeine reaches the same level in fetal tissues as in maternal tissues and is associated with fetal loss, premature deliveries and low birth weights, it is advisable to avoid caffeine throughout pregnancy.

Advisability of Use if Breast-Feeding

Presence of this drug in breast milk: Yes, in small amounts.
Monitor nursing infant closely and discontinue drug or nursing if adverse effects develop.

Habit-Forming Potential: Varying degrees of tolerance and psychological dependence (see Glossary) may occur with prolonged use.

Effects of Overdosage: Nervousness, restlessness, insomnia (followed by depression in some individuals), tremor, sweating, ringing in ears, spots before eyes, heart palpitation, diarrhea, excitement, delirium, hallucinations, seizures.

Possible Effects of Long-Term Use: Development of tolerance and psychological dependence; stomach irritation (gastritis), peptic ulcer.

Suggested Periodic Examinations While Taking This Drug (at physician's discretion)
None.

▷ **While Taking This Drug, Observe the Following**

Foods: No restrictions. Note: Chocolate contains 5 to 10 mg of caffeine per ounce.

Beverages: Keep in mind that caffeine beverages (coffee, tea, cola) will add to the total intake of caffeine taken in medicinal form. Avoid possible overdosage. The approximate caffeine content of popular beverages is as follows:
Regular coffee (average cup) 100–150 mg

Instant coffee (average cup) 80–100 mg
Coffee-grain blends (average cup) 14–37 mg
Decaffeinated coffee (average cup) 3–5 mg
Tea (average cup) 60–75 mg
Regular cola (6 ounces) 36 mg
Diet cola (6 ounces) 18 mg
Cocoa (6 ounces) 10 mg
▷ *Alcohol:* No interactions expected.
Tobacco Smoking: Consult physician regarding possible adverse effects of combined nicotine and caffeine. Smoking can hasten the elimination of caffeine and shorten its period of effectiveness.
▷ *Other Drugs*
Caffeine may **decrease** the effects of
• sedatives, tranquilizers, hypnotics and pain relievers.
The following drugs may **increase** the effects of caffeine
• cimetidine (tagamet).
• oral contraceptives.
▷ *Driving, Hazardous Activities:* No restrictions.
Aviation Note: No restrictions.
Exposure to Sun: No restrictions.
Discontinuation: Sudden discontinuation of this drug after extended use can produce a "caffeine-withdrawal" headache. This is readily relieved by coffee or caffeine in medicinal form.

CALCIUM CARBONATE
(KAL see um KAR boh nayt)

Other Name: Antacid

Introduced: 1825

Class: Antacid, calcium supplements

Prescription: USA: No
Canada: No

Controlled Drug: USA: No
Canada: No

Available as Generic: Yes

Brand Names: Alka-Mints, Alkets [CD], ✦Apo-Cal, BioCal, Bisodol Tablets [CD], ✦Calcite 500, ✦Calcium-Sandoz [CD], ✦Calsan, Cal.Sup, Caltrate 600, Camalox [CD], ✦DiCal-D [CD], Dicarbosil, Di-Gel Advanced Formula [CD], ✦Gramcal [CD], Marblen [CD], ✦Os-Cal, ✦Os-Cal D [CD], Os-Cal + D [CD], Os-Cal 500 + D [CD], Os-Cal 250 [CD], Os-Cal 500, Titralac, Tums, Tums Extra Strength, Tums with Simethicone [CD]

```
┌─────────────────────────────────────────────────────────────┐
│                   BENEFITS versus RISKS                       │
│                                                               │
│        Possible Benefits              Possible Risks          │
│   EFFECTIVE RELIEF OF ACID       Constipation                 │
│      INDIGESTION                 Predisposition to calcified kidney │
│   CORRECTION OF CALCIUM            stones and kidney damage    │
│      DEFICIENCY                    (excessive use)            │
└─────────────────────────────────────────────────────────────┘
```

▷ **Principal Uses**

As a Single Drug Product: Used primarily to (1) relieve acid indigestion, heartburn and sour stomach, and (2) supplement the diet to meet the body's requirements for calcium in the formation and maintenance of normal bone. Used primarily in children to prevent or treat rickets, and in adults to prevent or treat osteoporosis or osteomalacia.

As a Combination Drug Product [CD]: Often combined with other antacids to enhance the product's ability to neutralize stomach acids. Also combined with vitamin D, which increases the intestinal absorption of calcium. Also available in combination with the entire spectrum of essential vitamins and minerals.

How This Drug Works: By neutralizing some of the hydrochloric acid in the stomach and by reducing the action of the digestive enzyme pepsin, antacids lessen the irritant effect of digestive juices on inflamed tissues and create a more favorable environment for the healing of peptic ulcers.

Available Dosage Forms and Strengths

Capsules —	364 mg
Capsules, soft gel —	1512 mg
Chewing gum —	500 mg
Oral suspension —	1000 mg, 1250 mg per 5-ml teaspoonful
Tablets —	250 mg, 280 mg, 650 mg, 667 mg, 750 mg, 1250 mg, 1500 mg
Tablets, chewable —	350 mg, 420 mg, 500 mg, 625 mg, 650 mg, 750 mg, 850 mg, 1250 mg, 1500 mg

▷ **Usual Adult Dosage Range:**   (1) As antacid: 500 mg to 2 grams after meals and at bedtime, or as needed. Total daily dosage should not exceed 8 grams. (2) As supplement, the recommended daily dietary allowances are as follows:

Infants up to 6 months of age: 360 mg.

Infants 6 months to 1 year of age: 540 mg.

Children 1 to 10 years of age: 800 mg.

Males 11 to 18 years of age: 1200 mg.

Males 19 years of age and older: 800 mg.

Females 11 to 18 years of age: 1200 mg.

Females 19 to 50 years of age: 800 mg.

Females after 50 years of age (postmenopausal): 1500 mg.

During pregnancy: 1200 mg.

While breast-feeding: 1200 mg.
Note: For long-term use, actual dosage and administration schedule must be determined by the physician for each patient individually.

▷ **Dosing Instructions:** As antacid for treatment of peptic ulcer disease, take 1 to 3 hours after meals and at bedtime. As supplement, take 1 to 2 hours after meals. Chewable tablets should be chewed thoroughly before swallowing. Shake suspension well before measuring dose. Do not take within 2 hours of other oral medications.

Usual Duration of Use: If used for the treatment of peptic ulcer disease, continual use on a regular schedule is recommended for 4 to 6 weeks after all symptoms of ulcer activity have disappeared. Long-term use, as antacid or supplement, should be under physician supervision. Consult your physician on a regular basis.

▷ **This Drug Should Not Be Taken If**
• your calcium blood level is abnormally high.
• you have severe kidney disease.
• you have calcified kidney stones.
• you are immobilized for an extended period of time.

▷ **Inform Your Physician Before Taking This Drug If**
• you have a history of kidney stones or impaired kidney function.
• you have any form of heart disease.
• you have sarcoidosis.
• you have deficient or absent stomach acid.
• you are prone to constipation.
• you are taking any other oral medications at this time, especially thiazide diuretics, quinidine or tetracycline.

Possible Side-Effects (natural, expected and unavoidable drug actions)
Constipation (may be severe with large doses).

▷ **Possible Adverse Effects** (unusual, unexpected and infrequent reactions)
If any of the following develop, consult your physician promptly for guidance.
Mild Adverse Effects
Chalky taste in mouth, belching, intestinal gas.
Serious Adverse Effects
With normal dosage—none.
With excessive dosage—abnormally high level of blood calcium: headache, fatigue, weakness, loss of appetite, nausea, vomiting.

▷ **Possible Effects on Sexual Function:** None reported.

CAUTION
1. Calcium can interfere with the absorption of many drugs. Do not take any other oral medication within 2 hours of a dose of calcium carbonate.

2. Avoid large doses of vitamin D while taking any form of calcium. Ask physician for guidance regarding vitamin D dosage.

Precautions for Use

By Infants and Children: May cause constipation with frequent or chronic use. Limit use to short-term schedules.

By Those over 60 Years of Age: This drug should be avoided because of its potential for raising the blood calcium level and predisposing to kidney stones and impairment of kidney function.

▷ **Advisability of Use During Pregnancy**

Pregnancy Category: C (tentative). See Pregnancy Code inside back cover. Animal studies: No information available.

Human studies: Information from adequate studies of pregnant women is not available.

This drug is considered safe for use during the last 6 months of pregnancy in doses not to exceed 1200 mg daily. The calcium content of the diet must be considered.

Advisability of Use if Breast-Feeding

Presence of this drug in breast milk: Calcium is a normal constituent of breast milk. This drug does not increase the calcium content of milk to any significant degree, but does prevent deficiency.

Habit-Forming Potential: None.

Effects of Overdosage: Headache, fatigue, weakness, nervousness, muscle twitching, stomach pain, nausea, vomiting, constipation, mental disturbance, delirium, coma.

Possible Effects of Long-Term Use: Development of calcium-containing kidney stones.

Suggested Periodic Examinations While Taking This Drug (at physician's discretion)

Measurement of blood calcium levels (chronic use).

▷ **While Taking This Drug, Observe the Following**

Foods: Avoid frequent and excessive intake of spinach, rhubarb, bran and whole grain cereals; these can interfere with the absorption of calcium.

Beverages: Avoid large quantities of milk while taking calcium.

▷ *Alcohol:* No interactions.

Tobacco Smoking: No interactions.

▷ *Other Drugs*

Calcium may **increase** the effects of
• quinidine by delaying its elimination.

Calcium may **decrease** the effects of
• iron preparations.
• salicylates (aspirin, etc.).

- tetracyclines.

Calcium *taken concurrently* with

- thiazide diuretics (see Drug Class, Section Four) may cause abnormally high blood levels of calcium.

▷ *Driving, Hazardous Activities:* No restrictions.

CAPTOPRIL
(KAP toh pril)

Introduced: 1979

Class: Antihypertensive, ACE inhibitor

Prescription: USA: Yes
Canada: Yes

Controlled Drug: USA: No
Canada: No

Available as Generic: No

Brand Names: Capoten, Capozide [CD]

BENEFITS versus RISKS	
Possible Benefits	*Possible Risks*
EFFECTIVE CONTROL OF MILD TO SEVERE HIGH BLOOD PRESSURE	Rash, itching, fever (10%)
	Lost or altered taste (7%)
	Impaired white blood cell production (0.3%)
USEFUL ADJUNCTIVE TREATMENT FOR CONGESTIVE HEART FAILURE	Bone marrow depression (rare)
	Kidney damage (rare)
	Liver damage (rare)

▷ **Principal Uses**

As a Single Drug Product: Used primarily to treat all degrees of high blood pressure. Mild to moderate high blood pressure usually responds to low doses; severe high blood pressure requires higher doses, with greater risk of serious adverse effects. Also used to treat selected cases of advanced heart failure that have not responded to conventional treatment with digitalis and diuretics.

How This Drug Works: Not completely known. It is thought that by blocking certain enzyme systems that influence arterial function, this drug contributes to the relaxation of arterial walls throughout the body and thus lowers the resistance to blood flow that causes high blood pressure. This, in turn, reduces the workload of the heart and improves its performance.

Available Dosage Forms and Strengths
Tablets — 12.5 mg, 25 mg, 50 mg, 100 mg

▷ **Usual Adult Dosage Range:**   Initially 12.5 to 25 mg 2 or 3 times daily for 2 weeks. If necessary, dose may be increased to 50 mg 3 times daily. Usual maintenance dose is 50 to 100 mg 3 times daily. Total daily dose should not exceed 450 mg. **Note: Actual dosage and administration schedule must be determined by the physician for each patient individually.**

▷ **Dosing Instructions:**   Take on empty stomach, 1 hour before meals, at same time each day. Tablet may be crushed for administration.

Usual Duration of Use: Continual use on a regular schedule for several weeks is usually necessary to determine this drug's effectiveness in controlling high blood pressure. The proper treatment of high blood pressure usually requires the long-term use of effective medications. Consult your physician on a regular basis.

▷ **This Drug Should Not Be Taken If**
• you have had an allergic reaction to it previously.
• you currently have a blood cell or bone marrow disorder.
• you have active liver disease.
• you have an abnormally high level of blood potassium.

▷ **Inform Your Physician Before Taking This Drug If**
• you have a history of kidney disease or impaired kidney function.
• you have scleroderma or systemic lupus erythematosus.
• you have any form of heart disease.
• you have diabetes.
• you are taking any of the following drugs: other antihypertensives, diuretics, nitrates, allopurinol (Zyloprim), Indocin or potassium supplements.
• you plan to have surgery under general anesthesia in the near future.

Possible Side-Effects (natural, expected and unavoidable drug actions)
Dizziness, light-headedness, fainting (excessive drop in blood pressure).

▷ **Possible Adverse Effects** (unusual, unexpected and infrequent reactions)
If any of the following develop, consult your physician promptly for guidance.
Mild Adverse Effects
Allergic Reactions: Skin rash; swelling of face, hands or feet; fever.
Lost or altered taste, mouth or tongue sores.
Rapid heart rate, palpitation.
Serious Adverse Effects
Bone marrow depression—fatigue, weakness, fever, sore throat, abnormal bleeding or bruising.
Kidney damage—water retention (edema).
Liver damage—with or without jaundice.

▷ **Possible Effects on Sexual Function:**   Decreased male libido (20% to 30%) with recommended dosage.

CAUTION
1. If possible, it is advisable to discontinue all other antihypertensive drugs (especially diuretics) for 1 week before starting captopril.
2. **Report promptly** any indications of infection (fever, sore throat), and any indications of water retention (weight gain, puffiness, swollen feet or ankles).
3. Do not use a salt substitute without your physician's knowledge and approval. (Many salt substitutes contain potassium.)
4. It is advisable to obtain blood cell counts and urine analyses **before** starting this drug.

Precautions for Use
By Infants and Children: Safety and effectiveness for use by those in this age group have not been established.
By Those over 60 Years of Age: Small doses are advisable until tolerance has been determined. Sudden and excessive lowering of blood pressure can predispose to stroke or heart attack in those with impaired brain circulation or coronary artery heart disease.

▷ **Advisability of Use During Pregnancy**
Pregnancy Category: C (tentative). See Pregnancy Code inside back cover.
Animal studies: No birth defects found in rat, rabbit or hamster studies. However, this drug was shown to be toxic to the embryo and newborn.
Human studies: Information from adequate studies of pregnant women is not available.
Avoid during first 3 months if possible. Use only if clearly needed during last 6 months.

Advisability of Use if Breast-Feeding
Presence of this drug in breast milk: Yes, in small amounts.
Monitor nursing infant closely and discontinue drug or nursing if adverse effects develop.

Habit-Forming Potential: None.

Effects of Overdosage: Excessive drop in blood pressure—light-headedness, dizziness, fainting.

Possible Effects of Long-Term Use: Gradual increase in blood potassium level.

Suggested Periodic Examinations While Taking This Drug (at physician's discretion)
Before starting drug: Complete blood cell counts; urine analysis with measurement of protein content, blood potassium level. During use of drug: Blood cell counts every 2 weeks during the first 3 months of treatment, then periodically for duration of use. Urine protein meas-

urements every month during the first 9 months of treatment, then periodically for duration of use. Periodic measurements of blood potassium.

▷ **While Taking This Drug, Observe the Following**

Foods: Consult physician regarding salt intake.

Nutritional Support: **Do not take** potassium supplements unless directed by your physician.

Beverages: No restrictions. May be taken with milk.

▷ *Alcohol:* Use caution until combined effect has been determined. Alcohol may enhance the blood-pressure-lowering effect of this drug.

Tobacco Smoking: No interactions expected.

▷ *Other Drugs*

Captopril *taken concurrently* with

- potassium preparations (K-Lyte, Slow-K, etc.) may cause increased blood levels of potassium with risk of serious heart rhythm disturbances.
- potassium-sparing diuretics: amiloride (Moduretic), spironolactone (Aldactazide), triamterene (Dyazide) may cause increased blood levels of potassium with risk of serious heart rhythm disturbances.

The following drugs may *decrease* the effects of captopril

- indomethacin (Indocin).
- salicylates (aspirin, etc.).

▷ *Driving, Hazardous Activities:* Usually no restrictions. Be aware of possible drops in blood pressure with resultant dizziness or faintness.

Aviation Note: The use of this drug *may be a disqualification* for piloting. Consult a designated Aviation Medical Examiner.

Exposure to Sun: Caution advised. This drug can cause photosensitivity.

Exposure to Heat: Caution advised. Avoid excessive perspiring with resultant loss of body water and drop in blood pressure.

Occurrence of Unrelated Illness: Report promptly any disorder that causes nausea, vomiting or diarrhea. Fluid and chemical imbalances must be corrected as soon as possible.

CARBAMAZEPINE
(kar ba MAZ e peen)

Introduced: 1962

Class: Anticonvulsant, antineuralgic

Prescription: USA: Yes
Canada: Yes

Controlled Drug: USA: No
Canada: No

Available as Generic: Yes

Brand Names: ✦Apo-Carbamazepine, Epitol, ✦Mazepine, ✦PMS-Carbamazepine, Tegretol

```
┌──────────────────────────────────────────────────────────────┐
│                    BENEFITS versus RISKS                       │
│                                                                │
│        Possible Benefits              Possible Risks           │
│   RELIEF OF PAIN IN             RARE BONE MARROW               │
│     TRIGEMINAL NEURALGIA          DEPRESSION (reduced          │
│   EFFECTIVE CONTROL OF            formation of all blood cells)│
│     CERTAIN TYPES OF            Liver damage with jaundice     │
│     EPILEPTIC SEIZURES                                         │
│   Relief of pain in some rare forms                            │
│     of neuralgia                                               │
└──────────────────────────────────────────────────────────────┘
```

▷ **Principal Uses**

As a Single Drug Product: This drug is used primarily in the management of two uncommon but serious disorders: (1) for relief of pain in true trigeminal neuralgia (tic douloureux) and glossopharyngeal neuralgia; (2) for control of several types of epilepsy, namely grand mal, psychomotor or temporal lobe, and mixed seizure patterns. Because of its potential for serious toxic effects, precise diagnosis and careful management are mandatory for its proper use.

How This Drug Works: Not completely known. It is thought that by reducing the transmission of impulses at certain nerve terminals, this drug relieves or reduces pain (of trigeminal neuralgia) and also reduces the excitability of certain nerve fibers in the brain and thereby inhibits the repetitive spread of electrical impulses along nerve pathways. This action may prevent seizures altogether or reduce their frequency and severity.

Available Dosage Forms and Strengths
       Oral suspension — 100 mg per 5-ml teaspoonful
              Tablets — 200 mg
   Tablets, chewable — 100 mg

▷ **Usual Adult Dosage Range:**   Initially 200 mg/12 hours. Dose may be increased by 200 mg/24 hours as needed and tolerated. Total daily dosage should not exceed 1200 mg. **Note: Actual dosage and administration schedule must be determined by the physician for each patient individually.**

▷ **Dosing Instructions:**   Take at same time each day, with or following food to reduce stomach irritation. Tablet may be crushed for administration.

Usual Duration of Use: Continual use on a regular schedule for 3 months is usually necessary to determine this drug's effectiveness in relieving the pain of trigeminal neuralgia. Longer periods, with dosage adjustment, may be required to determine its ability to control epileptic seizures. Careful evaluation of each individual's tolerance and response should be made every 3 months during long-term treatment. Consult your physician on a regular basis.

▷ **This Drug Should Not Be Taken If**
- you have had an allergic reaction to it previously.
- you have active liver disease.
- you currently have a blood cell or bone marrow disorder.
- you are currently taking, or have taken within the past 14 days, any monoamine oxidase (MAO) type A inhibitor drug (see Drug Class, Section Four).

▷ **Inform Your Physician Before Taking This Drug If**
- you have had an allergic reaction to any tricyclic antidepressant drug (see Drug Class, Section Four).
- you have taken this drug in the past.
- you have a history of any kind of blood cell or bone marrow disorder, especially one due to a drug.
- you have a history of liver or kidney disease.
- you have had serious mental depression or other mental disorder.
- you have had thrombophlebitis.
- you have high blood pressure, heart disease or glaucoma.
- you take more than 2 alcoholic drinks a day.

Possible Side-Effects (natural, expected and unavoidable drug actions)
Dry mouth and throat, constipation, impaired urination.

▷ **Possible Adverse Effects** (unusual, unexpected and infrequent reactions)
If any of the following develop, consult your physician promptly for guidance.

Mild Adverse Effects
Allergic Reactions: Skin rash, hives, itching, drug fever.
Headache, dizziness, drowsiness, unsteadiness, fatigue, blurred vision, confusion.
Exaggerated hearing, ringing in ears.
Loss of appetite, nausea, vomiting, indigestion, diarrhea.
Water retention (edema), frequent urination.
Changes in skin pigmentation, hair loss.
Aching of muscles and joints, leg cramps.

Serious Adverse Effects
Allergic Reactions: Severe dermatitis with peeling of skin, irritation of mouth and tongue, swelling of lymph glands.
Idiosyncratic Reactions: Lung inflammation (pneumonitis): cough, shortness of breath.
Bone marrow depression (see Glossary)—fatigue, weakness, fever, sore throat, abnormal bleeding or bruising.
Liver damage with jaundice (see Glossary)—yellow eyes and skin, dark-colored urine, light-colored stools.
Kidney damage—reduced urine volume, uremic poisoning.
Mental depression and agitation.
Double vision, visual hallucinations, speech disturbances, peripheral neuritis (see Glossary).
Thrombophlebitis.

▷ **Possible Effects on Sexual Function**

Decreased libido and/or impotence (13%), male infertility.

This drug is used to control hypersexuality (exaggerated sexual behavior) that can result from injury to the temporal lobe of the brain.

▷ **Adverse Effects That May Mimic Natural Diseases or Disorders**

Liver reactions may suggest viral hepatitis.

Rare lung reactions may suggest interstitial pneumonitis.

Natural Diseases or Disorders That May Be Activated by This Drug

Latent psychosis, systemic lupus erythematosus.

CAUTION

1. Because this drug can cause serious adverse effects, it should be used only after a trial of less hazardous drugs has been ineffective.
2. *Before* the first dose is taken, pretreatment blood cell counts, liver function tests and kidney function tests should be performed.
3. Careful periodic testing for early indications of blood cell or bone marrow toxicity is *mandatory.*
4. During periods of spontaneous remission from trigeminal neuralgia, this drug *should not be used* to prevent recurrence.
5. If used to control epileptic seizures, *do not discontinue this drug suddenly.*

Precautions for Use

By Infants and Children: Because of the high frequency of adverse effects (up to 25%), careful testing of blood cell production, liver function and kidney function must be performed regularly. This drug can reduce the effectiveness of other anticonvulsant drugs. Blood levels of all anticonvulsant drugs should be monitored when this drug is added to the treatment program.

By Those over 60 Years of Age: This drug can cause confusion and agitation. Observe for the possible aggravation of glaucoma, coronary artery disease (angina) or prostatism (see Glossary).

▷ **Advisability of Use During Pregnancy**

Pregnancy Category: C (tentative). See Pregnancy Code inside back cover.

Animal studies: Rat studies reveal significant birth defects.

Human studies: Information from adequate studies of pregnant women is not available.

Avoid completely during the first 3 months. Use during the last 6 months only if clearly needed.

Advisability of Use if Breast-Feeding

Presence of this drug in breast milk: Yes.

Avoid drug or refrain from nursing.

Habit-Forming Potential: None.

Effects of Overdosage: Dizziness, unsteadiness, drowsiness, disorientation, tremor, involuntary movements, nausea, vomiting, flushed skin, dilated pupils, stupor progressing to coma.

Possible Effects of Long-Term Use: Water retention (edema), impaired kidney function, possible liver damage with jaundice.

Suggested Periodic Examinations While Taking This Drug (at physician's discretion)
Complete blood cell counts weekly during the first 3 months of treatment, and monthly thereafter until the drug is discontinued. Liver and kidney function tests. Complete eye examinations.

▷ **While Taking This Drug, Observe the Following**
Foods: No restrictions.
Beverages: No restrictions. May be taken with milk.
▷ *Alcohol:* Use caution until the combined effect has been determined. This drug may increase the sedative effect of alcohol.
Tobacco Smoking: No interactions expected.
▷ *Other Drugs*
Carbamazepine may *increase* the effects of
• sedatives, tranquilizers, hypnotics, narcotics, and enhance their sedative effects.
Carbamazepine may *decrease* the effects of
• doxycycline (Doxy-II, Vibramycin, etc.).
• warfarin (Coumadin, Panwarfin, etc.).
Carbamazepine *taken concurrently* with
• lithium may cause serious neurological disturbances: confusion, drowsiness, weakness, unsteadiness, tremors, muscle twitching.
• monoamine oxidase (MAO) type A inhibitor drugs (see Drug Class, Section Four) may cause severe toxic reactions.
The following drugs may *increase* the effects of carbamazepine
• erythromycin (E.E.S., E-Mycin, etc.).
• isoniazid (INH).
• propoxyphene (Darvon, Darvocet, etc.).
• troleandomycin (Tao).
▷ *Driving, Hazardous Activities:* This drug can cause dizziness and drowsiness. Adjust activities accordingly.
Aviation Note: The use of this drug *is a disqualification* for piloting. Consult a designated Aviation Medical Examiner.
Exposure to Sun: This drug can cause photosensitivity (see Glossary). Use caution until sensitivity to sun has been determined.
Heavy Exercise or Exertion: Use caution if you have coronary artery disease. This drug can intensify angina and reduce tolerance for physical activity.
Occurrence of Unrelated Illness: Because of this drug's potential for serious adverse effects, it is mandatory that you inform each physician and dentist you consult that you are taking carbamazepine.
Discontinuation: If used to treat trigeminal neuralgia, attempt should be made every 3 months to reduce the maintenance dose or to discontinue this drug altogether. If used to control epilepsy, this drug *must not be discontinued abruptly.*

CARBENICILLIN
(kar ben i SIL in)

Introduced: 1964

Class: Antibiotic, penicillins

Prescription: USA: Yes
  Canada: Yes

Controlled Drug: USA: No
  Canada: No

Available as Generic: No

Brand Names: Geocillin, Geopen, ✦Geopen Oral, Pyopen

BENEFITS versus RISKS

Possible Benefits	*Possible Risks*
EFFECTIVE TREATMENT OF INFECTIONS due to susceptible microorganisms	ALLERGIC REACTIONS, mild to severe Superinfections (yeast) Drug-induced colitis Rare blood cell disorders

---

▷ **Principal Uses**

As a Single Drug Product: Oral tablets are used to treat certain infections of the urinary tract and prostate gland. Injections are used to treat a wider variety of more serious infections.

How This Drug Works: This drug destroys susceptible infecting bacteria by interfering with their ability to produce new protective cell walls as they multiply and grow.

Available Dosage Forms and Strengths
      Injections — Vials of 1 gram, 2 grams, 5 grams
   Tablets, film-coated — 382 mg

▷ **Usual Adult Dosage Range:**   382 to 764 mg/6 hours (4 doses/24 hours). **Note: Actual dosage and administration schedule must be determined by the physician for each patient individually.**

▷ **Dosing Instructions:** Take on an empty stomach, 1 hour before or 2 hours after eating, at same times each day. Tablet be crushed for administration, but drug has a bitter taste.

Usual Duration of Use: For urinary tract infections—10 days. For prostate gland infections—2 to 4 weeks. Recurrent and chronic infections require longer periods of treatment.

▷ **This Drug Should Not Be Taken If**
   • you have had an allergic reaction to any dosage form of it previously.
   • you are certain you are allergic to *any* form of penicillin.

▷ **Inform Your Physician Before Taking This Drug If**
- you suspect you may be allergic to penicillin or you have a history of a previous "reaction" to penicillin.
- you are allergic to cephalosporin antibiotics (Ancef, Ceporan, Ceporex, Kafocin, Keflex, Keflin, Kefzol, Loridine).
- you are allergic by nature—hay fever, asthma, hives, eczema.
- you have a history of a bleeding disorder, kidney disease, regional enteritis or ulcerative colitis.

Possible Side-Effects (natural, expected and unavoidable drug actions)
Superinfections (see Glossary), often due to yeast organisms.

▷ **Possible Adverse Effects** (unusual, unexpected and infrequent reactions)
If any of the following develop, consult your physician promptly for guidance.
Mild Adverse Effects
Allergic Reactions: Skin rashes, hives, itching.
Irritations of mouth and tongue, unpleasant taste, nausea, vomiting, mild diarrhea.
Serious Adverse Effects
Allergic Reactions: Anaphylactic reaction (see Glossary), severe skin reactions, drug fever, swollen painful joints, sore throat, abnormal bleeding or bruising.
Hemolytic anemia (see Glossary).
Pseudomembranous colitis—severe diarrhea.

▷ **Possible Effects on Sexual Function:**   None reported.

CAUTION
1. Take the exact dose and the full course prescribed.
2. This drug should not be used concurrently with antibiotics like erythromycin or tetracycline.

Precautions for Use
By Infants and Children: Safety and effectiveness for use by those under 12 years of age have not been established.
By Those over 60 Years of Age: It is advisable to evaluate kidney function before and during use of this drug to determine the need for dosage adjustment. Natural changes in the skin may predispose to prolonged itching reactions in the genital and anal regions. Report such reactions promptly.

▷ **Advisability of Use During Pregnancy**
Pregnancy Category: B (tentative). See Pregnancy Code inside back cover.
Animal studies: No information available.
Human studies: Information from adequate studies of pregnant women indicates no increased risk of birth defects in 3546 pregnancies exposed to penicillin derivatives.
Ask physician for guidance.

Advisability of Use if Breast-Feeding
Presence of this drug in breast milk: Probably yes.
The nursing infant may be sensitized to penicillin and be at risk for developing diarrhea or yeast infections.
Avoid drug if possible or refrain from nursing.

Habit-Forming Potential: None.

Effects of Overdosage: Possible nausea, vomiting and/or diarrhea.

Possible Effects of Long-Term Use: Superinfections, often due to yeast organisms.

Suggested Periodic Examinations While Taking This Drug (at physician's discretion)
Complete blood cell counts. Liver and kidney function tests with long-term use.

▷ **While Taking This Drug, Observe the Following**
Foods: No restrictions.
Beverages: No restrictions.
▷ *Alcohol:* No interactions expected.
Tobacco Smoking: No interactions expected.
▷ *Other Drugs*
Carbenicillin may *decrease* the effects of
• oral contraceptives in some women, and impair their effectiveness in preventing pregnancy.
The following drugs may *decrease* the effects of carbenicillin
• antacids may reduce the absorption of carbenicillin.
• chloramphenicol (Chloromycetin).
• erythromycin (Erythrocin, E-Mycin, etc.).
• tetracyclines (Achromycin, Declomycin, Minocin, etc.). (See Drug Class, Section Four.)
▷ *Driving, Hazardous Activities:* Usually no restrictions.
Aviation Note: The use of this drug *may be a disqualification* for piloting.
Consult a designated Aviation Medical Examiner.
Exposure to Sun: No restrictions.

CEFACLOR
(SEF a klor)

Introduced: 1979

Class: Antibiotic, cephalosporins

Prescription: USA: Yes
Canada: Yes

Controlled Drug: USA: No
Canada: No

Available as Generic: No

Brand Name: Ceclor

BENEFITS versus RISKS

Possible Benefits	*Possible Risks*
EFFECTIVE TREATMENT OF INFECTIONS due to susceptible microorganisms	ALLERGIC REACTIONS mild to severe (up to 5% of general population, up to 16% of those allergic to penicillin) Drug-induced colitis (rare) Superinfections (see Glossary)

▷ **Principal Uses**

As a Single Drug Product: To treat certain infections of the skin and skin structures, the upper and lower respiratory tract (including middle ear infections and "strep" throat) and certain infections of the urinary tract.

How This Drug Works: This drug destroys susceptible infecting bacteria by interfering with their ability to produce new protective cell walls as they multiply and grow.

Available Dosage Forms and Strengths

Capsules — 250 mg, 500 mg

Oral suspension — 125 mg, 250 mg per 5-ml teaspoonful

▷ **Usual Adult Dosage Range:** 250 to 500 mg/8 hours. Total daily dose should not exceed 4 grams. **Note: Actual dosage and administration schedule must be determined by the physician for each patient individually.**

▷ **Dosing Instructions:** May be taken on an empty stomach or with food if stomach irritation occurs. Capsule may be opened for administration. Shake suspension well before measuring dose. Take the full course prescribed.

Usual Duration of Use: Continual use on a regular schedule for 3 to 5 days is usually necessary to determine this drug's effectiveness in controlling the infection under treatment. Response varies with the nature of the infection. Total treatment time will vary from 1 to 4 weeks. Certain infections require that this drug be taken for 10 consecutive days to prevent the development of rheumatic fever. Follow your physician's instructions regarding duration of use.

▷ **This Drug Should Not Be Taken If**
   • you are allergic to any cephalosporin antibiotic (see Drug Class, Section Four).

▷ **Inform Your Physician Before Taking This Drug If**
   • you have a history of allergy to any form of penicillin (see Drug Class, Section Four).

- you have a history of regional enteritis or ulcerative colitis.
- you have impaired kidney function.

Possible Side-Effects (natural, expected and unavoidable drug actions)
Superinfections (see Glossary).

▷ **Possible Adverse Effects** (unusual, unexpected and infrequent reactions)
If any of the following develop, consult your physician promptly for guidance.
Mild Adverse Effects
Allergic Reactions: Skin rash, itching, hives.
Nausea and vomiting (1 in 90), mild diarrhea (1 in 70), sore mouth or tongue.
Serious Adverse Effects
Allergic Reactions: Drug fever (see Glossary), joint aches and pains, anaphylactic reaction (see Glossary).
Idiosyncratic Reactions: Minor and temporary changes in white blood cell counts and liver function tests (infrequent).
Genital itching (may represent a fungus superinfection).
Severe diarrhea, possibly indicating a drug-induced form of colitis (rare).

▷ **Possible Effects on Sexual Function:**   None reported.

▷ **Adverse Effects That May Mimic Natural Diseases or Disorders**
Skin rash and fever may resemble measles.

CAUTION
In the management of diabetes it should be noted that this drug can cause a false positive test result for urine sugar when using Clinitest tablets, Benedict's solution or Fehling's solution, but not with Tes-Tape.

Precautions for Use
By Infants and Children: Not recommended for use in infants less than 1 month old. The maximal dose in children should not exceed 1 gram/24 hours.
By Those over 60 Years of Age: Dosage must be carefully individualized and based upon evaluation of kidney function. Natural changes in the skin may predispose to severe and prolonged itching reactions in the genital and anal regions. Such reactions should be reported promptly.

▷ **Advisability of Use During Pregnancy**
Pregnancy Category: B (tentative). See Pregnancy Code inside back cover.
Animal studies: No birth defects reported.
Human studies: Information from adequate studies of pregnant women is not available.
Generally considered to be safe. Ask physician for guidance.

Advisability of Use if Breast-Feeding
Presence of this drug in breast milk: Yes, in small amounts.
Avoid drug or refrain from nursing.

Habit-Forming Potential: None.

Effects of Overdosage: Nausea, vomiting, stomach cramps and/or diarrhea.

Possible Effects of Long-Term Use: Superinfections (see Glossary).

Suggested Periodic Examinations While Taking This Drug (at physician's discretion)
Complete blood cell counts.

▷ **While Taking This Drug, Observe the Following**
   Foods: No restrictions.
   Beverages: No restrictions. May be taken with milk.
▷ *Alcohol:* No interactions expected.
   Tobacco Smoking: No interactions expected.
▷ *Other Drugs*
      Cefaclor **taken concurrently** with
      • probenecid (Benemid) will slow the elimination of cefaclor, resulting in higher blood levels and prolonged effect.
▷ *Driving, Hazardous Activities:* Usually no restrictions.
   Aviation Note: The use of this drug **may be a disqualification** for piloting. Consult a designated Aviation Medical Examiner.
   Exposure to Sun: No restrictions.
   Special Storage Instructions: Oral suspension should be refrigerated.
   Observe the Following Expiration Times: Do not take the oral suspension of this drug if it is older than 14 days.

CEFADROXIL
(sef a DROX il)

Introduced: 1977

Class: Antibiotic, cephalosporins

Prescription: USA: Yes
      Canada: Yes

Controlled Drug: USA: No
      Canada: No

Available as Generic: No

Brand Names: Duricef, Ultracef

BENEFITS versus RISKS	
Possible Benefits	*Possible Risks*
EFFECTIVE TREATMENT OF INFECTIONS due to susceptible microorganisms	ALLERGIC REACTIONS mild to severe (up to 5% of general population, up to 16% of those allergic to penicillin) Drug-induced colitis (rare) Superinfections (see Glossary)

▷ **Principal Uses**

As a Single Drug Product: To treat certain infections of the skin and skin structures, the upper respiratory tract (including tonsillitis and "strep" throat) and certain infections of the urinary tract.

How This Drug Works: This drug destroys susceptible infecting bacteria by interfering with their ability to produce new protective cell walls as they multiply and grow.

Available Dosage Forms and Strengths

Capsules — 500 mg

Oral suspension — 125 mg, 250 mg, 500 mg per 5-ml teaspoonful

Tablets — 1000 mg (1 gram)

▷ **Usual Adult Dosage Range:** Skin infections—500 mg/12 hours, or 1 gram daily. "Strep" throat—500 mg/12 hours for 10 days. Urinary tract infections—500 mg to 1 gram/12 hours, or 1 to 2 grams daily. Total daily dosage should not exceed 6 grams. **Note: Actual dosage and administration schedule must be determined by the physician for each patient individually.**

▷ **Dosing Instructions:** May be taken on an empty stomach or with food if stomach irritation occurs. Capsule may be opened for administration. Shake suspension well before measuring dose. Take the full course prescribed.

Usual Duration of Use: Continual use on a regular schedule for 3 to 5 days is usually necessary to determine this drug's effectiveness in controlling the infection under treatment. Response varies with the nature of the infection. Total treatment time will vary from 1 to 4 weeks. Certain infections require that this drug be taken for 10 consecutive days to prevent the development of rheumatic fever. Follow your physician's instructions regarding duration of use.

▷ **This Drug Should Not Be Taken If**

• you are allergic to any cephalosporin antibiotic (see Drug Class, Section Four).

▷ **Inform Your Physician Before Taking This Drug If**

• you have a history of allergy to any form of penicillin (see Drug Class, Section Four).
• you have a history of regional enteritis or ulcerative colitis.
• you have impaired kidney function.

Possible Side-Effects (natural, expected and unavoidable drug actions)
Superinfections (see Glossary).

▷ **Possible Adverse Effects** (unusual, unexpected and infrequent reactions)
If any of the following develop, consult your physician promptly for guidance.

Mild Adverse Effects
Allergic Reactions: Skin rash, itching, hives, localized swellings.
Headache, drowsiness, dizziness.
Indigestion, stomach cramping, nausea, vomiting, mild diarrhea, sore mouth or tongue.

Serious Adverse Effects
Allergic Reactions: Drug fever (see Glossary), joint aches and pains, anaphylactic reaction (see Glossary).
Idiosyncratic Reactions: Minor and temporary changes in white blood cell counts and liver function tests (infrequent).
Genital itching (may represent a fungus superinfection).
Severe diarrhea, possibly indicating a drug-induced form of colitis (rare).

▷ **Possible Effects on Sexual Function:**   None reported.

▷ **Adverse Effects That May Mimic Natural Diseases or Disorders**
Skin rash and fever may resemble measles.

CAUTION
In the management of diabetes it should be noted that this drug can cause a false positive test result for urine sugar when using Clinitest tablets, Benedict's solution or Fehling's solution, but not with Tes-Tape.

Precautions for Use
By Infants and Children: Dosage is based upon weight, and must be determined by the physician for each individual. Follow your physician's instructions exactly.
By Those over 60 Years of Age: Dosage must be carefully individualized and based upon evaluation of kidney function. Natural changes in the skin may predispose to severe and prolonged itching reactions in the genital and anal regions. Such reactions should be reported promptly.

▷ **Advisability of Use During Pregnancy**
Pregnancy Category: B (tentative). See Pregnancy Code inside back cover.
Animal studies: No birth defects reported.
Human studies: Information from adequate studies of pregnant women is not available.
Generally considered to be safe. Ask physician for guidance.

Advisability of Use if Breast-Feeding
Presence of this drug in breast milk: Yes, in small amounts.
Avoid drug or refrain from nursing.

Habit-Forming Potential: None.

Effects of Overdosage: Nausea, vomiting, stomach cramps and/or diarrhea.

Possible Effects of Long-Term Use: Superinfections (see Glossary).

Suggested Periodic Examinations While Taking This Drug (at physician's discretion)

Complete blood cell counts. Liver and kidney function tests.

▷ **While Taking This Drug, Observe the Following**

Foods: No restrictions.

Beverages: No restrictions. May be taken with milk.

▷ *Alcohol:* No interactions expected.

Tobacco Smoking: No interactions expected.

▷ *Other Drugs*

Cefadroxil **taken concurrently** with

• probenecid (Benemid) will slow the elimination of cefadroxil, resulting in higher blood levels and prolonged effect.

▷ *Driving, Hazardous Activities:* Usually no restrictions. If drowsiness or dizziness occurs, restrict activities accordingly.

Aviation Note: The use of this drug **may be a disqualification** for piloting. Consult a designated Aviation Medical Examiner.

Exposure to Sun: No restrictions.

Special Storage Instructions: Oral suspension should be refrigerated.

Observe the Following Expiration Times: Do not take the oral suspension of this drug if it is older than 14 days.

CEFUROXIME
(sef yur OX eem)

Introduced: 1976

Class: Antibiotic, cephalosporins

Prescription: USA: Yes

Controlled Drug: USA: No

Available as Generic: No

Brand Name: Ceftin

BENEFITS versus RISKS	
Possible Benefits	*Possible Risks*
EFFECTIVE TREATMENT OF INFECTIONS due to susceptible microorganisms	ALLERGIC REACTIONS mild to severe (up to 1% of general population, up to 2.9% of those allergic to penicillin) Drug-induced colitis (rare) Superinfections (see Glossary)

▷ **Principal Uses**

As a Single Drug Product: Used primarily to treat certain infections of the middle ear, tonsils, throat, bronchial tubes, urinary tract and skin.

How This Drug Works: This drug destroys susceptible infecting bacteria by interfering with their ability to produce new protective cell walls as they multiply and grow.

Available Dosage Forms and Strengths
Tablets — 125 mg, 250 mg, 500 mg

▷ **Usual Adult Dosage Range:** 250 to 500 mg/12 hrs. Total daily dosage should not exceed 4 grams. **Note: Actual dosage and administration schedule must be determined by the physician for each patient individually.**

▷ **Dosing Instructions:** May be taken on an empty stomach or with food if stomach irritation occurs. The tablet may be crushed and mixed with food (such as applesauce or ice cream) if necessary to facilitate swallowing. (Note: The crushed tablet has a persistent, bitter taste.) Take the full course prescribed.

Usual Duration of Use: Continual use on a regular schedule for 3 to 5 days is usually necessary to determine this drug's effectiveness in controlling the infection under treatment. Response varies with the nature of the infection. Total treatment time will vary from 1 to 4 weeks. Certain infections require that this drug be taken for 10 consecutive days to prevent the development of rheumatic fever. Follow your physician's instructions regarding duration of use.

▷ **This Drug Should Not Be Taken If**
  • you are allergic to any cephalosporin antibiotic (see Drug Class, Section Four).

▷ **Inform Your Physician Before Taking This Drug If**
  • you have a history of allergy to any form of penicillin (see Drug Class, Section Four).
  • you have a history of regional enteritis or ulcerative colitis.
  • you have impaired kidney function.

Possible Side-Effects (natural, expected and unavoidable drug actions)
Superinfections (see Glossary): vaginitis (1.9%).

▷ **Possible Adverse Effects** (unusual, unexpected and infrequent reactions)
  If any of the following develop, consult your physician promptly for guidance.
  Mild Adverse Effects
  Allergic Reactions: Skin rash (0.6%), hives (0.2%), itching (0.3%).
  Nausea (2.4%), vomiting (2.0%), loose stools (1.3%), mild diarrhea (3.5%).
  Headache (0.7%), dizziness (0.2%).
  Serious Adverse Effects
  Severe diarrhea, possibly indicating a drug-induced form of colitis (rare).

▷ **Possible Effects on Sexual Function:** None reported.

▷ **Adverse Effects That May Mimic Natural Diseases or Disorders**
Skin rash may resemble measles.

CAUTION
In the management of diabetes it should be noted that this drug can cause a false positive test result for urine sugar when using Clinitest tablets, Benedict's solution or Fehling's solution, but not with Clinistix or Tes-Tape.

Precautions for Use
By Infants and Children: The usual dose is 125 mg/12 hours. For middle ear infection, the recommended dose for those under 2 years of age is 125 mg/12 hours, and 250 mg/12 hours for those over 2 years of age.
By Those over 60 Years of Age: Dosage must be carefully individualized and based upon evaluation of kidney function. Natural changes in the skin may predispose to severe and prolonged itching reactions in the genital and anal regions. Such reactions should be reported promptly.

▷ **Advisability of Use During Pregnancy**
Pregnancy Category: B (tentative). See Pregnancy Code inside back cover.
Animal studies: No birth defects due to this drug reported in mouse and rat studies.
Human studies: Information from adequate studies of pregnant women is not available.
Generally considered to be safe. Ask physician for guidance.

Advisability of Use if Breast-Feeding
Presence of this drug in breast milk: Yes, in small amounts.
Avoid drug or refrain from nursing.

Habit-Forming Potential: None.

Effects of Overdosage: Nausea, vomiting, stomach cramps and/or diarrhea.

Possible Effects of Long-Term Use: Superinfections (see Glossary).

Suggested Periodic Examinations While Taking This Drug (at physician's discretion)
None.

▷ **While Taking This Drug, Observe the Following**
Foods: No restrictions. Food enhances the absorption of this drug.
Beverages: No restrictions. May be taken with milk.
▷ *Alcohol:* No interactions expected.
Tobacco Smoking: No interactions expected.
▷ *Other Drugs*
Cefuroxime *taken concurrently* with
• probenecid (Benemid) will slow the elimination of cefuroxime, resulting in higher blood levels and prolonged effect.

▷ *Driving, Hazardous Activities:* Usually no restrictions. Observe for the rare occurrence of dizziness.

Aviation Note: The use of this drug **may be a disqualification** for piloting. Consult a designated Aviation Medical Examiner.

Exposure to Sun: No restrictions.

CEPHALEXIN
(sef a LEX in)

Introduced: 1969

Class: Antibiotic, cephalosporins

Prescription: USA: Yes
Canada: Yes

Controlled Drug: USA: No
Canada: No

Available as Generic: Yes

Brand Names: ✦Ceporex, Keflet, Keflex, Keftab, ✦Novolexin

BENEFITS versus RISKS	
Possible Benefits	*Possible Risks*
EFFECTIVE TREATMENT OF INFECTIONS due to susceptible microorganisms	ALLERGIC REACTIONS mild to severe (up to 5% of general population, up to 16% of those allergic to penicillin) Drug-induced colitis (rare) Superinfections (see Glossary)

▷ **Principal Uses**

As a Single Drug Product: To treat certain infections of the skin and skin structures, the upper respiratory tract (including middle ear infections and "strep" throat), the genitourinary tract and certain infections involving bones and joints.

How This Drug Works: This drug destroys susceptible infecting bacteria by interfering with their ability to produce new protective cell walls as they multiply and grow.

Available Dosage Forms and Strengths
Capsules — 250 mg, 500 mg
Oral suspension — 125 mg, 250 mg per 5-ml teaspoonful
Pediatric oral suspension — 100 mg per ml
Tablets — 250 mg, 500 mg, 1000 mg (1 gram)

▷ **Usual Adult Dosage Range:** 250 to 500 mg/6 hours. Total daily dose should not exceed 4 grams. **Note: Actual dosage and administration schedule must be determined by the physician for each patient individually.**

▷ **Dosing Instructions:**   May be taken on an empty stomach or with food if stomach irritation occurs. Capsule may be opened and tablet may be crushed for administration. Shake suspension well before measuring dose. Take the full course prescribed.

Usual Duration of Use: Continual use on a regular schedule for 3 to 5 days is usually necessary to determine this drug's effectiveness in controlling the infection under treatment. Response varies with the nature of the infection. Total treatment time will vary from 1 to 4 weeks. Certain infections require that this drug be taken for 10 consecutive days to prevent the development of rheumatic fever. Follow your physician's instructions regarding duration of use.

▷ **This Drug Should Not Be Taken If**
  • you are allergic to any cephalosporin antibiotic (see Drug Class, Section Four).

▷ **Inform Your Physician Before Taking This Drug If**
  • you have a history of allergy to any form of penicillin (see Drug Class, Section Four).
  • you have a history of regional enteritis or ulcerative colitis.
  • you have impaired kidney function.

Possible Side-Effects (natural, expected and unavoidable drug actions)
  Superinfections (see Glossary).

▷ **Possible Adverse Effects** (unusual, unexpected and infrequent reactions)
  If any of the following develop, consult your physician promptly for guidance.
  Mild Adverse Effects
  Allergic Reactions: Skin rash (0.8%), itching, hives (0.3%).
  Headache, drowsiness, dizziness.
  Irritation of mouth or tongue, indigestion, stomach cramping, nausea, vomiting (1.8%), diarrhea (1.1%).
  Serious Adverse Effects
  Allergic Reactions: Drug fever (see Glossary), joint aches and pains, anaphylactic reaction (see Glossary).
  Idiosyncratic Reactions: Minor and temporary changes in white blood cell counts and liver function tests (infrequent).
  Genital itching (may represent a fungus superinfection).
  Severe diarrhea, possibly indicating a drug-induced form of colitis (rare).

▷ **Possible Effects on Sexual Function:**   None reported.

▷ **Adverse Effects That May Mimic Natural Diseases or Disorders**
  Skin rash and fever may resemble measles.

CAUTION
  1. In the management of diabetes it should be noted that this drug can cause a false positive test result for urine sugar when using

Clinitest tablets, Benedict's solution or Fehling's solution, but not with Tes-Tape.

2. Do not use this drug concurrently with other antibiotics such as erythromycin or tetracyclines.

Precautions for Use

By Infants and Children: Not recommended for use in infants less than 1 year old. Monitor allergic children closely for evidence of developing allergy to this drug.

By Those over 60 Years of Age: Dosage must be carefully individualized and based upon evaluation of kidney function. Natural changes in the skin may predispose to severe and prolonged itching reactions in the genital and anal regions. Such reactions should be reported promptly.

▷ **Advisability of Use During Pregnancy**

Pregnancy Category: B (tentative). See Pregnancy Code inside back cover. Animal studies: No birth defects reported.

Human studies: Information from adequate studies of pregnant women is not available.

Generally considered to be safe. Ask physician for guidance.

Advisability of Use if Breast-Feeding

Presence of this drug in breast milk: Yes, in small amounts. Avoid drug or refrain from nursing.

Habit-Forming Potential: None.

Effects of Overdosage: Nausea, vomiting, stomach cramps and/or diarrhea.

Possible Effects of Long-Term Use: Superinfections (see Glossary).

Suggested Periodic Examinations While Taking This Drug (at physician's discretion)

Complete blood cell counts. Liver and kidney function tests.

▷ **While Taking This Drug, Observe the Following**

Foods: No restrictions.

Beverages: No restrictions. May be taken with milk.

▷ *Alcohol:* No interactions expected.

Tobacco Smoking: No interactions expected.

▷ *Other Drugs*

Cephalexin **taken concurrently** with

• probenecid (Benemid) will slow the elimination of cephalexin, resulting in higher blood levels and prolonged effect.

▷ *Driving, Hazardous Activities:* Usually no restrictions. Use caution if drowsiness or dizziness occurs.

Aviation Note: The use of this drug **may be a disqualification** for piloting. Consult a designated Aviation Medical Examiner.

Exposure to Sun: No restrictions.

Special Storage Instructions: Oral suspension should be refrigerated.
Observe the Following Expiration Times: Do not take the oral suspension of this drug if it is older than 14 days.

CHLORAL HYDRATE
(klor al HI drayt)

Introduced: 1832

Class: Sedative, hypnotic

Prescription: USA: Yes
Canada: Yes

Controlled Drug: USA: C-IV*
Canada: No

Available as Generic: Yes

Brand Names: Aquachloral Supprettes, Noctec, ✦Novochlorhydrate

---

BENEFITS versus RISKS

Possible Benefits	*Possible Risks*
EFFECTIVE HYPNOTIC for short-term use (2 weeks)	DRUG DEPENDENCE with prolonged use
Effective daytime sedative for intermittent use	Severe allergic skin reactions
	Paradoxical excitement, delirium, psychotic behavior (infrequent)

▷ **Principal Uses**

As a Single Drug Product: Used primarily as a bedtime sedative in sufficient dosage to induce sleep. It is the drug of choice for use in the elderly because it produces less "hangover" effect and is less likely to cause the confusion so commonly seen with use of barbiturates.

How This Drug Works: Not completely known. It is converted into an alcohol, which is thought to have a sedative effect on the wake-sleep centers of the brain.

Available Dosage Forms and Strengths
Capsules — 250 mg, 500 mg
Suppositories — 324 mg, 500 mg, 648 mg
Syrup — 250 mg, 500 mg per 5-ml teaspoonful

▷ **Usual Adult Dosage Range:** As sedative—250 mg 3 times daily. As hypnotic—500 to 1000 mg, 15 to 30 minutes before bedtime. Total daily dosage should not exceed 2000 mg (2 grams). **Note: Actual dosage and administration schedule must be determined by the physician for each patient individually.**

*See Schedules of Controlled Drugs inside back cover.

▷ **Dosing Instructions:** Take capsules whole (unopened) with a full glass of water, fruit juice or ginger ale to prevent stomach irritation. Mix the elixir or syrup in half a glass of water, fruit juice or ginger ale. Daytime doses are best taken after meals.

Usual Duration of Use: As sedative, use intermittently and not on a regular basis. As hypnotic, limit use to periods of 7 to 10 days. Avoid continual and prolonged use. Duration of use should not exceed 14 days without drug-free periods of several days, and reappraisal of continued need.

▷ **This Drug Should Not Be Taken If**
- you have had an allergic or unfavorable reaction to it previously.
- you have severely impaired liver or kidney function.
- you have severe heart disease.
- you have active gastritis or peptic ulcer disease.
- you have a history of intermittent porphyria.

▷ **Inform Your Physician Before Taking This Drug If**
- you have a history of heart disease or peptic ulcer disease.
- you are taking other sedatives, hypnotics, tranquilizers or narcotic drugs of any kind.
- you plan to have surgery under general anesthesia in the near future.

Possible Side-Effects (natural, expected and unavoidable drug actions)
Light-headedness in upright position, unsteadiness, weakness.
"Hangover" effect following nighttime use as hypnotic.

▷ **Possible Adverse Effects** (unusual, unexpected and infrequent reactions)
If any of the following develop, consult your physician promptly for guidance.
Mild Adverse Effects
Allergic Reactions: Skin rashes, hives, conjunctivitis.
Dizziness, confusion, hallucinations, nightmares.
Unpleasant taste, stomach irritation, nausea, vomiting, diarrhea.
Serious Adverse Effects
Allergic Reactions: Severe forms of dermatitis.
Idiosyncratic Reactions: Sleepwalking, delirium, disorientation, paranoid behavior.
Double vision, temporary blindness.
Reduced formation of white blood cells.

▷ **Possible Effects on Sexual Function:** None reported.

Possible Delayed Adverse Effects: Allergic skin reactions may occur up to 10 days following the last dose.

▷ **Adverse Effects That May Mimic Natural Diseases or Disorders**
Paradoxical excitement or delirium may suggest latent psychosis.

Natural Diseases or Disorders That May Be Activated by This Drug
Intermittent porphyria.

CAUTION
1. Use with caution in the presence of bronchial asthma. Avoid high and frequent doses.
2. Take all doses well diluted with water, milk, fruit juice or ginger ale to prevent stomach irritation.

Precautions for Use
By Infants and Children: Avoid concurrent use with other drugs that have a sedative effect. Use very cautiously in asthmatic children.

By Those over 60 Years of Age: Small doses are advisable until your individual response has been determined. You may be more susceptible to the development of "hangover" effect, dizziness, confused thinking, impaired memory, unsteadiness, loss of bladder control or constipation.

▷ Advisability of Use During Pregnancy
Pregnancy Category: C (tentative). See Pregnancy Code inside back cover.
Animal studies: No information available.
Human studies: Information from adequate studies of pregnant women is not available.
Use this drug only if clearly needed. Continual use during pregnancy can cause withdrawal symptoms in the newborn infant.

Advisability of Use if Breast-Feeding
Presence of this drug in breast milk: Yes.
Monitor nursing infant closely and discontinue drug or nursing if adverse effects develop.

Habit-Forming Potential:
This drug can cause psychological and/or physical dependence (see Glossary). Avoid large doses and continual use.

Effects of Overdosage:
Marked drowsiness, confusion, incoordination, slurred speech, staggering gait, weakness, vomiting, stupor, deep sleep.

Possible Effects of Long-Term Use:
Psychological and/or physical dependence, toxic psychosis, liver and kidney damage.

Suggested Periodic Examinations While Taking This Drug (at physician's discretion)
Complete blood cell counts. Liver and kidney function tests.

▷ While Taking This Drug, Observe the Following
Foods: No restrictions.
Beverages: No restrictions. May be taken with milk.
▷ *Alcohol:* Avoid completely for at least 6 hours before taking this drug. Alcohol can greatly increase the sedative and depressant actions of this drug on brain function.
Tobacco Smoking: No interactions expected.
Marijuana Smoking: Increased drowsiness, impaired mental and physical performance.

▷ *Other Drugs*
Chloral hydrate may *increase* the effects of
- oral anticoagulants (Coumadin, etc.), and cause abnormal bleeding or hemorrhage. Consult physician regarding prothrombin time testing and dosage adjustment.

▷ *Driving, Hazardous Activities:* This drug can impair mental alertness, judgment, physical coordination and reaction time. Avoid hazardous activities until all sensation of drowsiness has disappeared.

Aviation Note: The use of this drug *is a disqualification* for piloting. Consult a designated Aviation Medical Examiner.

Exposure to Sun: No restrictions.

Discontinuation: If this drug has been used continually over an extended period of time, it should be discontinued gradually under physician supervision.

CHLORAMPHENICOL
(klor am FEN i kohl)

Introduced: 1947   **Class:** Antibiotic

Prescription: USA: Yes   **Controlled Drug:** USA: No
   Canada: Yes   Canada: No

Available as Generic: USA: Yes
   Canada: No

Brand Names: Ak-Chlor, Chloromycetin, Chloroptic, ✦Fenicol, ✦Isopto Fenicol, ✦Minims, ✦Nova-Phenicol, ✦Novochlorocap, Ophthochlor, ✦Pentamycetin

---

BENEFITS versus RISKS

Possible Benefits	*Possible Risks*
VERY EFFECTIVE TREATMENT OF INFECTIONS due to susceptible microorganisms	BONE MARROW DEPRESSION APLASTIC ANEMIA (see Glossary) Peripheral neuritis (see Glossary) Liver damage, jaundice

---

▷ **Principal Uses**
As a Single Drug Product: This drug is quite effective in a broad spectrum of serious infections. However, because of its potential for serious toxicity (fatal aplastic anemia), its use is now reserved for life-threatening infections caused by organisms that are resistant to safer antibiotics, and for infections in individuals who, for one reason or another, cannot take other appropriate anti-infective drugs.

How This Drug Works: This drug prevents the growth and multiplication of susceptible microorganisms by interfering with their formation of essential proteins.

Available Dosage Forms and Strengths
Capsules — 250 mg, 500 mg
Cream — 1%
Eye/ear solutions — 0.5%
Eye ointment — 1%
Injection — 100 mg per ml
Oral suspension — 150 mg per 5-ml teaspoonful

▷ **Usual Adult Dosage Range:** Total daily dose is 250 mg for each 10 pounds of body weight, given in 4 equally divided doses, 6 hours apart. Total daily dose should not exceed 500 mg for each 10 pounds of body weight. **Note: Actual dosage and administration schedule must be determined by the physician for each patient individually.**

▷ **Dosing Instructions:** Take with a full glass of water on an empty stomach, 1 hour before or 2 hours after eating. Capsule may be opened for administration. Shake oral suspension well before measuring dose.

Usual Duration of Use: Continual use on a regular schedule for 3 to 5 days is usually necessary to determine this drug's effectiveness in controlling the infection. Limit use to the time required to eradicate the infection. Avoid repeated courses of treatment if possible.

▷ **This Drug Should Not Be Taken If**
- you have had an allergic reaction to it previously.
- you have an active blood cell or bone marrow disorder.
- it is prescribed for a mild or trivial infection such as a cold, sore throat or "flulike" illness.
- it is prescribed for a premature or newborn infant (under 2 weeks of age).

▷ **Inform Your Physician Before Taking This Drug If**
- you have a history of a blood cell or bone marrow disorder.
- you have impaired liver or kidney function.
- you are taking anticoagulants.

Possible Side-Effects (natural, expected and unavoidable drug actions)
Superinfections (see Glossary).

▷ **Possible Adverse Effects** (unusual, unexpected and infrequent reactions)
If any of the following develop, consult your physician promptly for guidance.
Mild Adverse Effects
Allergic Reactions: Skin rashes, hives, swelling of face or extremities, fever.

Headache, confusion, peripheral neuritis (see Glossary)—numbness, pain, weakness in hands and/or feet.

Sore mouth or tongue, "black tongue," nausea, vomiting, diarrhea.

Serious Adverse Effects

Allergic Reactions: Anaphylactic reaction (see Glossary), liver damage with jaundice (rare).

Bone marrow depression (see Glossary)—fatigue, weakness, fever, sore throat, abnormal bleeding or bruising.

▷ **Possible Effects on Sexual Function:**   None reported.

▷ **Adverse Effects That May Mimic Natural Diseases or Disorders**
Liver reaction with jaundice may suggest viral hepatitis.

CAUTION
1. This drug can cause serious bone marrow depression and aplastic anemia (see Glossary). It must not be used to treat trivial infections or as a preventive medication under any circumstances. Its use must be restricted to the treatment of serious or life-threatening infections that fail to respond to other anti-infective drugs.
2. Troublesome and persistent diarrhea can develop in sensitive individuals. If diarrhea persists for more than 24 hours, discontinue this drug and consult your physician.

Precautions for Use
By Infants and Children: Follow prescribed dosage exactly. Blood cell counts should be monitored twice a week. Long-term use of this drug can cause optic neuritis. This may be prevented by taking supplemental vitamin B complex during treatment. Idiosyncratic aplastic anemia is rare (1 in 40,000 users), but may occur weeks or months after discontinuation of this drug.

By Those over 60 Years of Age: The natural decline in liver and kidney function after 60 may require reduction in dosage and adjustment of dosage interval. Natural changes in the skin after 60 may predispose to severe and prolonged itching reactions in the genital and anal regions. Report such reactions promptly.

▷ **Advisability of Use During Pregnancy**
Pregnancy Category: C (tentative). See Pregnancy Code inside back cover.
Animal studies: Results are inconclusive.
Human studies: Information from adequate studies of pregnant women is not available. Limited studies (348 exposures) indicate that this drug does not cause birth defects. However, it has been shown to be potentially toxic for the fetus and newborn. Ask physician for guidance.

Advisability of Use if Breast-Feeding
Presence of this drug in breast milk: Yes.
Avoid drug or refrain from nursing.

Habit-Forming Potential: None.

Effects of Overdosage: Possible nausea, vomiting, diarrhea.

Possible Effects of Long-Term Use: Superinfections, impaired vision, bone marrow depression.

Suggested Periodic Examinations While Taking This Drug (at physician's discretion)
Complete blood cell counts—before treatment is started and every 2 to 3 days during administration of drug.
Liver and kidney function tests.

▷ **While Taking This Drug, Observe the Following**
Foods: No restrictions.
Nutritional Support: Supplemental vitamins B-2, B-6 and B-12 are recommended.
Beverages: No restrictions. May be taken with milk.
▷ *Alcohol:* Avoid completely if you have liver disease. Use cautiously until the combined effect has been determined. Some sensitive individuals may develop a disulfiramlike reaction (see Glossary).
Tobacco Smoking: No interactions expected.
▷ *Other Drugs*
Chloramphenicol may ***increase*** the effects of
- oral anticoagulants (Coumadin, dicumarol, etc.), and increase the risk of bleeding.
- barbiturates (phenobarbital, etc.), and cause excessive sedation.
- phenytoin (Dilantin), and cause phenytoin toxicity.
- sulfonylureas (Diabinese, Dymelor, Orinase, Tolinase), and cause hypoglycemia (see Glossary).

Chloramphenicol may ***decrease*** the effects of
- iron preparations, used to treat anemia.
- penicillins.
- vitamin B-12.

The following drugs may ***decrease*** the effects of chloramphenicol
- barbiturates (phenobarbital, etc.).
- rifampin (Rifadin, Rimactane, etc.).

▷ *Driving, Hazardous Activities:* Usually no restrictions. Be alert to the rare occurrence of confusion, and restrict activities accordingly.
Aviation Note: The use of this drug ***may be a disqualification*** for piloting. Consult a designated Aviation Medical Examiner.
Exposure to Sun: No restrictions.

CHLORDIAZEPOXIDE
(klor di az e POX ide)

Introduced: 1960

Class: Mild tranquilizer, benzodiazepines

Prescription: USA: Yes
Canada: Yes

Controlled Drug: USA: C-IV*
Canada: No

Available as Generic: Yes

Brand Names: ✦Apo-Chlorax [CD], ✦Apo-Chlordiazepoxide, ✦Corium [CD], Librax [CD], Libritabs, Librium, Lidox [CD], Limbitrol [CD], Lipoxide, Menrium [CD], ✦Novopoxide, ✦Pentrium [CD], ✦Solium

---

BENEFITS versus RISKS

Possible Benefits	*Possible Risks*
RELIEF OF ANXIETY AND NERVOUS TENSION in 70% to 80% of users	Habit-forming potential with prolonged use
Wide margin of safety with therapeutic doses	Minor impairment of mental functions
Very few drug interactions	Very rare jaundice
	Very rare blood cell disorders

▷ **Principal Uses**

As a Single Drug Product: Used primarily to (1) provide short-term relief of mild to moderate anxiety, and (2) relieve the symptoms of acute alcohol withdrawal: agitation, tremors, hallucinations, incipient delirium tremens.

As a Combination Drug Product [CD]: Used in combination with amitriptyline (an antidepressant) to allay the anxiety that is often a troublesome feature in the agitated and depressed individual. Also used in combination with clidinium (a synthetic atropinelike antispasmodic) to treat peptic ulcer disease and irritable bowel syndrome.

How This Drug Works: It is thought that this drug produces a calming effect by enhancing the action of the nerve transmitter gamma-aminobutyric acid (GABA), which in turn blocks the arousal of higher brain centers.

Available Dosage Forms and Strengths
Capsules — 5 mg, 10 mg, 25 mg
Injection — 100 mg/ampul
Tablets — 5 mg, 10 mg, 25 mg

*See Schedules of Controlled Drugs inside back cover.

▷ **Usual Adult Dosage Range:**   5 to 25 mg, 3 or 4 times daily. Dose may be increased cautiously as needed and tolerated. After 1 week of continual use, the total daily dose may be taken at bedtime. Total daily dose should not exceed 150 mg for anxiety and tension, or 300 mg for alcohol withdrawal. **Note: Actual dosage and administration schedule must be determined by the physician for each patient individually.**

▷ **Dosing Instructions:**   May be taken on empty stomach or with food or milk. Capsule may be opened and tablet may be crushed for administration. Do not discontinue this drug abruptly if taken for more than 4 weeks.

Usual Duration of Use: Continual use on a regular schedule for 3 to 5 days is usually necessary to determine this drug's effectiveness in relieving moderate anxiety. Limit continual use to 1 to 3 weeks. Avoid uninterrupted and prolonged use.

▷ **This Drug Should Not Be Taken If**
- you have had an allergic reaction to any dosage form of it previously.
- you have acute narrow-angle glaucoma.
- it is prescribed for a child under 6 years of age.

▷ **Inform Your Physician Before Taking This Drug If**
- you are allergic to any benzodiazepine drug (see Drug Class, Section Four).
- you have a history of alcoholism or drug abuse.
- you are pregnant or planning pregnancy.
- you have impaired liver or kidney function.
- you have a history of serious depression or mental disorder.
- you have any of the following: asthma, emphysema, epilepsy, myasthenia gravis, porphyria.

Possible Side-Effects (natural, expected and unavoidable drug actions)
Drowsiness (3.9%), lethargy, unsteadiness; "hangover" effects on the day following bedtime use.

▷ **Possible Adverse Effects** (unusual, unexpected and infrequent reactions)
If any of the following develop, consult your physician promptly for guidance.
Mild Adverse Effects
Allergic Reactions: Rashes, fixed skin eruptions, bruising.
Dizziness, fainting, blurred vision, double vision, slurred speech, sweating, nausea.
Serious Adverse Effects
Allergic Reactions: Liver damage with jaundice (see Glossary), abnormally low blood platelet count.
Idiosyncratic Reaction: Acute hepatic porphyria.
Bone marrow depression—impaired production of red and white blood cells.
Paradoxical responses of excitement, agitation, anger, rage.

▷ **Possible Effects on Sexual Function**

Decreased libido with high doses, increased libido with low doses (antianxiety effect); rare report of inhibited ejaculation.

Altered timing and pattern of menstruation; female breast enlargement and milk production.

▷ **Adverse Effects That May Mimic Natural Diseases or Disorders**

Liver reaction with jaundice may suggest viral hepatitis.

Natural Diseases or Disorders That May Be Activated by This Drug

Acute intermittent hepatic porphyria, systemic lupus erythematosus—like syndrome.

CAUTION

1. This drug should not be discontinued abruptly if it has been taken continually for more than 4 weeks.
2. The concurrent use of some over-the-counter drug products that contain antihistamines (allergy and cold preparations, sleep aids) can cause excessive sedation in sensitive individuals.

Precautions for Use

By Infants and Children: Safety and effectiveness for use by those under 6 years of age have not been established. This drug should not be used in the hyperactive or psychotic child of any age.

By Those over 60 Years of Age: It is advisable to use smaller doses at longer intervals to avoid overdosage. Observe for the possible development of lethargy, indifference, fatigue, weakness, unsteadiness, disturbing dreams, nightmares and paradoxical reactions of excitement, agitation, anger, hostility and rage.

▷ **Advisability of Use During Pregnancy**

Pregnancy Category: D (tentative). See Pregnancy Code inside back cover.

Animal studies: Cleft palate reported in mice.

Human studies: Available information is conflicting and inconclusive. Some studies found a fourfold increase in serious birth defects associated with the use of this drug. Other studies have found no significant increase in birth defects.

Frequent use in late pregnancy can cause the "floppy infant" syndrome in the newborn: weakness, lethargy, unresponsiveness, depressed breathing, low body temperature.

Avoid use during entire pregnancy if possible.

Advisability of Use if Breast-Feeding

Presence of this drug in breast milk: Yes, in small amounts.

Monitor nursing infant closely and discontinue drug or nursing if adverse effects develop.

Habit-Forming Potential: This drug can produce psychological and/or physical dependence (see Glossary) if used in large doses for an extended period of time.

Effects of Overdosage: Marked drowsiness, weakness, feeling of drunkenness, staggering gait, tremor, stupor progressing to deep sleep or coma.

Possible Effects of Long-Term Use: Psychological and/or physical dependence, rare blood cell disorders.

Suggested Periodic Examinations While Taking This Drug (at physician's discretion)
Complete blood cell counts during long-term use.

▷ **While Taking This Drug, Observe the Following**
Foods: No restrictions.
Beverages: Avoid excessive intake of caffeine-containing beverages: coffee, tea, cola. May be taken with milk.
▷ *Alcohol:* Use with extreme caution until the combined effect is determined. Alcohol may increase the absorption of this drug and add to its depressant effects on the brain. It is advisable to avoid alcohol completely—throughout the day and night—if it is necessary to drive or to engage in any hazardous activity.
Tobacco Smoking: Heavy smoking may reduce the calming action of this drug.
Marijuana Smoking: Increased sedation and significant impairment of intellectual and physical performance.
▷ *Other Drugs*
Chlordiazepoxide may *increase* the effects of
• digoxin (Lanoxin), and cause digoxin toxicity.
Chlordiazepoxide may *decrease* the effects of
• levodopa (Sinemet, etc.), and reduce its effectiveness in treating Parkinson's disease.
The following drugs may *increase* the effects of chlordiazepoxide
• cimetidine (Tagamet).
• disulfiram (Antabuse).
• isoniazid (INH, Rifamate, etc.).
• oral contraceptives.
• valproic acid (Depakene).
The following drugs may *decrease* the effects of chlordiazepoxide
• rifampin (Rimactane, etc.).
• theophylline (aminophylline, Theo-Dur, etc.).
▷ *Driving, Hazardous Activities:* This drug can impair mental alertness, judgment, physical coordination and reaction time. Avoid hazardous activities accordingly.
Aviation Note: The use of this drug *is a disqualification* for piloting. Consult a designated Aviation Medical Examiner.
Exposure to Sun: Use caution until sensitivity is determined. A photoallergic skin reaction may occur rarely.
Discontinuation: Avoid sudden discontinuation if this drug has been taken for over 4 weeks. Dosage should be tapered gradually to prevent a withdrawal syndrome that could include depression, confusion, hal-

lucinations, tremor, seizures, muscle cramping, sweating and vomiting.

CHLOROTHIAZIDE
(klor oh THI a zide)

Introduced: 1957

Class: Antihypertensive, diuretic, thiazides

Prescription: USA: Yes

Controlled Drug: USA: No

Available as Generic: USA: Yes

Brand Names: Aldoclor [CD], Diachlor, Diupres [CD], Diurigen, Diuril

---

BENEFITS versus RISKS

Possible Benefits	*Possible Risks*
EFFECTIVE, WELL-TOLERATED DIURETIC	Loss of body potassium
POSSIBLY EFFECTIVE IN MILD HYPERTENSION	Increased blood sugar
ENHANCES EFFECTIVENESS OF OTHER ANTIHYPERTENSIVES	Increased blood uric acid
Beneficial in treatment of diabetes insipidus	Increased blood calcium
	Rare blood cell disorders

▷ **Principal Uses**

As a Single Drug Product: Thiazide diuretics are used primarily to (1) increase the volume of urine (diuresis) to correct the excessive fluid retention associated with congestive heart failure and certain types of liver and kidney disease; and (2) initiate treatment for high blood pressure (hypertension). They are often the first drugs tried in treating mild to moderate hypertension. Less frequent uses include the treatment of diabetes insipidus and the prevention of kidney stones that contain calcium.

As a Combination Drug Product [CD]: When this drug is used alone to treat hypertension, it is referred to as a "step 1" antihypertensive. Should it fail to reduce the blood pressure adequately, a "step 2" antihypertensive drug is added to be taken concurrently with the "step 1" drug. These drugs may be combined into one drug product. Thiazides are available in combination with beta blockers, hydralazine, methyldopa, reserpine and other diuretics to increase their effectiveness in treating hypertension.

How This Drug Works: By increasing the elimination of salt and water from the body (through increased urine production), this drug reduces the volume of fluid in the blood and body tissues and lowers the sodium content throughout the body. By relaxing the walls of smaller arteries and allowing them to expand, this drug increases the total capacity of the arterial system. The combined effect of these two actions (reduced blood volume in expanded space) results in lowering of the blood pressure.

Available Dosage Forms and Strengths
> Injection — 500 mg per 20 ml
> Oral suspension — 250 mg per 5-ml teaspoonful
> Tablets — 250 mg, 500 mg

▷ **Usual Adult Dosage Range:** As antihypertensive: 500 to 1000 mg/day initially; 500 to 2000 mg/day for maintenance. As diuretic: 500 to 2000 mg/day initially; the smallest effective dose should be determined. The total daily dose should not exceed 2000 mg. **Note: Actual dosage and administration schedule must be determined by the physician for each patient individually.**

▷ **Dosing Instructions:** May be taken with or following meals to reduce stomach irritation. Best taken in the morning to avoid nighttime urination. The tablet may be crushed for administration.

Usual Duration of Use: Continual use on a regular schedule for 2 to 3 weeks is usually necessary to determine this drug's effectiveness in lowering high blood pressure. Long-term use (months to years) requires periodic evaluation of response and possible dosage adjustment. Use as a diuretic should be intermittent with "drug holidays" (no drug taken) to reduce the risk of sodium and potassium imbalance. Consult your physician on a regular basis.

▷ **This Drug Should Not Be Taken If**
- you have had an allergic reaction to any dosage form of it previously.

▷ **Inform Your Physician Before Taking This Drug If**
- you are allergic to any form of "sulfa" drug.
- you are pregnant or planning pregnancy.
- you have a history of kidney or liver disease.
- you have diabetes, gout or lupus erythematosus.
- you are taking any form of cortisone, digitalis, oral antidiabetic drug or insulin.
- you plan to have surgery under general anesthesia in the near future.

Possible Side-Effects (natural, expected and unavoidable drug actions)
> Light-headedness on arising from sitting or lying position (see Orthostatic Hypotension in Glossary).
> Increase in blood sugar level, affecting control of diabetes.
> Increase in blood uric acid level, affecting control of gout.

Decrease in blood potassium level, causing muscle weakness and cramping.

▷ **Possible Adverse Effects** (unusual, unexpected and infrequent reactions)
If any of the following develop, consult your physician promptly for guidance.
Mild Adverse Effects
Allergic Reactions: Skin rashes, hives, drug fever.
Headache, dizziness, blurred or yellow vision.
Reduced appetite, indigestion, nausea, vomiting, diarrhea.
Serious Adverse Effects
Allergic Reactions: Hepatitis with jaundice (see Glossary), anaphylactic reaction (see Glossary), severe skin reactions.
Inflammation of the pancreas—severe abdominal pain.
Bone marrow depression (see Glossary)—fatigue, weakness, fever, sore throat, abnormal bleeding or bruising.

▷ **Possible Effects on Sexual Function:**   Impotence (500 to 2000 mg/day).

▷ **Adverse Effects That May Mimic Natural Diseases or Disorders**
Liver reaction may suggest viral hepatitis.

Natural Diseases or Disorders That May Be Activated by This Drug
Diabetes, gout, systemic lupus erythematosus.

CAUTION
1. Do not exceed recommended doses. Increased dosage can cause excessive loss of sodium and potassium, with resultant loss of appetite, nausea, fatigue, weakness, confusion and tingling in the extremities.
2. If you are also taking a digitalis preparation (digitoxin, digoxin), ensure an adequate intake of high-potassium foods to prevent potassium deficiency—a potential cause of digitalis toxicity. (See Table of High Potassium Foods in Section Six.)

Precautions for Use
By Infants and Children: Avoid overdosage that could cause serious dehydration. Significant potassium loss can occur within the first 2 weeks of drug use.
By Those over 60 Years of Age: Small doses are advisable until your individual response has been determined. You may be more susceptible to the development of impaired thinking, orthostatic hypotension, potassium loss and blood sugar increase. Overdosage and extended use of this drug can cause excessive loss of body water, thickening (increased viscosity) of the blood and an increased tendency for the blood to clot—predisposing to stroke, heart attack or thrombophlebitis (vein inflammation with blood clot).

▷ **Advisability of Use During Pregnancy**
Pregnancy Category: D (tentative). See Pregnancy Code inside back cover.
Animal studies: No birth defects found in rat studies.

Human studies: Reports are conflicting and inconclusive. This drug does not seem to carry the risk of birth defects that has been found with other related diuretics. However, other types of fetal injury are possible with this drug. It should not be used during pregnancy unless a very serious complication occurs for which this drug is significantly beneficial. Ask physician for guidance.

Advisability of Use if Breast-Feeding
Presence of this drug in breast milk: Yes, in small amounts.
Avoid drug or refrain from nursing.

Habit-Forming Potential: None.

Effects of Overdosage: Dry mouth, thirst, lethargy, weakness, muscle cramping, nausea, vomiting, drowsiness progressing to stupor or coma.

Possible Effects of Long-Term Use: Impaired balance of water, salt and potassium in blood and body tissues. Development of diabetes in predisposed individuals. Pathological changes in parathyroid glands with increased blood calcium levels and decreased blood phosphate levels.

Suggested Periodic Examinations While Taking This Drug (at physician's discretion)
Complete blood cell counts, measurements of blood levels of sodium, potassium, chloride, sugar and uric acid.
Kidney and liver function tests.

▷ **While Taking This Drug, Observe the Following**
Foods: Consult your physician regarding the advisability of eating foods rich in potassium. If so advised, see the Table of High Potassium Foods in Section Six. Follow physician's advice regarding the use of salt.
Beverages: No restrictions. This drug may be taken with milk.
▷ *Alcohol:* Use with caution until the combined effects have been determined. Alcohol may exaggerate the blood-pressure-lowering effects of this drug and cause orthostatic hypotension.
Tobacco Smoking: No interactions expected. Follow physician's advice.
▷ *Other Drugs*
Chlorothiazide may *increase* the effects of
• other antihypertensive drugs; dosage adjustments may be necessary to prevent excessive lowering of blood pressure.
• lithium, and cause lithium toxicity.
Chlorothiazide may *decrease* the effects of
• oral antidiabetic drugs (sulfonylureas); dosage adjustments may be necessary for proper control of blood sugar.
Chlorothiazide *taken concurrently* with
• digitalis preparations (digitoxin, digoxin) requires very careful monitoring and dosage adjustments to prevent fluctuations of blood potassium levels and serious disturbances of heart rhythm.

The following drugs may **decrease** the effects of chlorothiazide
- cholestyramine (Cuemid, Questran) may interfere with its absorption.
- colestipol (Colestid) may interfere with its absorption.

Take cholestyramine and colestipol 1 hour before any oral diuretic.

▷ *Driving, Hazardous Activities:* Use caution until the possible occurrence of orthostatic hypotension, dizziness or impaired vision has been determined.

Aviation Note: The use of this drug **may be a disqualification** for piloting. Consult a designated Aviation Medical Examiner.

Exposure to Sun: Use caution until sensitivity has been determined. This drug can cause photosensitivity (see Glossary).

Exposure to Heat: Avoid excessive perspiring, which could cause additional loss of salt and water from the body.

Heavy Exercise or Exertion: Avoid exertion that produces light-headedness, excessive fatigue or muscle cramping. Isometric exercises—the "overload" technique for strengthening individual muscles—can raise blood pressure significantly. Ask physician for guidance regarding participation in this form of exercise.

Occurrence of Unrelated Illness: Illnesses that cause vomiting or diarrhea can produce a serious imbalance of important body chemistry. Consult your physician for guidance.

Discontinuation: This drug should not be stopped abruptly following long-term use; serious thiazide-withdrawal fluid retention (edema) can develop after sudden withdrawal. The dose should be reduced gradually. It may be advisable to discontinue this drug 5 to 7 days before major surgery. Ask your physician, surgeon and/or anesthesiologist for guidance regarding dosage adjustment or drug withdrawal.

CHLORPHENIRAMINE
(klor fen IR a meen)

Introduced: 1949

Class: Antihistamines

Prescription: USA: Varies
Canada: No

Controlled Drug: USA: No
Canada: No

Available as Generic: USA: Yes
Canada: Yes

Brand Names: Alka-Seltzer Plus [CD], Allerest Tablets [CD], Chlor-Tri-
meton, ✦Chlor-Tripolon, ✦Chlor-Tripolon Decongestant [CD], Contac
Severe Cold Formula Caplets [CD], Contac 12-Hour Capsules [CD],
✦Corsym [CD], CoTylenol Children's Liquid Cold Formula [CD],
CoTylenol Cold Caplets & Tablets [CD], CoTylenol Liquid [CD],
CoTylenol Tablets [CD], Deconamine [CD], Demazin [CD], Fedahist
[CD], Fedahist Expectorant [CD], 4-Way Cold Tablets [CD],
✦Histapan-P [CD], Hycomine Compound [CD], Isoclor [CD], Naldecon
[CD], ✦Neo-Nasol [CD], Novafed A [CD], ✦Novahistex Cold Capsules
[CD], ✦Novopheniram, Ornade [CD], ✦Ornade-A.F. [CD], ✦Ornade-DM
[CD], ✦Ornade Expectorant [CD], Penntuss [CD], Polaramine*, Ry-
natan [CD], Sine-Off Extra Strength Capsules [CD], Sine-Off Tablets
[CD], Singlet [CD], Sinutab Maximum Strength Capsules & Tablets
[CD], Sinutab Tablets [CD], Sudafed Plus [CD], Teldrin, Triaminic
Allergy Tablets [CD], Triaminic Chewable Tablets [CD], Triaminic
Cold Syrup & Tablets [CD], Tiaminicin [CD]

BENEFITS versus RISKS

Possible Benefits	*Possible Risks*
EFFECTIVE RELIEF OF	Mild sedation
ALLERGIC RHINITIS AND	Atropinelike effects
ALLERGIC SKIN DISORDERS	Very rare blood cell disorders

▷ **Principal Uses**

As a Single Drug Product: Used primarily to provide symptomatic relief
in allergic and related disorders: seasonal and perennial allergic rhinitis (hay fever), allergic conjunctivitis and vasomotor rhinitis; also in
hives and localized swellings (angioedema) of allergic origin.

As a Combination Drug Product [CD]: This drug is combined with a decongestant drug to enhance its ability to reduce tissue swelling and
secretions in allergic and infectious disorders of the upper respiratory
tract—hay fever, head colds and sinusitis. It is also combined with
decongestants, expectorants and codeine to increase their effectiveness in the symptomatic treatment of allergic and infectious disorders
of the lower respiratory tract, often with associated coughing.

How This Drug Works: Antihistamines reduce the intensity of the allergic
response by blocking the action of histamine after it has been released
from sensitized tissue cells in the eyes, nose, respiratory passages and
skin.

Available Dosage Forms and Strengths
Capsules, prolonged-action — 8 mg, 12 mg
Injection — 10 mg, 100 mg per ml
Syrup — 2 mg per 5-ml teaspoonful (7% alcohol)

*A brand of the closely related generic drug dexchlorpheniramine.

Tablets — 4 mg
Tablets, chewable — 2 mg
Tablets, prolonged-action — 8 mg, 12 mg

▷ **Usual Adult Dosage Range:**   4 mg/4 to 6 hours, or 8 to 12 mg (prolonged-action form)/12 hours. Total daily dosage should not exceed 24 mg. **Note: Actual dosage and administration schedule must be determined by the physician for each patient individually.**

▷ **Dosing Instructions:**   Take with food or milk to prevent stomach irritation. The prolonged-action forms should be swallowed whole (not crushed or chewed).

Usual Duration of Use: Continual use on a regular schedule for 2 to 3 days is usually necessary to determine this drug's effectiveness in relieving the symptoms of allergic rhinitis and dermatosis. It may be necessary to take this drug throughout the entire pollen season, depending upon individual sensitivity. However, antihistamines should not be taken continually (without interruption) for long-term use. Limit their use to periods that require symptomatic relief.

▷ **This Drug Should Not Be Taken If**
  • you have had an allergic reaction to any dosage form of it previously.
  • you are currently undergoing allergy skin tests.
  • you are taking, or have taken within the past 14 days, any monoamine oxidase (MAO) type A inhibitor drug (see Drug Class, Section Four).

▷ **Inform Your Physician Before Taking This Drug If**
  • you have had any allergic reactions or unfavorable responses to the previous use of antihistamines.
  • you have glaucoma (narrow-angle type) or asthma.
  • you have epilepsy or a seizure disorder.
  • you have difficulty emptying the urinary bladder, especially if due to prostate gland enlargement.
  • you plan to have surgery under general anesthesia in the near future.

Possible Side-Effects (natural, expected and unavoidable drug actions)
  Drowsiness; sense of weakness; blurred vision; dryness of the nose, mouth and throat; impaired urination.

▷ **Possible Adverse Effects** (unusual, unexpected and infrequent reactions)
  If any of the following develop, consult your physician promptly for guidance.
  Mild Adverse Effects
  Allergic Reactions: Skin rash, hives.
  Headache, nervous agitation, dizziness, confusion, tremor, blurred or double vision, ringing in ears.
  Reduced tolerance for contact lenses.
  Thickening of bronchial secretions in asthma or bronchitis.
  Indigestion, nausea, vomiting, diarrhea.

Serious Adverse Effects
Allergic Reaction: Anaphylactic reaction (see Glossary).
Idiosyncratic Reactions: Euphoria, hysteria, depression, nightmares.
Hemolytic anemia (see Glossary).
Abnormally low white blood cell count—fever, sore throat, infections.
Abnormally low blood platelet count—abnormal bleeding or bruising.

▷ **Possible Effects on Sexual Function:** Shortened menstrual cycle (early arrival of expected menstrual onset).

Natural Diseases or Disorders That May Be Activated by This Drug
Latent epilepsy, glaucoma, prostatism (see Glossary).

CAUTION
1. Discontinue this drug 4 days before diagnostic skin testing procedures in order to prevent false negative test results.
2. Do not use this drug if you have active bronchial asthma, bronchitis or pneumonia. It can thicken bronchial mucus and make it more difficult to remove (by absorption or coughing).

Precautions for Use
By Infants and Children: This drug should not be used in premature or full-term newborn infants. Doses for children should be small. The young child is especially sensitive to the effects of antihistamines on the brain and nervous system.
By Those over 60 Years of Age: You may be more susceptible to the development of drowsiness, dizziness and unsteadiness, and to impairment of thinking, judgment and memory. This drug can increase the degree of impaired urination associated with prostate gland enlargement (prostatism). The sedative effects of antihistamines in the elderly can cause a syndrome of underactivity that may be misinterpreted as senility or emotional depression.

▷ **Advisability of Use During Pregnancy**
Pregnancy Category: B (tentative). See Pregnancy Code inside back cover.
Animal studies: No birth defects reported in mice.
Human studies: Information from studies of pregnant women indicates no significant increase in defects in 3931 exposures to this drug. However, this drug may cause seizures and other adverse effects in newborn infants if used during pregnancy.
Use this drug only if clearly needed. Avoid during the last 3 months. Ask physician for guidance.

Advisability of Use if Breast-Feeding
Presence of this drug in breast milk: Yes, in small amounts.
Avoid drug or refrain from nursing.

Habit-Forming Potential: None.

Effects of Overdosage: Drowsiness; unsteadiness; faintness; marked dryness of mouth, nose and throat; flushing of face; shortness of breath; hallucinations; convulsions; stupor progressing to coma.

Possible Effects of Long-Term Use: Tardive dyskinesia (see Glossary) has been reported in association with the long-term use of several widely used antihistamines. It is advisable to avoid the prolonged, continual use of antihistamines without interruption.

Suggested Periodic Examinations While Taking This Drug (at physician's discretion)
Complete blood cell counts.

▷ **While Taking This Drug, Observe the Following**
   Foods: No restrictions.
   Beverages: No restrictions. May be taken with milk.
▷ *Alcohol:* Use with extreme caution until the combined effects have been determined. The combination of antihistamine and alcohol can produce rapid and marked sedation.
   Tobacco Smoking: No interactions expected.
▷ *Other Drugs*
   Chlorpheniramine may ***increase*** the effects of
   • all sedatives, sleep-inducing drugs, tranquilizers, analgesics and narcotic drugs, and produce oversedation.
   Chlorpheniramine ***taken concurrently*** with
   • phenytoin (Dantoin, Dilantin) may cause phenytoin toxicity, and may alter the pattern of seizures. Dosage adjustments may be necessary.
   The following drugs may ***increase*** the effects of chlorpheniramine
   • monoamine oxidase (MAO) type A inhibitor drugs (see Drug Class, Section Four) may prolong the action of antihistamines.
▷ *Driving, Hazardous Activities:* This drug can impair mental alertness, judgment, coordination and reaction time. Avoid hazardous activities until the full sedative effects have been determined.
   Aviation Note: The use of this drug *is a disqualification* for piloting. Consult a designated Aviation Medical Examiner.
   Exposure to Sun: Use caution. Some drugs of this class can cause photosensitivity (see Glossary).

CHLORPROMAZINE
(klor PROH ma zeen)

Introduced: 1952

Class: Strong tranquilizer, phenothiazines

Prescription: USA: Yes
   Canada: Yes

Controlled Drug: USA: No
   Canada: No

Available as Generic: Yes

Brand Names: ✦Chlorpromanyl, ✦Largactil, ✦Novochlorpromazine, Promapar, Sonazine, Thorazine

---

BENEFITS versus RISKS

Possible Benefits	*Possible Risks*
EFFECTIVE CONTROL OF ACUTE MENTAL DISORDERS in the majority of patients	SERIOUS TOXIC EFFECTS ON BRAIN with long-term use
Beneficial effects on thinking, mood and behavior	Liver damage with jaundice (less than 0.5%)
Moderately effective control of nausea and vomiting	Rare blood cell disorders: hemolytic anemia, abnormally low white blood cell count

---

▷ **Principal Uses**

As a Single Drug Product: This antipsychotic drug is used primarily to treat acute and chronic psychotic disorders such as agitated depression, schizophrenia and similar states of mental dysfunction. It may be used as a tranquilizer in the management of agitated and disruptive behavior in the absence of true psychosis. Less frequently it may be used to relieve severe nausea or vomiting.

How This Drug Works: Not completely established. Present theory is that by inhibiting the action of dopamine, this drug acts to correct an imbalance of nerve impulse transmissions that is thought to be responsible for certain mental disorders.

Available Dosage Forms and Strengths

Capsules, prolonged-action — 30 mg, 75 mg, 150 mg, 200 mg, 300 mg
Concentrate — 30 mg per ml, 100 mg per ml
Injection — 25 mg per ml
Suppositories — 25 mg, 100 mg
Syrup — 10 mg per 5-ml teaspoonful
Tablets — 10 mg, 25 mg, 50 mg, 100 mg, 200 mg

▷ **Usual Adult Dosage Range:**   Initially 10 to 25 mg 3 or 4 times daily. Dose may be increased by 20 to 50 mg at 3- to 4-day intervals as needed and tolerated. Usual dosage range is 300 to 800 mg daily. Extreme range is 25 to 2000 mg daily. Total daily dosage should not exceed 2000 mg. **Note: Actual dosage and administration schedule must be determined by the physician for each patient individually.**

▷ **Dosing Instructions:**   May be taken with or following meals to reduce stomach irritation. Tablets may be crushed for administration. Prolonged-action capsules may be opened, but do not crush or chew contents.

Usual Duration of Use: Continual use on a regular schedule for several weeks is usually necessary to determine this drug's effectiveness in controlling psychotic disorders. If not significantly beneficial within 6 weeks, it should be discontinued. Long-term use (months to years) requires periodic evaluation of response, appropriate dosage adjustment and consideration of continued need. Consult your physician on a regular basis.

▷ **This Drug Should Not Be Taken If**
  • you are allergic to any of the drugs bearing the brand names listed above.
  • you have active liver disease.
  • you have cancer of the breast.
  • you have a current blood cell or bone marrow disorder.

▷ **Inform Your Physician Before Taking This Drug If**
  • you are allergic or abnormally sensitive to any phenothiazine drug (see Drug Class, Section Four).
  • you have impaired liver or kidney function.
  • you have any type of seizure disorder.
  • you have diabetes, glaucoma or heart disease.
  • you have a history of lupus erythematosus.
  • you are taking any drug with sedative effects.
  • you plan to have surgery under general or spinal anesthesia in the near future.

Possible Side-Effects (natural, expected and unavoidable drug actions)
  Drowsiness (usually during the first 2 weeks), orthostatic hypotension (see Glossary), blurred vision, dry mouth, nasal congestion, constipation, impaired urination.
  Pink or purple coloration of urine, of no significance.

▷ **Possible Adverse Effects** (unusual, unexpected and infrequent reactions)
  If any of the following develop, consult your physician promptly for guidance.
  Mild Adverse Effects
  Allergic Reactions: Skin rash, hives, low-grade fever.
  Lowering of body temperature, especially in the elderly.
  Increased appetite and weight gain.
  Weakness, agitation, insomnia, impaired day and night vision.
  Chronic constipation, fecal impaction.
  Serious Adverse Effects
  Allergic Reactions: Hepatitis with jaundice (see Glossary), usually between second and fourth week; high fever; asthma; anaphylactic reaction (see Glossary).
  Depression, disorientation, seizures.
  Disturbances of heart rhythm, rapid heart rate.
  Hemolytic anemia (see Glossary), impaired production of white blood cells—fever, sore throat, infections.
  Parkinson-like disorders (see Glossary); muscle spasms of face, jaw, neck, back, extremities.
  Prolonged drop in blood pressure with weakness, perspiration and fainting.

▷ **Possible Effects on Sexual Function**
  Decreased libido and impotence (1200 mg/day); inhibited ejaculation (400 mg/day); priapism (see Glossary) (250 mg/day); male infertility

(30 to 800 mg/day); enlargement of male breasts, enlargement of female breasts with milk production, cessation of menstruation (30 to 800 mg/day).

This drug may also cause a false positive pregnancy test.

▷ **Adverse Effects That May Mimic Natural Diseases or Disorders**
Nervous system reactions may suggest Parkinson's disease.
Liver reactions may suggest viral hepatitis.
Reactions resembling systemic lupus erythematosus can occur.

Natural Diseases or Disorders That May Be Activated by This Drug
Latent epilepsy, glaucoma, diabetes mellitus (25%), prostatism (see Glossary).

CAUTION
1. Many over-the-counter medications (see OTC Drugs in Glossary) for allergies, colds and coughs contain drugs that can interact unfavorably with this drug. Ask your physician or pharmacist for guidance before using any such medications.
2. Antacids that contain aluminum and/or magnesium can prevent the absorption of this drug and reduce its effectiveness.
3. Obtain prompt evaluation of any change or disturbance of vision.
4. This drug can cause false positive pregnancy tests.

Precautions for Use
By Infants and Children: Do not use this drug in infants under 6 months of age, or in children of any age with symptoms suggestive of Reye syndrome (see Glossary). Monitor carefully for blood cell changes.
By Those over 60 Years of Age: Small doses are advisable until individual response has been determined. You may be more susceptible to the development of drowsiness, lethargy, constipation, lowering of body temperature (hypothermia) and orthostatic hypotension (see Glossary). This drug can enhance existing prostatism (see Glossary). You may also be more susceptible to the development of Parkinson-like reactions and/or tardive dyskinesia (see discussion of these terms in Glossary). These reactions must be recognized early since they may become unresponsive to treatment and irreversible.

▷ **Advisability of Use During Pregnancy**
Pregnancy Category: C (tentative). See Pregnancy Code inside back cover.
Animal studies: No birth defects reported in rodent studies. However, rodent studies suggest possible permanent neurological damage to the fetus.
Human studies: No increase in birth defects reported in 284 exposures. Information from adequate studies of pregnant women is not available.
Limit use to small and infrequent doses only when clearly needed. Avoid drug during the last month because of possible adverse effects on the newborn infant.

Advisability of Use if Breast-Feeding
Presence of this drug in breast milk: Yes, in small amounts.
Avoid drug or refrain from nursing.

Habit-Forming Potential: None.

Effects of Overdosage: Marked drowsiness, weakness, tremor, agitation, unsteadiness, deep sleep, coma, convulsions.

Possible Effects of Long-Term Use: Tardive dyskinesia in 10% to 20% (see Glossary); eye changes—cataracts and pigmentation of retina; gray to violet pigmentation of skin in exposed areas, more common in women; severe ulcerative colitis.

Suggested Periodic Examinations While Taking This Drug (at physician's discretion)
Complete blood cell counts, especially between the fourth and tenth weeks of treatment.
Liver function tests, electrocardiograms.
Complete eye examinations—eye structures and vision.
Careful inspection of the tongue for early evidence of fine, involuntary, wavelike movements that could indicate the beginning of tardive dyskinesia.

▷ **While Taking This Drug, Observe the Following**
Foods: No restrictions.
Nutritional Support: A riboflavin (vitamin B-2) supplement should be taken with long-term use.
Beverages: No restrictions. May be taken with milk.

▷ *Alcohol:* Avoid completely. Alcohol can increase the sedative action of phenothiazines and accentuate their depressant effects on brain function and blood pressure. Phenothiazines can increase the intoxicating effects of alcohol.

Tobacco Smoking: Possible reduction of drowsiness from drug.
Marijuana Smoking: Moderate increase in drowsiness; accentuation of orthostatic hypotension; increased risk of precipitating latent psychoses, confusing the interpretation of mental status and drug responses.

▷ *Other Drugs*
Chlorpromazine may *increase* the effects of
- all sedative drugs, especially meperidine (Demerol), and cause excessive sedation.
- all atropinelike drugs, and cause nervous system toxicity.

Chlorpromazine may *decrease* the effects of
- guanethidine (Ismelin, Esimil), and reduce its effectiveness in lowering blood pressure.

Chlorpromazine *taken concurrently* with
- propranolol (Inderal) may cause increased effects of both drugs; monitor drug effects closely and adjust dosages as necessary.

The following drugs may *decrease* the effects of chlorpromazine

- antacids containing aluminum and/or magnesium.
- benztropine (Cogentin).
- trihexyphenidyl (Artane).

▷ *Driving, Hazardous Activities:* This drug can impair mental alertness, judgment and physical coordination. Avoid hazardous activities.

Aviation Note: The use of this drug *is a disqualification* for piloting. Consult a designated Aviation Medical Examiner.

Exposure to Sun: Use caution until sensitivity has been determined. Some phenothiazines can cause photosensitivity (see Glossary).

Exposure to Heat: Use caution and avoid excessive heat as much as possible. This drug may impair the regulation of body temperature and increase the risk of heat stroke.

Exposure to Cold: Use caution and dress warmly. This drug can increase the risk of hypothermia in the elderly.

Discontinuation: After a period of long-term use, do not discontinue this drug suddenly. Gradual withdrawal over 2 to 3 weeks under physician supervision is recommended. Do not discontinue this drug without your physician's knowledge and approval. The relapse rate of schizophrenia after discontinuation is 50% to 60%.

CHLORPROPAMIDE
(klor PROH pa mide)

Introduced: 1958

Class: Antidiabetic, sulfonylureas

Prescription: USA: Yes
Canada: Yes

Controlled Drug: USA: No
Canada: No

Available as Generic: Yes

Brand Names: ✦Apo-Chlorpropamide, ✦Chloronase, Diabinese, ✦Novopropamide

BENEFITS versus RISKS	
Possible Benefits	*Possible Risks*
Assistance in regulating blood sugar in noninsulin-dependent diabetes (adjunctive to appropriate diet and weight control)	HYPOGLYCEMIA, severe and prolonged Allergic skin reactions (some severe) Water retention Liver damage Rare blood cell and bone marrow disorders

▷ **Principal Uses**

As a Single Drug Product: To assist in the control of mild to moderately severe type II diabetes mellitus (adult, maturity-onset) that does not require insulin, but that cannot be adequately controlled by diet alone.

How This Drug Works: It is thought that this drug (1) stimulates the secretion of insulin (by a pancreas that is capable of responding to stimulation), and (2) enhances the utilization of insulin by appropriate tissues.

Available Dosage Forms and Strengths
Tablets — 100 mg, 250 mg

▷ **Usual Adult Dosage Range:**   Initially 250 mg daily with breakfast. After 5 to 7 days, dose may be increased to 500 mg daily if needed and tolerated. Total daily dosage should not exceed 750 mg. A "loading" or priming dose is not necessary and should not be given. **Note: Actual dosage and administration schedule must be determined by the physician for each patient individually.**

▷ **Dosing Instructions:**   May be taken with food to reduce stomach irritation. Tablet may be crushed for administration.

Usual Duration of Use: Continual use on a regular schedule for 1 to 2 weeks is usually necessary to determine this drug's effectiveness in controlling diabetes. Failure to respond to maximal doses within 1 month constitutes a primary failure. Up to 15% of those who respond initially may develop secondary failure of the drug within the first year of use. The duration of effective use can only be determined by periodic measurement of the blood sugar. Consult your physician on a regular basis.

▷ **This Drug Should Not Be Taken If**
  • you have had an allergic reaction to it previously.
  • you have severe impairment of liver or kidney function.
  • you are pregnant.

▷ **Inform Your Physician Before Taking This Drug If**
  • you are allergic to other sulfonylurea drugs or to "sulfa" drugs.
  • your diabetes has been unstable or "brittle" in the past.
  • you do not know how to recognize or treat hypoglycemia (see Glossary).
  • you have a history of congestive heart failure, peptic ulcer disease, cirrhosis of the liver, hypothyroidism or porphyria.

Possible Side-Effects (natural, expected and unavoidable drug actions)
If drug dosage is excessive or food intake is delayed or inadequate, abnormally low blood sugar (hypoglycemia) will occur as a predictable drug effect.

▷ **Possible Adverse Effects** (unusual, unexpected and infrequent reactions)
If any of the following develop, consult your physician promptly for guidance.
Mild Adverse Effects
Allergic Reactions: Skin rash, hives, itching, drug fever.
Headache, ringing in ears, weakness, numbness and tingling.
Indigestion, nausea, vomiting, diarrhea (may be severe).
Serious Adverse Effects
Allergic Reactions: Hepatitis with jaundice (see Glossary), severe skin reactions.
Idiosyncratic Reaction: Hemolytic anemia (see Glossary).
Disulfiramlike reaction with concurrent use of alcohol (see Glossary).
Water retention (edema), weight gain.
Bone marrow depression (see Glossary)—fatigue, weakness, fever, sore throat, abnormal bleeding or bruising.

▷ **Possible Effects on Sexual Function:** None reported.

▷ **Adverse Effects That May Mimic Natural Diseases or Disorders**
Liver reactions may suggest viral hepatitis.

Natural Diseases or Disorders That May Be Activated by This Drug
Acute intermittent porphyria, congestive heart failure (in predisposed individuals), peptic ulcer disease.

CAUTION
1. This drug must be regarded as only one part of the total program for the management of your diabetes. It is not a substitute for a properly prescribed diet and regular exercise.
2. Over a period of time (usually several months), this drug may lose its effectiveness in controlling blood sugar levels. Periodic follow-up examinations are necessary to monitor all aspects of response to drug treatment.
3. This drug has a long duration of action (up to 60 hours) and therefore can be cumulative in its effects. It can produce severe and prolonged hypoglycemia in some individuals, especially the elderly.

Precautions for Use
By Infants and Children: This drug is not effective in type I (juvenile, growth-onset) insulin-dependent diabetes.
By Those over 60 Years of Age: This drug is best avoided in this age group. Due to its long duration of action it can accumulate and cause marked and prolonged hypoglycemia. Repeated episodes of hypoglycemia in the elderly can cause brain damage.

▷ **Advisability of Use During Pregnancy**
Pregnancy Category: X (tentative). See Pregnancy Code inside back cover.
Animal studies: This class of drugs has been shown to cause birth defects in animals.

Human studies: Information from adequate studies of pregnant women is not available.

The manufacturer states that this drug is contraindicated during entire pregnancy.

Advisability of Use if Breast-Feeding

Presence of this drug in breast milk: Yes.

Avoid drug or refrain from nursing.

Habit-Forming Potential: None.

Effects of Overdosage: Symptoms of mild to severe hypoglycemia: headache, light-headedness, faintness, nervousness, confusion, tremor, sweating, heart palpitation, weakness, hunger, nausea, vomiting, stupor progressing to coma.

Possible Effects of Long-Term Use: Reduced function of the thyroid gland (hypothyroidism). Reports of increased frequency and severity of heart and blood vessel diseases associated with long-term use of this class of drugs are highly controversial and inconclusive. A direct cause-and-effect relationship (see Glossary) is tenuous. Ask your physician for guidance.

Suggested Periodic Examinations While Taking This Drug (at physician's discretion)

Complete blood cell counts, liver function tests, thyroid function tests, periodic evaluation of heart and circulatory system.

▷ **While Taking This Drug, Observe the Following**

Foods: Follow the diabetic diet prescribed by your physician.

Beverages: As directed in the diabetic diet. May be taken with milk.

▷ *Alcohol:* Use with extreme caution until the combined effect has been determined. Alcohol can exaggerate this drug's hypoglycemic effect. This drug can cause a marked intolerance of alcohol resulting in a disulfiramlike reaction (see Glossary): facial flushing, sweating, palpitation.

Tobacco Smoking: No interactions expected.

▷ *Other Drugs*

The following drugs may *increase* the effects of chlorpropamide

• ammonium chloride.
• aspirin, and other salicylates.
• chloramphenicol (Chloromycetin).
• clofibrate (Atromid S).
• dicumarol.
• fenfluramine (Pondimin).
• monoamine oxidase (MAO) type A inhibitor drugs (see Drug Class, Section Four).
• phenylbutazone (Butazolidin).
• some "sulfa" drugs: sulfamethoxazole (Gantanol), sulfisoxazole (Gantrisin).

The following drugs may *decrease* the effects of chlorpropamide
- diazoxide (Proglycem).
- propranolol (Inderal).
- rifampin (Rifidin, Rimactane).
- sodium bicarbonate.
- thiazide diuretics (see Drug Class, Section Four).

▷ *Driving, Hazardous Activities:* Regulate your dosage schedule, eating schedule and physical activities very carefully to prevent hypoglycemia. Be able to recognize the early symptoms of hypoglycemia so you can avoid hazardous activities and take corrective measures.

Aviation Note: Diabetes *is a disqualification* for piloting. Consult a designated Aviation Medical Examiner.

Exposure to Sun: Use caution until sensitivity has been determined. Some drugs of this class can cause photosensitivity (see Glossary).

Occurrence of Unrelated Illness: Acute infections, illnesses causing vomiting or diarrhea, serious injuries and surgical procedures can interfere with diabetic control and may require the use of insulin. If any of these conditions occur, consult your physician promptly.

Discontinuation: It is estimated that no more than 12% of patients remain well controlled by this drug for more than 6 to 7 years. Because of the high incidence of secondary failures, it is advisable to evaluate the continued benefit of this drug every 6 months.

CHLORTHALIDONE
(klor THAL i dohn)

Introduced: 1960   **Class:** Antihypertensive, diuretic

Prescription: USA: Yes   **Controlled Drug:** USA: No
Canada: Yes   Canada: No

Available as Generic: USA: Yes
Canada: Yes

Brand Names: ✦Apo-Chlorthalidone, Combipres [CD], Demi-Regroton [CD], Hygroton, ✦Hygroton-Reserpine [CD], Hylidone, ✦Novothalidone, Regroton [CD], Tenoretic [CD], Thalitone, ✦Uridon

---

BENEFITS versus RISKS

Possible Benefits	*Possible Risks*
EFFECTIVE, WELL-TOLERATED DIURETIC	Loss of body potassium
POSSIBLY EFFECTIVE IN MILD HYPERTENSION	Increased blood sugar
ENHANCES EFFECTIVENESS OF OTHER ANTIHYPERTENSIVES	Increased blood uric acid
Beneficial in treatment of diabetes insipidus	Increased blood calcium
	Rare blood cell disorders

▷ **Principal Uses**

> *As a Single Drug Product:* Thiazidelike diuretics are used primarily to (1) increase the volume of urine (diuresis) to correct the excessive fluid retention associated with congestive heart failure and certain types of liver and kidney disease; and (2) initiate treatment for high blood pressure (hypertension). They are often the first drugs tried in treating mild to moderate hypertension. Less frequent uses include the treatment of diabetes insipidus and the prevention of kidney stones that contain calcium.

> *As a Combination Drug Product* [CD]: When this drug is used alone to treat hypertension, it is referred to as a "step 1" antihypertensive. Should it fail to reduce the blood pressure adequately, a "step 2" antihypertensive drug is added to be taken concurrently with the "step 1" drug. These drugs may be combined into one drug product. This drug is available in combination with atenolol, clonidine and reserpine to increase their effectiveness in treating hypertension.

How This Drug Works: By increasing the elimination of salt and water from the body (through increased urine production), this drug reduces the volume of fluid in the blood and body tissues and lowers the sodium content throughout the body. By relaxing the walls of smaller arteries and allowing them to expand, this drug increases the total capacity of the arterial system. The combined effect of these two actions (reduced blood volume in expanded space) results in lowering of blood pressure.

Available Dosage Forms and Strengths
> Tablets — 25 mg, 50 mg, 100 mg

▷ **Usual Adult Dosage Range:** As antihypertensive: 25 to 50 mg/day initially; 50 to 100 mg/day for maintenance. As diuretic: 50 to 100 mg/day initially; the smallest effective dose should be determined. The total daily dose should not exceed 200 mg. **Note: Actual dosage and administration schedule must be determined by the physician for each patient individually.**

▷ **Dosing Instructions:** May be taken with or following meals to reduce stomach irritation. Best taken in the morning to avoid nighttime urination. The tablet may be crushed for administration.

Usual Duration of Use: Continual use on a regular schedule for 2 to 3 weeks is usually necessary to determine this drug's effectiveness in lowering high blood pressure. Long-term use (months to years) requires periodic evaluation of response and possible dosage adjustment. Use as a diuretic should be intermittent with "drug holidays" (no drug taken) to reduce the risk of sodium and potassium imbalance. Consult your physician on a regular basis.

▷ **This Drug Should Not Be Taken If**
> • you have had an allergic reaction to it previously.

▷ **Inform Your Physician Before Taking This Drug If**
- you are allergic to any form of "sulfa" drug.
- you are pregnant or planning pregnancy.
- you have a history of kidney or liver disease.
- you have diabetes, gout or lupus erythematosus.
- you are taking any form of cortisone, digitalis, oral antidiabetic drug or insulin.
- you plan to have surgery under general anesthesia in the near future.

Possible Side-Effects (natural, expected and unavoidable drug actions)
Light-headedness on arising from sitting or lying position (see Orthostatic Hypotension in Glossary).
Increase in blood sugar level, affecting control of diabetes.
Increase in blood uric acid level, affecting control of gout.
Decrease in blood potassium level, causing muscle weakness and cramping.

▷ **Possible Adverse Effects** (unusual, unexpected and infrequent reactions)
If any of the following develop, consult your physician promptly for guidance.
Mild Adverse Effects
Allergic Reactions: Skin rashes, hives, drug fever.
Headache, dizziness, blurred or yellow vision.
Reduced appetite, indigestion, nausea, vomiting, diarrhea.
Serious Adverse Effects
Allergic Reactions: Hepatitis with jaundice (see Glossary), anaphylactic reaction (see Glossary), severe skin reactions.
Inflammation of the pancreas—severe abdominal pain.
Bone marrow depression (see Glossary)—fatigue, weakness, fever, sore throat, abnormal bleeding or bruising.

▷ **Possible Effects on Sexual Function:** Decreased libido and impotence, beginning from 2 weeks to several months after starting drug (100 mg/day).

▷ **Adverse Effects That May Mimic Natural Diseases or Disorders**
Liver reaction may suggest viral hepatitis.

Natural Diseases or Disorders That May Be Activated by This Drug
Diabetes, gout, systemic lupus erythematosus (questionable).

CAUTION
1. Do not exceed recommended doses. Increased dosage can cause excessive loss of sodium and potassium, with resultant loss of appetite, nausea, fatigue, weakness, confusion and tingling in the extremities.
2. If you are also taking a digitalis preparation (digitoxin, digoxin), ensure an adequate intake of high-potassium foods to prevent potassium deficiency, a potential cause of digitalis toxicity. (See Table of High Potassium Foods in Section Six.)

Precautions for Use

By Infants and Children: Avoid overdosage that could cause serious de-hydration. Significant potassium loss can occur within the first 2 weeks of drug use.

By Those over 60 Years of Age: Small doses are advisable until your individual response has been determined. You may be more susceptible to the development of fatigue (40%), low blood potassium (10%), elevated blood uric acid (30%), impaired thinking, orthostatic hypotension and blood sugar increase. Overdosage and extended use of this drug can cause excessive loss of body water, thickening (increased viscosity) of the blood, and an increased tendency for the blood to clot—predisposing to stroke, heart attack, or thrombophlebitis (vein inflammation with blood clot). Report promptly any type of skin reaction.

▷ **Advisability of Use During Pregnancy**

Pregnancy Category: D (tentative). See Pregnancy Code inside back cover. Animal studies: No birth defects reported.

Human studies: Information from adequate studies of pregnant women is not available.

It should not be used during pregnancy unless a very serious complication occurs for which this drug is significantly beneficial. This drug can cause serious adverse effects in the newborn infant. Ask physician for guidance.

Advisability of Use if Breast-Feeding

Presence of this drug in breast milk: Yes.

Avoid drug or refrain from nursing.

Habit-Forming Potential: None.

Effects of Overdosage: Dry mouth, thirst, lethargy, weakness, muscle cramping, nausea, vomiting, drowsiness progressing to stupor or coma.

Possible Effects of Long-Term Use: Impaired balance of water, salt and potassium in blood and body tissues. Development of diabetes in predisposed individuals. Pathological changes in parathyroid glands with increased blood calcium levels and decreased blood phosphate levels.

Suggested Periodic Examinations While Taking This Drug (at physician's discretion)

Complete blood cell counts; measurements of blood levels of sodium, potassium, chloride, sugar and uric acid.

Kidney and liver function tests.

▷ **While Taking This Drug, Observe the Following**

Foods: Consult your physician regarding the advisability of eating foods rich in potassium. If so advised, see the Table of High Potassium

Foods in Section Six. Follow physician's advice regarding the use of salt.

Beverages: No restrictions. This drug may be taken with milk.

▷ *Alcohol:* Use with caution until the combined effects have been determined. Alcohol may exaggerate the blood-pressure-lowering effects of this drug and cause orthostatic hypotension (see Glossary).

Tobacco Smoking: No interactions expected. Follow physician's advice.

▷ *Other Drugs*

Chlorthalidone may **increase** the effects of

- other antihypertensive drugs; dosage adjustments may be necessary to prevent excessive lowering of blood pressure.
- lithium, and cause lithium toxicity.

Chlorthalidone may **decrease** the effects of

- oral antidiabetic drugs (sulfonylureas); dosage adjustments may be necessary for proper control of blood sugar.

Chlorthalidone **taken concurrently** with

- digitalis preparations (digitoxin, digoxin) requires very careful monitoring and dosage adjustments to prevent fluctuations of blood potassium levels and serious disturbances of heart rhythm.

The following drugs may **decrease** the effects of chlorthalidone

- cholestyramine (Cuemid, Questran) may interfere with its absorption.
- colestipol (Colestid) may interfere with its absorption.

Take cholestyramine and colestipol 1 hour before any oral diuretic.

▷ *Driving, Hazardous Activities:* Use caution until the possible occurrence of orthostatic hypotension, dizziness or impaired vision has been determined.

Aviation Note: The use of this drug **may be a disqualification** for piloting. Consult a designated Aviation Medical Examiner.

Exposure to Sun: Use caution until sensitivity has been determined. This drug can cause photosensitivity (see Glossary).

Exposure to Heat: Avoid excessive perspiring which could cause additional loss of salt and water from the body.

Heavy Exercise or Exertion: Avoid exertion that produces light-headedness, excessive fatigue or muscle cramping. Isometric exercises—the "overload" technique for strengthening individual muscles—can raise the blood pressure significantly. Ask physician for guidance regarding participation in this form of exercise.

Occurrence of Unrelated Illness: Illnesses that cause vomiting or diarrhea can produce a serious imbalance of important body chemistry. Consult your physician for guidance.

Discontinuation: It may be advisable to discontinue this drug 5 to 7 days before major surgery. Ask your physician, surgeon and/or anesthesiologist for guidance regarding dosage adjustment or drug withdrawal. Following long-term use, this drug should be withdrawn gradually to prevent the occurrence of rebound edema.

CHLORZOXAZONE
(klor ZOX a zohn)

Introduced: 1958

Class: Muscle relaxant

Prescription: USA: Yes
  Canada: No

Controlled Drug: USA: No
  Canada: No

Available as Generic: USA: Yes
  Canada: No

Brand Names: Paraflex, Parafon Forte [CD]

BENEFITS versus RISKS

Possible Benefits	*Possible Risks*
Mild to moderate relief of discomfort due to spasm of voluntary muscles	Red and white blood cell disorders Gastrointestinal bleeding Liver damage, jaundice (questionable) (All rare)

▷ **Principal Uses**

As a Single Drug Product: Used primarily to relieve the pain and stiffness associated with spasm of voluntary muscles, such as that resulting from accidental injury of musculoskeletal structures. It is often necessary to supplement the use of this drug with other treatment measures, such as rest, support and physiotherapy.

As a Combination Drug Product [CD]: It is combined with acetaminophen to enhance its effectiveness in relieving discomfort. Acetaminophen is an effective analgesic and may be necessary to control the pain that is not relieved by chlorzoxazone alone.

How This Drug Works: Not completely established. It is thought that this drug may relieve muscle spasm and pain by blocking the transmission of nerve impulses over reflex pathways and/or by producing a sedative effect that decreases the perception of pain.

Available Dosage Forms and Strengths
  Caplets — 500 mg
  Tablets — 250 mg

▷ **Usual Adult Dosage Range:** 250 to 750 mg, 3 or 4 times daily; adjust dosage as needed and tolerated. **Note: Actual dosage and administration schedule must be determined by the physician for each patient individually.**

▷ **Dosing Instructions:** Take either on empty stomach or with food to prevent stomach irritation. Tablet may be crushed for administration.

Usual Duration of Use: Continual use on a regular schedule for 2 to 3 days is usually necessary to determine this drug's effectiveness in relieving the discomfort of muscle spasm. Evaluate need for continued use after periods of 7 to 10 days.

▷ **This Drug Should Not Be Taken If**
- you have had an allergic reaction to it previously.
- you have active liver disease.

▷ **Inform Your Physician Before Taking This Drug If**
- you have experienced any unfavorable reactions to muscle relaxants in the past.
- you have a history of liver or kidney disease.

Possible Side-Effects (natural, expected and unavoidable drug actions)
Drowsiness, orange or reddish purple discoloration of the urine (of no significance).

▷ **Possible Adverse Effects** (unusual, unexpected and infrequent reactions)
If any of the following develop, consult your physician promptly for guidance.
Mild Adverse Effects
Allergic Reactions: Skin rash, hives, itching, spontaneous bruising.
Light-headedness, dizziness, lethargy.
Indigestion, heartburn, nausea.
Serious Adverse Effects
Idiosyncratic Reactions: Nervousness, excitement, irritability.
Anemia, abnormally low white blood cell count—weakness, fever, sore throat.
Gastrointestinal bleeding—black- or dark-colored stools.
Liver reaction with or without jaundice (see Glossary)—yellow eyes and skin, dark-colored urine, light-colored stools.

▷ **Possible Effects on Sexual Function:** None reported.

▷ **Adverse Effects That May Mimic Natural Diseases or Disorders**
Liver reaction may suggest viral hepatitis.

Precautions for Use
By Infants and Children: Dosage is based on the child's age and weight. Consult your physician for exact dosage schedule.
By Those over 60 Years of Age: Small doses are advisable initially. You may be more susceptible to the development of drowsiness, dizziness, weakness, unsteadiness and falling.

▷ **Advisability of Use During Pregnancy**
Pregnancy Category: C (tentative). See Pregnancy Code inside back cover.
Animal studies: No data available.
Human studies: Information from adequate studies of pregnant women is not available.
Avoid drug if possible; use only if clearly needed.

Advisability of Use if Breast-Feeding
   Presence of this drug in breast milk: Yes.
   Avoid drug or refrain from nursing.

Habit-Forming Potential: None.

Effects of Overdosage: Nausea, vomiting, diarrhea, headache, drowsiness, dizziness, marked weakness, sense of paralysis of arms and legs, rapid and irregular breathing.

Possible Effects of Long-Term Use: None reported.

Suggested Periodic Examinations While Taking This Drug (at physician's discretion)
   Complete blood cell counts. Liver function tests.

▷ **While Taking This Drug, Observe the Following**
   Foods: No restrictions.
   Beverages: No restrictions. May be taken with milk.
▷   *Alcohol:* Use with caution until the combined effect has been determined. This drug may add to the depressant action of alcohol on the brain.
   Tobacco Smoking: No interactions expected.
   Marijuana Smoking: Moderate to marked drowsiness, muscle weakness, incoordination, accentuation of orthostatic hypotension (see Glossary).
▷   *Other Drugs*
   The following drug may *decrease* the effects of chlorzoxazone
   • testosterone is reported to reduce its ability to relax muscles in spasm.
▷   *Driving, Hazardous Activities:* This drug can cause drowsiness, light-headedness or dizziness in susceptible individuals. Avoid hazardous activities if these drug effects occur.
   Aviation Note: The use of this drug *is a disqualification* for piloting. Consult a designated Aviation Medical Examiner.
   Exposure to Sun: No restrictions.

CHOLESTYRAMINE
(koh LES tir a meen)

Introduced: 1959   **Class:** Anticholesterol

Prescription: USA: Yes   **Controlled Drug:** USA: No
   Canada: No   Canada: No

Available as Generic: USA: No
   Canada: No

Brand Names: Cholybar, Questran

```
┌─────────────────────────────────────────────────────────────┐
│                   BENEFITS versus RISKS                     │
│                                                             │
│      Possible Benefits              Possible Risks          │
│   EFFECTIVE REDUCTION OF       Constipation (may be severe) │
│     TOTAL CHOLESTEROL AND      Reduced absorption of fat, fat-│
│     LOW DENSITY                  soluble vitamins (A, D, E and│
│     CHOLESTEROL IN TYPE IIa      K) and folic acid          │
│     CHOLESTEROL DISORDERS      Reduced formation of         │
│     (15% to 25% reduction of total  prothrombin with resultant│
│     cholesterol, 25% to 35%       bleeding                  │
│     reduction of LDL cholesterol)                           │
│   EFFECTIVE RELIEF OF                                       │
│     ITCHING associated with                                 │
│     biliary obstruction                                     │
└─────────────────────────────────────────────────────────────┘
```

▷ **Principal Uses**

As a Single Drug Product: Used primarily to (1) reduce abnormally high blood levels of total cholesterol and low density (LDL) cholesterol in Type IIa cholesterol disorders; (2) relieve the itching due to the deposit of bile acids in the skin associated with partial biliary obstruction.

How This Drug Works: By combining with bile acids and bile salts in the intestinal tract, this drug forms insoluble complexes that are excreted in the feces. This removal of bile acids (which are necessary for food digestion) stimulates the conversion of cholesterol to bile acids to replace the loss; this in turn reduces the blood levels of cholesterol. By reducing the blood levels of bile acids, this drug hastens the absorption and clearance of bile acids deposited in the skin and thus relieves itching.

Available Dosage Forms and Strengths

Bars — 4 grams
Cans — 378 grams
Packets — 9 grams

▷ **Usual Adult Dosage Range:** 9 grams of powder (equivalent to 4 grams of cholestyramine) 3 times daily. Dose may be increased slowly as needed and tolerated. The total daily dosage should not exceed 72 grams of powder (32 grams of cholestyramine). **Note: Actual dosage and administration schedule must be determined by the physician for each patient individually.**

▷ **Dosing Instructions:** Always take just before or with a meal; this drug is ineffective when taken without food. Mix the powder thoroughly in 4 to 6 ounces of water, fruit juice, milk, thin soup or a soft food like applesauce; do not use carbonated beverages. **Do not take it in its dry form.**

Usual Duration of Use: Continual use on a regular schedule for 4 to 6 weeks is usually necessary to determine this drug's effectiveness in

lowering excessively high blood levels of cholesterol. Duration of use should not exceed 3 months if an adequate response does not occur. Long-term use (months to years) requires periodic evaluation of response and dosage adjustment. Consult your physician on a regular basis.

Currently a "Drug of Choice" for initiating treatment of elevated LDL cholesterol. See Cholesterol Disorders in Section Two.

▷ **This Drug Should Not Be Taken If**
- you have had an allergic reaction to it previously.
- you have complete biliary obstruction.

▷ **Inform Your Physician Before Taking This Drug If**
- you are prone to constipation.
- you have peptic ulcer disease.
- you have a bleeding disorder of any kind.
- you have impaired kidney function.

Possible Side-Effects (natural, expected and unavoidable drug actions)
Constipation (25%); interference with normal fat digestion and absorption; reduced absorption of vitamins A, D, E and K and folic acid.

▷ **Possible Adverse Effects** (unusual, unexpected and infrequent reactions)
If any of the following develop, consult your physician promptly for guidance.
Mild Adverse Effects
Allergic Reactions: Skin rash, hives, tongue irritation, anal itching.
Loss of appetite, indigestion, heartburn, abdominal discomfort, excessive gas, nausea, vomiting, diarrhea.
Serious Adverse Effects
Allergic Reaction: Asthmalike wheezing.
Vitamin K deficiency with resultant deficiency of prothrombin and increased bleeding tendency.
Impaired absorption of calcium; predisposition to osteoporosis.
Gallbladder colic.

▷ **Possible Effects on Sexual Function:**   Increased libido (questionable).

Natural Diseases or Disorders That May Be Activated by This Drug
Peptic ulcer disease; steatorrhea (excessive fat in stools) with large doses.

CAUTION
1. The powder should never be taken in its dry form; always mix it thoroughly with a suitable liquid before swallowing.
2. Observe carefully for the development of constipation; use stool softeners and laxatives as needed.
3. This drug may bind other drugs taken concurrently and impair their absorption. It is advisable to take *all other drugs* 1 to 2 hours before or 4 to 6 hours after taking this drug.

Precautions for Use

By Infants and Children: Safety and effectiveness for use by those under 6 years of age have not been established. Observe carefully for the possible development of acidosis and vitamin A or folic acid deficiency. (Ask your physician for guidance.)

By Those over 60 Years of Age: There may be increased risk of developing severe constipation. Impaired kidney function may predispose to the development of acidosis.

▷ **Advisability of Use During Pregnancy**

Pregnancy Category: C (tentative). See Pregnancy Code inside back cover.

Animal studies: No information available.

Human studies: Information from adequate studies of pregnant women is not available.

Use this drug only if clearly needed. Ensure adequate intake of vitamins and minerals since this drug can reduce their availability to both mother and fetus. Ask physician for guidance.

Advisability of Use if Breast-Feeding

Presence of this drug in breast milk: No.

Breast-feeding is permitted.

Habit-Forming Potential: None.

Effects of Overdosage: Progressive constipation.

Possible Effects of Long-Term Use

Deficiencies of vitamins A, D, E and K and folic acid.

Calcium deficiency, osteoporosis.

Acidosis due to excessive retention of chloride.

Suggested Periodic Examinations While Taking This Drug (at physician's discretion)

Measurements of blood levels of total cholesterol, low density (LDL) cholesterol and high density (HDL) cholesterol.

Hemoglobin and red blood cell studies for possible anemia.

▷ **While Taking This Drug, Observe the Following**

Foods: Avoid foods that tend to constipate (cheeses, etc.).

Nutritional Support: Consult your physician regarding the need for supplements of vitamins A, D, E and K, folic acid and calcium.

Beverages: Avoid carbonated beverages. Ensure adequate liquid intake (up to 2 quarts daily). This drug may be taken with milk.

▷ *Alcohol:* No interactions expected.

Tobacco Smoking: No interactions expected.

▷ *Other Drugs*

Cholestyramine may *decrease* the effects of

- acetaminophen; give 2 hours before cholestyramine.
- digitoxin and digoxin; give 2 hours before.
- iron preparations; give 2 to 3 hours before.

- phenobarbital; give 2 hours before.
- thiazide diuretics (see Drug Class, Section Four); give 2 hours before.
- thyroxin; give 5 hours before.
- warfarin; give 6 hours after.

▷ *Driving, Hazardous Activities:* No restrictions.

   Aviation Note: The use of this drug *is usually not a disqualification* for piloting. Consult a designated Aviation Medical Examiner.

   Exposure to Sun: No restrictions.

   Discontinuation: The dose of any potentially toxic drug taken concurrently must be reduced appropriately when this drug is discontinued.

CIMETIDINE
(si MET i deen)

Introduced: 1976

Class: Antiulcer, H-2 receptor blocker

Prescription: USA: Yes
Canada: Yes

Controlled Drug: USA: No
Canada: No

Available as Generic: No

Brand Names: ✦Apo-Cimetidine, ✦Novocimetine, ✦Peptol, Tagamet

---

BENEFITS versus RISKS

Possible Benefits	*Possible Risks*
EFFECTIVE TREATMENT OF PEPTIC ULCER DISEASE: relief of symptoms, acceleration of healing, prevention of recurrence	CONFUSIONAL STATES in the elderly and debilitated
	Rare blood cell and bone marrow disorders
CONTROL OF HYPERSECRETORY STOMACH DISORDERS	Rare pancreatitis
	Rare liver damage
Beneficial in treatment of reflux esophagitis	Rare kidney damage

---

▷ **Principal Uses**

   As a Single Drug Product: Used primarily in the treatment of peptic ulcer disease, specifically to hasten the healing of duodenal ulcer and to prevent its recurrence. Also used to control the excessive production of stomach acid in Zollinger-Ellison syndrome. Though its effectiveness has not been fully established, this drug is also widely used in the management of stomach (gastric) ulcer, esophagitis (as with hiatal hernia) and upper gastrointestinal bleeding.

How This Drug Works: By blocking the action of histamine, this drug effectively inhibits the secretion of stomach acid and thus creates a more favorable environment for the healing of peptic ulcers.

Available Dosage Forms and Strengths
Injection — 300 mg per 2 ml
Liquid — 300 mg per 5-ml teaspoonful (2.8% alcohol)
Tablets — 200 mg, 300 mg, 400 mg, 800 mg

▷ **Usual Adult Dosage Range:** For active peptic ulcer and hypersecretory states—300 mg, 4 times daily, taken with meals and at bedtime. For prevention of recurrent ulcer—400 mg at bedtime. Total daily dosage should not exceed 1200 mg. **Note: Actual dosage and administration schedule must be determined by the physician for each patient individually.**

▷ **Dosing Instructions:** To obtain the longest period of stomach acid reduction, this drug should be taken with or immediately following meals. The tablet may be crushed for administration.

Usual Duration of Use: Continual use on a regular schedule for 4 to 6 weeks is usually necessary to determine this drug's effectiveness in healing active peptic ulcer. Continual use for up to 1 year is recommended for prevention of ulcer recurrence. Consult your physician on a regular basis.

▷ **This Drug Should Not Be Taken If**
- you have had an allergic reaction to any dosage form of it previously.

▷ **Inform Your Physician Before Taking This Drug If**
- you have impaired liver or kidney function.
- you have a low sperm count.
- you are taking any oral anticoagulant, propranolol or quinidine.

Possible Side-Effects (natural, expected and unavoidable drug actions)
None reported.

▷ **Possible Adverse Effects** (unusual, unexpected and infrequent reactions)
If any of the following develop, consult your physician promptly for guidance.
Mild Adverse Effects
Allergic Reactions: Skin rash, hives, drug fever (see Glossary).
Headache, dizziness, double vision, fatigue, muscular pains, diarrhea.
Serious Adverse Effects
Allergic Reactions: Pancreatitis, kidney damage.
Idiosyncratic Reactions: Nervous agitation, confusion, delirium, hallucinations, coma.
Slowed heart rate, liver damage.
Bone marrow depression (see Glossary)—weakness, fever, sore throat, abnormal bleeding or bruising.

▷ **Possible Effects on Sexual Function:**   Decreased libido (600 mg/day); impaired erection and impotence (1000 mg/day); decreased male fertility (1200 mg/day); male breast enlargement (1000 mg/day); female breast enlargement with milk production (1600 mg/day).

▷ **Adverse Effects That May Mimic Natural Diseases or Disorders**
Liver reactions may suggest viral hepatitis.

Natural Diseases or Disorders That May Be Activated by This Drug
Psoriasis (questionable).

CAUTION
1. Do not discontinue this drug abruptly. Ulcer activation and perforation have occurred following abrupt cessation.
2. Hemodialysis can remove from 8% to 14% of this drug. Schedule the dosage to follow completion of each dialysis treatment.

Precautions for Use
By Infants and Children: Safety and effectiveness for use by those under 16 years of age have not been established. If use of this drug is deemed necessary, observe for sedation, confusion, breast enlargement, milk secretion and possible kidney damage.
By Those over 60 Years of Age: Initiate treatment with one-half the usual dose. Observe for the development of nervous agitation, depression, confusion, slurred speech or excessive drowsiness. This drug can contribute to the formation of stomach phytobezoars (masses of undigested vegetable fibers). Individuals with poor chewing ability (missing teeth) and those who have had partial gastrectomy or vagotomy (stomach surgery) are most susceptible. Observe for loss of appetite, stomach fullness, nausea and vomiting.

▷ **Advisability of Use During Pregnancy**
Pregnancy Category: B (tentative). See Pregnancy Code inside back cover.
Animal studies: No birth defects reported.
Human studies: Information from adequate studies of pregnant women is not available.
Use this drug only if clearly needed. Ask physician for guidance.

Advisability of Use if Breast-Feeding
Presence of this drug in breast milk: Yes, in large amounts.
Avoid drug or refrain from nursing.

Habit-Forming Potential: None.

Effects of Overdosage: Confusion, delirium, slurred speech, flushing, sweating, drowsiness, muscle twitching, seizures, coma.

Possible Effects of Long-Term Use: Liver damage (reversible), swelling and tenderness of breast tissue in men.

Suggested Periodic Examinations While Taking This Drug (at physician's discretion)

Complete blood cell counts, liver and kidney function tests, sperm counts, prothrombin times if an anticoagulant is taken concurrently.

▷ **While Taking This Drug, Observe the Following**

Foods: Protein-rich foods produce maximal stomach acid secretion. Follow the diet prescribed to derive optimal benefit from this drug.

Nutritional Support: This drug may inhibit the absorption of vitamin B-12. Consult physician regarding the need for B-12 supplement.

Beverages: No restrictions. May be taken with milk.

▷ *Alcohol:* No interactions with drug. However, alcoholic beverages increase stomach acidity and can reduce the effectiveness of this drug.

Marijuana Smoking: Possible accentuation of reduced sperm production due to this drug.

▷ *Other Drugs*

Cimetidine may *increase* the effects of
- oral anticoagulants, and increase the risk of bleeding.
- benzodiazepines (Librium, Valium, etc.), see Drug Class, Section Four.
- phenytoin (Dilantin).
- procainamide (Procan, Pronestyl).
- propranolol (Inderal).
- quinidine (Quinaglute, etc.).
- theophylline (Theo-Dur, Bronkodyl, Slo-bid, etc.).

Cimetidine *taken concurrently* with
- carmustine (BCNU) may cause severe bone marrow depression. Do not use these drugs concurrently.

▷ *Driving, Hazardous Activities:* This drug can cause erratic driving behavior. Use caution until it has been determined that dizziness, confusion or double vision does not occur.

Aviation Note: The use of this drug *may be a disqualification* for piloting. Consult a designated Aviation Medical Examiner.

Exposure to Sun: No restrictions.

Discontinuation: Do not discontinue this drug suddenly if taken for peptic ulcer disease. Consult physician for withdrawal instructions. This drug does not provide an extended protective effect. Be alert to the possibility of ulcer recurrence anytime after discontinuation.

CIPROFLOXACIN
(sip roh FLOX a sin)

Introduced: 1984

Prescription: USA: Yes

Available as Generic: USA: No

Class: Anti-infective

Controlled Drug: USA: No

Brand Name: Cipro

BENEFITS versus RISKS

Possible Benefits	*Possible Risks*
HIGHLY EFFECTIVE TREATMENT FOR INFECTIONS OF THE LOWER RESPIRATORY TRACT, URINARY TRACT, BONES, JOINTS AND SKIN TISSUES due to susceptible organisms	Nausea (1.6%), diarrhea (1.5%), very rare drug-induced colitis
Effective treatment for some forms of bacterial gastroenteritis (diarrhea)	Mild allergic reactions (1.4%) Very rare hallucination or seizure

---

▷ **Principal Uses**

As a Single Drug Product: Used primarily to treat responsive infections (in adults) of: (1) the lower respiratory tract (lungs and bronchial tubes); (2) the urinary tract (kidneys, bladder, urethra and prostate gland); (3) the digestive tract (small intestine and colon); (4) bones and joints; (5) skin and related tissues.

How This Drug Works: By interfering with the bacterial enzyme DNA gyrase (which is required for DNA synthesis and cell reproduction), this drug arrests bacterial growth (in low concentrations) and destroys bacteria (in high concentrations).

Available Dosage Forms and Strengths
Tablets — 250 mg, 500 mg, 750 mg

▷ **Usual Adult Dosage Range:** 250 mg to 750 mg/12 hours, depending upon the nature and severity of the infection. The total daily dosage should not exceed 1500 mg. **Note: Actual dosage and administration schedule must be determined by the physician for each patient individually.**

▷ **Dosing Instructions:** May be taken with or without food. Preferably it should be taken 2 hours after eating. Drink fluids liberally during the entire course of treatment. Avoid antacids containing aluminum or magnesium for 2 hours before and after dosing. The tablet may be crushed for administration.

Usual Duration of Use: Continual use on a regular schedule for 7 to 14 days is usually necessary to determine this drug's effectiveness in eradicating the infection. The drug should be continued for at least 2 days after all indications of infection have disappeared. Bone and joint infections may require treatment for 6 weeks or longer. Long-term use requires periodic evaluation of response and dosage adjustment. Consult your physician on a regular basis.

Possible Advantages of This Drug

The most potent anti-infective action of the drugs in this class (quinolones).

Highly effective in treating numerous types of infection caused by a wide spectrum of bacteria (overall clinical response rate of 96%).

Capable of establishing effective drug levels throughout the prostate gland (clinical response rate of 83% in treating prostatitis).

Effective one-dose treatment for uncomplicated gonorrheal infection of the urethra.

No significant effect on kidney function.

Currently a "Drug of Choice" for (1) starting treatment of urinary tract infections prior to obtaining the results of urine bacterial culture and sensitivity tests; (2) treating infections due to *Pseudomonas aeruginosa*, a bacterial strain often resistant to other anti-infective drugs.

▷ **This Drug Should Not Be Taken If**

- you have had an allergic reaction to it previously.
- you are pregnant or breast-feeding.
- you have a seizure disorder that is not adequately controlled.
- it is prescribed for a person under 18 years of age.

▷ **Inform Your Physician Before Taking This Drug If**

- you are allergic to cinoxacin (Cinobac), nalidixic acid (NegGram) or norfloxacin (Noroxin).
- you have a history of a seizure disorder or a circulatory disorder of the brain.
- you have impaired liver or kidney function.
- you are taking any form of probenecid or theophylline.

Possible Side-Effects (natural, expected and unavoidable drug actions)

Superinfections (5%). (See Superinfection in the Glossary.)

▷ **Possible Adverse Effects** (unusual, unexpected and infrequent reactions)

If any of the following develop, consult your physician promptly for guidance.

Mild Adverse Effects

Allergic Reactions: Rash (0.83%), itching (0.47%), localized swelling (0.12%).

Dizziness (0.53%), headache (0.30%), weakness (0.36%), migraine (0.06%), anxiety (0.06%), abnormal vision (0.06%).

Nausea (1.6%), diarrhea (1.5%), vomiting (0.7%), indigestion (0.36%).

Serious Adverse Effects

Allergic Reactions: None reported.

Idiosyncratic Reactions: None reported.

Central nervous system stimulation: restlessness, tremor, confusion, hallucinations, seizures (all very rare).

▷ **Possible Effects on Sexual Function:** None reported.

▷ **Natural Diseases or Disorders That May Be Activated by This Drug**
Latent epilepsy, latent gout.

CAUTION
1. With high doses or prolonged use, crystal formation in the kidney may occur. This can be prevented by drinking copious amounts of water, up to 2 quarts/24 hours.
2. Drugs of this class may decrease the formation of saliva and predispose to the development of dental cavities or gum disease. Consult your dentist if dry mouth persists.

Precautions for Use
By Infants and Children: Avoid the use of this drug completely. It can impair normal bone growth and development.
By Those over 60 Years of Age: Impaired kidney function may require dosage reduction.
If you are taking theophylline concurrently with this drug, observe closely for possible theophylline accumulation and toxicity.

▷ **Advisability of Use During Pregnancy**
Pregnancy Category: C (tentative). See Pregnancy Code inside back cover.
Animal studies: No birth defects due to this drug found in mouse, rat or rabbit studies. However, this drug can impair normal bone development in immature dogs.
Human studies: Information from adequate studies of pregnant women is not available. However, the potential for adverse effects on fetal bone development contraindicates the use of this drug during entire pregnancy.

Advisability of Use if Breast-Feeding
Presence of this drug in breast milk: Probably yes.
Avoid drug or refrain from nursing.

Habit-Forming Potential: None.

Effects of Overdosage: No information available.

Possible Effects of Long-Term Use: Superinfections (see Glossary); crystal formation in kidneys.

Suggested Periodic Examinations While Taking This Drug (at physician's discretion)
Liver function tests, urine analysis.

▷ **While Taking This Drug, Observe the Following**
Foods: No restrictions.
Beverages: No restrictions. May be taken with milk.
▷ *Alcohol:* No interactions expected.
Tobacco Smoking: No interactions expected.
▷ *Other Drugs*
Ciprofloxacin may *increase* the effects of

- theophylline, and cause theophylline toxicity.

The following drug may *increase* the effects of ciprofloxacin

- probenecid (Benemid).

The following drugs may *decrease* the effects of ciprofloxacin

- antacids containing aluminum or magnesium can reduce the absorption of ciprofloxacin and lessen its effectiveness.

▷ *Driving, Hazardous Activities:* This drug may cause dizziness and impair vision. Restrict activities as necessary.

Aviation Note: The use of this drug *may be a disqualification* for piloting. Consult a designated Aviation Medical Examiner.

Exposure to Sun: This drug may rarely cause photosensitivity (see Glossary). Sunglasses are advised if eyes are overly sensitive to bright light.

Discontinuation: If you experience no adverse effects from this drug, take the full course prescribed for maximal results. Consult your physician regarding termination of treatment.

CLEMASTINE
(KLEM as teen)

Introduced: 1968

Class: Antihistamines

Prescription: USA: Yes
　　　　　Canada: No

Controlled Drug: USA: No
　　　　　　Canada: No

Available as Generic: USA: No
　　　　　　Canada: No

Brand Names: Tavist, Tavist-D [CD], Tavist-1

BENEFITS versus RISKS	
Possible Benefits	*Possible Risks*
EFFECTIVE RELIEF OF ALLERGIC RHINITIS AND ALLERGIC SKIN DISORDERS	Mild sedation Atropinelike effects Very rare blood cell disorders

▷ **Principal Uses**

As a Single Drug Product: Used primarily to provide symptomatic relief in allergic and related disorders: seasonal and perennial allergic rhinitis (hay fever), allergic conjunctivitis and vasomotor rhinitis; also in hives and localized swellings (angioedema) of allergic origin.

As a Combination Drug Product [CD]: This drug is combined with a decongestant drug (phenylpropanolamine) to enhance its ability to reduce tissue swelling and secretions in allergic and infectious disorders of the upper respiratory tract—hay fever, head colds and sinusitis.

How This Drug Works: Antihistamines reduce the intensity of the allergic response by blocking the action of histamine after it has been released from sensitized tissue cells in the eyes, nose, respiratory passages and skin.

Available Dosage Forms and Strengths
Syrup — 0.67 mg per 5-ml teaspoonful (5.5% alcohol)
Tablets — 1.34 mg, 2.68 mg

▷ **Usual Adult Dosage Range:**   1.34 mg twice daily, or 2.68 mg 3 times daily. The total daily dosage should not exceed 8.04 mg. **Note: Actual dosage and administration schedule must be determined by the physician for each patient individually.**

▷ **Dosing Instructions:**   Take with food or milk to prevent stomach irritation. The tablet may be crushed for administration.

Usual Duration of Use: Continual use on a regular schedule for 2 to 3 days is usually necessary to determine this drug's effectiveness in relieving the symptoms of allergic rhinitis and dermatosis. It may be necessary to take this drug throughout the entire pollen season, depending upon individual sensitivity. However, antihistamines should not be taken continually (without interruption) for long-term use. Limit their use to periods that require symptomatic relief.

▷ **This Drug Should Not Be Taken If**
• you have had an allergic reaction to any dosage form of it previously.
• you are currently undergoing allergy skin tests.
• you are taking, or have taken within the past 14 days, any monoamine oxidase (MAO) type A inhibitor drug (see Drug Class, Section Four).

▷ **Inform Your Physician Before Taking This Drug If**
• you have had any allergic reactions or unfavorable responses to the previous use of antihistamines.
• you have glaucoma (narrow-angle type) or asthma.
• you have epilepsy or a seizure disorder.
• you have difficulty emptying the urinary bladder, especially if due to prostate gland enlargement (see Prostatism in Glossary).
• you plan to have surgery under general anesthesia in the near future.

Possible Side-Effects (natural, expected and unavoidable drug actions)
Drowsiness; sense of weakness; blurred vision; dryness of the nose, mouth and throat; impaired urination.

▷ **Possible Adverse Effects** (unusual, unexpected and infrequent reactions)
If any of the following develop, consult your physician promptly for guidance.
Mild Adverse Effects
Allergic Reactions: Skin rash, hives.
Headache, nervous agitation, dizziness, confusion, tremor, blurred or double vision, altered color vision, ringing in ears.

Reduced tolerance for contact lenses.

Thickening of bronchial secretions in asthma or bronchitis.

Indigestion, nausea, vomiting, diarrhea.

Serious Adverse Effects

Allergic Reaction: Anaphylactic reaction (see Glossary).

Idiosyncratic Reactions: Euphoria, hysteria, depression, nightmares.

Hemolytic anemia (see Glossary).

Abnormally low white blood cell count—fever, sore throat, infections.

Abnormally low blood platelet count—abnormal bleeding or bruising.

▷ **Possible Effects on Sexual Function:** Shortened menstrual cycle (early arrival of expected menstrual onset).

Natural Diseases or Disorders That May Be Activated by This Drug

Latent epilepsy, glaucoma, prostatism (see Glossary).

CAUTION

1. Discontinue this drug 4 days before diagnostic skin testing procedures in order to prevent false negative test results.
2. Do not use this drug if you have active bronchial asthma, bronchitis or pneumonia. It can thicken bronchial mucus and make it more difficult to remove (by absorption or coughing).

Precautions for Use

By Infants and Children: This drug should not be used in premature or full-term newborn infants. Doses for children should be small. The young child is especially sensitive to the effects of antihistamines on the brain and nervous system.

By Those over 60 Years of Age: You may be more susceptible to the development of drowsiness, dizziness and unsteadiness, and to impairment of thinking, judgment and memory. This drug can increase the degree of impaired urination associated with prostate gland enlargement (prostatism). The sedative effects of antihistamines in the elderly can cause a syndrome of underactivity that may be misinterpreted as senility or emotional depression.

▷ **Advisability of Use During Pregnancy**

Pregnancy Category: B (tentative). See Pregnancy Code inside back cover.

Animal studies: No birth defects due to this drug reported in rat and rabbit studies.

Human studies: Information from adequate studies of pregnant women is not available. However, drugs of this class can cause seizures and other adverse effects on the newborn infant.

Use this drug only if clearly needed. Avoid during the last 3 months. Ask physician for guidance.

Advisability of Use if Breast-Feeding

Presence of this drug in breast milk: Probably yes.

Avoid drug or refrain from nursing.

Habit-Forming Potential: None.

Effects of Overdosage: Drowsiness; unsteadiness; faintness; marked dryness of mouth, nose and throat; flushing of face; shortness of breath; hallucinations; convulsions; stupor progressing to coma.

Possible Effects of Long-Term Use: Tardive dyskinesia (see Glossary) has been reported in association with the long-term use of several widely used antihistamines. It is advisable to avoid the prolonged, continual use of antihistamines without interruption.

Suggested Periodic Examinations While Taking This Drug (at physician's discretion)
    Complete blood cell counts.

▷ **While Taking This Drug, Observe the Following**
    Foods: No restrictions.
    Beverages: No restrictions. May be taken with milk.
▷   *Alcohol:* Use with extreme caution until the combined effects have been determined. The combination of antihistamine and alcohol can produce rapid and marked sedation.
    Tobacco Smoking: No interactions expected.
▷   *Other Drugs*
        Clemastine may *increase* the effects of
        • all sedatives, sleep-inducing drugs, tranquilizers, analgesics and narcotic drugs, and produce oversedation.
        Clemastine *taken concurrently* with
        • phenytoin (Dantoin, Dilantin) may alter the pattern of seizures. Dosage adjustments of the anticonvulsant may be necessary.
        The following drugs may *increase* the effects of clemastine
        • monoamine oxidase (MAO) type A inhibitor drugs (see Drug Class, Section Four) may prolong the action of antihistamines.
▷   *Driving, Hazardous Activities:* This drug can impair mental alertness, judgment, coordination and reaction time. Avoid hazardous activities until the full sedative effects have been determined.
    Aviation Note: The use of this drug *is a disqualification* for piloting. Consult a designated Aviation Medical Examiner.
    Exposure to Sun: Use caution. Some drugs of this class can cause photosensitivity (see Glossary).

CLIDINIUM
(kli DIN ee um)

Introduced: 1961   **Class:** Antispasmodic, atropinelike

Prescription: USA: Yes   **Controlled Drug:** USA: No
    Canada: Yes   Canada: No

Available as Generic: No

Brand Names: ✦Apo-Chlorax [CD], ✦Corium [CD], Librax [CD], Lidox [CD], Quarzan

---

BENEFITS versus RISKS

Possible Benefits	*Possible Risks*
RELIEF OF SYMPTOMS DUE TO GASTROINTESTINAL SPASM AND OVERACTIVITY as in peptic ulcer disease and irritable bowel syndrome	Skin rash, hives Dizziness, unsteadiness Confusion, delirium

---

▷ **Principal Uses**

As a Single Drug Product: This atropinelike antispasmodic drug is used primarily in the management of peptic ulcer disease and the irritable bowel syndrome. Because it has been replaced by more effective drugs, it is seldom used alone.

As a Combination Drug Product [CD]: The major use of this drug is in combination with chlordiazepoxide. When combined, the tranquilizing effect of chlordiazepoxide and the atropinelike effects of clidinium are more effective than either drug used alone. Their actions complement each other in the treatment of peptic ulcer and functional disorders of the gastrointestinal tract.

How This Drug Works: By blocking the action of the chemical (acetylcholine) that transmits impulses at parasympathetic nerve endings, this drug prevents stimulation of muscular contraction and glandular secretion within the organs involved. This results in reduced overall activity, including the prevention or relief of muscle spasms.

Available Dosage Forms and Strengths

Capsules — 2.5 mg, 5 mg

Capsules [CD] — 2.5 mg and 5 mg of chlordiazepoxide

Note: In Canada this drug is available only in combination with chlordiazepoxide. To be fully informed on the use of Librax, read the Drug Profiles of both components.

▷ **Usual Adult Dosage Range:** For Librax—1 or 2 capsules from 1 to 4 times daily, as needed and tolerated. Total daily dosage should not exceed 8 capsules. **Note: Actual dosage and administration schedule must be determined by the physician for each patient individually.**

▷ **Dosing Instructions:** Take 30 to 60 minutes before meals and also at bedtime if necessary. The capsule may be opened for administration.

Usual Duration of Use: Continual use on a regular schedule for 3 to 5 days is usually necessary to determine this drug's effectiveness in relieving the symptoms of gastrointestinal spasm and overactivity. Long-term use (weeks to months) requires physician supervision and guidance. Consult your physician on a regular basis.

▷ **This Drug Should Not Be Taken If**
- you have had an allergic reaction to it previously.
- your stomach cannot empty properly into the intestine (pyloric obstruction).
- you are unable to empty the urinary bladder completely.
- you have narrow-angle-type glaucoma.
- you have severe ulcerative colitis.

▷ **Inform Your Physician Before Taking This Drug If**
- you have open-angle type glaucoma.
- you have angina or coronary heart disease.
- you have a history of peptic ulcer disease.
- you have chronic bronchitis, a hiatal hernia, myasthenia gravis or prostatism (see Glossary).
- you plan to have surgery under general anesthesia in the near future.

Possible Side-Effects (natural, expected and unavoidable drug actions)
Blurred vision (impaired focus), dry mouth and throat, constipation, impaired urination. (Nature and degree of side-effects depend upon individual sensitivity and drug dosage.)

▷ **Possible Adverse Effects** (unusual, unexpected and infrequent reactions)
If any of the following develop, consult your physician promptly for guidance.
Mild Adverse Effects
Allergic Reactions: Skin rash, hives.
Light-headedness, dizziness, unsteadiness.
Dilation of pupils, causing sensitivity to light.
Flushing and dryness of skin, reduced sweating.
Rapid heart action.
Serious Adverse Effects
Idiosyncratic Reactions: Confusion, delirium, abnormal behavior.
Development of acute glaucoma (in susceptible individuals).

▷ **Possible Effects on Sexual Function:**   Impotence; suppressed milk production (7.5 to 20 mg/day).

CAUTION
1. Many over-the-counter medications (see OTC Drugs in Glossary) for allergies, colds and coughs contain drugs that can interact unfavorably with this drug. Ask your physician or pharmacist for guidance before taking these drugs together.
2. Constipation should be treated promptly with stool softeners and effective laxatives.

Precautions for Use
By Infants and Children: Safety, effectiveness and dosage for use by those under 12 years of age have not been established. Ask physician for guidance.

By Those over 60 Years of Age: Initial dosage should be 1 capsule twice a day until tolerance has been determined. This drug can accentuate the symptoms of prostatism (see Glossary).

▷ **Advisability of Use During Pregnancy**
Pregnancy Category: B (tentative). See Pregnancy Code inside back cover.
Animal studies: No birth defects reported.
Human studies: Information from adequate studies of pregnant women is not available.
Note: If this drug is taken in its combination form (Librax [CD]), see the pregnancy category in the Drug Profile of Chlordiazepoxide. Ask physician for guidance.

Advisability of Use if Breast-Feeding
Presence of this drug in breast milk: Yes.
Avoid drug or refrain from nursing.

Habit-Forming Potential: For clidinium—none. For Librax—see Drug Profile of Chlordiazepoxide.

Effects of Overdosage: Dilated pupils, dry mouth, headache, excitement, confusion, hallucinations, delirium, hot skin, high fever, convulsions, coma.

Possible Effects of Long-Term Use: Chronic constipation, severe enough to cause fecal impaction.

Suggested Periodic Examinations While Taking This Drug (at physician's discretion)
Measurement of internal eye pressure to detect significant increase that could indicate developing glaucoma.

▷ **While Taking This Drug, Observe the Following**
Foods: No interactions with drug. Follow prescribed diet.
Beverages: As allowed by prescribed diet. Drug may be taken with milk.
▷ *Alcohol:* Use caution and observe for increased sedation or dizziness.
Tobacco Smoking: No interactions with clidinium. For Librax—see Drug Profile of Chlordiazepoxide.
▷ *Other Drugs*
Clidinium may *increase* the effects of
• atenolol (Tenormin), and require reduction of its dosage.
• other drugs with atropinelike actions (see Drug Class, Section Four).
▷ *Driving, Hazardous Activities:* This drug may cause drowsiness, dizziness or blurred vision. Avoid hazardous activities if these drug effects occur.
Aviation Note: The use of this drug *may be a disqualification* for piloting. Consult a designated Aviation Medical Examiner.
Exposure to Sun: No restrictions.

Exposure to Heat: Use extreme caution. The use of this drug in hot environments may impair the regulation of body temperature and increase the risk of heat stroke.

CLINDAMYCIN
(klin da MI sin)

Introduced: 1973

Class: Antibiotic

Prescription: USA: Yes
Canada: Yes

Controlled Drug: USA: No
Canada: No

Available as Generic: USA: Yes
Canada: No

Brand Names: Cleocin, Cleocin T, ✦Dalacin C

BENEFITS versus RISKS

Possible Benefits	*Possible Risks*
EFFECTIVE TREATMENT FOR SERIOUS INFECTIONS OF THE LOWER RESPIRATORY TRACT, ABDOMINAL CAVITY, GENITAL TRACT IN WOMEN, BLOOD STREAM (SEPTICEMIA), SKIN AND RELATED TISSUES caused by susceptible organisms	SEVERE DRUG-INDUCED COLITIS (fatalities reported) Rare liver injury with jaundice Rare reduction in white blood cell and platelet counts
SPECIFIC PREVENTION AND TREATMENT FOR PNEUMOCYSTIS CARINII PNEUMONIA (PCP) ASSOCIATED WITH AIDS	
Possibly effective for the local treatment of acne	

▷ **Principal Uses**

As a Single Drug Product

Used primarily to treat serious and unusual infections of the lungs and bronchial tubes, organs and tissues within the abdominal cavity, the genital tract and pelvic organs in women, the skin and soft tissue structures and generalized infections involving the bloodstream.

A more recent use has been the prevention and treatment of pneumocystis carinii pneumonia, a frequent infection associated with AIDS.

How This Drug Works: By interfering with the formation of proteins necessary for cell growth and reproduction, this drug (in low concentrations) arrests the multiplication of bacteria and (in high concentrations) destroys bacteria.

Available Dosage Forms and Strengths
Capsules — 75 mg, 150 mg, 300 mg
Injection — 150 mg per ml
Oral solution — 75 mg per 5-ml teaspoonful
Topical solution — 10 mg per ml

▷ **Usual Adult Dosage Range:** For infections of average severity: 150 to 300 mg/6 hours; for more severe infections: 300 to 450 mg/6 hours. The total daily dosage should not exceed 1800 mg. **Note: Actual dosage and administration schedule must be determined by the physician for each patient individually.**

▷ **Dosing Instructions:** Take the capsule with a full glass of water or with food to prevent irritation of the esophagus. The capsule may be opened and the contents mixed with food for administration. Shake the oral solution well before measuring the dose. Do not refrigerate the oral solution; chilling can cause it to thicken, making administration difficult.

Usual Duration of Use: Continual use on a regular schedule for 3 to 5 days is usually necessary to determine this drug's effectiveness in controlling responsive infections. The duration of use should not exceed the time required to eliminate the infection.

Possible Advantages of This Drug: Bacterial sensitivity testing may show this drug to be more effective than commonly used antibiotics in treating some severe and unusual infections.

Currently a "Drug of Choice" for preventing and treating pneumonia due to pneumocystis carinii, a frequent complication of AIDS.

▷ **This Drug Should Not Be Taken If**
• you are allergic to either clindamycin or lincomycin.
• it is prescribed for a mild or trivial infection such as a cold, sore throat or "flulike" illness.
• you have a history of Crohn's disease or ulcerative colitis.

▷ **Inform Your Physician Before Taking This Drug If**
• you have a history of allergy to any drug.
• you have a history of drug-induced colitis.
• you are allergic by nature: hay fever, asthma, hives, eczema.
• you have a history of previous yeast infections.
• you have myasthenia gravis.
• you have impaired liver or kidney function.
• you plan to have surgery under general anesthesia in the near future.

Possible Side-Effects (natural, expected and unavoidable drug actions)
Superinfections (see Glossary).

▷ **Possible Adverse Effects** (unusual, unexpected and infrequent reactions)
If any of the following develop, consult your physician promptly for guidance.
Mild Adverse Effects
Allergic Reactions: Skin rashes (3% to 5%), hives.
Nausea, vomiting, mild diarrhea (3% to 30%), stomach pain.
Multiple joint pains (rare).
Serious Adverse Effects
Allergic Reactions: Severe skin reactions: erythema multiforme (Stevens-Johnson syndrome).
Toxic liver reaction with jaundice (see Glossary).
Severe colitis with persistent diarrhea (0.01% to 10%); stools may contain blood and/or mucus.
Rare reduction of white blood cell and platelet counts.

▷ **Possible Effects on Sexual Function:** None reported.

Possible Delayed Adverse Effects: Severe colitis with diarrhea (pseudomembranous colitis) may begin several weeks after discontinuing this drug.

▷ **Adverse Effects That May Mimic Natural Diseases or Disorders**
Liver reactions may suggest viral hepatitis.
Multiple joint pains may suggest the onset of arthritis.

▷ **Natural Diseases or Disorders That May Be Activated by This Drug**
Crohn's disease, ulcerative colitis, myasthenia gravis.

CAUTION
1. Troublesome and persistent diarrhea can develop in sensitive individuals. If diarrhea persists longer than 24 hours, discontinue this drug and consult your physician for guidance.
2. If surgery under general anesthesia is planned while taking this drug, the choice of anesthetic must be considered carefully to prevent excessive muscle relaxation and associated impairment of breathing.

Precautions for Use
By Infants and Children: Safety and effectiveness for use by those under 1 month of age have not been established. Use with caution.
By Those over 60 Years of Age: Observe closely for the possible development of diarrhea (more common in this age group). Also observe for the possible development of yeast infection of the skin in the genital and anal regions, a form of superinfection (see Glossary). Report such developments promptly to your physician.

▷ **Advisability of Use During Pregnancy**
Pregnancy Category: B (tentative). See Pregnancy Code inside back cover.
Animal studies: No birth defects due to this drug found in mouse or
rat studies.
Human studies: Information from adequate studies of pregnant women
is not available. Use this drug only if clearly needed. Ask your physician for guidance.

Advisability of Use if Breast-Feeding
Presence of this drug in breast milk: Yes.
Avoid drug or refrain from nursing.

Habit-Forming Potential: None.

Effects of Overdosage: Nausea, vomiting, cramping, diarrhea.

Possible Effects of Long-Term Use
Superinfections, especially from yeast organisms.
Severe colitis with persistent diarrhea.

Suggested Periodic Examinations While Taking This Drug (at physician's
discretion)
Complete blood cell counts, liver function tests.

▷ **While Taking This Drug, Observe the Following**
Foods: No restrictions.
Beverages: No restrictions. May be taken with milk.
▷   *Alcohol:* No interactions expected.
Tobacco Smoking: No interactions expected.
▷   *Other Drugs*
Clindamycin **taken concurrently** with
• antidiarrheal drugs (diphenoxylate, loperamide, paregoric) may re-
sult in worsening of the underlying colitis because of impaired elim-
ination of causative toxins.
• antimyasthenic drugs (ambenonium, neostigmine, pyridostigmine)
may reduce their effectiveness in relieving the muscle weakness of
myasthenia gravis.
The following drugs may **decrease** the effects of clindamycin
• chloramphenicol (Chloromycetin).
• erythromycin (E.E.S., E-Mycin, etc.).
▷   *Driving, Hazardous Activities:* This drug may cause nausea and diarrhea.
Restrict activities as necessary.
Aviation Note: The use of this drug **may be a disqualification** for piloting.
Consult a designated Aviation Medical Examiner.
Exposure to Sun: Use caution until sensitivity is determined.
Discontinuation: If tolerated satisfactorily, take the full course prescribed.
When used to treat infections that may predispose to rheumatic fever
or nephritis, take continually in full dosage for no less than 10 days.
Special Storage Instructions: Oral solution should be kept at room tem-
perature; do not refrigerate.

Observe the Following Expiration Time: Do not take the oral solution if it is older than 14 days.

CLONIDINE
(KLOH ni deen)

Introduced: 1969

Class: Antihypertensive

Prescription: USA: Yes
Canada: Yes

Controlled Drug: USA: No
Canada: No

Available as Generic: USA: Yes
Canada: No

Brand Names: Catapres, Catapres-TTS, Combipres [CD], ✦Dixarit

---

BENEFITS versus RISKS

Possible Benefits	*Possible Risks*
EFFECTIVE ANTIHYPERTEN-SIVE in mild to moderate high blood pressure	ACUTE WITHDRAWAL SYNDROME and hypertensive "overshoot" with abrupt discontinuation
Effective control of menopausal hot flashes (in selected cases)	Raynaud's phenomenon (cold fingers or toes)

▷ **Principal Uses**

As a Single Drug Product: This antihypertensive drug is often used as a "step 2" drug in the treatment of mild to moderate high blood pressure. It is generally not used to initiate treatment, but is added when a "step 1" drug proves to be inadequate. It may also be used as a "step 3 or 4" drug in place of drugs that cause marked orthostatic hypotension (see Glossary). It is sometimes used to prevent migraine headache, to prevent hot flashes of the menopause and to treat menstrual cramps.

As a Combination Drug Product [CD]: This "step 2" antihypertensive is available in combination with the "step 1" antihypertensive drug chlorthalidone, a diuretic. The differing methods of action complement each other to make the combination a more effective antihypertensive.

How This Drug Works: By decreasing the activity of the vasomotor center in the brain, this drug reduces the ability of the sympathetic nervous system to maintain the degree of blood vessel constriction responsible for the elevation of blood pressure. This change results in relaxation of blood vessel walls and lowering of blood pressure.

Available Dosage Forms and Strengths
Patches — 0.1 mg, 0.2 mg, 0.3 mg
Tablets — 0.1 mg, 0.2 mg, 0.3 mg

▷ **Usual Adult Dosage Range:** Tablets—initially 0.1 mg twice daily. Increase by 0.1 to 0.2 mg daily as needed and tolerated. Usual range is 0.2 to 0.8 mg daily, taken in 2 doses. Total daily dosage should not exceed 2.4 mg. Medicated patches are applied once a week. **Note: Actual dosage and administration schedule must be determined by the physician for each patient individually.**

▷ **Dosing Instructions:** Tablets may be taken without regard to eating. The tablet may be crushed for administration.

Usual Duration of Use: Continual use on a regular schedule for 2 to 3 weeks is usually necessary to determine this drug's effectiveness in controlling high blood pressure. Long-term use (months to years) requires supervision and guidance by the physician. Consult your physician on a regular basis.

▷ **This Drug Should Not Be Taken If**
- you have had an allergic reaction to it previously.

▷ **Inform Your Physician Before Taking This Drug If**
- you have a circulatory disorder of the brain.
- you have angina or coronary artery disease.
- you have or have had serious emotional depression.
- you have Buerger's disease or Raynaud's phenomenon.
- you are taking any sedative or hypnotic drugs or an antidepressant.
- you plan to have surgery under general anesthesia in the near future.

Possible Side-Effects (natural, expected and unavoidable drug actions)
Drowsiness (35%), dry nose and mouth (40%), constipation (common), decreased heart rate, mild orthostatic hypotension (see Glossary).

▷ **Possible Adverse Effects** (unusual, unexpected and infrequent reactions)
If any of the following develop, consult your physician promptly for guidance.
Mild Adverse Effects
Allergic Reactions: Skin rash, hives, localized swellings, itching.
Headache, dizziness, fatigue, anxiety, nervousness, dryness and burning of eyes.
Painful parotid (salivary) gland, nausea, vomiting.
Weight gain, urinary retention.
Serious Adverse Effects
Idiosyncratic Reaction: Raynaud's phenomenon (see Glossary).
Aggravation of congestive heart failure, heart rhythm disorders, vivid dreaming, nightmares, depression, hallucinations.
Corneal ulcers (rare). Acute pancreatitis (rare).

▷ **Possible Effects on Sexual Function:** Decreased libido in 10% (0.2 to 0.8 mg/day); impotence in 8% to 24% (0.5 to 3.6 mg/day); impaired ejaculation (rare); enlargement of male breasts (0.2 to 0.8 mg/day).

CAUTION
1. *Do not discontinue this drug suddenly.* Sudden withdrawal can produce a severe and possibly fatal reaction.
2. Hot weather and the fever associated with infection can reduce blood pressure significantly. Dosage adjustments may be necessary.
3. Report the development of any tendency to emotional depression.

Precautions for Use
By Infants and Children: Safety and effectiveness for use by those under 12 years of age have not been established.
By Those over 60 Years of Age: Proceed cautiously with the use of any antihypertensive drug. Unacceptably high blood pressure should be reduced without creating the risks associated with excessively low blood pressure. Start treatment with small doses and monitor the blood pressure response frequently. Observe for the development of light-headedness, dizziness, unsteadiness, fainting and falling. Sedation and dry mouth occur in 50% of elderly users. Report promptly any changes in mood or behavior: depression, delusions, hallucinations.

▷ **Advisability of Use During Pregnancy**
Pregnancy Category: C (tentative). See Pregnancy Code inside back cover.
Animal studies: No birth defects reported. However, this drug is toxic to the embryo in low dosage.
Human studies: Information from adequate studies of pregnant women is not available.
The manufacturer recommends that this drug be avoided by women who are or who may become pregnant. Ask physician for guidance.

Advisability of Use if Breast-Feeding
Presence of this drug in breast milk: Yes.
This drug may impair milk production. Monitor nursing infant closely and discontinue drug or nursing if adverse effects develop.

Habit-Forming Potential: None.

Effects of Overdosage: Marked drowsiness, weakness, dry mouth, slow pulse, low blood pressure, vomiting, stupor progressing to coma.

Possible Effects of Long-Term Use: Development of tolerance (see Glossary) with loss of drug effectiveness; weight gain due to salt and water retention; temporary sexual impotence.

Suggested Periodic Examinations While Taking This Drug (at physician's discretion)
Blood pressure measurements, monitoring of body weight.

▷ **While Taking This Drug, Observe the Following**
> *Foods:* Avoid excessive salt. Ask physician for guidance regarding degree
> of salt restriction.
>
> *Beverages:* No restrictions. May be taken with milk.

▷ *Alcohol:* Use with extreme caution. The combined effects can cause
> marked drowsiness and exaggerated reduction of blood pressure.
>
> *Tobacco Smoking:* No interactions expected. Follow your physician's ad-
> vice regarding use of tobacco.

▷ *Other Drugs*
> Clonidine may *decrease* the effects of
> - levodopa (Larodopa, Sinemet, etc.), causing an increase in parkin-
> sonism symptoms.
>
> Clonidine *taken concurrently* with
> - beta-adrenergic-blocking drugs (Inderal, Lopressor, etc.) may increase
> the risk of serious rebound hypertension if clonidine is discontinued
> first. It is advisable to discontinue the beta blocker first and then
> withdraw clonidine gradually.
>
> The following drugs may *decrease* the effects of clonidine
> - tricyclic antidepressants (Elavil, Sinequan, etc.) may reduce its ef-
> fectiveness in lowering blood pressure.

▷ *Driving, Hazardous Activities:* Use caution. This drug can cause drowsiness
> and can impair mental alertness, judgment and coordination.
>
> *Aviation Note:* Hypertension (high blood pressure) *is a disqualification* for
> piloting. Consult a designated Aviation Medical Examiner.
>
> *Exposure to Sun:* No restrictions.
>
> *Exposure to Heat:* Use caution. Hot environments may reduce the blood
> pressure significantly; be alert to the possibility of orthostatic hy-
> potension (see Glossary).
>
> *Exposure to Cold:* Use caution. This drug may cause painful blanching and
> numbness of the hands and feet on exposure to cold air or water
> (Raynaud's phenomenon).
>
> *Heavy Exercise or Exertion:* Use caution. Isometric exercises—the "over-
> load" technique for strengthening individual muscles—can raise
> blood pressure significantly. The use of this drug may intensify the
> hypertensive response to isometric exercise. Ask physician for guid-
> ance.
>
> *Occurrence of Unrelated Illness:* Fever associated with infections may lower
> the blood pressure significantly. Repeated vomiting may prevent the
> regular use of this drug and result in an acute withdrawal reaction.
> Consult your physician.
>
> *Discontinuation:* **Do not discontinue this drug suddenly.** A severe with-
> drawal reaction can occur within 12 to 48 hours after the last dose.
> The dose should be reduced gradually over 3 to 4 days, with periodic
> monitoring of the blood pressure.

CLORAZEPATE
(klor AZ e payt)

Introduced: 1968

Class: Mild tranquilizer, benzodi-azepines

Prescription: USA: Yes
Canada: Yes

Controlled Drug: USA: C-IV*
Canada: No

Available as Generic: Yes

Brand Names: Gen-Xene, ♦Novoclopate, Tranxene, Tranxene-SD, Tranxene-SD Half Strength

---

BENEFITS versus RISKS

Possible Benefits	*Possible Risks*
RELIEF OF ANXIETY AND NERVOUS TENSION in 70% to 80% of users	Habit-forming potential with prolonged use
Wide margin of safety with therapeutic doses	Minor impairment of mental functions
Very few drug interactions	

▷ **Principal Uses**

As a Single Drug Product: Used primarily to (1) provide short-term relief of mild to moderate anxiety, and (2) provide adjunctive treatment in controlling "partial" seizures, a type of epilepsy.

How This Drug Works: It is thought that this drug produces a calming effect by enhancing the action of the nerve transmitter gamma-aminobutyric acid (GABA), which in turn blocks the arousal of higher brain centers.

Available Dosage Forms and Strengths

Capsules — 3.75 mg, 7.5 mg, 15 mg
Tablets — 3.75 mg, 7.5 mg, 15 mg
Tablets, single dose — 11.25 mg, 22.5 mg

▷ **Usual Adult Dosage Range:** 15 to 60 mg/24 hours, in 2 to 4 divided doses or as a single dose at bedtime. The usual dose is 30 mg/24 hours. Total daily dose should not exceed 90 mg. **Note: Actual dosage and administration schedule must be determined by the physician for each patient individually.**

▷ **Dosing Instructions:** May be taken on empty stomach or with food or milk. Capsule may be opened and regular tablet may be crushed for admin-

*See Schedules of Controlled Drugs inside back cover.

istration; the single-dose tablet should not be crushed. Do not discontinue this drug abruptly if taken for more than 4 weeks.

Usual Duration of Use: Continual use on a regular schedule for 5 to 7 days is usually necessary to determine this drug's effectiveness in relieving moderate anxiety. Limit continual use to 1 to 3 weeks. Avoid uninterrupted and prolonged use.

▷ **This Drug Should Not Be Taken If**
- you have had an allergic reaction to any dosage form of it previously.
- you have acute narrow-angle glaucoma.

▷ **Inform Your Physician Before Taking This Drug If**
- you are allergic to any benzodiazepine drug (see Drug Class, Section Four).
- you have a history of alcoholism or drug abuse.
- you are pregnant or planning pregnancy.
- you have impaired liver or kidney function.
- you have a history of serious depression or mental disorder.
- you have any of the following: asthma, emphysema, epilepsy, myasthenia gravis.

Possible Side-Effects (natural, expected and unavoidable drug actions)
Drowsiness, lethargy, unsteadiness; "hangover" effects on the day following bedtime use.

▷ **Possible Adverse Effects** (unusual, unexpected and infrequent reactions)
If any of the following develop, consult your physician promptly for guidance.
Mild Adverse Effects
Allergic Reactions: Skin rash, hives.
Dizziness, fainting, blurred vision, double vision, slurred speech, sweating, nausea.
Serious Adverse Effects
Idiosyncratic Reactions: Paradoxical responses of excitement, agitation, anger, rage.

▷ **Possible Effects on Sexual Function:**   Altered timing and pattern of menstruation.

CAUTION
1. This drug should not be discontinued abruptly if it has been taken continually for more than 4 weeks.
2. The concurrent use of some over-the-counter drug products that contain antihistamines (allergy and cold preparations, sleep aids) can cause excessive sedation in sensitive individuals.
3. If this drug is taken at bedtime as a hypnotic (see Glossary), significant impairment of intellectual and physical skills may persist into the following day; avoid alcohol and hazardous activities (driving, etc.).

Precautions for Use
By Infants and Children: Safety and effectiveness for use by those under 9 years of age have not been established. This drug should not be used in the hyperactive or psychotic child of any age.

By Those over 60 Years of Age: It is advisable to use smaller doses at longer intervals to avoid overdosage. Observe for the possible development of lethargy, indifference, fatigue, weakness, unsteadiness, disturbing dreams, nightmares and paradoxical reactions of excitement, agitation, anger, hostility and rage.

▷ ## Advisability of Use During Pregnancy
Pregnancy Category: D (tentative). See Pregnancy Code inside back cover.
Animal studies: No birth defects reported in mouse, rat and rabbit studies.
Human studies: Information from adequate studies of pregnant women is not available.
There has been one report of multiple birth defects in a fetus exposed to this drug during the first 3 months. Frequent use in late pregnancy can cause the "floppy infant" syndrome in the newborn: weakness, lethargy, unresponsiveness, depressed breathing, low body temperature. Avoid use during entire pregnancy.

Advisability of Use if Breast-Feeding
Presence of this drug in breast milk: Yes, in small amounts.
Avoid drug or refrain from nursing.

Habit-Forming Potential: This drug can produce psychological and/or physical dependence (see Glossary) if used in large doses for an extended period of time.

Effects of Overdosage: Marked drowsiness, weakness, feeling of drunkenness, staggering gait, tremor, stupor progressing to deep sleep or coma.

Possible Effects of Long-Term Use: Psychological and/or physical dependence.

Suggested Periodic Examinations While Taking This Drug (at physician's discretion)
During long-term use: Complete blood cell counts.

▷ ## While Taking This Drug, Observe the Following
Foods: No restrictions.
Beverages: Avoid excessive intake of caffeine-containing beverages: coffee, tea, cola. May be taken with milk.
▷ *Alcohol:* Use with extreme caution until the combined effect is determined. Alcohol may increase the absorption of this drug and add to its depressant effects on the brain. It is advisable to avoid alcohol completely—throughout the day and night—if it is necessary to drive or to engage in any hazardous activity.

Tobacco Smoking: Heavy smoking may reduce the calming action of this drug.

Marijuana Smoking: Increased sedation and significant impairment of intellectual and physical performance.

▷ *Other Drugs*

Clorazepate may *increase* the effects of
- digoxin (Lanoxin), and cause digoxin toxicity.

Clorazepate may *decrease* the effects of
- levodopa (Sinemet, etc.), and reduce its effectiveness in treating Parkinson's disease.

The following drugs may *increase* the effects of clorazepate
- cimetidine (Tagamet).
- disulfiram (Antabuse).
- isoniazid (INH, Rifamate, etc.).
- oral contraceptives.
- valproic acid (Depakene).

The following drugs may *decrease* the effects of clorazepate
- rifampin (Rimactane, etc.).
- theophylline (aminophylline, Theo-Dur, etc.).

▷ *Driving, Hazardous Activities:* This drug can impair mental alertness, judgment, physical coordination and reaction time. Avoid hazardous activities accordingly.

Aviation Note: The use of this drug *is a disqualification* for piloting. Consult a designated Aviation Medical Examiner.

Exposure to Sun: No restrictions.

Discontinuation: Avoid sudden discontinuation if this drug has been taken for more than 4 weeks. Dosage should be tapered gradually to prevent a withdrawal syndrome that could include depression, confusion, hallucinations, tremor, seizures, muscle cramping, sweating and vomiting.

CLOXACILLIN
(klox a SIL in)

Introduced: 1962

Class: Antibiotic, penicillins

Prescription: USA: Yes
Canada: Yes

Controlled Drug: USA: No
Canada: No

Available as Generic: USA: Yes
Canada: No

Brand Names: ✦Apo-Cloxi, ✦Bactopen, Cloxapen, ✦Novocloxin, ✦Orbenin, Tegopen

---

BENEFITS versus RISKS

Possible Benefits	*Possible Risks*
EFFECTIVE TREATMENT OF INFECTIONS due to susceptible microorganisms	ALLERGIC REACTIONS, mild to severe Superinfections (yeast) Drug-induced colitis Rare blood cell disorders

---

▷ **Principal Uses**

As a Single Drug Product: Used primarily to treat infections that are caused by bacteria (principally staphylococcus) that have developed resistance to the original types of penicillin. It is of value in treating infections of the skin and skin structures, the upper and lower respiratory tract (including "strep" throat) and infections that are widely scattered throughout the body.

How This Drug Works: This drug destroys susceptible infecting bacteria by interfering with their ability to produce new protective cell walls as they multiply and grow.

Available Dosage Forms and Strengths
Capsules — 250 mg, 500 mg
Oral solution — 125 mg per 5-ml teaspoonful

▷ **Usual Adult Dosage Range:** 250 to 500 mg/6 hours (4 doses/24 hours). The maximal dose is 6000 mg/24 hours. **Note: Actual dosage and administration schedule must be determined by the physician for each patient individually.**

▷ **Dosing Instructions:** Take on empty stomach, 1 hour before or 2 hours after eating, at same times each day. Capsule may be opened for administration.

Usual Duration of Use: As long as necessary to eradicate the infection. For all streptococcal infections: not less than 10 consecutive days (without interruption) to reduce the possibility of developing rheumatic fever or glomerulonephritis.

▷ **This Drug Should Not Be Taken If**
- you have had an allergic reaction to any dosage form of it previously.
- you are certain you are allergic to *any* form of penicillin.

▷ **Inform Your Physician Before Taking This Drug If**
- you suspect you may be allergic to penicillin or you have a history of a previous "reaction" to penicillin.
- you are allergic to cephalosporin antibiotics (Ancef, Ceporan, Ceporex, Duricef, Kafocin, Keflex, Keflin, Kefzol, Loridine).
- you are allergic by nature—hay fever, asthma, hives, eczema.

- you have a history of kidney disease, regional enteritis or ulcerative colitis.

Possible Side-Effects (natural, expected and unavoidable drug actions)
Superinfections (see Glossary), often due to yeast organisms.

▷ **Possible Adverse Effects** (unusual, unexpected and infrequent reactions)
If any of the following develop, consult your physician promptly for guidance.
Mild Adverse Effects
Allergic Reactions: Skin rashes, hives, itching.
Irritations of mouth and tongue, unpleasant taste, nausea, vomiting, mild diarrhea.
Serious Adverse Effects
Allergic Reactions: Anaphylactic reaction (see Glossary), severe skin reactions, drug fever, swollen painful joints, sore throat.
Pseudomembranous colitis—severe diarrhea.

▷ **Possible Effects on Sexual Function:** None reported.

CAUTION
1. Take the exact dose and the full course prescribed.
2. This drug should not be used concurrently with antibiotics like erythromycin or tetracycline.

Precautions for Use
By Infants and Children: Dosage is based on age and weight. Consult your physician for precise dosage schedule.
By Those over 60 Years of Age: It is advisable to evaluate kidney function before and during use of this drug to determine the need for dosage adjustment. Natural changes in the skin may predispose to prolonged itching reactions in the genital and anal regions. Report such reactions promptly.

▷ **Advisability of Use During Pregnancy**
Pregnancy Category: B (tentative). See Pregnancy Code inside back cover.
Animal studies: No birth defects reported in rabbit studies.
Human studies: Information from adequate studies of pregnant women indicates no increased risk of birth defects in 3546 pregnancies exposed to penicillin derivatives.
Use only if clearly needed. Ask physician for guidance.

Advisability of Use if Breast-Feeding
Presence of this drug in breast milk: Probably yes.
The nursing infant may be sensitized to penicillin and may be at risk for diarrhea or yeast infections. Avoid drug if possible or refrain from nursing.

Habit-Forming Potential: None.

Effects of Overdosage: Possible nausea, vomiting and/or diarrhea.

Possible Effects of Long-Term Use: Superinfections, often due to yeast organisms.

Suggested Periodic Examinations While Taking This Drug (at physician's discretion)
Complete blood cell counts. Liver and kidney function tests with long-term use.

▷ **While Taking This Drug, Observe the Following**
Foods: No restrictions.
Beverages: No restrictions.
▷ *Alcohol:* No interactions expected.
Tobacco Smoking: No interactions expected.
▷ *Other Drugs*
Cloxacillin may *decrease* the effects of
  • oral contraceptives in some women, and impair their effectiveness in preventing pregnancy.
The following drugs may *decrease* the effects of cloxacillin
  • antacids may reduce the absorption of cloxacillin.
  • chloramphenicol (Chloromycetin).
  • erythromycin (Erythrocin, E-Mycin, etc.).
  • tetracyclines (Achromycin, Declomycin, Minocin, etc.). (See Drug Class, Section Four.)
▷ *Driving, Hazardous Activities:* Usually no restrictions.
Aviation Note: The use of this drug *may be a disqualification* for piloting. Consult a designated Aviation Medical Examiner.
Exposure to Sun: No restrictions.
Special Storage Instructions: Keep capsules in a tightly closed container at room temperature. Keep oral solution in the refrigerator.
Observe the Following Expiration Times: Oral solution kept refrigerated is good for 14 days; when kept at room temperature, it is good for only 3 days.

CODEINE
(KOH deen)

Introduced: 1886

Class: Analgesic, narcotic

Prescription: USA: Yes
Canada: Yes

Controlled Drug: USA: C-II*
Canada: <N>

Available as Generic: Yes

*See Schedules of Controlled Drugs inside back cover.

Brand Names: Actifed w/Codeine [CD], Ambenyl Expectorant [CD], Ambenyl Syrup [CD], Atasol-8, -15, -30 [CD], Benylin Syrup w/Codeine [CD], Bufferin w/Codeine [CD], ✦Coryphen-Codeine [CD], Dimetane Cough Syrup-DC [CD], Dimetane Expectorant-C [CD], Dimetapp-C [CD], Dimetapp w/Codeine [CD], Empirin w/Codeine No. 2, 4 [CD], Empracet w/Codeine No. 3, 4 [CD], ✦Empracet-30, -60 [CD], ✦Emtec-30 [CD], ✦Exdol [CD], ✦Exdol-8, -15, -30 [CD], ✦Fiorinal-C 1/4, -C 1/2 [CD], Fiorinal w/Codeine No. 1, 2, 3 [CD], Isoclor Expectorant [CD], ✦Lenoltec w/Codeine No. 1, 2, 3, 4 [CD], Naldecon-CX [CD], ✦Novahistex C [CD], ✦Paveral, Penntuss [CD], ✦Phenaphen No. 2, 3, 4 [CD], Phenaphen w/Codeine No. 2, 3, 4 [CD], Phenergan w/Codeine [CD], Robaxisal-C [CD], ✦Rounox w/Codeine [CD], Triaminic Expectorant w/Codeine [CD], ✦Tylenol w/Codeine [CD], Tylenol w/Codeine No. 1, 2, 3, 4 [CD], ✦Tylenol w/Codeine Elixir [CD]

BENEFITS versus RISKS

Possible Benefits	*Possible Risks*
EFFECTIVE RELIEF OF MODERATE TO SEVERE PAIN	Low potential for habit formation (dependence)
EFFECTIVE CONTROL OF COUGH	Mild allergic reactions (infrequent)
	Nausea, constipation

▷ **Principal Uses**

As a Single Drug Product: Used primarily to (1) relieve moderate to severe pain; (2) control cough; (3) control diarrhea. Its widest use is as an ingredient in analgesic preparations and cough remedies. Its constipating effect is sometimes used to treat diarrhea, though better drugs are now available for this purpose.

As a Combination Drug Product [CD]: Codeine is commonly combined with other milder analgesics to enhance their effectiveness, notably aspirin and acetaminophen. It is frequently added to cough mixtures containing antihistamines, decongestants and expectorants to make these "shotgun" preparations more effective in reducing the frequency and severity of cough.

How This Drug Works: Acting primarily as a depressant of certain brain functions, this drug suppresses the perception of pain, calms the emotional response to pain, reduces the sensitivity of the cough reflex and inhibits the activity of brain centers that regulate the intestinal tract.

Available Dosage Forms and Strengths

Injection — 30 mg per ml, 60 mg per ml
Tablets — 15 mg, 30 mg, 60 mg
Tablets, soluble — 15 mg, 30 mg, 60 mg

▷ **Usual Adult Dosage Range:** As analgesic—15 to 60 mg/3 to 6 hours as needed. For cough—10 to 20 mg/4 to 6 hours as needed. For diarrhea—30 mg/6 hours as needed. Total daily dosage should not exceed 200 mg for pain or 120 mg for cough or diarrhea. **Note: Actual dosage and administration schedule must be determined by the physician for each patient individually.**

▷ **Dosing Instructions:**   May be taken with or following food to reduce stomach irritation or nausea. Tablet may be crushed for administration.

Usual Duration of Use: As required to control pain, cough or diarrhea. Continual use should not exceed 5 to 7 days without interruption and reassessment of need.

▷ **This Drug Should Not Be Taken If**
- you have had an allergic reaction to any dosage form of it previously.
- you are having an acute attack of asthma.

▷ **Inform Your Physician Before Taking This Drug If**
- you have a history of drug abuse or alcoholism.
- you have impaired liver or kidney function.
- you have gall-bladder disease, a seizure disorder or an underactive thyroid gland.
- you are taking any other drugs that have a sedative effect.
- you plan to have surgery under general anesthesia in the near future.

Possible Side-Effects (natural, expected and unavoidable drug actions)
Drowsiness, light-headedness, dry mouth, urinary retention, constipation.

▷ **Possible Adverse Effects** (unusual, unexpected and infrequent reactions)
If any of the following develop, consult your physician promptly for guidance.
Mild Adverse Effects
Allergic Reactions: Skin rash, hives, itching.
Dizziness, impaired concentration, sensation of drunkenness, confusion, depression, blurred or double vision.
Nausea, vomiting.
Serious Adverse Effects
Allergic Reactions: Anaphylaxis (rare), severe skin reactions.
Idiosyncratic Reactions: Delirium, hallucinations, excitement, increased sensitivity to pain after the analgesic effect has worn off.
Seizures (rare), impaired breathing.

▷ **Possible Effects on Sexual Function:**   None reported.

▷ **Adverse Effects That May Mimic Natural Diseases or Disorders**
Paradoxical behavioral disturbances may suggest psychotic disorder.

CAUTION
1. If you have asthma, chronic bronchitis or emphysema, excessive use of this drug may cause significant respiratory difficulty, thickening of bronchial secretions and suppression of coughing.

2. The concurrent use of this drug with atropinelike drugs can increase the risk of urinary retention and reduced intestinal function.
3. Do not take this drug following acute head injury.

Precautions for Use
By Infants and Children: Do not use this drug in children under 2 years of age because of their vulnerability to life-threatening respiratory depression.
By Those over 60 Years of Age: Use small doses initially and increase dosage as needed and tolerated. Limit use to short-term treatment only. There may be increased susceptibility to the development of drowsiness, dizziness, unsteadiness, falling, urinary retention and constipation (often leading to fecal impaction).

▷ **Advisability of Use During Pregnancy**
Pregnancy Category: C (tentative). See Pregnancy Code inside back cover.
Animal studies: Skull defects reported in hamster studies.
Human studies: Information from adequate studies of pregnant women is not available. Some studies suggest a possible increase in significant birth defects when this drug is taken during the first 6 months of pregnancy. Codeine taken during the last few weeks before delivery can cause withdrawal symptoms in the newborn infant.
Use this drug only if clearly needed and in small, infrequent doses.

Advisability of Use if Breast-Feeding
Presence of this drug in breast milk: Yes, in small amounts.
Avoid drug or refrain from nursing.

Habit-Forming Potential: Psychological and/or physical dependence can develop with use of large doses for an extended period of time. However, true dependence is infrequent and unlikely with prudent use.

Effects of Overdosage: Drowsiness, restlessness, agitation, nausea, vomiting, dry mouth, vertigo, weakness, lethargy, stupor, coma, seizures.

Possible Effects of Long-Term Use: Psychological and physical dependence, chronic constipation.

Suggested Periodic Examinations While Taking This Drug (at physician's discretion)
None.

▷ **While Taking This Drug, Observe the Following**
Foods: No restrictions.
Beverages: No restrictions. May be taken with milk.
▷ *Alcohol:* Use extreme caution until the combined effects have been determined. Codeine can intensify the intoxicating effects of alcohol, and alcohol can intensify the depressant effects of codeine on brain function, breathing and circulation.
Tobacco Smoking: No interactions expected.

Marijuana Smoking: Increase in drowsiness and pain relief; impairment of mental and physical performance.

▷ *Other Drugs*

Codeine may *increase* the effects of
* other drugs with sedative effects.
* atropinelike drugs, and increase the risk of constipation and urinary retention.

▷ *Driving, Hazardous Activities:* This drug can impair mental alertness, judgment, reaction time and physical coordination. Avoid hazardous activities accordingly.

Aviation Note: The use of this drug *is a disqualification* for piloting. Consult a designated Aviation Medical Examiner.

Exposure to Sun: No restrictions.

Discontinuation: It is advisable to limit this drug to short-term use. If it is necessary to use it for extended periods of time, discontinuation should be gradual to minimize possible effects of withdrawal (usually mild with codeine).

COLCHICINE
(KOL chi seen)

Introduced: 1763

Class: Antigout

Prescription: USA: Yes
Canada: No

Controlled Drug: USA: No
Canada: No

Available as Generic: Yes

Brand Names: Colabid [CD], ColBENEMID [CD], Proben-C [CD], ♦Verban [CD]

BENEFITS versus RISKS	
Possible Benefits	*Possible Risks*
EFFECTIVE RELIEF OF ACUTE GOUT SYMPTOMS	Loss of hair
Prevention of recurrent gout attacks	Rare bone marrow depression (see Glossary)
Prevention of attacks of Mediterranean fever	Rare peripheral neuritis (see Glossary)
	Rare liver damage

▷ **Principal Uses**

As a Single Drug Product: Used primarily to reduce the pain, swelling and inflammation associated with acute attacks of gout. It is also used in smaller doses to prevent recurrent gout attacks. An infrequent use is the prevention and control of attacks of familial Mediterranean fever.

As a Combination Drug Product [CD]: Colchicine is combined with pro-benecid to enhance its ability to prevent recurrent attacks of gout. While colchicine is most effective in relieving the symptoms of acute gout, it has some effect in preventing recurrent and chronic discomfort. Probenecid increases the elimination of uric acid by the kidneys and thereby reduces the blood level of uric acid to a point at which acute episodes of gout will not occur. This dual action is more effective than either drug used alone in the long-term management of gout.

How This Drug Works: It is thought that by decreasing the acidity of joint tissues, this drug reduces the deposit of uric acid crystals that cause acute inflammation and pain. (Colchicine does not lower the level of uric acid in the blood or increase the level of uric acid in the urine.)

Available Dosage Forms and Strengths
  Injection — 1 mg per 2 ml
  Tablets — 0.5 mg, 0.6 mg

▷ **Usual Adult Dosage Range:** For acute attack—0.5 to 1.3 mg initially, followed by 0.5 to 0.65 mg/1 to 2 hours until pain is relieved or nausea, vomiting or diarrhea occurs. The total dose should not exceed 10 mg. For prevention of recurrent attacks—0.5 to 0.65 mg, 1 to 3 times/day. **Note: Actual dosage and administration schedule must be determined by the physician for each patient individually.**

▷ **Dosing Instructions:** May be taken either on an empty stomach or with food to reduce nausea or stomach irritation. Start treatment at the earliest indication of an acute attack. Take the exact dose prescribed. The tablet may be crushed for administration.

Usual Duration of Use: For acute attack—discontinue when pain is relieved or when nausea, vomiting or diarrhea occurs; do not resume this drug for 3 days without consulting your physician. For prevention—use the smallest effective dose for long-term management; consult your physician regarding dosage schedule and duration.

▷ **This Drug Should Not Be Taken If**
  • you have had an allergic reaction to it previously.
  • you have an active stomach or duodenal ulcer.
  • you have active ulcerative colitis.

▷ **Inform Your Physician Before Taking This Drug If**
  • you have a history of peptic ulcer disease or ulcerative colitis.
  • you have any type of heart disease.
  • you have impaired liver or kidney function.
  • you plan to have surgery in the near future.

Possible Side-Effects (natural, expected and unavoidable drug actions)
Nausea, vomiting, abdominal cramping, diarrhea.

▷ **Possible Adverse Effects** (unusual, unexpected and infrequent reactions)
   If any of the following develop, consult your physician promptly for guidance.
   Mild Adverse Effects
   Allergic Reactions: Skin rash, hives, fever.
   Serious Adverse Effects
   Allergic Reaction: Anaphylactic reaction (see Glossary).
   Loss of hair.
   Bone marrow depression (see Glossary)—fatigue, weakness, fever, sore throat, abnormal bleeding or bruising.
   Peripheral neuritis (see Glossary)—numbness, tingling, pain, weakness in hands and/or feet.
   Inflammation of colon with bloody diarrhea.
   Liver damage.

▷ **Possible Effects on Sexual Function:**   None reported.

   Possible Delayed Adverse Effects: Impaired production of sperm, possibly resulting in birth defects of child that was conceived while father was taking this drug.

   Natural Diseases or Disorders That May Be Activated by This Drug
   Peptic ulcer disease, ulcerative colitis.

   CAUTION
   1. If this drug causes vomiting and/or diarrhea before relief of joint pain, discontinue it and inform your physician.
   2. Try to limit each course of treatment for acute gout to 4 to 8 mg. Do not exceed 3 mg/24 hours or a total of 10 mg/course.
   3. Omit drug for 3 days between courses to avoid toxicity.
   4. Carry this drug with you while traveling if you are subject to attacks of acute gout.
   5. It is advisable to take colchicine preventively prior to and following surgery if you have recurrent gout. (Surgery often precipitates acute attacks of gout.) Ask your physician for proper dosage schedule.

   Precautions for Use
   By Infants and Children: Dosage has not been established. Ask physician for guidance.
   By Those over 60 Years of Age: This drug has a very narrow margin of safety. Because the total dosage required to relieve the pain of acute gout often causes vomiting and/or diarrhea, extreme caution is advised when this drug is used by anyone with heart or circulatory disorders, reduced liver or kidney function or general debility.

▷ **Advisability of Use During Pregnancy**
   Pregnancy Category: D (tentative). See Pregnancy Code inside back cover.
   Animal studies: This drug causes significant birth defects in hamsters and rabbits.

Human studies: Information from adequate studies of pregnant women is not available. However, it is reported that colchicine can cause harm to the fetus.

Avoid during entire pregnancy if possible. Ask physician for guidance.

Advisability of Use if Breast-Feeding

Presence of this drug in breast milk: Unknown.

Avoid drug or refrain from nursing.

Habit-Forming Potential: None.

Effects of Overdosage: Nausea, vomiting, abdominal cramping, diarrhea (may be bloody), burning sensation in throat and skin, weak and rapid pulse, progressive paralysis, inability to breathe.

Possible Effects of Long-Term Use: Hair loss, aplastic anemia (see Glossary), peripheral neuritis (see Glossary).

Suggested Periodic Examinations While Taking This Drug (at physician's discretion)

Complete blood cell counts, uric acid blood levels to monitor status of gout, sperm analysis for quantity and condition, liver function tests.

▷ **While Taking This Drug, Observe the Following**

Foods: Follow physician's advice regarding the need for a low-purine diet.

Beverages: It is advisable to drink no less than 3 quarts of liquids/24 hours. This drug may be taken with milk. Some "herbal teas" (promoted as being beneficial for arthritis) contain phenylbutazone and other potentially toxic ingredients. Avoid herbal teas if you are not certain of their source, content and medicinal effects.

▷ *Alcohol:* No interactions expected. However, alcohol may increase the risk of gastrointestinal irritation or bleeding. It also raises uric acid blood levels and could interfere with gout management.

Tobacco Smoking: No interactions expected.

▷ *Other Drugs*

Colchicine **taken concurrently** with

• allopurinol (Zyloprim), probenecid (Benemid) or sulfinpyrazone (Anturane) can prevent attacks of acute gout that often occur when treatment with these drugs is first started.

▷ *Driving, Hazardous Activities:* Usually no restrictions when taken continually in small (preventive) doses. Be alert to the possible occurrence of nausea, vomiting and/or diarrhea when taken in larger (treatment) doses.

Aviation Note: The use of this drug **may be a disqualification** for piloting. Consult a designated Aviation Medical Examiner.

Exposure to Sun: No restrictions.

Exposure to Cold: This drug can lower body temperature. Use caution to prevent excessive lowering (hypothermia), especially if you are over 60 years of age.

Occurrence of Unrelated Illness: Inform your physician if you are injured or if you develop any new illness or disorder. During periods of such stress you may be subject to acute attacks of gout, and it may be necessary to adjust your medication schedule.

COLESTIPOL
(koh LES ti pohl)

Introduced: 1974

Class: Anticholesterol

Prescription: USA: Yes
Canada: Yes

Controlled Drug: USA: No
Canada: No

Available as Generic: USA: No
Canada: No

Brand Name: Colestid

BENEFITS versus RISKS

Possible Benefits	*Possible Risks*
EFFECTIVE REDUCTION OF TOTAL CHOLESTEROL AND LOW DENSITY CHOLESTEROL IN TYPE IIa CHOLESTEROL DISORDERS (15% to 25% reduction of total cholesterol, 25% to 35% reduction of LDL cholesterol) EFFECTIVE RELIEF OF ITCHING associated with biliary obstruction	Constipation (may be severe) Reduced absorption of fat, fat-soluble vitamins (A, D, E and K) and folic acid Reduced formation of prothrombin with resultant bleeding

---

▷ **Principal Uses**

As a Single Drug Product: Used primarily to (1) reduce abnormally high blood levels of total cholesterol and low density (LDL) cholesterol in Type IIa cholesterol disorders; (2) relieve the itching due to the deposit of bile acids in the skin associated with partial biliary obstruction.

How This Drug Works: By combining with bile acids and bile salts in the intestinal tract, this drug forms insoluble complexes that are excreted in the feces. This removal of bile acids (which are necessary for food digestion) stimulates the conversion of cholesterol to bile acids to replace the loss; this in turn reduces the blood levels of cholesterol. By reducing the blood levels of bile acids, this drug hastens the absorption and clearance of bile acids deposited in the skin and thus relieves itching.

Available Dosage Forms and Strengths
Bottles — 250 grams, 500 grams
Packets — 5 grams

▷ **Usual Adult Dosage Range:**   Initially 5 grams of powder 3 times daily. Dose may be increased slowly as needed and tolerated to 30 grams daily in 2 to 4 divided doses. **Note: Actual dosage and administration schedule must be determined by the physician for each patient individually.**

▷ **Dosing Instructions:**   Always take just before or with a meal; this drug is ineffective when taken without food. Mix the powder thoroughly in 4 to 6 ounces of water, fruit juice, tomato juice, milk, thin soup or a soft food like applesauce. **Do not take it in its dry form.**

Usual Duration of Use: Continual use on a regular schedule for 4 to 6 weeks is usually necessary to determine this drug's effectiveness in lowering excessively high blood levels of cholesterol. Duration of use should not exceed 3 months if an adequate response does not occur. Long-term use (months to years) requires periodic evaluation of response and dosage adjustment. Consult your physician on a regular basis.

Currently a "Drug of Choice" for initiating treatment of elevated LDL cholesterol. See Cholesterol Disorders in Section Two.

▷ **This Drug Should Not Be Taken If**
- you have had an allergic reaction to it previously.
- you have complete biliary obstruction.

▷ **Inform Your Physician Before Taking This Drug If**
- you are prone to constipation.
- you have peptic ulcer disease.
- you have a bleeding disorder of any kind.
- you have impaired kidney function.

Possible Side-Effects (natural, expected and unavoidable drug actions)
Constipation (10%); interference with normal fat digestion and absorption; reduced absorption of vitamins A, D, E and K and folic acid.

▷ **Possible Adverse Effects** (unusual, unexpected and infrequent reactions)
If any of the following develop, consult your physician promptly for guidance.
Mild Adverse Effects
Allergic Reactions: Skin rash (0.1%), hives, tongue irritation, anal itching.
Headache, dizziness, weakness, muscle and joint pains.

Loss of appetite, indigestion, heartburn, abdominal discomfort, excessive gas, nausea, vomiting, diarrhea.

Serious Adverse Effects

Vitamin K deficiency with resultant deficiency of prothrombin and increased bleeding tendency.

Impaired absorption of calcium; predisposition to osteoporosis.

Gallbladder colic (questionable).

▷ **Possible Effects on Sexual Function:**   None reported.

Natural Diseases or Disorders That May Be Activated by This Drug

Peptic ulcer disease; steatorrhea (excessive fat in stools) with large doses.

CAUTION

1. The powder should never be taken in its dry form; always mix it thoroughly with a suitable liquid before swallowing.
2. Observe carefully for the development of constipation; use stool softeners and laxatives as needed.
3. This drug may bind other drugs taken concurrently and impair their absorption. It is advisable to take *all other drugs* 1 to 2 hours before or 4 to 6 hours after taking this drug.

Precautions for Use

By Infants and Children: Safety and effectiveness for use by those under 12 years of age have not been established. Observe carefully for the possible development of acidosis and vitamin A or folic acid deficiency. (Ask your physician for guidance.)

By Those over 60 Years of Age: There may be increased risk of developing severe constipation. Impaired kidney function may predispose to the development of acidosis.

▷ **Advisability of Use During Pregnancy**

Pregnancy Category: C (tentative). See Pregnancy Code inside back cover.

Animal studies: No information available.

Human studies: Information from adequate studies of pregnant women is not available.

Use this drug only if clearly needed. Ensure adequate intake of vitamins and minerals to satisfy needs of mother and fetus.

Advisability of Use if Breast-Feeding

Presence of this drug in breast milk: No.

Breast-feeding is permitted.

Habit-Forming Potential: None.

Effects of Overdosage: Progressive constipation.

Possible Effects of Long-Term Use: Deficiencies of vitamins A, D, E and K and folic acid. Calcium deficiency, osteoporosis. Acidosis due to excessive retention of chloride.

Suggested Periodic Examinations While Taking This Drug (at physician's discretion)

Measurements of blood levels of total cholesterol, low density (LDL) cholesterol and high density (HDL) cholesterol.

Hemoglobin and red blood cell studies for possible anemia.

▷ **While Taking This Drug, Observe the Following**

Foods: Avoid foods that tend to constipate (cheeses, etc.).

Nutritional Support: Consult your physician regarding the need for supplements of vitamins A, D, E and K, folic acid and calcium.

Beverages: Ensure adequate liquid intake (up to 2 quarts daily). This drug may be taken with milk.

▷ *Alcohol:* No interactions expected.

Tobacco Smoking: No interactions expected.

▷ *Other Drugs*

Colestipol may *decrease* the effects of

- acetaminophen; give 2 hours before colestipol.
- aspirin; give 2 hours before.
- digitoxin and digoxin; give 2 hours before.
- iron preparations; give 2 to 3 hours before.
- penicillin G; give 2 hours before.
- phenobarbital; give 2 hours before.
- tetracycline; give 2 hours before.
- thiazide diuretics (see Drug Class, Section Four); give 2 hours before.
- thyroxin; give 5 hours before.
- warfarin; give 6 hours after.

▷ *Driving, Hazardous Activities:* No restrictions.

Aviation Note: The use of this drug **is usually not a disqualification** for piloting. Consult a designated Aviation Medical Examiner.

Exposure to Sun: No restrictions.

Discontinuation: The dose of any potentially toxic drug taken concurrently must be reduced appropriately when this drug is discontinued. Following discontinuation of this drug, cholesterol blood levels usually return to pretreatment levels in approximately 1 month.

CROMOLYN
(KROH moh lin)

Other Names: Cromolyn sodium, sodium cromoglycate

Introduced: 1968

Class: Asthma preventive, rhinitis preventive

Prescription: USA: Yes
Canada: Yes

Controlled Drug: USA: No
Canada: No

Available as Generic: USA: No
Canada: No

Brand Names: ✦Fivent, Intal, ✦Nalcrom, Nasalcrom, Opticrom, ✦Rynacrom, ✦Vistacrom

---

BENEFITS versus RISKS

Possible Benefits	*Possible Risks*
LONG-TERM PREVENTION OF RECURRENT ASTHMA ATTACKS (70% to 75% effective)	Rare anaphylactic reaction (see Glossary)
Prevention of acute asthma due to allergens or exercise	Rare spasm of bronchial tubes, increased wheezing
Prevention and treatment of allergic rhinitis	Rare allergic pneumonitis (allergic reaction in lung tissue)
Relief of allergic conjunctivitis	

▷ **Principal Uses**

As a Single Drug Product: Used primarily to *prevent* allergic reactions in the nose (allergic rhinitis, hay fever) and allergic reactions in the bronchial tubes (bronchial asthma). (It is of no value in relieving asthma after the attack has begun.) It is also used to treat the symptoms of allergic rhinitis (70% effective) and conjunctivitis.

How This Drug Works: By blocking the release of histamine (and other substances) that normally occurs in allergic reactions, this drug acts to prevent the sequence of tissue changes that leads to swelling and itching of nasal membranes (allergic rhinitis) and to constriction of bronchial tubes (asthma).

Available Dosage Forms and Strengths

Eye drops — 2%, 4%
Inhalation aerosol — 0.8 mg per metered spray
Inhalation capsules (powder) — 20 mg
Inhalation solution — 20 mg per ampul
Nasal insufflation (powder) — 10 mg per cartridge
Nasal solution — 20 mg per ml, 40 mg per ml

▷ **Usual Adult Dosage Range**

Eye drops: 1 drop 4 to 6 times daily at regular intervals.
Inhalation aerosol: 1.6 mg (2 inhalations) 4 times daily at regular intervals for long-term prevention of asthma, or as a single dose 10 to 15 minutes before exposure to prevent acute allergen-induced or exercise-induced asthma.
Inhalation powder: 20 mg (1 capsule) 4 times daily at regular intervals for long-term prevention of asthma; 20 mg (1 capsule) as a single dose 10 to 15 minutes before exposure to prevent acute allergen-induced

or exercise-induced asthma. Total daily dosage should not exceed 160 mg (8 capsules).

Inhalation solution: Same as inhalation powder.

Nasal insufflation: Initially 10 mg in each nostril every 4 to 6 hours as needed; reduce to every 8 to 12 hours for maintenance.

Nasal solution: 2.6 mg to 5.2 mg in each nostril 3 to 6 times daily as needed.

Note: Actual dosage and administration schedule must be determined by the physician for each patient individually.

▷ **Dosing Instructions:** Follow carefully the dosing instructions provided with each of the above dosage forms, especially the inhalers. Do not swallow the capsules; the powder is intended for inhalation into the air passages of the lungs. (If the capsule is swallowed inadvertently, the drug will cause no beneficial or adverse effects.)

Usual Duration of Use: Continual use on a regular schedule for 4 to 6 weeks is usually necessary to determine this drug's effectiveness in preventing recurrent attacks of asthma or allergic rhinitis. Long-term use (months to years) requires periodic evaluation of response and dosage adjustment. Consult your physician on a regular basis.

Possible Advantages of This Drug
May be quite effective in the young asthmatic.
Usually well tolerated.
Serious adverse effects are very rare.

▷ **This Drug Should Not Be Taken If**
- you have had an allergic reaction to any dosage form of it previously.

▷ **Inform Your Physician Before Taking This Drug If**
- you are allergic to milk, milk products or lactose. (The inhalation powder contains lactose.)
- you have impaired liver or kidney function.
- you have angina or a heart rhythm disorder. (The inhalation aerosol contains propellants that could be hazardous.)

Possible Side-Effects (natural, expected and unavoidable drug actions)
Unpleasant taste with use of inhalation aerosol.
Mild throat irritation, hoarseness, cough. (These can be minimized by a few swallows of water after each inhalation of powder.)

▷ **Possible Adverse Effects** (unusual, unexpected and infrequent reactions)
If any of the following develop, consult your physician promptly for guidance.
Mild Adverse Effects
Allergic Reactions: Skin rash, hives, itching.
Headache, dizziness.
Nausea, vomiting, urinary urgency and pain, joint and muscle pain.

Serious Adverse Effects
Allergic Reactions: Anaphylactic reaction (see Glossary). Allergic pneumonitis (allergic reaction in lung tissue).

▷ **Possible Effects on Sexual Function:**   None reported.

CAUTION
1. Remember that this drug acts solely as a *preventive* in the management of bronchial asthma; its effectiveness is limited to the pretreatment phase of asthma—*before* the onset of acute bronchial constriction (asthmatic wheezing).
2. *Do not* use this drug during an acute attack of asthma; it could worsen and prolong asthmatic wheezing.
3. This drug does *not* interfere with the actions of those drugs used to relieve the acute asthma attack after it has begun. Cromolyn is used *before and between* acute attacks to prevent their development; bronchodilators are used *during* acute attacks to relieve them.
4. If you are also using a bronchodilator drug by inhalation, it is advisable to take it about 5 minutes before inhaling cromolyn.

Precautions for Use
By Infants and Children: Safety and effectiveness for use by those under 5 years of age have not been established. Young children may find it easier to use the nebulized solution than the powder.
By Those over 60 Years of Age: This drug is not effective in the management of chronic bronchitis or emphysema.

▷ **Advisability of Use During Pregnancy**
Pregnancy Category: B (tentative). See Pregnancy Code inside back cover.
Animal studies: Mouse, rat and rabbit studies revealed no birth defects due to this drug.
Human studies: Information from adequate studies of pregnant women is not available.
Use this drug only if clearly needed.

Advisability of Use if Breast-Feeding
Presence of this drug in breast milk: Unknown.
Avoid drug or refrain from nursing.

Habit-Forming Potential: None.

Effects of Overdosage: No significant effects reported.

Possible Effects of Long-Term Use: Allergic reaction of lung tissue (allergic pneumonitis, very rare).

Suggested Periodic Examinations While Taking This Drug (at physician's discretion)
Examination of lungs by sputum analysis and X-ray if symptoms suggest allergic pneumonitis.

▷ **While Taking This Drug, Observe the Following**

Foods: Follow diet prescribed by your physician. Avoid all foods to which you may be allergic.

Beverages: Avoid all beverages to which you may be allergic.

▷ *Alcohol:* No interactions expected.

Tobacco Smoking: Follow your physician's advice regarding smoking.

▷ *Other Drugs:* Cromolyn may make it possible to reduce the dosage of cortisonelike drugs in the management of chronic asthma. Consult your physician regarding dosage adjustment.

▷ *Driving, Hazardous Activities:* This drug may cause dizziness. Restrict activities as necessary.

Aviation Note: The use of this drug **may be a disqualification** for piloting. Consult a designated Aviation Medical Examiner.

Exposure to Sun: No restrictions.

Heavy Exercise or Exertion: This drug may be effective in preventing exercise-induced asthma if taken 10 to 15 minutes before exertion. It is most effective in young individuals.

Discontinuation: If the regular use of cromolyn has made it possible to reduce or discontinue maintenance doses of cortisonelike drugs, and you find it necessary to discontinue cromolyn for any reason, observe closely for a sudden return of asthma. It may be necessary to resume a cortisonelike drug and to institute other measures for satisfactory control of asthma.

Special Storage Instructions: Keep the powder cartridges in a dry, tightly closed container. Store in a cool place but not in the refrigerator. Do not handle the cartridges or the inhaler when hands are wet.

CYCLOBENZAPRINE
(si kloh BENZ a preen)

Introduced: 1977

Class: Muscle relaxant

Prescription: USA: Yes
Canada: Yes

Controlled Drug: USA: No
Canada: No

Available as Generic: USA: No
Canada: No

Brand Name: Flexeril

BENEFITS versus RISKS	
Possible Benefits	*Possible Risks*
Mild to moderate relief of discomfort due to spasm of voluntary muscles	Confusion, depression Impaired urination Allergic reactions: skin rash, hives, swelling of face or tongue

▷ **Principal Uses**

As a Single Drug Product: Used primarily to relieve the pain and stiffness associated with spasm of voluntary muscles, such as that resulting from accidental injury of musculoskeletal structures. It is often necessary to supplement the use of this drug with other treatment measures, such as rest, support and physiotherapy.

How This Drug Works: Not completely established. It is thought that this drug may relieve muscle spasm and pain by blocking the transmission of nerve impulses over reflex pathways and/or by producing a sedative effect that decreases the perception of pain.

Available Dosage Forms and Strengths
Tablets — 10 mg

▷ **Usual Adult Dosage Range:**   10 mg, 2 to 4 times daily; adjust dosage as needed and tolerated. Total daily dosage should not exceed 60 mg. **Note: Actual dosage and administration schedule must be determined by the physician for each patient individually.**

▷ **Dosing Instructions:**   Take either on empty stomach or with food to prevent stomach irritation. Tablet may be crushed for administration.

Usual Duration of Use: Continual use on a regular schedule for 7 to 10 days is usually necessary to determine this drug's effectiveness in relieving the discomfort of muscle spasm. Evaluate need for continued use after periods of 2 to 3 weeks.

▷ **This Drug Should Not Be Taken If**
• you have had an allergic reaction to it previously.
• you have taken any monoamine oxidase (MAO) type A inhibitor drug within the past 14 days (see Drug Class, Section Four).
• you are recovering from a recent heart attack.
• you have congestive heart failure or a serious heart rhythm disorder.
• you have uncorrected hyperthyroidism (overactive thyroid function).

▷ **Inform Your Physician Before Taking This Drug If**
• you have experienced any unfavorable reactions to other muscle relaxants or to tricyclic antidepressants (see Drug Class, Section Four) in the past.
• you have a history of heart disease or heart rhythm disorder.
• you have glaucoma or prostatism (see Glossary).
• you are currently taking any drugs with atropinelike effects or sedative effects.

Possible Side-Effects (natural, expected and unavoidable drug actions)
Drowsiness (40%), dizziness (11%), dry mouth (28%), constipation (3%).

▷ **Possible Adverse Effects** (unusual, unexpected and infrequent reactions)
If any of the following develop, consult your physician promptly for guidance.

Mild Adverse Effects
Allergic Reactions: Skin rash, hives, swelling of face and tongue.
Headache, fatigue, weakness, numbness, blurred vision, slurred speech, unsteadiness.
Unpleasant taste, indigestion, nausea.
Serious Adverse Effects
Idiosyncratic Reactions: Euphoria, confusion, disorientation, hallucinations, depression.
Impaired urination (urine retention).

▷ **Possible Effects on Sexual Function:** Increased or decreased libido, impotence, swelling of testicles, enlargement of male breasts, enlargement of female breasts with milk production. (Any effect may occur with dosage of 30 to 60 mg/day.)

▷ **Adverse Effects That May Mimic Natural Diseases or Disorders**
Mental and behavioral reactions may suggest acute psychosis.

Precautions for Use
By Infants and Children: Safety and effectiveness for use by those under 15 years of age have not been established.
By Those over 60 Years of Age: Small doses are advisable initially. You may be more susceptible to the development of drowsiness, dizziness, weakness, unsteadiness and falling. This drug can aggravate existing prostatism (see Glossary).

▷ **Advisability of Use During Pregnancy**
Pregnancy Category: B (tentative). See Pregnancy Code inside back cover.
Animal studies: No birth defects reported in mice, rats or rabbits.
Human studies: Information from adequate studies of pregnant women is not available.
Avoid drug if possible; use only if clearly needed.

Advisability of Use if Breast-Feeding
Presence of this drug in breast milk: Probably yes.
Avoid drug or refrain from nursing.

Habit-Forming Potential: None.

Effects of Overdosage: Excessive drowsiness, confusion, impaired concentration, visual disturbances, vomiting, stupor progressing to coma, seizures, weak and rapid pulse.

Possible Effects of Long-Term Use: None reported.

Suggested Periodic Examinations While Taking This Drug (at physician's discretion)
Measurements of internal eye pressure (if any predisposition to glaucoma).

▷ **While Taking This Drug, Observe the Following**
Foods: No restrictions.
Beverages: No restrictions. May be taken with milk.
▷   *Alcohol:* Use with caution until the combined effect has been determined. This drug may add to the depressant action of alcohol on the brain.
Tobacco Smoking: No interactions expected.
Marijuana Smoking: Moderate to marked drowsiness, muscle weakness, incoordination, impairment of intellectual and physical performance. All hazardous activities should be avoided.
▷   *Other Drugs*
Cyclobenzaprine may *increase* the effects of
- atropinelike drugs (see Drug Class, Section Four).
- all drugs with sedative effects, and cause excessive sedation.

Cyclobenzaprine *taken concurrently* with
- monoamine oxidase (MAO) type A inhibitor drugs may cause high fever, seizures and life-threatening reactions (theoretical).
▷   *Driving, Hazardous Activities:* This drug may cause drowsiness, dizziness and incoordination in susceptible individuals. Avoid hazardous activities if these drug effects occur.
Aviation Note: The use of this drug *is a disqualification* for piloting. Consult a designated Aviation Medical Examiner.
Exposure to Sun: Use caution until sensitivity to sun has been determined. Other drugs closely related to this drug can cause photosensitivity (see Glossary).
Exposure to Heat: Use caution in hot environments. This drug may increase the risk of heat stroke.

CYCLOPHOSPHAMIDE
(si kloh FOSS fa mide)

Introduced: 1959

Class: Anticancer, immunosuppressive

Prescription: USA: Yes
Canada: Yes

Controlled Drug: USA: No
Canada: No

Available as Generic: No

Brand Names: Cytoxan, Neosar, ✦Procytox

BENEFITS versus RISKS

Possible Benefits	*Possible Risks*
CURE OR CONTROL OF CERTAIN TYPES OF CANCER	REDUCED WHITE BLOOD CELL COUNT
PREVENTION OF REJECTION IN ORGAN TRANSPLANTATION	SECONDARY INFECTION
	URINARY BLADDER BLEEDING
	HEART, LUNG, LIVER OR KIDNEY DAMAGE
Possibly beneficial in the treatment of rheumatoid arthritis and lupus erythematosus	Loss of hair
Possibly beneficial in selected cases of nephrotic syndrome in children	

▷ **Principal Uses**

As a Single Drug Product: Used primarily in the treatment of various forms of cancer, notably malignant lymphomas, multiple myeloma, leukemias and cancers of the breast and ovary. Because this drug exerts a suppressant effect on the immune system, it is also used to prevent rejection in organ transplantation and to treat certain autoimmune disorders. It is also approved for treating certain resistant forms of nephrotic syndrome in children.

How This Drug Works: Not completely known. Because of its ability to kill cancer cells during all phases of their development and reproduction, this drug suppresses the primary growth and secondary spread (metastasis) of certain types of cancer.

Available Dosage Forms and Strengths
   Injection — vials of 100 mg, 200 mg, 500 mg, 1 gram, 2 grams
   Tablets — 25 mg, 50 mg

▷ **Usual Adult Dosage Range:**   1 to 5 mg per kg of body weight daily. **Note: Actual dosage and administration schedule must be determined by the physician for each patient individually.**

▷ **Dosing Instructions:**   It is preferable to take the tablet on an empty stomach. However, if nausea or indigestion occurs, this drug may be taken with or following food. The total liquid intake should be no less than 3 quarts/24 hours to reduce the risk of bladder irritation. Tablets may be crushed for administration.

Usual Duration of Use: Continual use on a regular schedule is required to achieve and maintain a significant remission of the cancer under treatment. Actual duration of use depends upon the response of the cancer and the tolerance of the patient to the effects of the drug. Consult your physician on a regular basis.

▷ **This Drug Should Not Be Taken If**
- you have had an allergic reaction to any dosage form of it previously.
- you have an active infection of any kind.
- you have bloody urine for any reason.

▷ **Inform Your Physician Before Taking This Drug If**
- you have impaired liver or kidney function.
- you have a blood cell or bone marrow disorder.
- you have had previous chemotherapy or X-ray therapy for any type of cancer.
- you are now taking, or have taken within the past year, any cortisonelike drug (adrenal corticosteroids).
- you have diabetes.
- you plan to have surgery under general anesthesia in the near future.

Possible Side-Effects (natural, expected and unavoidable drug actions)
Bone marrow depression (see Glossary)—impaired production of primarily white blood cells and, to a lesser degree, red blood cells and blood platelets (see Glossary). Possible effects include fever, chills, sore throat, fatigue, weakness, abnormal bleeding or bruising.
Impairment of natural resistance (immunity) to infection.

▷ **Possible Adverse Effects** (unusual, unexpected and infrequent reactions)
If any of the following develop, consult your physician promptly for guidance.
Mild Adverse Effects
Allergic Reaction: Skin rash (rare).
Headache, dizziness.
Loss of scalp hair (50% of users), darkening of skin and fingernails, transverse ridging of nails.
Loss of appetite, nausea (30%), vomiting (25%), ulceration of mouth, diarrhea (may be bloody).
Serious Adverse Effects
Idiosyncratic Reaction: Hemolytic anemia (see Glossary).
Liver damage with jaundice—yellow eyes and skin, dark-colored urine, light-colored stools.
Kidney damage—impaired kidney function, reduced urine volume, bloody urine.
Severe inflammation of bladder (10%)—painful urination, bloody urine.
Drug-induced damage of heart and lung tissue.

▷ **Possible Effects on Sexual Function**
Suppression of ovarian function—irregular menstrual pattern or cessation of menstruation (18% to 57% of users depending upon dosage and duration of use).
Suppression of testicular function—reduction or cessation of sperm production (100% of users).

Possible Delayed Adverse Effects
Development of other types of cancer (secondary malignancies).
Development of severe cystitis with bleeding from the bladder wall. (This may occur many months after the last dose.)

CAUTION
1. This drug may interfere with the normal healing of wounds.
2. This drug can cause significant changes (mutations) in the chromosome structure of both sperm and eggs (ova). Any man or woman taking this drug should understand its potential for causing serious defects in children that are conceived during or following the course of medication.
3. This drug can suppress natural resistance (immunity) to infection, resulting in life-threatening illness.
4. Avoid live-virus vaccines while taking this drug.

Precautions for Use
By Infants and Children: This drug should not be given if the child is dehydrated. Provide adequate fluid intake to ensure a copious urine volume for 4 hours following each dose. Prevent exposure of child to anyone with active chicken pox or shingles. This drug may cause ovarian or testicular sterility.
By Those over 60 Years of Age: To reduce the risk of developing serious chemical cystitis, it is necessary to maintain a copious volume of urine. This may increase the risk of urinary retention in the man with prostatism (see Glossary).

▷ **Advisability of Use During Pregnancy**
Pregnancy Category: D (tentative). See Pregnancy Code inside back cover.
Animal studies: Significant birth defects reported in mice, rat and rabbit studies.
Human studies: Information from studies of pregnant women indicates that this drug can cause serious birth defects or fetal death.
Avoid completely during the first 3 months. Use of this drug during the last 6 months must be carefully individualized.

Advisability of Use if Breast-Feeding
Presence of this drug in breast milk: Yes.
Avoid drug or refrain from nursing.

Habit-Forming Potential: None.

Effects of Overdosage: Nausea, vomiting, diarrhea, bloody urine, water retention, weight gain, severe bone marrow depression, severe infections.

Possible Effects of Long-Term Use: Development of fibrous tissue in lungs; secondary malignancies.

Suggested Periodic Examinations While Taking This Drug (at physician's discretion)

Complete blood cell counts, every 2 to 4 days during initial treatment; then every 3 to 4 weeks during maintenance treatment.

Liver and kidney function tests.

Thyroid function tests (if symptoms warrant).

▷ **While Taking This Drug, Observe the Following**

Foods: No restrictions.

Beverages: No restrictions. May be taken with milk.

▷ *Alcohol:* No interactions expected.

Tobacco Smoking: No interactions expected.

▷ *Other Drugs*

Cyclophosphamide ***taken concurrently*** with

• allopurinol (Zyloprim) may increase the degree of bone marrow depression.

▷ *Driving, Hazardous Activities:* Use caution if dizziness occurs.

Aviation Note: The use of this drug ***may be a disqualification*** for piloting. Consult a designated Aviation Medical Examiner.

Exposure to Sun: No restrictions.

Occurrence of Unrelated Illness: Report promptly the development of any indications of infection—fever, chills, sore throat, cough, flulike symptoms. It may be necessary to discontinue this drug until the infection is controlled. Consult your physician.

DEMECLOCYCLINE
(dem e kloh SI kleen)

Introduced: 1959

Class: Antibiotic, tetracyclines

Prescription: USA: Yes
Canada: Yes

Controlled Drug: USA: No
Canada: No

Available as Generic: No

Brand Name: Declomycin

BENEFITS versus RISKS	
Possible Benefits	*Possible Risks*
EFFECTIVE TREATMENT OF INFECTIONS due to susceptible microorganisms	Allergic reactions
	Drug-induced colitis
	Drug-induced diabetes insipidus (water diabetes)
	Fungal superinfections

▷ **Principal Uses**

As a Single Drug Product: This member of the tetracycline drug class is used primarily to (1) treat a broad range of infections caused by susceptible bacteria and protozoa and (2) treat the syndrome of inappropriate secretion of antidiuretic hormone, a condition that reduces the normal production of urine.

How This Drug Works: This drug prevents the growth and multiplication of susceptible bacteria by interfering with their formation of essential proteins.

Available Dosage Forms and Strengths
Capsules — 150 mg
Tablets, film-coated — 150 mg, 300 mg

▷ **Usual Adult Dosage Range:** 150 mg/6 hours or 300 mg/12 hours. Total daily dosage should not exceed 2400 mg. **Note: Actual dosage and administration schedule must be determined by the physician for each patient individually.**

▷ **Dosing Instructions:** Preferably taken on an empty stomach, 1 hour before or 2 hours after eating. However, if stomach irritation occurs, it may be taken with crackers or light food (not milk or milk products). Take at same time each day, with a full glass of water. Take the full course prescribed. The tablet may be crushed and the capsule may be opened for administration.

Usual Duration of Use: The time required to control the infection and be free of fever and symptoms for 48 hours. This varies with the nature of the infection.

▷ **This Drug Should Not Be Taken If**
- you are allergic to any tetracycline drug (see Drug Class, Section Four).
- you are pregnant or breast-feeding.

▷ **Inform Your Physician Before Taking This Drug If**
- it is prescribed for a child under 8 years of age.
- you have a history of liver or kidney disease.
- you have systemic lupus erythematosus.
- you are taking any penicillin drug.
- you are taking any anticoagulant drug.
- you plan to have surgery under general anesthesia in the near future.

Possible Side-Effects (natural, expected and unavoidable drug actions)
Superinfections (see Glossary), often due to yeast organisms. These can occur in the mouth, intestinal tract, rectum and/or vagina, resulting in rectal and vaginal itching.

▷ **Possible Adverse Effects** (unusual, unexpected and infrequent reactions)
If any of the following develop, consult your physician promptly for guidance.

Mild Adverse Effects
Allergic Reactions: Skin rash, hives, itching of hands and feet, swelling of face or extremities.
Loss of appetite, nausea, vomiting, diarrhea.
Irritation of mouth or tongue, "black tongue," sore throat, abdominal cramping or pain.

Serious Adverse Effects
Allergic Reactions: Anaphylactic reaction (see Glossary), asthma, fever, swollen joints, abnormal bleeding or bruising, jaundice (see Glossary).
Permanent discoloration and/or malformation of teeth when taken under 8 years of age, including unborn child and infant.
Drug-induced diabetes insipidus (water diabetes).

▷ **Possible Effects on Sexual Function:**   Questionable decrease of libido (1 report only).

Natural Diseases or Disorders That May Be Activated by This Drug
Systemic lupus erythematosus.

CAUTION
1. Antacids, dairy products and preparations containing aluminum, bismuth, calcium, iron, magnesium or zinc can prevent adequate absorption of this drug and reduce its effectiveness significantly.
2. Troublesome and persistent diarrhea can develop in sensitive individuals. If diarrhea persists for more than 24 hours, discontinue this drug and consult your physician.
3. If surgery under general anesthesia is required while taking this drug, the choice of anesthetic agent must be considered carefully to prevent serious kidney damage.

Precautions for Use
By Infants and Children: If possible, tetracyclines should not be given to children under 8 years of age because of the risk of permanent discoloration and deformity of the teeth. Rarely, young infants may develop increased intracranial pressure within the first 4 days of receiving this drug. Tetracyclines may inhibit normal bone growth and development.
By Those over 60 Years of Age: Dosage must be carefully individualized and based upon determinations of kidney function. Natural skin changes may predispose to severe and prolonged itching reactions in the genital and anal regions.

▷ **Advisability of Use During Pregnancy**
Pregnancy Category: D (tentative). See Pregnancy Code inside back cover.
Animal studies: Tetracycline causes limb defects in rats, rabbits and chickens.
Human studies: Information from studies of pregnant women indicates that this drug can cause impaired development and discoloration of teeth and other developmental defects.
It is advisable to avoid this drug completely during entire pregnancy.

Advisability of Use if Breast-Feeding
Presence of this drug in breast milk: Yes.
Avoid drug or refrain from nursing.

Habit-Forming Potential: None.

Effects of Overdosage: Nausea, vomiting, diarrhea, acute liver damage (rare).

Possible Effects of Long-Term Use: Superinfections; rarely, impairment of bone marrow, liver or kidney function.

Suggested Periodic Examinations While Taking This Drug (at physician's discretion)
Complete blood cell counts, liver and kidney function tests.
During extended use, sputum and stool examinations may detect early superinfection due to yeast organisms.

▷ **While Taking This Drug, Observe the Following**
Foods: Avoid cheeses, yogurt, ice cream, iron-fortified cereals and supplements and meats for 2 hours before and after taking this drug.
Beverages: Avoid all forms of milk for 2 hours before and after taking this drug.
▷ *Alcohol:* No interactions expected. However, it is best avoided if you have active liver disease.
Tobacco Smoking: No interactions expected.
▷ *Other Drugs*
Tetracyclines may *increase* the effects of
- oral anticoagulants, and make it necessary to reduce their dosage.
- digoxin (Lanoxin), and cause digitalis toxicity.
- lithium (Eskalith, Lithane, etc.), and increase the risk of lithium toxicity.
Tetracyclines may *decrease* the effects of
- oral contraceptives, and impair their effectiveness in preventing pregnancy.
- penicillins, and impair their effectiveness in treating infections.
Tetracyclines *taken concurrently* with
- methoxyflurane anesthesia may impair kidney function.
The following drugs may *decrease* the effects of tetracyclines
- antacids (aluminum and magnesium preparations, sodium bicarbonate, etc.) may reduce drug absorption.
- iron and mineral preparations may reduce drug absorption.
▷ *Driving, Hazardous Activities:* Usually no restrictions. Be alert to the possible occurrence of nausea or diarrhea.
Aviation Note: The use of this drug *may be a disqualification* for piloting. Consult a designated Aviation Medical Examiner.
Exposure to Sun: Use caution until sensitivity has been determined. Tetracyclines can cause photosensitivity (see Glossary).

DESIPRAMINE
(des IP ra meen)

Introduced: 1964

Class: Antidepressant

Prescription: USA: Yes
Canada: Yes

Controlled Drug: USA: No
Canada: No

Available as Generic: USA: No
Canada: No

Brand Names: Norpramin, Pertofrane

BENEFITS versus RISKS

Possible Benefits	*Possible Risks*
EFFECTIVE RELIEF OF ENDOGENOUS DEPRESSION	ADVERSE BEHAVIORAL EFFECTS: confusion, disorientation, delusions, hallucinations
Possibly beneficial in other depressive disorders	CONVERSION OF DEPRESSION TO MANIA in bipolar affective disorders
	Aggravation of paranoia and schizophrenia
	Drug-induced heart rhythm disorders
	Abnormally low white blood cell and platelet counts

▷ **Principal Uses**

As a Single Drug Product: Used primarily to relieve severe emotional depression and to initiate gradual restoration of normal mood. This drug is more likely to be effective in primary (endogenous) depression than in secondary, reactive (exogenous) depression. It is also being used to treat attention deficit disorder in children over 6 years of age and in adolescents.

How This Drug Works: Not completely established. It is thought that by increasing brain tissue concentrations of certain nerve impulse transmitters (norepinephrine and serotonin), this drug relieves the symptoms associated with depression.

Available Dosage Forms and Strengths
Capsules — 25 mg, 50 mg
Tablets — 10 mg, 25 mg, 50 mg, 75 mg, 100 mg, 150 mg

▷ **Usual Adult Dosage Range:** Initially 25 mg 2 to 4 times daily. Dose may be increased cautiously as needed and tolerated by 25 mg daily at intervals of 1 week. The usual maintenance dose is 100 mg to 200 mg/24 hours. The total daily dosage should not exceed 300 mg. (When determined, the optimal daily requirement may be given at bedtime as a single dose.) **Note: Actual dosage and administration schedule must be determined by the physician for each patient individually.**

▷ **Dosing Instructions:** May be taken without regard to meals. The capsule may be opened and the tablet may be crushed for administration.

Usual Duration of Use: Continual use on a regular schedule for 3 to 4 weeks is usually necessary to determine this drug's effectiveness in relieving depression; optimal response may require 3 months of use. Long-term use (months to years) requires periodic evaluation of response and dosage adjustment. Consult your physician on a regular basis.

▷ **This Drug Should Not Be Taken If**
- you have had an allergic reaction to it previously.
- you are taking, or have taken within the past 14 days, any monoamine oxidase (MAO) type A inhibitor drug (see Drug Class, Section Four).
- you have had a recent heart attack (myocardial infarction).
- you have narrow-angle glaucoma.

▷ **Inform Your Physician Before Taking This Drug If**
- you have had an adverse reaction to any other antidepressant drug.
- you have any type of seizure disorder.
- you have increased internal eye pressure.
- you have any type of heart disease, especially a heart rhythm disorder.
- you have any type of thyroid disorder or are taking thyroid medication.
- you have diabetes or sugar intolerance.
- you have prostatism (see Glossary).
- you plan to have surgery under general anesthesia in the near future.

Possible Side-Effects (natural, expected and unavoidable drug actions)
Mild drowsiness, light-headedness (low blood pressure), blurred vision, dry mouth, constipation, impaired urination.

▷ **Possible Adverse Effects** (unusual, unexpected and infrequent reactions)
If any of the following develop, consult your physician promptly for guidance.
Mild Adverse Effects
Allergic Reactions: Skin rash, hives, swelling of face or tongue, drug fever (see Glossary).
Headache, dizziness, weakness, unsteadiness, tremors, fainting.
Irritation of tongue or mouth, altered taste, indigestion, nausea.
Fluctuations of blood sugar.
Serious Adverse Effects
Allergic Reactions: Drug-induced hepatitis, with or without jaundice; anaphylactoid reaction (see terms in Glossary).

Adverse behavioral effects: confusion, disorientation, delusions, hallucinations.

Seizures; reduced control of epilepsy.

Aggravation of paranoid psychoses and schizophrenia.

Heart rhythm disturbances.

Parkinsonlike disorders, peripheral neuritis (see both terms in Glossary).

Abnormally low white blood cell and platelet counts: fever, sore throat, infections, abnormal bleeding or bruising.

▷ **Possible Effects on Sexual Function:** Decreased libido, increased libido (antidepressant effect), impotence, painful male orgasm, male breast enlargement, female breast enlargement with milk production, swelling of testicles.

▷ **Adverse Effects That May Mimic Natural Diseases or Disorders**
Liver toxicity may suggest viral hepatitis.

Natural Diseases or Disorders That May Be Activated by This Drug
Latent diabetes, epilepsy, glaucoma, prostatism.

CAUTION
1. This drug should be used only when a true, primary, endogenous depression has been diagnosed. It should *not* be used to treat the symptoms of reactive depression that may be associated with many life situations in the absence of a true bona fide affective illness.
2. Observe for early indications of toxicity or overdosage: confusion, agitation, rapid heart rate, heart irregularity. Measurement of the blood level of the drug will clarify the situation.
3. It is advisable to withhold this drug if electroconvulsive therapy (ECT) is to be used to treat the depression.

Precautions for Use
By Infants and Children: Safety and effectiveness for use by those under 6 years of age have not been established. This drug is being used experimentally to treat children who have attention deficit syndrome, with or without hyperactivity. Dosage and management must be supervised by a properly trained pediatrician.
By Those over 60 Years of Age: Initiate treatment with 25 mg 1 or 2 times daily to evaluate tolerance. During the first 2 weeks of treatment, observe for confusional reactions—restlessness, agitation, forgetfulness, disorientation, delusions or hallucinations. Also observe for unsteadiness and instability that may predispose to falling. This drug may aggravate prostatism.

▷ **Advisability of Use During Pregnancy**
Pregnancy Category: C (tentative). See Pregnancy Code inside back cover.
Animal studies: Birth defects reported in rat and rabbit studies.
Human studies: Information from adequate studies of pregnant women is not available.
Use only if clearly needed. Avoid during the first 3 months if possible.

Advisability of Use if Breast-Feeding
Presence of this drug in breast milk: Yes, in small amounts.
Monitor nursing infant closely and discontinue drug or nursing if adverse effects develop.

Habit-Forming Potential: Psychological or physical dependence is rare and unexpected. This drug is not liable to abuse.

Effects of Overdosage: Confusion, hallucinations, drowsiness, tremors, heart irregularity, seizures, stupor, hypothermia (see Glossary).

Possible Effects of Long-Term Use: None reported.

Suggested Periodic Examinations While Taking This Drug (at physician's discretion)
Complete blood cell counts, liver function tests.
Serial blood pressure readings and electrocardiograms.

▷ **While Taking This Drug, Observe the Following**
Foods: No specific restrictions. May need to limit food intake to avoid excessive weight gain.
Beverages: No restrictions. May be taken with milk.
▷ *Alcohol:* Avoid completely. This drug can markedly increase the intoxicating effects of alcohol; the combination can depress brain function significantly.
Tobacco Smoking: May accelerate the elimination of this drug and require increased dosage.
Marijuana Smoking
Occasional (once or twice weekly): Transient increase in drowsiness and mouth dryness.
Daily: Persistent drowsiness and mouth dryness; possible reduced effectiveness of this drug.
▷ *Other Drugs*
Desipramine may *increase* the effects of
• all drugs with sedative effects; observe for excessive sedation.
• all drugs with atropinelike effects (see Drug Class, Section Four).
Desipramine may *decrease* the effects of
• clonidine (Catapres).
• guanethidine (Ismelin, Esimil).
Desipramine *taken concurrently* with
• anticonvulsants requires careful monitoring for changes in seizure patterns and need to adjust anticonvulsant dosage.
• ethchlorvynol (Placidyl) may cause delirium; avoid concurrent use.
• monoamine oxidase (MAO) type A inhibitor drugs (see Drug Class, Section Four) may cause high fever, seizures and excessive rise in blood pressure; avoid concurrent use of these drugs and provide periods of 14 days between administration of either.
• stimulant drugs (amphetamine, cocaine, epinephrine, phenylpropanolamine, etc.) may cause severe high blood pressure and/or high fever.
• thyroid preparations may increase the risk of heart rhythm disorders.

The following drugs may *increase* the effects of desipramine
- methylphenidate (Ritalin).
- phenothiazines (see Drug Class, Section Four).

The following drugs may *decrease* the effects of desipramine
- barbiturates (see Drug Class, Section Four).
- chloral hydrate (Noctec, Somnos, etc.).
- estrogen (see Drug Profile for brand names).
- lithium (Lithobid, Lithotab, etc.).
- oral contraceptives (see Drug Profile for brand names).
- reserpine (Serpasil, Ser-Ap-Es, etc.).

▷ *Driving, Hazardous Activities:* This drug may impair mental alertness, judgment, physical coordination and reaction time. Restrict activities as necessary.

Aviation Note: The use of this drug *is a disqualification* for piloting. Consult a designated Aviation Medical Examiner.

Exposure to Sun: Use caution until sensitivity has been determined. This drug may cause photosensitivity (see Glossary).

Exposure to Heat: Use caution. This drug can inhibit sweating and impair the body's adaptation to hot environments, increasing the risk of heat stroke. Avoid saunas.

Exposure to Cold: The elderly should use caution and avoid conditions conducive to hypothermia (see Glossary).

Exposure to Environmental Chemicals: This drug may mask the symptoms of poisoning due to handling certain insecticides (organophosphorus types). Read their labels carefully.

Discontinuation: It is advisable to discontinue this drug gradually. Abrupt withdrawal after prolonged use may cause headache, malaise and nausea. When this drug is stopped, it may be necessary to adjust the dosages of other drugs taken concurrently.

DEXAMETHASONE
(dex a METH a sohn)

Introduced: 1958

Class: Cortisonelike drugs

Prescription: USA: Yes
Canada: Yes

Controlled Drug: USA: No
Canada: No

Available as Generic: USA: Yes
Canada: Yes

Brand Names: ♣Ak-Dex, Decaderm, Decadron, Decadron-LA, Decadron Phosphate Ophthalmic, Decadron Phosphate Respihaler, Decadron Phosphate Turbinaire, Decadron w/Xylocaine [CD], Decaspray, ♣Deronil, Dexasone, Dexone, Hexadrol, Maxidex

```
┌─────────────────────────────────────────────────────────────┐
│                    BENEFITS versus RISKS                      │
│                                                               │
│      *Possible Benefits*              *Possible Risks*        │
│   EFFECTIVE RELIEF OF          Short-term use (up to 10 days) is │
│     SYMPTOMS IN A WIDE            usually well tolerated       │
│     VARIETY OF INFLAMMATORY    Long-term use (exceeding 2     │
│     AND ALLERGIC DISORDERS       weeks) is associated with many │
│   EFFECTIVE                      possible adverse effects:    │
│     IMMUNOSUPPRESSION in       ALTERED MOOD AND               │
│     selected benign and malignant  PERSONALITY                │
│     disorders                  CATARACTS, GLAUCOMA           │
│                                HYPERTENSION                   │
│                                OSTEOPOROSIS                   │
│                                ASEPTIC BONE NECROSIS         │
│                                INCREASED SUSCEPTIBIL-        │
│                                  ITY TO INFECTIONS           │
│                                (See Possible Adverse Effects │
│                                  and Possible Effects of Long-│
│                                  Term Use below)             │
└─────────────────────────────────────────────────────────────┘
```

▷ **Principal Uses**

As a Single Drug Product: This potent drug of the cortisone class is used in the treatment of a wide variety of allergic and inflammatory conditions. It is used most commonly in the management of serious skin disorders, asthma, regional enteritis, ulcerative colitis and all types of major rheumatic disorders including bursitis, tendonitis and most forms of arthritis.

How This Drug Works: Not fully established. It is thought that this drug's anti-inflammatory effect is due to its ability to inhibit the normal defensive functions of certain white blood cells. Its immunosuppressant effect is attributed to a reduced production of lymphocytes and antibodies.

Available Dosage Forms and Strengths

Aerosol — 0.01%, 0.04%

Aerosol inhaler — 84 mcg per spray

Cream — 0.1%

Elixir — 0.5 mg per 5-ml teaspoonful

Eye ointment — 0.05%

Gel — 0.1%

Injection — 4 mg per ml, 8 mg per ml, 10 mg per ml, 16 mg per ml, 20 mg per ml, 24 mg per ml

Oral solution — 0.5 mg per 0.5 ml, 0.5 mg per 5 ml

Solution — 0.1%

Suspension — 0.1%

Tablets — 0.25 mg, 0.5 mg, 0.75 mg, 1 mg, 1.5 mg, 2 mg, 4 mg, 6 mg

▷ **Usual Adult Dosage Range:** 0.5 to 9 mg daily as a single dose or in divided doses. **Note: Actual dosage and administration schedule must be determined by the physician for each patient individually.**

▷ **Dosing Instructions:** Take with or following food to prevent stomach irritation, preferably in the morning. The tablet may be crushed for administration.

Usual Duration of Use: For acute disorders: 4 to 10 days. For chronic disorders: according to individual requirements. The duration of use should not exceed the time necessary to obtain adequate symptomatic relief in acute self-limiting conditions; or the time required to stabilize a chronic condition and permit gradual withdrawal. Because of its long duration of action, this drug is not appropriate for alternate day administration. Consult your physician on a regular basis.

▷ **This Drug Should Not Be Taken If**
- you have had an allergic reaction to any dosage form of it previously.
- you have active peptic ulcer disease.
- you have an active infection of the eye caused by the herpes simplex virus.
- you have active tuberculosis.

▷ **Inform Your Physician Before Taking This Drug If**
- you have had an unfavorable reaction to any cortisonelike drug in the past.
- you have a history of peptic ulcer disease, thrombophlebitis or tuberculosis.
- you have any of the following: diabetes, glaucoma, high blood pressure, deficient thyroid function or myasthenia gravis.
- you plan to have surgery of any kind in the near future.

Possible Side-Effects (natural, expected and unavoidable drug actions)
Increased appetite, weight gain, retention of salt and water, excretion of potassium, increased susceptibility to infection.

▷ **Possible Adverse Effects** (unusual, unexpected and infrequent reactions)
If any of the following develop, consult your physician promptly for guidance.
Mild Adverse Effects
Allergic Reaction: Skin rash.
Headache, dizziness, insomnia.
Acid indigestion, abdominal distention.
Muscle cramping and weakness.
Acne, excessive growth of facial hair.
Serious Adverse Effects
Mental and emotional disturbances of serious magnitude.
Reactivation of latent tuberculosis.
Development of peptic ulcer.
Increased blood pressure.

Development of inflammation of the pancreas.

Thrombophlebitis (inflammation of a vein with the formation of blood clot)—pain or tenderness in thigh or leg, with or without swelling of the foot, ankle or leg.

Pulmonary embolism (movement of a blood clot to the lung)—sudden shortness of breath, pain in the chest, coughing, bloody sputum.

▷ **Possible Effects on Sexual Function:** Altered timing and pattern of menstruation.

▷ **Adverse Effects That May Mimic Natural Diseases or Disorders**

Pattern of symptoms and signs resembling Cushing's syndrome.

Natural Diseases or Disorders That May Be Activated by This Drug

Latent diabetes, glaucoma, peptic ulcer disease, tuberculosis.

CAUTION

1. It is advisable to carry a card of personal identification with a notation that you are taking this drug, if your course of treatment is to exceed 1 week.
2. Do not discontinue this drug abruptly if you are using it for long-term treatment.
3. If vaccination against measles, rabies, smallpox or yellow fever is required, discontinue this drug 72 hours before vaccination and do not resume it for at least 14 days after vaccination.

Precautions for Use

By Infants and Children: Avoid prolonged use if possible. During long-term use, observe for suppression of normal growth and the possibility of increased intracranial pressure. Following long-term use, the child may be at risk for adrenal gland deficiency during stress for as long as 18 months after cessation of this drug.

By Those over 60 Years of Age: Cortisonelike drugs should be used very sparingly after 60 and only when the disorder under treatment is unresponsive to adequate trials of unrelated drugs. Avoid prolonged use of this drug. Continual use (even in small doses) can increase the severity of diabetes, enhance fluid retention, raise blood pressure, weaken resistance to infection, induce stomach ulcer and accelerate the development of cataract and osteoporosis.

▷ **Advisability of Use During Pregnancy**

Pregnancy Category: C (tentative). See Pregnancy Code inside back cover.

Animal studies: Birth defects reported in mice, rats and rabbits.

Human studies: Information from adequate studies of pregnant women is not available.

Avoid completely during the first 3 months. Limit use during the last 6 months as much as possible. If used, examine infant for possible deficiency of adrenal gland function.

Advisability of Use if Breast-Feeding
Presence of this drug in breast milk: Yes.
Avoid drug or refrain from nursing.

Habit-Forming Potential: Use of this drug to suppress symptoms over an extended period of time may produce a state of functional dependence (see Glossary). In the treatment of conditions like asthma and rheumatoid arthritis, it is advisable to keep the dose as small as possible and to attempt drug withdrawal after periods of reasonable improvement. Such procedures may reduce the degree of "steroid rebound"—the return of symptoms as the drug is withdrawn.

Effects of Overdosage: Fatigue, muscle weakness, stomach irritation, acid indigestion, excessive sweating, facial flushing, fluid retention, swelling of extremities, increased blood pressure.

Possible Effects of Long-Term Use: Increased blood sugar (possible diabetes), increased fat deposits on the trunk of the body ("buffalo hump"), rounding of the face ("moon face"), thinning and fragility of skin, loss of texture and strength of bones (osteoporosis, aseptic necrosis), cataracts, glaucoma, retarded growth and development in children.

Suggested Periodic Examinations While Taking This Drug (at physician's discretion)
Measurements of blood pressure, blood sugar and potassium levels.
Complete eye examinations at regular intervals.
Chest X-ray if history of tuberculosis.
Determination of the rate of development of the growing child to detect retardation of normal growth.

▷ **While Taking This Drug, Observe the Following**
Foods: No interactions expected. Ask physician regarding need to restrict salt intake or to eat potassium-rich foods. During long-term use of this drug, it is advisable to eat a high-protein diet.
Nutritional Support: During long-term use, take a vitamin D supplement. During wound repair, take a zinc supplement.
Beverages: No restrictions. Drink all forms of milk liberally.
▷ *Alcohol:* No interactions expected. Use caution if you are prone to peptic ulcer disease.
Tobacco Smoking: Nicotine increases the blood levels of naturally produced cortisone and related hormones. Heavy smoking may add to the expected actions of this drug and requires close observation for excessive effects.
Marijuana Smoking: May cause additional impairment of immunity.
▷ *Other Drugs*
Dexamethasone may **decrease** the effects of
- isoniazid (INH, Niconyl, etc.)
- salicylates (aspirin, sodium salicylate, etc.)

Dexamethasone *taken concurrently* with
- oral anticoagulants may either increase or decrease their effectiveness; consult physician regarding the need for prothrombin time testing and dosage adjustment.

The following drugs may *decrease* the effects of dexamethasone
- antacids may reduce its absorption.
- barbiturates (Amytal, Butisol, phenobarbital, etc.).
- phenytoin (Dilantin, etc.).
- rifampin (Rifadin, Rimactane, etc.).

▷ *Driving, Hazardous Activities:* Usually no restrictions. Be alert to the rare occurrence of dizziness.

Aviation Note: The use of this drug *may be a disqualification* for piloting. Consult a designated Aviation Medical Examiner.

Exposure to Sun: No restrictions.

Occurrence of Unrelated Illness: This drug may decrease natural resistance to infection. Inform your physician if you develop an infection of any kind. It may also reduce your body's ability to respond to the stress of acute illness, injury or surgery. Keep your physician fully informed of any significant changes in your state of health.

Discontinuation: If you have been taking this drug for an extended period of time, do not discontinue it abruptly. Ask physician for guidance regarding gradual withdrawal. For a period of 2 years after discontinuing this drug, it is essential in the event of illness, injury or surgery that you inform attending medical personnel that you have used this drug in the past. The period of impaired response to stress following the use of cortisonelike drugs may last for 1 to 2 years.

DIAZEPAM
(di AZ e pam)

Introduced: 1963

Class: Mild tranquilizer, benzodiazepines

Prescription: USA: Yes
Canada: Yes

Controlled Drug: USA: C-IV*
Canada: No

Available as Generic: Yes

Brand Names: ✦Apo-Diazepam, ✦Diazemuls, Diazepam Intensol, ✦E-Pam, ✦Meval, ✦Novodipam, ✦Rival, Valium, Valrelease, Vazepam, ✦Vivol

*See Schedules of Controlled Drugs inside back cover.

```
┌─────────────────────────────────────────────────────────────────┐
│                    BENEFITS versus RISKS                          │
│                                                                   │
│       Possible Benefits              Possible Risks               │
│   RELIEF OF ANXIETY AND         Habit-forming potential with      │
│     NERVOUS TENSION in 70% to     prolonged use                   │
│     80% of users                Minor impairment of mental        │
│   Wide margin of safety with      functions                       │
│     therapeutic doses           Very rare jaundice                │
│   Very few drug interactions    Very rare blood cell disorders    │
└─────────────────────────────────────────────────────────────────┘
```

▷ **Principal Uses**

As a Single Drug Product: Used primarily to (1) provide short-term relief of mild to moderate anxiety; (2) relieve the symptoms of acute alcohol withdrawal: agitation, tremors, hallucinations, incipient delirium tremens; (3) relieve skeletal muscle spasm; (4) provide short-term control of certain types of seizures (epilepsy).

How This Drug Works: It is thought that this drug produces a calming effect by enhancing the action of the nerve transmitter gamma-aminobutyric acid (GABA), which in turn blocks the arousal of higher brain centers.

Available Dosage Forms and Strengths

Capsules, prolonged-action — 15 mg
Concentrate — 5 mg per ml
Injection — 5 mg per ml
Oral solution — 5 mg per ml, 5 mg per 5-ml teaspoonful
Tablets — 2 mg, 5 mg, 10 mg

▷ **Usual Adult Dosage Range:** 2 to 10 mg, 2 to 4 times daily. Dose may be increased cautiously as needed and tolerated. After 1 week of continual use, the total daily dose may be taken at bedtime. Total daily dose should not exceed 60 mg. **Note: Actual dosage and administration schedule must be determined by the physician for each patient individually.**

▷ **Dosing Instructions:** May be taken on empty stomach or with food or milk. The prolonged-action capsule should not be opened, but the tablet may be crushed for administration. Do not discontinue this drug abruptly if taken for more than 4 weeks.

Usual Duration of Use: Continual use on a regular schedule for 3 to 5 days is usually necessary to determine this drug's effectiveness in relieving moderate anxiety. Limit continual use to 1 to 3 weeks. Avoid uninterrupted and prolonged use.

▷ **This Drug Should Not Be Taken If**
- you have had an allergic reaction to any dosage form of it previously.
- you have acute narrow-angle glaucoma.
- it is prescribed for a child under 6 months of age.

▷ **Inform Your Physician Before Taking This Drug If**
- you are allergic to any benzodiazepine drug (see Drug Class, Section Four).
- you have a history of alcoholism or drug abuse.
- you are pregnant or planning pregnancy.
- you have impaired liver or kidney function.
- you have a history of serious depression or mental disorder.
- you have any of the following: asthma, emphysema, epilepsy, myasthenia gravis.

Possible Side-Effects (natural, expected and unavoidable drug actions)
Drowsiness (5%), lethargy, unsteadiness (0.2%), "hangover" effects on the day following bedtime use.

▷ **Possible Adverse Effects** (unusual, unexpected and infrequent reactions)
If any of the following develop, consult your physician promptly for guidance.
Mild Adverse Effects
Allergic Reactions: Rashes (0.4%), hives.
Dizziness, fainting, blurred vision, double vision, slurred speech, sweating, nausea.
Serious Adverse Effects
Allergic Reactions: Liver damage with jaundice (see Glossary), abnormally low blood platelet count.
Bone marrow depression—impaired production of white blood cells, fever, sore throat.
Paradoxical responses of excitement, agitation, anger, rage.

▷ **Possible Effects on Sexual Function**
Altered timing and pattern of menstruation.
Small doses (2 to 5 mg/day) are used to allay the anxiety that accounts for many cases of impotence in the male and inhibited sexual responsiveness in the female.
Larger doses (10 mg/day or more) can decrease libido, impair potency in the male and inhibit orgasm in the female.

▷ **Adverse Effects That May Mimic Natural Diseases or Disorders**
Liver reaction with jaundice may suggest viral hepatitis.

CAUTION
1. This drug should not be discontinued abruptly if it has been taken continually for more than 4 weeks.
2. The concurrent use of some over-the-counter drug products that contain antihistamines (allergy and cold preparations, sleep aids) can cause excessive sedation in sensitive individuals.

Precautions for Use
By Infants and Children: Safety and effectiveness for use by those under 6 months of age have not been established. This drug should not be

used in the hyperactive or psychotic child of any age. Observe for excessive sedation and incoordination.

By Those over 60 Years of Age: It is advisable to use smaller doses at longer intervals to avoid overdosage. Observe for the possible development of lethargy, indifference, fatigue, weakness, unsteadiness, disturbing dreams, nightmares and paradoxical reactions of excitement, agitation, anger, hostility and rage.

▷ **Advisability of Use During Pregnancy**
Pregnancy Category: D (tentative). See Pregnancy Code inside back cover.
Animal studies: Cleft palate reported in mice; skeletal defects reported in rats.

Human studies: Available information is conflicting and inconclusive. Some studies found an increase in serious birth defects associated with the use of this drug. Other studies have found no significant increase in birth defects.

Frequent use in late pregnancy can cause the "floppy infant" syndrome in the newborn: weakness, lethargy, unresponsiveness, depressed breathing, low body temperature.

Avoid use during entire pregnancy.

Advisability of Use if Breast-Feeding
Presence of this drug in breast milk: Yes.
Avoid drug or refrain from nursing.

Habit-Forming Potential: This drug can produce psychological and/or physical dependence (see Glossary) if used in large doses for an extended period of time.

Effects of Overdosage: Marked drowsiness, weakness, feeling of drunkenness, staggering gait, tremor, stupor progressing to deep sleep or coma.

Possible Effects of Long-Term Use: Psychological and/or physical dependence, rare blood cell disorders.

Suggested Periodic Examinations While Taking This Drug (at physician's discretion)
Complete blood cell counts during long-term use.

▷ **While Taking This Drug, Observe the Following**
Foods: No restrictions.
Beverages: Avoid excessive intake of caffeine-containing beverages: coffee, tea, cola. May be taken with milk.
▷ *Alcohol:* Use with extreme caution until the combined effect is determined. Alcohol may increase the absorption of this drug and add to its depressant effects on the brain. It is advisable to avoid alcohol completely—throughout the day and night—if it is necessary to drive or to engage in any hazardous activity.
Tobacco Smoking: Heavy smoking may reduce the calming action of this drug.

Marijuana Smoking: Increased sedation and significant impairment of intellectual and physical performance.

▷ *Other Drugs*

Diazepam may *increase* the effects of
- digoxin (Lanoxin), and cause digoxin toxicity.
- phenytoin (Dilantin), and cause phenytoin toxicity.

Diazepam may *decrease* the effects of
- levodopa (Sinemet, etc.), and reduce its effectiveness in treating Parkinson's disease.

The following drugs may *increase* the effects of diazepam
- cimetidine (Tagamet).
- disulfiram (Antabuse).
- isoniazid (INH, Rifamate, etc.).
- oral contraceptives.
- valproic acid (Depakene).

The following drugs may *decrease* the effects of diazepam
- rifampin (Rimactane, etc.).
- theophylline (aminophylline, Theo-Dur, etc.).

▷ *Driving, Hazardous Activities:* This drug can impair mental alertness, judgment, physical coordination and reaction time. Avoid hazardous activities accordingly.

Aviation Note: The use of this drug *is a disqualification* for piloting. Consult a designated Aviation Medical Examiner.

Exposure to Sun: No restrictions.

Exposure to Heat: Use caution until the effect of excessive perspiration is determined. Because of reduced urine volume, this drug may accumulate in the body and produce effects of overdosage.

Discontinuation: Avoid sudden discontinuation if this drug has been taken for over 4 weeks without interruption. Dosage should be tapered gradually to prevent a withdrawal syndrome that could include depression, confusion, hallucinations, tremor, seizures, muscle cramping, sweating and vomiting.

DICLOFENAC
(di KLOH fen ak)

Introduced: 1976

Class: Mild analgesic, anti-inflammatory

Prescription: USA: Yes
Canada: Yes

Controlled Drug: USA: No
Canada: No

Available as Generic: USA: No
Canada: No

Brand Name: Voltaren

BENEFITS versus RISKS

Possible Benefits	*Possible Risks*
EFFECTIVE RELIEF OF SYMPTOMS ASSOCIATED WITH MAJOR TYPES OF ARTHRITIS	PEPTIC ULCER DISEASE (less than 2%); associated bleeding and perforation
Effective relief of symptoms associated with bursitis, tendinitis and related conditions	Liver toxicity with jaundice (less than 1%)
	Rare aplastic anemia (see Glossary)
Effective relief of menstrual cramps	Water retention
	Rare kidney toxicity

▷ **Principal Uses**

As a Single Drug Product: Used primarily to relieve the symptoms associated with (1) rheumatoid arthritis, osteoarthritis and ankylosing spondylitis; (2) bursitis, tendinitis, capsulitis and tenosynovitis; (3) painful menstruation.

How This Drug Works: Not completely established. It is thought that this drug reduces the tissue concentrations of prostaglandins (and related compounds), chemicals involved in the production of inflammation and pain.

Available Dosage Forms and Strengths

Suppositories (Canada) — 50 mg, 100 mg
Tablets, enteric-coated — 25 mg, 50 mg, 75 mg
Tablets, prolonged-action (Canada) — 100 mg

▷ **Usual Adult Dosage Range:** Initially 100 to 200 mg/24 hours, in 2 to 5 divided doses. After a satisfactory response has been achieved, dosage should be reduced to the minimum that will sustain adequate relief. The usual maintenance dose is 50 to 100 mg/24 hours. **Note: Actual dosage and administration schedule must be determined by the physician for each patient individually.**

▷ **Dosing Instructions:** Take either on an empty stomach or with food or milk if necessary to prevent stomach irritation. Take with a full glass of water and remain upright (do not lie down) for 15 to 30 minutes to prevent lodging of the tablet in the esophagus (food tube). Take the tablet whole; do not crush for administration.

Usual Duration of Use: Continual use on a regular schedule for 1 to 2 weeks is usually necessary to determine this drug's effectiveness in relieving the symptoms of arthritis, bursitis, etc. Severe arthritis may require continual use for 3 to 4 weeks to obtain maximal relief. Long-term use (months to years) requires periodic evaluation of response and dosage adjustment. Consult your physician on a regular basis.

▷ **This Drug Should Not Be Taken If**
  • you have had an allergic reaction to it previously.
  • you are subject to asthma or nasal polyps caused by aspirin.
  • you have active peptic ulcer disease or any form of gastrointestinal bleeding.
  • you have active liver disease.
  • you have a bleeding disorder or a blood cell disorder.
  • you have severe impairment of kidney function.
  • you have porphyria (see Glossary).

▷ **Inform Your Physician Before Taking This Drug If**
  • you are allergic to aspirin or to other aspirin substitutes.
  • you have a history of peptic ulcer disease or any type of bleeding disorder.
  • you have impaired liver or kidney function.
  • you have high blood pressure or a history of heart failure.
  • you have systemic lupus erythematosus (SLE).
  • you are taking any of the following drugs: acetaminophen, aspirin or other aspirin substitutes, anticoagulants, cyclosporine, digoxin, diuretics, insulin, lithium, methotrexate, oral antidiabetic drugs.

Possible Side-Effects (natural, expected and unavoidable drug actions)
  Fluid retention (weight gain).

▷ **Possible Adverse Effects** (unusual, unexpected and infrequent reactions)
  If any of the following develop, consult your physician promptly for guidance.
  Mild Adverse Effects
  Allergic Reactions: Skin rash, hives, itching.
  Headache, dizziness, drowsiness, depression, anxiety, insomnia, blurred vision, double vision, reversible hearing loss, ear ringing, altered taste.
  Mouth soreness, stomach discomfort, nausea, vomiting, indigestion, constipation, diarrhea.
  Serious Adverse Effects
  Allergic Reactions: Severe skin reactions, eczema, bruising, erythema multiforme, Stevens-Johnson syndrome, hair loss; swelling of lips, tongue, vocal cords; anaphylactoid reaction (see Glossary).
  Drug-induced peptic ulcers, with bleeding and perforation; colitis with bloody diarrhea.
  Abnormally low red blood cell, white blood cell and blood platelet counts; rare aplastic anemia (see Glossary).
  Liver injury with jaundice.
  Kidney injury with significantly impaired function.

▷ **Possible Effects on Sexual Function:** Impotence reported (less than 1%), but causal relationship not established.

Possible Delayed Adverse Effects: Mild anemia due to "silent" blood loss from the stomach (less than that caused by aspirin).

▷ **Adverse Effects That May Mimic Natural Diseases or Disorders**
Liver reactions may suggest viral hepatitis.

▷ **Natural Diseases or Disorders That May Be Activated by This Drug**
Peptic ulcer disease, Crohn's disease, ulcerative colitis, porphyria, kidney failure associated with systemic lupus erythematosus.

CAUTION
1. Dosage should always be limited to the smallest amount that produces reasonable improvement.
2. This drug may mask early indications of infection. Inform your physician if you think you are developing an infection of any kind.
3. Observe for a pattern of symptoms that may indicate the development of liver toxicity: fatigue, lethargy, "flulike" symptoms, nausea, itching, tenderness under the right rib cage, jaundice (see Glossary). Report such symptoms promptly.
4. Observe for possible drug-induced bleeding in the gastrointestinal tract: bloody (reddish) or tarry (black) stools.

Precautions for Use
By Infants and Children: Safety and effectiveness for use by those under 12 years of age have not been established.
By Those over 60 Years of Age: Small doses are advisable initially until tolerance is determined. Observe for any indications of liver or kidney toxicity, fluid retention, dizziness, confusion, impaired memory, stomach bleeding or constipation.

▷ **Advisability of Use During Pregnancy**
Pregnancy Category: B (tentative). See Pregnancy Code inside back cover.
Animal studies: Mouse, rat and rabbit studies reveal toxic effects on the embryo but no birth defects due to this drug.
Human studies: Information from adequate studies of pregnant women is not available.
Avoid this drug completely during the last 3 months. Use it during the first 6 months only if clearly needed. Ask your physician for guidance.

Advisability of Use if Breast-Feeding
Presence of this drug in breast milk: Yes.
Avoid drug or refrain from nursing.

Habit-Forming Potential: None.

Effects of Overdosage: Probable drowsiness, dizziness, ear ringing, nausea, vomiting, diarrhea, confusion, unsteadiness, stupor.

Possible Effects of Long-Term Use: Secondary anemia (chronic blood loss from stomach), fluid retention, elevated blood pressure.

Suggested Periodic Examinations While Taking This Drug (at physician's discretion)

Complete blood cell counts; liver function tests within the first 8 weeks of use and periodically thereafter; kidney function tests.

Complete eye examinations if vision is altered in any way.

▷ **While Taking This Drug, Observe the Following**

Foods: No restrictions.

Nutritional Support: Supplemental iron if anemia develops.

Beverages: No restrictions. May be taken with milk.

▷ *Alcohol:* Use sparingly and with caution. The irritant action of alcohol on the stomach lining, added to the irritant action of this drug in sensitive individuals, can increase the risk of stomach ulceration and/or bleeding.

Tobacco Smoking: No interactions expected.

▷ *Other Drugs*

Diclofenac may *increase* the effects of

- acetaminophen (Tylenol, etc.), and increase the risk of liver or kidney damage; avoid prolonged use of this combination.
- anticoagulants (Coumadin, etc.), and increase the risk of bleeding; monitor prothrombin time, adjust dose accordingly.
- aspirin, and increase the risk of stomach ulceration and/or bleeding; avoid this combination.

Diclofenac may *decrease* the effects of

- amiloride (Midamor, Moduretic), and raise blood potassium levels.
- oral antidiabetic drugs (see Drug Class, Section Four), and alter control of blood sugar unpredictably.
- bumetanide (Bumex).
- chlorthalidone (Hygroton, etc.).
- ethacrynic acid (Edecrin).
- furosemide (Lasix).
- indapamide (Lozol).
- metolazone (Diulo, Zaroxolyn).
- spironolactone (Aldactone, Aldactazide), and raise blood potassium levels.
- thiazide diuretics (see Drug Class, Section Four).
- triamterene (Dyazide, Maxzide), and raise blood potassium levels.

Diclofenac *taken concurrently* with the following drugs may increase the risk of bleeding (antiplatelet effect); monitor these combinations closely:

- aspirin.
- colchicine (ColBenemid, etc.).
- dipyridamole (Persantine).
- indomethacin (Indocin).
- sulfinpyrazone (Anturane).
- valproic acid (Depakene).

Diclofenac *taken concurrently* with the following drugs may increase their toxicity; monitor these combinations closely:

- cyclosporine (Sandimmune).
- digoxin (Lanoxin).
- lithium (Lithane, etc.).
- methotrexate (Folex, Mexate).

The following drug may **increase** the effects of diclofenac

- probenecid (Benemid), by slowing its elimination.

▷ *Driving, Hazardous Activities:* This drug may cause dizziness, drowsiness or blurred vision. Restrict activities as necessary.

Aviation Note: The use of this drug **may be a disqualification** for piloting. Consult a designated Aviation Medical Examiner.

Exposure to Sun: Use caution until sensitivity is determined. Photosensitivity (see Glossary) has been reported.

DICYCLOMINE
(di SI kloh meen)

Introduced: 1952

Class: Antispasmodic, atropinelike drugs

Prescription: USA: Yes
Canada: No

Controlled Drug: USA: No
Canada: No

Available as Generic: Yes

Brand Names: Bentyl, ✦Bentylol, Byclomine, ✦Formulex, ✦Lomine, ✦Protylol, ✦Spasmoban, ✦Viscerol

---

BENEFITS versus RISKS

Possible Benefits	*Possible Risks*
EFFECTIVE RELIEF OF GASTROINTESTINAL SPASM	Increased internal eye pressure (important in glaucoma) Constipation Urinary retention (in predisposed persons)

▷ **Principal Uses**

As a Single Drug Product: Used primarily for its atropinelike antispasmodic effect in the management of functional disorders of the gastrointestinal tract, notably the irritable bowel syndrome (spastic colon). It is also used to relieve cramping and pain in infant colic.

How This Drug Works: Not completely established. It has been suggested that this drug may relax gastrointestinal muscle by means of a local anesthetic action that blocks reflex activity responsible for contraction and motility.

Available Dosage Forms and Strengths
  Capsules — 10 mg, 20 mg
  Injection — 10 mg per ml
    Syrup — 10 mg per 5-ml teaspoonful
  Tablets — 20 mg

▷ **Usual Adult Dosage Range:**   10 to 20 mg, 3 or 4 times daily. Total daily dosage should not exceed 160 mg. **Note: Actual dosage and administration schedule must be determined by the physician for each patient individually.**

▷ **Dosing Instructions:**   May be taken with or following food to prevent stomach irritation. The syrup may be diluted with an equal amount of water. The capsule may be opened and the tablet may be crushed for administration.

  Usual Duration of Use: Continual use on a regular schedule for 2 to 5 days is usually necessary to determine this drug's effectiveness in relieving the symptoms of spastic disorders of the digestive system. Limit use to the relief of symptoms as necessary. Ask physician for guidance regarding long-term use.

▷ **This Drug Should Not Be Taken If**
  • you have had an allergic reaction to any dosage form of it previously.
  • your stomach cannot empty properly into the intestine (pyloric obstruction).
  • you are unable to empty the urinary bladder completely.
  • you have ulcerative colitis.

▷ **Inform Your Physician Before Taking This Drug If**
  • you have a history of peptic ulcer disease.
  • you have impaired liver or kidney function.
  • you have glaucoma, myasthenia gravis or prostatism (see Glossary).

  Possible Side-Effects (natural, expected and unavoidable drug actions)
  Dryness of the mouth, blurred vision, constipation.

▷ **Possible Adverse Effects** (unusual, unexpected and infrequent reactions)
  If any of the following develop, consult your physician promptly for guidance.
  Mild Adverse Effects
  Allergic Reactions: Skin rash, hives.
  Headache, dizziness, drowsiness, weakness.
  Reduced appetite, nausea, vomiting.
  Difficult urination.
  Serious Adverse Effects
  Allergic Reaction: Anaphylactic reaction (see Glossary).
  Idiosyncratic Reactions: Excitement, confusion, disturbed behavior.
  Increased internal eye pressure (significant in glaucoma).

▷ **Possible Effects on Sexual Function**
Impotence (6-hour effect following dosage).
Suppression of milk production.

Natural Diseases or Disorders That May Be Activated by This Drug
Glaucoma, prostatism (see Glossary).

CAUTION
Many over-the-counter medications (see OTC drugs in Glossary) for allergies, colds and coughs contain drugs that can interact unfavorably with this drug. Ask your physician or pharmacist for guidance before using any such medications.

Precautions for Use
By Infants and Children: Use extreme care in giving syrup to infants so as to prevent aspiration (inhalation) of the drug. Serious reactions have occurred as a result of this accident during administration.
By Those over 60 Years of Age: Begin treatment with small doses until tolerance is determined. You may be more susceptible to the development of confusion, excitement, constipation and prostatism.

▷ **Advisability of Use During Pregnancy**
Pregnancy Category: B (tentative). See Pregnancy Code inside back cover.
Animal studies: No birth defects reported.
Human studies: Information from adequate studies of pregnant women is not available.
Use only if clearly needed. Ask physician for guidance.

Advisability of Use if Breast-Feeding
Presence of this drug in breast milk: Unknown.
Avoid drug or refrain from nursing.

Habit-Forming Potential: None.

Effects of Overdosage: Headache, dizziness, nausea, dry mouth, difficulty in swallowing, excitement, restlessness, dilated pupils, hot and dry skin.

Possible Effects of Long-Term Use: None reported.

Suggested Periodic Examinations While Taking This Drug (at physician's discretion)
Measurements of internal eye pressure (in presence of glaucoma or suspected glaucoma).

▷ **While Taking This Drug, Observe the Following**
Foods: No interactions. Follow prescribed diet.
Beverages: No interactions. May be taken with milk.
▷ *Alcohol:* Use caution until combined effects have been determined. Observe for increased drowsiness.
Tobacco Smoking: No interactions expected. Follow physician's advice regarding smoking.

Marijuana Smoking: Possible increase in drowsiness and dryness of mouth.

▷ *Other Drugs*

Dicyclomine may *increase* the effects of
- other drugs that have atropinelike actions (see Drug Class, Section Four).

Dicyclomine may *decrease* the effects of
- levodopa (Larodopa, Sinemet, etc.).

▷ *Driving, Hazardous Activities:* This drug may cause drowsiness, dizziness or blurred vision. Restrict activities accordingly.

Aviation Note: The use of this drug *may be a disqualification* for piloting. Consult a designated Aviation Medical Examiner.

Exposure to Sun: No restrictions.

Exposure to Heat: Use caution. The use of this drug in hot environments may impair normal perspiration and interfere with the regulation of body temperature, thus increasing the risk of heat stroke.

DIFLUNISAL
(di FLOO ni sal)

Introduced: 1977

Class: Mild analgesic, anti-inflammatory

Prescription: USA: Yes
Canada: Yes

Controlled Drug: USA: No
Canada: No

Available as Generic: No

Brand Name: Dolobid

BENEFITS versus RISKS	
Possible Benefits	*Possible Risks*
EFFECTIVE RELIEF OF MILD TO MODERATE PAIN AND INFLAMMATION	Gastrointestinal pain, ulceration, bleeding (rare)
	Rare liver or kidney damage
	Rare fluid retention

▷ **Principal Uses**

As a Single Drug Product: Used primarily to relieve mild to moderately severe pain associated with (1) musculoskeletal injuries; (2) acute and chronic rheumatoid arthritis and osteoarthritis; and (3) dental, obstetrical and orthopedic surgery.

How This Drug Works: Not completely established. It is thought that this drug reduces the tissue concentrations of prostaglandins (and related compounds), chemicals involved in the production of inflammation and pain.

Available Dosage Forms and Strengths
Tablets — 250 mg, 500 mg

▷ **Usual Adult Dosage Range:** Initially 500 to 1000 mg (loading dose), then 250 to 500 mg/8 to 12 hours. Total daily dosage should not exceed 1500 mg. **Note: Actual dosage and administration schedule must be determined by the physician for each patient individually.**

▷ **Dosing Instructions:** Take either on an empty stomach or with food or milk to prevent stomach irritation. Swallow tablets whole; do not crush or chew. Take with a full glass of water and remain upright (do not lie down) for 30 minutes.

Usual Duration of Use: Continual use on a regular schedule for 1 to 2 weeks is usually necessary to determine this drug's effectiveness in relieving the discomfort of arthritis. Long-term use requires supervision and periodic evaluation by the physician. Consult your physician on a regular basis.

▷ **This Drug Should Not Be Taken If**
- you have had an allergic reaction to it previously.
- you are subject to asthma or nasal polyps caused by aspirin.
- you have active peptic ulcer disease or any form of gastrointestinal bleeding.

▷ **Inform Your Physician Before Taking This Drug If**
- you are allergic to aspirin or to other aspirin substitutes.
- you have a history of peptic ulcer disease or any type of bleeding disorder.
- you have impaired liver or kidney function.
- you have high blood pressure or a history of heart failure.
- you are pregnant.
- you are taking any of the following: acetaminophen, aspirin or other aspirin substitutes, anticoagulants, oral antidiabetic drugs.

Possible Side-Effects (natural, expected and unavoidable drug actions)
Drowsiness, ringing in ears, fluid retention.

▷ **Possible Adverse Effects** (unusual, unexpected and infrequent reactions)
If any of the following develop, consult your physician promptly for guidance.
Mild Adverse Effects
Allergic Reactions: Skin rash, hives, itching.
Headache, dizziness, altered or blurred vision, depression.
Mouth sores, indigestion, nausea, vomiting, constipation, diarrhea.
Serious Adverse Effects
Allergic Reactions: Severe skin reactions, swollen lymph glands, drug fever (see Glossary), asthma, anaphylaxis (see Glossary).

Active peptic ulcer, with or without bleeding.

Liver damage with jaundice (see Glossary).

Kidney damage with painful urination, bloody urine, reduced urine formation.

Reduced blood platelet (see Glossary) count with abnormal bleeding or bruising.

▷ **Possible Effects on Sexual Function:**   None reported.

▷ **Adverse Effects That May Mimic Natural Diseases or Disorders**
Liver reaction may suggest viral hepatitis.

Natural Diseases or Disorders That May Be Activated by This Drug
Peptic ulcer disease, ulcerative colitis.

CAUTION
1. Inform your physician promptly if flulike symptoms develop in association with a skin rash; this could represent a serious allergic reaction.
2. This drug may mask early indications of infection. Inform your physician if you think you are developing an infection of any kind.

Precautions for Use
By Infants and Children: Safety and effectiveness for use by those under 12 years of age have not been established.
By Those over 60 Years of Age: Small doses are advisable until tolerance is determined. Observe for any indications of liver or kidney toxicity.

▷ **Advisability of Use During Pregnancy**
Pregnancy Category: C (tentative). See Pregnancy Code inside back cover.
Animal studies: Skeletal birth defects reported in rabbits.
Human studies: Information from adequate studies of pregnant women is not available.
Avoid this drug during the first and last 3 months. Use it during the middle 3 months only if clearly needed. Ask physician for guidance.

Advisability of Use if Breast-Feeding
Presence of this drug in breast milk: Yes.
Avoid drug or refrain from nursing.

Habit-Forming Potential: None.

Effects of Overdosage: Drowsiness, confusion, disorientation, nausea, vomiting, stupor.

Possible Effects of Long-Term Use: None reported.

Suggested Periodic Examinations While Taking This Drug (at physician's discretion)
Complete blood cell counts, liver and kidney function tests.
Complete eye examinations if vision is altered in any way.

▷ **While Taking This Drug, Observe the Following**

Foods: No restrictions.

Beverages: No restrictions. May be taken with milk.

▷ *Alcohol:* Use with caution. The irritant action of alcohol on the stomach lining, added to the irritant action of this drug in sensitive individuals, can increase the risk of stomach ulceration and/or bleeding.

Tobacco Smoking: No interactions expected.

▷ *Other Drugs*

Diflunisal may ***increase*** the effects of
- acetaminophen (Tylenol, etc.), and increase the risk of liver damage; avoid this combination.
- anticoagulants (Coumadin, etc.), and increase the risk of bleeding; monitor prothrombin time, adjust dose accordingly.
- hydrochlorothiazide (Esidrix, HydroDiuril, etc.).

Diflunisal ***taken concurrently*** with the following drugs may increase the risk of bleeding; avoid these combinations:
- aspirin.
- dipyridamole (Persantine).
- indomethacin (Indocin).
- sulfinpyrazone (Anturane).
- valproic acid (Depakene).

The following drugs may ***decrease*** the effects of diflunisal
- aluminum antacids may decrease its absorption.

▷ *Driving, Hazardous Activities:* This drug may cause drowsiness, dizziness or altered vision. Restrict activities as necessary.

Aviation Note: The use of this drug ***may be a disqualification*** for piloting. Consult a designated Aviation Medical Examiner.

Exposure to Sun: Use caution until sensitivity is determined. This drug may cause photosensitivity (see Glossary).

DIGOXIN
(di JOX in)

Introduced: 1934

Class: Digitalis preparations

Prescription: USA: Yes
Canada: No

Controlled Drug: USA: No
Canada: No

Available as Generic: Yes

Brand Names: Lanoxicaps, Lanoxin, ✦Novodigoxin

```
┌─────────────────────────────────────────────────────────────────┐
│                    BENEFITS versus RISKS                         │
│                                                                   │
│      Possible Benefits                  Possible Risks           │
│  EFFECTIVE HEART STIMULANT      NARROW TREATMENT RANGE            │
│    IN CONGESTIVE HEART            (treatment dose is 60% of toxic │
│    FAILURE                        dose)                          │
│  EFFECTIVE PREVENTION AND       Frequent and sometimes serious   │
│    TREATMENT OF CERTAIN           disturbances of heart rhythm   │
│    HEART RHYTHM DISORDERS                                        │
└─────────────────────────────────────────────────────────────────┘
```

▷ **Principal Uses**

As a Single Drug Product: This drug has two primary uses: (1) the treatment of congestive heart failure; (2) the restoration and maintenance of normal heart rate and rhythm in such disorders as atrial fibrillation, atrial flutter and atrial/supraventricular tachycardia.

How This Drug Works: By increasing the availability of calcium within the heart muscle, this drug improves the efficiency of the conversion of chemical energy to mechanical energy, thus increasing the force of heart muscle contraction. By slowing the activity of the pacemaker and delaying the transmission of electrical impulses through the conduction system of the heart, this drug assists in restoring normal heart rate and rhythm.

Available Dosage Forms and Strengths
Elixir, pediatric — 0.05 mg per ml
Capsules — 0.05 mg, 0.1 mg, 0.2 mg
Injection — 0.1 mg per ml, 0.25 mg per ml
Tablets — 0.125 mg, 0.25 mg, 0.5 mg

▷ **Usual Adult Dosage Range:** Rapid digitalization—1 to 1.5 mg divided into 2 or 3 doses given every 6 to 8 hours in 1 day. Slow digitalization— 0.125 to 0.5 mg/day for 7 days. Maintenance—0.125 to 0.5 mg/day. Total daily dosage should not exceed 2 mg. **Note: Actual dosage and administration schedule must be determined by the physician for each patient individually.**

▷ **Dosing Instructions:** Take at the same time each day, or preferably on an empty stomach to ensure uniform absorption. May be taken with or following food if desired (not milk or dairy products). The tablet may be crushed for administration; the capsule should be swallowed whole.

Usual Duration of Use: Continual use on a regular schedule for 7 to 10 days is usually necessary to determine this drug's effectiveness in relieving heart failure or controlling heart rhythm disorders. Long-term use requires physician supervision and periodic assessment of continued need. The use of this drug is not necessarily "for life." Consult your physician on a regular basis.

▷ **This Drug Should Not Be Taken If**
  • you have had an allergic reaction to any dosage form of it previously.

▷ **Inform Your Physician Before Taking This Drug If**
  • you have experienced any unfavorable reaction to a digitalis preparation in the past.
  • you have taken any digitalis preparation within the past 2 weeks.
  • you are now taking (or have recently taken) any diuretic (urine-producing) drug.
  • you have impaired liver or kidney function.
  • you have a history of thyroid function disorder.

Possible Side-Effects (natural, expected and unavoidable drug actions)
  Slow heart rate, rare enlargement and/or sensitivity of the male breast tissue.

▷ **Possible Adverse Effects** (unusual, unexpected and infrequent reactions)
  If any of the following develop, consult your physician promptly for guidance.
  Mild Adverse Effects
  Allergic Reactions: Skin rash, hives.
  Headache, drowsiness, lethargy, confusion, changes in vision: "halo" effect, blurring, spots, double vision, yellow-green vision.
  Loss of appetite, nausea, vomiting, diarrhea—early indications of toxicity in adults.
  Serious Adverse Effects
  Idiosyncratic Reactions: Hallucinations, facial neuralgias, peripheral neuralgias, blindness (very rare).
  Disorientation, most common in the elderly.
  Heart rhythm disturbances.

▷ **Possible Effects on Sexual Function**
  Decreased libido and impotence in 35% of male users.
  Enlargement and tenderness of male breasts.
  Both effects are attributed to digoxin's estrogenlike action.

▷ **Adverse Effects That May Mimic Natural Diseases or Disorders**
  Drug-induced mental disturbances in the elderly may be mistaken for senile dementia or psychosis.

Natural Diseases or Disorders That May Be Activated by This Drug
  Digitalis may induce a systemic lupus erythematosus–like syndrome.

CAUTION
  1. This drug has a narrow margin of safe use. Adhere strictly to prescribed dosage schedules. Do not raise or lower the dose without first consulting your physician.
  2. If you are taking calcium supplements, ask your physician for guidance. Avoid large doses.
  3. It is advisable to carry a card of personal identification with a notation that you are taking this drug.

4. Avoid taking over-the-counter antacids and cold, cough and allergy remedies without consulting your physician.

Precautions for Use

By Infants and Children: Observe carefully for indications of toxicity: slow heart rate (below 60 beats/minute), irregular heart rhythms.

By Those over 60 Years of Age: You may have a reduced tolerance for this drug; smaller doses are advisable. Observe for indications of early toxicity: headache, dizziness, fatigue, weakness, lethargy, depression, confusion, nervousness, agitation, delusions, difficulty with reading. Report the development of any of these effects promptly to your physician.

▷ **Advisability of Use During Pregnancy**

Pregnancy Category: C (tentative). See Pregnancy Code inside back cover.

Animal studies: No birth defects reported.

Human studies: Information from adequate studies of pregnant women is not available. However, no birth defects attributable to the therapeutic use of this drug have been reported.

Use this drug only if clearly needed. Overdosage can be harmful to the fetus.

Advisability of Use if Breast-Feeding

Presence of this drug in breast milk: Yes.

Monitor nursing infant closely and discontinue drug or nursing if adverse effects develop.

Habit-Forming Potential: None.

Effects of Overdosage: Loss of appetite, excessive saliva, nausea, vomiting, diarrhea, serious disturbances of heart rate and rhythm, intestinal bleeding, drowsiness, headache, confusion, delirium, hallucinations, convulsions.

Possible Effects of Long-Term Use: None reported.

Suggested Periodic Examinations While Taking This Drug (at physician's discretion)

Measurements of blood levels of digoxin, calcium, magnesium and potassium; electrocardiograms.

▷ **While Taking This Drug, Observe the Following**

Foods: Avoid all cheeses, yogurt and ice cream for 2 hours before and after taking this drug. Consult physician regarding the advisability of eating high-potassium foods.

Beverages: Avoid all forms of milk for 2 hours before and after taking this drug. Avoid excessive amounts of caffeine-containing beverages: coffee, tea, cola.

▷ *Alcohol:* No interactions expected.

Tobacco Smoking: Nicotine can cause irritability of the heart muscle and can predispose to serious rhythm disturbances. It is advisable to abstain from all forms of tobacco.

Marijuana Smoking: Possible accentuation of heart failure; reduced digoxin effect; possible changes in electrocardiogram, confusing interpretation.

▷ *Other Drugs*

Digoxin *taken concurrently* with

- diuretics (other than spironolactone and triamterene) may result in serious heart rhythm disturbances due to excessive loss of potassium.
- quinidine may result in decreased digoxin effectiveness and increased digoxin toxicity; careful dosage adjustments are necessary.

The following drugs may *increase* the effects of digoxin

- amiodarone (Cordarone).
- benzodiazepines (Librium, Valium, etc.; see Drug Class, Section Four).
- captopril (Capoten, Capazide).
- diltiazem (Cardizem).
- erythromycin (EES, Erythrocin, etc.).
- flecainide (Tambocor).
- hydroxychloroquine.
- ibuprofen (Advil, Medipren, Motrin, Nuprin, etc.).
- indomethacin (Indocin).
- methimazole (Tapazole).
- nifedipine (Adalat, Procardia).
- propylthiouracil (Propacil).
- quinine.
- tetracyclines (see Drug Class, Section Four).
- tolbutamide (Orinase).
- verapamil (Isoptin).

The following drugs may *decrease* the effects of digoxin

- aluminum-containing antacids (Amphojel, Maalox, etc.).
- bleomycin (Blenoxane).
- carmustine (Bicnu).
- cholestyramine (Questran).
- colestipol (Colestid).
- cyclophosphamide (Cytoxan).
- cytarabine (Cytosar).
- doxorubicin (Adriamycin).
- methotrexate (Mexate).
- penicillamine (Cuprimine, Depen).
- procarbazine (Matulane).
- thyroid hormones.
- vincristine (Oncovin).

▷ *Driving, Hazardous Activities:* Usually no restrictions. However, this drug may cause drowsiness, vision changes and nausea. Restrict activities as necessary.

Aviation Note: Heart function disorders *are a disqualification* for piloting. Consult a designated Aviation Medical Examiner.

Exposure to Sun: No restrictions.

Occurrence of Unrelated Illness: Any illness that causes vomiting or diarrhea can seriously alter this drug's effectiveness. Notify your physician promptly.

Discontinuation: This drug must be continued indefinitely. Do not discontinue it without consulting your physician.

DILTIAZEM
(dil TI a zem)

Introduced: 1977

Class: Antianginal, antihypertensive, calcium channel blocker

Prescription: USA: Yes
Canada: Yes

Controlled Drug: USA: No
Canada: No

Available as Generic: No

Brand Names: Cardizem, Cardizem SR

BENEFITS versus RISKS	
Possible Benefits	*Possible Risks*
EFFECTIVE PREVENTION OF BOTH MAJOR TYPES OF ANGINA	Depression, confusion
	Low blood pressure
	Heart rhythm disturbance (2%)
EFFECTIVE CONTROL OF MILD TO MODERATE HYPERTENSION	Fluid retention (2.4%)
	Liver damage (very rare)

▷ **Principal Uses**

As a Single Drug Product: Used primarily to treat (1) angina pectoris due to coronary artery spasm (Prinzmetal's variant angina) that occurs spontaneously and is not associated with exertion; (2) classical angina-of-effort (due to atherosclerotic disease of the coronary arteries) in individuals who have not responded to or cannot tolerate the nitrates and beta blocker drugs customarily used to treat this disorder; (3) mild to moderately severe hypertension.

How This Drug Works: Not completely established. It is thought that by blocking the normal passage of calcium through certain cell walls (which is necessary for the function of nerve and muscle tissue), this drug slows the spread of electrical activity through the conduction system of the heart and inhibits the contraction of coronary arteries and peripheral arterioles. As a result of these combined effects, this drug

- prevents spontaneous spasm of the coronary arteries (Prinzmetal's type of angina).
- reduces the rate and contraction force of the heart during exertion, thus lowering the oxygen requirement of the heart muscle; this reduces the occurrence of effort-induced angina (classical angina pectoris).
- reduces the degree of contraction of peripheral arterial walls, resulting in their relaxation and consequent lowering of blood pressure. This further reduces the work load of the heart during exertion and contributes to the prevention of angina.

Available Dosage Forms and Strengths
Tablets — 30 mg, 60 mg, 90 mg, 120 mg
Capsules, prolonged-action — 60 mg, 90 mg, 120 mg

▷ **Usual Adult Dosage Range:**   Initially 30 mg, 3 or 4 times daily. Dose may be increased gradually at 1- to 2-day intervals as needed and tolerated. Total daily dosage should not exceed 360 mg. **Note: Actual dosage and administration schedule must be determined by the physician for each patient individually.**

▷ **Dosing Instructions:**   Preferably taken before meals and at bedtime. Tablet may be crushed for administration.

Usual Duration of Use: Continual use on a regular schedule for 2 to 4 weeks is usually necessary to determine this drug's effectiveness in reducing the frequency and severity of angina and in lowering elevated blood pressure. For long-term use (months to years), determine the smallest effective dose. Consult your physician on a regular basis.

Possible Advantages of This Drug
Often effective as single drug therapy.
Does not reduce blood supply to kidneys.
Does not raise blood cholesterol levels.
Does not induce asthma in susceptible individuals.

▷ **This Drug Should Not Be Taken If**
- you have had an allergic reaction to it previously.
- you have a "sick sinus" syndrome (and are not wearing an artificial pacemaker).
- you have been told that you have a second-degree or third-degree heart block.
- you have low blood pressure—systolic pressure below 90.

▷ **Inform Your Physician Before Taking This Drug If**
- you have had an unfavorable response to any calcium blocker drug in the past.
- you are currently taking any form of digitalis or a beta blocker drug (see Drug Class, Section Four).

- you have a history of congestive heart failure.
- you have impaired liver or kidney function.
- you have a history of drug-induced liver damage.

Possible Side-Effects (natural, expected and unavoidable drug actions)
Fatigue (1.2%), light-headedness, heart rate and rhythm changes in pre-disposed individuals (1.1%).

▷ **Possible Adverse Effects** (unusual, unexpected and infrequent reactions)
If any of the following develop, consult your physician promptly for guidance.
Mild Adverse Effects
Allergic Reactions: Skin rash (1.3%), hives, itching.
Headache (2.1%), drowsiness, dizziness (1.5%), nervousness, insomnia, depression, confusion, hallucinations.
Flushing, palpitations, fainting, slow heart rate, low blood pressure.
Nausea (1.9%), indigestion, heartburn, vomiting, diarrhea, constipation.
Serious Adverse Effects
Serious disturbances of heart rate and/or rhythm, fluid retention (edema) (2.4%), congestive heart failure.
Drug-induced liver damage (very rare).

▷ **Possible Effects on Sexual Function:** Impotence is reported in less than 1% of users.

CAUTION
1. Be sure to inform all physicians and dentists you consult that you are taking this drug. Note the use of this drug on your card of personal identification.
2. You may use nitroglycerin and other nitrate drugs as needed to relieve acute episodes of angina pain. However, if you detect that your angina attacks are becoming more frequent or intense, notify your physician promptly.

Precautions for Use
By Infants and Children: Safety and effectiveness for use by those under 12 years of age have not been established.
By Those over 60 Years of Age: You may be more susceptible to the development of weakness, dizziness, fainting and falling. Take necessary precautions to prevent injury. Report promptly any changes in your pattern of thirst and urination.

▷ **Advisability of Use During Pregnancy**
Pregnancy Category: C (tentative). See Pregnancy Code inside back cover.
Animal studies: Embryo and fetal deaths and skeletal birth defects reported in mice, rats and rabbits.
Human studies: Information from adequate studies of pregnant women is not available.
Avoid this drug during the first 3 months.

Use during the last 6 months only if clearly needed. Ask physician for guidance.

Advisability of Use if Breast-Feeding
Presence of this drug in breast milk: Yes.
Avoid drug or refrain from nursing.

Habit-Forming Potential: None.

Effects of Overdosage: Weakness, light-headedness, fainting, slow pulse, low blood pressure, shortness of breath, congestive heart failure.

Possible Effects of Long-Term Use: None reported.

Suggested Periodic Examinations While Taking This Drug (at physician's discretion)
Evaluations of heart function, including electrocardiograms; liver and kidney function tests, with long-term use.

▷ **While Taking This Drug, Observe the Following**
Foods: No restrictions. Avoid excessive salt intake.
Beverages: No restrictions. May be taken with milk.
▷ *Alcohol:* Use with caution until combined effects have been determined. Alcohol may exaggerate the drop in blood pressure experienced by some individuals.
Tobacco Smoking: Nicotine may reduce the effectiveness of this drug. Follow your physician's advice regarding smoking.
Marijuana Smoking: Possible reduced effectiveness of this drug; mild to moderate increase in angina; possible changes in electrocardiogram, confusing interpretation.
▷ *Other Drugs*
Diltiazem *taken concurrently* with
• beta blocker drugs or digitalis preparations (see Drug Classes, Section Four) may affect heart rate and rhythm adversely. Careful monitoring by your physician is necessary if these drugs are taken concurrently.
The following drugs may *increase* the effects of diltiazem
• cimetidine (Tagamet).
▷ *Driving, Hazardous Activities:* Usually no restrictions. This drug may cause drowsiness or dizziness. Restrict activities as necessary.
Aviation Note: Coronary artery disease *is a disqualification* for piloting. Consult a designated Aviation Medical Examiner.
Exposure to Sun: Use caution until sensitivity has been determined. This drug may cause photosensitivity (see Glossary).
Exposure to Heat: Caution advised. Hot environments can exaggerate the blood-pressure-lowering effects of this drug. Observe for light-headedness or weakness.
Heavy Exercise or Exertion: This drug may improve your ability to be more active without resulting angina pain. Use caution and avoid excessive exercise that could impair heart function in the absence of warning pain.

Discontinuation: Do not discontinue this drug abruptly. Consult your physician regarding gradual withdrawal.

DIPHENHYDRAMINE
(di fen HI dra meen)

Introduced: 1946

Class: Hypnotic, antihistamines

Prescription: USA: Varies
Canada: No

Controlled Drug: USA: No*
Canada: No

Available as Generic: Yes

Brand Names: ✦Allerdryl, ✦Ambenyl Expectorant [CD], Ambenyl Syrup [CD], Benadryl, Benadryl 25, Benylin, ✦Benylin Decongestant [CD], ✦Benylin Pediatric Syrup, ✦Benylin Syrup w/Codeine [CD], ✦Caladryl [CD], Compoz, ✦Ergodryl [CD], Excedrin P.M. [CD], Genahist, ✦Insomnal, ✦Mandrax [CD], Nytol, Sleep-Eze 3, Sominex 2, Twilite, Valdrene

---

BENEFITS versus RISKS

Possible Benefits	*Possible Risks*
EFFECTIVE RELIEF OF ALLERGIC RHINITIS AND ALLERGIC SKIN DISORDERS	Marked sedation (50%)
	Atropinelike effects
EFFECTIVE, NONADDICTIVE SEDATIVE AND HYPNOTIC	Accentuation of prostatism (see Glossary)
Prevention and relief of motion sickness	Rare blood cell disorders: abnormally low white blood cell and platelet counts
Partial relief of symptoms of Parkinson's disease	

▷ **Principal Uses**

As a Single Drug Product: This versatile antihistamine is used primarily for (1) the safe and effective induction of sleep (mild to moderate sedation); (2) the prevention and treatment of motion sickness (control of dizziness, nausea and vomiting); (3) the relief of symptoms associated with Parkinson's disease; (4) the treatment of drug-induced parkinsonian reactions, especially in children and the elderly.

As a Combination Drug Product [CD]: This drug may have a mild suppressant effect on coughing, but its actual effectiveness is questionable. It is combined with expectorants and either codeine or dextromethorphan in some cough preparations.

*Ambenyl Syrup is C-V. See Schedules of Controlled Drugs inside back cover.

How This Drug Works: This drug reduces the intensity of allergic response by blocking the action of histamine after it has been released from sensitized tissue cells. Its natural side-effects are used to advantage: its sedative action is used to induce drowsiness and sleep; its atropinelike action is used in the management of motion sickness and Parkinson-related disorders.

Available Dosage Forms and Strengths
> Capsules — 25 mg, 50 mg
> Cream — 1%
> Elixir — 12.5 mg per 5-ml teaspoonful (14% alcohol)
> Syrup — 12.5 mg, 13.3 mg per 5-ml teaspoonful
> Tablets — 25 mg, 50 mg

▷ **Usual Adult Dosage Range:**   25 to 50 mg/4 to 6 hours. Total daily dosage should not exceed 300 mg. **Note: Actual dosage and administration schedule must be determined by the physician for each patient individually.**

▷ **Dosing Instructions:**   Preferably taken with or following food to reduce stomach irritation. Tablet may be crushed and capsule may be opened for administration.

Usual Duration of Use: Continual use on a regular schedule for 2 to 3 days is usually necessary to determine this drug's effectiveness in relieving the symptoms of allergic rhinitis and dermatosis. If not effective after 5 days, this drug should be discontinued. As a bedtime sedative (hypnotic), use only as needed. Avoid long-term use without interruption.

▷ **This Drug Should Not Be Taken If**
- you have had an allergic reaction to any dosage form of it previously.
- you are taking, or have taken during the past 2 weeks, any monoamine oxidase (MAO) type A inhibitor drug (see Drug Class, Section Four).

▷ **Inform Your Physician Before Taking This Drug If**
- you have had an unfavorable response to any antihistamine drug in the past.
- you have narrow-angle glaucoma.
- you have peptic ulcer disease, with any degree of pyloric obstruction.
- you have prostatism (see Glossary).
- you are subject to bronchial asthma or seizures (epilepsy).

Possible Side-Effects (natural, expected and unavoidable drug actions)
Drowsiness; sense of weakness; dryness of nose, mouth and throat; constipation.

▷ **Possible Adverse Effects** (unusual, unexpected and infrequent reactions)
If any of the following develop, consult your physician promptly for guidance.

Mild Adverse Effects
 Allergic Reactions: Skin rash, hives.
 Headache, dizziness, inability to concentrate, nervousness, blurred or double vision, difficult urination.
 Reduced tolerance for contact lenses.
 Nausea, vomiting, diarrhea.
Serious Adverse Effects
 Allergic Reaction: Anaphylactic reaction (see Glossary).
 Idiosyncratic Reactions: Insomnia, excitement, confusion.
 Hemolytic anemia (see Glossary).
 Reduced white blood cell count—fever, sore throat, infections.
 Blood platelet destruction (see Glossary)—abnormal bleeding or bruising.

▷ **Possible Effects on Sexual Function:** Shortened menstrual cycle (early arrival of expected menstrual onset).

Natural Diseases or Disorders That May Be Activated by This Drug
 Latent epilepsy, glaucoma, prostatism.

CAUTION
 1. Discontinue this drug 5 days before diagnostic skin testing procedures in order to prevent false negative test results.
 2. Do not use this drug if you have active bronchial asthma, bronchitis or pneumonia. It can thicken bronchial mucous and make it more difficult to remove (by absorption or coughing).

Precautions for Use
 By Infants and Children: This drug should not be used in premature or full-term newborn infants. Doses for children should be small. The young child is especially sensitive to the effects of antihistamines on the brain and nervous system. Avoid the use of this drug in the child with chicken pox or a flulike infection; although unproven, this drug may adversely affect the course of Reye syndrome should the child develop it during the course of illness.
 By Those over 60 Years of Age: You may be more susceptible to the development of drowsiness, dizziness and unsteadiness, and to impairment of thinking, judgment and memory. This drug can increase the degree of impaired urination associated with prostate gland enlargement (prostatism). The sedative effects of antihistamines in the elderly can cause a syndrome of underactivity that may be misinterpreted as senility or emotional depression.

▷ **Advisability of Use During Pregnancy**
 Pregnancy Category: B (tentative). See Pregnancy Code inside back cover.
 Animal studies: No birth defects reported in rats or rabbits.
 Human studies: Information from studies of pregnant women indicates no significant increase in birth defects in 2948 exposures to this drug. A withdrawal syndrome of tremor and diarrhea has been reported in

a 5-day-old infant whose mother used this drug (150 mg daily) during pregnancy.

Avoid drug during the last 3 months. Use sparingly during the first 6 months only if clearly needed.

Advisability of Use if Breast-Feeding

Presence of this drug in breast milk: Yes.
Avoid drug or refrain from nursing.

Habit-Forming Potential: None.

Effects of Overdosage: Marked drowsiness, confusion, incoordination, unsteadiness, muscle tremors, stupor, coma, seizures, fever, flushed face, dilated pupils, weak pulse, shallow breathing.

Possible Effects of Long-Term Use: The development of tolerance (see Glossary) and reduced effectiveness of drug.

Suggested Periodic Examinations While Taking This Drug (at physician's discretion)

Complete blood cell counts.

▷ **While Taking This Drug, Observe the Following**
Foods: No restrictions.
Beverages: No restrictions. May be taken with milk.
▷   *Alcohol:* Use with extreme caution until the combined effect has been determined. The combination of alcohol and antihistamines can cause rapid and marked sedation.
Tobacco Smoking: No interactions expected.
Marijuana Smoking: Increased drowsiness and mouth dryness; possible accentuation of impaired thinking.
▷   *Other Drugs*
Diphenhydramine may ***increase*** the effects of
• all drugs with a sedative effect, and cause oversedation.
• atropine and atropinelike drugs (see Drug Class, Section Four).
The following drugs may ***increase*** the effects of diphenhydramine
• monoamine oxidase (MAO) type A inhibitor drugs (see Drug Class, Section Four) may delay its elimination, thus exaggerating and prolonging its action.
▷   *Driving, Hazardous Activities:* This drug may impair mental alertness, judgment, physical coordination and reaction time. Restrict activities as necessary.
Aviation Note: The use of this drug ***is a disqualification*** for piloting. Consult a designated Aviation Medical Examiner.
Exposure to Sun: Use caution until sensitivity has been determined. This drug may cause photosensitivity (see Glossary).
Exposure to Environmental Chemicals: The insecticides Aldrin, Dieldrin and Chlordane may decrease the effectiveness of this drug. The insecticide Sevin may increase the sedative effects of this drug.

DIPHENOXYLATE
(di fen OX i layt)

Introduced: 1960

Prescription: USA: Yes
Canada: Yes

Available as Generic: USA: Yes
Canada: No

Brand Names: Lomotil [CD], ✦Lomotil

Class: Antidiarrheal

Controlled Drug: USA: C-V*
Canada: <N>

BENEFITS versus RISKS

Possible Benefits	*Possible Risks*
EFFECTIVE RELIEF OF INTESTINAL CRAMPING AND DIARRHEA	Drowsiness Constipation Low habit-forming potential

---

▷ **Principal Uses**

As a Single Drug Product: Used primarily for the control of overactivity of the intestinal tract, cramping and diarrhea. Because of its potential for abuse, this drug is not marketed as a single-entity product in the USA.

As a Combination Drug Product [CD]: This drug, in therapeutically effective dosage, is combined with a small amount of atropine to discourage abusive overdosage. The accumulative effects of atropine overdosage would make the combination intolerable.

How This Drug Works: Not completely established. It is thought that this drug acts directly on the nerve supply of the gastrointestinal tract to reduce its motility and propulsive contractions, thus relieving cramping and diarrhea.

Available Dosage Forms and Strengths
Liquid — 2.5 mg (+ 0.025 mg atropine) per 5-ml teaspoonful
Tablets — 2.5 mg (+ 0.025 mg atropine)

▷ **Usual Adult Dosage Range:** Initially 2.5 to 5 mg/4 hours as needed for acute diarrhea; then 2.5 mg/6 to 8 hours as needed for chronic diarrhea. **Note: Actual dosage and administration schedule must be determined by the physician for each patient individually.**

▷ **Dosing Instructions:** May be taken on an empty stomach or with food if stomach irritation occurs. Tablet may be crushed for administration.

Usual Duration of Use: Continual use on a regular schedule for 24 to 36 hours is usually necessary to determine this drug's effectiveness in

*See Schedules of Controlled Drugs inside back cover.

controlling acute diarrhea. If diarrhea persists, consult your physician. Avoid prolonged and uninterrupted use.

▷ **This Drug Should Not Be Taken If**
- you are allergic to either component of this combination drug (single component in Canada).
- you have active liver disease.
- it is prescribed for a child under 2 years of age.

▷ **Inform Your Physician Before Taking This Drug If**
- you have a history of liver disease or impaired liver function.
- you have regional enteritis or ulcerative colitis.
- you have chronic lung disease of any kind.

Possible Side-Effects (natural, expected and unavoidable drug actions)
Drowsiness, constipation.

▷ **Possible Adverse Effects** (unusual, unexpected and infrequent reactions)
If any of the following develop, consult your physician promptly for guidance.
Mild Adverse Effects
Allergic Reactions: Skin rash, hives, localized swellings, itching.
Headache, dizziness, weakness, euphoria.
Reduced appetite, nausea, vomiting, bloating.
Serious Adverse Effects
"Toxic megacolon" (distended, immobile colon with fluid retention) may develop in acute ulcerative colitis.

▷ **Possible Effects on Sexual Function:**   None reported.

CAUTION
1. Do not exceed recommended doses.
2. Use with caution in the presence of chronic lung disease (asthma, bronchitis, emphysema). This drug may impair respiration.
3. If used to treat chronic diarrhea, report promptly any development of bloating, abdominal distension, nausea, vomiting, constipation or abdominal pain.

Precautions for Use
By Infants and Children: Do not use in those under 2 years of age. Use with caution (especially in children with Down's syndrome); observe closely for any indications of atropine overdosage: excitement, over-activity, hallucinations, fever, flushed face, dilated pupils.
By Those over 60 Years of Age: Start treatment with small doses. You may be more sensitive to the sedative and constipating effects of this drug.

▷ **Advisability of Use During Pregnancy**
Pregnancy Category: C (tentative). See Pregnancy Code inside back cover.
Animal studies: No information available.

Human studies: Information from adequate studies of pregnant women is not available.
Use sparingly and only if clearly needed. Ask physician for guidance.

Advisability of Use if Breast-Feeding
Presence of this drug in breast milk: Yes.
Avoid drug or refrain from nursing.

Habit-Forming Potential: Because of its similarity to meperidine, this drug may cause physical dependence (see Glossary) if used in large doses over an extended period of time.

Effects of Overdosage: Marked drowsiness, lethargy, depression, numbness in arms and legs, dry skin and mouth, flushing, fever, rapid pulse, slow and shallow breathing, stupor progressing to coma.

Possible Effects of Long-Term Use: The development of tolerance with loss of drug effectiveness. Physical dependence is a remote possibility.

Suggested Periodic Examinations While Taking This Drug (at physician's discretion)
None required.

▷ **While Taking This Drug, Observe the Following**
Foods: No restrictions. Follow prescribed diet.
Beverages: No restrictions. May be taken with milk.
▷ *Alcohol:* Use with extreme caution until combined effects have been determined. This drug may increase the depressant action of alcohol on the brain.
Tobacco Smoking: No interactions expected.
▷ *Other Drugs*
Diphenoxylate may *increase* the effects of
• all drugs with a sedative effect, and cause oversedation.
Diphenoxylate *taken concurrently* with
• monoamine oxidase (MAO) type A inhibitor drugs (see Drug Class, Section Four) will require close observation for excessive rise in blood pressure.
▷ *Driving, Hazardous Activities:* This drug may cause drowsiness or dizziness. Restrict activities as necessary.
Aviation Note: The use of this drug *is a disqualification* for piloting. Consult a designated Aviation Medical Examiner.
Exposure to Sun: No restrictions.

DIPYRIDAMOLE
(di peer ID a mohl)

Introduced: 1959

Prescription: USA: Yes
Canada: No

Class: Platelet inhibitor

Controlled Drug: USA: No
Canada: No

Available as Generic: USA: Yes
Canada: No

Brand Names: ✦Apo-Dipyridamole, ✦Asasantine [CD], Persantine, Pyridamole

---

BENEFITS versus RISKS

Possible Benefits	*Possible Risks*
EFFECTIVE PREVENTION OF THROMBOEMBOLISM (BLOOD CLOTS) FOLLOWING HEART VALVE SURGERY	Mild low blood pressure with dizziness and fainting (infrequent) Mild indigestion

---

▷ **Principal Uses**

As a Single Drug Product: This drug is used primarily for (1) the prevention of thromboembolism (blood clot formation and migration) following heart valve surgery; (2) the prevention of thromboembolism thought to be responsible for transient ischemic attacks in brain circulation (ministrokes). It may be used together with aspirin or with anticoagulants such as warfarin (Coumadin).

How This Drug Works: Not completely established. It is thought that by inhibiting the actions of certain enzymes, this drug prevents the aggregation of blood platelets (see Glossary) and thereby reduces the tendency to blood clot formation.

Available Dosage Forms and Strengths
Tablets — 25 mg, 50 mg, 75 mg

▷ **Usual Adult Dosage Range:**   50 to 100 mg, 3 or 4 times daily. Total daily dosage should not exceed 400 mg. **Note: Actual dosage and administration schedule must be determined by the physician for each patient individually.**

▷ **Dosing Instructions:**   Preferably taken with a full glass of water on an empty stomach, 1 hour before or 2 hours after eating. However, it may be taken with or following food to reduce stomach irritation. The tablet may be crushed for administration.

Usual Duration of Use: Significant reduction in platelet aggregation is thought to occur in 1 week. Long-term use (months to years) requires supervision and periodic evaluation by your physician.

▷ **This Drug Should Not Be Taken If**
  • you have had an allergic reaction to it previously.
  • you have just experienced an acute heart attack (myocardial infarction).
  • you have uncontrolled high blood pressure.

▷ **Inform Your Physician Before Taking This Drug If**
- you have low blood pressure.
- you have impaired liver function.
- you have any type of bleeding disorder.

Possible Side-Effects (natural, expected and unavoidable drug actions)
Flushing, light-headedness, weakness.

▷ **Possible Adverse Effects** (unusual, unexpected and infrequent reactions)
If any of the following develop, consult your physician promptly for guidance.
Mild Adverse Effects
Allergic Reaction: Skin rash.
Headache, dizziness, fainting.
Stomach irritation, nausea, diarrhea.
Serious Adverse Effects
Significant low blood pressure with large doses.
Paradoxical increase in angina on starting treatment (infrequent).
Aggravation of migraine headaches.

▷ **Possible Effects on Sexual Function:** None reported.

CAUTION
1. Occasionally this drug may cause an *increase* in the frequency and/ or severity of preexisting angina. If this response occurs, inform your physician promptly.
2. Anyone with low blood pressure should avoid large doses of this drug.

Precautions for Use
By Infants and Children: Observe closely for indications of excessively low blood pressure.
By Those over 60 Years of Age: Begin treatment with small doses (25 mg twice daily) to evaluate effect on blood pressure. Avoid doses that cause excessively low blood pressure. Observe for any tendency to develop hypothermia (see Glossary) in cold environments.

▷ **Advisability of Use During Pregnancy**
Pregnancy Category: B (tentative). See Pregnancy Code inside back cover.
Animal studies: Mouse, rat and rabbit studies show no birth defects due to this drug.
Human studies: Information from adequate studies of pregnant women is not available.
Use this drug only if clearly needed. If possible, avoid use during the last month of pregnancy and during labor and delivery because of possible prolongation of bleeding following delivery.

Advisability of Use if Breast-Feeding
Presence of this drug in breast milk: Yes, in small amounts.
Monitor nursing infant closely and discontinue drug or nursing if adverse effects develop.

Habit-Forming Potential: None.

Effects of Overdosage: Flushing, stomach irritation, nausea, vomiting, stomach cramps, diarrhea, rapid heart rate, low blood pressure, weakness, fainting.

Possible Effects of Long-Term Use: None reported.

Suggested Periodic Examinations While Taking This Drug (at physician's discretion)
Measurements of blood pressure in lying, sitting and standing positions.

▷ **While Taking This Drug, Observe the Following**
Foods: No restrictions.
Beverages: No restrictions. May be taken with milk.
▷ *Alcohol:* Use with caution until the combined effect has been determined. Alcohol may enhance the ability of this drug to lower blood pressure.
Tobacco Smoking: Nicotine can reduce the effectiveness of this drug. Follow physician's advice regarding smoking.
Marijuana Smoking: Possible reduced effectiveness of this drug; mild to moderate increase in angina; possible changes in electrocardiogram, confusing interpretation.
▷ *Other Drugs*
Dipyridamole may *increase* the effects of
• oral anticoagulants (warfarin, etc.), when doses of dipyridamole approach or exceed 400 mg/day; observe for abnormal bleeding or bruising.
• other drugs that inhibit platelet activity; observe for abnormal bleeding or bruising.
Dipyridamole *taken concurrently* with
• aspirin makes it possible to reduce the dose of dipyridamole and thus lessen any side-effects that may occur.
▷ *Driving, Hazardous Activities:* This drug may cause light-headedness or dizziness. Restrict activities as necessary.
Aviation Note: The use of this drug *may be a disqualification* for piloting. Consult a designated Aviation Medical Examiner.
Exposure to Sun: No restrictions.
Exposure to Heat: Use caution. Hot environments can cause significant drop in blood pressure.
Exposure to Cold: Use caution. This drug may increase the risk of hypothermia (see Glossary) in the elderly.
Discontinuation: Following long-term use, this drug should not be discontinued abruptly. It should be withdrawn gradually over a period of 2 to 3 weeks. Ask your physician for guidance.

DISOPYRAMIDE
(di so PEER a mide)

Introduced: 1969

Class: Antiarrhythmic

Prescription: USA: Yes
Canada: Yes

Controlled Drug: USA: No
Canada: No

Available as Generic: USA: Yes
Canada: No

Brand Names: Napamide, Norpace, Norpace CR, ✦Rythmodan, ✦Rythmodan-LA

BENEFITS versus RISKS

Possible Benefits	*Possible Risks*
EFFECTIVE TREATMENT OF SELECTED HEART RHYTHM DISORDERS	NARROW TREATMENT RANGE FREQUENT ADVERSE EFFECTS (10–40%) LOW BLOOD PRESSURE CONGESTIVE HEART FAILURE Heart conduction and rhythm abnormalities Frequent atropinelike side-effects

---

▷ **Principal Uses**

As a Single Drug Product: This drug is classified as a Type 1 antiarrhythmic agent, similar to procainamide and quinidine in its actions. It is used primarily to abolish and prevent the recurrence of premature beats arising in the atria (upper chambers) and the ventricles (lower chambers) of the heart. It is also useful in the treatment and prevention of abnormally rapid heart rates (tachycardia) that originate in the atria or the ventricles.

How This Drug Works: By slowing the activity of the pacemaker and delaying the transmission of electrical impulses through the conduction system and muscle of the heart, this drug assists in restoring normal heart rate and rhythm.

Available Dosage Forms and Strengths
Capsules — 100 mg, 150 mg
Capsules, prolonged-action — 100 mg, 150 mg

▷ **Usual Adult Dosage Range:** 100 to 200 mg/6 hours. Dosage should not exceed 200 mg/6 hours or 800 mg/24 hours (1600 mg/24 hours have been used occasionally). **Note: Actual dosage and administration schedule must be determined by the physician for each patient individually.**

▷ **Dosing Instructions:** Preferably taken on an empty stomach, 1 hour before or 2 hours after eating. However, it may be taken with or following food to reduce stomach irritation. The regular capsules may be opened for administration; however, the prolonged-action capsules should not be opened, chewed or crushed.

Usual Duration of Use: Continual use on a regular schedule for 2 to 4 days is usually necessary to determine this drug's effectiveness in correcting or preventing responsive rhythm disorders. Long-term use requires supervision and periodic evaluation by your physician.

▷ **This Drug Should Not Be Taken If**
- you have had an allergic reaction to it previously.
- you have second-degree or third-degree heart block (determined by electrocardiogram).

▷ **Inform Your Physician Before Taking This Drug If**
- you have had any unfavorable reactions to other antiarrhythmic drugs in the past.
- you have a history of heart disease of any kind, especially "heart block."
- you have a history of low blood pressure.
- you have impaired liver or kidney function.
- you have glaucoma, or a family history of glaucoma.
- you have an enlarged prostate gland.
- you have myasthenia gravis.
- you are taking any form of digitalis or any diuretic drug that can cause excessive loss of body potassium (ask physician).

Possible Side-Effects (natural, expected and unavoidable drug actions)
Drop in blood pressure in susceptible individuals.
Dry mouth (32%), constipation (11%), blurred vision (3–9%), impaired urination (14%).

▷ **Possible Adverse Effects** (unusual, unexpected and infrequent reactions)
If any of the following develop, consult your physician promptly for guidance.
Mild Adverse Effects
Allergic Reactions: Skin rash (1–3%), itching.
Headache, nervousness, fatigue, muscular weakness, mild aches.
Loss of appetite, indigestion, nausea, vomiting, diarrhea.
Lowered blood sugar level (hypoglycemia).
Serious Adverse Effects
Idiosyncratic Reaction: Acute psychotic behavior (rare).
Severe drop in blood pressure, fainting.
Progressive heart weakness, predisposing to congestive heart failure.
Inability to empty urinary bladder, prostatism (see Glossary).
Jaundice (see Glossary).
Abnormally low white blood cell count (rare).

▷ **Possible Effects on Sexual Function:** Rare reports of impotence (300 mg/ day); enlargement and tenderness of male breasts.

▷ **Adverse Effects That May Mimic Natural Diseases or Disorders**
Reversible jaundice may suggest viral hepatitis.

Natural Diseases or Disorders That May Be Activated by This Drug
Glaucoma, myasthenia gravis.

CAUTION
1. Thorough evaluation of your heart function (including electrocardiograms) is necessary prior to using this drug.
2. Periodic evaluation of your heart function is necessary to determine your response to this drug. Some individuals may experience worsening of their heart rhythm disorder and/or deterioration of heart function. Close monitoring of heart rate, rhythm and overall performance is essential.
3. Dosage must be adjusted carefully for each individual. Do not change your dosage without the knowledge and supervision of your physician.
4. Do not take any other antiarrhythmic drug while taking this drug unless directed to do so by your physician.

Precautions for Use
By Infants and Children: Safety and effectiveness for use by those under 12 years of age have not been established. Initial use of this drug requires hospitalization and supervision by a qualified pediatrician.
By Those over 60 Years of Age: Reduced kidney function may require reduction in dosage. This drug can aggravate existing prostatism (see Glossary) and promote constipation. Observe carefully for light-headedness, dizziness, unsteadiness and tendency to fall.

▷ **Advisability of Use During Pregnancy**
Pregnancy Category: B (tentative). See Pregnancy Code inside back cover.
Animal studies: No birth defects reported in rats and rabbits.
Human studies: Information from adequate studies of pregnant women is not available. It has been reported that this drug can cause contractions of the pregnant uterus.
Use this drug only if clearly needed. Ask your physician for guidance.

Advisability of Use if Breast-Feeding
Presence of this drug in breast milk: Yes.
Avoid drug or refrain from nursing.

Habit-Forming Potential: None.

Effects of Overdosage: Dryness of eyes, nose, mouth and throat; impaired urination; constipation; marked drop in blood pressure; abnormal heart rhythms; congestive heart failure.

Possible Effects of Long-Term Use: None reported.

Suggested Periodic Examinations While Taking This Drug (at physician's discretion)

Electrocardiograms, complete blood cell counts, measurements of potassium blood levels.

▷ **While Taking This Drug, Observe the Following**

Foods: No restrictions. Ask physician regarding need for salt restriction and advisability of eating potassium-rich foods.

Beverages: No restrictions. May be taken with milk.

▷ *Alcohol:* Use caution until the combined effects have been determined. Alcohol can increase the blood-pressure-lowering effects and the blood-sugar-lowering effects of this drug.

Tobacco Smoking: Nicotine can cause irritability of the heart and reduce the effectiveness of this drug. Follow physician's advice regarding smoking.

▷ *Other Drugs*

Disopyramide may ***increase*** the effects of

- antihypertensive drugs, and cause excessive lowering of blood pressure.
- atropinelike drugs (see Drug Class, Section Four).
- warfarin (Coumadin, etc.); monitor prothrombin times, adjust dosage accordingly.

Disopyramide may ***decrease*** the effects of

- ambenonium (Mytelase).
- neostigmine (Prostigmin).
- pyridostigmine (Mestinon).

The beneficial effects of these three drugs in the treatment of myasthenia gravis may be reduced.

The following drugs may ***decrease*** the effects of disopyramide

- all diuretics that promote potassium loss.
- rifampin (Rimactane, Rifadin).

▷ *Driving, Hazardous Activities:* This drug may cause dizziness or blurred vision. Restrict activities as necessary.

Aviation Note: The use of this drug ***may be a disqualification*** for piloting. Consult a designated Aviation Medical Examiner.

Exposure to Sun: Use caution. This drug is reported to cause photosensitization (see Glossary) in susceptible individuals.

Exposure to Heat: Use caution. The use of this drug in hot environments may increase the risk of heat stroke.

Occurrence of Unrelated Illness: Disorders that cause vomiting, diarrhea or dehydration can affect this drug's action adversely. Report such developments promptly.

Discontinuation: This drug should not be discontinued abruptly following long-term use. Ask your physician for guidance regarding gradual dose reduction.

DISULFIRAM
(di SULF i ram)

Introduced: 1948

Class: Antialcoholism

Prescription: USA: Yes
Canada: Yes

Controlled Drug: USA: No
Canada: No

Available as Generic: USA: Yes
Canada: No

Brand Name: Antabuse

BENEFITS versus RISKS

Possible Benefits	*Possible Risks*
EFFECTIVE ADJUNCT IN THE TREATMENT OF CHRONIC ALCOHOLISM	DANGEROUS REACTIONS WITH ALCOHOL INGESTION Acute psychotic reactions (uncommon) Drug-induced liver damage (rare) Drug-induced optic and/or peripheral neuritis (rare)

▷ **Principal Uses**

As a Single Drug Product: This drug is used for one purpose only—to deter the abusive drinking of alcoholic beverages. It does not abolish the craving or impulse to drink. It is of value in the treatment of alcoholism because of the psychological reinforcement it provides by reminding the patient of the dire consequences of ingesting alcohol.

How This Drug Works: Following the ingestion of alcohol, this drug interrupts normal liver enzyme activity after the conversion of alcohol to acetaldehyde. This causes excessive accumulation of acetaldehyde, a highly toxic substance that produces the disulfiram (Antabuse) reaction (see Glossary).

Available Dosage Forms and Strengths
Tablets — 250 mg, 500 mg

▷ **Usual Adult Dosage Range:** In the absence of all signs of alcoholic intoxication and no less than 12 hours after the last ingestion of alcohol, treatment is started with a single dose of 500 mg/day for 1 to 2 weeks. This is followed by a maintenance dose of 250 mg/day. The range of the maintenance dose is 125 mg to 500 mg/day and is determined by experience with each patient individually. The total daily dosage should not exceed 1000 mg. **Note: Actual dosage and administration schedule must be determined by the physician for each patient individually.**

▷ **Dosing Instructions:** May be taken with or following food to reduce stomach irritation. Tablet may be crushed for administration.

Usual Duration of Use: Continual use on a regular schedule for several months is usually necessary to determine this drug's effectiveness in deterring the drinking of alcohol. If tolerated well, use should continue until a basis for permanent self-control and sobriety is established. Consult your physician on a regular basis.

▷ **This Drug Should Not Be Taken If**
- you have experienced a severe allergic reaction to disulfiram in the past. (Note: The interaction of disulfiram and alcohol is ***not an allergic*** reaction.)
- you have ingested any form of alcohol in any amount within the past 12 hours.
- you are pregnant.
- you are taking (or have taken recently) metronidazole (Flagyl).
- you have coronary heart disease or a serious heart rhythm disorder.

▷ **Inform Your Physician Before Taking This Drug If**
- you have used disulfiram in the past.
- you do not intend to avoid alcohol completely while taking this drug.
- you have not been given a full explanation of the reaction you will experience if you drink alcohol while taking this drug.
- you are planning pregnancy in the near future.
- you have a history of diabetes, epilepsy, kidney or liver disease.
- you are currently taking oral anticoagulants, digitalis, isoniazid, paraldehyde or phenytoin (Dilantin).
- you plan to have surgery under general anesthesia while taking this drug.

Possible Side-Effects (natural, expected and unavoidable drug actions)
Drowsiness, lethargy during early use.
Offensive breath and body odor.

▷ **Possible Adverse Effects** (unusual, unexpected and infrequent reactions)
If any of the following develop, consult your physician promptly for guidance.
Mild Adverse Effects
Allergic Reactions: Skin rash, hives.
Headache, dizziness, restlessness, tremor.
Metallic or garliclike taste, indigestion. (These usually subside after 2 weeks of use.)
Serious Adverse Effects
Allergic Reactions: Severe skin rashes, drug-induced hepatitis (rare).
Idiosyncratic Reaction: Acute toxic effect on brain; psychotic behavior.
Optic or peripheral neuritis (see Glossary).

▷ **Possible Effects on Sexual Function:** Decreased libido and/or impaired erection in 30% of users taking recommended doses of 125 to 500 mg/day.

▷ **Adverse Effects That May Mimic Natural Diseases or Disorders**

Liver reaction may suggest viral hepatitis.

Brain toxicity may suggest spontaneous psychosis.

CAUTION

1. This drug should never be taken by anyone who is in a state of alcoholic intoxication.
2. The patient should be fully informed regarding the purpose and actions of this drug *before* treatment is started.
3. During long-term use of this drug, examine for any indication of reduced thyroid function.
4. Carry a card of personal identification with the notation that you are taking this drug.

Precautions for Use

By Infants and Children: Safety and effectiveness for use by those under 12 years of age have not been established.

By Those over 60 Years of Age: Observe for excessive sedation during the early use of this drug. *Do not* perform an "alcohol trial" to determine the effects of this drug.

▷ **Advisability of Use During Pregnancy**

Pregnancy Category: X (tentative). See Pregnancy Code inside back cover.

Animal studies: No defects reported in rats and hamsters.

Human studies: Two reports indicate that 4 of 8 fetuses exposed to this drug had serious birth defects. Information from adequate studies of pregnant women is not available.

Avoid this drug completely if possible.

Advisability of Use if Breast-Feeding

Presence of this drug in breast milk: Unknown.

Avoid drug or refrain from nursing.

Habit-Forming Potential: None.

Effects of Overdosage: Marked lethargy, impaired memory, altered behavior, confusion, unsteadiness, weakness, stomach pain, nausea, vomiting, diarrhea.

Possible Effects of Long-Term Use: Decreased function of thyroid gland.

Suggested Periodic Examinations While Taking This Drug (at physician's discretion)

Visual acuity, liver function tests.

▷ **While Taking This Drug, Observe the Following**

Foods: Avoid all foods prepared with alcohol, including sauces, marinades, vinegars, desserts, etc. Inquire when dining out regarding the use of alcohol in food preparation.

Beverages: Avoid all punches, fruit drinks, etc., that may contain alcohol. This drug may be taken with milk.

▷ *Alcohol:* **Avoid completely in all forms** while taking this drug and for 14 days following the last dose. The combination of disulfiram and alcohol—even in small amounts—produces the disulfiram (Antabuse) reaction. This begins within 5 to 10 minutes after ingesting alcohol and consists of intense flushing and warming of the face, a severe throbbing headache, shortness of breath, chest pains, nausea, repeated vomiting, sweating and weakness. If the amount of alcohol ingested is large enough, the reaction may progress to blurred vision, vertigo, confusion, marked drop in blood pressure and loss of consciousness. Severe reactions may lead to convulsions and death. The reaction may last from 30 minutes to several hours, depending upon the amount of alcohol and disulfiram in the body. As the symptoms subside, the individual is exhausted and usually sleeps for several hours.

Tobacco Smoking: No interactions expected.

Marijuana Smoking: Possible increase in drowsiness and lethargy.

▷ *Other Drugs*

Disulfiram may **increase** the effects of

- oral anticoagulants (warfarin, etc.), and increase the risk of bleeding; dosage adjustments may be necessary.
- barbiturates, and cause oversedation (see Drug Class, Section Four).
- chlordiazepoxide (Librium) and diazepam (Valium), and cause oversedation.
- paraldehyde, and cause excessive depression of brain function.
- phenytoin (Dilantin), and cause toxic effects on the brain; dosage adjustments may be necessary.

Disulfiram may **decrease** the effects of

- perphenazine (Tilafon, etc.).

Disulfiram **taken concurrently** with

- isoniazid (INH, etc.) may cause acute mental disturbance and incoordination, making it necessary to discontinue treatment.
- metronidazole (Flagyl) may cause acute mental and behavioral disturbances, making it necessary to discontinue treatment.
- OTC cough syrups, tonics, etc., containing alcohol may cause a disulfiram (Antabuse) reaction; avoid concurrent use. (See OTC Drugs in Glossary.)

The following drugs may **increase** the effects of disulfiram

- amitriptyline (Elavil) may enhance the disulfiram + alcohol interaction; avoid concurrent use of these drugs.

▷ *Driving, Hazardous Activities:* This drug may cause drowsiness or dizziness. Restrict activities as necessary.

Aviation Note: Alcoholism **is a disqualification** for piloting. Consult a designated Aviation Medical Examiner.

Exposure to Sun: No restrictions.

Exposure to Environmental Chemicals: Thiram, a pesticide, and carbon disulfide, a pesticide and industrial solvent, can have additive toxic effects during use of this drug. Observe for toxic effects on the brain and nervous system.

Discontinuation: Treatment with this drug is only part of your total treatment program. Do not discontinue it without the knowledge and guidance of your physician. Abrupt withdrawal does not cause any symptoms. However, no alcohol should be ingested for 14 days following discontinuation.

DOXEPIN
(DOX e pin)

Introduced: 1969

Class: Antidepressant

Prescription: USA: Yes
Canada: Yes

Controlled Drug: USA: No
Canada: No

Available as Generic: USA: Yes
Canada: No

Brand Names: Adapin, Sinequan, ✦Triadapin

BENEFITS versus RISKS	
Possible Benefits	*Possible Risks*
EFFECTIVE RELIEF OF ENDOGENOUS DEPRESSION	ADVERSE BEHAVIORAL EFFECTS: confusion, disorientation, hallucinations, delusions
EFFECTIVE RELIEF OF ANXIETY AND NERVOUS TENSION	CONVERSION OF DEPRESSION TO MANIA in manic-depressive disorder
Possibly beneficial in other depressive disorders	Aggravation of schizophrenia and paranoia
	Rare blood cell disorders

▷ **Principal Uses**

As a Single Drug Product: To relieve the symptoms associated with spontaneous (endogenous) depression, and to initiate the restoration of normal mood. This drug should be used only when a diagnosis of a true, primary depression of significant degree has been established. It should not be used to treat the symptoms of mild and transient (reactive) depression that may be associated with many life situations in the absence of a bona fide affective illness.

How This Drug Works: Not completely established. It is thought that this drug relieves depression by slowly restoring to normal levels certain constituents of brain tissue (norepinephrine and serotonin) that transmit nerve impulses.

Available Dosage Forms and Strengths
       Capsules — 10 mg, 25 mg, 50 mg, 75 mg, 100 mg, 150 mg
    Oral concentrate — 10 mg per ml

▷ **Usual Adult Dosage Range:**   Initially 25 mg 2 to 4 times daily. Dose may be increased cautiously as needed and tolerated by 10 to 25 mg daily at intervals of 1 week. Usual maintenance dose is 75 to 150 mg/24 hours. Total dose should not exceed 300 mg/24 hours. When the optimal requirement is determined, it may be taken at bedtime as one dose. **Note: Actual dosage and administration schedule must be determined by the physician for each patient individually.**

▷ **Dosing Instructions:**   May be taken without regard to meals. Capsule may be opened for administration.

Usual Duration of Use: Some benefit may be apparent within 1 to 2 weeks, but adequate response may require continual use for 10 to 12 weeks or longer. Long-term use should not exceed 6 months without evaluation regarding the need for continuation of the drug. Consult your physician on a regular basis.

▷ **This Drug Should Not Be Taken If**
- you have had an allergic reaction to it previously.
- you are taking or have taken within the past 14 days any monoamine oxidase (MAO) type A inhibitor drug (see Drug Class, Section Four).
- you are recovering from a recent heart attack.
- you have narrow-angle glaucoma.

▷ **Inform Your Physician Before Taking This Drug If**
- you are allergic or sensitive to any other tricyclic antidepressant (see Drug Class, Section Four).
- you have a history of any of the following: diabetes, epilepsy, glaucoma, heart disease, prostate gland enlargement or overactive thyroid function.
- you plan to have surgery under general anesthesia in the near future.

Possible Side-Effects (natural, expected and unavoidable drug actions)
Drowsiness, blurred vision, dry mouth, constipation, impaired urination.

▷ **Possible Adverse Effects** (unusual, unexpected and infrequent reactions)
If any of the following develop, consult your physician promptly for guidance.
Mild Adverse Effects
Allergic Reactions: Skin rash, hives, swelling of face or tongue, drug fever (see Glossary).
Headache, dizziness, weakness, fainting, unsteady gait, tremors.
Peculiar taste, irritation of tongue or mouth, nausea, indigestion.
Fluctuation of blood sugar levels.

Serious Adverse Effects

Allergic Reactions: Hepatitis, with or without jaundice (see Glossary).

Confusion, hallucinations, agitation, restlessness, delusions.

Bone marrow depression (see Glossary)—fatigue, weakness, fever, sore throat, abnormal bleeding or bruising (reported for other drugs of this class).

Peripheral neuritis (see Glossary)—numbness, tingling, pain, loss of strength in arms and legs.

Parkinson-like disorders (see Glossary)—usually mild and infrequent; more likely to occur in the elderly.

▷ **Possible Effects on Sexual Function:** Female breast enlargement with milk production; swelling of testicles.

▷ **Adverse Effects That May Mimic Natural Diseases or Disorders**

Liver toxicity may suggest viral hepatitis.

Natural Diseases or Disorders That May Be Activated by This Drug

Latent diabetes, epilepsy, glaucoma, impaired urination due to prostate gland enlargement (prostatism, see Glossary).

CAUTION

1. Dosage must be adjusted for each person individually. Report for follow-up evaluation and laboratory tests as directed by your physician.
2. It is advisable to withhold this drug if electroconvulsive therapy (ECT, "shock" treatment) is to be used to treat your depression.

Precautions for Use

By Infants and Children: Safety and effectiveness for use by those under 12 years of age have not been established.

By Those over 60 Years of Age: During the first 2 weeks of treatment, observe for the development of confusion, agitation, forgetfulness, disorientation, delusions and hallucinations. Reduction of dosage or discontinuation may be necessary. Unsteadiness may predispose to falling and injury. This drug can increase the degree of impaired urination associated with prostate gland enlargement (prostatism).

▷ **Advisability of Use During Pregnancy**

Pregnancy Category: B (tentative). See Pregnancy Code inside back cover.

Animal studies: No birth defects reported in rats, rabbits, dogs or monkeys.

Human studies: Information from adequate studies of pregnant women is not available.

Use this drug only if clearly needed. If possible, avoid use during the first 3 months and the last month. Ask physician for guidance.

Advisability of Use if Breast-Feeding

Presence of this drug in breast milk: Yes, in small amounts.

Monitor nursing infant closely and discontinue drug or nursing if adverse effects develop.

Habit-Forming Potential: None.

Effects of Overdosage: Confusion, hallucinations, marked drowsiness, heart palpitations, dilated pupils, tremors, stupor, deep sleep, coma, convulsions.

Suggested Periodic Examinations While Taking This Drug (at physician's discretion)
Complete blood cell counts, liver function tests, serial blood pressure readings and electrocardiograms.

▷ **While Taking This Drug, Observe the Following**
Foods: No restrictions. This drug may increase the appetite and cause excessive weight gain.
Beverages: No restrictions. May be taken with milk.
▷ *Alcohol:* Avoid completely. This drug can markedly increase the intoxicating effects of alcohol and accentuate its depressant action on brain function.
Tobacco Smoking: May hasten the elimination of this drug. Higher doses may be necessary.
▷ *Other Drugs*
Doxepin may *increase* the effects of
• atropinelike drugs (see Drug Class, Section Four).
• dicumarol, and increase the risk of bleeding; dosage adjustments may be necessary.
• thyroid hormones.
Doxepin may *decrease* the effects of
• clonidine (Catapres).
• guanethidine (Ismelin).
Doxepin *taken concurrently* with
• monoamine oxidase (MAO) type A inhibitor drugs may cause high fever, delirium and convulsions (see Drug Class, Section Four).
▷ *Driving, Hazardous Activities:* This drug may impair mental alertness, judgment, physical coordination and reaction time. Avoid hazardous activities.
Aviation Note: The use of this drug *is a disqualification* for piloting. Consult a designated Aviation Medical Examiner.
Exposure to Sun: Use caution until sensitivity to sun has been determined. This drug may cause photosensitivity (see Glossary).
Exposure to Heat: This drug can inhibit sweating and impair the body's adaptation to hot environments, increasing the risk of heat stroke. Avoid saunas.
Exposure to Cold: The elderly should use caution and avoid conditions conducive to hypothermia (see Glossary).
Discontinuation: It is advisable to discontinue this drug gradually. Abrupt withdrawal after long-term use can cause headache, malaise and nausea.

DOXYCYCLINE
(dox ee SI kleen)

Introduced: 1967

Class: Antibiotic, tetracyclines

Prescription: USA: Yes
Canada: Yes

Controlled Drug: USA: No
Canada: No

Available as Generic: USA: Yes
Canada: No

Brand Names: Doryx, Doxychel, Vibramycin, Vibra-Tabs, Vivox

BENEFITS versus RISKS

Possible Benefits	*Possible Risks*
EFFECTIVE TREATMENT OF INFECTIONS due to susceptible microorganisms	ALLERGIC REACTIONS, mild to severe Liver reaction with jaundice (rare) Fungal superinfections Drug-induced colitis Blood cell disorders

---

▷ **Principal Uses**

As a Single Drug Product: This member of the tetracycline drug class is used primarily to (1) treat a broad range of infections caused by susceptible bacteria and protozoa; (2) treat and prevent "traveler's diarrhea." It is often used to treat acute and chronic sinusitis and bronchitis.

How This Drug Works: This drug prevents the growth and multiplication of susceptible bacteria by interfering with their formation of essential proteins.

Available Dosage Forms and Strengths

Capsules — 50 mg, 100 mg
Capsules, coated pellets — 100 mg
Injection — 100 mg per vial, 200 mg per vial
Oral suspension — 25 mg per 5-ml teaspoonful
Syrup — 50 mg per 5-ml teaspoonful
Tablets — 50 mg, 100 mg

▷ **Usual Adult Dosage Range:** 100 mg/12 hours the first day; then 100 to 200 mg once daily or 50 to 100 mg/12 hours. Total daily dosage should not exceed 300 mg. **Note: Actual dosage and administration schedule must be determined by the physician for each patient individually.**

▷ **Dosing Instructions:** Preferably taken on an empty stomach, 1 hour before or 2 hours after eating. However, if stomach irritation occurs, it may be taken with food or milk. Take at same time each day, with a full glass of water. Take the full course prescribed. The tablet may be crushed and the capsule may be opened for administration.

Usual Duration of Use: The time required to control the infection and be free of fever and symptoms for 48 hours. This varies with the nature of the infection.

▷ **This Drug Should Not Be Taken If**
- you are allergic to any tetracycline drug (see Drug Class, Section Four).
- you are pregnant or breast-feeding.

▷ **Inform Your Physician Before Taking This Drug If**
- it is prescribed for a child under 8 years of age.
- you have a history of liver or kidney disease.
- you have systemic lupus erythematosus.
- you are taking any penicillin drug.
- you are taking any anticoagulant drug.
- you plan to have surgery under general anesthesia in the near future.

Possible Side-Effects (natural, expected and unavoidable drug actions)
Superinfections (see Glossary), often due to yeast organisms. These can occur in the mouth, intestinal tract, rectum and/or vagina, resulting in rectal and vaginal itching.

▷ **Possible Adverse Effects** (unusual, unexpected and infrequent reactions)
If any of the following develop, consult your physician promptly for guidance.
Mild Adverse Effects
Allergic Reactions: Skin rash, hives, itching of hands and feet, swelling of face or extremities.
Loss of appetite, nausea, vomiting, diarrhea.
Irritation of mouth or tongue, "black tongue," sore throat, abdominal cramping or pain.
Serious Adverse Effects
Allergic Reactions: Anaphylactic reaction (see Glossary), asthma, fever, swollen joints, abnormal bleeding or bruising, jaundice (see Glossary).
Permanent discoloration and/or malformation of teeth when taken by children under 8 years of age, including unborn child and infant.

▷ **Possible Effects on Sexual Function:**   None reported.

Natural Diseases or Disorders That May Be Activated by This Drug
Systemic lupus erythematosus.

CAUTION
1. Antacids and preparations containing aluminum, bismuth, iron, magnesium or zinc can prevent adequate absorption of this drug and reduce its effectiveness significantly.

2. Troublesome and persistent diarrhea can develop in sensitive individuals. If diarrhea persists for more than 24 hours, discontinue this drug and consult your physician.

Precautions for Use
By Infants and Children: If possible, tetracyclines should not be given to children under 8 years of age because of the risk of permanent discoloration and deformity of the teeth. Rarely, young infants may develop increased intracranial pressure within the first 4 days of receiving this drug. Tetracyclines may inhibit normal bone growth and development.

By Those over 60 Years of Age: Natural skin changes may predispose to severe and prolonged itching reactions in the genital and anal regions.

▷ **Advisability of Use During Pregnancy**
Pregnancy Category: D (tentative). See Pregnancy Code inside back cover.
Animal studies: Tetracycline causes limb defects in rats, rabbits and chickens.
Human studies: Information from studies of pregnant women indicates that drugs of this class can cause impaired development and discoloration of teeth and other developmental defects.
It is advisable to avoid this drug completely during entire pregnancy.

Advisability of Use if Breast-Feeding
Presence of this drug in breast milk: Yes.
Avoid drug or refrain from nursing.

Habit-Forming Potential: None.

Effects of Overdosage: Nausea, vomiting, diarrhea, acute liver damage (rare).

Possible Effects of Long-Term Use: Superinfections (see Glossary), prolongation of prothrombin time.

Suggested Periodic Examinations While Taking This Drug (at physician's discretion)
Complete blood cell counts, liver and kidney function tests.
During extended use, sputum and stool examinations may detect early superinfection due to yeast organisms.

▷ **While Taking This Drug, Observe the Following**
Foods: Avoid meats and iron-fortified cereals and supplements for 2 hours before and after taking this drug.
Beverages: No restrictions. May be taken with milk.
▷ *Alcohol:* No interactions expected. However, it is best avoided if you have active liver disease.
Tobacco Smoking: No interactions expected.

▷   *Other Drugs*

Doxycycline may ***increase*** the effects of
- oral anticoagulants, and make it necessary to reduce their dosage.
- digoxin (Lanoxin), and cause digitalis toxicity.
- lithium (Eskalith, Lithane, etc.), and increase the risk of lithium toxicity.

Doxycycline may ***decrease*** the effects of
- oral contraceptives, and impair their effectiveness in preventing pregnancy.
- penicillins, and impair their effectiveness in treating infections.

The following drugs may ***decrease*** the effects of doxycycline
- antacids (aluminum and magnesium preparations, sodium bicarbonate, etc.) may reduce drug absorption.
- barbiturates (see Drug Class, Section Four).
- bismuth preparations (Pepto-Bismol, etc.).
- carbamazepine (Tegretol).
- cimetidine (Tagamet).
- phenytoin (Dilantin).
- iron and mineral preparations may reduce drug absorption.

▷   *Driving, Hazardous Activities:* Usually no restrictions. Be alert to the possible occurrence of nausea or diarrhea.

Aviation Note: The use of this drug ***may be a disqualification*** for piloting. Consult a designated Aviation Medical Examiner.

Exposure to Sun: Use caution until sensitivity has been determined. Tetracyclines can cause photosensitivity (see Glossary).

ENALAPRIL
(e NAL a pril)

Introduced: 1981

Class: Antihypertensive, ACE inhibitor

Prescription: USA: Yes

Controlled Drug: USA: No

Available as Generic: No

Brand Names: Vaseretic [CD], Vasotec

BENEFITS versus RISKS

Possible Benefits	*Possible Risks*
EFFECTIVE CONTROL OF MILD TO SEVERE HIGH BLOOD PRESSURE	Headache (4.8%), dizziness (4.6%), fatigue (2.8%)
Possibly beneficial as adjunctive treatment in selected cases of congestive heart failure	Low blood pressure (2.3%)
	Bone marrow depression (rare)
	Allergic swelling of face, tongue or vocal cords (0.2%)

▷ **Principal Uses**

As a Single Drug Product

Used primarily to treat all degrees of high blood pressure. Mild to moderate high blood pressure usually responds to low doses; severe high blood pressure may require higher doses, with greater risk of serious adverse effects.

This drug is also used adjunctively to treat heart failure that is not responding adequately to digitalis and diuretics.

How This Drug Works: Not completely known. It is thought that by blocking certain enzyme systems that influence arterial function, this drug contributes to the relaxation of arterial walls throughout the body and thus lowers the resistance to blood flow that causes high blood pressure. This, in turn, reduces the workload of the heart and improves its performance.

Available Dosage Forms and Strengths

Tablets — 5 mg, 10 mg, 20 mg

▷ **Usual Adult Dosage Range:**   Initially 5 mg once daily for 2 weeks. Usual maintenance dose is 10 to 40 mg/day in a single dose or in 2 divided doses. Total daily dose should not exceed 40 mg if kidney function is impaired. **Note: Actual dosage and administration schedule must be determined by the physician for each patient individually.**

▷ **Dosing Instructions:**   Take on an empty stomach or with food, at same time each day. Tablet may be crushed for administration.

Usual Duration of Use: Continual use on a regular schedule for several weeks is usually necessary to determine this drug's effectiveness in controlling high blood pressure. The proper treatment of high blood pressure usually requires the long-term use of effective medications. Consult your physician on a regular basis.

▷ **This Drug Should Not Be Taken If**
- you have had an allergic reaction to it previously.
- you currently have a blood cell or bone marrow disorder.
- you have active liver disease.
- you have an abnormally high level of blood potassium.

▷ **Inform Your Physician Before Taking This Drug If**
- you have a history of kidney disease or impaired kidney function.
- you have scleroderma or systemic lupus erythematosus.
- you have any form of heart disease.
- you have diabetes.
- you are taking any of the following drugs: other antihypertensives, diuretics, nitrates or potassium supplements.
- you plan to have surgery under general anesthesia in the near future.

Possible Side-Effects (natural, expected and unavoidable drug actions)

Dizziness, light-headedness, fainting (excessive drop in blood pressure).

▷ **Possible Adverse Effects** (unusual, unexpected and infrequent reactions)
  If any of the following develop, consult your physician promptly for guidance.
  Mild Adverse Effects
  Allergic Reactions: Skin rash, itching.
  Headache, fatigue, drowsiness, nervousness, numbness and tingling, insomnia.
  Rapid heart rate, palpitation.
  Indigestion, stomach pain, nausea, vomiting, diarrhea.
  Excessive sweating, muscle cramps.
  Serious Adverse Effects
  Allergic Reactions: Swelling (angioedema) of face, tongue and/or vocal cords: can be life threatening.
  Bone marrow depression—fatigue, weakness, fever, sore throat, abnormal bleeding or bruising.

▷ **Possible Effects on Sexual Function:**   Rare report of impotence.

  CAUTION
    1. Consult your physician regarding the advisability of discontinuing other antihypertensive drugs (especially diuretics) for 1 week before starting this drug.
    2. **Report promptly** any indications of infection (fever, sore throat), and any indications of water retention (weight gain, puffiness, swollen feet or ankles).
    3. Do not use a salt substitute without your physician's knowledge and approval. (Many salt substitutes contain potassium.)
    4. It is advisable to obtain blood cell counts and urine analyses **before** starting this drug.

  Precautions for Use
  By Infants and Children: Safety and effectiveness for use by those in this age group have not been established.
  By Those over 60 Years of Age: Small doses are advisable until tolerance has been determined. Sudden and excessive lowering of blood pressure can predispose to stroke or heart attack in those with impaired brain circulation or coronary artery heart disease.

▷ **Advisability of Use During Pregnancy**
  Pregnancy Category: C (tentative). See Pregnancy Code inside back cover.
  Animal studies: No birth defects found in rat or rabbit studies.
  Human studies: Information from adequate studies of pregnant women is not available.
  Avoid during first 3 months if possible.

  Advisability of Use if Breast-Feeding
  Presence of this drug in breast milk: Not known.
  Monitor nursing infant closely and discontinue drug or nursing if adverse effects develop.

Habit-Forming Potential: None.

Effects of Overdosage: Excessive drop in blood pressure—light-headedness, dizziness, fainting.

Possible Effects of Long-Term Use: Gradual increase in blood potassium level.

Suggested Periodic Examinations While Taking This Drug (at physician's discretion)

Before starting drug: Complete blood cell counts; urine analysis with measurement of protein content; blood potassium level.

During use of drug: Blood cell counts; measurements of blood potassium.

▷ **While Taking This Drug, Observe the Following**

Foods: Consult physician regarding salt intake.

Nutritional Support: **Do not take** potassium supplements unless directed by your physician.

Beverages: No restrictions. May be taken with milk.

▷ *Alcohol:* Use caution until combined effect has been determined. Alcohol may enhance the blood-pressure-lowering effect of this drug.

Tobacco Smoking: No interactions expected.

▷ *Other Drugs*

Enalapril *taken concurrently* with

- potassium preparations (K-Lyte, Slow-K, etc.) may cause increased blood levels of potassium with risk of serious heart rhythm disturbances.
- potassium-sparing diuretics: amiloride (Moduretic), spironolactone (Aldactazide), triamterene (Dyazide) may cause increased blood levels of potassium with risk of serious heart rhythm disturbances.

▷ *Driving, Hazardous Activities:* Usually no restrictions. Be aware of possible drops in blood pressure with resultant dizziness or faintness.

Aviation Note: The use of this drug **may be a disqualification** for piloting. Consult a designated Aviation Medical Examiner.

Exposure to Sun: Caution advised. A similar drug of this class can cause photosensitivity.

Exposure to Heat: Caution advised. Avoid excessive perspiring with resultant loss of body water and drop in blood pressure.

Occurrence of Unrelated Illness: Report promptly any disorder that causes nausea, vomiting or diarrhea. Fluid and chemical imbalances must be corrected as soon as possible.

EPINEPHRINE
(ep i NEF rin)

Other Name: Adrenaline

Introduced: 1900

Class: Antiasthmatic, antiglaucoma, decongestant

Prescription: USA: Varies
Canada: No

Controlled Drug: USA: No
Canada: No

Available as Generic: USA: Yes
Canada: No

Brand Names: Adrenalin, Bronkaid Mist, ✦Bronkaid Mistometer, ✦Dysne-
Inhal, Epifrin, E-Pilo Preparations [CD], Epitrate, Glaucon, Medihaler-Epi Preparations, Primatene Mist, Sus-Phrine, Vaponefrin

---

BENEFITS versus RISKS

Possible Benefits	*Possible Risks*
EFFECTIVE RELIEF OF SEVERE ALLERGIC (ANAPHYLACTIC) REACTIONS	Significant increase in blood pressure (in sensitive individuals)
TEMPORARY RELIEF OF ACUTE BRONCHIAL ASTHMA	Idiosyncratic reaction: pulmonary edema (fluid formation in lungs)
Reduction of internal eye pressure (treatment of glaucoma)	Heart rhythm disorders (in sensitive individuals)
Relief of allergic congestion of the nose and sinuses	

▷ **Principal Uses**

As a Single Drug Product: This drug is used most commonly by inhalation to relieve acute attacks of bronchial asthma. It is used less frequently as a decongestant for symptomatic relief of allergic nasal congestion and as eye drops in the management of glaucoma.

How This Drug Works: By stimulating certain sympathetic nerve terminals, this drug acts to

- contract blood vessel walls and raise the blood pressure.
- inhibit the release of harmful amounts of histamine into the skin and internal organs.
- dilate those bronchial tubes that are in sustained constriction, thereby increasing the size of the airways and improving the ability to breathe.
- decrease the formation of fluid within the eye, increase its outflow from the eye and thereby reduce internal eye pressure.
- decrease the volume of blood in nasal tissue, thereby shrinking the tissue mass (decongestion) and expanding the nasal airway.

Available Dosage Forms and Strengths

Aerosol — 0.2 mg, 0.27 mg, 0.3 mg per spray
Eye drops — 0.1%, 0.25%, 0.5%, 1%, 2%

Injection — 0.01 mg, 0.1 mg, 1 mg, 5 mg per ml
Nose drops — 0.1%
Solution for nebulizer — 1%, 1.25%, 2.25%

▷ **Usual Adult Dosage Range:** Aerosols: 1 inhalation, repeated in 1 to 2 minutes if needed; wait 4 hours before next inhalation. Eye drops: 1 drop/ 12 hours. Dosage may vary with product; follow printed instructions and label directions. **Note: Actual dosage and administration schedule must be determined by the physician for each patient individually.**

▷ **Dosing Instructions:** Aerosols and inhalation solutions: After first inhalation, wait 1 to 2 minutes to determine if a second inhalation is necessary. If relief does not occur within 20 minutes of use, and difficult breathing persists, discontinue this drug and seek medical attention promptly. Avoid prolonged and excessive use. Eye drops: During instillation of drops and for 2 minutes following, press finger against the tear sac (inner corner of eye) to prevent rapid absorption of drug into body circulation.

Usual Duration of Use: According to individual needs. Long-term use requires supervision and periodic evaluation by your physician.

▷ **This Drug Should Not Be Taken If**
- you have had an allergic reaction to any dosage form of it previously.
- you have narrow-angle glaucoma.
- you have experienced a recent stroke or heart attack.

▷ **Inform Your Physician Before Taking This Drug If**
- you have any degree of high blood pressure.
- you have any form of heart disease, especially coronary heart disease (with or without angina), or a heart rhythm disorder.
- you have diabetes or overactive thyroid function (hyperthyroidism).
- you have a history of stroke.
- you are taking any of the following drugs: monoamine oxidase (MAO) type A inhibitors, phenothiazines (see Drug Classes, Section Four), digitalis preparations or quinidine.

Possible Side-Effects (natural, expected and unavoidable drug actions)
In sensitive individuals—restlessness, anxiety, headache, tremor, palpitation, coldness of hands and feet, dryness of mouth and throat (with use of aerosol).

▷ **Possible Adverse Effects** (unusual, unexpected and infrequent reactions)
If any of the following develop, consult your physician promptly for guidance.
Mild Adverse Effects
Allergic Reactions: Skin rash; eye drops may cause redness, swelling and itching of the eyelids.
Weakness, dizziness, pallor.

Serious Adverse Effects

Idiosyncratic Reaction: Sudden development of excessive fluid in the lungs (pulmonary edema).

In predisposed individuals—excessive rise in blood pressure with risk of stroke (cerebral hemorrhage).

▷ **Possible Effects on Sexual Function:**   None reported.

CAUTION

1. The frequently repeated use of this drug at short intervals can produce a condition of unresponsiveness and result in medication failure. If this develops, avoid use completely for 12 hours, at which time a normal response should return.
2. Excessive use of aerosol preparations in the treatment of asthma has been associated with sudden death.
3. This drug can cause significant irritability of the nerve pathways (conduction system) and muscles of the heart, predisposing to serious heart rhythm disorders. If you have any form of heart disorder, consult your physician.
4. This drug can increase the blood sugar level. If you have diabetes, test for urine sugar frequently to detect significant changes.
5. If you become unresponsive to this drug and you intend to substitute isoproterenol (Isuprel), allow an interval of 4 hours between using these two drugs.
6. Promptly discard all preparations of this drug at the first appearance of discoloration (pink to red to brown) or cloudiness (precipitation). Such changes indicate drug deterioration.

Precautions for Use

By Infants and Children: Use cautiously in small doses until tolerance is determined. Observe for any indications of weakness, light-headedness or inclination to faint.

By Those over 60 Years of Age: Use cautiously in small doses until tolerance is determined. Observe for excessive stimulation: nervousness, headache, tremor, rapid heart rate. If you have hardening of the arteries (arteriosclerosis), heart disease, high blood pressure, Parkinson's disease or prostatism (see Glossary), this drug may aggravate your disorder. Ask your physician for guidance.

▷ **Advisability of Use During Pregnancy**

Pregnancy Category: C (tentative). See Pregnancy Code inside back cover.

Animal studies: Birth defects reported in rats.

Human studies: Information from adequate studies of pregnant women is not available.

This drug can cause significant reduction of oxygen supply to the fetus. Use it only if clearly needed and in small, infrequent doses. Avoid during the first 3 months and during labor and delivery.

Advisability of Use if Breast-Feeding

Presence of this drug in breast milk: Yes.

Avoid drug or refrain from nursing.

Habit-Forming Potential: Tolerance to this drug can develop with frequent use (see Glossary), but dependence does not occur.

Effects of Overdosage: Nervousness, throbbing headache, dizziness, tremor, palpitation, disturbance of heart rhythm, difficult breathing, abdominal pain, vomiting of blood.

Possible Effects of Long-Term Use: "Epinephrine-fastness": loss of ability to respond to this drug's bronchodilator effect. With long-term treatment of glaucoma: pigment deposits on eyeball and eyelids, possible damage to retina, impaired vision, blockage of tear ducts.

Suggested Periodic Examinations While Taking This Drug (at physician's discretion)
Blood pressure measurements; blood or urine sugar measurements in presence of diabetes; vision testing and measurement of internal eye pressure in presence of glaucoma.

▷ **While Taking This Drug, Observe the Following**
Foods: No restrictions, except those that have been shown to cause you to have asthma.
Beverages: No restrictions.
▷ *Alcohol:* Alcoholic beverages can increase the urinary excretion of this drug.
Tobacco Smoking: No interactions expected. Follow physician's advice regarding smoking as it affects the condition under treatment.
▷ *Other Drugs*
Epinephrine *taken concurrently* with
- certain beta blocker drugs (nadolol, propranolol) may cause increased blood pressure and decreased heart rate.
- chlorpromazine (Thorazine) may cause decreased blood pressure and increased heart rate.
- furazolidone (Furoxone) may cause increased blood pressure and high fever.
- guanethidine (Esimil, Ismelin) may cause increased blood pressure.
- tricyclic antidepressants (amitriptyline, etc.) may cause increased blood pressure and heart rhythm disturbances.
▷ *Driving, Hazardous Activities:* This drug may cause dizziness or excessive nervousness. Restrict activities as necessary.
Aviation Note: The use of this drug *may be a disqualification* for piloting. Consult a designated Aviation Medical Examiner.
Exposure to Sun: No restrictions.
Heavy Exercise or Exertion: No interactions expected. However, exercise can induce asthma in sensitive individuals.
Occurrence of Unrelated Illness: Use caution in presence of severe burns. This drug can increase drainage from burned tissue and cause significant loss of tissue fluids and blood proteins.
Discontinuation: If this drug fails to provide relief after an adequate trial, discontinue it and consult your physician. It is dangerous to increase the dosage or frequency of use.

Special Storage Instructions: Protect drug from exposure to air, light and heat. Keep in a cool place, preferably in the refrigerator.

ERGOLOID MESYLATES
(ER goh loyd MESS i lates)

Other Name: Dihydrogenated ergot alkaloids

Introduced: 1949   **Class:** Ergot preparations

Prescription: USA: Yes   **Controlled Drug:** USA: No
    Canada: Yes   Canada: No

Available as Generic: USA: Yes
    Canada: No

Brand Names: Deapril-ST, Hydergine, Hydergine LC

BENEFITS versus RISKS	
Possible Benefits	*Possible Risks*
Limited relief of symptoms associated with deteriorating brain function (in some individuals)	Low blood pressure, fainting Slow heart rate Worsening of symptoms (instead of relief)

▷ **Principal Uses**

As a Single Drug Product: The use of this drug is limited to the treatment of the aging individual with symptoms indicative of deteriorating brain function. Its benefit is unpredictable, and its use must be monitored carefully and adjusted appropriately for each individual.

How This Drug Works: Not completely established. Present theory is that by stimulating brain cell metabolism, this drug increases the brain's ability to utilize oxygen and nutrients. The resulting improvement in brain function is thought to contribute to the benefit seen in responsive individuals.

Available Dosage Forms and Strengths
        Capsules, liquid — 1 mg
                Liquid — 1 mg per ml
                Tablets — 1 mg
        Tablets, sublingual — 0.5 mg, 1 mg

▷ **Usual Adult Dosage Range:**   1 to 2 mg, 3 times/day. **Note: Actual dosage and administration schedule must be determined by the physician for each patient individually.**

▷ **Dosing Instructions:** May be taken on an empty stomach or with food to reduce stomach irritation. The regular tablet may be crushed for administration. The sublingual tablet should be dissolved under the tongue and not swallowed. The liquid capsule should be taken whole (unopened).

Usual Duration of Use: Continual use on a regular schedule for 3 to 4 weeks is usually necessary to determine this drug's effectiveness in relieving the symptoms of mental deterioration. Long-term use requires supervision and periodic evaluation by your physician. Consult your physician on a regular basis.

▷ **This Drug Should Not Be Taken If**
- you have had an allergic reaction to any dosage form of it previously.
- your pulse rate is below 60 beats/minute or your systolic blood pressure is consistently below 100.
- you have an active psychosis.

▷ **Inform Your Physician Before Taking This Drug If**
- you have a history of low blood pressure.
- you are taking any of the following: antihypertensive drugs, a beta blocker drug or any form of digitalis.

Possible Side-Effects (natural, expected and unavoidable drug actions)
Orthostatic hypotension (see Glossary).

▷ **Possible Adverse Effects** (unusual, unexpected and infrequent reactions)
If any of the following develop, consult your physician promptly for guidance.
Mild Adverse Effects
Allergic Reactions: Skin rash, drug fever (see Glossary).
Headache, dizziness, flushing, blurred vision.
Nasal stuffiness, reduced appetite, nausea, vomiting, stomach cramping.
Serious Adverse Effects
Marked drop in blood pressure, falling, fainting.
Marked slowing of the heart rate (40 to 50 beats/minute).
Reduced activity, sluggishness, drowsiness, emotional withdrawal, apathy.

▷ **Possible Effects on Sexual Function:** None reported.

Natural Diseases or Disorders That May Be Activated by This Drug
Ergot alkaloids can precipitate attacks of acute intermittent porphyria in susceptible individuals.

CAUTION
While numerous studies have demonstrated that this drug can be beneficial in relieving many complaints of the elderly related to memory, intellectual performance and social adjustment, others have not con-

firmed this. It is important to remember that the causes of such symptoms are poorly understood, that they can occur whether or not drugs are being taken and that behavioral changes in the elderly are often frequent and unpredictable. It is therefore advisable to monitor the response to this drug very closely and to notify the physician if any significant adverse personality changes occur. In some instances, the development of nervousness, hostility, confusion and depression may be related to the use of this drug.

Precautions for Use
By Those over 60 Years of Age: It is not possible to predict in advance the nature of your response to this drug. It may relieve your symptoms, have no significant effect or make your symptoms worse. Dosage must be carefully individualized.

Habit-Forming Potential: None.

Effects of Overdosage: Headache, flushing, nasal stuffiness, weakness, nausea, vomiting, collapse, coma.

Possible Effects of Long-Term Use: None reported.

Suggested Periodic Examinations While Taking This Drug (at physician's discretion)
Pulse counts and blood pressure measurements on a regular basis.

▷ **While Taking This Drug, Observe the Following**
Foods: No restrictions.
Beverages: No restrictions.
▷ *Alcohol:* Use with caution until the combined effects have been determined. Sensitive individuals may experience an excessive drop in blood pressure.
Tobacco Smoking: No interactions expected.
▷ *Other Drugs*
Ergoloid mesylates may ***increase*** the effects of
• antihypertensive drugs, and cause excessive lowering of blood pressure.
Ergoloid mesylates ***taken concurrently*** with
• beta blocker drugs (see Drug Class, Section Four) may cause excessive slowing of heart rate and/or excessive lowering of blood pressure.
• digitalis preparations (Lanoxin, etc.) may cause excessive slowing of heart rate.
▷ *Driving, Hazardous Activities:* This drug may cause dizziness or blurred vision. Restrict activities as necessary.
Aviation Note: Brain function disorder ***is a disqualification*** for piloting. Consult a designated Aviation Medical Examiner.
Exposure to Sun: No restrictions.
Exposure to Cold: Use caution. Avoid exposure that could lower body temperature, impair metabolism and induce hypothermia (see Glossary).

ERGOTAMINE
(er GOT a meen)

Introduced: 1926

Class: Antimigraine, ergot preparations

Prescription: USA: Yes
Canada: Yes

Controlled Drug: USA: No
Canada: No

Available as Generic: No

Brand Names: ✦Bellergal [CD], Bellergal-S [CD], ✦Bellergal Spacetabs [CD], Cafergot [CD], Cafergot P-B [CD], Ercaf [CD], ✦Ergodryl [CD], Ergomar, Ergostat, ✦Gynergen, Medihaler Ergotamine, Wigraine [CD], Wigrettes

---

BENEFITS versus RISKS

Possible Benefits	*Possible Risks*
PREVENTION AND RELIEF OF VASCULAR HEADACHES: MIGRAINE, MIGRAINELIKE AND HISTAMINE HEADACHES	GANGRENE OF THE FINGERS, TOES OR INTESTINE AGGRAVATION OF CORONARY ARTERY DISEASE (ANGINA) ABORTION

▷ **Principal Uses**

As a Single Drug Product: This drug is used primarily in the treatment of vascular headaches, especially migraine and "cluster" headaches. It should not be used on a continual basis to prevent migraine attacks, but it is often effective in terminating the headache if taken within the first hour following the onset of pain. It may be used on a short-term basis in an attempt to prevent or abort "cluster" headaches during the period of their occurrence. The inhalation form provides rapid onset of action.

As a Combination Drug Product [CD]: This drug is combined with caffeine to take advantage of caffeine's ability to enhance its absorption. This permits a smaller dose of ergotamine to be effective and reduces the risk of adverse effects with repeated use. This drug is also combined with belladonna (atropine) and one of the barbiturates to provide preparations that are useful in relieving the symptoms of premenstrual tension and the menopausal syndrome: nervousness, nausea, hot flushes and sweating.

How This Drug Works: Not completely established. It is thought that by constricting the walls of blood vessels in the head, this drug prevents or relieves the excessive expansion (dilation) that is responsible for the pain of migrainelike headaches.

Available Dosage Forms and Strengths
Aerosol — 9 mg per ml (0.36 mg/inhalation)
Suppositories — 2 mg (in combination with caffeine)
Tablets, sublingual — 2 mg

▷ **Usual Adult Dosage Range:**   Inhalation: 1 spray (0.36 mg) at the onset of headache; repeat 1 spray every 5 to 10 minutes as needed for relief, up to a maximum of 6 sprays/24 hours. Do not exceed 15 sprays/week. Sublingual tablets: Dissolve 1 mg under tongue at the onset of headache; repeat 1 mg every 30 to 60 minutes as needed, up to a maximum of 5 mg/attack. Do not exceed 5 mg/24 hours or 10 mg/week. Try to determine the optimal dose required (up to 5 mg) that will abort the headache when taken as a single dose at the onset of pain. **Note: Actual dosage and administration schedule must be determined by the physician for each patient individually.**

▷ **Dosing Instructions:**   Follow written instructions carefully. Do not exceed prescribed doses. The regular tablets (combination drug) may be crushed for administration; the sustained-release tablets should be taken whole (not crushed). Sublingual tablets should be dissolved under the tongue, not swallowed.

Usual Duration of Use: Continual use on a regular schedule for several episodes of headache is usually necessary to determine this drug's effectiveness in aborting or relieving the pain of vascular headache. Do not exceed recommended dosage schedules. If headaches are not controlled after several trials of maximal doses, consult your physician for alternative treatment.

▷ **This Drug Should Not Be Taken If**
- you have had an allergic reaction to any dosage form of it previously.
- you are pregnant.
- you have a severe infection.
- you have any of the following conditions:
angina pectoris (coronary artery disease)
Buerger's disease
hardening of the arteries (arteriosclerosis)
high blood pressure (severe hypertension)
kidney disease or impaired kidney function
liver disease or impaired liver function
Raynaud's phenomenon
thrombophlebitis
severe itching

▷ **Inform Your Physician Before Taking This Drug If**
- you are allergic or overly sensitive to *any* ergot preparation.

Possible Side-Effects (natural, expected and unavoidable drug actions)
Usually infrequent and mild with recommended doses.
Susceptible individuals may notice a sensation of cold hands and feet, with mild numbness and tingling.

▷ **Possible Adverse Effects** (unusual, unexpected and infrequent reactions)
If any of the following develop, consult your physician promptly for guidance.
Mild Adverse Effects
Allergic Reactions: Localized swellings (angioedema), itching.
Headache, drowsiness, dizziness, confusion.
Chest pain, numbness and tingling of fingers and toes, muscle pains in arms or legs.
Nausea, vomiting, diarrhea.
Serious Adverse Effects
Gangrene of the extremities—coldness; numbness; pain; dark discoloration; eventual loss of fingers, toes or feet.
Gangrene of the intestine—severe abdominal pain and swelling; emergency surgery required.

▷ **Possible Effects on Sexual Function:**   None reported.

Natural Diseases or Disorders That May Be Activated by This Drug
Angina pectoris (coronary artery insufficiency), Buerger's disease, Raynaud's syndrome.

CAUTION
1. The excessive use of this drug can actually provoke migraine headache and increase the frequency of its occurrence.
2. Do not exceed a total dose of 5 mg/24 hours or 10 mg/week.
3. Individual sensitivity to the effects of this drug vary greatly. Some may experience early toxic effects even while taking recommended doses. Report promptly any indications of impaired circulation: numbness in fingers or toes, muscle cramping, chest pain.

Precautions for Use
By Infants and Children: Safety and effectiveness for use by those under 12 years of age have not been established.
By Those over 60 Years of Age: Natural changes in blood vessels and circulation may make you more susceptible to the serious adverse effects of this drug. See the preceding list of disorders that are contraindications for the use of this drug.

▷ **Advisability of Use During Pregnancy**
Pregnancy Category: X. See Pregnancy Code inside back cover.
Animal studies: Fetal deaths reported due to this drug.
Human studies: Information from studies of pregnant women indicates that this drug can cause abortion.
This drug should be avoided during the entire pregnancy.

Advisability of Use if Breast-Feeding
Presence of this drug in breast milk: Yes.
Avoid drug or refrain from nursing.

Habit-Forming Potential: None.

Effects of Overdosage: Manifestations of "ergotism": coldness of skin, severe muscle pains, tingling and burning pain in hands and feet, loss of blood supply to extremities resulting in tissue death (gangrene) in fingers and toes. Acute ergot poisoning: nausea, vomiting, diarrhea, cold skin, numbness extremities, confusion, seizures, coma.

Possible Effects of Long-Term Use: A form of functional dependence (see Glossary) may develop, resulting in withdrawal headaches when the drug is discontinued.

Suggested Periodic Examinations While Taking This Drug (at physician's discretion)

Evaluation of circulation (blood flow) to the extremities.

▷ **While Taking This Drug, Observe the Following**

Foods: No interactions expected. Avoid all foods to which you are allergic; some migraine headaches are due to food allergies.

Beverages: No restrictions.

▷ *Alcohol:* Best avoided; alcohol can intensify vascular headache.

Tobacco Smoking: Best avoided; nicotine can further reduce the restricted blood flow produced by this drug.

Marijuana Smoking: Best avoided; additive effects can increase the coldness of hands and feet.

▷ *Other Drugs*

Ergotamine may ***decrease*** the effects of

• nitroglycerin, and reduce its effectiveness in preventing or relieving angina pain.

The following drugs may ***increase*** the effects of ergotamine

• erythromycin (E-Mycin, Eryc, etc.).

• troleandomycin (TAO).

▷ *Driving, Hazardous Activities:* This drug may cause drowsiness or dizziness. Restrict activities as necessary.

Aviation Note: Vascular headache ***is a disqualification*** for piloting. Consult a designated Aviation Medical Examiner.

Exposure to Sun: No restrictions.

Exposure to Cold: Avoid as much as possible. Cold environments and handling cold objects will further reduce the restricted blood flow to the extremities.

Discontinuation: Following long-term use, it may be necessary to withdraw this drug gradually to prevent withdrawal headache. Ask physician for guidance.

ERYTHROMYCIN
(er ith roh MY sin)

Introduced: 1952

Class: Antibiotic, erythromycins

Prescription: USA: Yes
Canada: Yes

Controlled Drug: USA: No
Canada: No

Available as Generic: Yes

Brand Names: ✦Apo-Erythro Base, ✦Apo-Erythro-ES, ✦Apo-Erythro-S, E.E.S., E-Mycin, E-Mycin E, E-Mycin 333, Eryc, Eryderm, Erypar, EryPed, Ery-Tab, Erythrocin, ✦Erythromid, Ilosone, Ilotycin, ✦Novorythro, PCE Dispertab, Pediamycin, Pediazole [CD], Robimycin, Wyamycin E, Wyamycin S

BENEFITS versus RISKS

Possible Benefits	*Possible Risks*
EFFECTIVE TREATMENT OF INFECTIONS DUE TO SUSCEPTIBLE MICROORGANISMS	Allergic reactions, mild and infrequent Liver reaction (most common with erythromycin estolate) Drug-induced colitis (rare) Superinfections (rare)

▷ **Principal Uses**

As a Single Drug Product: This well-tolerated and versatile antibiotic is used to treat a broad variety of common infections. The more important among these are (1) skin and skin structure infections; (2) upper and lower respiratory tract infections, including "strep" throat, diphtheria and several types of pneumonia; (3) gonorrhea and syphilis; and (4) amebic dysentery. It is also used for the long-term prevention of recurrences of rheumatic fever. Effective use requires the precise identification of the causative organism and determination of its sensitivity to erythromycin.

How This Drug Works: This drug prevents the growth and multiplication of susceptible organisms by interfering with their formation of essential proteins.

Available Dosage Forms and Strengths

Capsules —	125 mg, 250 mg
Capsules, enteric-coated —	125 mg, 250 mg
Drops —	100 mg per ml
Eye ointment —	5 mg per gram
Oral suspension —	125 mg, 250 mg per 5-ml teaspoonful
Skin ointment —	2%
Tablets —	500 mg
Tablets, chewable —	125 mg, 250 mg
Tablets, enteric-coated —	250 mg, 333 mg, 500 mg
Tablets, film-coated —	250 mg, 500 mg
Topical solution —	1.5%, 2%

▷ **Usual Adult Dosage Range:**   250 to 1000 mg/6 hours, according to nature and severity of infection. Total daily dosage should not exceed 8 grams. For endocarditis prophylaxis: 1 gram 2 hours before procedure and 500 mg 6 hours later. **Note: Actual dosage and administration schedule must be determined by the physician for each patient individually.**

▷ **Dosing Instructions:** Nonenteric-coated preparations should be taken 1 hour before or 2 hours after eating. Enteric-coated preparations may be taken without regard to food. Regular uncoated capsules may be opened and tablets may be crushed for administration; coated and prolonged-action preparations should be swallowed whole. Ask pharmacist for guidance.

Usual Duration of Use: Continual use on a regular schedule for 3 to 5 days is usually necessary to determine this drug's effectiveness in controlling responsive infections. For streptococcal infections: not less than 10 consecutive days (without interruption) to reduce the possibility of developing rheumatic fever or glomerulonephritis. The duration of use should not exceed the time required to eliminate the infection.

▷ **This Drug Should Not Be Taken If**
- you have had an allergic reaction to any form of erythromycin previously.
- you have active liver disease.

▷ **Inform Your Physician Before Taking This Drug If**
- you have a history of a previous "reaction" to erythromycin.
- you are allergic by nature: hay fever, asthma, hives, eczema.
- you have taken the estolate form of erythromycin previously.

Possible Side-Effects (natural, expected and unavoidable drug actions)
Superinfections (see Glossary).

▷ **Possible Adverse Effects** (unusual, unexpected and infrequent reactions)
If any of the following develop, consult your physician promptly for guidance.
Mild Adverse Effects
Allergic Reactions: Skin rash, hives, itching.
Nausea, vomiting, diarrhea, abdominal cramping.
Serious Adverse Effects
Allergic Reaction: Rare anaphylactic reaction (see Glossary).
Idiosyncratic Reactions: Liver reaction—nausea, vomiting, fever, jaundice (usually but not exclusively associated with erythromycin estolate).
Drug-induced colitis, transient loss of hearing.

▷ **Possible Effects on Sexual Function:** None reported.

▷ **Adverse Effects That May Mimic Natural Diseases or Disorders**
Liver toxicity may resemble acute gallbladder disease or viral hepatitis.

CAUTION

1. Take the full dosage prescribed to prevent the possible emergence of resistant bacterial strains.
2. If you have a history of liver disease or impaired liver function, avoid any form of erythromycin estolate.
3. If diarrhea develops and continues for more than 24 hours, consult your physician promptly.

Precautions for Use

By Infants and Children: Observe allergic children closely for indications of developing allergy to this drug. Observe also for evidence of gastrointestinal irritation.

By Those over 60 Years of Age: Observe for indications of itching reactions in the genital and anal regions, often due to yeast superinfections. Observe also for evidence of hearing loss. Report such developments promptly.

▷ **Advisability of Use During Pregnancy**

Pregnancy Category: B (tentative). See Pregnancy Code inside back cover.
Animal studies: Studies of rats are inconclusive.
Human studies: No increase in birth defects reported in 230 exposures. Information from adequate studies of pregnant women is not available.
Generally thought to be safe during entire pregnancy, *except for erythromycin estolate*; this form of erythromycin can cause toxic liver reactions during pregnancy and should be avoided.

Advisability of Use if Breast-Feeding

Presence of this drug in breast milk: Yes.
Monitor nursing infant closely and discontinue drug or nursing if adverse effects develop.

Habit-Forming Potential: None.

Effects of Overdosage: Possible nausea, vomiting, diarrhea and abdominal discomfort.

Possible Effects of Long-Term Use: Superinfections (see Glossary).

Suggested Periodic Examinations While Taking This Drug (at physician's discretion)
Liver function tests if the estolate form is used.

▷ **While Taking This Drug, Observe the Following**

Foods: No restrictions.
Beverages: Avoid fruit juices and carbonated beverages for 1 hour after taking any nonenteric-coated preparation. May be taken with milk.
▷ *Alcohol:* Avoid if you have impaired liver function or are taking the estolate form of this drug.
Tobacco Smoking: No interactions expected.

▷ *Other Drugs*
Erythromycin may *increase* the effects of
- carbamazepine (Tegretol), and cause toxicity.
- digoxin (Lanoxin), and cause toxicity.
- ergotamine (Cafergot, Ergostat, etc.), and cause impaired circulation to extremities.
- methylprednisolone (Medrol), and cause excess steroid effects.
- theophylline (aminophylline, Theo-Dur, etc.), and cause toxicity.
- warfarin (Coumadin), and increase the risk of bleeding.

Erythromycin may *decrease* the effects of
- clindamycin.
- lincomycin.
- penicillins.

▷ *Driving, Hazardous Activities:* This drug may cause nausea and/or diarrhea. Restrict activities as necessary.

Aviation Note: The use of this drug *may be a disqualification* for piloting. Consult a designated Aviation Medical Examiner.

Exposure to Sun: No restrictions.

Special Storage Instructions: Keep liquid forms refrigerated.

Observe the Following Expiration Times: Freshly mixed oral suspension—14 days. Premixed oral suspension—18 months. Ask pharmacist for guidance.

ESTROGENS
(ES troh jenz)

Other Names: Chlorotrianisene, conjugated estrogens, esterified estrogens, estradiol, estriol, estrone, estropipate, quinestrol

Introduced: 1933　　**Class:** Female sex hormones

Prescription: USA: Yes　　**Controlled Drug:** USA: No
　　Canada: Yes　　　　　　　　　Canada: No

Available as Generic: USA: Yes
　　Canada: No

Brand Names: ✦C.E.S., ✦Climestrone, ✦Delestrogen, DV, Estinyl, Estrace, Estraderm, Estraguard, Estratab, Estrovis, Feminone, ✦Femogen, ✦Femogex, Menest, Menrium [CD], Milprem [CD], ✦Oestrilin, Ogen, PMB [CD], Premarin, TACE

BENEFITS versus RISKS

Possible Benefits	*Possible Risks*
EFFECTIVE RELIEF OF MENOPAUSAL HOT FLUSHES AND NIGHT SWEATS	INCREASED RISK OF CANCER OF THE UTERUS with 3+ years of continual use
PREVENTION OR RELIEF OF ATROPHIC VAGINITIS, ATROPHY OF THE VULVA AND URETHRA	Increased frequency of gallstones
	Accelerated growth of preexisting fibroid tumors of the uterus
	Fluid retention
PREVENTION OF OSTEOPOROSIS	Postmenopausal bleeding
Prevention of thinning of the skin	Deep vein thrombophlebitis and thromboembolism (less likely with conjugated estrogens, more likely with synthetic unconjugated hormones)
Mental tonic effect	Increased blood pressure (rare)
	Decreased sugar tolerance (rare)

▷ **Principal Uses**

As a Single Drug Product: This widely used hormone is very effective when administered in proper dosage and carefully supervised. Its primary use is supplemental ("replacement" therapy) when used to treat the following conditions: (1) ovarian failure or removal in the young woman; (2) the menopausal syndrome; (3) postmenopausal atrophy of genital tissues; and (4) postmenopausal osteoporosis. It is also used in selected cases of breast cancer and prostate cancer.

As a Combination Drug Product [CD]: Estrogen is available in combination with chlordiazepoxide (Librium) and with meprobamate (Equanil, Miltown). These mild tranquilizers are added to provide a calming effect that makes the combination more effective in treating selected cases of the menopausal syndrome. See the Drug Profile of the Oral Contraceptives for a discussion of the combination of estrogens and progestins.

How This Drug Works: When used to correct hormonal deficiency states, estrogens restore normal cellular activity by increasing the synthesis of chromatin, RNA and cellular proteins. The frequency and intensity of menopausal symptoms are significantly reduced when normal tissue levels of estrogen are restored.

Available Dosage Forms and Strengths

Capsules — 12 mg, 25 mg, 72 mg (TACE)

Tablets — 0.02 mg, 0.05 mg, 0.1 mg, 0.3 mg, 0.5 mg, 0.625 mg, 0.9 mg, 1.25 mg, 2.5 mg, 5 mg

Transdermal patch — 0.05 mg, 0.1 mg

Vaginal cream — 0.1 mg, 0.625 mg, 1.5 mg per gram

▷ **Usual Adult Dosage Range:**   For conjugated and esterified estrogens: 0.3 to 1.25 mg daily for 21 days. Omit for 7 days. Repeat cyclically as needed. For other forms of estrogen: consult your physician. **Note: Actual dosage and administration schedule must be determined by the physician for each patient individually.**

▷ **Dosing Instructions:**   May be taken without regard to food. The tablets may be crushed for administration. The capsules should be taken whole.

Usual Duration of Use: Continual use on a regular schedule for 10 to 20 days is usually necessary to determine this drug's effectiveness in relieving menopausal symptoms. Long-term use requires supervision and periodic evaluation by your physician every 6 months. Consult your physician on a regular basis.

▷ **This Drug Should Not Be Taken If**
  • you have had a significant allergic reaction to any dosage form of it previously.
  • you have a history of thrombophlebitis, embolism, heart attack or stroke.
  • you have seriously impaired liver function.
  • you have abnormal and unexplained vaginal bleeding.
  • you have sickle cell disease.
  • you are pregnant.

▷ **Inform Your Physician Before Taking This Drug If**
  • you have had an unfavorable reaction to estrogen therapy previously.
  • you have a history of cancer of the breast or reproductive organs.
  • you have any of the following conditions: fibrocystic breast changes, fibroid tumors of the uterus, endometriosis, migrainelike headaches, epilepsy, asthma, heart disease, high blood pressure, gallbladder disease, diabetes or porphyria.
  • you smoke tobacco on a regular basis.
  • you plan to have surgery in the near future.

Possible Side-Effects (natural, expected and unavoidable drug actions)
  Fluid retention, weight gain, "breakthrough" bleeding (spotting in middle of menstrual cycle), altered menstrual pattern, resumption of menstrual flow (bleeding from the uterus) after a period of natural cessation (postmenopausal bleeding), increased susceptibility to yeast infection of the genital tissues.

▷ **Possible Adverse Effects** (unusual, unexpected and infrequent reactions)
  If any of the following develop, consult your physician promptly for guidance.
  Mild Adverse Effects
  Allergic Reactions: Skin rash, hives, itching.
  Headache, nervous tension, irritability, accentuation of migraine headaches.

Nausea, vomiting, bloating, diarrhea.

Tannish pigmentation of the face.

Serious Adverse Effects

Idiosyncratic Reaction: Cutaneous porphyria—fragility and scarring of the skin.

Emotional depression, rise in blood pressure (in susceptible individuals).

Gallbladder disease, benign liver tumors, jaundice, rise in blood sugar.

Erosion of uterine cervix, enlargement of uterine fibroid tumors.

Thrombophlebitis (inflammation of a vein with formation of blood clot)—pain or tenderness in thigh or leg, with or without swelling of foot or leg.

Pulmonary embolism (movement of blood clot to lung)—sudden shortness of breath, pain in chest, coughing, bloody sputum.

Stroke (blood clot in brain)—headaches, blackout, sudden weakness or paralysis of any part of the body, severe dizziness, altered vision, slurred speech, inability to speak.

Retinal thrombosis (blood clot in eye vessels)—sudden impairment or loss of vision.

Heart attack (blood clot in coronary artery)—sudden pain in chest, neck, jaw or arm; weakness; sweating; nausea.

▷ **Possible Effects on Sexual Function**

Swelling and tenderness of breasts, milk production.

Increased vaginal secretions.

Possible Delayed Adverse Effects: Estrogens taken during pregnancy can predispose the female child to the later development of cancer of the vagina or cervix following puberty.

▷ **Adverse Effects That May Mimic Natural Diseases or Disorders**

Liver reactions may suggest viral hepatitis.

Natural Diseases or Disorders That May Be Activated by This Drug

Latent hypertension, diabetes mellitus, acute intermittent porphyria.

CAUTION

1. To avoid prolonged (uninterrupted) stimulation of breast and uterine tissues, estrogen should be taken in cycles of 3 weeks on and 1 week off of medication.
2. The estrogen in estrogen vaginal creams is absorbed systemically by the woman. It may also be absorbed through the penis during sexual intercourse and can cause enlargement and tenderness of male breast tissue.

Precautions for Use

By Those over 60 Years of Age: This drug has very limited usefulness after 60. Its use should be restricted to those women who are at increased risk for developing osteoporosis. In this age group, it is advisable to attempt relief of hot flushes with nonestrogenic medications. During use, report promptly any indications of impaired circulation: speech disturbances, altered vision, sudden hearing loss, vertigo, sudden weakness or paralysis, angina, leg pains.

▷ **Advisability of Use During Pregnancy**

Pregnancy Category: X. See Pregnancy Code inside back cover.

Animal studies: Genital defects reported in mice and guinea pigs; cleft palate reported in rodents.

Human studies: Information from studies of pregnant women indicates that estrogens can masculinize the female fetus. In addition, limb defects and heart malformations have been reported.

It is now known that estrogens taken during pregnancy can predispose the female child to the development of cancer of the vagina or cervix following puberty. *Avoid estrogens completely during entire pregnancy.*

Advisability of Use if Breast-Feeding

Presence of this drug in breast milk: Yes, in minute amounts.

Estrogens in large doses can suppress milk formation.

Breast-feeding is considered to be safe during the use of estrogens.

Habit-Forming Potential: None.

Effects of Overdosage: Headache, drowsiness, nausea, vomiting, fluid retention, abnormal vaginal bleeding, breast enlargement and discomfort.

Possible Effects of Long-Term Use: High blood pressure, gallbladder disease with gallstone formation, increased growth of benign fibroid tumors of the uterus. Several reports suggest possible association between the long-term use (3 + years) of estrogens and the development of cancer of the lining of the uterus. Further studies are needed to establish a definite cause-and-effect relationship (see Glossary). Prudence dictates that women with uterus intact should use estrogens only when symptoms justify it and with proper supervision. See the profile of menopause in Section Two.

Suggested Periodic Examinations While Taking This Drug (at physician's discretion)

Regular (every 6 months) evaluation of the breasts and pelvic organs, including Pap smears. Liver function tests as indicated.

▷ **While Taking This Drug, Observe the Following**

Foods: Avoid excessive use of salt if fluid retention occurs.

Beverages: No restrictions. May be taken with milk.

▷ *Alcohol:* No interactions expected.

Tobacco Smoking: Recent studies indicate that heavy smoking (15 or more cigarettes daily) in association with the use of estrogen-containing oral contraceptives significantly increases the risk of heart attack (coronary thrombosis). Avoid heavy smoking during long-term estrogen therapy.

▷ *Other Drugs*

Estrogens *taken concurrently* with
- antidiabetic drugs may cause unpredictable fluctuations of blood sugar.
- tricyclic antidepressants (Elavil, Sinequan, etc.) may enhance their adverse effects and reduce their antidepressant effectiveness.
- warfarin (Coumadin) may cause unpredictable alterations of pro-thrombin activity.

The following drugs may *decrease* the effects of estrogens
- carbamazepine (Tegretol).
- phenobarbital.
- phenytoin (Dilantin).
- primidone (Mysoline).
- rifampin (Rifadin, Rimactane).

▷ *Driving, Hazardous Activities:* Usually no restrictions. Consult your physician for assessment of individual risk and for guidance regarding specific restrictions.

Aviation Note: Usually no restrictions. However, it is advisable to observe for the rare occurrence of disturbed vision and to restrict activities accordingly. Consult a designated Aviation Medical Examiner.

Exposure to Sun: Use caution until full effect is known. These drugs can cause photosensitivity (see Glossary).

Discontinuation: It is advisable to discontinue estrogens periodically to determine if a need for them still exists. Reduce the dose gradually to prevent acute withdrawal hot flushes. Avoid continual, uninterrupted use of large doses. Discontinue altogether when a definite indication for replacement therapy no longer exists. Ask your physician for guidance.

ETHOSUXIMIDE
(eth oh SUX i mide)

Introduced: 1960

Class: Anticonvulsant, succinimides

Prescription: USA: Yes
Canada: Yes

Controlled Drug: USA: No
Canada: No

Available as Generic: No

Brand Name: Zarontin

BENEFITS versus RISKS	
Possible Benefits	*Possible Risks*
EFFECTIVE CONTROL OF ABSENCE SEIZURES (PETIT MAL EPILEPSY) in 70% of cases	RARE APLASTIC ANEMIA (See Aplastic Anemia and Bone Marrow Depression in Glossary)
EFFECTIVE CONTROL OF MYOCLONIC AND AKINETIC EPILEPSY in some individuals	Rare decrease in white blood cells and blood platelets

▷ **Principal Uses**

As a Single Drug Product: This is the drug of first choice by many physicians for the management of absence seizures. It causes serious adverse effects less frequently than other drugs used for this disorder, and it is quite effective in the presence of structural abnormalities of the brain.

How This Drug Works: Not completely established. It is thought that by altering the transmission of certain nerve impulses, this drug suppresses the abnormal showers of electrical activity responsible for the absence seizures of petit mal epilepsy.

Available Dosage Forms and Strengths

Capsules — 250 mg
Syrup — 250 mg per 5-ml teaspoonful

▷ **Usual Adult Dosage Range:**   20 to 40 mg per kilogram of body weight/24 hours. Initially 500 mg/24 hours. Dosage may be increased cautiously by 250 mg every 4 to 7 days until satisfactory control is achieved. The total daily dosage should not exceed 1500 mg. **Note: Actual dosage and administration schedule must be determined by the physician for each patient individually.**

▷ **Dosing Instructions:**   May be taken with food to reduce stomach irritation. Capsule may be opened for administration.

Usual Duration of Use: Continual use on a regular schedule for 1 to 2 weeks is usually necessary to determine this drug's effectiveness in reducing the frequency of absence seizures. Long-term use requires supervision and periodic evaluation by your physician. Consult your physician on a regular basis.

▷ **This Drug Should Not Be Taken If**

- you are allergic to this or any other succinimide: methsuximide (Celontin), phenfuximide (Milontin).
- you have active liver disease.
- you currently have a blood cell or bone marrow disorder.

▷ **Inform Your Physician Before Taking This Drug If**
- you have a history of liver or kidney disease.
- you have a history of any type of blood cell disorder, especially one induced by drugs.
- you have a history of serious depression or other mental illness.

Possible Side-Effects (natural, expected and unavoidable drug actions)
Drowsiness, lethargy, fatigue.

▷ **Possible Adverse Effects** (unusual, unexpected and infrequent reactions)
If any of the following develop, consult your physician promptly for guidance.
Mild Adverse Effects
Allergic Reactions: Skin rash, hives.
Headache, dizziness, unsteadiness, euphoria, impaired vision, numbness and tingling in extremities.
Loss of appetite, nausea, vomiting, hiccups, stomach pain, diarrhea.
Excessive growth of hair.
Serious Adverse Effects
Allergic Reaction: Swelling of tongue.
Thickening and overgrowth of gums.
Nervousness, hyperactivity, disturbed sleep, night terrors.
Aggravation of emotional depression and paranoid mental disorders.
Severe bone marrow depression—fatigue, weakness, fever, sore throat, abnormal bleeding or bruising.

▷ **Possible Effects on Sexual Function:**   Increased libido (questionable); nonmenstrual vaginal bleeding.

Natural Diseases or Disorders That May Be Activated by This Drug
Latent psychosis, systemic lupus erythematosus.

CAUTION
1. This drug may increase the frequency of grand mal seizures in individuals with mixed seizure disorders.
2. It is mandatory that you comply with your physician's request for periodic blood counts and other tests that are deemed necessary.

Precautions for Use
By Infants and Children: If a single daily dose causes nausea or vomiting, give in 2 or 3 divided doses 8 to 12 hours apart. Marked individual variation in response occurs; the use of blood levels for monitoring is advised. Observe for a possible lupuslike reaction: fever, rash, arthritis.
By Those over 60 Years of Age: Rarely used in this age group.

▷ **Advisability of Use During Pregnancy**
Pregnancy Category: C (tentative). See Pregnancy Code inside back cover.
Animal studies: Bone defects reported in rodents.

Human studies: Three instances of birth defects have been reported. Information from adequate studies of pregnant women is not available.

Avoid during first 3 months. Use only if clearly needed during the last 6 months.

Advisability of Use if Breast-Feeding

Presence of this drug in breast milk: Yes.

Monitor nursing infant closely and discontinue drug or nursing if adverse effects develop. If mother requires high doses, refrain from nursing. Ask physician for guidance.

Habit-Forming Potential: None.

Effects of Overdosage: Increased drowsiness, lethargy, weakness, dizziness, unsteadiness, nausea, vomiting, stupor progressing to coma.

Possible Effects of Long-Term Use: Systemic lupus erythematosus.

Suggested Periodic Examinations While Taking This Drug (at physician's discretion)

Complete blood cell counts every 2 weeks during the first 3 months of use, then monthly thereafter; liver and kidney function tests.

▷ **While Taking This Drug, Observe the Following**

Foods: No restrictions.

Beverages: No restrictions. May be taken with milk.

▷   *Alcohol:* Use caution until the combined effects have been determined. This drug may increase the sedative effects of alcohol. Excessive alcohol may precipitate seizures.

Tobacco Smoking: No interactions expected.

▷   *Other Drugs*

Ethosuximide may *increase* the effects of

• phenytoin (Dilantin), by slowing its elimination.

Ethosuximide *taken concurrently* with

• valproic acid (Depakene) may alter the effects of ethosuximide unpredictably.

The following drugs may *increase* the effects of ethosuximide

• isoniazid (INH, Niconyl, etc.).

▷   *Driving, Hazardous Activities:* This drug may cause drowsiness, dizziness, unsteadiness and impaired vision. Restrict activities as necessary.

Aviation Note: Seizure disorders and the use of this drug **are disqualifications** for piloting. Consult a designated Aviation Medical Examiner.

Exposure to Sun: No restrictions.

Discontinuation: Do not stop taking this drug abruptly. Ask your physician for guidance regarding gradual reduction of dosage.

ETRETINATE
(e TRET i nayt)

Introduced: 1976

Class: Antipsoriasis

Prescription: USA: Yes
Canada: Yes

Controlled Drug: USA: No
Canada: No

Available as Generic: USA: No
Canada: No

Brand Name: Tegison

BENEFITS versus RISKS	
Possible Benefits	*Possible Risks*
EFFECTIVE TREATMENT FOR SEVERE, RESISTANT PSORIASIS in the majority of all cases treated	MAJOR DRUG-INDUCED BIRTH DEFECTS RARE DRUG-INDUCED HEPATITIS Adverse effects on eyes and vision Adverse effects on musculoskeletal structures Adverse effects on blood cholesterol and triglycerides Increased intracranial pressure (very rare)

▷ **Principal Uses**

As a Single Drug Product: Used primarily to treat severe, generalized forms of psoriasis (and related skin disorders) that have failed to respond to conventional, less hazardous treatments.

How This Drug Works: Not completely established. Its principal action is the regulation of cell differentiation in the skin; this results in a more normal pattern of cell growth, with reduction of inflammation and scale formation.

Available Dosage Forms and Strengths
Capsules — 10 mg, 25 mg

▷ **Usual Adult Dosage Range:**   Initially 0.75 to 1 mg/kg/day, in divided doses, until satisfactory response is obtained (usually 8 to 16 weeks). Maintenance: 0.5 to 0.75 mg/kg/day, beginning after initial response. Total daily dosage should not exceed 75 mg. **Note: Actual dosage and administration schedule must be determined by the physician for each patient individually.**

▷ **Dosing Instructions:**   Take with or immediately following meals, preferably with whole milk. Do not suck or chew the capsule; swallow it whole.

Usual Duration of Use: Continual use on a regular schedule for 2 to 4 weeks is usually necessary to determine this drug's effectiveness in reversing the skin changes of psoriasis. The full effect of treatment may not be apparent until after 2 to 3 months of continual use. Long-term use (months to years) requires periodic evaluation of response and dosage adjustment. Due to the potential for drug accumulation and toxicity with long-term use, this drug should be temporarily discontinued after 18 months of treatment; it may be resumed as needed. Consult your physician on a regular basis.

Possible Advantages of This Drug: When used in conjunction with other antipsoriasis drugs and procedures, this drug can enhance the therapeutic response and reduce the total dosage and length of treatment required for satisfactory management.

▷ **This Drug Should Not Be Taken If**
- you have had an allergic reaction to any dosage form of it previously.
- you are pregnant or breast-feeding.
- you plan to donate blood in the near future.

▷ **Inform Your Physician Before Taking This Drug If**
- you are allergic to vitamin A or other vitamin A derivatives: isotretinoin (Accutane), tretinoin (Retin-A).
- you are allergic to parabens (preservatives).
- you have cerebral or coronary artery disease.
- you have high blood cholesterol or triglyceride levels.
- you have diabetes.
- you have impaired liver or kidney function.
- you have alcoholism.
- you have a history of Crohn's disease or ulcerative colitis.

Possible Side-Effects (natural, expected and unavoidable drug actions)
Dry nose, nosebleed, dry lips, sore mouth and tongue, bleeding gums.
Loss of hair, skin peeling of hands and feet, dry skin, itching, bruising, nail deformities.
Thickening of bone (hyperostosis), calcification of tendons and ligaments, bone and joint pain.

▷ **Possible Adverse Effects** (unusual, unexpected and infrequent reactions)
If any of the following develop, consult your physician promptly for guidance.
Mild Adverse Effects
Allergic Reactions: Skin rash, hives, itching.
Headache, dizziness, fatigue, fever, emotional irritability.
Eye irritation, blurred or double vision, sensitivity to bright light, decreased tolerance for contact lenses, earache, impaired hearing.
Altered taste, loss of appetite, nausea, stomach pain, constipation, diarrhea.
Painful urination.

Serious Adverse Effects

Increased intracranial pressure (less than 1%): headache, nausea, vomiting, visual disturbances.

Hepatitis (1.5%); 4 reported deaths worldwide.

Eye reactions: corneal erosion, abrasion, staining; cataract; retinal hemorrhage; visual field defects; reduced night vision.

Inflammatory bowel disease (Crohn's disease), rare.

Altered blood fat levels: increased triglycerides (45%), increased total cholesterol (16%), decreased HDL cholesterol (37%); any of these changes may increase the risk for the development of atherosclerotic heart disease.

▷ **Possible Effects on Sexual Function:**   Altered timing and pattern of menstruation.

Possible Delayed Adverse Effects: This drug has been found in the blood 2.9 years following termination of its use and has the potential for inducing birth defects during this time. It has not been determined how long pregnancy should be avoided after discontinuation of treatment.

▷ **Adverse Effects That May Mimic Natural Diseases or Disorders**

Increased intracranial pressure may suggest brain tumor.

Liver reactions may suggest viral hepatitis.

Joint pains due to calcification of ligaments and tendons may suggest the onset of arthritis.

Natural Diseases or Disorders That May Be Activated by This Drug

Angina may develop in the presence of coronary artery heart disease. Heart attack (myocardial infarction) has been associated with the use of this drug.

CAUTION

1. *This drug should not be taken during pregnancy.* A pregnancy test should be performed within 2 weeks prior to taking this drug. In the absence of pregnancy, the drug should be started on the second or third day of the next normal menstrual period. An effective form of contraception should be used for 1 month before the drug is started, during the entire period of treatment, and for an indefinite period (minimum of 3 years) after the drug is discontinued. If pregnancy does occur, discontinue this drug immediately and consult your physician.

2. *Do not donate blood to a blood bank if you are taking this drug.* Blood containing this drug could pose a serious risk to the developing fetus of a pregnant patient who received it. Avoid blood donation for a minimum of 3 years if use of the blood is beyond your control.

3. *Comply fully with your physician's recommendations for periodic examinations before, during and following treatment with this drug.* These are mandatory for safe and effective use.
4. Avoid the concurrent use of vitamin A supplements while taking this drug.
5. If you experience significant eye reactions or altered vision, consult your physician promptly.
6. Your psoriasis may appear to worsen during the early period of treatment with this drug. This is a common response. Consult your physician if symptoms become severe or prolonged.
7. If dry mouth or sore and bleeding gums persist, consult your dentist.

Precautions for Use

By Infants and Children: This drug should be used only after all less hazardous treatments have failed. It is advisable to obtain pretreatment X-rays to determine bone age and to monitor bone growth and development by yearly X-ray studies. This drug can impair normal bone maturation.

By Those over 60 Years of Age: Monitor for the possible development of anemia, impaired kidney function and fluctuation of blood potassium levels.

▷ ## Advisability of Use During Pregnancy

Pregnancy Category: X. See Pregnancy Code inside back cover.

Animal studies: No information available.

Human studies: Major birth defects occur in association with the use of this drug: malformations of the skull, vertebrae, face, extremities, brain and spinal cord.

Avoid this drug completely during entire pregnancy. See *CAUTION.*

Advisability of Use if Breast-Feeding

Presence of this drug in breast milk: Unknown.

Avoid drug or refrain from nursing.

Habit-Forming Potential: None.

Effects of Overdosage: Severe headache, irritability, drowsiness, itching, nausea, vomiting.

Possible Effects of Long-Term Use: Hyperostosis (84%): abnormal thickening of bone (pelvis), calcification of ligaments and tendons (knees and ankles).

Suggested Periodic Examinations While Taking This Drug (at physician's discretion)

Complete blood cell counts; measurements of blood sugar, potassium, sodium and chloride.

Blood cholesterol profiles, before and during treatment.
Liver and kidney function tests.
Complete eye examinations.
Bone X-rays, especially children.

▷ **While Taking This Drug, Observe the Following**
Foods: No restrictions. High-fat foods increase absorption of this drug.
Beverages: No restrictions. Whole milk increases absorption of this drug.
▷ *Alcohol:* No interactions expected. Use moderately; excessive intake can increase blood triglyceride levels.
Tobacco Smoking: No interactions expected.
▷ *Other Drugs*
Etretinate may *increase* the effects of
• vitamin A and its derivatives (isotretinoin and tretinoin) and increase the risk of vitamin A toxicity.
Etretinate *taken concurrently* with
• methotrexate may increase the risk of liver toxicity.
• tetracyclines may increase the risk of elevated intracranial pressure.
▷ *Driving, Hazardous Activities:* This drug may cause dizziness and blurred vision. Restrict activities as necessary.
Aviation Note: The use of this drug *may be a disqualification* for piloting. Consult a designated Aviation Medical Examiner.
Exposure to Sun: Use caution. This drug can cause photosensitivity (see Glossary).
Discontinuation: If this drug is not significantly beneficial after 4 months of continual use, it should be discontinued. If response is adequate to justify its long-term use, it should be discontinued temporarily ("drug holiday") after 18 months of continual treatment. Once the skin has cleared satisfactorily, this drug should be discontinued. The majority of individuals will experience some degree of recurrence by the end of 2 months. Subsequent treatment courses of 4 to 9 months can be instituted as required.

FAMOTIDINE
(fa MOH te deen)

Introduced: 1986

Class: Antiulcer, H-2 receptor blocker

Prescription: USA: Yes

Controlled Drug: USA: No

Available as Generic: USA: No

Brand Name: Pepcid

BENEFITS versus RISKS

Possible Benefits	*Possible Risks*
EFFECTIVE TREATMENT OF PEPTIC ULCER DISEASE: relief of symptoms, acceleration of healing, prevention of recurrence	Headache, dizziness
CONTROL OF HYPERSECRETORY STOMACH DISORDERS	
Beneficial in treatment of reflux esophagitis	

▷ **Principal Uses**

As a Single Drug Product: Used primarily in the treatment of peptic ulcer disease, both benign stomach (gastric) ulcer and duodenal ulcer. It is used specifically to hasten the healing of ulcer and to prevent recurrence. Also used to control the excessive production of stomach acid in the Zollinger-Ellison syndrome. Though its effectiveness has not been fully established, this drug is also used in the management of esophagitis (as with hiatal hernia) and upper gastrointestinal bleeding.

How This Drug Works: By blocking the action of histamine, this drug effectively inhibits the secretion of stomach acid and thus creates a more favorable environment for the healing of peptic ulcers.

Available Dosage Forms and Strengths
           Injection — 10 mg per ml
Oral suspension — 40 mg per 5-ml teaspoonful
           Tablets — 20 mg, 40 mg

▷ **Usual Adult Dosage Range:** For active peptic ulcer: 20 mg twice daily, or 40 mg at bedtime. For prevention of recurrent ulcer: 20 mg at bedtime. For hypersecretory states: 20 mg/6 hours. **Note: Actual dosage and administration schedule must be determined by the physician for each patient individually.**

▷ **Dosing Instructions:** To obtain the longest period of stomach acid reduction, this drug should be taken with or immediately following food. The tablet may be crushed for administration. If needed, antacids may be taken concurrently with this drug to relieve ulcer pain.

Usual Duration of Use: Continual use on a regular schedule for 4 to 6 weeks is usually necessary to determine this drug's effectiveness in healing active peptic ulcer. Long-term use (months to years) for prevention of ulcer recurrence requires individual consideration by your physician.

▷ **This Drug Should Not Be Taken If**
- you have had an allergic reaction to any dosage form of it previously.

▷ **Inform Your Physician Before Taking This Drug If**
- you are allergic to cimetidine (Tagamet) or ranitidine (Zantac).
- you have impaired liver or kidney function.

Possible Side-Effects (natural, expected and unavoidable drug actions)
None reported.

▷ **Possible Adverse Effects** (unusual, unexpected and infrequent reactions)
If any of the following develop, consult your physician promptly for guidance.
Mild Adverse Effects
Allergic Reactions: Skin rash, swelling of eyelids.
Headache (4.7%), dizziness (1.3%), fatigue.
Nausea, constipation (1.2%), diarrhea (1.7%).
Serious Adverse Effects
Rare decrease in blood platelet counts: abnormal bleeding or bruising (questionable).

▷ **Possible Effects on Sexual Function:**   Decreased libido.

CAUTION
1. Do not discontinue this drug abruptly. (Ulcer activation and perforation have occurred following abrupt cessation of cimetidine, a closely related drug.)
2. After discontinuation of this drug, inform your physician promptly if you experience a return of symptoms indicative of ulcer reactivation.
3. Inform your allergist that you are taking this drug if allergy skin tests are to be done; this drug may interfere with skin testing and cause false negative results.

Precautions for Use
By Infants and Children: Safety and effectiveness for use by those under 12 years of age have not been established.
By Those over 60 Years of Age: This drug may contribute to the formation of stomach phytobezoars (masses of undigested vegetable fibers). Individuals with poor chewing ability (missing teeth) and those who have had partial gastrectomy or vagotomy (stomach surgery) are most susceptible. Observe for loss of appetite, stomach fullness, nausea and vomiting.

▷ **Advisability of Use During Pregnancy**
Pregnancy Category: B (tentative). See Pregnancy Code inside back cover.
Animal studies: No birth defects reported.
Human studies: Information from adequate studies of pregnant women is not available.
Use this drug only if clearly needed. Ask physician for guidance.

Advisability of Use if Breast-Feeding
Presence of this drug in breast milk: Probably yes.
Avoid drug or refrain from nursing.

Habit-Forming Potential: None.

Effects of Overdosage: Related drugs (cimetidine, ranitidine) may cause confusion, delirium, slurred speech, flushing, sweating, drowsiness, muscle twitching, seizures, coma.

Possible Effects of Long-Term Use: Impaired absorption of vitamin B-12.

Suggested Periodic Examinations While Taking This Drug (at physician's discretion)
Complete blood cell counts.

▷ **While Taking This Drug, Observe the Following**
Foods: Protein-rich foods produce maximal stomach acid secretion. Follow the diet prescribed to derive optimal benefit from this drug.
Beverages: No restrictions. May be taken with milk.
▷   *Alcohol:* No interactions with drug. However, alcoholic beverages increase stomach acidity and can reduce the effectiveness of this drug.
Tobacco Smoking: Decreased effectiveness of this drug, especially in its ability to reduce nocturnal stomach acid secretion. Avoid smoking during periods of active peptic ulcer disease.
▷   *Other Drugs:* No significant drug interactions reported to date.
▷   *Driving, Hazardous Activities:* This drug may cause dizziness. Restrict activities as necessary.
Aviation Note: The use of this drug **may be a disqualification** for piloting. Consult a designated Aviation Medical Examiner.
Exposure to Sun: No restrictions.
Discontinuation: Do not discontinue this drug suddenly if taken for peptic ulcer disease. Consult physician for withdrawal instructions. This drug does not provide an extended protective effect. Be alert to the possibility of ulcer recurrence anytime after discontinuation.

FENOPROFEN
(fen oh PROH fen)

Introduced: 1976

Class: Mild analgesic, anti-inflammatory

Prescription: USA: Yes
Canada: Yes

Controlled Drug: USA: No
Canada: No

Available as Generic: Yes

Brand Name: Nalfon

```
+-----------------------------------------------------------+
|                 BENEFITS versus RISKS                      |
|                                                            |
|   Possible Benefits              Possible Risks            |
|  EFFECTIVE RELIEF OF MILD    Gastrointestinal pain, ulceration,|
|   TO MODERATE PAIN AND        bleeding (rare)              |
|   INFLAMMATION               Rare liver or kidney damage   |
|                              Rare fluid retention          |
|                              Rare bone marrow depression   |
+-----------------------------------------------------------+
```

▷ **Principal Uses**

As a Single Drug Product: Used primarily to relieve mild to moderately severe pain associated with (1) musculoskeletal injuries; (2) acute and chronic gout, rheumatoid arthritis and osteoarthritis; (3) dental, obstetrical and orthopedic surgery; (4) menstrual cramps; and (5) vascular (migrainelike) headaches.

How This Drug Works: Not completely established. It is thought that this drug reduces the tissue concentrations of prostaglandins (and related compounds), chemicals involved in the production of inflammation and pain.

Available Dosage Forms and Strengths
Capsules — 200 mg, 300 mg
Tablets — 600 mg

▷ **Usual Adult Dosage Range:**   300 to 600 mg 3 or 4 times/day. Total daily dosage should not exceed 3200 mg. **Note: Actual dosage and administration schedule must be determined by the physician for each patient individually.**

▷ **Dosing Instructions:**   Take either on an empty stomach or with food or milk to prevent stomach irritation. Take with a full glass of water and remain upright (do not lie down) for 30 minutes. The tablet may be crushed and the capsule may be opened for administration.

Usual Duration of Use: Continual use on a regular schedule for 2 to 3 weeks is usually necessary to determine this drug's effectiveness in relieving the discomfort of arthritis. Long-term use requires supervision and periodic evaluation by the physician. Consult your physician on a regular basis.

▷ **This Drug Should Not Be Taken If**
• you have had an allergic reaction to it previously.
• you are subject to asthma or nasal polyps caused by aspirin.
• you have active peptic ulcer disease or any form of gastrointestinal bleeding.
• you have a bleeding disorder or a blood cell disorder.
• you have severe impairment of kidney function.

▷ **Inform Your Physician Before Taking This Drug If**
- you are allergic to aspirin or to other aspirin substitutes.
- you have a history of peptic ulcer disease or any type of bleeding disorder.
- you have impaired liver or kidney function.
- you have high blood pressure or a history of heart failure.
- you are taking any of the following: acetaminophen, aspirin or other aspirin substitutes, anticoagulants, oral antidiabetic drugs.

Possible Side-Effects (natural, expected and unavoidable drug actions)
Drowsiness (15%), ringing in ears, fluid retention.

▷ **Possible Adverse Effects** (unusual, unexpected and infrequent reactions)
If any of the following develop, consult your physician promptly for guidance.
Mild Adverse Effects
Allergic Reactions: Skin rash, hives, itching (9%).
Headache (15%), dizziness, altered or blurred vision, depression.
Mouth sores, indigestion, nausea, vomiting, constipation, diarrhea.
Serious Adverse Effects
Allergic Reaction: Anaphylaxis (see Glossary).
Blurred vision, impaired hearing.
Active peptic ulcer, with or without bleeding.
Liver damage with jaundice (see Glossary).
Kidney damage with painful urination, bloody urine, reduced urine formation.
Rare bone marrow depression (see Glossary)—fatigue, weakness, fever, sore throat, abnormal bleeding or bruising.

▷ **Possible Effects on Sexual Function:**   None reported.

Possible Delayed Adverse Effects: Mild anemia due to "silent" blood loss from the stomach (less than that caused by aspirin).

▷ **Adverse Effects That May Mimic Natural Diseases or Disorders**
Liver reaction may suggest viral hepatitis.

Natural Diseases or Disorders That May Be Activated by This Drug
Peptic ulcer disease, ulcerative colitis.

CAUTION
1. Dosage should always be limited to the smallest amount that produces reasonable improvement.
2. This drug may mask early indications of infection. Inform your physician if you think you are developing an infection of any kind.

Precautions for Use
By Infants and Children: Safety and effectiveness for use by those under 12 years of age have not been established.
By Those over 60 Years of Age: Small doses are advisable until tolerance is determined. Observe for any indications of liver or kidney toxicity,

fluid retention, dizziness, confusion, impaired memory, stomach bleeding or constipation.

▷ **Advisability of Use During Pregnancy**
Pregnancy Category: B (tentative). See Pregnancy Code inside back cover.
Animal studies: No birth defects reported.
Human studies: Information from adequate studies of pregnant women is not available.
Avoid this drug during the last 3 months. Use it during the first 6 months only if clearly needed. Ask physician for guidance.
The manufacturer does not recommend the use of this drug during pregnancy.

Advisability of Use if Breast-Feeding
Presence of this drug in breast milk: Yes, in minute amounts.
Avoid drug or refrain from nursing.

Habit-Forming Potential: None.

Effects of Overdosage: Drowsiness, nausea, vomiting, diarrhea.

Possible Effects of Long-Term Use: Cataracts have been reported, but a definite cause-and-effect relationship (see Glossary) has not been established.

Suggested Periodic Examinations While Taking This Drug (at physician's discretion)
Complete blood cell counts, liver and kidney function tests, complete eye examinations if vision is altered in any way.

▷ **While Taking This Drug, Observe the Following**
Foods: No restrictions.
Beverages: No restrictions. May be taken with milk.
▷ *Alcohol:* Use with caution. The irritant action of alcohol on the stomach lining, added to the irritant action of this drug in sensitive individuals, can increase the risk of stomach ulceration and/or bleeding.
Tobacco Smoking: No interactions expected.
▷ *Other Drugs*
Fenoprofen may *increase* the effects of
• acetaminophen (Tylenol, etc.), and increase the risk of kidney damage; avoid prolonged use of this combination.
• anticoagulants (Coumadin, etc.), and increase the risk of bleeding; monitor prothrombin time, adjust dose accordingly.
Fenoprofen *taken concurrently* with the following drugs may increase the risk of bleeding; avoid these combinations:
• aspirin.
• dipyridamole (Persantine).
• indomethacin (Indocin).
• sulfinpyrazone (Anturane).
• valproic acid (Depakene).

▷ *Driving, Hazardous Activities:* This drug may cause drowsiness or dizziness. Restrict activities as necessary.
Aviation Note: The use of this drug *may be a disqualification* for piloting. Consult a designated Aviation Medical Examiner.
Exposure to Sun: No restrictions.

FLECAINIDE
(FLEK a nide)

Introduced: 1982   **Class:** Antiarrhythmic

Prescription: USA: Yes   **Controlled Drug:** USA: No

Available as Generic: USA: No

Brand Name: Tambocor

BENEFITS versus RISKS	
Possible Benefits	*Possible Risks*
EFFECTIVE TREATMENT (72%) OF SELECTED HEART RHYTHM DISORDERS	DRUG-INDUCED HEART RHYTHM DISORDERS (7%) CONGESTIVE HEART FAILURE (5%) Rare blood cell disorders Rare liver damage with jaundice

▷ **Principal Uses**
As a Single Drug Product: This drug is classified as a Type 1 antiarrhythmic agent, similar to procainamide and quinidine in its actions. It is used primarily to correct and prevent the recurrence of life-threatening rapid heart rates (tachycardia) that arise in the ventricles (lower heart chambers).

How This Drug Works: By slowing the transmission of electrical impulses throughout the conduction system of the heart, this drug assists in restoring normal heart rate and rhythm.

Available Dosage Forms and Strengths
Tablets — 50 mg, 100 mg, 150 mg

▷ **Usual Adult Dosage Range:** Do not take a loading dose. Initiate treatment with 100 mg/12 hours. At intervals of 4 days, increase dose by 50-mg increments to 150 mg/12 hours, then to 200 mg/12 hours if necessary. Total daily dosage should not exceed 400 mg. Measurement of drug blood levels is advised to determine the optimal dose and schedule.

Note: Actual dosage and administration schedule must be determined by the physician for each patient individually.

▷ **Dosing Instructions:** May be taken without regard to meals. Take at same time each day to obtain uniform results. Tablet may be crushed for administration.

Usual Duration of Use: Continual use on a regular schedule for 1 to 2 weeks is usually necessary to determine this drug's effectiveness in correcting or preventing responsive rhythm disorders. Long-term use requires supervision and periodic evaluation by your physician. Consult your physician on a regular basis.

▷ **This Drug Should Not Be Taken If**
- you have had an allergic reaction to it previously.
- you have second-degree or third-degree heart block (determined by electrocardiogram).

▷ **Inform Your Physician Before Taking This Drug If**
- you have had any unfavorable reactions to other antiarrhythmic drugs in the past.
- you have a history of heart disease of any kind, especially "heart block."
- you have impaired liver or kidney function.
- you are taking any form of digitalis, a potassium supplement or any diuretic drug that can cause excessive loss of body potassium (ask physician).

Possible Side-Effects (natural, expected and unavoidable drug actions)
Flushing, increased sweating, light-headedness.

▷ **Possible Adverse Effects** (unusual, unexpected and infrequent reactions)
If any of the following develop, consult your physician promptly for guidance.
Mild Adverse Effects
Allergic Reactions: Skin rash (1% to 3%), hives, itching.
Headache (9%), dizziness (18%), visual disturbance (15%), fatigue (7%), weakness (4%), tremor (4%).
Loss of appetite, indigestion, nausea (8%), vomiting, constipation (4%), abdominal pain (3%).
Serious Adverse Effects
Idiosyncratic Reactions: Depression, confusion, amnesia, euphoria (less than 1%).
Drug-induced heart rhythm disorders (7%), congestive heart failure (5%), shortness of breath (10%), palpitations (6%), chest pain (5%), swelling of feet (3%).
Urinary retention.
Jaundice (see Glossary).
Abnormally low white blood cell and blood platelet counts (rare): fever, sore throat, abnormal bleeding or bruising.

▷ **Possible Effects on Sexual Function:**   Decreased libido; impaired erection with doses of 200 mg/day; complete impotence with doses of 400 mg/day.

▷ **Adverse Effects That May Mimic Natural Diseases or Disorders**
Reversible jaundice may suggest viral hepatitis.

CAUTION
1. Thorough evaluation of your heart function (including electrocardiograms) is necessary prior to using this drug.
2. Periodic evaluation of your heart function is necessary to determine your response to this drug. Some individuals may experience worsening of their heart rhythm disorder and/or deterioration of heart function. Close monitoring of heart rate, rhythm and overall performance is essential.
3. Dosage must be adjusted carefully for each individual. Do not change your dosage without the knowledge and supervision of your physician.
4. Do not take any other antiarrhythmic drug while taking this drug unless directed to do so by your physician.

Precautions for Use
By Infants and Children: Safety and effectiveness for use by those under 18 years of age have not been established. Initial use of this drug requires hospitalization and supervision by a qualified cardiologist.
By Those over 60 Years of Age: Reduced kidney function may require reduction in dosage. Observe carefully for light-headedness, dizziness, unsteadiness and tendency to fall.

▷ **Advisability of Use During Pregnancy**
Pregnancy Category: C (tentative). See Pregnancy Code inside back cover.
Animal studies: Birth defects reported in one species of rabbit.
Human studies: Information from adequate studies of pregnant women is not available.
Avoid during first 3 months. Use this drug only if clearly needed. Ask physician for guidance.

Advisability of Use if Breast-Feeding
Presence of this drug in breast milk: Unknown.
Avoid drug or refrain from nursing.

Habit-Forming Potential: None.

Effects of Overdosage: Impaired urination, constipation, marked drop in blood pressure, abnormal heart rhythms, slow heart rate, congestive heart failure.

Possible Effects of Long-Term Use: None reported.

Suggested Periodic Examinations While Taking This Drug (at physician's discretion)

Electrocardiograms, complete blood cell counts, measurements of potassium blood levels.

▷ **While Taking This Drug, Observe the Following**

Foods: No restrictions. Ask physician regarding need for salt restriction and advisability of eating potassium-rich foods.

Beverages: No restrictions. May be taken with milk.

▷ *Alcohol:* Use caution until the combined effects have been determined. Alcohol can increase the blood-pressure-lowering effects of this drug.

Tobacco Smoking: Nicotine can cause irritability of the heart and reduce the effectiveness of this drug. Follow physician's advice regarding smoking.

▷ *Other Drugs*

Flecainide may *increase* the effects of

- antihypertensive drugs, and cause excessive lowering of blood pressure.
- beta blocker drugs (see Drug Class, Section Four).

The following drugs may *decrease* the effects of flecainide

- diuretics that promote potassium loss.

▷ *Driving, Hazardous Activities:* This drug may cause drowsiness, dizziness or blurred vision. Restrict activities as necessary.

Aviation Note: The use of this drug *may be a disqualification* for piloting. Consult a designated Aviation Medical Examiner.

Exposure to Sun: No restrictions.

Occurrence of Unrelated Illness: Disorders that cause vomiting, diarrhea or dehydration can affect this drug's action adversely. Report such developments promptly.

Discontinuation: This drug should not be discontinued abruptly following long-term use. Ask your physician for guidance regarding gradual dose reduction.

FLUOXETINE
(flu OX e teen)

Introduced: 1978   **Class:** Antidepressant

Prescription: USA: Yes   **Controlled Drug:** USA: No

Available as Generic: USA: No

Brand Name: Prozac

```
┌─────────────────────────────────────────────────────────────────┐
│                    BENEFITS versus RISKS                          │
│                                                                   │
│        Possible Benefits                    Possible Risks        │
│   EFFECTIVE TREATMENT OF            Serious allergic reactions (4%)│
│     MAJOR DEPRESSIVE               Conversion of depression to     │
│     DISORDERS in 60% to 75% of       mania in manic-depressive     │
│     cases                            disorders (1%)                │
│   Possibly effective in relieving the   Seizures (0.2%)            │
│     symptoms of obsessive-                                         │
│     compulsive disorder                                           │
└─────────────────────────────────────────────────────────────────┘
```

▷ **Principal Uses**

As a Single Drug Product: Used primarily to treat major forms of depression that have not responded well to other therapies. This drug should be used only when a diagnosis of a true, primary depression of significant degree has been established. It should not be used to treat the symptoms of mild and transient (reactive) depression that may be associated with many life situations in the absence of a bona fide affective illness.

How This Drug Works: It is thought that this drug relieves depression by slowly restoring to normal levels a specific constituent of brain tissue (serotonin) that transmits nerve impulses.

Available Dosage Forms and Strengths
Capsules — 20 mg

▷ **Usual Adult Dosage Range:** Initially 20 mg daily as a single morning dose; if no improvement after 3 weeks of treatment, the dose may be increased by 20 mg/day as needed and tolerated. Doses over 20 mg/day should be taken in 2 divided doses, early morning and noon. Total daily dosage should not exceed 80 mg. **Note: Actual dosage and administration schedule must be determined by the physician for each patient individually.**

▷ **Dosing Instructions:** May be taken without regard to food. The capsule may be opened for administration and the contents mixed with any convenient food.

Usual Duration of Use: Continual use on a regular schedule for up to 3 weeks is usually necessary to determine this drug's effectiveness in relieving depression. Long-term use (months to years) requires periodic evaluation of response and dosage adjustment. Consult your physician on a regular basis.

Possible Advantages of This Drug
Does not cause weight gain, a common side-effect of tricyclic antidepressants.

Less likely to cause dry mouth, constipation, urinary retention, orthostatic hypotension (see Glossary) and heart rhythm disturbances than tricyclic antidepressants.

Does not cause Parkinson-like reactions.

▷ **This Drug Should Not Be Taken If**
- you have had an allergic reaction to any dosage form of it previously.
- you are currently taking or have taken within the past 14 days any monoamine oxidase (MAO) type A inhibitor drug (see Drug Class, Section Four).

▷ **Inform Your Physician Before Taking This Drug If**
- you have experienced any adverse effects from antidepressant drugs used in the past.
- you have impaired liver or kidney function.
- you have a seizure disorder.

Possible Side-Effects (natural, expected and unavoidable drug actions)
Decreased appetite (8.7%), weight loss (13%).

▷ **Possible Adverse Effects** (unusual, unexpected and infrequent reactions)
If any of the following develop, consult your physician promptly for guidance.
Mild Adverse Effects
Allergic Reactions: Skin rash (2.7%), hives (2%), itching (2.4%).
Headache (20%), nervousness (14%), insomnia (13%), drowsiness (11%), tremor (7%), dizziness (5%), fatigue (4%), impaired concentration (1.5%).
Altered taste (1.8%), nausea (21%), vomiting (2.4%), diarrhea (12%).
Serious Adverse Effects
Allergic Reactions: Serum sickness–like syndrome (2% to 3%): fever, weakness, joint pain and swelling, swollen lymph glands, fluid retention, skin rash and/or hives.
Drug-induced seizures (0.2%).

▷ **Possible Effects on Sexual Function:** Impaired erection (1.9%).

Natural Diseases or Disorders That May Be Activated by This Drug
Latent epilepsy.

CAUTION
1. If any type of skin reaction develops (rash, hives, etc.), discontinue this drug and inform your physician promptly.
2. If dryness of the mouth develops and persists for more than 2 weeks, consult your dentist for guidance.
3. Consult your physician before taking any other prescription or over-the-counter drug while taking this drug.
4. If you are advised to take any monoamine oxidase (MAO) type A inhibitor drug (see Drug Class, Section Four), allow an interval of 5 weeks after discontinuing this drug before starting the MAO inhibitor.

5. It is advisable to withhold this drug if electroconvulsive therapy (ECT, "shock" treatment) is to be used to treat your depression.

Precautions for Use
By Infants and Children: Safety and effectiveness for use by those under 12 years of age have not been established.

By Those over 60 Years of Age: Total daily dosage should not exceed 60 mg.

▷ **Advisability of Use During Pregnancy**
Pregnancy Category: B (tentative). See Pregnancy Code inside back cover.
Animal studies: No birth defects due to this drug found in rat or rabbit studies.
Human studies: Information from adequate studies of pregnant women is not available.
Use this drug only if clearly needed.

Advisability of Use if Breast-Feeding
Presence of this drug in breast milk: Unknown.
Avoid drug or refrain from nursing.

Habit-Forming Potential: None.

Effects of Overdosage: Agitation, restlessness, excitement, nausea, vomiting, seizures.

Possible Effects of Long-Term Use: None reported.

Suggested Periodic Examinations While Taking This Drug (at physician's discretion)
None.

▷ **While Taking This Drug, Observe the Following**
Foods: No restrictions.
Beverages: No restrictions. May be taken with milk.
▷   *Alcohol:* Avoid completely.
Tobacco Smoking: No interactions expected.
▷   *Other Drugs*
Fluoxetine may ***increase*** the effects of
• diazepam (Valium).
• digitalis preparations (digitoxin, digoxin).
• warfarin (Coumadin) and related oral anticoagulants.
Fluoxetine ***taken concurrently*** with
• monoamine oxidase (MAO) type A inhibitor drugs may cause confusion, agitation, high fever, seizures and dangerous elevations of blood pressure. Avoid the concurrent use of these drugs.
▷   *Driving, Hazardous Activities:* This drug may cause drowsiness, dizziness, impaired judgment and delayed reaction time. Restrict activities as necessary.
Aviation Note: The use of this drug ***is a disqualification*** for piloting. Consult a designated Aviation Medical Examiner.

Exposure to Sun: No restrictions.

Discontinuation: The slow elimination of this drug from the body makes it unlikely that any withdrawal effects will result from abrupt discontinuation. However, consult your physician if you plan to discontinue this drug for any reason.

FLUPHENAZINE
(flu FEN a zeen)

Introduced: 1959

Class: Strong tranquilizer, phenothiazines

Prescription: USA: Yes
Canada: Yes

Controlled Drug: USA: No
Canada: No

Available as Generic: USA: No
Canada: Yes

Brand Names: ✦Apo-Fluphenazine, ✦Modecate, ✦Moditen, Permitil, Prolixin

```
                    BENEFITS versus RISKS

      Possible Benefits                    Possible Risks
EFFECTIVE CONTROL OF              SERIOUS TOXIC EFFECTS ON
  ACUTE MENTAL DISORDERS            BRAIN with long-term use
  in the majority of patients     Liver damage with jaundice (less
Beneficial effects on thinking,     than 0.5%)
  mood and behavior               Rare blood cell disorders:
                                    abnormally low white blood
                                    cell counts
```

▷ **Principal Uses**

As a Single Drug Product: This antipsychotic drug is used primarily to treat acute and chronic psychotic disorders such as schizophrenia, mania and similar states of mental dysfunction.

How This Drug Works: Not completely established. Present theory is that by inhibiting the action of dopamine, this drug acts to correct an imbalance of nerve impulse transmissions that is thought to be responsible for certain mental disorders.

Available Dosage Forms and Strengths
    Concentrate — 5 mg per ml (1% alcohol)
        Elixir — 2.5 mg per 5-ml teaspoonful (14% alcohol)
    Injection — 2.5 mg per ml
        Tablets — 1 mg, 2.5 mg, 5 mg, 10 mg

▷ **Usual Adult Dosage Range:**   0.5 to 2.5 mg 1 to 4 times/day; adjust dosage as needed and tolerated. Total daily dosage should not exceed 20 mg. **Note: Actual dosage and administration schedule must be determined by the physician for each patient individually.**

▷ **Dosing Instructions:**   May be taken with or following meals to reduce stomach irritation. Regular tablets may be crushed for administration. Prolonged-action tablets should be swallowed whole (not crushed). The concentrate must be diluted in 4 to 6 ounces of water, milk, fruit juice or carbonated beverage.

  Usual Duration of Use: Continual use on a regular schedule for several weeks is usually necessary to determine this drug's effectiveness in controlling psychotic disorders. If not significantly beneficial within 6 weeks, it should be discontinued. Long-term use (months to years) requires periodic evaluation of response, appropriate dosage adjustment and consideration of continued need. Consult your physician on a regular basis.

▷ **This Drug Should Not Be Taken If**
  • you are allergic to any of the drugs bearing the brand names listed above.
  • you have a history of brain damage.
  • you have active liver disease.
  • you have cancer of the breast.
  • you have a current blood cell or bone marrow disorder.

▷ **Inform Your Physician Before Taking This Drug If**
  • you are allergic or abnormally sensitive to any phenothiazine drug (see Drug Class, Section Four).
  • you have impaired liver or kidney function.
  • you have any type of seizure disorder.
  • you have diabetes, glaucoma, heart disease or chronic lung disease.
  • you have a history of lupus erythematosus.
  • you are taking any drug with sedative effects.
  • you plan to have surgery under general or spinal anesthesia in the near future.

  Possible Side-Effects (natural, expected and unavoidable drug actions)
  Drowsiness (usually during the first 2 weeks), orthostatic hypotension (see Glossary), blurred vision, dry mouth, nasal congestion, constipation, impaired urination (all mild).

▷ **Possible Adverse Effects** (unusual, unexpected and infrequent reactions)
  If any of the following develop, consult your physician promptly for guidance.
  Mild Adverse Effects
  Allergic Reactions: Skin rash, hives, itching.
  Lowering of body temperature, especially in the elderly.

Headache, dizziness, weakness, excitement, restlessness, unusual dreaming.

Increased appetite and weight gain.

Serious Adverse Effects

Allergic Reactions: Hepatitis with jaundice (see Glossary), usually between second and fourth week; anaphylactic reaction (see Glossary).

Idiosyncratic Reaction: High fever.

Impaired production of white blood cells—fever, sore throat, infections.

Parkinson-like disorders (see Glossary); muscle spasms of face, jaw, neck, back, extremities.

Prolonged drop in blood pressure with weakness, perspiration and fainting.

▷ **Possible Effects on Sexual Function**

Decreased male libido; increased female libido.

Impaired erection (38% to 42%); complete impotence.

Inhibited male orgasm (58%); inhibited female orgasm (22% to 33%).

Inhibited ejaculation (46%).

Altered timing and pattern of menstruation (91%).

Female breast enlargement and milk production.

Male breast enlargement and tenderness.

▷ **Adverse Effects That May Mimic Natural Diseases or Disorders**

Nervous system reactions may suggest Parkinson's disease.

Liver reactions may suggest viral hepatitis.

Reactions resembling systemic lupus erythematosus may occur.

Natural Diseases or Disorders That May Be Activated by This Drug

Latent epilepsy, glaucoma, prostatism (see Glossary).

CAUTION

1. Many over-the-counter medications (see OTC Drugs in Glossary) for allergies, colds and coughs contain drugs that can interact unfavorably with this drug. Ask your physician or pharmacist for guidance before using any such medications.
2. Antacids that contain aluminum and/or magnesium can prevent the absorption of this drug and reduce its effectiveness.
3. Obtain prompt evaluation of any change or disturbance of vision.

Precautions for Use

By Infants and Children: Do not use this drug in infants under 6 months of age, or in children of any age with symptoms suggestive of Reye syndrome (see Glossary). Monitor carefully for blood cell changes.

By Those over 60 Years of Age: Small doses are advisable until individual response has been determined. You may be more susceptible to the development of drowsiness, lethargy, constipation, lowering of body temperature (hypothermia) and orthostatic hypotension (see Glossary). This drug can enhance existing prostatism (see Glossary). You may also be more susceptible to the development of Parkinson-like reactions and/or tardive dyskinesia (see discussion of these terms in

Glossary). These reactions must be recognized early since they may become unresponsive to treatment and irreversible.

▷ **Advisability of Use During Pregnancy**
Pregnancy Category: C (tentative). See Pregnancy Code inside back cover.
Animal studies: Significant birth defects reported in mice.
Human studies: Information from adequate studies of pregnant women is not available.
Avoid drug during the first 3 months and during the last month because of possible effects on the newborn infant.

Advisability of Use if Breast-Feeding
Presence of this drug in breast milk: Unknown.
Avoid drug or refrain from nursing.

Habit-Forming Potential: None.

Effects of Overdosage: Marked drowsiness, weakness, tremor, agitation, unsteadiness, deep sleep, coma, convulsions.

Possible Effects of Long-Term Use: Tardive dyskinesia (see Glossary); eye changes—cataracts and pigmentation of retina; gray to violet pigmentation of skin in exposed areas, more common in women.

Suggested Periodic Examinations While Taking This Drug (at physician's discretion)
Complete blood cell counts, especially between the fourth and tenth weeks of treatment.
Liver function tests, electrocardiograms.
Complete eye examinations—eye structures and vision.
Careful inspection of the tongue for early evidence of fine, involuntary, wavelike movements that could indicate the beginning of tardive dyskinesia.

▷ **While Taking This Drug, Observe the Following**
Foods: No restrictions.
Beverages: No restrictions. May be taken with milk.
▷ *Alcohol:* Avoid completely. Alcohol can increase the sedative action of phenothiazines and accentuate their depressant effects on brain function and blood pressure. Phenothiazines can increase the intoxicating effects of alcohol.
Tobacco Smoking: Possible reduction of drowsiness from drug.
Marijuana Smoking: Moderate increase in drowsiness; accentuation of orthostatic hypotension; increased risk of precipitating latent psychoses, confusing the interpretation of mental status and drug responses.
▷ *Other Drugs*
Fluphenazine may ***increase*** the effects of
• all sedative drugs, and cause excessive sedation.
• all atropinelike drugs, and cause nervous system toxicity.

Fluphenazine may *decrease* the effects of
- guanethidine (Ismelin, Esimil), and reduce its effectiveness in lowering blood pressure.

Fluphenazine *taken concurrently* with
- beta blocker drugs (see Drug Class, Section Four) may cause increased effects of both drugs; monitor drug effects closely and adjust dosages as necessary.

The following drugs may *decrease* the effects of fluphenazine
- antacids containing aluminum and/or magnesium.
- benztropine (Cogentin).
- trihexyphenidyl (Artane).

▷ *Driving, Hazardous Activities:* This drug can impair mental alertness, judgment and physical coordination. Avoid hazardous activities.

Aviation Note: The use of this drug *is a disqualification* for piloting. Consult a designated Aviation Medical Examiner.

Exposure to Sun: Use caution until sensitivity has been determined. Some phenothiazines can cause photosensitivity (see Glossary).

Exposure to Heat: Use caution and avoid excessive heat as much as possible. This drug may impair the regulation of body temperature and increase the risk of heat stroke.

Exposure to Cold: Use caution and dress warmly. This drug can increase the risk of hypothermia in the elderly.

Discontinuation: After a period of long-term use, do not discontinue this drug suddenly. Gradual withdrawal over 2 to 3 weeks under physician supervision is recommended. Do not discontinue this drug without your physician's knowledge and approval. The relapse rate of schizophrenia after discontinuation is 50% to 60%.

FLURAZEPAM
(floor AZ e pam)

Introduced: 1970

Class: Hypnotic, benzodiazepines

Prescription: USA: Yes
Canada: Yes

Controlled Drug: USA: C-IV*
Canada: No

Available as Generic: USA: Yes
Canada: No

Brand Names: ✦Apo-Flurazepam, Dalmane, Durapam, ✦Novoflupam, ✦Somnol, ✦Som-Pam

*See Schedules of Controlled Drugs inside back cover.

BENEFITS versus RISKS

Possible Benefits	*Possible Risks*
EFFECTIVE HYPNOTIC after 2 weeks of continual use	Habit-forming potential with long-term use
NO SUPPRESSION OF REM (RAPID EYE MOVEMENT) SLEEP	Minor impairment of mental functions ("hangover" effect)
NO REM SLEEP REBOUND after discontinuation	Very rare jaundice
Wide margin of safety with therapeutic doses	Very rare blood cell disorder
	Suppression of stage-4 sleep with reduced "quality" of sleep

---

▷ **Principal Uses**

As a Single Drug Product: This member of the benzodiazepine class of "minor tranquilizers" is used exclusively as a bedtime sedative to induce sleep.

How This Drug Works: It is thought that this drug produces calming effect by enhancing the action of the nerve transmitter gamma-aminobutyric acid (GABA), which in turn blocks the arousal of higher brain centers and helps to induce sleep.

Available Dosage Forms and Strengths
Capsules — 15 mg, 30 mg

▷ **Usual Adult Dosage Range:**   15 to 30 mg at bedtime. Total daily dosage should not exceed 90 mg. **Note: Actual dosage and administration schedule must be determined by the physician for each patient individually.**

▷ **Dosing Instructions:**   May be taken on an empty stomach or with food or milk. The capsule may be opened for administration. Do not discontinue this drug abruptly if taken for more than 4 weeks.

Usual Duration of Use: Periods of 3 to 5 nights intermittently, repeated as needed with appropriate dosage adjustment. Avoid uninterrupted and prolonged use. The duration of use should not exceed 2 weeks without reappraisal of continued need.

▷ **This Drug Should Not Be Taken If**
- you have had an allergic reaction to it previously.
- you have acute narrow-angle glaucoma.

▷ **Inform Your Physician Before Taking This Drug If**
- you are allergic to any benzodiazepine drug (see Drug Class, Section Four).
- you have a history of alcoholism or drug abuse.
- you are pregnant or planning pregnancy.
- you have impaired liver or kidney function.

- you have a history of serious depression or mental disorder.
- you are taking other drugs with sedative effects.
- you have any of the following: asthma, emphysema, epilepsy, myasthenia gravis.

Possible Side-Effects (natural, expected and unavoidable drug actions)
"Hangover" effects on arising: drowsiness, lethargy and unsteadiness.

▷ **Possible Adverse Effects** (unusual, unexpected and infrequent reactions)
If any of the following develop, consult your physician promptly for guidance.
Mild Adverse Effects
Allergic Reactions: Skin rash, hives, burning eyes, swelling of tongue.
Dizziness, fainting, blurred vision, double vision, slurred speech, nausea, indigestion.
Serious Adverse Effects
Allergic Reactions: Liver damage with jaundice (see Glossary).
Idiosyncratic Reactions: Nervousness, talkativeness, irritability, apprehension, euphoria, excitement, hallucinations.
Bone marrow depression—impaired production of white blood cells, fever, sore throat.

▷ **Possible Effects on Sexual Function:** None reported.

▷ **Adverse Effects That May Mimic Natural Diseases or Disorders**
Liver reaction with jaundice may suggest viral hepatitis.

CAUTION
1. This drug should not be discontinued abruptly if it has been taken continually for more than 4 weeks.
2. The concurrent use of some over-the-counter drug products that contain antihistamines (allergy and cold preparations, sleep aids) can cause excessive sedation in sensitive individuals.
3. Regular nightly use of any hypnotic drug should be avoided.
4. This drug is transformed by the liver into long-acting forms that can persist in the body for 24 hours or more. With continual use of this drug daily, these active drug forms accumulate and produce increasing sedation. If you experience a "hangover" effect, avoid hazardous activities (driving, etc.) and the use of alcohol.

Precautions for Use
By Infants and Children: Safety and effectiveness for use by those under 15 years of age have not been established.
By Those over 60 Years of Age: It is advisable to use smaller doses at longer intervals to avoid overdosage. Observe for the possible development of lethargy, indifference, fatigue, weakness, unsteadiness, disturbing dreams, nightmares and paradoxical reactions of excitement, agitation, anger, hostility and rage.

▷ **Advisability of Use During Pregnancy**

Pregnancy Category: C (tentative). See Pregnancy Code inside back cover.

Animal studies: No birth defects reported in rat and rabbit studies.

Human studies: Information from adequate studies of pregnant women is not available.

Frequent use in late pregnancy can cause the "floppy infant" syndrome in the newborn: weakness, lethargy, unresponsiveness, depressed breathing, low body temperature.

Avoid use during entire pregnancy if possible. Ask physician for guidance.

Advisability of Use if Breast-Feeding

Presence of this drug in breast milk: Probably yes.

Avoid drug or refrain from nursing.

Habit-Forming Potential: This drug can produce psychological and/or physical dependence (see Glossary) if used in large doses for an extended period of time. Avoid continual use.

Effects of Overdosage: Marked drowsiness, weakness, feeling of drunkenness, staggering gait, tremor, stupor progressing to deep sleep or coma.

Possible Effects of Long-Term Use: Psychological and/or physical dependence, impaired liver function.

Suggested Periodic Examinations While Taking This Drug (at physician's discretion)

Complete blood cell counts and liver function tests during long-term use.

▷ **While Taking This Drug, Observe the Following**

Foods: No restrictions.

Beverages: Avoid excessive intake of caffeine-containing beverages (coffee, tea, cola) within 4 hours of taking this drug. May be taken with milk.

▷ *Alcohol:* Use with extreme caution until the combined effect is determined. Alcohol may increase the absorption of this drug and add to its depressant effects on the brain. It is advisable to avoid alcohol completely—throughout the day and night—if it is necessary to drive or to engage in any hazardous activity.

Tobacco Smoking: Heavy smoking may reduce the hypnotic action of this drug.

Marijuana Smoking: Increased sedation and significant impairment of intellectual and physical performance.

▷ *Other Drugs*

Flurazepam may *increase* the effects of

• digoxin (Lanoxin), and cause digoxin toxicity.

• phenytoin (Dilantin), and cause phenytoin toxicity.

Flurazepam may *decrease* the effects of

- levodopa (Sinemet, etc.), and reduce its effectiveness in treating Parkinson's disease.

The following drugs may *increase* the effects of flurazepam

- cimetidine (Tagamet).
- disulfiram (Antabuse).
- isoniazid (INH, Rifamate, etc.).
- oral contraceptives.
- valproic acid (Depakene).

The following drugs may *decrease* the effects of flurazepam

- rifampin (Rimactane, etc.).
- theophylline (aminophylline, Theo-Dur, etc.).

▷ *Driving, Hazardous Activities:* This drug can impair mental alertness, judgment, physical coordination and reaction time. Avoid hazardous activities accordingly.

Aviation Note: The use of this drug *is a disqualification* for piloting. Consult a designated Aviation Medical Examiner.

Exposure to Sun: No restrictions.

Exposure to Heat: Use caution until the effect of excessive perspiration is determined. Because of reduced urine volume, this drug may accumulate in the body and produce effects of overdosage.

Discontinuation: Avoid sudden discontinuation if this drug has been taken for over 4 weeks without interruption. Dosage should be tapered gradually to prevent a withdrawal syndrome that could include depression, confusion, hallucinations, tremor, seizures, muscle cramping, sweating and vomiting.

FLURBIPROFEN
(floor BI pro fen)

Introduced: 1977

Class: Mild analgesic, anti-inflammatory

Prescription: USA: Yes
Canada: Yes

Controlled Drug: USA: No
Canada: No

Available as Generic: USA: No
Canada: No

Brand Names: Ansaid, ✦Froben

```
┌─────────────────────────────────────────────────────────────────┐
│                    BENEFITS versus RISKS                          │
│                                                                   │
│      Possible Benefits                    Possible Risks          │
│  EFFECTIVE RELIEF OF            PEPTIC ULCER DISEASE (1% to        │
│    SYMPTOMS ASSOCIATED           4%) with associated bleeding      │
│    WITH MAJOR TYPES OF           and perforation                  │
│    ARTHRITIS                   Liver toxicity with jaundice (less  │
│  Effective relief of symptoms    than 1%)                         │
│    associated with bursitis,   Water retention                    │
│    tendinitis and related      Rare kidney toxicity               │
│    conditions                  Rare aplastic anemia (see          │
│  Effective relief of menstrual   Glossary)                        │
│    cramps                                                         │
└─────────────────────────────────────────────────────────────────┘
```

▷ **Principal Uses**

As a Single Drug Product: Used primarily to relieve the symptoms associated with (1) rheumatoid arthritis, osteoarthritis and ankylosing spondylitis; (2) bursitis, tendinitis, capsulitis and tenosynovitis; (3) painful menstruation.

How This Drug Works: Not completely established. It is thought that this drug reduces the tissue concentrations of prostaglandins (and related compounds), chemicals involved in the production of inflammation and pain.

Available Dosage Forms and Strengths

Tablets — 50 mg (Canada), 100 mg

▷ **Usual Adult Dosage Range:**   Initially 100 to 200 mg/24 hours, in 2 to 4 divided doses. After a satisfactory response has been achieved, dosage should be reduced to the minimum that will sustain adequate relief. Total daily dosage should not exceed 300 mg. **Note: Actual dosage and administration schedule must be determined by the physician for each patient individually.**

▷ **Dosing Instructions:**   Take either on an empty stomach or with food or milk if necessary to prevent stomach irritation. Take with a full glass of water and remain upright (do not lie down) for 15 to 30 minutes to prevent lodging of the tablet in the esophagus (food tube). The tablet may be crushed for administration.

Usual Duration of Use: Continual use on a regular schedule for 1 to 2 weeks is usually necessary to determine this drug's effectiveness in relieving the symptoms of arthritis, bursitis, etc. Severe arthritis may require continual use for 3 to 4 weeks to obtain maximal relief. Long-term use (months to years) requires periodic evaluation of response and dosage adjustment. Consult your physician on a regular basis.

▷ **This Drug Should Not Be Taken If**
  • you have had an allergic reaction to it previously.
  • you are subject to asthma or nasal polyps caused by aspirin.

- you have active peptic ulcer disease or any form of gastrointestinal bleeding.
- you have active liver disease.
- you have a bleeding disorder or a blood cell disorder.
- you have severe impairment of kidney function.

▷ **Inform Your Physician Before Taking This Drug If**
- you are allergic to aspirin or to other aspirin substitutes.
- you have a history of peptic ulcer disease or any type of bleeding disorder.
- you have a history of gout.
- you have impaired liver or kidney function.
- you have high blood pressure or a history of heart failure.
- you have systemic lupus erythematosus (SLE).
- you are taking any of the following drugs: acetaminophen, aspirin or other aspirin substitutes, anticoagulants, diuretics, insulin, lithium, methotrexate, oral antidiabetic drugs.

Possible Side-Effects (natural, expected and unavoidable drug actions)
Fluid retention (1%), increased blood uric acid levels.

▷ **Possible Adverse Effects** (unusual, unexpected and infrequent reactions)
If any of the following develop, consult your physician promptly for guidance.
Mild Adverse Effects
Allergic Reactions: Skin rash (1.4%), hives (0.1%), itching (0.6%).
Headache (1%), dizziness (1%), drowsiness, depression (0.1%), anxiety (0.1%), insomnia (0.3%), blurred vision (1.6%), double vision, reversible hearing loss, ear ringing (1.7%), altered taste (0.2%).
Mouth soreness (0.4%), stomach discomfort (4%), nausea (3.5%), vomiting (0.5%), indigestion (6.9%), constipation (2%), diarrhea (3.8%).
Serious Adverse Effects
Allergic Reactions: Severe skin reactions, eczema, bruising (0.1%), erythema multiforme, Stevens-Johnson syndrome, hair loss; swelling of lips, tongue, vocal cords; anaphylactoid reaction (see Glossary).
Drug-induced gastrointestinal ulceration, with bleeding and perforation (1% after 3 to 6 months of use, up to 4% after 1 year); colitis with bloody diarrhea.
Abnormally low red blood cell (0.3%), white blood cell and blood platelet counts; rare aplastic anemia (see Glossary).
Liver injury with jaundice (0.2%).
Kidney injury with significantly impaired function.

▷ **Possible Effects on Sexual Function:** None reported to date.

Possible Delayed Adverse Effects: Mild anemia due to "silent" blood loss from the stomach (less than that caused by aspirin).

▷ **Adverse Effects That May Mimic Natural Diseases or Disorders**
Liver reactions may suggest viral hepatitis.

▷ **Natural Diseases or Disorders That May Be Activated by This Drug**

Peptic ulcer disease, Crohn's disease, ulcerative colitis, gout, kidney failure associated with systemic lupus erythematosus.

CAUTION

1. Dosage should always be limited to the smallest amount that produces reasonable improvement.
2. This drug may mask early indications of infection. Inform your physician if you think you are developing an infection of any kind.
3. Observe for a pattern of symptoms that may indicate the development of liver toxicity: fatigue, lethargy, "flulike" symptoms, nausea, itching, tenderness under the right rib cage, jaundice (see Glossary). Report such symptoms promptly.
4. Observe for possible drug-induced bleeding in the gastrointestinal tract: bloody (reddish) or tarry (black) stools.

Precautions for Use

By Infants and Children: Safety and effectiveness for use by those under 12 years of age have not been established.

By Those over 60 Years of Age: Small doses are advisable initially until tolerance is determined. Observe for any indications of liver or kidney toxicity, fluid retention, dizziness, confusion, impaired memory, stomach bleeding or constipation.

▷ **Advisability of Use During Pregnancy**

Pregnancy Category: B (tentative). See Pregnancy Code inside back cover.

Animal studies: Mouse, rat and rabbit studies reveal no birth defects due to this drug.

Human studies: Information from adequate studies of pregnant women is not available.

The manufacturer does not recommend the use of this drug during pregnancy.

Advisability of Use if Breast-Feeding

Presence of this drug in breast milk: Unknown.

Avoid drug or refrain from nursing.

Habit-Forming Potential: None.

Effects of Overdosage: Probable drowsiness, dizziness, ear ringing, nausea, vomiting, diarrhea, confusion, unsteadiness, stupor.

Possible Effects of Long-Term Use: Secondary anemia (chronic blood loss from stomach), fluid retention, elevated blood pressure.

Suggested Periodic Examinations While Taking This Drug (at physician's discretion)

Complete blood cell counts; liver function tests within the first 8 weeks of use and periodically thereafter; kidney function tests.

Complete eye examinations if vision is altered in any way.

▷ **While Taking This Drug, Observe the Following**
  Foods: No restrictions.
  Nutritional Support: Supplemental iron if anemia develops.
  Beverages: No restrictions. May be taken with milk.
▷   *Alcohol:* Use sparingly and with caution. The irritant action of alcohol on
    the stomach lining, added to the irritant action of this drug in sen-
    sitive individuals, can increase the risk of stomach ulceration and/or
    bleeding.
  Tobacco Smoking: No interactions expected.
▷   *Other Drugs*
    Flurbiprofen may *increase* the effects of
    • acetaminophen (Tylenol, etc.), and increase the risk of liver or kidney
      damage; avoid prolonged use of this combination.
    • anticoagulants (Coumadin, etc.), and increase the risk of bleeding;
      monitor prothrombin and bleeding times, adjust dose accordingly.
    • oral antidiabetic drugs, and alter control of blood sugar levels un-
      predictably.
    • aspirin, and increase the risk of stomach ulceration and/or bleeding;
      avoid this combination.
    Flurbiprofen may *decrease* the effects of
    • amiloride (Midamor, Moduretic).
    • bumetanide (Bumex).
    • chlorthalidone (Hygroton, etc.).
    • ethacrynic acid (Edecrin).
    • furosemide (Lasix).
    • indapamide (Lozol).
    • metolazone (Diulo, Zaroxolyn).
    • spironolactone (Aldactone, Aldactazide).
    • thiazide diuretics (see Drug Class, Section Four).
    • triamterene (Dyazide, Maxzide).
    Flurbiprofen *taken concurrently* with the following drugs may increase
    the risk of bleeding (antiplatelet effect); monitor these combinations
    closely:
    • aspirin.
    • colchicine (ColBenemid, etc.).
    • dipyridamole (Persantine).
    • indomethacin (Indocin).
    • sulfinpyrazone (Anturane).
    • valproic acid (Depakene).
    Flurbiprofen *taken concurrently* with the following drugs may increase
    their toxicity; monitor these combinations closely:
    • lithium (Lithane, etc.).
    • methotrexate (Folex, Mexate).
    The following drug may *increase* the effects of flurbiprofen
    • probenecid (Benemid), by slowing its elimination.
▷   *Driving, Hazardous Activities:* This drug may cause dizziness, drowsiness
    or blurred vision. Restrict activities as necessary.

Aviation Note: The use of this drug **may be a disqualification** for piloting. Consult a designated Aviation Medical Examiner.

Exposure to Sun: Use caution until sensitivity is determined. Photosensitivity (see Glossary) has been reported.

FUROSEMIDE
(fur OH se mide)

Introduced: 1964

Class: Antihypertensive, diuretic

Prescription: USA: Yes
    Canada: Yes

Controlled Drug: USA: No
    Canada: No

Available as Generic: USA: Yes
    Canada: Yes

Brand Names: ✦Apo-Furosemide, ✦Furoside, Lasix, ✦Novosemide, ✦Uritol

BENEFITS versus RISKS	
Possible Benefits	*Possible Risks*
PROMPT, EFFECTIVE, RELIABLE DIURETIC	WATER AND ELECTROLYTE DEPLETION with excessive use
MODEST ANTIHYPERTENSIVE IN MILD TO MODERATE HYPERTENSION	Excessive potassium loss
	Increased blood sugar level
	Increased blood uric acid level
ENHANCES EFFECTIVENESS OF OTHER ANTIHYPERTENSIVES	Decreased blood calcium level
	Rare liver damage
	Rare blood cell disorder

▷ **Principal Uses**

As a Single Drug Product: This powerful diuretic is used primarily to increase the volume of urine and thereby relieve the body of excessive water retention (edema) that is commonly associated with congestive heart failure and some forms of liver disease and kidney disease. It is also used in the treatment of high blood pressure, but usually in conjunction with other antihypertensive drugs. A less frequent use is to increase the amount of calcium excreted the urine when the blood level of calcium is abnormally high.

How This Drug Works: By increasing the elimination of salt and water from the body (through increased urine production), this drug reduces the volume of fluid in the blood and body tissues and lowers the sodium content throughout the body. These changes contribute to lowering blood pressure.

Available Dosage Forms and Strengths
Injection — 10 mg per ml
Solution — 10 mg per ml, 40 mg per 5-ml teaspoonful
Tablets — 20 mg, 40 mg, 80 mg

▷ **Usual Adult Dosage Range:**   As antihypertensive: 40 mg/12 hours initially; increase dose as needed and tolerated. As diuretic: 20 to 80 mg in a single dose initially; if necessary, increase the dose by 20 to 40 mg/ 6 to 8 hours. The smallest effective dose should be determined. The total daily dose should not exceed 600 mg. **Note: Actual dosage and administration schedule must be determined by the physician for each patient individually.**

▷ **Dosing Instructions:**   May be taken with or following meals to reduce stomach irritation. Best taken in the morning to avoid nighttime urination. The tablet may be crushed for administration.

Usual Duration of Use: Continual use on a regular schedule for 2 to 3 weeks is usually necessary to determine this drug's effectiveness in lowering high blood pressure. Long-term use (months to years) requires periodic evaluation of response and possible dosage adjustment. Use as a diuretic should be intermittent with "drug holidays" (no drug taken) to reduce the risk of sodium and potassium imbalance. Consult your physician on a regular basis.

▷ **This Drug Should Not Be Taken If**
  • you have had an allergic reaction to any dosage form of it previously.

▷ **Inform Your Physician Before Taking This Drug If**
  • you are allergic to any form of "sulfa" drug.
  • you are pregnant or planning pregnancy.
  • you have a history of kidney or liver disease.
  • you have diabetes, gout or lupus erythematosus.
  • you are taking any form of cortisone, digitalis, oral antidiabetic drug or insulin.
  • you plan to have surgery under general anesthesia in the near future.

Possible Side-Effects (natural, expected and unavoidable drug actions)
Light-headedness on arising from sitting or lying position (see Orthostatic Hypotension in Glossary).
Increase in blood sugar level, affecting control of diabetes.
Increase in blood uric acid level, affecting control of gout.
Decrease in blood potassium level, causing muscle weakness and cramping.

▷ **Possible Adverse Effects** (unusual, unexpected and infrequent reactions)
  If any of the following develop, consult your physician promptly for guidance.

Mild Adverse Effects
   Allergic Reactions: Skin rashes, hives, drug fever.
   Headache, dizziness, blurred or yellow vision, ringing in ears, numbness and tingling.
   Reduced appetite, indigestion, nausea, vomiting, diarrhea.
Serious Adverse Effects
   Allergic Reactions: Hepatitis with jaundice (see Glossary), anaphylactic reaction (see Glossary), severe skin reactions.
   Idiosyncratic Reaction: Fluid accumulation in lungs.
   Temporary hearing loss.
   Inflammation of the pancreas—severe abdominal pain.
   Bone marrow depression (see Glossary)—fatigue, weakness, fever, sore throat, abnormal bleeding or bruising.

▷ **Possible Effects on Sexual Function:**   Impotence (5%) using recommended dosage of 20 to 80 mg/day.

▷ **Adverse Effects That May Mimic Natural Diseases or Disorders**
   Liver reaction may suggest viral hepatitis.

Natural Diseases or Disorders That May Be Activated by This Drug
   Diabetes, gout, systemic lupus erythematosus.

CAUTION
   1. Do not exceed recommended doses. Increased dosage can cause excessive loss of sodium and potassium, with resultant loss of appetite, nausea, fatigue, weakness, confusion and tingling in the extremities.
   2. If you are also taking a digitalis preparation (digitoxin, digoxin), ensure an adequate intake of high-potassium foods to prevent potassium deficiency—a potential cause of digitalis toxicity. (See Table of High Potassium Foods in Section Six.)

Precautions for Use
   By Infants and Children: Avoid overdosage that could cause serious dehydration. Significant potassium loss can occur within the first 2 weeks of drug use.
   By Those over 60 Years of Age: Small doses are advisable until your individual response has been determined. You may be more susceptible to the development of impaired thinking, orthostatic hypotension, potassium loss and blood sugar increase. Overdosage and extended use of this drug can cause excessive loss of body water, thickening (increased viscosity) of the blood and an increased tendency for the blood to clot—predisposing to stroke, heart attack or thrombophlebitis (vein inflammation with blood clot).

▷ **Advisability of Use During Pregnancy**
   Pregnancy Category: C (tentative). See Pregnancy Code inside back cover.
   Animal studies: Significant birth defects have been reported.

Human studies: Information from adequate studies of pregnant women is not available.

It should not be used during pregnancy unless a very serious complication occurs for which this drug is significantly beneficial. Avoid completely during the first 3 months. Ask physician for guidance.

Advisability of Use if Breast-Feeding
Presence of this drug in breast milk: Yes.
Avoid drug or refrain from nursing.

Habit-Forming Potential: None.

Effects of Overdosage: Dry mouth, thirst, lethargy, weakness, muscle cramping, nausea, vomiting, drowsiness progressing to stupor or coma.

Possible Effects of Long-Term Use: Impaired balance of water, salt and potassium in blood and body tissues; dehydration and increased blood coagulability, with predisposition to thromboembolic disorders. Development of diabetes in predisposed individuals.

Suggested Periodic Examinations While Taking This Drug (at physician's discretion)
Complete blood cell counts, measurements of blood levels of sodium, potassium, chloride, sugar and uric acid.
Kidney and liver function tests.

▷ **While Taking This Drug, Observe the Following**
Foods: Consult your physician regarding the advisability of eating foods rich in potassium. If so advised, see the Table of High Potassium Foods in Section Six. Follow physician's advice regarding the use of salt.
Beverages: No restrictions. This drug may be taken with milk.
▷ *Alcohol:* Use with caution until the combined effects have been determined. Alcohol may exaggerate the blood-pressure-lowering effects of this drug and cause orthostatic hypotension.
Tobacco Smoking: No interactions expected. Follow physician's advice.
▷ *Other Drugs*
Furosemide may ***increase*** the effects of
• other antihypertensive drugs; dosage adjustments may be necessary to prevent excessive lowering of blood pressure.
• lithium, and cause lithium toxicity.
Furosemide may ***decrease*** the effects of
• oral antidiabetic drugs (sulfonylureas); dosage adjustments may be necessary for proper control of blood sugar.
Furosemide ***taken concurrently*** with
• digitalis preparations (digitoxin, digoxin) requires very careful monitoring and dosage adjustments to prevent fluctuations of blood potassium levels and serious disturbances of heart rhythm.

The following drug may *decrease* the effects of furosemide
- indomethacin (Indocin).

▷ *Driving, Hazardous Activities:* Use caution until the possible occurrence of orthostatic hypotension, dizziness or impaired vision has been determined.

Aviation Note: The use of this drug *may be a disqualification* for piloting. Consult a designated Aviation Medical Examiner.

Exposure to Sun: Use caution until sensitivity has been determined. This drug may cause photosensitivity (see Glossary).

Exposure to Heat: Avoid excessive perspiring, which could cause additional loss of salt and water from the body.

Heavy Exercise or Exertion: Avoid exertion that produces light-headedness, excessive fatigue or muscle cramping. Isometric exercises—the "overload" technique for strengthening individual muscles—can raise blood pressure significantly. Ask physician for guidance regarding participation in this form of exercise.

Occurrence of Unrelated Illness: Illnesses that cause vomiting or diarrhea can produce a serious imbalance of important body chemistry. Consult your physician for guidance.

Discontinuation: It may be advisable to discontinue this drug 5 to 7 days before major surgery. Ask your physician, surgeon and/or anesthesiologist for guidance regarding dosage adjustment or drug withdrawal.

GEMFIBROZIL
(jem FI broh zil)

Introduced: 1976

Prescription: USA: Yes
Canada: Yes

Available as Generic: USA: No
Canada: No

Brand Name: Lopid

Class: Anticholesterol

Controlled Drug: USA: No
Canada: No

BENEFITS versus RISKS

Possible Benefits	*Possible Risks*
EFFECTIVE REDUCTION OF TRIGLYCERIDE BLOOD LEVELS AND ELEVATION OF HIGH DENSITY (HDL) CHOLESTEROL BLOOD LEVELS (40% to 50% reduction of triglycerides; 25% to 30% elevation of HDL cholesterol)	May elevate total cholesterol levels in one third of users Gallstone formation with long-term use Increased susceptibility to viral and bacterial infections

▷ **Principal Uses**

As a Single Drug Product: Used primarily to reduce abnormally high blood levels of triglycerides in Types IV and V blood lipid (fat) disorders. Its use is recommended as an adjunct to appropriate dietary adjustment in those individuals who are considered to be at high risk for developing coronary artery heart disease.

How This Drug Works: Not completely known. It is thought that this drug reduces blood levels of triglycerides by inhibiting their production in the liver. It addition, it may hasten removal of cholesterol from the liver and increase its excretion in the stool.

Available Dosage Forms and Strengths
Capsules — 300 mg
Tablets — 600 mg

▷ **Usual Adult Dosage Range:**   900 mg to 1500 mg daily in 2 divided doses. The average dose is 1200 mg/24 hours. Dose increases should be made gradually over a period of 2 to 3 months. **Note: Actual dosage and administration schedule must be determined by the physician for each patient individually.**

▷ **Dosing Instructions:**   Take 30 minutes before the morning and evening meals. The capsule may be opened for administration.

Usual Duration of Use: Continual use on a regular schedule for 4 to 8 weeks is usually necessary to determine this drug's effectiveness in reducing blood levels of triglycerides. Long-term use (months to years) requires periodic evaluation of response and dosage adjustment. Consult your physician on a regular basis.

Currently a "Drug of Choice" for initiating treatment of elevated LDL cholesterol and VLDL triglycerides. See Cholesterol Disorders in Section Two.

▷ **This Drug Should Not Be Taken If**
- you have had an allergic reaction to it previously.
- you have biliary cirrhosis of the liver.

▷ **Inform Your Physician Before Taking This Drug If**
- you have impaired liver or kidney function.
- you have gallbladder disease or gallstones.

Possible Side-Effects (natural, expected and unavoidable drug actions)
Moderate increase in blood sugar levels.

▷ **Possible Adverse Effects** (unusual, unexpected and infrequent reactions)
If any of the following develop, consult your physician promptly for guidance.
Mild Adverse Effects
Allergic Reactions: Skin rash, hives, itching.
Headache, dizziness, blurred vision, fatigue, muscle aches and cramps.

Indigestion, excessive gas, stomach discomfort (6%), nausea (4%), vomiting (1.6%), diarrhea (5%).

Serious Adverse Effects

Abnormally low white blood cell count: fever, chills, sore throat.

Formation of gallstones with long-term use.

▷ **Possible Effects on Sexual Function:** Decreased libido.

Natural Diseases or Disorders That May Be Activated by This Drug

Latent diabetes, latent urinary tract infections.

CAUTION

1. This drug should be used only after nondrug methods (primarily diet) have been ineffective in lowering triglyceride levels.
2. If you used the drug clofibrate (Atromid-S) in the past, inform your physician fully regarding your experience.
3. Comply fully with all recommendations for periodic measurements of blood triglyceride and cholesterol levels. These are essential to the proper management of drug therapy for your disorder.

Precautions for Use

By Infants and Children: Safety and effectiveness for use by those under 12 years of age have not been established.

By Those over 60 Years of Age: Observe for any increased tendency to infection; treat all infections promptly.

▷ **Advisability of Use During Pregnancy**

Pregnancy Category: B (tentative). See Pregnancy Code inside back cover.

Animal studies: No significant birth defects found due to this drug.

Human studies: Information from adequate studies of pregnant women is not available.

Use only if clearly needed. Ask your physician for guidance.

Advisability of Use if Breast-Feeding

Presence of this drug in breast milk: Unknown.

Avoid drug or refrain from nursing.

Habit-Forming Potential: None.

Effects of Overdosage: Abdominal pain, nausea, vomiting, diarrhea.

Possible Effects of Long-Term Use: Formation of gallstones.

Suggested Periodic Examinations While Taking This Drug (at physician's discretion)

Complete blood cell counts.

Measurements of blood levels of total cholesterol, HDL and LDL cholesterol fractions, triglycerides and sugar.

Liver function tests.

▷ **While Taking This Drug, Observe the Following**

Foods: Follow the diet prescribed by your physician.

Beverages: No restrictions. May be taken with milk.

▷   *Alcohol:* No interactions expected.
      Tobacco Smoking: No interactions expected.
▷   *Other Drugs*
      Gemfibrozil may ***increase*** the effects of
      • warfarin (Coumadin), and increase the risk of bleeding; frequent pro-
        thrombin time measurements and dosage adjustments are necessary.
      Gemfibrozil may ***decrease*** the effects of
      • chenodiol (Chenix), and reduce its effectiveness in the treatment of
        gallstones.
▷   *Driving, Hazardous Activities:* This drug may cause dizziness and blurred
      vision. Restrict activities as necessary.
      Aviation Note: The use of this drug ***is usually not a disqualification*** for
      piloting. Consult a designated Aviation Medical Examiner.
      Exposure to Sun: No restrictions.
      Discontinuation: If adequate reduction of triglycerides does not occur
      after 3 months of treatment, this drug should be discontinued. Fol-
      lowing withdrawal, blood cholesterol and triglyceride will return to
      pretreatment levels.

GLIPIZIDE
(GLIP i zide)

Introduced: 1972   **Class:** Antidiabetic, sulfonylureas

Prescription: USA: Yes   **Controlled Drug:** USA: No

Available as Generic: No

Brand Name: Glucotrol

BENEFITS versus RISKS

Possible Benefits	*Possible Risks*
Assistance in regulating blood sugar in noninsulin-dependent diabetes (adjunctive to appropriate diet and weight control)	HYPOGLYCEMIA, severe and prolonged Allergic skin reactions (some severe) Water retention Rare liver damage Rare blood cell and bone marrow disorders

---

▷ **Principal Uses**
      As a Single Drug Product: To assist in the control of mild to moderately
      severe type II diabetes mellitus (adult, maturity-onset) that does not

require insulin, but that cannot be adequately controlled by diet alone.

How This Drug Works: It is thought that this drug (1) stimulates the secretion of insulin (by a pancreas that is capable of responding to stimulation), and (2) enhances the utilization of insulin by appropriate tissues.

Available Dosage Forms and Strengths
Tablets — 5 mg, 10 mg

▷ **Usual Adult Dosage Range:** Initially 5 mg daily with breakfast. At 7 day intervals, the dose may be increased by increments of 2.5 to 5 mg daily as needed and tolerated. Total daily dosage should not exceed 40 mg. A "loading" or priming dose is not necessary and should not be given. **Note: Actual dosage and administration schedule must be determined by the physician for each patient individually.**

▷ **Dosing Instructions:** If the daily maintenance dose is found to be 15 mg or more, the total dose should be divided into 2 equal doses: the first taken with the morning meal, the second with the evening meal. The tablet may be crushed for administration.

Usual Duration of Use: Continual use on a regular schedule for 1 to 2 weeks is usually necessary to determine this drug's effectiveness in controlling diabetes. Failure to respond to maximal doses within 1 month constitutes a primary failure. Up to 10% of those who respond initially may develop secondary failure of the drug later. The duration of effective use can only be determined by periodic measurement of the blood sugar. Consult your physician on a regular basis.

Possible Advantages of This Drug
Effective with once-daily dosing.
Onset of action within 30 minutes.
Near-normal insulin response to eating.
Well tolerated by the elderly diabetic.

Currently a "Drug of Choice" for initiating treatment in noninsulin-dependent diabetes when diet and weight control fail.

▷ **This Drug Should Not Be Taken If**
  • you have had an allergic reaction to it previously.
  • you have severe impairment of liver or kidney function.
  • you are pregnant.

▷ **Inform Your Physician Before Taking This Drug If**
  • you are allergic to other sulfonylurea drugs or to "sulfa" drugs.
  • your diabetes has been unstable or "brittle" in the past.
  • you do not know how to recognize or treat hypoglycemia (see Glossary).

- you have a history of congestive heart failure, peptic ulcer disease, cirrhosis of the liver, hypothyroidism or porphyria.

Possible Side-Effects (natural, expected and unavoidable drug actions)
If drug dosage is excessive or food intake is delayed or inadequate, abnormally low blood sugar (hypoglycemia) will occur as a predictable drug effect.

▷ **Possible Adverse Effects** (unusual, unexpected and infrequent reactions)
If any of the following develop, consult your physician promptly for guidance.
Mild Adverse Effects
Allergic Reactions: Skin rash, hives, itching.
Headache (1.25%), drowsiness (1.75%), dizziness (2.25%), fatigue (2.13%), sweating (1.25%).
Indigestion, nausea (1.38%), vomiting, diarrhea (1.25%).
Serious Adverse Effects
Allergic Reactions: Hepatitis with jaundice (see Glossary), severe skin reactions.
Idiosyncratic Reaction: Hemolytic anemia (see Glossary).
Disulfiramlike reaction with concurrent use of alcohol (see Glossary), infrequent with this drug.
Water retention (edema), weight gain.
Bone marrow depression (see Glossary)—fatigue, weakness, fever, sore throat, abnormal bleeding or bruising.

▷ **Possible Effects on Sexual Function:**   None reported.

▷ **Adverse Effects That May Mimic Natural Diseases or Disorders**
Liver reactions may suggest viral hepatitis.

CAUTION
1. This drug must be regarded as only one part of the total program for the management of your diabetes. It is not a substitute for a properly prescribed diet and regular exercise.
2. Over a period of time (usually several months), this drug may lose its effectiveness in controlling blood sugar levels. Periodic followup examinations are necessary to monitor all aspects of response to drug treatment.

Precautions for Use
By Infants and Children: This drug is not effective in type I (juvenile, growth-onset) insulin-dependent diabetes.
By Those over 60 Years of Age: This drug should be used with caution in this age group. Start treatment with 2.5 mg/day; increase dosage cautiously and monitor closely to prevent hypoglycemic reactions. Repeated episodes of hypoglycemia in the elderly can cause brain damage.

▷ **Advisability of Use During Pregnancy**
Pregnancy Category: C (tentative). See Pregnancy Code inside back cover.
Animal studies: No birth defects reported in rats and rabbits.
Human studies: Information from adequate studies of pregnant women is not available.
Because uncontrolled blood sugar levels during pregnancy are associated with a higher incidence of birth defects, many experts recommend that insulin (instead of an oral agent) be used as necessary to control diabetes during the entire pregnancy.

Advisability of Use if Breast-Feeding
Presence of this drug in breast milk: Unknown.
Avoid drug or refrain from nursing.

Habit-Forming Potential: None.

Effects of Overdosage: Symptoms of mild to severe hypoglycemia: headache, light-headedness, faintness, nervousness, confusion, tremor, sweating, heart palpitation, weakness, hunger, nausea, vomiting, stupor progressing to coma.

Possible Effects of Long-Term Use: Reduced function of the thyroid gland (hypothyroidism). Reports of increased frequency and severity of heart and blood vessel diseases associated with long-term use of this class of drugs are highly controversial and inconclusive. A direct cause-and-effect relationship (see Glossary) is tenuous. Ask your physician for guidance.

Suggested Periodic Examinations While Taking This Drug (at physician's discretion)
Complete blood cell counts, liver function tests, thyroid function tests, periodic evaluation of heart and circulatory system.

▷ **While Taking This Drug, Observe the Following**
Foods: Follow the diabetic diet prescribed by your physician.
Beverages: As directed in the diabetic diet. May be taken with milk.
▷   *Alcohol:* Use with extreme caution until the combined effect has been determined. Alcohol can exaggerate this drug's hypoglycemic effect. This drug infrequently causes a marked intolerance of alcohol, resulting in a disulfiramlike reaction (see Glossary): facial flushing, sweating, palpitation.
Tobacco Smoking: No interactions expected.
▷   *Other Drugs*
The following drugs may *increase* the effects of glipizide
• aspirin, and other salicylates.
• cimetidine (Tagamet).
• clofibrate (Atromid S).
• fenfluramine (Pondimin).
• monoamine oxidase (MAO) type A inhibitor drugs (see Drug Class, Section Four).

- phenylbutazone (Butazolidin).
- ranitidine (Zantac).

The following drugs may *decrease* the effects of glipizide
- beta blocker drugs (see Drug Class, Section Four).
- bumetanide (Bumex).
- diazoxide (Proglycem).
- ethacrynic acid (Edecrin).
- furosemide (Lasix).
- phenytoin (Dilantin).
- thiazide diuretics (see Drug Class, Section Four).

▷ *Driving, Hazardous Activities:* Regulate your dosage schedule, eating schedule and physical activities very carefully to prevent hypoglycemia. Be able to recognize the early symptoms of hypoglycemia so you can avoid hazardous activities and take corrective measures.

Aviation Note: Diabetes *is a disqualification* for piloting. Consult a designated Aviation Medical Examiner.

Exposure to Sun: Use caution until sensitivity has been determined. Some drugs of this class can cause photosensitivity (see Glossary).

Occurrence of Unrelated Illness: Acute infections, illnesses causing vomiting or diarrhea, serious injuries and surgical procedures can interfere with diabetic control and may require the use of insulin. If any of these conditions occur, consult your physician promptly.

Discontinuation: Because of the possibility of secondary failure, it is advisable to evaluate the continued benefit of this drug every 6 months.

GLYBURIDE
(GLI byoor ide)

Other Name: Glibenclamide

Introduced: 1970   **Class:** Antidiabetic, sulfonylureas

Prescription: USA: Yes   **Controlled Drug:** USA: No
    Canada: Yes   Canada: No

Available as Generic: No

Brand Names: DiaBeta, ✦Euglucon, Micronase

BENEFITS versus RISKS
Possible Benefits   *Possible Risks*

Possible Benefits	*Possible Risks*
Assistance in regulating blood sugar in noninsulin-dependent diabetes (adjunctive to appropriate diet and weight control)	HYPOGLYCEMIA, severe and prolonged Allergic skin reactions (some severe) Rare liver damage Rare blood cell and bone marrow disorders

▷ **Principal Uses**

As a Single Drug Product: To assist in the control of mild to moderately severe type II diabetes mellitus (adult, maturity-onset) that does not require insulin, but that cannot be adequately controlled by diet alone.

How This Drug Works: It is thought that this drug (1) stimulates the secretion of insulin (by a pancreas that is capable of responding to stimulation), and (2) enhances the utilization of insulin by appropriate tissues.

Available Dosage Forms and Strengths
Tablets — 1.25 mg, 2.5 mg, 5 mg

▷ **Usual Adult Dosage Range:** Initially 2.5 to 5 mg daily with breakfast. At 7-day intervals the dose may be increased by increments of 2.5 mg daily as needed and tolerated. Total daily dosage should not exceed 20 mg. A "loading" or priming dose is not necessary and should not be given. **Note: Actual dosage and administration schedule must be determined by the physician for each patient individually.**

▷ **Dosing Instructions:** If the daily maintenance dose is found to be 10 mg or more, the total dose should be divided into 2 equal doses: the first taken with the morning meal, the second with the evening meal. The tablet may be crushed for administration.

Usual Duration of Use: Continual use on a regular schedule for 1 to 2 weeks is usually necessary to determine this drug's effectiveness in controlling diabetes. Failure to respond to maximal doses within 1 month constitutes a primary failure. Up to 10% of those who respond initially may develop secondary failure of the drug later. The duration of effective use can only be determined by periodic measurement of the blood sugar. Consult your physician on a regular basis.

▷ **This Drug Should Not Be Taken If**
- you have had an allergic reaction to it previously.
- you have severe impairment of liver and kidney function.
- you are pregnant.

▷ **Inform Your Physician Before Taking This Drug If**
- you are allergic to other sulfonylurea drugs or to "sulfa" drugs.
- your diabetes has been unstable or "brittle" in the past.
- you do not know how to recognize or treat hypoglycemia (see Glossary).
- you have a history of congestive heart failure, peptic ulcer disease, cirrhosis of the liver, hypothyroidism or porphyria.

Possible Side-Effects (natural, expected and unavoidable drug actions)
If drug dosage is excessive or food intake is delayed or inadequate, abnormally low blood sugar (hypoglycemia) will occur as a predictable drug effect.

▷ **Possible Adverse Effects** (unusual, unexpected and infrequent reactions)
If any of the following develop, consult your physician promptly for guidance.
Mild Adverse Effects
Allergic Reactions: Skin rash, hives, itching.
Headache, drowsiness, dizziness, fatigue.
Indigestion, heartburn, nausea.
Serious Adverse Effects
Allergic Reactions: Hepatitis with jaundice (see Glossary), severe skin reactions.
Idiosyncratic Reaction: Hemolytic anemia (see Glossary).
Disulfiramlike reaction with concurrent use of alcohol (see Glossary), infrequent with this drug.
Bone marrow depression (see Glossary)—fatigue, weakness, fever, sore throat, abnormal bleeding or bruising.

▷ **Possible Effects on Sexual Function:** None reported.

▷ **Adverse Effects That May Mimic Natural Diseases or Disorders**
Liver reactions may suggest viral hepatitis.

CAUTION
1. This drug must be regarded as only one part of the total program for the management of your diabetes. It is not a substitute for a properly prescribed diet and regular exercise.
2. Over a period of time (usually several months), this drug may lose its effectiveness in controlling blood sugar levels. Periodic follow-up examinations are necessary to monitor all aspects of response to drug treatment.

Precautions for Use
By Infants and Children: This drug is not effective in type I (juvenile, growth-onset) insulin-dependent diabetes.
By Those over 60 Years of Age: This drug should be used with caution in this age group. Start treatment with 1.25 mg/day; increase dosage cautiously and monitor closely to prevent hypoglycemic reactions. Repeated episodes of hypoglycemia in the elderly can cause brain damage.

▷ **Advisability of Use During Pregnancy**
Pregnancy Category: B (tentative). See Pregnancy Code inside back cover.
Animal studies: No birth defects reported in rats and rabbits.
Human studies: Information from adequate studies of pregnant women is not available.
Because uncontrolled blood sugar levels during pregnancy are associated with a higher incidence of birth defects, many experts recommend that insulin (instead of an oral agent) be used as necessary to control diabetes during the entire pregnancy.

Advisability of Use if Breast-Feeding
Presence of this drug in breast milk: Unknown.
Avoid drug or refrain from nursing.

Habit-Forming Potential: None.

Effects of Overdosage: Symptoms of mild to severe hypoglycemia: headache, light-headedness, faintness, nervousness, confusion, tremor, sweating, heart palpitation, weakness, hunger, nausea, vomiting, stupor progressing to coma.

Possible Effects of Long-Term Use: Reduced function of the thyroid gland (hypothyroidism). Reports of increased frequency and severity of heart and blood vessel diseases associated with long-term use of this class of drugs are highly controversial and inconclusive. A direct cause-and-effect relationship (see Glossary) is tenuous. Ask your physician for guidance.

Suggested Periodic Examinations While Taking This Drug (at physician's discretion)
Complete blood cell counts, liver function tests, thyroid function tests, periodic evaluation of heart and circulatory system.

▷ **While Taking This Drug, Observe the Following**
Foods: Follow the diabetic diet prescribed by your physician.
Beverages: As directed in the diabetic diet. May be taken with milk.
▷   *Alcohol:* Use with extreme caution until the combined effect has been determined. Alcohol can exaggerate this drug's hypoglycemic effect. This drug infrequently causes a marked intolerance of alcohol, resulting in a disulfiramlike reaction (see Glossary): facial flushing, sweating, palpitation.
Tobacco Smoking: No interactions expected.
▷   *Other Drugs*
The following drugs may **increase** the effects of glyburide
- aspirin, and other salicylates.
- cimetidine (Tagamet).
- clofibrate (Atromid S).
- fenfluramine (Pondimin).
- monoamine oxidase (MAO) type A inhibitor drugs (see Drug Class, Section Four).
- phenylbutazone (Butazolidin).
- ranitidine (Zantac).
The following drugs may **decrease** the effects of glyburide
- beta blocker drugs (see Drug Class, Section Four).
- bumetanide (Bumex).
- diazoxide (Proglycem).
- ethacrynic acid (Edecrin).
- furosemide (Lasix).
- phenytoin (Dilantin).
- thiazide diuretics (see Drug Class, Section Four).

▷ *Driving, Hazardous Activities:* Regulate your dosage schedule, eating schedule and physical activities very carefully to prevent hypoglycemia. Be able to recognize the early symptoms of hypoglycemia so you can avoid hazardous activities and take corrective measures.

Aviation Note: Diabetes *is a disqualification* for piloting. Consult a designated Aviation Medical Examiner.

Exposure to Sun: Use caution until sensitivity has been determined. Some drugs of this class can cause photosensitivity (see Glossary).

Occurrence of Unrelated Illness: Acute infections, illnesses causing vomiting or diarrhea, serious injuries and surgical procedures can interfere with diabetic control and may require the use of insulin. If any of these conditions occur, consult your physician promptly.

Discontinuation: Because of the possibility of secondary failure, it is advisable to evaluate the continued benefit of this drug every 6 months.

GUANFACINE
(GWAHN fa seen)

Introduced: 1980

Class: Antihypertensive

Prescription: USA: Yes

Controlled Drug: USA: No

Available as Generic: USA: No

Brand Name: Tenex

BENEFITS versus RISKS	
Possible Benefits	*Possible Risks*
EFFECTIVE ANTIHYPERTENSIVE in mild to moderate high blood pressure	Amnesia, confusion, mental depression (3% or less)

▷ **Principal Uses**

As a Single Drug Product: This antihypertensive drug is often used as a "step 2" drug in the treatment of mild to moderate high blood pressure. It is generally not used to initiate treatment, but is added when a "step 1" drug proves to be inadequate. It may also be used as a "step 3 or 4" drug in place of drugs that cause marked orthostatic hypotension (see Glossary).

How This Drug Works: By decreasing the activity of the vasomotor center in the brain, this drug reduces the ability of the sympathetic nervous system to maintain the degree of blood vessel constriction responsible for the elevation of blood pressure. This change results in relaxation of blood vessel walls and lowering of blood pressure.

Available Dosage Forms and Strengths
Tablets — 1 mg

▷ **Usual Adult Dosage Range:** Initially 1 mg once daily taken at bedtime. The dose may be increased after 3 to 4 weeks to 2 mg daily, as needed and tolerated. If needed, the dose may be increased again after 3 to 4 weeks to 3 mg daily. The total daily requirement may be taken in 2 divided doses if necessary for stable blood pressure control. **Note: Actual dosage and administration schedule must be determined by the physician for each patient individually.**

▷ **Dosing Instructions:** Tablets may be taken without regard to eating. It is recommended that the daily dose be taken at bedtime to reduce the side-effect of daytime drowsiness. The tablet may be crushed for administration.

Usual Duration of Use: Continual use on a regular schedule for 4 to 6 weeks is usually necessary to determine this drug's effectiveness in controlling high blood pressure. Long-term use (months to years) requires supervision and guidance by the physician. Consult your physician on a regular basis.

▷ **This Drug Should Not Be Taken If**
- you have had an allergic reaction to it previously.

▷ **Inform Your Physician Before Taking This Drug If**
- you have a circulatory disorder of the brain.
- you have angina or coronary artery disease.
- you have or have had serious emotional depression.
- you have impaired liver or kidney function.
- you are taking any sedative or hypnotic drugs or an antidepressant.
- you plan to have surgery under general anesthesia in the near future.

Possible Side-Effects (natural, expected and unavoidable drug actions)
Drowsiness (21%), dry nose and mouth (30%), constipation (10%), decreased heart rate, mild orthostatic hypotension (see Glossary).

▷ **Possible Adverse Effects** (unusual, unexpected and infrequent reactions)
If any of the following develop, consult your physician promptly for guidance.
Mild Adverse Effects
Allergic Reactions: Skin rash, itching.
Headache (4%), dizziness (11%), fatigue (9%), insomnia (4%).
Indigestion, nausea, diarrhea.

Serious Adverse Effects
Amnesia, confusion, depression.

▷ **Possible Effects on Sexual Function:** Decreased libido, impotence.

CAUTION
1. *Do not discontinue this drug suddenly.* Sudden withdrawal can produce anxiety, nervousness, tremors, fast or irregular heart action, nausea, stomach cramps, vomiting and rebound hypertension.
2. Hot weather and the fever associated with infection can reduce blood pressure significantly. Dosage adjustments may be necessary.
3. Report the development of any tendency to emotional depression.

Precautions for Use
By Infants and Children: Safety and effectiveness for use by those under 12 years of age have not been established.
By Those over 60 Years of Age: Proceed cautiously with the use of any antihypertensive drug. Unacceptably high blood pressure should be reduced without creating the risks associated with excessively low blood pressure. Start treatment with small doses and monitor the blood pressure response frequently. Observe for the development of light-headedness, dizziness, unsteadiness, fainting and falling. Sedation and dry mouth occur commonly in elderly users. Report promptly any changes in mood or behavior: depression, delusions, hallucinations.

▷ **Advisability of Use During Pregnancy**
Pregnancy Category: B (tentative). See Pregnancy Code inside back cover.
Animal studies: No birth defects due to this drug reported in rat and rabbit studies.
Human studies: Information from adequate studies of pregnant women is not available.
Use this drug only if clearly needed. Ask your physician for guidance.

Advisability of Use if Breast-Feeding
Presence of this drug in breast milk: Probably yes.
Avoid drug or refrain from nursing.

Habit-Forming Potential: None.

Effects of Overdosage: Marked drowsiness, weakness, dry mouth, slow pulse, low blood pressure, vomiting, stupor progressing to coma.

Possible Effects of Long-Term Use: Development of tolerance (see Glossary) with loss of drug effectiveness.

Suggested Periodic Examinations While Taking This Drug (at physician's discretion)
Blood pressure measurements.

▷ **While Taking This Drug, Observe the Following**

Foods: Avoid excessive salt. Ask physician for guidance regarding degree of salt restriction.

Beverages: No restrictions. May be taken with milk.

▷ *Alcohol:* Use with extreme caution. The combined effects can cause marked drowsiness and exaggerated reduction of blood pressure.

Tobacco Smoking: No interactions expected. Follow your physician's advice regarding use of tobacco.

▷ *Other Drugs:* No significant drug interactions reported to date.

▷ *Driving, Hazardous Activities:* Use caution. This drug can cause drowsiness and can impair mental alertness, judgment and coordination.

Aviation Note: Hypertension (high blood pressure) ***is a disqualification*** for piloting. Consult a designated Aviation Medical Examiner.

Exposure to Sun: No restrictions.

Exposure to Heat: Use caution. Hot environments may reduce the blood pressure significantly; be alert to the possibility of orthostatic hypotension (see Glossary).

Heavy Exercise or Exertion: Use caution. Isometric exercises—the "overload" technique for strengthening individual muscles—can raise blood pressure significantly. The use of this drug may intensify the hypertensive response to isometric exercise. Ask physician for guidance.

Occurrence of Unrelated Illness: Fever associated with infections may lower the blood pressure significantly. Repeated vomiting may prevent the regular use of this drug and result in an acute withdrawal reaction. Consult your physician.

Discontinuation: **Do not discontinue this drug suddenly.** A significant withdrawal reaction can occur within 2 to 7 days after the last dose. The dose should be reduced gradually over 3 to 4 days, with periodic monitoring of the blood pressure.

HALOPERIDOL
(hal oh PER i dohl)

Introduced: 1958

Class: Strong tranquilizer, butyrophenones

Prescription: USA: Yes
Canada: Yes

Controlled Drug: USA: No
Canada: No

Available as Generic: USA: Yes
Canada: No

Brand Names: ✦Apo-Haloperidol, Haldol, ✦Haldol LA, Halperon, ✦Novoperidol, ✦Peridol

```
┌─────────────────────────────────────────────────────────────┐
│                    BENEFITS versus RISKS                     │
│                                                              │
│      Possible Benefits                Possible Risks         │
│  EFFECTIVE CONTROL OF           FREQUENT PARKINSON-LIKE      │
│    ACUTE FREQUENT                 SIDE-EFFECTS               │
│    PSYCHOSES in majority of     SERIOUS TOXIC EFFECTS ON     │
│    patients: beneficial effects on  BRAIN with long-term use │
│    thinking, mood and behavior  Rare blood cell disorders    │
│  EFFECTIVE CONTROL OF SOME      Abnormally low white blood cell│
│    CASES OF TOURETTE'S            count                      │
│    DISORDER                                                  │
│  Beneficial in the management of                             │
│    the hyperactive child                                     │
└─────────────────────────────────────────────────────────────┘
```

▷ **Principal Uses**

As a Single Drug Product: Used primarily to control the psychotic thinking and abnormal behavior associated with acute psychosis of unknown nature, acute schizophrenia, paranoid states and the manic phase of manic-depressive disorders. It is also used to treat the hyperactivity syndrome in children. A less frequent use is to control the tics and offensive language characteristic of Gilles de la Tourette's syndrome.

How This Drug Works: Not completely established. It is thought that by interfering with the action of dopamine as nerve impulse transmitter in certain areas of the brain, this drug reduces anxiety and agitation, improves coherence and organization of thinking and abolishes delusions and hallucinations.

Available Dosage Forms and Strengths
    Concentrate — 2 mg per ml
      Injection — 5 mg per ml, 50 mg per ml
      Tablets — 0.5 mg, 1 mg, 2 mg, 5 mg, 10 mg, 20 mg

▷ **Usual Adult Dosage Range:**   Initially 0.5 to 2 mg 2 or 3 times daily. Dose may be increased by 0.5 mg/day at 3- to 4-day intervals as needed and tolerated. The usual dosage range is 0.5 to 30 mg/24 hours. The total daily dosage should not exceed 100 mg. **Note: Actual dosage and administration schedule must be determined by the physician for each patient individually.**

▷ **Dosing Instructions:**   May be taken with or following food to reduce stomach irritation. The concentrate may be diluted in 2 ounces of water or fruit juice; do not add it to coffee or tea. The tablet may be crushed for administration.

Usual Duration of Use: Continual use on a regular schedule for several weeks is usually necessary to determine this drug's effectiveness in controlling the symptoms of psychotic or psychoneurotic behavior. If not significantly beneficial within 6 weeks, it should be discontinued.

Long-term use requires supervision and periodic evaluation by your physician. Consult your physician on a regular basis.

▷ **This Drug Should Not Be Taken If**
- you have had an allergic reaction to any dosage form of it previously.
- you are experiencing mental depression.
- you have any form of Parkinson's disease.
- you have cancer of the breast.
- you have active liver disease.
- you currently have a bone marrow or blood cell disorder.

▷ **Inform Your Physician Before Taking This Drug If**
- you are allergic or abnormally sensitive to phenothiazine drugs.
- you have a history of mental depression.
- you have any type of heart disease.
- you have impaired liver or kidney function.
- you have low blood pressure, epilepsy or glaucoma.
- you are taking any drugs with a sedative effect.
- you plan to have surgery under general or spinal anesthesia in the near future.

Possible Side-Effects (natural, expected and unavoidable drug actions)
Mild drowsiness, low blood pressure, blurred vision, dry mouth, constipation, marked and frequent Parkinson-like reactions (see Glossary).

▷ **Possible Adverse Effects** (unusual, unexpected and infrequent reactions)
If any of the following develop, consult your physician promptly for guidance.
Mild Adverse Effects
Allergic Reactions: Skin rash, hives.
Dizziness, weakness, agitation, insomnia.
Loss of appetite, indigestion, nausea, vomiting, diarrhea.
Urinary retention.
Serious Adverse Effects
Allergic Reactions: Rare liver reaction with jaundice, asthma, spasm of vocal cords.
Idiosyncratic Reactions: High fever, weakness, fast heart rate, muscle stiffness, seizures (rare neuroleptic malignant syndrome).
Depression, disorientation, eye damage (deposits in cornea, lens and retina).
Blood cell disorders: anemia, fluctuation in number of white blood cells.
Nervous system reactions: rigidity of extremities, tremors, restlessness, constant movement, facial grimacing, eye-rolling, spasm of neck muscles, tardive dyskinesia (see Glossary).

▷ **Possible Effects on Sexual Function**
Decreased libido; impotence (10% to 20%); painful ejaculation; priapism (see Glossary).

Male breast enlargement and tenderness; female breast enlargement
with milk production.
Altered timing and pattern of menstruation.

▷ **Adverse Effects That May Mimic Natural Diseases or Disorders**
Liver reaction may suggest viral hepatitis.
Nervous system reactions may suggest Parkinson's disease or Reye syndrome.

Natural Diseases or Disorders That May Be Activated by This Drug
Latent epilepsy, glaucoma, diabetes.

CAUTION
1. It is advisable to use the smallest dose that is effective for long-term treatment.
2. Use with extreme caution in epilepsy; this drug can alter the pattern of seizures.
3. Individuals with lupus erythematosus and those taking prednisone are more susceptible to nervous system reactions.
4. Do not use levodopa to treat Parkinson-like reactions; it can cause agitation and worsening of the psychotic disorder.
5. Obtain prompt evaluation of any change or disturbance in vision.

Precautions for Use
By Infants and Children: This drug should not be used in children under 3 years of age or 15 kilograms in weight. Avoid this drug in the presence of symptoms suggestive of Reye syndrome. Children are quite susceptible to nervous system reactions induced by this drug.
By Those over 60 Years of Age: Initiate treatment with small doses. This drug can cause significant changes in mood and behavior; observe for confusion, disorientation, agitation, restlessness, aggression and paranoia. You may be more susceptible to the development of drowsiness, lethargy, orthostatic hypotension (see Glossary), hypothermia (see Glossary), Parkinson-like reactions and prostatism (see Glossary).

▷ **Advisability of Use During Pregnancy**
Pregnancy Category: C (tentative). See Pregnancy Code inside back cover.
Animal studies: Cleft palate reported in mouse studies.
Human studies: No increase in birth defects reported in 100 exposures. Information from adequate studies of pregnant women is not available.
Avoid during the first trimester. Use only if clearly needed. Ask physician for guidance.

Advisability of Use if Breast-Feeding
Presence of this drug in breast milk: Yes.
Monitor nursing infant closely and discontinue drug or nursing if adverse effects develop.

Habit-Forming Potential: None.

Effects of Overdosage: Marked drowsiness, weakness, tremor, unsteadiness, agitation, stupor, coma, convulsions.

Possible Effects of Long-Term Use: Eye damage: deposits in cornea, lens or retina; tardive dyskinesia (see Glossary).

Suggested Periodic Examinations While Taking This Drug (at physician's discretion)

Complete blood cell counts, liver function tests, eye examinations, electrocardiograms.

Careful inspection of the tongue for early evidence of fine, involuntary, wavelike movements that could indicate the beginning of tardive dyskinesia.

▷ **While Taking This Drug, Observe the Following**

Foods: No restrictions.

Beverages: No restrictions. May be taken with milk.

▷ *Alcohol:* Avoid completely. Alcohol can increase the sedative action of haloperidol and accentuate its depressant effects on brain function. Haloperidol can increase the intoxicating effects of alcohol.

Tobacco Smoking: No interactions expected.

Marijuana Smoking: Moderate increase in drowsiness; accentuation of orthostatic hypotension; increased risk of precipitating latent psychosis, confusing interpretation of mental status and of drug response.

▷ *Other Drugs*

Haloperidol may *increase* the effects of

- all drugs with sedative actions, and cause excessive sedation.
- some antihypertensive drugs, and cause excessive lowering of blood pressure; monitor the combined effects carefully.

Haloperidol may *decrease* the effects of

- guanethidine (Esimil, Ismelin), and reduce its antihypertensive effect.

Haloperidol *taken concurrently* with

- beta blocker drugs may cause excessive lowering of blood pressure.
- lithium may cause toxic effects on the brain and nervous system.
- methyldopa (Aldomet) may cause serious dementia.

The following drugs may *decrease* the effects of haloperidol

- antacids containing aluminum and/or magnesium may reduce its absorption.
- barbiturates.
- benztropine (Cogentin).
- phenytoin (Dilantin).
- trihexyphenidyl (Artane).

▷ *Driving, Hazardous Activities:* This drug may impair mental alertness, judgment and physical coordination. Restrict activities as necessary.

Aviation Note: The use of this drug *is a disqualification* for piloting. Consult a designated Aviation Medical Examiner.

Exposure to Sun: Use caution until sensitivity has been determined. This drug can cause photosensitivity.

Exposure to Heat: Use caution in hot environments. This drug may impair the regulation of body temperature and increase the risk of heat stroke.

Exposure to Cold: The elderly are advised to use caution; this drug can increase the risk of hypothermia (see Glossary).

Discontinuation: This drug should not be discontinued abruptly following long-term use. Gradual withdrawal over a period of 2 to 3 weeks is advised. Ask physician for guidance.

HYDRALAZINE
(hi DRAL a zeen)

Introduced: 1950	**Class:** Antihypertensive
Prescription: USA: Yes Canada: Yes	**Controlled Drug:** USA: No Canada: No
Available as Generic: USA: Yes Canada: No	

Brand Names: Alazine, Apresazide [CD], Apresoline, Apresoline-Esidrix [CD], Ser-Ap-Es [CD], Serpasil-Apresoline [CD], Unipres [CD]

BENEFITS versus RISKS

Possible Benefits	*Possible Risks*
EFFECTIVE STEP 2 OR 3 ANTIHYPERTENSIVE FOR MODERATE TO SEVERE HYPERTENSION when used adjunctively with other antihypertensive drugs Possibly beneficial in the management of severe congestive heart failure	DRUG-INDUCED LUPUS ERYTHEMATOSUS–LIKE SYNDROME (up to 13%) Intensification of angina pectoris Rare blood cell disorders Rare liver damage

---

▷ **Principal Uses**

As a Single Drug Product: Used primarily as a step 2 or antihypertensive drug in conjunction with other antihypertensives in the treatment of moderate to severe high blood pressure.

As a Combination Drug Product [CD]: This drug is available in combination with hydrochlorothiazide (a diuretic) and with reserpine (another type of antihypertensive). When used in combination, several different types of drug action occur concurrently to reduce blood pressure: hydralazine relaxes and expands blood vessel walls; the diuretic reduces the amount of water and sodium in the body; reserpine reduces the rate and contraction force of the heart and enhances the expansion of blood vessels.

How This Drug Works: By causing direct relaxation of arterial walls (mechanism unknown), this drug dilates peripheral blood vessels, with resultant lowering of blood pressure. The dilation of blood vessels can also be beneficial in some cases of heart failure by reducing the workload of the heart and increasing its output.

Available Dosage Forms and Strengths
Tablets — 10 mg, 25 mg, 50 mg, 100 mg

▷ **Usual Adult Dosage Range:** Initially 10 mg 4 times daily for 2 to 4 days; then increase to 25 mg 4 times daily for the balance of the first week. During the second week the dose may be increased to 50 mg 4 times daily if needed and tolerated. The total daily dosage should not exceed 300 mg for fast acetylators or 200 mg for slow acetylators. Ask your physician for guidance. **Note: Actual dosage and administration schedule must be determined by the physician for each patient individually.**

▷ **Dosing Instructions:** Preferably taken with or following meals to enhance absorption and reduce stomach irritation. The tablet may be crushed and the capsule [CD] may be opened for administration.

Usual Duration of Use: Continual use on a regular schedule for several weeks is usually necessary to determine this drug's effectiveness in lowering blood pressure. Long-term use requires supervision and periodic evaluation by your physician. Consult your physician on a regular basis.

▷ **This Drug Should Not Be Taken If**
- you have had an allergic reaction to it previously.
- you have active angina pectoris.
- you have mitral valvular heart disease.

▷ **Inform Your Physician Before Taking This Drug If**
- you have a history of any type of heart disease.
- you have lupus erythematosus.
- you have impaired brain circulation.
- you are subject to migraine headaches.
- you have impaired kidney function.
- you have a history of liver sensitivity to other drugs.
- you plan to have surgery under general anesthesia in the near future.

Possible Side-Effects (natural, expected and unavoidable drug actions)
Orthostatic hypotension (see Glossary), nasal congestion, constipation, delayed or impaired urination, increased heart rate of 10 to 25 beats/minute.

▷ **Possible Adverse Effects** (unusual, unexpected and infrequent reactions)
If any of the following develop, consult your physician promptly for guidance.

Mild Adverse Effects

Allergic Reactions: Skin rash, hives, itching, drug fever.

Headache, dizziness, flushing of face, palpitation.

Loss of appetite, nausea, vomiting, diarrhea.

Tremors, muscle cramps.

Serious Adverse Effects

Allergic Reactions: Liver reaction, with or without jaundice.

Idiosyncratic Reactions: Behavioral changes: nervousness, confusion, emotional depression. Bleeding into lung tissue: densities found on X-ray examination. A syndrome resembling rheumatoid arthritis or lupus erythematosus (see Glossary).

Intensification of coronary artery disease.

Peripheral neuropathy (see Glossary): weakness, numbness and/or pain in extremities.

Rare bone marrow depression (see Glossary): fatigue, weakness, fever, sore throat, abnormal bleeding or bruising.

▷ **Possible Effects on Sexual Function:**   Rare reports of impotence and priapism (see Glossary).

▷ **Adverse Effects That May Mimic Natural Diseases or Disorders**

Drug fever may suggest systemic infection. Liver reaction may suggest viral hepatitis. Skin and joint symptoms may suggest lupus erythematosus.

Natural Diseases or Disorders That May Be Activated by This Drug

Latent coronary artery disease.

CAUTION

1. Toxic reactions are more likely to occur with large doses. Adhere strictly to prescribed dosage schedules. Keep appointments for periodic follow-up examinations.
2. Report the development of any tendency to emotional depression.
3. This drug can cause salt and water retention if a diuretic is not taken concurrently.
4. This drug can provoke migraine headache.

Precautions for Use

By Infants and Children: Dosage is based upon age, weight and kidney function status. Observe for the possible development of a lupus erythematosus–like reaction.

By Those over 60 Years of Age: Initiate treatment with low doses and proceed cautiously. Unacceptably high blood pressure should be reduced without creating the risks associated with excessively low blood pressure. Sudden, rapid and excessive reduction of blood pressure can predispose to stroke or heart attack. Observe for possible dizziness, unsteadiness, fainting or falling. Headache, palpitation and rapid heart rates are more common in the elderly and can mimic acute anxiety states.

▷ **Advisability of Use During Pregnancy**

Pregnancy Category: C (tentative). See Pregnancy Code inside back cover.
Animal studies: Birth defects of head and facial bones reported in mice.
Human studies: Information from adequate studies of pregnant women is not available.
Avoid use during the first and last 3 months; if taken late in pregnancy, this drug can cause a deficiency of blood platelets (see Glossary) in the newborn infant.

Advisability of Use if Breast-Feeding

Presence of this drug in breast milk: Yes.
Avoid drug or refrain from nursing.

Habit-Forming Potential: None.

Effects of Overdosage: Marked light-headedness, dizziness, headache, flushing of skin, nausea, vomiting, collapse of circulation: loss of consciousness, cold and sweaty skin, weak and rapid pulse, irregular heart rhythm.

Possible Effects of Long-Term Use: An acute or subacute syndrome resembling rheumatoid arthritis or lupus erythematosus, usually seen in slow acetylators taking daily doses of over 200 mg.

Suggested Periodic Examinations While Taking This Drug (at physician's discretion)

Complete blood cell counts, liver function tests, blood tests for evidence of lupus erythematosus.

▷ **While Taking This Drug, Observe the Following**

Foods: No restrictions.
Nutritional Support: Monitor for peripheral neuropathy and take a supplement of pyridoxine (vitamin B-6) as needed. Ask physician for guidance.
Beverages: No restrictions. May be taken with milk.
▷ *Alcohol:* Use with extreme caution until the combined effect has been determined. Alcohol can exaggerate the blood-pressure-lowering effect of this drug and cause excessive reduction.
Tobacco Smoking: Avoid completely. Nicotine can contribute significantly to this drug's ability to intensify angina in susceptible individuals.
▷ *Other Drugs*

Hydralazine may *increase* the effects of
• metoprolol (Lopressor).
• oxprenolol (Trasicor).
• propranolol (Inderal).
▷ *Driving, Hazardous Activities:* This drug may cause light-headedness or dizziness. Restrict activities as necessary.

Aviation Note: Hypertension and the use of this drug *are disqualifications* for piloting. Consult a designated Aviation Medical Examiner.

Exposure to Sun: No restrictions.

Exposure to Heat: Caution advised. Hot environments may reduce blood pressure significantly.

Exposure to Cold: Caution advised. Cold environments may increase this drug's ability to cause angina in susceptible individuals.

Heavy Exercise or Exertion: Caution advised. Excessive exertion can increase this drug's ability to cause angina in susceptible individuals. Also, isometric exercises can raise blood pressure significantly.

HYDROCHLOROTHIAZIDE
(hi droh klor oh THI a zide)

Introduced: 1959

Class: Antihypertensive, diuretic, thiazides

Prescription: USA: Yes
Canada: Yes

Controlled Drug: USA: No
Canada: No

Available as Generic: USA: Yes
Canada: Yes

Brand Names: Aldactazide [CD], Aldoril-15/25 [CD], Aldoril D30/D50 [CD], ✦Apo-Hydro, ✦Apo-Methazide [CD], ✦Apo-Triazide [CD], Apresazide [CD], Apresoline-Esidrix [CD], Capozide [CD], ✦Co-Betaloc [CD], ✦Diuchlor H, Dyazide [CD], Esidrix, Hydral [CD], HydroDIURIL, Hydropres [CD], Hydro-Z-50, Inderide [CD], Inderide LA [CD], ✦Ismelin-Esidrix [CD], Lopressor HCT [CD], Maxzide [CD], Maxzide-25 [CD], ✦Moduret [CD], Moduretic [CD], ✦Natrimax, ✦Neo-Codema, Normozide [CD], ✦Novodoparil [CD], ✦Novohydrazide, ✦Novospirozine [CD], ✦Novotriamzide [CD], Oretic, Oreticyl [CD], ✦PMS Dopazide [CD], Prinzide [CD], Ser-Ap-Es [CD], Serpasil-Esidrix [CD], Thiuretic, Timolide [CD], Trandate HCT [CD], Unipres [CD], ✦Urozide, Vaseretic [CD], ✦Viskazide [CD], Zestoretic [CD], Zide

---

BENEFITS versus RISKS

Possible Benefits	*Possible Risks*
EFFECTIVE, WELL-TOLERATED DIURETIC	Loss of body potassium
POSSIBLY EFFECTIVE IN MILD HYPERTENSION	Increased blood sugar
ENHANCES EFFECTIVENESS OF OTHER ANTIHYPERTENSIVES	Increased blood uric acid
Beneficial in treatment of diabetes insipidus	Increased blood calcium
	Rare blood cell disorders

▷ **Principal Uses**

As a Single Drug Product: Thiazide diuretics are used primarily to (1) increase the volume of urine (diuresis) to correct the excessive fluid retention associated with congestive heart failure and certain types of liver and kidney disease; and (2) initiate treatment for high blood pressure (hypertension). They are often the first drugs tried in treating mild to moderate hypertension. Less frequent uses include the treatment of diabetes insipidus and the prevention of kidney stones that contain calcium.

As a Combination Drug Product [CD]: When this drug is used alone to treat hypertension, it is referred to as a "step 1" antihypertensive. Should it fail to reduce the blood pressure adequately, a "step 2" antihypertensive drug is added to be taken concurrently with the "step 1" drug. These drugs may be combined into one drug product. Thiazides are available in combination with beta blockers, hydralazine, methyldopa, reserpine and other diuretics to increase their effectiveness in treating hypertension.

How This Drug Works: By increasing the elimination of salt and water from the body (through increased urine production), this drug reduces the volume of fluid in the blood and body tissues and lowers the sodium content throughout the body. By relaxing the walls of smaller arteries and allowing them to expand, this drug increases the total capacity of the arterial system. The combined effect of these two actions (reduced blood volume in expanded space) results in lowering of the blood pressure.

Available Dosage Forms and Strengths

Solution — 50 mg per 5-ml teaspoonful
Solution, intensol — 100 mg per ml
Tablets — 25 mg, 50 mg, 100 mg

▷ **Usual Adult Dosage Range:** As antihypertensive: 50 to 100 mg/day initially; 50 to 200 mg/day for maintenance. As diuretic: 50 to 200 mg/day initially; the smallest effective dose should be determined. The total daily dose should not exceed 200 mg. **Note: Actual dosage and administration schedule must be determined by the physician for each patient individually.**

▷ **Dosing Instructions:** May be taken with or following meals to reduce stomach irritation. Best taken in the morning to avoid nighttime urination. The tablet may be crushed for administration.

Usual Duration of Use: Continual use on a regular schedule for 2 to 3 weeks is usually necessary to determine this drug's effectiveness in lowering high blood pressure. Long-term use (months to years) requires periodic evaluation of response and possible dosage adjustment. Use as a diuretic should be intermittent with "drug holidays" (no drug taken) to reduce the risk of sodium and potassium imbalance. Consult your physician on a regular basis.

▷ **This Drug Should Not Be Taken If**
- you have had an allergic reaction to any dosage form of it previously.

▷ **Inform Your Physician Before Taking This Drug If**
- you are allergic to any form of "sulfa" drug.
- you are pregnant or planning pregnancy.
- you have a history of kidney or liver disease.
- you have a history of pancreatitis.
- you have diabetes, gout or lupus erythematosus.
- you are taking any form of cortisone, digitalis, oral antidiabetic drug or insulin.
- you plan to have surgery under general anesthesia in the near future.

Possible Side-Effects (natural, expected and unavoidable drug actions)
Light-headedness on arising from sitting or lying position (see Orthostatic Hypotension in Glossary).
Increase in blood sugar level, affecting control of diabetes.
Increase in blood uric acid level, affecting control of gout.
Decrease in blood potassium level, causing muscle weakness and cramping.

▷ **Possible Adverse Effects** (unusual, unexpected and infrequent reactions)
If any of the following develop, consult your physician promptly for guidance.
Mild Adverse Effects
Allergic Reactions: Skin rashes, hives, drug fever.
Headache, dizziness, blurred or yellow vision.
Reduced appetite, indigestion, nausea, vomiting, diarrhea.
Serious Adverse Effects
Allergic Reactions: Hepatitis with jaundice (see Glossary), anaphylactic reaction (see Glossary), severe skin reactions.
Inflammation of the pancreas—severe abdominal pain.
Bone marrow depression (see Glossary)—fatigue, weakness, fever, sore throat, abnormal bleeding or bruising.

▷ **Possible Effects on Sexual Function:** Decreased libido (12%); impotence (3%).

▷ **Adverse Effects That May Mimic Natural Diseases or Disorders**
Liver reaction may suggest viral hepatitis.

Natural Diseases or Disorders That May Be Activated by This Drug
Diabetes, gout, systemic lupus erythematosus.

CAUTION
1. Do not exceed recommended doses. Increased dosage can cause excessive loss of sodium and potassium, with resultant loss of appetite, nausea, fatigue, weakness, confusion and tingling in the extremities.
2. If you are also taking a digitalis preparation (digitoxin, digoxin), ensure an adequate intake of high-potassium foods to prevent po-

tassium deficiency—a potential cause of digitalis toxicity. (See Table of High Potassium Foods in Section Six.)

Precautions for Use

By Infants and Children: Avoid overdosage that could cause serious dehydration. Significant potassium loss can occur within the first 2 weeks of drug use.

By Those over 60 Years of Age: Small doses are advisable until your individual response has been determined. You may be more susceptible to the development of impaired thinking, orthostatic hypotension, potassium loss and blood sugar increase. Overdosage and extended use of this drug can cause excessive loss of body water, thickening (increased viscosity) of the blood and an increased tendency for the blood to clot—predisposing to stroke, heart attack or thrombophlebitis (vein inflammation with blood clot).

▷ **Advisability of Use During Pregnancy**

Pregnancy Category: D (tentative). See Pregnancy Code inside back cover.

Animal studies: No birth defects found in rat studies.

Human studies: Reports are conflicting and inconclusive. This drug does not seem to carry the risk of birth defects that has been found with other related diuretics. However, other types of fetal injury are possible with this drug. It should not be used during pregnancy unless a very serious complication occurs for which this drug is significantly beneficial. Ask physician for guidance.

Advisability of Use if Breast-Feeding

Presence of this drug in breast milk: Yes.

Avoid drug or refrain from nursing.

Habit-Forming Potential: None.

Effects of Overdosage: Dry mouth, thirst, lethargy, weakness, muscle cramping, nausea, vomiting, drowsiness progressing to stupor or coma.

Possible Effects of Long-Term Use: Impaired balance of water, salt and potassium in blood and body tissues. Development of diabetes in predisposed individuals. Pathological changes in parathyroid glands with increased blood calcium levels and decreased blood phosphate levels.

Suggested Periodic Examinations While Taking This Drug (at physician's discretion)

Complete blood cell counts, measurements of blood levels of sodium, potassium, chloride, sugar and uric acid.

Kidney and liver function tests.

▷ **While Taking This Drug, Observe the Following**

Foods: Consult your physician regarding the advisability of eating foods rich in potassium. If so advised, see the Table of High Potassium

Foods in Section Six. Follow physician's advice regarding the use of salt.

Beverages: No restrictions. This drug may be taken with milk.

▷ *Alcohol:* Use with caution until the combined effects have been determined. Alcohol may exaggerate the blood-pressure-lowering effects of this drug and cause orthostatic hypotension.

Tobacco Smoking: No interactions expected. Follow physician's advice.

▷ *Other Drugs*

Hydrochlorothiazide may *increase* the effects of

- other antihypertensive drugs; dosage adjustments may be necessary to prevent excessive lowering of blood pressure.
- lithium, and cause lithium toxicity.

Hydrochlorothiazide may *decrease* the effects of

- oral antidiabetic drugs (sulfonylureas); dosage adjustments may be necessary for proper control of blood sugar.

Hydrochlorothiazide *taken concurrently* with

- digitalis preparations (digitoxin, digoxin) requires very careful monitoring and dosage adjustments to prevent fluctuations of blood potassium levels and serious disturbances of heart rhythm.

The following drugs may *decrease* the effects of hydrochlorothiazide

- cholestyramine (Cuemid, Questran) may interfere with its absorption.
- colestipol (Colestid) may interfere with its absorption.

Take cholestyramine and colestipol 1 hour before any oral diuretic.

▷ *Driving, Hazardous Activities:* Use caution until the possible occurrence of orthostatic hypotension, dizziness or impaired vision has been determined.

Aviation Note: The use of this drug *may be a disqualification* for piloting. Consult a designated Aviation Medical Examiner.

Exposure to Sun: Use caution until sensitivity has been determined. This drug can cause photosensitivity (see Glossary).

Exposure to Heat: Avoid excessive perspiring, which could cause additional loss of salt and water from the body.

Heavy Exercise or Exertion: Avoid exertion that produces light-headedness, excessive fatigue or muscle cramping. Isometric exercises—the "overload" technique for strengthening individual muscles—can raise blood pressure significantly. Ask physician for guidance regarding participation in this form of exercise.

Occurrence of Unrelated Illness: Illnesses that cause vomiting or diarrhea can produce a serious imbalance of important body chemistry. Consult your physician for guidance.

Discontinuation: This drug should not be stopped abruptly following long-term use; sudden discontinuation can cause serious thiazide-withdrawal fluid retention (edema). The dose should be reduced gradually. It may be advisable to discontinue this drug 5 to 7 days before major surgery. Ask your physician, surgeon and/or anesthesiologist for guidance regarding dosage adjustment or drug withdrawal.

HYDROCODONE
(hi droh KOH dohn)

Other Name: Dihydrocodeinone

Introduced: 1951

Class: Analgesic, narcotic; cough suppressant

Prescription: USA: Yes
Canada: Yes

Controlled Drug: USA: C-III*
Canada: <N>

Available as Generic: USA: Yes
Canada: No

Brand Names: Anexsia [CD], Anexsia 7.5 [CD], Azdone, ✦Biohisdex DHC [CD], ✦Biohisdine DHC [CD], Dimetane Expectorant-DC [CD], ✦Hycodan, Hycodan [CD], ✦Hycomine [CD], Hycomine Compound [CD], Hycomine Pediatric Syrup [CD], ✦Hycomine-S [CD], Hycomine Syrup [CD], Hycotuss Expectorant [CD], Lorcet Plus [CD], Lortab [CD], Lortab ASA [CD], ✦Novahistex DH [CD], ✦Novahistine DH [CD], ✦Robidone, Triaminic Expectorant DH [CD], Tussend [CD], Tussend Expectorant [CD], Tussionex [CD], Tycolet [CD], Vicodin [CD], Vicodin ES [CD], Zydone [CD]

BENEFITS versus RISKS	
Possible Benefits	*Possible Risks*
EFFECTIVE RELIEF OF MILD TO MODERATE PAIN	Low potential for habit formation (dependence)
EFFECTIVE CONTROL OF COUGH	Mild allergic reactions (infrequent)
	Nausea, constipation

▷ **Principal Uses**

As a Single Drug Product: Used primarily to (1) control cough; (2) relieve mild to moderate pain. Its widest use is as an ingredient in cough remedies.

As a Combination Drug Product [CD]: Hydrocodone is frequently added to cough mixtures containing antihistamines, decongestants and expectorants to make these "shotgun" preparations more effective in reducing the frequency and severity of cough. It is also combined with milder analgesics, such as acetaminophen and aspirin, to enhance pain relief.

How This Drug Works: Acting primarily as a depressant of certain brain functions, this drug suppresses the perception of pain, calms the emotional response to pain and reduces the sensitivity of the cough reflex.

*See Schedules of Controlled Drugs inside back cover.

Available Dosage Forms and Strengths
   Syrup — 5 mg per 5-ml teaspoonful
   Tablets — 5 mg

▷ **Usual Adult Dosage Range:** As analgesic—5 to 10 mg/4 to 6 hours as needed. For cough—5 mg/4 to 6 hours as needed. Total daily dosage should not exceed 60 mg. **Note: Actual dosage and administration schedule must be determined by the physician for each patient individually.**

▷ **Dosing Instructions:** May be taken with or following food to reduce stomach irritation or nausea. Tablet may be crushed for administration.

Usual Duration of Use: As required, to control pain or cough. Continual use should not exceed 5 to 7 days without interruption and reassessment of need.

▷ **This Drug Should Not Be Taken If**
   • you have had an allergic reaction to any dosage form of it previously.
   • you are having an acute attack of asthma.

▷ **Inform Your Physician Before Taking This Drug If**
   • you have had an unfavorable reaction to any narcotic drug in the past.
   • you have a history of drug abuse or alcoholism.
   • you have chronic lung disease with impaired breathing.
   • you have impaired liver or kidney function.
   • you have gallbladder disease, a seizure disorder or an underactive thyroid gland.
   • you have difficulty emptying the urinary bladder.
   • you are taking any other drugs that have a sedative effect.
   • you plan to have surgery under general anesthesia in the near future.

Possible Side-Effects (natural, expected and unavoidable drug actions)
   Drowsiness, light-headedness, dry mouth, urinary retention, constipation.

▷ **Possible Adverse Effects** (unusual, unexpected and infrequent reactions)
   If any of the following develop, consult your physician promptly for guidance.
   Mild Adverse Effects
   Allergic Reactions: Skin rash, hives, itching.
   Dizziness, impaired concentration, sensation of drunkenness, confusion, depression, blurred or double vision, facial flushing, sweating.
   Nausea, vomiting.
   Serious Adverse Effects
   Allergic Reactions: Anaphylaxis (rare), severe skin reactions.
   Idiosyncratic Reactions: Delirium, hallucinations, excitement, increased sensitivity to pain after the analgesic effect has worn off.
   Seizures (rare), impaired breathing.

▷ **Possible Effects on Sexual Function:**   None reported.

▷ **Adverse Effects That May Mimic Natural Diseases or Disorders**
Paradoxical behavioral disturbances may suggest psychotic disorder.

CAUTION
1. If you have asthma, chronic bronchitis or emphysema, the excessive use of this drug may cause significant respiratory difficulty, thickening of bronchial secretions and suppression of coughing.
2. The concurrent use of this drug with atropinelike drugs can increase the risk of urinary retention and reduced intestinal function.
3. Do not take this drug following acute head injury.

Precautions for Use
By Infants and Children: Do not use this drug in children under 2 years of age because of their vulnerability to life-threatening respiratory depression.
By Those over 60 Years of Age: Use small doses initially and increase dosage as needed and tolerated. Limit use to short-term treatment only. There may be increased susceptibility to the development of drowsiness, dizziness, unsteadiness, falling, urinary retention and constipation (often leading to fecal impaction).

▷ **Advisability of Use During Pregnancy**
Pregnancy Category: C (tentative). See Pregnancy Code inside back cover.
Animal studies: Birth defects reported in hamster studies.
Human studies: Information from adequate studies of pregnant women is not available. Hydrocodone taken repeatedly during the last few weeks before delivery may cause withdrawal symptoms in the newborn infant.
Use this drug only if clearly needed and in small, infrequent doses.

Advisability of Use if Breast-Feeding
Presence of this drug in breast milk: Unknown.
Monitor nursing infant closely and discontinue drug or nursing if adverse effects develop. Ask physician for guidance.

Habit-Forming Potential: Psychological and/or physical dependence can develop with use of large doses for an extended period of time. However, true dependence is infrequent and unlikely with prudent use.

Effects of Overdosage: Drowsiness, restlessness, agitation, nausea, vomiting, dry mouth, vertigo, weakness, lethargy, stupor, coma, seizures.

Possible Effects of Long-Term Use: Psychological and physical dependence, chronic constipation.

Suggested Periodic Examinations While Taking This Drug (at physician's discretion)
None.

▷ **While Taking This Drug, Observe the Following**
Foods: No restrictions.
Beverages: No restrictions. May be taken with milk.

▷ *Alcohol:* Use extreme caution until the combined effects have been determined. Hydrocodone can intensify the intoxicating effects of alcohol, and alcohol can intensify the depressant effects of hydrocodone on brain function, breathing and circulation.
Tobacco Smoking: No interactions expected.
Marijuana Smoking: Increase in drowsiness and pain relief; impairment of mental and physical performance.

▷ *Other Drugs*
Hydrocodone may **increase** the effects of
• other drugs with sedative effects.
• atropinelike drugs, and increase the risk of constipation and urinary retention.

▷ *Driving, Hazardous Activities:* This drug can impair mental alertness, judgment, reaction time and physical coordination. Avoid hazardous activities accordingly.
Aviation Note: The use of this drug **is a disqualification** for piloting. Consult a designated Aviation Medical Examiner.
Exposure to Sun: No restrictions.
Discontinuation: It is advisable to limit this drug to short-term use. If it is necessary to use it for extended periods of time, discontinuation should be gradual to minimize possible effects of withdrawal (usually mild with this drug).

HYDROXYZINE
(hi DROX i zeen)

Introduced: 1953

Class: Mild tranquilizer, antihistamines

Prescription: USA: Yes
Canada: Yes

Controlled Drug: USA: No
Canada: No

Available as Generic: USA: Yes
Canada: No

Brand Names: ✦Apo-Hydroxyzine, Atarax, Marax [CD], Marax DF [CD], ✦Multipax, Vistaril, Vistrax [CD],

---

BENEFITS versus RISKS

Possible Benefits	*Possible Risks*
EFFECTIVE RELIEF OF ITCHING DUE TO HIVES	Mild atropinelike effects
Moderately effective relief of itching due to allergic skin disorders	Potentiation of other sedative drugs
Moderately effective relief of mild to moderate anxiety and nervous tension	Impaired control of seizure disorders (epilepsy)

▷ **Principal Uses**

As a Single Drug Product: Used primarily as a mild tranquilizer to relieve anxiety and nervous tension, whether occurring independently or in association with a physical disorder. Also used frequently to relieve itching due to allergic skin conditions.

As a Combination Drug Product [CD]: Combined with antispasmodic drugs, this drug helps to allay the anxiety that is conducive to functional disorders of the gastrointestinal tract. Combined with ephedrine and theophylline (bronchodilator drugs), this drug controls the anxiety that is often associated with bronchial spasm in asthma, bronchitis and emphysema.

How This Drug Works: Not completely established. It is thought that this drug may reduce excessive activity in those brain systems that determine the emotional state.

Available Dosage Forms and Strengths

Capsules — 25 mg, 50 mg, 100 mg
Injection — 25 mg per ml, 50 mg per ml
Oral suspension — 25 mg per 5-ml teaspoonful
Syrup — 10 mg per 5-ml teaspoonful
Tablets — 10 mg, 25 mg, 50 mg, 100 mg

▷ **Usual Adult Dosage Range:** 25 to 100 mg 3 or 4 times daily. The total daily dosage should not exceed 600 mg. **Note: Actual dosage and administration schedule must be determined by the physician for each patient individually.**

▷ **Dosing Instructions:** May be taken without regard to eating. The tablet may be crushed and the capsule may be opened for administration.

Usual Duration of Use: Continual use on a regular schedule for 1 to 3 weeks is usually necessary to determine this drug's effectiveness in relieving anxiety and tension. Relief of itching is usually apparent in 2 to 3 days. Duration of use as a tranquilizer should not exceed 4 months without reappraisal of continued need. Consult your physician on a regular basis.

▷ **This Drug Should Not Be Taken If**
  • you have had an allergic reaction to any dosage form of it previously.

▷ **Inform Your Physician Before Taking This Drug If**
  • you have a seizure disorder (epilepsy).
  • you have prostatism (see Glossary).
  • you are taking any drugs with sedative effects.
  • you plan to have surgery under general anesthesia in the near future.

Possible Side-Effects (natural, expected and unavoidable drug actions)
  Drowsiness (may subside with continued use); "hangover" effect if taken at bedtime for sleep; dry mouth.

▷ **Possible Adverse Effects** (unusual, unexpected and infrequent reactions)
  If any of the following develop, consult your physician promptly for guidance.
  Mild Adverse Effects
  Allergic Reaction: Itching.
  Headache.
  Serious Adverse Effects
  Idiosyncratic Reactions: Involuntary movements, tremors, seizures (with excessive dosage).

▷ **Possible Effects on Sexual Function:** None reported.

Natural Diseases or Disorders That May Be Activated by This Drug
  Latent epilepsy.

CAUTION
  1. This drug can cause excessive sedation if taken concurrently with other sedative drugs.
  2. Use very cautiously if you have a seizure disorder. This drug may increase the frequency of seizures.
  3. If pregnancy occurs, discontinue this drug immediately and inform your physician.

Precautions for Use
  By Infants and Children: Observe for evidence of excessive sedation.
  By Those over 60 Years of Age: There may be increased susceptibility to the development of drowsiness, dizziness and lethargy, and to impairment of thinking, judgment and memory. A pattern of underactivity may be misinterpreted as senility or emotional depression. Observe also for orthostatic hypotension and prostatism (see Glossary).

▷ **Advisability of Use During Pregnancy**
  Pregnancy Category: C (tentative). See Pregnancy Code inside back cover.
  Animal studies: Facial bone defects reported in mice, rats and dogs.
  Human studies: Information from adequate studies of pregnant women is not available.
  Avoid completely during the first 3 months. During the last 6 months, use only if clearly needed. Ask physician for guidance.

Advisability of Use if Breast-Feeding
   Presence of this drug in breast milk: Yes.
   Monitor nursing infant closely and discontinue drug or nursing if adverse effects (sedation, poor feeding) develop.

Habit-Forming Potential: None.

Effects of Overdosage: Drowsiness, unsteadiness, dry mouth, delirium, stupor, tremors, seizures.

Possible Effects of Long-Term Use: Loss of drug effectiveness due to development of tolerance (see Glossary).

Suggested Periodic Examinations While Taking This Drug (at physician's discretion)
   None required.

▷ **While Taking This Drug, Observe the Following**
   Foods: No restrictions.
   Beverages: Avoid large amounts of caffeine-containing beverages: coffee, tea, cola, chocolate. May be taken with milk.
▷ *Alcohol:* Use with extreme caution until the combined effects have been determined. Alcohol can increase the sedative action of hydroxyzine. Hydroxyzine can increase the intoxicating effect of alcohol.
   Tobacco Smoking: No interactions expected.
   Marijuana Smoking: Increased sedative effects.
▷ *Other Drugs*
   Hydroxyzine may *increase* the effects of
   • ketamine (intravenous anesthetic), and prolong the recovery time.
   • other drugs with sedative effects, and cause excessive sedation.
   Hydroxyzine may *decrease* the effects of
   • phenothiazines (see Drug Class, Section Four), and reduce their antipsychotic effectiveness.
▷ *Driving, Hazardous Activities:* This drug may impair mental alertness, judgment, coordination and reaction time. Restrict activities as necessary.
   Aviation Note: The use of this drug *is a disqualification* for piloting. Consult a designated Aviation Medical Examiner.
   Exposure to Sun: No restrictions.

IBUPROFEN
(i BYU proh fen)

Introduced: 1969

Class: Mild analgesic, anti-inflammatory

Prescription: USA: Varies
   Canada: Yes

Controlled Drug: USA: No
   Canada: No

Available as Generic: Yes

Brand Names: Advil, ✦Amersol, ✦Apo-Ibuprofen, Haltran, Ibu-Tab, Medi-pren, Motrin, ✦Novoprofen, Nuprin, Rufen

---

BENEFITS versus RISKS

Possible Benefits	*Possible Risks*
EFFECTIVE RELIEF OF MILD TO MODERATE PAIN AND INFLAMMATION	Gastrointestinal pain, ulceration, bleeding (rare) Rare kidney damage Rare fluid retention Rare bone marrow depression (less than 1%)

▷ **Principal Uses**

As a Single Drug Product: Used primarily to relieve mild to moderately severe pain associated with (1) musculoskeletal injuries; (2) acute and chronic gout, rheumatoid arthritis and osteoarthritis; (3) dental, obstetrical and orthopedic surgery; (4) menstrual cramps; (5) vascular (migrainelike) headaches; and (6) to reduce fever.

How This Drug Works: Not completely established. It is thought that this drug reduces the tissue concentrations of prostaglandins (and related compounds), chemicals involved in the production of inflammation and pain.

Available Dosage Forms and Strengths
Tablets — 200 mg, 300 mg, 400 mg, 600 mg, 800 mg

▷ **Usual Adult Dosage Range:**   200 to 800 mg 3 or 4 times/day. Total daily dosage should not exceed 3200 mg (3600 mg in selected individuals). **Note: Actual dosage and administration schedule must be determined by the physician for each patient individually.**

▷ **Dosing Instructions:**   Take either on an empty stomach or with food or milk to prevent stomach irritation. Take with a full glass of water and remain upright (do not lie down) for 30 minutes. The tablet may be crushed for administration.

Usual Duration of Use: Continual use on a regular schedule for 1 to 2 weeks is usually necessary to determine this drug's effectiveness in relieving the discomfort of arthritis. Long-term use requires supervision and periodic evaluation by the physician. Consult your physician on a regular basis.

▷ **This Drug Should Not Be Taken If**
   • you have had an allergic reaction to it previously.
   • you are subject to asthma or nasal polyps caused by aspirin.
   • you have active peptic ulcer disease or any form of gastrointestinal bleeding.

- you have a bleeding disorder or a blood cell disorder.
- you have severe impairment of kidney function.

▷ **Inform Your Physician Before Taking This Drug If**
- you are allergic to aspirin or to other aspirin substitutes.
- you have a history of peptic ulcer disease or any type of bleeding disorder.
- you have impaired liver or kidney function.
- you have high blood pressure or a history of heart failure.
- you are taking any of the following: acetaminophen, aspirin or other aspirin substitutes, anticoagulants, oral antidiabetic drugs.

Possible Side-Effects (natural, expected and unavoidable drug actions)
Fluid retention (weight gain); pink, red, purple or rust coloration of urine (of no significance).

▷ **Possible Adverse Effects** (unusual, unexpected and infrequent reactions)
If any of the following develop, consult your physician promptly for guidance.
Mild Adverse Effects
Allergic Reactions: Skin rash, hives, itching.
Headache, dizziness, altered or blurred vision, ringing in the ears, depression.
Mouth sores, indigestion, nausea, vomiting, constipation, diarrhea.
Serious Adverse Effects
Allergic Reactions: Anaphylaxis (see Glossary), severe skin reactions.
Idiosyncratic Reactions: Drug-induced meningitis with fever and coma.
Active peptic ulcer, with or without bleeding.
Liver damage with jaundice (see Glossary).
Kidney damage with painful urination, bloody urine, reduced urine formation.
Rare bone marrow depression (see Glossary)—fatigue, weakness, fever, sore throat, abnormal bleeding or bruising.

▷ **Possible Effects on Sexual Function**
Altered timing and pattern of menstruation (30%); excessive menstrual bleeding.
Male breast enlargement and tenderness.

Possible Delayed Adverse Effects: Mild anemia due to "silent" blood loss from the stomach (less than that caused by aspirin).

▷ **Adverse Effects That May Mimic Natural Diseases or Disorders**
Liver reaction may suggest viral hepatitis.

Natural Diseases or Disorders That May Be Activated by This Drug
Peptic ulcer disease, ulcerative colitis.

CAUTION
1. Dosage should always be limited to the smallest amount that produces reasonable improvement.

2. This drug may mask early indications of infection. Inform your physician if you think you are developing an infection of any kind.

Precautions for Use
By Infants and Children: Safety and effectiveness for use by those under 12 years of age have not been established.

By Those over 60 Years of Age: Small doses are advisable until tolerance is determined. Observe for any indications of liver or kidney toxicity, fluid retention, dizziness, confusion, impaired memory, stomach bleeding or constipation.

▷ Advisability of Use During Pregnancy
Pregnancy Category: B (tentative). See Pregnancy Code inside back cover.
Animal studies: No birth defects reported in rats or rabbits.
Human studies: Information from adequate studies of pregnant women is not available.
Avoid this drug during the last 3 months. Use it during the first 6 months only if clearly needed. Ask physician for guidance.
The manufacturer does not recommend the use of this drug during pregnancy.

Advisability of Use if Breast-Feeding
Presence of this drug in breast milk: Yes, in minute amounts.
Avoid drug or refrain from nursing.

Habit-Forming Potential: None.

Effects of Overdosage: Drowsiness, dizziness, ringing in the ears, nausea, vomiting, diarrhea, confusion, unsteadiness, stupor progressing to coma.

Possible Effects of Long-Term Use: Fluid retention.

Suggested Periodic Examinations While Taking This Drug (at physician's discretion)
Complete blood cell counts, liver and kidney function tests, complete eye examinations if vision is altered in any way.

▷ While Taking This Drug, Observe the Following
Foods: No restrictions.
Beverages: No restrictions. May be taken with milk.
▷ *Alcohol:* Use with caution. The irritant action of alcohol on the stomach lining, added to the irritant action of this drug in sensitive individuals, can increase the risk of stomach ulceration and/or bleeding.
Tobacco Smoking: No interactions expected.
▷ *Other Drugs*
Ibuprofen may ***increase*** the effects of
- acetaminophen (Tylenol, etc.), and increase the risk of kidney damage; avoid prolonged use of this combination.
- anticoagulants (Coumadin, etc.), and increase the risk of bleeding; monitor prothrombin time, adjust dose accordingly.

Ibuprofen *taken concurrently* with the following drugs may increase the risk of bleeding; avoid these combinations:

- aspirin.
- dipyridamole (Persantine).
- indomethacin (Indocin).
- sulfinpyrazone (Anturane).
- valproic acid (Depakene).

▷ *Driving, Hazardous Activities:* This drug may cause drowsiness or dizziness. Restrict activities as necessary.

Aviation Note: The use of this drug *may be a disqualification* for piloting. Consult a designated Aviation Medical Examiner.

Exposure to Sun: Use caution until sensitivity is determined. Questionable photosensitivity (see Glossary) has been reported.

INDAPAMIDE
(in DAP a mide)

Introduced: 1974

Class: Antihypertensive, diuretic

Prescription: USA: Yes
Canada: Yes

Controlled Drug: USA: No
Canada: No

Available as Generic: No

Brand Names: ✦Lozide, Lozol

BENEFITS versus RISKS	
Possible Benefits	*Possible Risks*
EFFECTIVE ONCE-A-DAY TREATMENT OF MILD TO MODERATE HYPERTENSION	Excessive loss of blood potassium (14%)
EFFECTIVE, MILD DIURETIC	Increased blood sugar level
	Increased blood uric acid level

▷ **Principal Uses**

As a Single Drug Product: Used primarily to (1) increase the volume of urine (diuresis) to correct the excessive fluid retention associated with congestive heart failure; and (2) initiate treatment for high blood pressure (hypertension). It may be the first drug tried in treating mild to moderate hypertension.

How This Drug Works: By increasing the elimination of salt and water from the body (through increased urine production), this drug reduces the volume of fluid in the blood and body tissues and lowers the sodium content throughout the body. By relaxing the walls of smaller arteries and allowing them to expand, this drug increases the total capacity of the arterial system. The combined effect of these two actions (reduced blood volume in expanded space) results in lowering of blood pressure.

Available Dosage Forms and Strengths
Tablets — 2.5 mg

▷ **Usual Adult Dosage Range:**   Initially 2.5 mg/day, taken as a single dose in the morning. If necessary, the dose may be increased to 5 mg/day after 1 week (for diuresis) or after 4 weeks (for hypertension). The total daily dosage should not exceed 5 mg. (In Canada, the total daily dosage limit is given as 2.5 mg.) **Note: Actual dosage and administration schedule must be determined by the physician for each patient individually.**

▷ **Dosing Instructions:**   May be taken with or following food to reduce stomach irritation. Best taken in the morning to avoid nighttime urination. The tablet may be crushed for administration.

Usual Duration of Use: Continual use on a regular schedule for 2 to 4 weeks is usually necessary to determine this drug's effectiveness in lowering high blood pressure. Long-term use (months to years) requires periodic evaluation of response and possible dosage adjustment. Use as a diuretic should be intermittent with "drug holidays" (no drug taken) to reduce the risk of sodium and potassium imbalance. Consult your physician on a regular basis.

Possible Advantages of This Drug
Causes no significant increase in blood cholesterol levels.
Less likely to cause significant loss of potassium.

▷ **This Drug Should Not Be Taken If**
  • you have had an allergic reaction to it previously.

▷ **Inform Your Physician Before Taking This Drug If**
  • you are allergic to any form of "sulfa" drug.
  • you are pregnant or planning pregnancy.
  • you have a history of kidney or liver disease.
  • you have diabetes, gout or lupus erythematosus.
  • you are taking any form of cortisone, digitalis, oral antidiabetic drug or insulin.
  • you plan to have surgery under general anesthesia in the near future.

Possible Side-Effects (natural, expected and unavoidable drug actions)
Light-headedness on arising from sitting or lying position (see Orthostatic Hypotension in Glossary).
Increase in blood sugar level, affecting control of diabetes.
Increase in blood uric acid level, affecting control of gout.
Decrease in blood potassium level, causing muscle weakness and cramping.

▷ **Possible Adverse Effects** (unusual, unexpected and infrequent reactions)
If any of the following develop, consult your physician promptly for guidance.

Mild Adverse Effects

Allergic Reactions: Skin rashes, hives, itching.

Headache, dizziness, drowsiness, weakness, lethargy, visual disturbance.

Reduced appetite, indigestion, nausea, vomiting, diarrhea.

Serious Adverse Effects

None reported.

▷ **Possible Effects on Sexual Function:** Decreased libido (4%); impotence (less than 1%).

Natural Diseases or Disorders That May Be Activated by This Drug

Diabetes, gout, systemic lupus erythematosus.

CAUTION

1. Do not exceed recommended doses. Increased dosage can cause excessive loss of sodium and potassium, with resultant loss of appetite, nausea, fatigue, weakness, confusion and tingling in the extremities.
2. If you are also taking a digitalis preparation (digitoxin, digoxin), ensure an adequate intake of high-potassium foods to prevent potassium deficiency—a potential cause of digitalis toxicity. (See Table of High Potassium Foods in Section Six.)

Precautions for Use

By Infants and Children: Safety and effectiveness for use by those under 12 years of age have not been established.

By Those over 60 Years of Age: Small doses are advisable until your individual response has been determined. You may be more susceptible to the development of impaired thinking, orthostatic hypotension, potassium loss and blood sugar increase. Overdosage and extended use of this drug can cause excessive loss of body water, thickening (increased viscosity) of the blood and an increased tendency for the blood to clot—predisposing to stroke, heart attack or thrombophlebitis (vein inflammation with blood clot).

▷ **Advisability of Use During Pregnancy**

Pregnancy Category: B (tentative). See Pregnancy Code inside back cover.

Animal studies: No birth defects reported.

Human studies: Information from adequate studies of pregnant women is not available.

This drug should not be used during pregnancy unless a very serious complication occurs for which this drug is significantly beneficial. Ask physician for guidance.

Advisability of Use if Breast-Feeding

Presence of this drug in breast milk: Unknown.

Avoid drug or refrain from nursing.

Habit-Forming Potential: None.

Effects of Overdosage: Dry mouth, thirst, lethargy, weakness, muscle cramping, nausea, vomiting, drowsiness progressing to stupor or coma.

Possible Effects of Long-Term Use: Impaired balance of water, salt and potassium in blood and body tissues. Development of diabetes in predisposed individuals.

Suggested Periodic Examinations While Taking This Drug (at physician's discretion)
Measurements of blood levels of sodium, potassium, chloride, sugar and uric acid.

▷ **While Taking This Drug, Observe the Following**
Foods: Consult your physician regarding the advisability of eating foods rich in potassium. If so advised, see the Table of High Potassium Foods in Section Six. Follow physician's advice regarding the use of salt.
Beverages: No restrictions. This drug may be taken with milk.
▷ *Alcohol:* Use with caution until the combined effects have been determined. Alcohol may exaggerate the blood-pressure-lowering effects of this drug and cause orthostatic hypotension.
Tobacco Smoking: No interactions expected. Follow physician's advice.
▷ *Other Drugs*
Indapamide may *increase* the effects of
• other antihypertensive drugs; dosage adjustments may be necessary to prevent excessive lowering of blood pressure.
• lithium, and cause lithium toxicity.
Indapamide may *decrease* the effects of
• oral antidiabetic drugs (sulfonylureas); dosage adjustments may be necessary for proper control of blood sugar.
Indapamide *taken concurrently* with
• digitalis preparations (digitoxin, digoxin) requires very careful monitoring and dosage adjustments to prevent fluctuations of blood potassium levels and serious disturbances of heart rhythm.
The following drugs may *decrease* the effects of indapamide
• cholestyramine (Cuemid, Questran) may interfere with its absorption.
• colestipol (Colestid) may interfere with its absorption.
Take cholestyramine and colestipol 1 hour before any oral diuretic.
▷ *Driving, Hazardous Activities:* Use caution until the possible occurrence of orthostatic hypotension, drowsiness, dizziness or impaired vision has been determined.
Aviation Note: The use of this drug *may be a disqualification* for piloting. Consult a designated Aviation Medical Examiner.
Exposure to Sun: No restrictions.
Exposure to Heat: Avoid excessive perspiring, which could cause additional loss of salt and water from the body.

Heavy Exercise or Exertion: Avoid exertion that produces light-headedness, excessive fatigue or muscle cramping. Isometric exercises—the "overload" technique for strengthening individual muscles—can raise blood pressure significantly. Ask physician for guidance regarding participation in this form of exercise.

Occurrence of Unrelated Illness: Illnesses that cause vomiting or diarrhea can produce a serious imbalance of important body chemistry. Consult your physician for guidance.

Discontinuation: It may be advisable to discontinue this drug 5 to 7 days before major surgery. Ask your physician, surgeon and/or anesthesiologist for guidance regarding dosage adjustment or drug withdrawal.

INDOMETHACIN
(in doh METH a sin)

Introduced: 1963

Class: Mild analgesic, anti-inflammatory

Prescription: USA: Yes
Canada: Yes

Controlled Drug: USA: No
Canada: No

Available as Generic: USA: Yes
Canada: No

Brand Names: ✦Apo-Indomethacin, Indameth, ✦Indocid, ✦Indocid PDA, Indocin, Indocin-SR, ✦Novomethacin

BENEFITS versus RISKS	
Possible Benefits	*Possible Risks*
EFFECTIVE RELIEF OF MILD TO MODERATE PAIN AND INFLAMMATION	Gastrointestinal pain, ulceration, bleeding (rare)
	Rare liver or kidney damage
	Rare fluid retention
	Rare bone marrow depression
	Mental depression, confusion

▷ **Principal Uses**

As a Single Drug Product: Used primarily to relieve mild to moderately severe pain associated with (1) musculoskeletal injuries; (2) acute and chronic gout, rheumatoid arthritis and osteoarthritis; (3) dental, obstetrical and orthopedic surgery; (4) menstrual cramps; and (5) vascular (migrainelike) headaches.

How This Drug Works: Not completely established. It is thought that this drug reduces the tissue concentrations of prostaglandins (and related compounds), chemicals involved in the production of inflammation and pain.

Available Dosage Forms and Strengths

Capsules — 25 mg, 50 mg, 75 mg

Capsules, prolonged-action — 75 mg

Oral suspension — 25 mg per 5-ml teaspoonful

Suppositories — 50 mg

▷ **Usual Adult Dosage Range:**   For arthritis and related conditions: 25 to 50 mg 2 to 4 times daily. If needed and tolerated, dose may be increased by 25 or 50 mg/day at intervals of 1 week. For acute gout: 100 mg initially; then 50 mg 3 times/day until pain is relieved. Total daily dosage should not exceed 200 mg. **Note: Actual dosage and administration schedule must be determined by the physician for each patient individually.**

▷ **Dosing Instructions:**   Take with or following food to prevent stomach irritation. Take with a full glass of water and remain upright (do not lie down) for 30 minutes. The regular capsule may be opened for administration, but not the prolonged-action capsule.

Usual Duration of Use: Continual use on a regular schedule for 1 to 2 weeks is usually necessary to determine this drug's effectiveness in relieving the discomfort of arthritis. The usual length of treatment for bursitis or tendinitis is 7 to 14 days. Long-term use requires supervision and periodic evaluation by the physician. Consult your physician on a regular basis.

▷ **This Drug Should Not Be Taken If**
- you have had an allergic reaction to it previously.
- you are subject to asthma or nasal polyps caused by aspirin.
- you are pregnant or breast-feeding.
- you have active peptic ulcer disease or any form of gastrointestinal ulceration or bleeding.
- you have a bleeding disorder or a blood cell disorder.
- you have severe impairment of kidney function.

▷ **Inform Your Physician Before Taking This Drug If**
- you are allergic to aspirin or to other aspirin substitutes.
- you have a history of peptic ulcer disease, Crohn's disease, ulcerative colitis or any type of bleeding disorder.
- you have a history of epilepsy, Parkinson's disease or mental illness (psychosis).
- you have impaired liver or kidney function.
- you have high blood pressure or a history of heart failure.
- you are taking any of the following: acetaminophen, aspirin or other aspirin substitutes, anticoagulants, oral antidiabetic drugs.

Possible Side-Effects (natural, expected and unavoidable drug actions)
Drowsiness, ringing in ears, fluid retention.

▷ **Possible Adverse Effects** (unusual, unexpected and infrequent reactions)
If any of the following develop, consult your physician promptly for guidance.
Mild Adverse Effects
Allergic Reactions: Skin rash, hives, itching, localized swellings of face and/or extremities.
Headache, dizziness, feelings of detachment.
Mouth sores, indigestion, nausea, vomiting, diarrhea.
Temporary loss of hair.
Serious Adverse Effects
Allergic Reactions: Asthma, difficult breathing, mouth irritation.
Blurred vision, confusion, depression.
Active peptic ulcer, with or without bleeding.
Liver damage with jaundice (see Glossary).
Kidney damage with painful urination, bloody urine, reduced urine formation.
Rare bone marrow depression (see Glossary)—fatigue, weakness, fever, sore throat, abnormal bleeding or bruising.
Peripheral neuritis (see Glossary)—numbness, pain or weakness in extremities.

▷ **Possible Effects on Sexual Function**
Enlargement and tenderness of both male and female breasts.
Nonmenstrual vaginal bleeding.

Possible Delayed Adverse Effects: Mild anemia due to "silent" blood loss from the stomach (less than that caused by aspirin).

▷ **Adverse Effects That May Mimic Natural Diseases or Disorders**
Liver reaction may suggest viral hepatitis.

Natural Diseases or Disorders That May Be Activated by This Drug
Peptic ulcer disease, ulcerative colitis.

CAUTION
1. Dosage should always be limited to the smallest amount that produces reasonable improvement.
2. This drug may mask early indications of infection. Inform your physician if you think you are developing an infection of any kind.

Precautions for Use
By Infants and Children: This drug frequently causes impairment of kidney function in infants. Fatal liver reactions have occurred in children between 6 and 12 years of age; avoid the use of this drug in this age group.
By Those over 60 Years of Age: Adverse effects are very common in this age group. Small doses are advisable until tolerance is determined. Observe for any indications of liver or kidney toxicity, fluid retention, dizziness, confusion, impaired memory, depression, peptic ulcer or diarrhea, often with rectal bleeding.

▷ **Advisability of Use During Pregnancy**
Pregnancy Category: D (tentative). See Pregnancy Code inside back cover.
Animal studies: Significant toxicity and birth defects reported in mice and rats.
Human studies: Information from adequate studies of pregnant women is not available. However, birth defects have been attributed to the use of this drug during pregnancy.
The manufacturer recommends that this drug not be taken during pregnancy.

Advisability of Use if Breast-Feeding
Presence of this drug in breast milk: Yes.
Avoid drug or refrain from nursing.
The manufacturer recommends that this drug not be taken while breast-feeding.

Habit-Forming Potential: None.

Effects of Overdosage: Drowsiness, agitation, confusion, nausea, vomiting, diarrhea, disorientation, seizures, coma.

Possible Effects of Long-Term Use: Eye changes: deposits in the cornea, alterations in the retina.

Suggested Periodic Examinations While Taking This Drug (at physician's discretion)
Complete blood cell counts, liver and kidney function tests, complete eye examinations if vision is altered in any way.

▷ **While Taking This Drug, Observe the Following**
Foods: No restrictions.
Nutritional Support: Take 50 mg of vitamin C (ascorbic acid) daily.
Beverages: No restrictions. May be taken with milk.
▷ *Alcohol:* Use with caution. The irritant action of alcohol on the stomach lining, added to the irritant action of this drug in sensitive individuals, can increase the risk of stomach ulceration and/or bleeding.
Tobacco Smoking: No interactions expected.
▷ *Other Drugs*
Indomethacin may ***increase*** the effects of
- acetaminophen (Tylenol, etc.), and increase the risk of kidney damage; avoid prolonged use of this combination.
- anticoagulants (Coumadin, etc.), and increase the risk of bleeding; monitor prothrombin time, adjust dose accordingly.
- lithium, and cause lithium toxicity.
Indomethacin may ***decrease*** the effects of
- beta blocker drugs (see Drug Class, Section Four), and reduce their antihypertensive effectiveness.
- bumetanide (Bumex).
- captopril (Capoten).
- ethacrynic acid (Edecrin).

- furosemide (Lasix).

Indomethacin **taken concurrently** with the following drugs may increase the risk of bleeding; avoid these combinations:

- aspirin.
- diflunisal (Dolobid).
- dipyridamole (Persantine).
- sulfinpyrazone (Anturane).
- valproic acid (Depakene).

▷ *Driving, Hazardous Activities:* This drug may cause drowsiness, dizziness or impaired vision. Restrict activities as necessary.

Aviation Note: The use of this drug **may be a disqualification** for piloting. Consult a designated Aviation Medical Examiner.

Exposure to Sun: No restrictions.

INSULIN
(IN suh lin)

Introduced: 1922

Class: Antidiabetic

Prescription: USA: No
Canada: No

Controlled Drug: USA: No
Canada: No

Available as Generic: Yes

Brand Names: Humulin BR, Humulin L, Humulin N, Humulin R, Humulin U, Humulin U Ultralente, Iletin I NPH, ✦Initard, Insulatard NPH, ✦Insulin-Toronto, Lente Iletin I, Lente Iletin II Beef, Lente Iletin II Pork, Lente Insulin, Mixtard, Novolin L, Novolin N, NovolinPen, Novolin R, ✦Novolin-Lente, ✦Novolin-NPH, ✦Novolin-30/70, ✦Novolin-Toronto, ✦Novolin-Ultralente, NPH Iletin I, NPH Iletin II Beef, NPH Iletin II Pork, NPH Insulin, NPH Purified Pork, Protamine, Zinc & Iletin I, Protamine, Zinc & Iletin II Beef, Protamine, Zinc & Iletin II Pork, Regular Iletin I, Regular Iletin II Beef, Regular Iletin II Pork, Regular Iletin II U-500, Regular Insulin, Regular Purified Pork Insulin, Semilente Iletin I, Semilente Insulin, Semilente Purified Pork, Ultralente Iletin I, Ultralente Insulin, Ultralente Purified Beef, Velosulin

BENEFITS versus RISKS	
Possible Benefits	*Possible Risks*
EFFECTIVE CONTROL OF TYPE I (INSULIN-DEPENDENT) DIABETES MELLITUS	HYPOGLYCEMIA WITH EXCESSIVE DOSAGE Infrequent allergic reactions

▷ **Principal Uses**

As a Single Drug Product: Insulin is used to control diabetes mellitus in those individuals whose diabetes has been shown to be insulin-dependent. Proper use involves selection of the most appropriate type of insulin for the individual and determination of the optimal dosage schedule for the continuous regulation of blood sugar levels.

How This Drug Works: Not completely established. By direct action on certain cell membranes, insulin facilitates the transport of sugar through the cell wall to the interior of the cell where it is utilized. This occurs primarily in the brain, the voluntary muscles, the heart muscle and the liver.

Available Dosage Forms and Strengths

Injections — 40 units, 100 units, 500 units per ml
PenFil cartridges — 150 units

▷ **Usual Adult Dosage Range:** According to individual requirements for the optimal regulation of blood sugar on a 24-hour basis. **Note: Actual dosage and administration schedule must be determined by the physician for each patient individually.**

▷ **Dosing Instructions:** Inject insulin subcutaneously according to the schedule prescribed by your physician. The timing and frequency of injections will vary with the type of insulin precribed. The following table of insulin actions (according to type) will help you understand the treatment schedule prescribed for you.

Insulin Type	Action Onset	Peak	Duration
Regular	0.5–1 hr	2–4 hrs	5–7 hrs
Isophane (NPH)	3–4 hrs	6–12 hrs	18–28 hrs
Regular 30%/NPH 70%	0.5 hr	4–8 hrs	24 hrs
Semilente	1–3 hrs	2–8 hrs	12–16 hrs
Lente	1–3 hrs	8–12 hrs	18–28 hrs
Ultralente	4–6 hrs	18–24 hrs	36 hrs
Protamine Zinc	4–6 hrs	14–24 hrs	36 hrs

Usual Duration of Use: Type I insulin-dependent (juvenile-onset) diabetes mellitus usually requires insulin treatment for life. Type II noninsulin-dependent (maturity-onset) diabetes is usually controlled by oral antidiabetic drugs and/or diet but may, on occasion, require insulin for adequate control. Such occasions include serious infections, injuries, burns, surgical procedures and other forms of physical stress. Insulin is used as needed on a temporary basis to regulate and normalize the body's use of sugar until recovery is complete and basic health is restored. Consult your physician on a regular basis.

▷ **This Drug Should Not Be Taken If**

• the need for it and its correct dosage schedule have not been established by a properly qualified physician.

▷ **Inform Your Physician Before Taking This Drug If**
- you have a history of allergic reaction to any form of insulin on previous use.
- you do not know how to recognize and treat abnormally low blood sugar (see Hypoglycemia in Glossary).
- you are taking any of the following drugs: aspirin, beta blockers, fenfluramine (Pondimin), monoamine oxidase (MAO) type A inhibitors (see respective Drug Classes, Section Four).

Possible Side-Effects (natural, expected and unavoidable drug actions)
In the management of stable diabetes, no side-effects occur when insulin dose, diet and physical activity are correctly balanced and maintained.
In the management of unstable ("brittle") diabetes, unexpected drops in blood sugar levels can occur, resulting in periods of hypoglycemia (see Glossary).

▷ **Possible Adverse Effects** (unusual, unexpected and infrequent reactions)
If any of the following develop, consult your physician promptly for guidance.
Mild Adverse Effects
Allergic Reactions: Local redness, swelling and itching at site of injection. Occasional hives.
Thinning of subcutaneous tissue at sites of injection.
Serious Adverse Effects
Allergic Reaction: Anaphylactic reactions (see Glossary).
Severe, prolonged hypoglycemia.

▷ **Possible Effects on Sexual Function:**   None reported.

▷ **Adverse Effects That May Mimic Natural Diseases or Disorders**
The early manifestations of hypoglycemia may be mistaken for alcoholic intoxication.

CAUTION
1. It is most important that you carry with you a card of personal identification with a notation that you have diabetes and are taking insulin.
2. Be sure that you know how to recognize the onset of hypoglycemia and how to treat it. Always carry with you a readily available form of sugar, such as hard candy or sugar cubes. Report all episodes of hypoglycemia to your physician; it may be necessary to adjust your insulin dosage or schedule.
3. Improvement in vision may occur during the first several weeks of insulin treatment. It is advisable to defer examination for glasses for 6 weeks after starting insulin.
4. The rates of insulin absorption vary significantly from one anatomic site to another. Absorption is 80% greater from the abdominal wall than from the leg, and 30% greater than from the arm. Individuals with unstable diabetes may achieve better control of

blood sugar levels by rotating the injection site within the same anatomic region rather than by rotating from one anatomic region to another.

Precautions for Use

By Infants and Children: Insulin dosages and schedules are modified according to patient size. Adhere strictly to the physician's prescribed routine.

By Those over 60 Years of Age: Insulin requirements may change with aging. Periodic evaluation of individual status is necessary to determine correct insulin dosage and scheduling. The aging brain adapts well to higher blood sugar levels. Attempts to maintain strictly "normal" blood sugar levels may result in episodes of unrecognized hypoglycemia that is manifested by confusion and abnormal behavior. Repeated episodes of hypoglycemia (especially if severe) in the elderly may cause brain damage.

▷ **Advisability of Use During Pregnancy**

Pregnancy Category: B (tentative). See Pregnancy Code inside back cover. Animal studies: Inconclusive.

Human studies: Information from adequate studies of pregnant women is not available. It is known that birth defects occur 2 to 4 times more frequently in infants of diabetic mothers than in infants of mothers who do not have diabetes. The exact causes of this are not known.

Insulin is the drug of choice for managing diabetes during pregnancy. To preserve the health of the mother and the welfare of the fetus, every effort must be made to establish the optimal dosage of insulin necessary for "good control" and to prevent episodes of hypoglycemia.

Advisability of Use if Breast-Feeding

Presence of this drug in breast milk: No.

Insulin treatment of the mother has no adverse effect on the nursing infant.

Breast-feeding may decrease insulin requirements; dosage adjustment may be necessary.

Habit-Forming Potential: None.

Effects of Overdosage: Hypoglycemia: fatigue, weakness, headache, nervousness, irritability, sweating, tremors, hunger, confusion, delirium, abnormal behavior (resembling alcoholic intoxication), loss of consciousness, seizures.

Possible Effects of Long-Term Use: Thinning of subcutaneous fat tissue at sites of insulin injection.

Suggested Periodic Examinations While Taking This Drug (at physician's discretion)

Monitoring of urine sugar content as a guide to adjustment of diet and insulin dosage. Measurement of blood sugar levels at intervals recommended by physician.

▷ **While Taking This Drug, Observe the Following**

Foods: Follow your prescribed diabetic diet conscientiously. Do not omit snack foods in midafternoon or at bedtime if they are prescribed to prevent hypoglycemia.

Beverages: According to prescribed diabetic diet.

▷ *Alcohol:* Use with caution until the combined effect has been determined. Used excessively, alcohol can induce severe hypoglycemia, resulting in brain damage.

Tobacco Smoking: Regular smoking can decrease insulin absorption and increase insulin requirements by 30%. It is advisable to refrain from smoking altogether.

Marijuana Smoking: Possible increase in blood sugar levels.

▷ *Other Drugs*

The following drugs may *increase* the effects of insulin

- aspirin, and other salicylates.
- some beta blocker drugs (especially the nonselective ones) may prolong insulin-induced hypoglycemia. (See Drug Class, Section Four.)
- fenfluramine (Pondimin).
- monoamine oxidase (MAO) type A inhibitor drugs (see Drug Class, Section Four).

The following drugs may *decrease* the effects of insulin (by raising blood sugar levels)

- chlorthalidone (Hygroton).
- cortisonelike drugs (see Drug Class, Section Four).
- furosemide (Lasix).
- oral contraceptives.
- phenytoin (Dilantin, etc.).
- thiazide diuretics (see Drug Class, Section Four).
- thyroid preparations.

▷ *Driving, Hazardous Activities:* Usually no restrictions. However, be prepared to stop and take corrective action if indications of impending hypoglycemia develop.

Aviation Note: Diabetes and the use of this drug **are disqualifications** for piloting. Consult a designated Aviation Medical Examiner.

Exposure to Sun: No restrictions.

Exposure to Heat: Use caution. Sauna baths can signficantly increase the rate of insulin absorption and cause hypoglycemia.

Heavy Exercise or Exertion: Use caution. Periods of unusual or unplanned heavy physical activity will hasten the utilization of blood sugar and predispose to hypoglycemia.

Occurrence of Unrelated Illness: Report all illnesses that prevent regular eating. The omission of meals as a result of nausea, vomiting or injury may lead to hypoglycemia. Untreated infections can increase insulin requirements. Consult physician for guidance.

Discontinuation: Do not discontinue this drug without consulting your physician. Diabetes that is insulin-dependent requires continual treatment on a regular basis. Omission of insulin may result in life-threatening coma.

Special Storage Instructions: Keep in a cool place, preferably in the refrigerator. Protect from freezing. Protect from strong light and high
temperatures when not refrigerated.

Observe the Following Expiration Times: Do not use this drug if it is older
than the expiration date on the vial. Always use fresh, "within date"
insulin.

ISONIAZID
(i soh NI a zid)

Other Names: Isonicotinic acid hydrazide, INH

Introduced: 1956   **Class:** Antitubercular

Prescription: USA: Yes   **Controlled Drug:** USA: No
       Canada: Yes   Canada: No

Available as Generic: USA: Yes
       Canada: No

Brand Names: ✦Isotamine, Laniazid, Nydrazid, P-I-N Forte [CD], ✦PMS
Isoniazid, Rifamate [CD], Rimactane/INH Dual Pack [CD], Teebaconin, Teebaconin and Vitamin B-6 [CD]

BENEFITS versus RISKS

Possible Benefits	*Possible Risks*
EFFECTIVE PREVENTION AND TREATMENT OF ACTIVE TUBERCULOSIS	ALLERGIC LIVER REACTION (1% to 2%)
	Peripheral neuropathy (see Glossary)
	Bone marrow depression (see Glossary)
	Mental and behavioral disturbances

▷ **Principal Uses**

As a Single Drug Product: Used alone to prevent the development of active
tuberculous infection in individuals who are considered to be at high
risk because of known exposure to infection or recent conversion of
a negative tuberculin skin test to positive.

As a Combination Drug Product [CD]: This drug is available in combination with rifampin, another antitubercular drug that has a different
mechanism of action. This combination is more effective than either
drug used alone. Isoniazid can cause a deficiency of pyridoxine (vitamin B-6); for this reason, a combination of the two drugs is available in tablet form.

How This Drug Works: Not completely established. It is thought that this drug destroys susceptible tuberculosis organisms by interfering with several of their essential metabolic activities and by disrupting their cell wall.

Available Dosage Forms and Strengths
  Injection — 100 mg per ml
   Syrup — 50 mg per 5-ml teaspoonful
   Tablets — 50 mg, 100 mg, 300 mg

▷ **Usual Adult Dosage Range:**   For prevention: 300 mg once daily. For treatment: 5 mg per kilogram of body weight daily. The total daily dosage should not exceed 600 mg. **Note: Actual dosage and administration schedule must be determined by the physician for each patient individually.**

▷ **Dosing Instructions:**   May be taken with food to prevent stomach irritation. The tablet may be crushed for administration.

Usual Duration of Use: Continual use on a regular schedule for 1 or more years is often necessary, depending upon the nature of the infection. Shorter courses of intermittent high dosage may be adequate in some cases. Consult your physician on a regular basis.

▷ **This Drug Should Not Be Taken If**
  • you have had an allergic reaction (especially a liver reaction) to any dosage form of it previously.
  • you have active liver disease.

▷ **Inform Your Physician Before Taking This Drug If**
  • you have serious impairment of liver or kidney function.
  • you drink an alcoholic beverage daily.
  • you have a seizure disorder.
  • you are taking any other drugs on a long-term basis, especially phenytoin (Dilantin).
  • you plan to have surgery under general anesthesia in the near future.

Possible Side-Effects (natural, expected and unavoidable drug actions)
  None.

▷ **Possible Adverse Effects** (unusual, unexpected and infrequent reactions)
  If any of the following develop, consult your physician promptly for guidance.
  Mild Adverse Effects
  Allergic Reactions: Skin rash, fever, swollen glands, painful muscles and joints.
  Dizziness, indigestion, nausea, vomiting.
  Serious Adverse Effects
  Allergic Reactions: Drug-induced hepatitis (see Glossary): loss of appetite, nausea, fatigue, fever, itching, dark-colored urine, yellow discoloration of eyes and skin.

Peripheral neuritis (see Glossary): numbness, tingling, pain, weakness in hands and/or feet.

Acute mental and behavioral disturbances, impaired vision, increase in epileptic seizures.

Bone marrow depression (see Glossary): fatigue, weakness, fever, sore throat, abnormal bleeding or bruising.

▷ **Possible Effects on Sexual Function:** Male breast enlargement and tenderness.

Possible Delayed Adverse Effects: An increase in the frequency of cirrhosis of the liver has been reported.

▷ **Adverse Effects That May Mimic Natural Diseases or Disorders**
Drug-induced hepatitis may suggest viral hepatitis.

Natural Diseases or Disorders That May Be Activated by This Drug
Latent epilepsy, systemic lupus erythematosus (questionable).

CAUTION
1. Consult your physician regarding the advisability of determining if you are a "slow" or "rapid" inactivator (acetylator) of isoniazid. This has a bearing on your predisposition to developing adverse effects from this drug.
2. Copper sulfate tests for urine sugar may give a false positive test result. (Diabetics please note.)

Precautions for Use
By Infants and Children: Use with caution in children with seizure disorders. "Slow acetylators" are more prone to adverse drug effects. It is advisable to give supplemental pyridoxine (vitamin B-6).
By Those over 60 Years of Age: There is a greater incidence of liver damage in this age group; the liver status should be monitored carefully. Observe for any indications of an "acute brain syndrome" consisting of confusion, delirium and seizures.

▷ **Advisability of Use During Pregnancy**
Pregnancy Category: C (tentative). See Pregnancy Code inside back cover.
Animal studies: No birth defects reported in mice, rats or rabbits.
Human studies: Information from adequate studies of pregnant women is not available.
Earlier reports of human birth defects due to this drug have not been substantiated by later studies. If clearly needed, this drug is now used at any time during pregnancy. Ask your physician for guidance.

Advisability of Use if Breast-Feeding
Presence of this drug in breast milk: Yes.
Avoid drug or refrain from nursing.

Habit-Forming Potential: None.

Effects of Overdosage: Nausea, vomiting, dizziness, blurred vision, hallucinations, slurred speech, stupor, coma, seizures.

Possible Effects of Long-Term Use: Peripheral neuritis due to a deficiency of pyridoxine (vitamin B-6).

Suggested Periodic Examinations While Taking This Drug (at physician's discretion)
Complete blood cell counts, liver function tests, complete eye examinations.

▷ **While Taking This Drug, Observe the Following**
Foods: Eat the following foods cautiously until your tolerance is determined: Swiss and Cheshire cheeses, tuna fish, skipjack fish and Sardinella species. These may interact with the drug to produce skin rash, itching, sweating, chills, headache, light-headedness or rapid heart rate.
Nutritional Support: It is advisable to take a supplement of pyridoxine (vitamin B-6) to prevent peripheral neuritis. Ask your physician for dosage.
Beverages: No restrictions. May be taken with milk.
▷ *Alcohol:* Avoid completely or use very sparingly. Alcohol may reduce the effectiveness of this drug and increase the risk of liver toxicity.
Tobacco Smoking: No interactions expected.
▷ *Other Drugs*
Isoniazid may **increase** the effects of
• carbamazepine (Tegretol), and cause toxicity.
• phenytoin (Dilantin), and cause toxicity.
The following drugs may **decrease** the effects of isoniazid
• cortisonelike drugs (see Drug Class, Section Four).
▷ *Driving, Hazardous Activities:* Usually no restrictions. This drug may cause dizziness. Restrict activities as necessary.
Aviation Note: The use of this drug **may be a disqualification** for piloting. Consult a designated Aviation Medical Examiner.
Exposure to Sun: No restrictions.
Discontinuation: Long-term treatment is required. Do not discontinue this drug without consulting your physician.

ISOSORBIDE DINITRATE
(i soh SOHR bide di NI trayt)

Other Name: Sorbide nitrate

Introduced: 1959

Class: Antianginal, nitrates

Prescription: USA: Yes
Canada: No

Controlled Drug: USA: No
Canada: No

Available as Generic: USA: Yes
      Canada: No

Brand Names: ✦Apo-ISDN, ✦Coronex, Dilatrate-SR, Isonate, Isordil, Isordil Tembids, Isordil Titradose, ✦Novosorbide, Sorbitrate

---

BENEFITS versus RISKS

Possible Benefits	*Possible Risks*
EFFECTIVE RELIEF AND PREVENTION OF ANGINA	Orthostatic hypotension (see Glossary)
EFFECTIVE ADJUNCTIVE TREATMENT IN SELECTED CASES OF CONGESTIVE HEART FAILURE	Rare skin reactions (severe peeling)

▷ **Principal Uses**

As a Single Drug Product: The sublingual (under-the-tongue) tablets and the chewable tablets are used to prevent and to relieve acute attacks of anginal pain. The longer-acting tablets and capsules are used to prevent the development of angina, but are not effective in relieving acute episodes of anginal pain. This drug is also used to improve heart function in selected cases of congestive heart failure.

How This Drug Works: By direct action on the muscle in blood vessel walls, this drug relaxes and dilates both arteries and veins. It is thought that its beneficial effects in treating angina and heart failure are due to (1) dilation of coronary arteries, and (2) dilation of systemic veins with consequent reduction of volume and pressure of blood in the heart. The net effects are improved blood flow to the heart muscle and reduced workload of the heart.

Available Dosage Forms and Strengths
                    Capsules — 40 mg
    Capsules, prolonged-action — 40 mg
                      Tablets — 5 mg, 10 mg, 20 mg, 30 mg, 40 mg
          Tablets, chewable — 5 mg, 10 mg
      Tablets, prolonged-action — 40 mg
        Tablets, sublingual — 2.5 mg, 5 mg, 10 mg

▷ **Usual Adult Dosage Range**

Sublingual tablets: 5 to 10 mg dissolved under tongue every 2 to 3 hours; use for relief of acute attack and for prevention of anticipated attack.

Chewable tablets: Initially, 5 mg chewed to evaluate tolerance; increase dose to 5 or 10 mg every 2 to 3 hours as needed and tolerated; use for relief of acute attack and for prevention of anticipated attack.

Tablets: 5 to 30 mg 4 times daily to prevent acute attack; usual dose is 10 to 20 mg 4 times/day.

Prolonged-action capsules and tablets: 40 mg/6 to 12 hours as needed to prevent acute attacks.

The total daily dosage should not exceed 120 mg.

Note: Actual dosage and administration schedule must be determined by the physician for each patient individually.

▷ **Dosing Instructions:**   Capsules and tablets to be swallowed are best taken on an empty stomach to achieve maximal blood levels. Regular tablets may be crushed for administration; prolonged-action capsules and tablets should be taken whole and not altered.

Usual Duration of Use: Continual use on a regular schedule for 3 to 7 days is usually necessary to (1) determine this drug's effectiveness in preventing or relieving acute anginal pain, and (2) establish the optimal dosage sheldule. Long-term use (months to years) requires supervision and periodic evaluation by your physician. Consult your physician on a regular basis.

▷ **This Drug Should Not Be Taken If**
- you have had an allergic reaction to any dosage form of it previously.
- you have had a very recent heart attack (myocardial infarction).

▷ **Inform Your Physician Before Taking This Drug If**
- you have had an unfavorable response to other nitrate drugs or vasodilators in the past.
- you have a history of low blood pressure.
- you have any form of glaucoma.

Possible Side-Effects (natural, expected and unavoidable drug actions)
Flushing of face, throbbing in head, palpitation, rapid heart rate, orthostatic hypotension (see Glossary).

▷ **Possible Adverse Effects** (unusual, unexpected and infrequent reactions)
If any of the following develop, consult your physician promptly for guidance.
Mild Adverse Effects
Allergic Reaction: Skin rash.
Headache (may be severe and persistent), dizziness, fainting.
Nausea, vomiting.
Serious Adverse Effects
Allergic Reaction: Severe dermatitis with peeling of skin.
Transient ischemic attacks (TIAs) in presence of impaired circulation within the brain: dizziness, fainting, impaired vision or speech, localized numbness or weakness.

▷ **Possible Effects on Sexual Function:**   None reported.

▷ **Adverse Effects That May Mimic Natural Diseases or Disorders**
Spells of low blood pressure (due to this drug) may be mistaken for late-onset epilepsy.

CAUTION
1. The development of tolerance (see Glossary) to long-acting forms of nitrates may render the sublingual tablets of nitroglycerin less effective for the relief of acute anginal attacks. Antianginal effectiveness is restored after 1 week of abstinence from long-acting nitrates.
2. Many over-the-counter (OTC) medications for allergies, colds and coughs contain drugs that may counteract the desired effects of this drug. Ask your physician or pharmacist for guidance before using such medications.

Precautions for Use
By Those over 60 Years of Age: Small doses are advisable until your tolerance has been determined. You may be more susceptible to the development of low blood pressure and associated "blackout" spells, fainting and falling. Throbbing headaches and flushing may be more apparent.

▷ **Advisability of Use During Pregnancy**
Pregnancy Category: C (tentative). See Pregnancy Code inside back cover.
Animal studies: No information available.
Human studies: Information from adequate studies of pregnant women is not available.
Use this drug only if clearly needed.

Advisability of Use if Breast-Feeding
Presence of this drug in breast milk: Unknown.
If drug is thought to be necessary, monitor the nursing infant for low blood pressure and poor feeding.

Habit-Forming Potential: None.

Effects of Overdosage: Headache, dizziness, marked flushing of face and skin, vomiting, weakness, fainting, difficult breathing, coma.

Possible Effects of Long-Term Use: Development of tolerance with temporary loss of effectiveness at recommended doses. Development of abnormal hemoglobin (red blood cell pigment).

Suggested Periodic Examinations While Taking This Drug (at physician's discretion)
Measurement of internal eye pressure. Red blood cell counts and hemoglobin evaluation.

▷ **While Taking This Drug, Observe the Following**
Foods: No restrictions.
Beverages: No restrictions. May be taken with milk.
▷ *Alcohol:* Use extreme caution until the combined effects have been determined. Avoid alcohol completely in the presence of any side-effects or adverse effects of this drug. Alcohol may exaggerate the blood-pressure-lowering effect of this drug.

Tobacco Smoking: Nicotine can reduce the effectiveness of this drug. Avoid all forms of tobacco.

Marijuana Smoking: Possible reduced effectiveness of this drug; mild to moderate increase in angina; possible changes in electrocardiogram, confusing interpretation.

▷ *Other Drugs*

Isosorbide dinitrate *taken concurrently* with

- antihypertensive drugs may cause excessive lowering of blood pressure; dosage adjustments may be necessary.

▷ *Driving, Hazardous Activities:* Usually no restrictions. This drug may cause dizziness or spells of low blood pressure. Restrict activities as necessary.

Aviation Note: Coronary artery disease *is a disqualification* for piloting. Consult a designated Aviation Medical Examiner.

Exposure to Sun: No restrictions.

Exposure to Heat: Use caution. Hot environments can cause a significant drop in blood pressure.

Exposure to Cold: Cold environments can increase the need for this drug and limit its effectiveness.

Heavy Exercise or Exertion: This drug may improve your ability to be more active without anginal pain. Use caution and avoid excessive exertion.

Discontinuation: It is advisable to withdraw this drug gradually after long-term use. The dosage and frequency of prolonged-action dosage forms should be reduced gradually over a period of 4 to 6 weeks.

ISOTRETINOIN
(i soh TRET i noin)

Introduced: 1979

Class: Antiacne

Prescription: USA: Yes
Canada: Yes

Controlled Drug: USA: No
Canada: No

Available as Generic: No

Brand Name: Accutane

BENEFITS versus RISKS	
Possible Benefits	*Possible Risks*
EFFECTIVE TREATMENT OF SEVERE CYSTIC ACNE	MAJOR BIRTH DEFECTS
	Initial worsening of acne (transient)
	Inflammation of lips (90%)
	Dry skin, nose and mouth
	Musculoskeletal discomfort
	Corneal opacities (rare)

▷ **Principal Uses**

  As a Single Drug Product: This drug is reserved to treat severe nodular and cystic acne that has failed to respond to all other forms of standard therapy. ***It should not be used to treat mild forms of acne.*** It is also used to treat some less common conditions of the skin that are due to disorders of keratin production.

  How This Drug Works: Not completely established. By an unknown action, this drug reduces the size of sebaceous glands and inhibits their production of sebum (skin oil). This helps to correct the major feature of acne and its complications.

Available Dosage Forms and Strengths
  Capsules — 10 mg, 20 mg, 40 mg

▷ **Usual Adult Dosage Range:** Initial dosage is individualized according to the patient's weight and the severity of the acne; the usual dose is 1 to 2 mg per kilogram of body weight daily, taken in 2 divided doses for 15 to 20 weeks. After 2 weeks of treatment, the dose should be adjusted according to the response of the acne and the development of adverse effects. **Note: Actual dosage and administration schedule must be determined by the physician for each patient individually.**

▷ **Dosing Instructions:** Take with meals (morning and evening) to achieve optimal blood levels. The capsule should not be opened for administration.

  Usual Duration of Use: Continual use on a regular schedule for 15 to 20 weeks is usually necessary to determine this drug's effectiveness in clearing or improving severe cystic acne. The drug may be discontinued earlier if the total cyst count is reduced by more than 70%. If a repeat course of treatment is necessary, it should not be started until after a period of 2 months without this drug. Long-term use (months to years) requires supervision and periodic evaluation by your physician. Consult your physician on a regular basis.

▷ **This Drug Should Not Be Taken If**
  • you are allergic to parabens, additives that are used to preserve the drug product.
  • you are pregnant, or planning pregnancy.

▷ **Inform Your Physician Before Taking This Drug If**
  • you have had an allergic reaction to any form of vitamin A in the past.
  • you have diabetes mellitus.
  • you have a cholesterol or triglyceride disorder.
  • you have a history of liver or kidney disease.

  Possible Side-Effects (natural, expected and unavoidable drug actions)
  Dryness of the nose and mouth (80%), inflammation of the lips (90%), dryness of the skin with itching (80%), peeling of the palms and soles (5%).

▷ **Possible Adverse Effects** (unusual, unexpected and infrequent reactions)
  If any of the following develop, consult your physician promptly for guidance.
  Mild Adverse Effects
  Allergic Reaction: Skin rash (less than 10%).
  Thinning of hair, conjunctivitis, intolerance of contact lenses, muscular and joint aches, headache, fatigue, indigestion.
  Serious Adverse Effects
  Skin infections, worsening of arthritis, inflammatory bowel disorders.
  Abnormal acceleration of bone development in children.
  Development of opacities in the cornea of the eye.
  Reduced red blood cell and white blood cell counts; increased blood platelet count.
  Increased pressure within the head, with associated headache, visual disturbances, nausea and vomiting.

▷ **Possible Effects on Sexual Function**
  Decreased male libido (7%), decreased female libido (13%) beginning after 1 month of drug use.
  Impotence (3%) beginning after 3 months of drug use.
  Decreased vaginal secretions (43%).
  Altered timing and pattern of menstruation (22%).
  Female breast discharge (rare).

CAUTION
  1. This drug should not be used to treat mild forms of acne.
  2. A transient worsening of your acne may occur during the first few weeks of treatment; this will subside with continued use of the drug.
  3. Do not take any other form of vitamin A while taking this drug. (Observe contents of multiple vitamin preparations.)
  4. Women with potential for pregnancy should have a pregnancy test before taking this drug and should use an effective form of contraception during its use. It is recommended that contraception be continued until normal menstruation resumes after discontinuing this drug.
  5. This drug may cause increased blood levels of cholesterol and triglycerides.
  6. If repeated courses of this drug are prescribed, wait a minimum of 2 months between courses before resuming medication.

Precautions for Use
  By Infants and Children: Long-term use (6 to 12 months) may cause abnormal acceleration of bone growth and development. Your physician can monitor this possibility by periodic X-ray examination of long bones.

▷ **Advisability of Use During Pregnancy**
   Pregnancy Category: X. See Pregnancy Code inside back cover.
     Animal studies: Birth defects of skull, brain and vertebral column found
       in rats; skeletal birth defects found in rabbits.
     Human studies: Information from adequate studies of pregnant women
       is not available. However, serious birth defects of fetal brain devel-
       opment (thought to be due to this drug) have been reported.
     Avoid this drug completely during entire pregnancy.

Advisability of Use if Breast-Feeding
   Presence of this drug in breast milk: Unknown.
   Avoid drug or refrain from nursing.

Habit-Forming Potential: None.

Effects of Overdosage: No experience with overdosage in humans to date.

Suggested Periodic Examinations While Taking This Drug (at physician's
       discretion)
   Complete blood cell counts, including platelet counts.
   Measurements of blood cholesterol and triglyceride levels.
   Complete eye examinations.
   Liver and kidney function tests.

▷ **While Taking This Drug, Observe the Following**
   Foods: No restrictions.
   Beverages: No restrictions.
▷ *Alcohol:* No interactions expected.
   Tobacco Smoking: No interactions expected.
▷ *Other Drugs:* No interactions reported to date.
▷ *Driving, Hazardous Activities:* No restrictions.
   Exposure to Sun: This drug can cause photosensitivity (see Glossary).
       Avoid excessive exposure to sun until your sensitivity is determined.

KETOPROFEN
(kee toh PROH fen)

Introduced: 1973

Class: Mild analgesic, anti-
inflammatory

Prescription: USA: Yes
Canada: Yes

Controlled Drug: USA: No
Canada: No

Available as Generic: No

Brand Names: Orudis, ✦Orudis E-50

```
┌─────────────────────────────────────────────────────────────────┐
│                    BENEFITS versus RISKS                         │
│                                                                   │
│      Possible Benefits                   Possible Risks           │
│   EFFECTIVE RELIEF OF MILD        Gastrointestinal pain, ulceration, │
│   TO MODERATE PAIN AND              bleeding (rare)               │
│   INFLAMMATION                    Rare liver or kidney damage     │
│                                   Rare fluid retention           │
│                                   Rare bone marrow depression    │
└─────────────────────────────────────────────────────────────────┘
```

▷ **Principal Uses**

As a Single Drug Product: Used primarily to relieve mild to moderately severe pain associated with (1) rheumatoid arthritis and osteoarthritis; (2) acute gouty arthritis; (3) acute bursitis, tendinitis and related conditions; and (4) menstrual cramps.

How This Drug Works: Not completely established. It is thought that this drug reduces the tissue concentrations of prostaglandins (and related compounds), chemicals involved in the production of inflammation and pain.

Available Dosage Forms and Strengths
Capsules — 50 mg, 75 mg
Suppositories — 100 mg (in Canada)
Tablets, enteric-coated — 50 mg (in Canada)

▷ **Usual Adult Dosage Range:**   Initially, 75 mg 3 times/day or 50 mg 4 times/day. Usual daily dose is 150 to 300 mg divided into 3 or 4 doses. Total daily dosage should not exceed 300 mg. **Note: Actual dosage and administration schedule must be determined by the physician for each patient individually.**

▷ **Dosing Instructions:**   Take either on an empty stomach or with food or milk to prevent stomach irritation. Take with a full glass of water and remain upright (do not lie down) for 30 minutes. The capsule may be opened for administration; the tablet should not be crushed or altered.

Usual Duration of Use: Continual use on a regular schedule for 1 to 3 weeks is usually necessary to determine this drug's effectiveness in relieving the discomfort of arthritis. Long-term use (months to years) requires supervision and periodic evaluation by the physician. Consult your physician on a regular basis.

▷ **This Drug Should Not Be Taken If**
- you have had an allergic reaction to it previously.
- you are subject to asthma or nasal polyps caused by aspirin.
- you have active peptic ulcer disease or any form of gastrointestinal ulceration or bleeding.
- you have a bleeding disorder or a blood cell disorder.
- you have severe impairment of kidney function.
- you have active liver disease.

▷ **Inform Your Physician Before Taking This Drug If**
- you are allergic to aspirin or to other aspirin substitutes.
- you have a history of peptic ulcer disease or any type of bleeding disorder.
- you have impaired liver or kidney function.
- you have high blood pressure or a history of heart failure.
- you are taking any of the following: acetaminophen, aspirin or other aspirin substitutes, anticoagulants, oral antidiabetic drugs, or probenecid.

Possible Side-Effects (natural, expected and unavoidable drug actions)
Drowsiness (1% to 3%), ringing in ears (1% to 3%), fluid retention (3%).

▷ **Possible Adverse Effects** (unusual, unexpected and infrequent reactions)
If any of the following develop, consult your physician promptly for guidance.
Mild Adverse Effects
Allergic Reactions: Skin rash (1% to 3%), hives, itching.
Headache (less than 1%), dizziness, altered or blurred vision, depression, confusion, impaired memory.
Mouth sores, indigestion (11%), nausea, vomiting, constipation, diarrhea.
Serious Adverse Effects
Allergic Reaction: Anaphylaxis (see Glossary).
Impaired hearing.
Active peptic ulcer, with or without bleeding (2%).
Rare liver damage with jaundice (see Glossary).
Kidney damage with painful urination, bloody urine, reduced urine formation.
Rare bone marrow depression (see Glossary)—fatigue, weakness, fever, sore throat, abnormal bleeding or bruising.

▷ **Possible Effects on Sexual Function**
Decreased libido, impotence, male breast enlargement.
Altered timing and pattern of menstruation, excessive menstrual bleeding.

Possible Delayed Adverse Effects: Mild anemia due to "silent" blood loss from the stomach (less than that caused by aspirin).

▷ **Adverse Effects That May Mimic Natural Diseases or Disorders**
Liver reaction may suggest viral hepatitis.

Natural Diseases or Disorders That May Be Activated by This Drug
Peptic ulcer disease, ulcerative colitis.

CAUTION
1. Dosage should always be limited to the smallest amount that produces reasonable improvement.
2. This drug may mask early indications of infection. Inform your physician if you think you are developing an infection of any kind.

Precautions for Use

By Infants and Children: Safety and effectiveness for use by those under 12 years of age have not been established.

By Those over 60 Years of Age: Small doses are advisable until tolerance is determined. Observe for any indications of liver or kidney toxicity, fluid retention, dizziness, confusion, impaired memory, stomach bleeding or constipation.

▷ ## Advisability of Use During Pregnancy

Pregnancy Category: B (tentative). See Pregnancy Code inside back cover.

Animal studies: No birth defects reported in mouse, rat or rabbit studies.

Human studies: Information from adequate studies of pregnant women is not available.

Avoid this drug during the last 3 months. Use it during the first 6 months only if clearly needed. Ask physician for guidance.

Advisability of Use if Breast-Feeding

Presence of this drug in breast milk: Unknown.

Avoid drug or refrain from nursing.

Habit-Forming Potential: None.

Effects of Overdosage: Drowsiness, nausea, vomiting, diarrhea.

Possible Effects of Long-Term Use: None reported.

Suggested Periodic Examinations While Taking This Drug (at physician's discretion)

Complete blood cell counts, liver and kidney function tests, complete eye examinations if vision is altered in any way.

▷ ## While Taking This Drug, Observe the Following

Foods: No restrictions.

Beverages: No restrictions. May be taken with milk.

▷   *Alcohol:* Use with caution. The irritant action of alcohol on the stomach lining, added to the irritant action of this drug in sensitive individuals, can increase the risk of stomach ulceration and/or bleeding.

Tobacco Smoking: No interactions expected.

▷   *Other Drugs*

Ketoprofen may *increase* the effects of
- acetaminophen (Tylenol, etc.), and increase the risk of kidney damage; avoid prolonged use of this combination.
- anticoagulants (Coumadin, etc.), and increase the risk of bleeding; monitor prothrombin time, adjust dose accordingly.

Ketoprofen *taken concurrently* with the following drugs may increase the risk of bleeding; avoid these combinations:
- aspirin.
- dipyridamole (Persantine).
- indomethacin (Indocin).

- sulfinpyrazone (Anturane).
- valproic acid (Depakene).

▷ Driving, *Hazardous Activities:* This drug may cause drowsiness or dizziness. Restrict activities as necessary.

Aviation Note: The use of this drug *may be a disqualification* for piloting. Consult a designated Aviation Medical Examiner.

Exposure to Sun: This drug can cause photosensitivity (see Glossary). Avoid excessive exposure to sun until tolerance has been determined.

LABETALOL
(la BET a lohl)

Introduced: 1978

Class: Antihypertensive, alpha- and beta-adrenergic blocker

Prescription: USA: Yes
Canada: Yes

Controlled Drug: USA: No
Canada: No

Available as Generic: No

Brand Names: Normodyne, Normozide [CD], Trandate, Trandate HCT [CD]

BENEFITS versus RISKS

Possible Benefits	*Possible Risks*
EFFECTIVE, WELL-TOLERATED ANTIHYPERTENSIVE in mild to moderate high blood pressure	CONGESTIVE HEART FAILURE in advanced heart disease Worsening of angina in coronary heart disease (if drug is abruptly withdrawn) Masking of low blood sugar (hypoglycemia) in drug-treated diabetes

---

▷ **Principal Uses**

As a Single Drug Product: The treatment of mild to moderately severe high blood pressure. May be used alone or concurrently with other antihypertensive drugs, such as diuretics.

How This Drug Works: By blocking certain actions of the sympathetic nervous system, this drug

- reduces the rate and contraction force of the heart, thus lowering the ejection pressure of blood leaving the heart.
- reduces the degree of contraction of blood vessel walls, resulting in their relaxation and expansion and consequent lowering of blood pressure.

Available Dosage Forms and Strengths
Injection — 5 mg per ml
Tablets — 100 mg, 200 mg, 300 mg

▷ **Usual Adult Dosage Range:**   Initially, 100 mg twice daily, 12 hours apart;
the dose may be increased by 100 mg twice daily every 2 to 3 days
as required to reduce blood pressure. The usual maintenance dose is
200 to 400 mg twice daily. The total dose should not exceed 2400 mg/
24 hours, given as 800 mg 3 times daily. **Note: Actual dosage and
administration schedule must be determined by the physician for
each patient individually.**

▷ **Dosing Instructions:**   Take at the same times each day, preferably following
the morning and evening meals. The tablet may be crushed for
administration. Do not discontinue this drug abruptly.

Usual Duration of Use: Continual use on a regular schedule for 10 to 14
days is usually necessary to determine this drug's effectiveness in lowering blood pressure. The long-term use (months to years) of this drug
will be determined by the course of your blood pressure over time
and your response to the overall treatment program (weight reduction, salt restriction, smoking cessation, etc.). Consult your physician
on a regular basis.

Possible Advantages of This Drug
Decreases blood pressure more promptly than other beta blocker drugs.
Can be used to treat hypertensive emergencies.

Currently a "Drug of Choice" for initiating treatment of hypertension with
a single drug.

▷ **This Drug Should Not Be Taken If**
• you have had an allergic reaction to it previously.
• you have active bronchial asthma.
• you have congestive heart failure.
• you have an abnormally slow heart rate or a serious form of heart
block.

▷ **Inform Your Physician Before Taking This Drug If**
• you have had an adverse reaction to any beta blocker drug in the
past (see Drug Class, Section Four).
• you have a history of serious heart disease, with or without episodes
of heart failure.
• you have a history of hay fever (allergic rhinitis), asthma, chronic
bronchitis or emphysema.
• you have a history of overactive thyroid function (hyperthyroidism).
• you have a history of low blood sugar (hypoglycemia).
• you have impaired liver or kidney function.
• you have diabetes or myasthenia gravis.

- you are currently taking any form of digitalis, quinidine or reserpine, or any calcium blocker drug (see Drug Class, Section Four).
- you plan to have surgery under general anesthesia in the near future.

Possible Side-Effects (natural, expected and unavoidable drug actions)
Lethargy and fatigability (11%), light-headedness in upright position (see Orthostatic Hypotension in Glossary).

▷ **Possible Adverse Effects** (unusual, unexpected and infrequent reactions)
If any of the following develop, consult your physician promptly for guidance.
Mild Adverse Effects
Allergic Reactions: Skin rash, itching.
Headache, drowsiness, dizziness (20%), scalp tingling (during early treatment).
Indigestion, nausea, diarrhea.
Joint and muscle discomfort, fluid retention (edema).
Serious Adverse Effects
Chest pain, shortness of breath, precipitation of congestive heart failure.
Induction of bronchial asthma (in asthmatic individuals).
Liver damage with jaundice (rare).
Difficult urination (urinary bladder retention).

▷ **Possible Effects on Sexual Function**
Impotence (10%), inhibited ejaculation (10%), prolonged erection following orgasm (related to higher doses), Peyronie's disease (see Glossary).
Decreased vaginal secretions (with low doses), inhibited female orgasm (related to higher doses).

CAUTION
1. **Do not discontinue this drug suddenly** without the knowledge and guidance of your physician. Carry a notation on your person that you are taking this drug.
2. Consult your physician or pharmacist before using nasal decongestants usually present in over-the-counter cold preparations and nose drops. These can cause sudden increases in blood pressure when taken concurrently with beta blocker drugs.
3. Report the development of any tendency to emotional depression.

Precautions for Use
By Infants and Children: Safety and effectiveness for use by those under 12 years of age have not been established. However, if this drug is used, observe for the development of low blood sugar (hypoglycemia) during periods of reduced food intake.
By Those over 60 Years of Age: Proceed *cautiously* with all antihypertensive drugs. Unacceptably high blood pressure should be reduced without creating the risks associated with excessively low blood pressure. Start treatment with small doses, and monitor the blood pressure response frequently. Sudden, rapid and excessive reduction of blood

pressure can predispose to stroke or heart attack. Observe for dizziness, unsteadiness, tendency to fall, confusion, hallucinations, depression or urinary frequency.

▷ **Advisability of Use During Pregnancy**
Pregnancy Category: C (tentative). See Pregnancy Code inside back cover.
Animal studies: No significant increase in birth defects found in rats or rabbits; some increase in fetal deaths reported.
Human studies: Information from adequate studies of pregnant women is not available.
Use this drug only if clearly needed. Ask physician for guidance.

Advisability of Use if Breast-Feeding
Presence of this drug in breast milk: Yes, in very small amounts.
Avoid drug or refrain from nursing.

Habit-Forming Potential: None.

Effects of Overdosage: Weakness, slow pulse, low blood pressure, fainting, cold and sweaty skin, congestive heart failure, possible coma and convulsions.

Possible Effects of Long-Term Use: Reduced heart reserve and eventual heart failure in susceptible individuals with advanced heart disease.

Suggested Periodic Examinations While Taking This Drug (at physician's discretion)
Measurements of blood pressure, evaluation of heart function.

▷ **While Taking This Drug, Observe the Following**
Foods: No restrictions. Avoid excessive salt intake.
Beverages: No restrictions. May be taken with milk.
▷   *Alcohol:* Use with caution until the combined effect has been determined. Alcohol may exaggerate this drug's ability to lower blood pressure and may increase its mild sedative effect.
Tobacco Smoking: Nicotine may reduce this drug's effectiveness in treating high blood pressure. In addition, high doses of this drug may potentiate the constriction of the bronchial tubes caused by regular smoking.
▷   *Other Drugs*
Labetalol may *increase* the effects of
• other antihypertensive drugs and cause excessive lowering of blood pressure. Dosage adjustments may be necessary.
Labetalol *taken concurrently* with
• clonidine (Catapres) requires close monitoring for rebound high blood pressure if clonidine is withdrawn while labetalol is still being taken.
• insulin requires close monitoring to avoid undetected hypoglycemia (see Glossary).
▷   *Driving, Hazardous Activities:* Use caution until the full extent of fatigue, dizziness and blood pressure change has been determined.

Aviation Note: The use of this drug *is a disqualification* for piloting. Consult a designated Aviation Medical Examiner.

Exposure to Sun: No restrictions.

Exposure to Heat: Caution advised. Hot environments can lower the blood pressure and exaggerate the effects of this drug.

Exposure to Cold: Caution advised. Cold environments can enhance the circulatory deficiency in the extremities that may occur with some beta blocker drugs. The elderly should take precautions to prevent hypothermia (see Glossary).

Heavy Exercise or Exertion: It is advisable to avoid exertion that produces light-headedness, excessive fatigue or muscle cramping. The use of this drug may intensify the hypertensive response to isometric exercise.

Occurrence of Unrelated Illness: The fever that accompanies systemic infections can lower the blood pressure and require adjustment of dosage. Illnesses that cause nausea or vomiting may interrupt the regular dosage schedule. Ask your physician for guidance.

Discontinuation: It is advisable to avoid sudden discontinuation of this drug in all situations. If possible, gradual reduction of dose over a period of 2 to 3 weeks is recommended. Ask your physician for specific guidance.

LEVODOPA
(lee voh DOH pa)

Introduced: 1967

Class: Antiparkinsonism

Prescription: USA: Yes
Canada: Yes

Controlled Drug: USA: No
Canada: No

Available as Generic: USA: Yes
Canada: No

Brand Names: Dopar, Larodopa, ✦Prolopa [CD], Sinemet [CD]

BENEFITS versus RISKS	
Possible Benefits	*Possible Risks*
EFFECTIVE RELIEF OF SYMPTOMS IN 80% OF CASES OF IDIOPATHIC PARKINSON'S DISEASE	Emotional depression, confusion, abnormal thinking and behavior Abnormal involuntary movements Heart rhythm disturbance Urinary bladder retention Induction of peptic ulcer (rare) Blood cell abnormalities: hemolytic anemia, reduced white blood cell count (both rare)

▷ **Principal Uses**

As a Single Drug Product: Used exclusively to treat the major types of Parkinson's disease: paralysis agitans ("shaking palsy" of unknown cause), the type that follows encephalitis, the parkinsonism that develops with aging (associated with hardening of the brain arteries), and the forms of parkinsonism that follow poisoning by carbon monoxide or manganese.

As a Combination Drug Product [CD]: This drug is available in combination with carbidopa, a chemical that prevents the decomposition of levodopa before it reaches its site of action in the brain. The addition of carbidopa reduces the amount of levodopa required by 75%. This combination is more effective in smaller doses and reduces the frequency and severity of adverse effects.

How This Drug Works: Not completely established. Present thinking is that levodopa enters the brain tissue and is converted to dopamine. After sufficient dosage, this corrects the deficiency of dopamine (that is thought to be the cause of parkinsonism) and restores a more normal balance of the chemicals responsible for transmission of nerve impulses in appropriate control centers of the brain.

Available Dosage Forms and Strengths
Capsules — 100 mg, 250 mg, 500 mg
Tablets — 100 mg, 250 mg, 500 mg

▷ **Usual Adult Dosage Range:** Initially, 250 mg 2 to 4 times/day. The dose may be increased cautiously by increments of 100 to 750 mg at 3- to 7-day intervals as needed and tolerated. The total dosage should not exceed 8000 mg/24 hours. If the combination drug Sinemet is used, the total levodopa requirement will be considerably less. **Note: Actual dosage and administration schedule must be determined by the physician for each patient individually.**

▷ **Dosing Instructions:** Preferably taken with or following carbohydrate foods to reduce stomach irritation; when possible, do not take this drug concurrently with high-protein foods. The tablet may be crushed for administration.

Usual Duration of Use: Continual use on a regular schedule for 3 to 6 weeks is usually necessary to determine this drug's effectiveness in relieving the major symptoms of parkinsonism. The determination of maximal effectiveness may require continual use for 6 months. Long-term use (months to years) requires supervision and periodic evaluation by your physician; dosage adjustments will be necessary and unavoidable during the course of the disorder. Consult your physician on a regular basis.

▷ **This Drug Should Not Be Taken If**
- you are allergic to any of the drugs bearing the brand names listed.
- you have narrow-angle glaucoma (inadequately controlled).

- you are taking, or have taken within the past 14 days, any monoamine oxidase (MAO) type A inhibitor drug (see Drug Class, Section Four).

▷ **Inform Your Physician Before Taking This Drug If**
- you have diabetes, epilepsy, heart disease, high blood pressure or chronic lung disease.
- you have impaired liver or kidney function.
- you have a history of peptic ulcer disease or malignant melanoma.
- you plan to have surgery under general anesthesia in the near future.

Possible Side-Effects (natural, expected and unavoidable drug actions)
Fatigue, lethargy, altered taste, offensive body odor, orthostatic hypotension (see Glossary).
Pink to red coloration of urine, turning black on exposure to air (of no significance).

▷ **Possible Adverse Effects** (unusual, unexpected and infrequent reactions)
If any of the following develop, consult your physician promptly for guidance.
Mild Adverse Effects
Allergic Reactions: Skin rash, itching.
Headache, dizziness, numbness, unsteadiness, insomnia, nightmares, blurred vision, double vision.
Loss of appetite, nausea, vomiting, dry mouth, difficult swallowing, excessive gas, diarrhea, constipation.
Loss of hair (rare).
Serious Adverse Effects
Idiosyncratic Reaction: Hemolytic anemia (see Glossary).
Confusion, delusions, hallucinations, agitation, paranoia, depression, psychotic episodes, seizures.
Abnormal involuntary movements of the head, face and extremities.
Disturbances of heart rhythm, high blood pressure (rare).
Development of peptic ulcer, gastrointestinal bleeding.
Urinary bladder retention.
Abnormally low white blood cell count—lowered resistance to infection, fever, sore throat.

▷ **Possible Effects on Sexual Function:** Increased libido reported by both males and females (24% to 36%); inhibited ejaculation (rare); priapism (see Glossary).

▷ **Adverse Effects That May Mimic Natural Diseases or Disorders**
Mental reactions may resemble idiopathic psychosis.

Natural Diseases or Disorders That May Be Activated by This Drug
Latent peptic ulcer.

CAUTION
1. To reduce the high frequency of serious adverse effects, it is advisable to begin treatment with small doses, and to increase dosage gradually until the desired response is achieved.

2. As improvement occurs, avoid excessive and hurried activity (which often causes falls and injury).

Precautions for Use

By Infants and Children: This drug can cause precocious puberty when taken by the prepubertal boy. Observe closely for hypersexual behavior and for premature growth of the genital organs.

By Those over 60 Years of Age: Treatment should begin with half of the usual adult dose; dosage increases should be made cautiously in small increments as needed and tolerated. Observe for the possible development of significant behavioral changes: depression or inappropriate elation, acute confusion, agitation, paranoia, dementia, nightmares and hallucinations. Abnormal involuntary movements may also occur.

▷ Advisability of Use During Pregnancy

Pregnancy Category: C (tentative). See Pregnancy Code inside back cover.

Animal studies: Significant birth defects reported in rodent studies.

Human studies: Information from adequate studies of pregnant women is not available.

Avoid use of drug during the first 3 months. Use only if clearly needed during the last 6 months.

Advisability of Use if Breast-Feeding

Presence of this drug in breast milk: Yes.

Avoid drug or refrain from nursing.

Habit-Forming Potential: None.

Effects of Overdosage: Muscle twitching, spastic closure of eyelids, nausea, vomiting, diarrhea, weakness, fainting, confusion, agitation, hallucinations.

Possible Effects of Long-Term Use: Development of abnormal involuntary movements involving the head, face, mouth and extremities. These may be reversible and may gradually subside as the drug is withdrawn.

Suggested Periodic Examinations While Taking This Drug (at physician's discretion)

Complete blood cell counts; measurements of internal eye pressure; blood pressure measurements in lying, sitting and standing positions.

▷ While Taking This Drug, Observe the Following

Foods: No restrictions. Insofar as possible, do not take concurrently with protein foods; proteins compete for absorption.

Nutritional Support: If taken alone (without carbidopa), monitor for the development of peripheral neuritis and take small supplements of pyridoxine (vitamin B-6) if needed: 10 mg or less; larger doses can decrease the effectiveness of levodopa. If taken in combination with carbidopa (Sinemet), supplemental pyridoxine is not required.

Beverages: No restrictions. May be taken with milk.
▷ *Alcohol:* No interactions expected.
Tobacco Smoking: No interactions expected.
Marijuana Smoking: Increased fatigue and lethargy; possible accentuation of orthostatic hypotension (see Glossary).
▷ *Other Drugs*
Levodopa *taken concurrently* with
- monoamine oxidase (MAO) type A inhibitor drugs (see Drug Class, Section Four) may cause a dangerous rise in blood pressure and body temperature. Do not use these drugs concurrently.

The following drugs may *decrease* the effects of levodopa
- papaverine (Cerespan, Pavabid, Vasospan, etc.).
- phenytoin (Dilantin, etc.).
- pyridoxine (vitamin B-6).

▷ *Driving, Hazardous Activities:* This drug may cause dizziness, impaired vision and orthostatic hypotension. Restrict activities as necessary.
Aviation Note: Parkinson's disease *is a disqualification* for piloting. Consult a designated Aviation Medical Examiner.
Exposure to Sun: No restrictions.
Exposure to Heat: Use caution. This drug can cause flushing and excessive sweating and predispose to heat exhaustion.
Occurrence of Unrelated Illness: Suspicious dark-colored skin lesions should be evaluated carefully to exclude the possibility of malignant melanoma. During the course of any intercurrent infection, monitor the white blood cell count carefully for normal response.

LISINOPRIL
(li SIN oh pril)

Introduced: 1988

Class: Antihypertensive, ACE inhibitor

Prescription: USA: Yes

Controlled Drug: USA: No

Available as Generic: No

Brand Names: Prinivil, Prinzide [CD], Zestoretic [CD], Zestril

BENEFITS versus RISKS	
Possible Benefits	*Possible Risks*
EFFECTIVE CONTROL OF MILD TO SEVERE HIGH BLOOD PRESSURE	Headache (5.3%), dizziness (6.3%), fatigue (3.3%)
	Low blood pressure (1.8%)
	Allergic swelling of face, tongue, throat, vocal cords (0.1%)

▷ **Principal Uses**

As a Single Drug Product: Used primarily to treat all degrees of high blood pressure. Mild to moderate high blood pressure usually responds to low doses; severe high blood pressure may require higher doses and the concurrent use of a thiazide or other class of antihypertensive drug.

How This Drug Works: Not completely known. It is thought that by blocking certain enzyme systems that influence arterial function, this drug contributes to the relaxation of arterial walls throughout the body and thus lowers the resistance to blood flow that causes high blood pressure. This, in turn, reduces the workload of the heart and improves its performance.

Available Dosage Forms and Strengths

Tablets — 5 mg, 10 mg, 20 mg, 40 mg

▷ **Usual Adult Dosage Range:**   Initially 10 mg once daily for those not taking a diuretic; 5 mg once daily for those taking a diuretic. Usual maintenance dose is 20 to 40 mg/day taken in a single dose. Total daily dosage should not exceed 80 mg. **Note: Actual dosage and administration schedule must be determined by the physician for each patient individually.**

▷ **Dosing Instructions:**   Take on an empty stomach or with food, at same time each day. The tablet may be crushed for administration.

Usual Duration of Use: Continual use on a regular schedule for several weeks is usually necessary to determine this drug's effectiveness in controlling high blood pressure. The proper treatment of high blood pressure usually requires the long-term use of effective medications. Consult your physician on a regular basis.

Possible Advantages of This Drug

Controls blood pressure effectively with one daily dose.
Relatively low incidence of adverse effects.
No adverse influence on asthma, cholesterol blood levels or diabetes.
Sudden withdrawal does not result in a rapid increase in blood pressure.

▷ **This Drug Should Not Be Taken If**

- you have had an allergic reaction to it previously.
- you currently have a blood cell or bone marrow disorder.
- you have an abnormally high level of blood potassium.

▷ **Inform Your Physician Before Taking This Drug If**

- you have a history of kidney disease or impaired kidney function.
- you have scleroderma or systemic lupus erythematosus.
- you have cerebral artery disease.
- you have any form of heart disease.

- you are taking any of the following drugs: other antihypertensives, diuretics, nitrates or potassium supplements.
- you plan to have surgery under general anesthesia in the near future.

Possible Side-Effects (natural, expected and unavoidable drug actions)
Dizziness (6.3%), orthostatic hypotension (1.4%) (see Glossary), increased blood potassium level (2.2%).

▷ **Possible Adverse Effects** (unusual, unexpected and infrequent reactions)
If any of the following develop, consult your physician promptly for guidance.
Mild Adverse Effects
Allergic Reactions: Skin rash (1.5%), itching (0.3% to 1.0%).
Headache (5.3%), fatigue (3.3%), numbness and tingling (0.8%), weakness (1.3%).
Chest pain (1.3%), palpitation (0.3% to 1.0%), cough (2.9%).
Indigestion (1.0%), nausea (2.3%), vomiting (1.3%), diarrhea (3.2%).
Serious Adverse Effects
Allergic Reactions: Swelling (angioedema) of face, tongue and/or vocal cords (less than 0.1%); can be life-threatening.
Impairment of kidney function (0.3% to 1.0%).

▷ **Possible Effects on Sexual Function:** Decreased libido (0.2%), impotence (0.7%).

CAUTION
1. Consult your physician regarding the advisability of discontinuing other antihypertensive drugs (especially diuretics) for 1 week before starting this drug.
2. **Report promptly** any indications of infection (fever, sore throat), and any indications of water retention (weight gain, puffiness, swollen feet or ankles).
3. Do not use a salt substitute without your physician's knowledge and approval. (Many salt substitutes contain potassium.)
4. It is advisable to obtain blood cell counts and urine analyses **before** starting this drug.

Precautions for Use
By Infants and Children: Safety and effectiveness for use by those in this age group have not been established.
By Those over 60 Years of Age: Small doses are advisable until tolerance has been determined. Sudden and excessive lowering of blood pressure can predispose to stroke or heart attack in those with impaired brain circulation or coronary artery heart disease.

▷ **Advisability of Use During Pregnancy**
Pregnancy Category: C (tentative). See Pregnancy Code inside back cover.
Animal studies: No birth defects found in mouse or rat studies. Impaired bone formation found in rabbit studies.

Human studies: Information from adequate studies of pregnant women is not available.
Avoid during first 3 months if possible.

Advisability of Use if Breast-Feeding
Presence of this drug in breast milk: Unknown.
Avoid drug or refrain from nursing.

Habit-Forming Potential: None.

Effects of Overdosage: Excessive drop in blood pressure, light-headedness, dizziness, fainting.

Possible Effects of Long-Term Use: Gradual increase in blood potassium level.

Suggested Periodic Examinations While Taking This Drug (at physician's discretion)
Before starting drug: Complete blood cell counts; urine analysis with measurement of protein content; blood potassium level.
During use of drug: Blood cell counts; measurements of blood potassium.

▷ **While Taking This Drug, Observe the Following**
Foods: Consult physician regarding salt intake.
Nutritional Support: **Do not take** potassium supplements unless directed by your physician.
Beverages: No restrictions. May be taken with milk.
▷   *Alcohol:* Use caution until combined effect has been determined. Alcohol may enhance the blood-pressure-lowering effect of this drug.
Tobacco Smoking: No interactions expected.
▷   *Other Drugs*
Lisinopril *taken concurrently* with
- potassium preparations (K-Lyte, Slow-K, etc.) may cause increased blood levels of potassium with risk of serious heart rhythm disturbances.
- potassium-sparing diuretics: amiloride (Moduretic), spironolactone (Aldactazide), triamterene (Dyazide) may cause increased blood levels of potassium with risk of serious heart rhythm disturbances.
▷   *Driving, Hazardous Activities:* Usually no restrictions. Be aware of possible drops in blood pressure with resultant dizziness or faintness.
Aviation Note: The use of this drug **may be a disqualification** for piloting. Consult a designated Aviation Medical Examiner.
Exposure to Sun: Caution advised. A similar drug of this class can cause photosensitivity.
Exposure to Heat: Caution advised. Avoid excessive perspiring with resultant loss of body water and drop in blood pressure.
Occurrence of Unrelated Illness: Report promptly any disorder that causes nausea, vomiting or diarrhea. Fluid and chemical imbalances must be corrected as soon as possible.

Discontinuation: This drug may be stopped abruptly without causing a sudden increase in blood pressure. However, you should consult your physician regarding withdrawal of this drug for any reason.

LITHIUM
(LITH i um)

Introduced: 1949

Prescription: USA: Yes
Canada: Yes

Available as Generic: USA: Yes
Canada: No

Class: Antidepressant, antimanic

Controlled Drug: USA: No
Canada: No

Brand Names: ♦Carbolith, Cibalith-S, ♦Duralith, Eskalith, Lithane, ♦Lithizine, Lithobid, Lithonate, Lithotabs

BENEFITS versus RISKS	
Possible Benefits	*Possible Risks*
RAPID REVERSAL OF ACUTE MANIA in 80% of users STABILIZATION OF MOOD in 60% to 70% of users with manic-depressive disorder Prevention of recurrent depression in "responders"	VERY NARROW MARGIN BETWEEN TREATMENT AND TOXIC BLOOD LEVELS POTENTIALLY FATAL TOXICITY with inadequate monitoring Infrequent induction of diabetes mellitus, hypothyroidism Diabetes insipidus–like syndrome (excessive dilute urine without sugar)

▷ **Principal Uses**

As a Single Drug Product: Used primarily in the management of manic-depressive disorders. While its principal use is the prompt correction of acute mania, it is also used to stabilize these disorders by reducing the frequency and severity of recurrent manic-depressive mood swings. It is also beneficial in treating the depression phase of these disorders in individuals who do not experience the manic phase. Additional uses (experimental) include the prevention of cluster headaches and the stimulation of production of white blood cells.

How This Drug Works: Not completely established. It is thought that lithium may act to correct chemical imbalances in certain nerve impulse transmitters (dopamine and norepinephrine) that influence emotional status and behavior.

Available Dosage Forms and Strengths
Capsules — 150 mg, 300 mg, 600 mg
Syrup — 8 mEq per 5-ml teaspoonful
Tablets — 300 mg
Tablets, prolonged-action — 300 mg, 450 mg

▷ **Usual Adult Dosage Range:** First day: 300 mg taken 3 times, 6 hours apart; second day and thereafter: increase dose to 1200 mg/24 hours and later to 1800 mg/24 hours if needed and tolerated. The usual maintenance dose is 600 to 1200 mg/24 hours taken in 3 divided doses. The total daily dosage should not exceed 3600 mg. **Note: Actual dosage and administration schedule must be determined by the physician for each patient individually.**

▷ **Dosing Instructions:** May be taken after meals to reduce stomach irritation. The capsules may be opened and the regular tablets may be crushed for administration; the prolonged-action tablets should be swallowed whole and not altered.

Usual Duration of Use: Continual use on a regular schedule for 1 to 3 weeks is usually necessary to determine this drug's effectiveness in correcting acute mania; several months of continual treatment may be required to correct depression. Long-term use (months to years) requires supervision and periodic evaluation by your physician. Consult your physician on a regular basis.

Currently a "Drug of Choice" for the treatment of acute mania in bipolar manic-depressive disorders.

▷ **This Drug Should Not Be Taken If**
- you have had an allergic reaction to any dosage form of it previously.
- you have uncontrolled diabetes or uncorrected hypothyroidism.
- you are breast-feeding.
- you will be unable to comply with the need for regular monitoring of lithium blood levels.

▷ **Inform Your Physician Before Taking This Drug If**
- you have a history of a schizophreniclike thought disorder.
- you have any type of organic brain disease, or a history of grand mal epilepsy.
- you have diabetes, heart disease, hypothyroidism or impaired kidney function.
- you are on a salt-restricted diet.
- you are pregnant or planning pregnancy.
- you are taking any diuretic drug or a cortisonelike steroid preparation.

Possible Side-Effects (natural, expected and unavoidable drug actions)
Increased thirst and urine volume may occur in 60% of initial users and in 20% of long-term maintenance users. Weight gain may occur in

first few months of use. Drowsiness and lethargy may occur in sensitive individuals.

▷ **Possible Adverse Effects** (unusual, unexpected and infrequent reactions)
If any of the following develop, consult your physician promptly for guidance.

Mild Adverse Effects
Allergic Reactions: Skin rashes, generalized itching.
Skin dryness, loss of hair.
Headache, dullness, dizziness, weakness, blurred vision, ringing in ears, fine hand tremor, unsteadiness.
Metallic taste, loss of appetite, stomach irritation, nausea, vomiting, diarrhea.

Serious Adverse Effects
"Blackout" spells, confusion, stupor, slurred speech, spasmodic movements of extremities, epilepticlike seizures.
Loss of bladder or rectal control.
Diabetes insipidus–like syndrome: loss of kidney concentrating power, excessive dilute urine.

▷ **Possible Effects on Sexual Function:**   Decreased libido (blood level of 0.7 to 0.9 meq/L); inhibited erection: 30% of users (0.6 to 0.8 meq/L); male infertility; female breast swelling with milk production.

▷ **Adverse Effects That May Mimic Natural Diseases or Disorders**
Painful discoloration and coldness of the hands and feet may resemble Raynaud's syndrome.

Natural Diseases or Disorders That May Be Activated by This Drug
Diabetes mellitus may be worsened. Psoriasis may be intensified. Myasthenia gravis may be induced (1 case).

CAUTION
1. This drug has a very narrow margin of safe use. The blood level of drug required to be effective is quite close to the level that can cause toxic effects. Periodic measurements of blood lithium levels are mandatory for appropriate adjustments of dosage. Follow instructions exactly regarding drug dosage and periodic blood examinations.
2. Lithium should be discontinued at the first signs of toxicity: drowsiness, sluggishness, muscle twitching, vomiting or diarrhea.
3. The major causes of lithium toxicity are
   • accidental overdose (sometimes due to inadequate monitoring of blood levels).
   • impaired kidney function.
   • salt restriction.
   • inadequate fluid intake, dehydration.
   • concurrent use of diuretics.
   • intercurrent illness.
   • childbirth (rapid decrease in kidney clearance of lithium).

- initiation of treatment with a new drug.
4. Over-the-counter preparations that contain iodides (some cough products and vitamin-mineral supplements) should be avoided because of the added antithyroid effect when taken with lithium.

Precautions for Use

By Infants and Children: Safety and effectiveness for use by those under 12 years of age have not been established. Follow physician's instructions exactly.

By Those over 60 Years of Age: Initial and maintenance doses should be smaller than standard doses for younger adults; treatment should start with a "test" dose of 75 to 150 mg daily. Observe closely for early indications of toxic effects, especially if on a low-salt diet and using diuretics. Parkinsonian reactions (abnormal gait and movements) occur with greater frequency; coma can develop without warning symptoms.

▷ **Advisability of Use During Pregnancy**

Pregnancy Category: D (tentative). See Pregnancy Code inside back cover.

Animal studies: Cleft palate reported in mice; eye, ear and palate defects reported in rats.

Human studies: Information from adequate studies of pregnant women is not available. However, cardiovascular defects and goiter in newborn infants (of mothers using lithium) have been reported. If the infant's blood level of lithium approaches the toxic range before delivery, the newborn may suffer the "floppy infant" syndrome: weakness, lethargy, unresponsiveness, low body temperature, weak cry and poor feeding ability.

Avoid use of drug during the first 3 months. Use only if clearly necessary during the last 6 months. Monitor mother's blood lithium levels carefully to avoid possible toxicity.

Advisability of Use if Breast-Feeding

Presence of this drug in breast milk: Yes, in significant amounts.
Avoid drug or refrain from nursing.

Habit-Forming Potential: None.

Effects of Overdosage: Drowsiness, weakness, lack of coordination, nausea, vomiting, diarrhea, muscle spasms, blurred vision, dizziness, staggering gait, slurred speech, confusion, stupor, coma, seizures.

Possible Effects of Long-Term Use: Hypothyroidism (5%), goiter, reduced sugar tolerance, diabetes insipidus–like syndrome, serious kidney damage.

Suggested Periodic Examinations While Taking This Drug (at physician's discretion)

Regular determinations of blood lithium levels are absolutely essential to the safe and effective use of this drug.

Periodic evaluation of thyroid gland size and function.
Complete blood cell counts; kidney function tests.

▷ **While Taking This Drug, Observe the Following**
  Foods: Maintain a normal diet; **do not** restrict your use of salt.
  Beverages: No restrictions. Drink at least 2.5 to 3 quarts of liquids/24 hours. This drug may be taken with milk.
▷ *Alcohol:* Use with caution until the combined effects have been determined. Avoid alcohol completely if any symptoms of lithium toxicity develop.
  Tobacco Smoking: No interactions expected.
  Marijuana Smoking: Possible increase in apathy, lethargy, drowsiness or sluggishness; accentuation of lithium-induced tremor; possible increased risk of precipitating psychotic behavior.
▷ *Other Drugs* Lithium *taken concurrently* with
  • carbamazepine (Tegretol) or with
  • chlorpromazine (Thorazine, etc.) or with
  • haloperidol (Haldol) is usually well tolerated; however, it may cause a severe neurotoxic reaction in susceptible individuals. These combinations should be used very cautiously.
  • diazepam (Valium) may cause hypothermia.
  The following drugs may *increase* the effects of lithium
  • indomethacin (Indocin).
  • piroxicam (Feldene).
  • thiazide diuretics (see Drug Class, Section Four).
  The following drugs may *decrease* the effects of lithium
  • sodium bicarbonate.
  • theophylline (Theo-Dur, etc.) and related drugs.
▷ *Driving, Hazardous Activities:* This drug may impair mental alertness, judgment, physical coordination and reaction time. Restrict activities as necessary.
  Aviation Note: The use of this drug *is a disqualification* for piloting. Consult a designated Aviation Medical Examiner.
  Exposure to Sun: No restrictions.
  Exposure to Heat: Excessive sweating can cause significant depletion of salt and water and resultant lithium toxicity. Avoid sauna baths.
  Occurrence of Unrelated Illness: Any illness that causes fever, sweating, vomiting or diarrhea can result in significant alterations of blood and tissue lithium concentrations. Close monitoring of your physical condition and blood lithium levels is necessary to prevent serious toxicity.
  Discontinuation: Sudden discontinuation does not cause withdrawal symptoms. Avoid premature discontinuation; some individuals may require continual treatment for up to a year to achieve maximal response. Discontinuation by "responders" may result in recurrence of either mania or depression. Lithium should be discontinued if symptoms of brain toxicity appear or if an uncorrectable diabetes insipidus–like syndrome develops.

LOPERAMIDE
(loh PER a mide)

Introduced: 1977   **Class:** Antidiarrheal

Prescription: USA: Yes   **Controlled Drug:** USA: No
    Canada: No   Canada: No

Available as Generic: No

Brand Names: Imodium, Imodium A-D

BENEFITS versus RISKS	
Possible Benefits	*Possible Risks*
EFFECTIVE RELIEF OF INTESTINAL CRAMPING AND DIARRHEA	Drowsiness Constipation Induction of toxic megacolon

▷ **Principal Uses**

As a Single Drug Product: Used primarily for the control of cramping and diarrhea associated with acute gastroenteritis and chronic enteritis and colitis. Also used to reduce the volume of discharge from ileostomies.

How This Drug Works: Not completely established. It is thought that this drug acts directly on the nerve supply of the gastrointestinal tract to reduce its motility and propulsive contractions, thus relieving cramping and diarrhea.

Available Dosage Forms and Strengths
    Capsules — 2 mg
    Liquid — 1 mg per 5-ml teaspoonful (alcohol 5.25%)

▷ **Usual Adult Dosage Range:**   For acute diarrhea: 4 mg initially, then 2 mg after each unformed stool until diarrhea is controlled. For chronic diarrhea: 4 to 8 mg/day in divided doses, taken 8 to 12 hours apart. The total daily dosage should not exceed 16 mg. **Note: Actual dosage and administration schedule must be determined by the physician for each patient individually.**

▷ **Dosing Instructions:**   May be taken on an empty stomach or with food if stomach irritation occurs. The capsule may be opened for administration.

Usual Duration of Use: Continual use on a regular schedule for 48 hours is usually necessary to determine this drug's effectiveness in controlling acute diarrhea; continual use for 10 days may be needed to evaluate its effectiveness in controlling chronic diarrhea. If diarrhea persists, consult your physician.

▷ **This Drug Should Not Be Taken If**
  • you have had an allergic reaction to it previously.
  • it is prescribed for a child under 2 years of age.

▷ **Inform Your Physician Before Taking This Drug If**
  • you have a history of liver disease or impaired liver function.
  • you have regional enteritis or ulcerative colitis.

  Possible Side-Effects (natural, expected and unavoidable drug actions)
  Drowsiness, constipation.

▷ **Possible Adverse Effects** (unusual, unexpected and infrequent reactions)
  If any of the following develop, consult your physician promptly for guidance.
  Mild Adverse Effects
  Allergic Reaction: Skin rash.
  Fatigue, dizziness.
  Reduced appetite, dry mouth, nausea, vomiting, stomach pain, bloating.
  Serious Adverse Effects
  "Toxic megacolon" (distended, immobile colon with fluid retention) may develop while treating acute ulcerative colitis.

▷ **Possible Effects on Sexual Function:** None reported.

  CAUTION
  1. Do not exceed recommended doses.
  2. If used to treat chronic diarrhea, report promptly any development of bloating, abdominal distension, nausea, vomiting, constipation or abdominal pain.

  Precautions for Use
  By Infants and Children: Do not use in those under 2 years of age. Follow physician's instructions exactly regarding dosage. Observe for drowsiness, irritability, personality changes and altered behavior.
  By Those over 60 Years of Age: Start treatment with small doses. You may be more sensitive to the sedative and constipating effects of this drug.

▷ **Advisability of Use During Pregnancy**
  Pregnancy Category: B (tentative). See Pregnancy Code inside back cover.
  Animal studies: No birth defects found in rat and rabbit studies.
  Human studies: Information from adequate studies of pregnant women is not available.
  Use sparingly and only if clearly needed. Ask physician for guidance.

  Advisability of Use if Breast-Feeding
  Presence of this drug in breast milk: Unknown.
  Avoid drug or refrain from nursing.

  Habit-Forming Potential: None.

  Effects of Overdosage: Drowsiness, lethargy, depression, dry mouth.

Possible Effects of Long-Term Use: None identified.

Suggested Periodic Examinations While Taking This Drug (at physician's discretion)
    None required.

▷ **While Taking This Drug, Observe the Following**
    Foods: No restrictions. Follow prescribed diet.
    Beverages: No restrictions. May be taken with milk.
▷ *Alcohol:* Use with caution until combined effects have been determined. This drug may increase the depressant action of alcohol on the brain.
    Tobacco Smoking: No interactions expected.
▷ *Other Drugs:* No significant drug interactions reported.
▷ *Driving, Hazardous Activities:* This drug may cause drowsiness or dizziness. Restrict activities as necessary.
    Aviation Note: The use of this drug *is a disqualification* for piloting. Consult a designated Aviation Medical Examiner.
    Exposure to Sun: No restrictions.

LORAZEPAM
(lor AZ e pam)

Introduced: 1971

Class: Mild tranquilizer, benzodiazepines

Prescription: USA: Yes
    Canada: Yes

Controlled Drug: USA: C-IV*
    Canada: No

Available as Generic: USA: Yes
    Canada: No

Brand Names: Alzapam, ✦Apo-Lorazepam, Ativan, Loraz, ✦Novolorazepam

---

BENEFITS versus RISKS

Possible Benefits	*Possible Risks*
RELIEF OF ANXIETY AND NERVOUS TENSION in 70% to 80% of users	Habit-forming potential with prolonged use
Wide margin of safety with therapeutic doses	Minor impairment of mental functions
Very few drug interactions	

---

*See Schedules of Controlled Drugs inside back cover.

▷ **Principal Uses**

As a Single Drug Product: Used primarily to provide short-term relief of mild to moderate anxiety. While it is less sedative than the barbiturates, it is also used at bedtime to produce a calming effect that permits natural sleep.

How This Drug Works: It is thought that this drug produces a calming effect by enhancing the action of the nerve transmitter gamma-aminobutyric acid (GABA), which in turn blocks the arousal of higher brain centers.

Available Dosage Forms and Strengths

Injection — 2 mg per ml, 4 mg per ml
Tablets — 0.5 mg, 1 mg, 2 mg

▷ **Usual Adult Dosage Range:** 1 to 10 mg/24 hours. For anxiety: 2 to 3 mg, 2 or 3 times/day. For insomnia: 2 to 4 mg at bedtime. The total daily dose should not exceed 10 mg. **Note: Actual dosage and administration schedule must be determined by the physician for each patient individually.**

▷ **Dosing Instructions:** May be taken on empty stomach or with food or milk. The tablet may be crushed for administration. Do not discontinue this drug abruptly if taken for more than 4 weeks.

Usual Duration of Use: Continual use on a regular schedule for 3 to 5 days is usually necessary to determine this drug's effectiveness in relieving moderate anxiety. Limit continual use to 1 to 3 weeks. Avoid uninterrupted and prolonged use.

▷ **This Drug Should Not Be Taken If**

• you have had an allergic reaction to any dosage form of it previously.
• you have acute narrow-angle glaucoma.
• it is prescribed for a child under 12 years of age.

▷ **Inform Your Physician Before Taking This Drug If**

• you are allergic to any benzodiazepine drug (see Drug Class, Section Four).
• you have a history of alcoholism or drug abuse.
• you are pregnant or planning pregnancy.
• you have impaired liver or kidney function.
• you have a history of serious depression or mental disorder.
• you have any of the following: asthma, emphysema, epilepsy, myasthenia gravis.

Possible Side-Effects (natural, expected and unavoidable drug actions)

Drowsiness, lethargy, unsteadiness, "hangover" effects on the day following bedtime use.

▷ **Possible Adverse Effects** (unusual, unexpected and infrequent reactions)

If any of the following develop, consult your physician promptly for guidance.

Mild Adverse Effects
Allergic Reaction: Skin rash.
Dizziness (6%), fainting, blurred vision, double vision, slurred speech, headache, sweating, nausea, indigestion.
Serious Adverse Effects
Disorientation, emotional depression, agitation, disturbed sleep, periodic amnesia.

▷ **Possible Effects on Sexual Function:**   Antianxiety effect can relieve nervous tension that is often responsible for male impotence and female vaginismus (painful spasm of vagina), thus improving sexual performance. (Impaired sexual functioning relieved in 40%.)

CAUTION
1. This drug should not be discontinued abruptly if it has been taken continually for more than 4 weeks.
2. The concurrent use of some over-the-counter drug products that contain antihistamines (allergy and cold preparations, sleep aids) can cause excessive sedation in sensitive individuals.
3. If this drug is taken at bedtime as a hypnotic, significant impairment of intellectual and motor functions may persist into the following day; avoid hazardous activities and the use of alcohol.

Precautions for Use
By Infants and Children: Safety and effectiveness for use by those under 12 years of age have not been established. This drug should not be used in the hyperactive or psychotic child of any age. Observe for excessive sedation and incoordination.
By Those over 60 Years of Age: It is advisable to use smaller doses at longer intervals to avoid overdosage. Observe for the possible development of lethargy, indifference, fatigue, weakness, unsteadiness, disturbing dreams, nightmares and paradoxical reactions of excitement, agitation, anger, hostility and rage.

▷ **Advisability of Use During Pregnancy**
Pregnancy Category: C (tentative). See Pregnancy Code inside back cover.
Animal studies: Skeletal and eye defects reported in rabbits.
Human studies: Information from adequate studies of pregnant women is not available. No birth defects have been reported with the use of this drug.
Avoid drug completely during the first 3 months; avoid during the last 6 months if possible. Frequent use in late pregnancy may cause the "floppy infant" syndrome in the newborn: weakness, lethargy, unresponsiveness, depressed breathing, low body temperature.

Advisability of Use if Breast-Feeding
Presence of this drug in breast milk: Yes, in small amounts.
Monitor nursing infant closely and discontinue drug or nursing if adverse effects develop.

Habit-Forming Potential: This drug can produce psychological and/or physical dependence (see Glossary) if used in large doses for an extended period of time.

Effects of Overdosage: Marked drowsiness, weakness, feeling of drunkenness, staggering gait, tremor, stupor progressing to deep sleep or coma.

Possible Effects of Long-Term Use: Psychological and/or physical dependence.

Suggested Periodic Examinations While Taking This Drug (at physician's discretion)
Complete blood cell counts and liver function tests during long-term use. (Other drugs of this class are known to cause blood cell and liver function disorders rarely.)

▷ **While Taking This Drug, Observe the Following**
Foods: No restrictions.
Beverages: Avoid excessive intake of caffeine-containing beverages: coffee, tea, cola. May be taken with milk.
▷ *Alcohol:* Use with extreme caution until the combined effect is determined. Alcohol may increase the absorption of this drug and add to its depressant effects on the brain. It is advisable to avoid alcohol completely—throughout the day and night—if it is necessary to drive or to engage in any hazardous activity.
Tobacco Smoking: Heavy smoking may reduce the calming action of this drug.
Marijuana Smoking: Increased sedation and significant impairment of intellectual and physical performance.
▷ *Other Drugs*
Lorazepam may *increase* the effects of
• other sedatives, hypnotics, tranquilizers, anticonvulsants and narcotic drugs; excessive sedation may result.
▷ *Driving, Hazardous Activities:* This drug can impair mental alertness, judgment, physical coordination and reaction time. Avoid hazardous activities accordingly.
Aviation Note: The use of this drug *is a disqualification* for piloting. Consult a designated Aviation Medical Examiner.
Exposure to Sun: No restrictions.
Exposure to Heat: Use caution until the effect of excessive perspiration is determined. Because of reduced urine volume, this drug may accumulate in the body and produce effects of overdosage.
Discontinuation: Avoid sudden discontinuation if this drug has been taken for over 4 weeks without interruption. Dosage should be tapered gradually to prevent a withdrawal syndrome that could include depression, confusion, hallucinations, tremor, seizures, muscle cramping, sweating and vomiting.

LOVASTATIN
(loh vah STA tin)

Introduced: 1987

Class: Anticholesterol

Prescription: USA: Yes

Controlled Drug: USA: No

Available as Generic: USA: No

Brand Name: Mevacor

BENEFITS versus RISKS

Possible Benefits	*Possible Risks*
EFFECTIVE REDUCTION OF TOTAL BLOOD CHOLESTEROL in selected individuals	Drug-induced hepatitis (without jaundice) 1.9% Drug-induced myositis (muscle inflammation) 0.5% Drug-induced stomach ulceration (rare)

▷ **Principal Uses**

As a Single Drug Product: Used primarily to reduce abnormally high total blood cholesterol levels in individuals with Types IIa and IIb hypercholesterolemia. It is used in conjunction with a cholesterol-lowering diet. It should not be used until a trial of nondrug methods for lowering cholesterol has proved to be inadequate.

How This Drug Works: This drug is converted in the body to mevolinic acid, which inhibits the liver enzyme that initiates the production of cholesterol. Its principal action is the reduction of low-density lipoproteins (LDL), the fraction of total blood cholesterol that is thought to increase the risk of coronary heart disease. This drug may or may not increase the level of high-density lipoproteins (HDL), the cholesterol fraction that is thought to reduce the risk of heart disease.

Available Dosage Forms and Strengths
Tablets — 20 mg, 40 mg

▷ **Usual Adult Dosage Range:**   Initially 20 mg once a day; dose may be increased up to 40 mg twice a day as needed and tolerated. Dosage adjustments should be made at 4-week intervals. The total daily dosage should not exceed 80 mg. **Note: Actual dosage and administration schedule must be determined by the physician for each patient individually.**

▷ **Dosing Instructions:**   Take with food, preferably with the evening meal for maximal effectiveness. (The highest rates of cholesterol production occur between midnight and 5 a.m.) The tablet may be crushed for administration.

Usual Duration of Use: Continual use on a regular schedule for 4 to 6 weeks is usually necessary to determine this drug's effectiveness in reducing blood levels of total and LDL cholesterol. Long-term use (months to years) requires periodic evaluation of response and dosage adjustment. Consult your physician on a regular basis.

Possible Advantages of This Drug: Recent studies indicate that this drug is more effective and better tolerated than other drugs currently available for reducing total and LDL cholesterol. Its long-term effects are yet to be determined. See Cholesterol Disorders in Section Two.

▷ **This Drug Should Not Be Taken If**
- you have had an allergic reaction to it previously.
- you have active liver disease.
- you have active peptic ulcer disease.
- you are pregnant or breast-feeding.

▷ **Inform Your Physician Before Taking This Drug If**
- you have a history of liver disease or impaired liver function.
- you have a history of peptic ulcer disease or upper gastrointestinal bleeding.
- you are not using any method of birth control, or you are planning pregnancy.
- you regularly consume substantial amounts of alcohol.
- you have cataracts or impaired vision.
- you have any type of chronic muscular disorder.

Possible Side-Effects (natural, expected and unavoidable drug actions)
Development of abnormal liver function tests without associated symptoms.

▷ **Possible Adverse Effects** (unusual, unexpected and infrequent reactions)
If any of the following develop, consult your physician promptly for guidance.
Mild Adverse Effects
Allergic Reactions: Skin rash, itching (5.2%).
Headache (9.3%), dizziness (2.0%), blurred vision (1.5%), altered taste (0.8%).
Indigestion (3.9%), stomach pain (5.7%), nausea (4.7%), excessive gas (6.4%), constipation (4.9%), diarrhea (5.5%).
Muscle cramps and/or pain (2.4%).
Serious Adverse Effects
Marked and persistent abnormal liver function tests with focal hepatitis (without jaundice) occurred in 1.9% after 1 year of use.
Acute myositis (muscle pain and tenderness) occurred in 0.5% during long-term use.
Cataracts occurred in 8% after 5 to 15 months of continual use; a cause-and-effect relationship (see Glossary) has not been established.
Stomach and duodenal ulceration with bleeding have been reported in a few cases.

▷ **Possible Effects on Sexual Function:**   None reported.

Possible Delayed Adverse Effects: None reported to date.

Natural Diseases or Disorders That May Be Activated by This Drug
Latent liver disease; latent peptic ulcer disease; latent cataracts (possibly).

CAUTION
1. If pregnancy occurs while taking this drug, discontinue it immediately and consult your physician.
2. Report promptly any development of muscle pain or tenderness, especially if accompanied by fever or malaise.
3. Report promptly the development of altered or impaired vision so that appropriate evaluation can be made.

Precautions for Use
By Infants and Children: Safety and effectiveness for use by those under 20 years of age have not been established.
By Those over 60 Years of Age: Inform your physician regarding any personal or family history of cataracts. Comply with all recommendations regarding periodic eye examinations. Report promptly any alterations in vision.

▷ **Advisability of Use During Pregnancy**
Pregnancy Category: X. See Pregnancy Code inside back cover.
Animal studies: Mouse and rat studies reveal skeletal birth defects due to this drug.
Human studies: Information from adequate studies of pregnant women is not available.
This drug should be avoided during entire pregnancy.

Advisability of Use if Breast-Feeding
Presence of this drug in breast milk: Probably yes.
Avoid drug or refrain from nursing.

Habit-Forming Potential: None.

Effects of Overdosage: Increased indigestion, stomach distress, nausea, diarrhea.

Possible Effects of Long-Term Use: Abnormal liver function with focal hepatitis.

Suggested Periodic Examinations While Taking This Drug (at physician's discretion)
Blood cholesterol studies: total cholesterol, HDL and LDL fractions.
Liver function tests every 4 to 6 weeks during the first 15 months of use and periodically thereafter.
Complete eye examination at beginning of treatment and periodically thereafter. Ask your physician for guidance.

▷ **While Taking This Drug, Observe the Following**
  Foods: Follow a standard low-cholesterol diet.
  Beverages: No restrictions. May be taken with milk.
▷ *Alcohol:* No interactions expected. Use sparingly.
  Tobacco Smoking: No interactions expected.
▷ *Driving, Hazardous Activities:* This drug may cause dizziness or impaired vision. Restrict activities as necessary.
  Aviation Note: The use of this drug **may be a disqualification** for piloting. Consult a designated Aviation Medical Examiner.
  Exposure to Sun: No restrictions.
  Discontinuation: Do not discontinue this drug without your physician's knowledge and guidance.

MAPROTILINE
(ma PROH ti leen)

Introduced: 1974

Class: Antidepressant

Prescription: USA: Yes
Canada: Yes

Controlled Drug: USA: No
Canada: No

Available as Generic: No

Brand Name: Ludiomil

BENEFITS versus RISKS

Possible Benefits	*Possible Risks*
EFFECTIVE RELIEF OF ALL TYPES OF DEPRESSION	ADVERSE BEHAVIORAL EFFECTS: confusion, disorientation, hallucinations
CONVERSION OF DEPRESSION TO MANIA in manic-depressive disorders
Irregular heart rhythms
Rare liver toxicity with jaundice

▷ **Principal Uses**
  As a Single Drug Product: To relieve the symptoms associated with spontaneous (endogenous) depression and with reactive depressions, and to initiate the restoration of normal mood. This drug should be used only when a diagnosis of true depression of significant degree has been established. It should not be used to treat mild and transient despondency that may be associated with many life situations in the absence of a bona fide affective illness.

How This Drug Works: It is thought that this drug relieves depression by slowly restoring the nerve impulse transmitter norepinephrine to normal levels within brain tissue.

Available Dosage Forms and Strengths
Tablets — 10 mg (in Canada), 25 mg, 50 mg, 75 mg

▷ **Usual Adult Dosage Range:**   Initially 25 mg 3 times daily. Dose may be increased cautiously as needed and tolerated by 10 to 25 mg daily at intervals of 1 week. Usual maintenance dose is 50 to 100 mg/24 hours. The total daily dose should not exceed 150 mg. When the optimal requirement is determined, it may be taken at bedtime as one dose. **Note: Actual dosage and administration schedule must be determined by the physician for each patient individually.**

▷ **Dosing Instructions:**   May be taken without regard to meals. Tablet may be crushed for administration.

Usual Duration of Use: Some benefit may be apparent within 1 to 2 weeks, but adequate response may require continual use for 4 to 6 weeks or longer. Long-term use should not exceed 6 months without evaluation regarding the need for continuation of the drug. Consult your physician on a regular basis.

▷ **This Drug Should Not Be Taken If**
- you have had an allergic reaction to it previously.
- you are taking or have taken within the past 14 days any monoamine oxidase (MAO) type A inhibitor drug (see Drug Class, Section Four).
- you are recovering from a recent heart attack.

▷ **Inform Your Physician Before Taking This Drug If**
- you are allergic or overly sensitive to any tricyclic antidepressant (see Drug Class, Section Four).
- you have a history of any of the following: alcoholism, asthma, epilepsy, glaucoma, heart disease, paranoia, prostate gland enlargement, schizophrenia or overactive thyroid function.
- you have impaired liver function.
- you plan to have surgery under general anesthesia in the near future.

Possible Side-Effects (natural, expected and unavoidable drug actions)
Drowsiness, blurred vision, dry mouth, constipation, impaired urination.

▷ **Possible Adverse Effects** (unusual, unexpected and infrequent reactions)
If any of the following develop, consult your physician promptly for guidance.
Mild Adverse Effects
Allergic Reactions: Skin rash, itching.
Insomnia, nervousness, palpitations, dizziness, unsteadiness, tremors, fainting, weakness.

Nausea, vomiting, acid indigestion, diarrhea.
Increased sweating.
Serious Adverse Effects
Behavioral effects: anxiety, confusion, hallucinations.
Aggravation of paranoid psychosis and schizophrenia.
Aggravation of seizure disorders (epilepsy).
Liver toxicity with jaundice (see Glossary).

▷ **Possible Effects on Sexual Function:** Decreased libido, increased libido (antidepressant effect), impotence, male breast enlargement and tenderness, female breast enlargement with milk production, swelling of testicles.

▷ **Adverse Effects That May Mimic Natural Diseases or Disorders**
The development of jaundice may suggest viral hepatitis.

Natural Diseases or Disorders That May Be Activated by This Drug
Latent epilepsy, glaucoma, prostatism (see Glossary).

CAUTION
1. Dosage must be adjusted for each person individually. Report for follow-up evaluation and laboratory tests as directed by your physician.
2. Observe for early indications of toxicity: confusion, agitation, rapid heartbeat.
3. It is advisable to withhold this drug if electroconvulsive therapy (ECT, "shock" treatment) is to be used to treat your depression.

Precautions for Use
By Infants and Children: Safety and effectiveness for use by those under 18 years of age have not been established.
By Those over 60 Years of Age: During the first 2 weeks of treatment, observe for the development of confusion, agitation, forgetfulness, disorientation, delusions and hallucinations. Reduction of dosage or discontinuation may be necessary. Unsteadiness may predispose to falling and injury. This drug can increase the degree of impaired urination associated with prostate gland enlargement (prostatism).

▷ **Advisability of Use During Pregnancy**
Pregnancy Category: B (tentative). See Pregnancy Code inside back cover.
Animal studies: No birth defects found in mouse, rat or rabbit studies.
Human studies: Information from adequate studies of pregnant women is not available.
Avoid use of drug during first 3 months. Use during the last 6 months only if clearly needed.

Advisability of Use if Breast-Feeding
Presence of this drug in breast milk: Yes.
Monitor nursing infant closely for drowsiness or failure to feed properly; discontinue drug or nursing if adverse effects develop.

Habit-Forming Potential: None.

Effects of Overdosage: Confusion, hallucinations, marked drowsiness, heart palpitations, dilated pupils, tremors, stupor, deep sleep, coma, convulsions.

Suggested Periodic Examinations While Taking This Drug (at physician's discretion)
Complete blood cell counts, liver function tests, serial blood pressure readings and electrocardiograms.

▷ **While Taking This Drug, Observe the Following**
Foods: No restrictions.
Beverages: No restrictions. May be taken with milk.
▷   *Alcohol:* Avoid completely. This drug can markedly increase the intoxicating effects of alcohol and accentuate its depressant action on brain function.
Tobacco Smoking: No interactions expected.
Marijuana Smoking: Increased drowsiness and dryness of mouth; possible reduced effectiveness of this drug.
▷   *Other Drugs*
Maprotiline may **increase** the effects of
   • atropinelike drugs (see Drug Class, Section Four).
   • all drugs with sedative effects, and cause excessive sedation.
Maprotiline may **decrease** the effects of
   • clonidine (Catapres).
   • guanethidine (Ismelin).
   • methyldopa (Aldomet).
   • reserpine (Serpasil, Ser-Ap-Es, etc.).
Maprotiline **taken concurrently** with
   • amphetaminelike drugs may cause severe high blood pressure and/or high fever (see Drug Class, Section Four).
   • antiseizure drugs requires careful monitoring for change in seizure patterns; dosage adjustments may be necessary.
   • ethchlorvynol (Placidyl) may cause delirium; avoid concurrent use.
   • monoamine oxidase (MAO) type A inhibitor drugs may cause high fever, delirium and convulsions (see Drug Class, Section Four).
   • thyroid preparations may impair heart rhythm and function.
Ask physician for guidance regarding adjustment of thyroid dose.
The following drugs may **decrease** the effects of maprotiline
   • estrogens.
   • oral contraceptives.
▷   *Driving, Hazardous Activities:* This drug may impair mental alertness, judgment, physical coordination and reaction time. Avoid hazardous activities.
Aviation Note: The use of this drug **is a disqualification** for piloting. Consult a designated Aviation Medical Examiner.
Exposure to Sun: Use caution until sensitivity to sun has been determined. This drug may cause photosensitivity (see Glossary).

Exposure to Heat: This drug can inhibit sweating and impair the body's adaptation to hot environments, increasing the risk of heat stroke. Avoid saunas.

Exposure to Cold: The elderly should use caution and avoid conditions conducive to hypothermia (see Glossary).

Discontinuation: It is advisable to discontinue this drug gradually. Abrupt withdrawal after long-term use may cause headache, malaise and nausea.

MECLIZINE
(MEK li zeen)

Other Name: Meclozine

Introduced: 1951

Class: Antinausea, antivertigo, antihistamines

Prescription: USA: Varies
Canada: Yes

Controlled Drug: USA: No
Canada: No

Available as Generic: USA: Yes
Canada: No

Brand Names: Antivert, ✦Bonamine, Bonine, Ru-Vert-M

BENEFITS versus RISKS	
Possible Benefits	*Possible Risks*
EFFECTIVE PREVENTION OF MOTION SICKNESS	Mild sedation
Moderately effective relief of nausea and vertigo	Mild atropinelike effects

▷ **Principal Uses**

As a Single Drug Product: Used primarily to control dizziness and vertigo associated with disorders of the inner ear. Also used to prevent or relieve the nausea, vomiting and dizziness characteristic of motion sickness.

As a Combination Drug Product [CD]: This drug is available in Canada in combination with niacin (nicotinic acid), which is added because of its ability to dilate blood vessels and (theoretically) improve circulation.

How This Drug Works: Not completely established. It is thought that this drug reduces the sensitivity of the nerve pathways connecting the organ of equilibrium in the inner ear with the vomiting center in the brain; this prevents or reduces the occurrence of nausea, vomiting and vertigo.

Available Dosage Forms and Strengths
Tablets — 12.5 mg, 25 mg, 50 mg
Tablets, chewable — 25 mg

▷ **Usual Adult Dosage Range:**   12.5 to 25 mg, once or twice daily as needed for vertigo. For motion sickness: 25 to 50 mg taken 1 hour before travel; repeat once daily if needed. Total daily dosage should not exceed 100 mg. **Note: Actual dosage and administration schedule must be determined by the physician for each patient individually.**

▷ **Dosing Instructions:**   May be taken without regard to food. The regular tablet may be crushed for administration.

Usual Duration of Use: Continual use on a regular schedule for 2 to 4 days is usually necessary to determine this drug's effectiveness in relieving vertigo or preventing motion sickness. Duration of use should not exceed 5 days if this drug is not effective.

▷ **This Drug Should Not Be Taken If**
- you have had an allergic reaction to it previously.
- you are taking, or have taken within the past 14 days, any monoamine oxidase (MAO) type A inhibitor drug (see Drug Class, Section Four).
- you are, or think you may be, pregnant.

▷ **Inform Your Physician Before Taking This Drug If**
- you have had an unfavorable response to any antihistamine drug in the past.
- you have any of the following: asthma, epilepsy, glaucoma, peptic ulcer disease, prostate gland enlargement.

Possible Side-Effects (natural, expected and unavoidable drug actions)
Mild drowsiness, lethargy, impaired concentration, dry mouth, constipation.

▷ **Possible Adverse Effects** (unusual, unexpected and infrequent reactions)
If any of the following develop, consult your physician promptly for guidance.
Mild Adverse Effects
Allergic Reactions: No significant reactions identified.
Blurred vision.
Serious Adverse Effects
Possible increase in prostatism (see Glossary).

▷ **Possible Effects on Sexual Function:**   None reported.

Natural Diseases or Disorders That May Be Activated by This Drug
Latent epilepsy, glaucoma, prostatism.

CAUTION
1. Discontinue this drug 5 days before diagnostic skin testing for allergies.
2. Avoid this drug completely in children with flulike infections or chicken pox. Although a cause-and-effect relationship has not been established, this drug may contribute to the development of Reye syndrome (see Glossary) in susceptible children.

Precautions for Use
By Infants and Children: Safety and effectiveness for use by those under 12 years of age have not been established. See *CAUTION.*

By Those over 60 Years of Age: Observe for increased susceptibility to drowsiness, dizziness and impaired thinking, judgment and memory; the antihistamine-sedative effect can cause a hypoactive syndrome that may be mistaken for emotional depression or senility.

▷ **Advisability of Use During Pregnancy**
Pregnancy Category: C (tentative). See Pregnancy Code inside back cover.
Animal studies: Significant birth defects reported in mouse, rat and ferret studies.
Human studies: Information from studies of pregnant women is inconclusive. No increase in birth defects was reported in 2076 exposures in 2 studies; 12 cleft lips or palates were reported in 3333 exposures in another study.
Avoid this drug completely during the first 3 months. Use it during the last 6 months only if clearly needed. **Note:** This drug is *contraindicated* during pregnancy by one manufacturer.

Advisability of Use if Breast-Feeding
Presence of this drug in breast milk: Unknown.
Avoid drug or refrain from nursing.

Habit-Forming Potential: None.

Effects of Overdosage: Marked drowsiness, confusion, unsteadiness, tremors, stupor progressing to coma; in children: excitement, hallucinations, overactivity, seizures.

Possible Effects of Long-Term Use: Development of tolerance and loss of effectiveness.

Suggested Periodic Examinations While Taking This Drug (at physician's discretion)
None required.

▷ **While Taking This Drug, Observe the Following**
Foods: No restrictions.
Beverages: No restrictions. May be taken with milk.
▷   *Alcohol:* Use with extreme caution until the combined effects have been determined. The combination of alcohol and antihistamines can cause rapid and marked sedation.

Tobacco Smoking: No interactions expected.

▷ *Other Drugs*

Meclizine may *increase* the effects of
- all other drugs with atropinelike effects.
- all other drugs with sedative effects.

The following drugs may *increase* the effects of meclizine:
- monoamine oxidase (MAO) type A inhibitor drugs may prolong its atropinelike effects (see Drug Class, Section Four).

▷ *Driving, Hazardous Activities:* This drug may impair mental alertness, judgment, physical coordination and reaction time. Restrict activities as necessary.

Aviation Note: The use of this drug *is a disqualification* for piloting. Consult a designated Aviation Medical Examiner.

Exposure to Sun: No restrictions.

MECLOFENAMATE
(me kloh fen AM ayt)

Introduced: 1977   **Class:** Mild analgesic, anti-inflammatory

Prescription: USA: Yes   **Controlled Drug:** USA: No

Available as Generic: Yes

Brand Names: Meclodium, Meclomen

BENEFITS versus RISKS	
Possible Benefits	*Possible Risks*
EFFECTIVE RELIEF OF MILD TO MODERATE PAIN AND INFLAMMATION	Gastrointestinal pain, ulceration, bleeding (rare)
	Rare liver or kidney damage
	Rare fluid retention
	Rare bone marrow depression

▷ **Principal Uses**

As a Single Drug Product: Used primarily to relieve mild to moderately severe pain and inflammation associated with acute and chronic rheumatoid arthritis and osteoarthritis. Also used to relieve mild to moderate pain of any cause.

How This Drug Works: Not completely established. It is thought that this drug reduces the tissue concentrations of prostaglandins (and related compounds), chemicals involved in the production of inflammation and pain.

Available Dosage Forms and Strengths
Capsules — 50 mg, 100 mg

▷ **Usual Adult Dosage Range:**   200 to 400 mg daily, in 3 or 4 divided doses. Total daily dosage should not exceed 400 mg. **Note: Actual dosage and administration schedule must be determined by the physician for each patient individually.**

▷ **Dosing Instructions:**   Take with food or milk to prevent stomach irritation. Take with a full glass of water and remain upright (do not lie down) for 30 minutes. The capsule may be opened for administration.

Usual Duration of Use: Continual use on a regular schedule for 2 to 3 weeks is usually necessary to determine this drug's effectiveness in relieving the discomfort of arthritis. Long-term use (months to years) requires supervision and periodic evaluation by your physician. Consult your physician on a regular basis.

▷ **This Drug Should Not Be Taken If**
  • you have had an allergic reaction to it previously.
  • you are subject to asthma or nasal polyps caused by aspirin.
  • you have active peptic ulcer disease, regional enteritis, ulcerative colitis or any form of gastrointestinal bleeding.
  • you have a bleeding disorder or a blood cell disorder.
  • you have severe impairment of kidney function.

▷ **Inform Your Physician Before Taking This Drug If**
  • you are allergic to aspirin or to other aspirin substitutes.
  • you have a history of peptic ulcer disease, regional enteritis or ulcerative colitis.
  • you have a history of any type of bleeding disorder.
  • you have impaired liver or kidney function.
  • you have high blood pressure or a history of heart failure.
  • you are taking any of the following: acetaminophen, aspirin or other aspirin substitutes, anticoagulants, oral antidiabetic drugs or cortisonelike drugs.

Possible Side-Effects (natural, expected and unavoidable drug actions)
Ringing in ears, fluid retention.

▷ **Possible Adverse Effects** (unusual, unexpected and infrequent reactions)
  If any of the following develop, consult your physician promptly for guidance.
  Mild Adverse Effects
  Allergic Reactions: Skin rash, hives, itching.
  Headache, dizziness, altered or blurred vision, depression.
  Mouth sores, indigestion, nausea, vomiting (11%), diarrhea (10% to 33%).
  Serious Adverse Effects
  Allergic Reactions: Severe skin reactions, drug fever (see Glossary).
  Active peptic ulcer, with or without bleeding.

Liver damage with jaundice (see Glossary).

Kidney damage with painful urination, bloody urine, reduced urine formation.

Rare bone marrow depression (see Glossary)—fatigue, weakness, fever, sore throat, abnormal bleeding or bruising.

▷ **Possible Effects on Sexual Function**   None reported.

Possible Delayed Adverse Effects: Mild anemia due to "silent" blood loss from the stomach (less than that caused by aspirin).

▷ **Adverse Effects That May Mimic Natural Diseases or Disorders**
Liver reaction may suggest viral hepatitis.

Natural Diseases or Disorders That May Be Activated by This Drug
Peptic ulcer disease, ulcerative colitis.

CAUTION
1. Dosage should always be limited to the smallest amount that produces reasonable improvement.
2. This drug may mask early indications of infection. Inform your physician if you think you are developing an infection of any kind.

Precautions for Use
By Infants and Children: Safety and effectiveness for use by those under 14 years of age have not been established.
By Those over 60 Years of Age: Small doses are advisable until tolerance is determined. Observe for any indications of liver or kidney toxicity, fluid retention, dizziness, confusion, impaired memory, stomach bleeding or diarrhea.

▷ **Advisability of Use During Pregnancy**
Pregnancy Category: B (tentative). See Pregnancy Code inside back cover.
Animal studies: Some minor birth defects reported in rodents.
Human studies: Information from adequate studies of pregnant women is not available.
Avoid this drug during the first and last 3 months. Use it during the second 3 months only if clearly needed. Ask physician for guidance.
The manufacturer does not recommend the use of this drug during pregnancy.

Advisability of Use if Breast-Feeding
Presence of this drug in breast milk: Unknown.
Avoid drug or refrain from nursing.

Habit-Forming Potential: None.

Effects of Overdosage: Drowsiness, nausea, vomiting, diarrhea, marked agitation, irrational behavior, seizures.

Possible Effects of Long-Term Use: None identified.

Suggested Periodic Examinations While Taking This Drug (at physician's discretion)
Complete blood cell counts, liver and kidney function tests, complete eye examinations if vision is altered in any way.

▷ **While Taking This Drug, Observe the Following**
Foods: No restrictions.
Beverages: No restrictions. May be taken with milk.
▷ *Alcohol:* Use with caution. The irritant action of alcohol on the stomach lining, added to the irritant action of this drug in sensitive individuals, can increase the risk of stomach ulceration and/or bleeding.
Tobacco Smoking: No interactions expected.
▷ *Other Drugs*
Meclofenamate may *increase* the effects of
- acetaminophen (Tylenol, etc.), and increase the risk of kidney damage; avoid prolonged use of this combination.
- anticoagulants (Coumadin, etc.), and increase the risk of bleeding; monitor prothrombin time, adjust dose accordingly.

Meclofenamate *taken concurrently* with the following drugs may increase the risk of bleeding; avoid these combinations:
- aspirin.
- dipyridamole (Persantine).
- sulfinpyrazone (Anturane).
- valproic acid (Depakene).

▷ *Driving, Hazardous Activities:* This drug may cause dizziness or altered vision. Restrict activities as necessary.
Aviation Note: The use of this drug *may be a disqualification* for piloting. Consult a designated Aviation Medical Examiner.
Exposure to Sun: No restrictions.

MEDROXYPROGESTERONE
(me DROX ee proh JESS te rohn)

Introduced: 1959

Class: Female sex hormones, progestins

Prescription: USA: Yes
Canada: Yes

Controlled Drug: USA: No
Canada: No

Available as Generic: Yes

Brand Names: Amen, Curretab, Provera

BENEFITS versus RISKS

Possible Benefits	*Possible Risks*
EFFECTIVE TREATMENT OF ABSENT OR ABNORMAL MENSTRUATION due to hormone imbalance	Thrombophlebitis (rare)
	Pulmonary embolism (rare)
	Liver reaction with jaundice (rare)
EFFECTIVE CONTRACEPTION when given by injection	Drug-induced birth defects
Useful adjunctive therapy in selected cases of uterine and kidney cancer	

▷ **Principal Uses**

As a Single Drug Product: Used primarily to initiate and regulate menstruation and to correct abnormal patterns of menstrual bleeding caused by hormonal imbalance (and not by organic disease). The injectable form of this drug is a very effective contraceptive (but is not approved for this use in the USA).

How This Drug Works: By inducing and maintaining a lining in the uterus that resembles pregnancy, this drug can prevent uterine bleeding until it is withdrawn. By suppressing the release of the pituitary gland hormone that induces ovulation, and by stimulating the secretion of mucus by the uterine cervix (to resist the passage of sperm), this drug can prevent pregnancy.

Available Dosage Forms and Strengths

Tablets — 2.5 mg, 5 mg, 10 mg

▷ **Usual Adult Dosage Range:** To initiate menstruation: 5 to 10 mg/day for 5 to 10 days, started at any time; to correct abnormal bleeding: 5 to 10 mg/day for 5 to 10 days, started on the sixteenth or twenty-first day of the menstrual cycle. Withdrawal bleeding usually begins within 3 to 7 days after stopping the drug. **Note: Actual dosage and administration schedule must be determined by the physician for each patient individually.**

▷ **Dosing Instructions:** Take on an empty stomach or with food to prevent nausea. The tablet may be crushed for administration.

Usual Duration of Use: Continual use on a regular schedule for 2 or 3 menstrual cycles is usually necessary to determine this drug's effectiveness in correcting abnormal patterns of menstrual bleeding. Consult your physician on a regular basis.

▷ **This Drug Should Not Be Taken If**
- you have had an allergic reaction to it previously.
- you are pregnant.
- you have seriously impaired liver function.

- you have a history of cancer of the breast or reproductive organs.
- you have a history of thrombophlebitis, embolism or stroke.
- you have abnormal and unexplained vaginal bleeding.

▷ **Inform Your Physician Before Taking This Drug If**
- you have impaired kidney function.
- you have any of the following disorders: asthma, diabetes, emotional depression, epilepsy, heart disease, migraine headaches.

Possible Side-Effects (natural, expected and unavoidable drug actions)
Fluid retention, weight gain, changes in menstrual timing and flow, spotting between periods.

▷ **Possible Adverse Effects** (unusual, unexpected and infrequent reactions)
If any of the following develop, consult your physician promptly for guidance.
Mild Adverse Effects
Allergic Reactions: Skin rash, hives, itching.
Fatigue, weakness, nausea.
Acne, excessive hair growth.
Serious Adverse Effects
Liver toxicity with jaundice (see Glossary): yellow eyes and skin, dark-colored urine, light-colored stools.
Thrombophlebitis (inflammation of a vein with blood clot formation): pain or tenderness in thigh or leg, with or without swelling of the foot, ankle or leg.
Pulmonary embolism (movement of blood clot to lung): sudden shortness of breath, chest pain, cough, bloody sputum.
Stroke (blood clot in the brain): sudden headache, blackouts, sudden weakness or paralysis of any part of the body, severe dizziness, double vision, slurred speech, inability to speak.
Retinal thrombosis (blood clot in principal blood vessel to the eye): sudden impairment or loss of vision.

▷ **Possible Effects on Sexual Function**
Altered timing and pattern of menstruation.
Female breast tenderness and secretion.
Decreased vaginal secretions.

▷ **Adverse Effects That May Mimic Natural Diseases or Disorders**
Liver toxicity may suggest viral hepatitis.

CAUTION
1. There is an increased risk of birth defects in children whose mothers take this drug during the first 4 months of pregnancy.
2. Inform your physician promptly if you think you may be pregnant.
3. This drug should not be used as a test for pregnancy.

Precautions for Use

By Infants and Children: Not used in this age group.

By Those over 60 Years of Age: Used selectively as adjunctive therapy in treating cancer of the breast, uterus and kidney. Observe for excessive fluid retention.

▷ **Advisability of Use During Pregnancy**

Pregnancy Category: X. See Pregnancy Code inside back cover.

Animal studies: Genital defects reported in rat and rabbit studies; masculinization of the female rodent fetus; various defects in chick embryo and rabbit.

Human studies: Masculinization of the female genitals: enlargement of the clitoris, fusion of the labia. Increased risk of heart, nervous system and limb defects also reported.

Avoid this drug completely during entire pregnancy.

Advisability of Use if Breast-Feeding

Presence of this drug in breast milk: Yes.

Avoid drug or refrain from nursing.

Habit-Forming Potential: None.

Effects of Overdosage: Nausea, vomiting, fluid retention, breast enlargement and discomfort, abnormal vaginal bleeding.

Possible Effects of Long-Term Use: None reported in humans.

Suggested Periodic Examinations While Taking This Drug (at physician's discretion)

Regular examinations (every 6 to 12 months) of the breasts and reproductive organs (pelvic examination of the uterus and ovaries, including Pap smear).

▷ **While Taking This Drug, Observe the Following**

Foods: No restrictions.

Beverages: No restrictions.

▷ *Alcohol:* No interactions expected.

Tobacco Smoking: It is advisable to smoke lightly or not at all.

▷ *Other Drugs*

The following drugs may **decrease** the effects of medroxyprogesterone
• rifampin (Rifadin, Rimactane, etc.) may hasten its elimination.

▷ *Driving, Hazardous Activities:* Usually no restrictions. Consult your physician for assessment of individual risk and for guidance regarding specific restrictions.

Aviation Note: The use of this drug **may be a disqualification** for piloting. Consult a designated Aviation Medical Examiner.

Exposure to Sun: No restrictions.

MEPERIDINE
(me PER i deen)

Other Name: Pethidine

Introduced: 1939   **Class:** Strong analgesic, opioids

Prescription: USA: Yes   **Controlled Drug:** USA: C-II*
     Canada: Yes   Canada: <N>

Available as Generic: Yes

Brand Names: Demerol, Demerol APAP [CD], Pethadol

BENEFITS versus RISKS	
Possible Benefits	*Possible Risks*
EFFECTIVE RELIEF OF MODERATE TO SEVERE PAIN	POTENTIAL FOR HABIT FORMATION (DEPENDENCE)
	Weakness, fainting
	Disorientation, hallucinations
	Interference with urination

▷ **Principal Uses**

As a Single Drug Product: This potent analgesic is used by mouth or injection to relieve moderate to severe pain of any cause.

As a Combination Drug Product [CD]: This drug is available in combination with acetaminophen (APAP) to create a dosage form that utilizes two pain relievers, one of which also reduces fever.

How This Drug Works: Acting primarily as a depressant of certain brain functions, this drug suppresses the perception of pain and calms the emotional response to pain.

Available Dosage Forms and Strengths
Injection — 10 mg per ml, 25 mg per ml, 50 mg per ml, 75 mg per ml, 100 mg per ml
Syrup — 50 mg per 5-ml teaspoonful
Tablets — 50 mg, 100 mg

▷ **Usual Adult Dosage Range:** Taken by mouth: 50 to 150 mg/3 to 4 hours as needed to relieve pain; the usual dose is 100 mg. The total daily dosage should not exceed 900 mg. **Note: Actual dosage and administration schedule must be determined by the physician for each patient individually.**

▷ **Dosing Instructions:** May be taken with or following food to reduce stomach irritation or nausea. The tablet may be crushed for administration. The syrup may be diluted in 4 ounces of water to reduce the numbing effect on the tongue and mouth tissues.

*See Schedules of Controlled Drugs inside back cover.

Usual Duration of Use: As required to control pain. Continual use should not exceed 5 to 7 days without interruption and reassessment of need.

▷ **This Drug Should Not Be Taken If**
   - you have had an allergic reaction to any dosage form of it previously.
   - you are having an acute attack of asthma.
   - you are taking, or have taken within the past 14 days, any monoamine oxidase (MAO) type A inhibitor drug (see Drug Class, Section Four).

▷ **Inform Your Physician Before Taking This Drug If**
   - you have a history of drug abuse or alcoholism.
   - you have impaired liver or kidney function.
   - you have a history of asthma, epilepsy or glaucoma.
   - you are taking any other drugs that have a sedative effect.
   - you plan to have surgery under general anesthesia in the near future.

Possible Side-Effects (natural, expected and unavoidable drug actions)
   Drowsiness, light-headedness, weakness, euphoria, dry mouth, urinary retention, constipation.

▷ **Possible Adverse Effects** (unusual, unexpected and infrequent reactions)
   If any of the following develop, consult your physician promptly for guidance.
   Mild Adverse Effects
   Allergic Reactions: Skin rash, hives, itching.
   Headache, dizziness, impaired concentration, sensation of drunkenness, confusion, depression, blurred or double vision.
   Facial flushing, sweating, heart palpitation.
   Nausea, vomiting.
   Serious Adverse Effects
   Drop in blood pressure, causing severe weakness and fainting.
   Disorientation, hallucinations, unstable gait, tremor, muscle twitching.

▷ **Possible Effects on Sexual Function:**   None reported.

▷ **Adverse Effects That May Mimic Natural Diseases or Disorders**
   Paradoxical behavioral disturbances may suggest psychotic disorder.

   CAUTION
   1. If you have asthma, chronic bronchitis or emphysema, the excessive use of this drug may cause significant respiratory difficulty, thickening of bronchial secretions and suppression of coughing.
   2. The concurrent use of this drug with atropinelike drugs can increase the risk of urinary retention and reduced intestinal function.
   3. Do not take this drug following acute head injury.

Precautions for Use
   By Infants and Children: Do not use this drug in infants under 1 year of age because of their vulnerability to life-threatening respiratory depression.

By Those over 60 Years of Age: Use small doses initially and increase dosage as needed and tolerated. Limit use to short-term treatment only if possible. There may be increased susceptibility to the development of drowsiness, dizziness, unsteadiness, falling, urinary retention and constipation (often leading to fecal impaction).

▷ **Advisability of Use During Pregnancy**

Pregnancy Category: C (tentative). See Pregnancy Code inside back cover.
Animal studies: Significant birth defects reported in hamster studies.
Human studies: Information from adequate studies of pregnant women is not available. However, no significant increase in birth defects was found in 1100 exposures to this drug.

Avoid during the first 3 months. Use sparingly and in small doses during the last 6 months only if clearly needed.

Advisability of Use if Breast-Feeding

Presence of this drug in breast milk: Yes.
Avoid drug or refrain from nursing.

Habit-Forming Potential: This drug can cause psychological and physical dependence (see Glossary).

Effects of Overdosage: Marked drowsiness, confusion, tremors, convulsions, stupor progressing to coma.

Possible Effects of Long-Term Use: Psychological and physical dependence, chronic constipation.

Suggested Periodic Examinations While Taking This Drug (at physician's discretion)

None.

▷ **While Taking This Drug, Observe the Following**

Foods: No restrictions.

Beverages: No restrictions. May be taken with milk.

▷   *Alcohol:* Use extreme caution until the combined effects have been determined. Opioid analgesics can intensify the intoxicating effects of alcohol, and alcohol can intensify the depressant effects of opioids on brain function, breathing and circulation. Alcohol is best avoided.

Tobacco Smoking: No interactions expected.

Marijuana Smoking: Increase in drowsiness and pain relief; impairment of mental and physical performance.

▷   *Other Drugs*

Meperidine may ***increase*** the effects of
- other drugs with sedative effects.
- atropinelike drugs, and increase the risk of constipation and urinary retention.

Meperidine ***taken concurrently*** with
- monoamine oxidase (MAO) type A inhibitor drugs (see Drug Class, Section Four) can cause the equivalent of an acute narcotic overdose:

unconsciousness; severe depression of breathing, heart action and circulation. A variation of this reaction can be excitability, convulsions, high fever and rapid heart action.

- phenothiazines (see Drug Class, Section Four) can cause excessive and prolonged depression of brain functions, breathing and circulation.

▷ *Driving, Hazardous Activities:* This drug can impair mental alertness, judgment, reaction time and physical coordination. Avoid hazardous activities.

Aviation Note: The use of this drug **is a disqualification** for piloting. Consult a designated Aviation Medical Examiner.

Exposure to Sun: No restrictions.

Discontinuation: It is advisable to limit this drug to short-term use. If it is necessary to use it for extended periods of time, discontinuation should be gradual to minimize possible effects of withdrawal.

METAPROTERENOL
(met a proh TER e nohl)

Other Name: Orciprenaline

Introduced: 1964

Class: Antiasthmatic, bronchodilator

Prescription: USA: Yes
Canada: Yes

Controlled Drug: USA: No
Canada: No

Available as Generic: Yes

Brand Names: Alupent, Metaprel

BENEFITS versus RISKS	
Possible Benefits	*Possible Risks*
VERY EFFECTIVE RELIEF OF BRONCHOSPASM	Increased blood pressure
	Fine hand tremor
	Irregular heart rhythm (with excessive use)

▷ **Principal Uses**

As a Single Drug Product: To relieve acute bronchial asthma and to reduce the frequency and severity of chronic, recurrent asthmatic attacks; also used to relieve reversible bronchospasm associated with chronic bronchitis and emphysema.

How This Drug Works: By stimulating certain sympathetic nerve terminals, this drug acts to dilate those bronchial tubes that are in sustained constriction, thereby increasing the size of the airway and improving the ability to breathe.

Available Dosage Forms and Strengths
Powder for inhalation — 0.65 mg/inhalation
Solution for nebulizer — 0.6%, 5%
Syrup — 10 mg per 5-ml teaspoonful
Tablets — 10 mg, 20 mg

▷ **Usual Adult Dosage Range:**   Inhaler: 2 or 3 inhalations/3 to 4 hours; do not exceed 12 inhalations/day. Hand nebulizer: 5 to 15 inhalations/4 hours; do not exceed 40 inhalations/day. Syrup and tablets: 20 mg/6 to 8 hours. **Note: Actual dosage and administration schedule must be determined by the physician for each patient individually.**

▷ **Dosing Instructions:**   May be taken on empty stomach or with food or milk. Tablets should not be crushed for administration. For aerosol and nebulizer, follow the written instructions carefully. Do not overuse.

Usual Duration of Use: According to individual requirements. Do not use beyond the time necessary to terminate episodes of asthma.

▷ **This Drug Should Not Be Taken If**
- you have had an allergic reaction to any dosage form of it previously.
- you currently have an irregular heart rhythm.
- you are taking, or have taken within the past 2 weeks, any monoamine oxidase (MAO) type A inhibitor drug (see Drug Class, Section Four).

▷ **Inform Your Physician Before Taking This Drug If**
- you are overly sensitive to other drugs that stimulate the sympathetic nervous system.
- you are currently using epinephrine (Adrenalin, Primatene Mist, etc.) to relieve asthmatic breathing.
- you have any type of heart or circulatory disorder, especially high blood pressure or coronary heart disease.
- you have diabetes or an overactive thyroid gland (hyperthyroidism).
- you are taking any form of digitalis or any stimulant drug.

Possible Side-Effects (natural, expected and unavoidable drug actions)
Aerosol—dryness or irritation of mouth or throat, altered taste.
Tablet—nervousness, palpitation.

▷ **Possible Adverse Effects** (unusual, unexpected and infrequent reactions)
If any of the following develop, consult your physician promptly for guidance.
Mild Adverse Effects
Headache, dizziness, restlessness, insomnia, fine tremor of hands.
Rapid, pounding heartbeat; increased sweating; muscle cramps in arms and legs.
Nausea, heartburn, vomiting.

Serious Adverse Effects

Rapid or irregular heart rhythm, intensification of angina, increased blood pressure.

▷ **Possible Effects on Sexual Function:** None reported.

Natural Diseases or Disorders That May Be Activated By This Drug

Latent coronary artery disease, diabetes or high blood pressure.

CAUTION

1. Concurrent use of this drug by aerosol inhalation with beclomethasone aerosol (Beclovent, Vanceril) may increase the risk of toxicity due to fluorocarbon propellants. It is advisable to use this aerosol 20 to 30 minutes *before* beclomethasone aerosol. This will reduce the risk of toxicity and will enhance the penetration of beclomethasone.

2. *Avoid excessive use of aerosol inhalation.* The excessive or prolonged use of this drug by inhalation can reduce its effectiveness and cause serious heart rhythm disturbances, including cardiac arrest.

3. Do not use this drug concurrently with epinephrine. These two drugs may be used alternately if an interval of 4 hours is allowed between doses.

4. If you do not respond to your usually effective dose, ask your physician for guidance. Do not increase the size or frequency of the dose without your physician's approval.

Precautions for Use

By Infants and Children: Safety and effectiveness of use of the aerosol and nebulized solution have not been established for children under 12 years of age. Safety and effectiveness of use of the syrup and tablet have not been established for children under 6 years of age.

By Those over 60 Years of Age: Avoid excessive and continual use. If acute asthma is not relieved promptly, other drugs will have to be tried. Observe for the development of nervousness, palpitations, irregular heart rhythm and muscle tremors. Use with extreme caution if you have hardening of the arteries, heart disease or high blood pressure.

▷ **Advisability of Use During Pregnancy**

Pregnancy Category: C (tentative). See Pregnancy Code inside back cover.

Animal studies: Significant birth defects reported in rabbit studies.

Human studies: Information from adequate studies of pregnant women is not available.

Avoid use during first 3 months. Use during the last 6 months only if clearly needed.

Advisability of Use if Breast-Feeding

Presence of this drug in breast milk: Unknown.

Avoid drug or refrain from nursing.

Habit-Forming Potential: None.

Effects of Overdosage: Nervousness, palpitation, rapid heart rate, sweating, headache, tremor, vomiting, chest pain.

Possible Effects of Long-Term Use: Loss of effectiveness. See *CAUTION* category.

Suggested Periodic Examinations While Taking This Drug (at physician's discretion)
Blood pressure measurements, evaluation of heart status.

▷ **While Taking This Drug, Observe the Following**
Foods: No restrictions.
Beverages: Avoid excessive use of caffeine-containing beverages: coffee, tea, cola, chocolate.
▷ *Alcohol:* No interactions expected.
Tobacco Smoking: No interactions expected.
▷ *Other Drugs*
Metaproterenol *taken concurrently* with
• monoamine oxidase (MAO) type A inhibitor drugs may cause excessive increase in blood pressure and undesirable heart stimulation.
▷ *Driving, Hazardous Activities:* Usually no restrictions. Use caution if excessive nervousness or dizziness occurs.
Aviation Note: The use of this drug *is a disqualification* for piloting. Consult a designated Aviation Medical Examiner.
Exposure to Sun: No restrictions.
Heavy Exercise or Exertion: Use caution. Excessive exercise can induce asthma in sensitive individuals.

METHADONE
(METH a dohn)

Introduced: 1948

Class: Strong analgesic, opioids

Prescription: USA: Yes

Controlled Drug: USA: C-II*

Available as Generic: Yes

Brand Name: Dolophine

BENEFITS versus RISKS	
Possible Benefits	*Possible Risks*
EFFECTIVE RELIEF OF MODERATE TO SEVERE PAIN	POTENTIAL FOR HABIT FORMATION (DEPENDENCE) Weakness, fainting Disorientation, hallucinations Interference with urination

*See Schedules of Controlled Drugs inside back cover.

▷ **Principal Uses**

As a Single Drug Product: This potent analgesic is used by mouth or injection to relieve moderate to severe pain of any cause. Its primary use today is to provide an appropriate substitute for heroin in treatment programs for drug addiction.

How This Drug Works: Acting primarily as a depressant of certain brain functions, this drug suppresses the perception of pain and calms the emotional response to pain.

Available Dosage Forms and Strengths

Concentrate — 10 mg per ml
Injection — 10 mg per ml
Oral solution — 5 mg, 10 mg per 5-ml teaspoonful (8% alcohol)
Tablets — 5 mg, 10 mg
Tablets, dispersible — 40 mg

▷ **Usual Adult Dosage Range:** Taken by mouth: 2.5 to 10 mg/3 to 4 hours as needed to relieve pain. The total daily dosage should not exceed 80 mg. (Dosage schedules for maintenance treatment during heroin withdrawal must be individualized.) **Note: Actual dosage and administration schedule must be determined by the physician for each patient individually.**

▷ **Dosing Instructions:** May be taken with or following food to reduce stomach irritation or nausea. The tablet may be crushed for administration. The concentrate must be diluted in 3 ounces (or more) of water before swallowing.

Usual Duration of Use: As required to control pain. Continual use should not exceed 5 to 7 days without interruption and reassessment of need.

▷ **This Drug Should Not Be Taken If**
 • you have had an allergic reaction to any dosage form of it previously.
 • you are having an acute attack of asthma.

▷ **Inform Your Physician Before Taking This Drug If**
 • you have a history of drug abuse or alcoholism.
 • you have impaired liver or kidney function.
 • you have a history of asthma or other chronic lung disease.
 • you are taking any other drugs that have a sedative effect.
 • you are taking, or have taken within the past 14 days, any monoamine oxidase (MAO) type A inhibitor drug (see Drug Class, Section Four).
 • you plan to have surgery under general anesthesia in the near future.

Possible Side-Effects (natural, expected and unavoidable drug actions)
Drowsiness, light-headedness, weakness, euphoria, dry mouth, urinary retention, constipation.

▷ **Possible Adverse Effects** (unusual, unexpected and infrequent reactions)
If any of the following develop, consult your physician promptly for guidance.

Mild Adverse Effects
Allergic Reactions: Skin rash, hives, itching.
Headache, dizziness, impaired concentration, sensation of drunkenness, confusion, depression, blurred or double vision.
Facial flushing, sweating, heart palpitation.
Nausea, vomiting.
Serious Adverse Effects
Drop in blood pressure, causing severe weakness and fainting.
Disorientation, hallucinations, unstable gait, tremor, muscle twitching.

▷ **Possible Effects on Sexual Function:** Decreased libido, impotence, delayed ejaculation, inhibited female orgasm, male infertility, loss of menstruation. (These effects do not occur with short-term use for pain relief; however, they are very common with long-term use and addiction.)

▷ **Adverse Effects That May Mimic Natural Diseases or Disorders**
Paradoxical behavioral disturbances may suggest psychotic disorder.

CAUTION
1. If you have asthma, chronic bronchitis or emphysema, the excessive use of this drug may cause significant respiratory difficulty, thickening of bronchial secretions and suppression of coughing.
2. The concurrent use of this drug with atropinelike drugs can increase the risk of urinary retention and reduced intestinal function.
3. Do not take this drug following acute head injury.

Precautions for Use
By Infants and Children: Do not use this drug in infants under 1 year of age because of their vulnerability to life-threatening respiratory depression.
By Those over 60 Years of Age: Use small doses initially and increase dosage as needed and tolerated. Limit use to short-term treatment only if possible. There may be increased susceptibility to the development of drowsiness, dizziness, unsteadiness, falling, urinary retention and constipation (often leading to fecal impaction).

▷ **Advisability of Use During Pregnancy**
Pregnancy Category: C (tentative). See Pregnancy Code inside back cover.
Animal studies: Significant birth defects reported in mice and hamster studies.
Human studies: Information from adequate studies of pregnant women is not available.
Avoid during the first 3 months. Use sparingly and in small doses during the last 6 months only if clearly needed.

Advisability of Use if Breast-Feeding
Presence of this drug in breast milk: Yes.
Avoid drug or refrain from nursing.

Habit-Forming Potential: This drug can cause psychological and physical dependence (see Glossary).

Effects of Overdosage: Marked drowsiness, confusion, tremors, convulsions, stupor progressing to coma.

Possible Effects of Long-Term Use: Psychological and physical dependence, chronic constipation.

Suggested Periodic Examinations While Taking This Drug (at physician's discretion)
None.

▷ **While Taking This Drug, Observe the Following**
Foods: No restrictions.
Beverages: No restrictions. May be taken with milk.

▷ *Alcohol:* Use extreme caution until the combined effects have been determined. Opioid analgesics can intensify the intoxicating effects of alcohol, and alcohol can intensify the depressant effects of opioids on brain function, breathing and circulation. Alcohol is best avoided.

Tobacco Smoking: No interactions expected.

Marijuana Smoking: Increase in drowsiness and pain relief; impairment of mental and physical performance.

▷ *Other Drugs*
Methadone may *increase* the effects of
• other drugs with sedative effects, and cause excessive sedation.
Methadone *taken concurrently* with
• monoamine oxidase (MAO) type A inhibitor drugs (see Drug Class, Section Four) requires cautious observation for indications of nervous system toxicity.
The following drugs may *decrease* the effects of methadone
• phenytoin (Dilantin, etc.).
• rifampin (Rifadin, Rimactane, etc.).

▷ *Driving, Hazardous Activities:* This drug can impair mental alertness, judgment, reaction time and physical coordination. Avoid hazardous activities.

Aviation Note: The use of this drug *is a disqualification* for piloting. Consult a designated Aviation Medical Examiner.

Exposure to Sun: No restrictions.

Discontinuation: It is advisable to limit this drug to short-term use. If it is necessary to use it for extended periods of time, discontinuation should be gradual to minimize possible effects of withdrawal (stomach cramps, tearing eyes, nasal discharge, chills and tremors.

METHOCARBAMOL
(meth oh KAR ba mohl)

Introduced: 1957

Class: Muscle relaxant

Prescription: USA: Yes
Canada: No

Controlled Drug: USA: No
Canada: No

Available as Generic: USA: Yes
Canada: No

Brand Names: ✦Robaxacet [CD], Robaxin, Robaxin-750, Robaxisal [CD], ✦Robaxisal-C [CD]

```
┌─────────────────────────────────────────────────────────────────┐
│                    BENEFITS versus RISKS                          │
│                                                                   │
│       Possible Benefits              Possible Risks               │
│   Mild to moderate relief of     White blood cell reduction (rare)│
│   discomfort due to spasm of     Drowsiness, weakness             │
│   voluntary muscles              Blurred or double vision         │
└─────────────────────────────────────────────────────────────────┘
```

▷ **Principal Uses**
As a Single Drug Product: Used primarily to relieve the pain and stiffness associated with spasm of voluntary muscles, such as that resulting from accidental injury of musculoskeletal structures. It is often necessary to supplement the use of this drug with other treatment measures, such as rest, support and physiotherapy.
As a Combination Drug Product [CD]: It is combined with aspirin (and with codeine in Canada) to enhance its effectiveness in relieving discomfort. Aspirin and codeine are effective analgesics and may be necessary to control the pain that is not relieved by methocarbamol alone.

How This Drug Works: Not completely established. It is thought that this drug may relieve muscle spasm and pain by blocking the transmission of nerve impulses over reflex pathways and/or by producing a sedative effect that decreases the perception of pain.

Available Dosage Forms and Strengths
Injection — 100 mg per ml
Tablets — 500 mg, 750 mg

▷ **Usual Adult Dosage Range:** Initially, 1500 mg 4 times/day for the first 2 to 3 days; for maintenance, 750 to 1000 mg 4 times/day, or 1500 mg 3 times/day. The total daily dose should not exceed 8000 mg. **Actual dosage and administration schedule must be determined by the physician for each patient individually.**

▷ **Dosing Instructions:** Take either on empty stomach or with food to prevent stomach irritation. The tablet may be crushed for administration.

Usual Duration of Use: Continual use on a regular schedule for 2 to 3 days is usually necessary to determine this drug's effectiveness in relieving the discomfort of muscle spasm. Evaluate need for continued use after periods of 7 to 10 days.

▷ **This Drug Should Not Be Taken If**
- you have had an allergic reaction to it previously.
- you have active liver disease.

▷ **Inform Your Physician Before Taking This Drug If**
- you have experienced any unfavorable reactions to muscle relaxants in the past.
- you have epilepsy or myasthenia gravis.
- you have a history of liver or kidney disease.

Possible Side-Effects (natural, expected and unavoidable drug actions)
Drowsiness, light-headedness, weakness.
Brown, black, green or blue discoloration of the urine (of no significance).

▷ **Possible Adverse Effects** (unusual, unexpected and infrequent reactions)
If any of the following develop, consult your physician promptly for guidance.
Mild Adverse Effects
Allergic Reactions: Skin rash, hives, itching, fever.
Headache, dizziness, faintness, unsteadiness, blurred or double vision, red eyes, congested nose.
Indigestion, heartburn, nausea, vomiting.
Serious Adverse Effects
Abnormally low white blood cell count: fever, sore throat, infections.

▷ **Possible Effects on Sexual Function:**   None reported.

CAUTION
All muscle relaxants cause some degree of sedation. Use caution if other sedatives, tranquilizers or pain relievers are taken concurrently with this drug.

Precautions for Use
By Infants and Children: Dosage is based on the child's age and weight. Consult your physician for exact dosage schedule.
By Those over 60 Years of Age: Small doses are advisable initially. You may be more susceptible to the development of drowsiness, dizziness, weakness, unsteadiness and falling.

▷ **Advisability of Use During Pregnancy**
Pregnancy Category: C (tentative). See Pregnancy Code inside back cover.
Animal studies: No data available.
Human studies: Information from adequate studies of pregnant women is not available.
Avoid drug if possible; use only if clearly needed.

Advisability of Use if Breast-Feeding
Presence of this drug in breast milk: Yes, in small amounts.
Avoid drug or refrain from nursing.

Habit-Forming Potential: None.

Effects of Overdosage: Nausea, vomiting, diarrhea, headache, drowsiness, dizziness, marked weakness, impaired coordination, sense of paralysis of arms and legs, rapid and weak pulse, shallow breathing, cold and sweaty skin.

Possible Effects of Long-Term Use: None reported.

Suggested Periodic Examinations While Taking This Drug (at physician's discretion)
Complete blood cell counts.

▷ **While Taking This Drug, Observe the Following**
Foods: No restrictions.
Beverages: No restrictions. May be taken with milk.
▷ *Alcohol:* Use with caution until the combined effect has been determined. This drug may add to the depressant action of alcohol on the brain.
Tobacco Smoking: No interactions expected.
Marijuana Smoking: Moderate to marked drowsiness, muscle weakness, incoordination, accentuation of orthostatic hypotension (see Glossary).
▷ *Other Drugs*
Methocarbamol may **increase** the effects of
• all other drugs with sedative effects and cause excessive sedation.
▷ *Driving, Hazardous Activities:* This drug may cause drowsiness, light-headedness or dizziness in susceptible individuals. Avoid hazardous activities if these drug effects occur.
Aviation Note: The use of this drug **is a disqualification** for piloting. Consult a designated Aviation Medical Examiner.
Exposure to Sun: No restrictions.

METHOTREXATE
(meth oh TREX ayt)

Other Names: Amethopterin, MTX

Introduced: 1948

Class: Anticancer drugs, antipsoriasis

Prescription: USA: Yes
Canada: Yes

Controlled Drug: USA: No
Canada: No

Available as Generic: Yes

Brand Names: Folex, Mexate, Rheumatrex Dose Pack

```
BENEFITS versus RISKS

    Possible Benefits                    Possible Risks
EFFECTIVE TREATMENT OF          GASTROINTESTINAL
  SOME CASES OF SEVERE            ULCERATION AND BLEEDING
  DISABLING PSORIASIS           MOUTH AND THROAT
EFFECTIVE TREATMENT OF            ULCERATION
  CERTAIN ADULT AND             SEVERE BONE MARROW
  CHILDHOOD CANCERS               DEPRESSION
PREVENTION OF REJECTION         DAMAGE TO LUNGS, LIVER
  OF BONE MARROW                  AND KIDNEYS
  TRANSPLANTS                   Loss of hair
Helpful adjunctive therapy in
  severe, refractory rheumatoid
  arthritis and related disorders
```

▷ **Principal Uses**

As a Single Drug Product: This very potent drug is used to treat (1) severe and widespread forms of disabling psoriasis that have failed to respond to all standard treatment procedures; (2) various types of both adult and childhood cancer. In addition, it is used to prevent rejection of transplanted bone marrow. More recently, it is being used in the treatment of connective tissue disorders such as rheumatoid arthritis, scleroderma and related conditions. Its use in rheumatoid arthritis is restricted to the treatment of selected adults with severe active disease that has failed to respond to conventional therapy.

How This Drug Works: By interfering with the normal utilization of folic acid in tissue cell reproduction, this drug retards abnormally rapid tissue growth (as in psoriasis and cancer).

Available Dosage Forms and Strengths

Injections — 2.5 mg per ml, 25 mg per ml

Injections (preservative-free) — 25 mg per ml

Tablets — 2.5 mg

▷ **Usual Adult Dosage Range**

For psoriasis (alternate schedules): (1) 10 to 50 mg once/week; (2) 2.5 to 5 mg/12 hours for 3 doses, or every 8 hours for 4 doses, once a week up to a maximum of 30 mg/week; (3) 2.5 mg/day for 5 days, followed by 2 days without drug, with gradual increase in dosage to a maximum of 6.25 mg/day.

For rheumatoid arthritis (alternate schedules): (1) single oral dose of 7.5 mg once weekly; (2) divided doses of 2.5 mg every 12 hours for 3 doses per week. Dosage may be increased gradually as needed and tolerated. Do not exceed a weekly dose of 20 mg.

Note: Actual dosage and administration schedule must be determined by the physician for each patient individually.

▷ **Dosing Instructions:** May be taken with food to reduce stomach irritation. Drink at least 2 to 3 quarts of liquids daily. The tablet may be crushed for administration.

Usual Duration of Use: Continual use on a regular schedule for several weeks is usually necessary to determine this drug's effectiveness in reducing the severity and extent of psoriasis. Response in rheumatoid arthritis usually begins after 3 to 6 weeks of treatment. When a favorable response has been achieved, the dosage should be reduced to the smallest amount that will maintain acceptable improvement. Long-term use (months to years) requires supervision and periodic evaluation by your physician. Consult your physician on a regular basis.

▷ **This Drug Should Not Be Taken If**
- you have had an allergic reaction to it previously.
- you currently have, or have had a recent exposure to, either chicken pox or shingles (herpes zoster).
- you are pregnant or planning pregnancy in the near future, and you are taking this drug to treat psoriasis or rheumatoid arthritis.
- you have active liver disease, peptic ulcer, regional enteritis or ulcerative colitis.
- you currently have a blood cell or bone marrow disorder.

▷ **Inform Your Physician Before Taking This Drug If**
- you have a chronic infection of any kind.
- you have impaired liver or kidney function.
- you have a history of bone marrow impairment of any kind, especially drug-induced bone marrow depression.
- you have a history of gout, peptic ulcer disease, regional enteritis or ulcerative colitis.

Possible Side-Effects (natural, expected and unavoidable drug actions)
The following are due to the pharmacological actions of this drug. **Report such developments to your physician promptly.**
Sores on the lips, in the mouth or throat; vomiting; intestinal cramping; diarrhea (may be bloody); painful urination; bloody urine.
Reduced resistance to infection, fatigue, weakness, fever, abnormal bleeding or bruising (bone marrow depression).

▷ **Possible Adverse Effects** (unusual, unexpected and infrequent reactions)
If any of the following develop, consult your physician promptly for guidance.
Mild Adverse Effects
Allergic Reactions: Skin rash, hives, itching.
Headache, drowsiness, blurred vision.
Loss of appetite, nausea, vomiting.
Loss of hair, loss of skin pigmentation, acne.

Serious Adverse Effects
Allergic Reactions: Drug-induced pneumonia: cough, chest pain, shortness of breath.
Nervous system toxicity: speech disturbances, paralysis, seizures.
Liver toxicity with jaundice (see Glossary).
Kidney toxicity: reduced urine volume, kidney failure.

▷ **Possible Effects on Sexual Function:** Altered timing and pattern of menstruation.

Possible Delayed Adverse Effects: Some reports suggest that methotrexate therapy may contribute to the later development of secondary cancers. Other studies have not confirmed this.

CAUTION
1. This drug has a high potential for serious toxicity. Its use must be monitored carefully and continually by a physician who is skilled in its proper administration. Request the Patient Package Insert that is available with this drug (Rheumatrex Dose Pack) and read it thoroughly.
2. Appropriate laboratory examinations, performed before and during the use of this drug, are mandatory. Comply fully with your physician's instructions regarding periodic studies.
3. Women with potential for pregnancy should have a pregnancy test before taking this drug and should use an effective form of contraception during its use and for 8 weeks following its discontinuation.
4. Administration of live virus vaccines should be avoided during use of this drug. Because immune functions are suppressed by this drug, live virus vaccines could actually produce infection rather than stimulate an immune response.

Precautions for Use
By Those over 60 Years of Age: Careful evaluation of kidney function should be made before starting treatment and during the entire course of therapy.

▷ **Advisability of Use During Pregnancy**
Pregnancy Category: D (tentative). See Pregnancy Code inside back cover.
Animal studies: Skull and facial defects reported in mice.
Human studies: This drug is known to cause fetal deaths and birth defects.
Its use during pregnancy to treat psoriasis or rheumatoid arthritis cannot be justified. If its use during pregnancy is deemed necessary to treat a responsive type of cancer, it should be avoided during the first 3 months if possible.

Advisability of Use if Breast-Feeding
Presence of this drug in breast milk: Yes.
Avoid drug or refrain from nursing.

Habit-Forming Potential: None.

Effects of Overdosage: The side-effects and adverse effects listed previously develop earlier and with greater severity.

Possible Effects of Long-Term Use: Liver fibrosis and cirrhosis occur in 3% to 5% of long-term users (35 to 49 months).

Suggested Periodic Examinations While Taking This Drug (at physician's discretion)
Complete blood cell counts, liver and kidney function tests, blood uric acid levels, chest X-ray examinations.

▷ **While Taking This Drug, Observe the Following**
Foods: Avoid highly seasoned foods that could be irritating. Between courses of treatment, eat liberally of the following foods: beef, chicken, lamb and pork liver, asparagus, navy beans, kale and spinach.
Beverages: No restrictions. This drug may be taken with milk.
▷ *Alcohol:* Avoid completely.
Tobacco Smoking: No interactions expected.
▷ *Other Drugs Methotrexate may **decrease** the effects of
 • digoxin (Lanoxin).
 • phenytoin (Dilantin).
The following drugs may **increase** the effects of methotrexate and enhance its toxicity
 • aspirin and other salicylates.
 • probenecid (Benemid).
▷ *Driving, Hazardous Activities:* This drug may cause drowsiness, dizziness or blurred vision. Restrict activities as necessary.
Aviation Note: The use of this drug **is a disqualification** for piloting. Consult a designated Aviation Medical Examiner.
Exposure to Sun: Use caution until skin sensitivity has been determined. This drug can cause photosensitivity. Avoid ultraviolet lamps.

METHYCLOTHIAZIDE
(METH ee kloh THI a zide)

Introduced: 1960

Class: Antihypertensive, diuretic, thiazides

Prescription: USA: Yes
Canada: Yes

Controlled Drug: USA: No
Canada: No

Available as Generic: USA: Yes
Canada: No

Brand Names: Aquatensen, Diutensen [CD], Diutensen-R [CD], ✦Duretic, ✦Dureticyl [CD], Enduron, Enduronyl [CD], Enduronyl Forte [CD]

BENEFITS versus RISKS

Possible Benefits	*Possible Risks*
EFFECTIVE, WELL-TOLERATED DIURETIC	Loss of body potassium
POSSIBLY EFFECTIVE IN MILD HYPERTENSION	Increased blood sugar
	Increased blood uric acid
ENHANCES EFFECTIVENESS OF OTHER ANTIHYPERTENSIVES	Increased blood calcium
	Rare blood cell disorders
Beneficial in treatment of diabetes insipidus	

▷ **Principal Uses**

As a Single Drug Product: Thiazide diuretics are used primarily to (1) increase the volume of urine (diuresis) to correct the excessive fluid retention associated with congestive heart failure and certain types of liver and kidney disease; and (2) initiate treatment for high blood pressure (hypertension). They are often the first drugs tried in treating mild to moderate hypertension. Less frequent uses include the treatment of diabetes insipidus and the prevention of kidney stones that contain calcium.

As a Combination Drug Product [CD]: When this drug is used alone to treat hypertension, it is referred to as a "step 1" antihypertensive. Should it fail to reduce the blood pressure adequately, a "step 2" antihypertensive drug is added to be taken concurrently with the step 1 drug. These drugs may be combined into one drug product. Thiazides are available in combination with beta blockers, hydralazine, methyldopa, reserpine and other diuretics to increase their effectiveness in treating hypertension.

How This Drug Works: By increasing the elimination of salt and water from the body (through increased urine production), this drug reduces the volume of fluid in the blood and body tissues and lowers the sodium content throughout the body. By relaxing the walls of smaller arteries and allowing them to expand, this drug increases the total capacity of the arterial system. The combined effect of these two actions (reduced blood volume in expanded space) results in lowering of blood pressure.

Available Dosage Forms and Strengths

Tablets — 2.5 mg, 5 mg

▷ **Usual Adult Dosage Range:** As antihypertensive: 2.5 to 5 mg/day initially; 2.5 to 10 mg/day for maintenance. As diuretic: 2.5 to 10 mg/day initially; the smallest effective dose should be determined. The total daily dose should not exceed 10 mg. **Note: Actual dosage and administration schedule must be determined by the physician for each patient individually.**

▷ **Dosing Instructions:**   May be taken with or following meals to reduce stomach irritation. Best taken in the morning to avoid nighttime urination. The tablet may be crushed for administration.

Usual Duration of Use: Continual use on a regular schedule for 2 to 3 weeks is usually necessary to determine this drug's effectiveness in lowering high blood pressure. Long-term use (months to years) requires periodic evaluation of response and possible dosage adjustment. Use as a diuretic should be intermittent with "drug holidays" (no drug taken) to reduce the risk of sodium and potassium imbalance. Consult your physician on a regular basis.

▷ **This Drug Should Not Be Taken If**
   • you have had an allergic reaction to any dosage form of it previously.

▷ **Inform Your Physician Before Taking This Drug If**
   • you are allergic to any form of "sulfa" drug.
   • you are pregnant or planning pregnancy.
   • you have a history of kidney or liver disease.
   • you have diabetes, gout or lupus erythematosus.
   • you are taking any form of cortisone, digitalis, oral antidiabetic drug or insulin.
   • you plan to have surgery under general anesthesia in the near future.

Possible Side-Effects (natural, expected and unavoidable drug actions)
   Light-headedness on arising from sitting or lying position (see Orthostatic Hypotension in Glossary).
   Increase in blood sugar level, affecting control of diabetes.
   Increase in blood uric acid level, affecting control of gout.
   Decrease in blood potassium level, causing muscle weakness and cramping.

▷ **Possible Adverse Effects** (unusual, unexpected and infrequent reactions)
   If any of the following develop, consult your physician promptly for guidance.
   Mild Adverse Effects
   Allergic Reactions: Skin rashes, hives, drug fever.
   Headache, dizziness, blurred or yellow vision.
   Reduced appetite, indigestion, nausea, vomiting, diarrhea.
   Serious Adverse Effects
   Allergic Reactions: Hepatitis with jaundice (see Glossary), anaphylactic reaction (see Glossary), severe skin reactions.
   Inflammation of the pancreas—severe abdominal pain.
   Bone marrow depression (see Glossary)—fatigue, weakness, fever, sore throat, abnormal bleeding or bruising.

▷ **Possible Effects on Sexual Function:**   Impotence (rare) with recommended dosage.

▷ **Adverse Effects That May Mimic Natural Diseases or Disorders**
   Liver reaction may suggest viral hepatitis.

Natural Diseases or Disorders That May Be Activated by This Drug
Diabetes, gout, systemic lupus erythematosus.

CAUTION
1. Do not exceed recommended doses. Increased dosage can cause excessive loss of sodium and potassium, with resultant loss of appetite, nausea, fatigue, weakness, confusion and tingling in the extremities.
2. If you are also taking a digitalis preparation (digitoxin, digoxin), ensure an adequate intake of high-potassium foods to prevent potassium deficiency—a potential cause of digitalis toxicity. (See Table of High Potassium Foods in Section Six.)

Precautions for Use
By Infants and Children: Avoid overdosage that could cause serious dehydration. Significant potassium loss can occur within the first 2 weeks of drug use.
By Those over 60 Years of Age: Small doses are advisable until your individual response has been determined. You may be more susceptible to the development of impaired thinking, orthostatic hypotension, potassium loss and blood sugar increase. Overdosage and extended use of this drug can cause excessive loss of body water, thickening (increased viscosity) of the blood and an increased tendency for the blood to clot—predisposing to stroke, heart attack or thrombophlebitis (vein inflammation with blood clot).

▷ **Advisability of Use During Pregnancy**
Pregnancy Category: D (tentative). See Pregnancy Code inside back cover.
Animal studies: No information available.
Human studies: Information from adequate studies of pregnant women is not available.
This drug should not be used during pregnancy unless a very serious complication occurs for which this drug is significantly beneficial. Ask physician for guidance.

Advisability of Use if Breast-Feeding
Presence of this drug in breast milk: Yes, in small amounts.
Avoid drug or refrain from nursing.

Habit-Forming Potential: None.

Effects of Overdosage: Dry mouth, thirst, lethargy, weakness, muscle cramping, nausea, vomiting, drowsiness progressing to stupor or coma.

Possible Effects of Long-Term Use: Impaired balance of water, salt and potassium in blood and body tissues. Development of diabetes in predisposed individuals. Pathological changes in parathyroid glands with increased blood calcium levels and decreased blood phosphate levels.

Suggested Periodic Examinations While Taking This Drug (at physician's discretion)

Complete blood cell counts, measurements of blood levels of sodium, potassium, chloride, sugar and uric acid.

Kidney and liver function tests.

▷ **While Taking This Drug, Observe the Following**

Foods: Consult your physician regarding the advisability of eating foods rich in potassium. If so advised, see the Table of High Potassium Foods in Section Six. Follow physician's advice regarding the use of salt.

Beverages: No restrictions. This drug may be taken with milk.

▷ *Alcohol:* Use with caution until the combined effects have been determined. Alcohol may exaggerate the blood-pressure-lowering effects of this drug and cause orthostatic hypotension.

Tobacco Smoking: No interactions expected. Follow physician's advice.

▷ *Other Drugs*

Methyclothiazide may *increase* the effects of

- other antihypertensive drugs; dosage adjustments may be necessary to prevent excessive lowering of blood pressure.
- lithium, and cause lithium toxicity.

Methyclothiazide may *decrease* the effects of

- oral antidiabetic drugs (sulfonylureas); dosage adjustments may be necessary for proper control of blood sugar.

Methyclothiazide *taken concurrently* with

- digitalis preparations (digitoxin, digoxin) requires very careful monitoring and dosage adjustments to prevent fluctuations of blood potassium levels and serious disturbances of heart rhythm.

The following drugs may *decrease* the effects of methyclothiazide

- cholestyramine (Cuemid, Questran) may interfere with its absorption.
- colestipol (Colestid) may interfere with its absorption.

Take cholestyramine and colestipol 1 hour before any oral diuretic.

▷ *Driving, Hazardous Activities:* Use caution until the possible occurrence of orthostatic hypotension, dizziness or impaired vision has been determined.

Aviation Note: The use of this drug *may be a disqualification* for piloting. Consult a designated Aviation Medical Examiner.

Exposure to Sun: Use caution until sensitivity has been determined. This drug can cause photosensitivity (see Glossary).

Exposure to Heat: Avoid excessive perspiring, which could cause additional loss of salt and water from the body.

Heavy Exercise or Exertion: Avoid exertion that produces light-headedness, excessive fatigue or muscle cramping. Isometric exercises—the "overload" technique for strengthening individual muscles—can raise blood pressure significantly. Ask physician for guidance regarding participation in this form of exercise.

Occurrence of Unrelated Illness: Illnesses that cause vomiting or diarrhea can produce a serious imbalance of important body chemistry. Consult your physician for guidance.

Discontinuation: This drug should not be stopped abruptly following long-term use; serious thiazide-withdrawal fluid retention (edema) can develop after sudden withdrawal. The dose should be reduced gradually. It may be advisable to discontinue this drug 5 to 7 days before major surgery. Ask your physician, surgeon and/or anesthesiologist for guidance regarding dosage adjustment or drug withdrawal.

METHYLDOPA
(meth il DOH pa)

Other Name: Alpha-methyldopa

Introduced: 1963   **Class:** Antihypertensive

Prescription: USA: Yes   **Controlled Drug:** USA: No
Canada: Yes   Canada: No

Available as Generic: Yes

Brand Names: Aldochlor-150/250 [CD], Aldomet, Aldoril-15/25 [CD], Aldoril D30/D50 [CD], ✤Apo-Methazide [CD], ✤Apo-Methyldopa, ✤Dopamet, ✤Medimet-250, ✤Novodoparil [CD], ✤Novomedopa, ✤PMS Dopazide [CD]

BENEFITS versus RISKS

Possible Benefits	*Possible Risks*
EFFECTIVE STEP-2 OR -3 ANTIHYPERTENSIVE IN 66% OF CASES OF MILD TO SEVERE HYPERTENSION when used adjunctively with other drugs	LIVER TOXICITY (may be severe) Mental depression Water retention Hemolytic anemia (less than 1%) Drug fever Blood cell disorders (rare)
Symptomatic relief in cases of Raynaud's disease	

▷ **Principal Uses**

As a Single Drug Product: Used as a "step 2" or "step 3" medication in conjunction with other antihypertensive drugs in the treatment of moderate to severe high blood pressure.

As a Combination Drug Product [CD]: This drug is available in combination with chlorothiazide and with hydrochlorothiazide, mild diuretics that represent "step 1" antihypertensive drugs. Combinations of "step 1" and "step 2" drugs are more effective and more convenient for long-term use.

How This Drug Works: By decreasing the activity of the vasomotor center in the brain, this drug reduces the ability of the sympathetic nervous system to maintain the degree of blood vessel constriction that is responsible for blood pressure elevation. This change results in relaxation of blood vessel walls and lowering of blood pressure.

Available Dosage Forms and Strengths

Injection — 250 mg per 5 ml
Oral suspension — 250 mg per 5-ml teaspoonful (1% alcohol)
Tablets — 125 mg, 250 mg, 500 mg

▷ **Usual Adult Dosage Range:**   Initially, 250 mg 2 or 3 times/day for 2 days; increase dose as needed and tolerated. For maintenance, 500 to 2000 mg/day in 2 to 4 divided doses. The total daily dose should not exceed 3000 mg. **Note: Actual dosage and administration schedule must be determined by the physician for each patient individually.**

▷ **Dosing Instructions:**   May be taken without regard to meals. The tablet may be crushed for administration.

Usual Duration of Use: Continual use on a regular schedule for 2 to 4 weeks is usually necessary to determine this drug's effectiveness in controlling high blood pressure. Long-term use (months to years) requires supervision and periodic evaluation by your physician. Consult your physician on a regular basis.

▷ **This Drug Should Not Be Taken If**
- you have had an allergic reaction to it previously.
- you have active liver disease.
- you have a mild and uncomplicated case of hypertension.

▷ **Inform Your Physician Before Taking This Drug If**
- you have a history of liver disease or impaired liver function.
- you have a history of mental depression or porphyria.
- you are taking any monoamine oxidase (MAO) type A inhibitor drugs, phenothiazines or tricyclic antidepressant drugs (see Drug Classes, Section Four).
- you plan to have surgery under general anesthesia in the near future.

Possible Side-Effects (natural, expected and unavoidable drug actions)
Drowsiness, lethargy and weakness; these may occur during the first few weeks and then subside.
Light-headedness in upright position (see Orthostatic Hypotension in Glossary).
Nasal stuffiness, dry mouth.

▷ **Possible Adverse Effects** (unusual, unexpected and infrequent reactions)
If any of the following develop, consult your physician promptly for guidance.

Mild Adverse Effects
Allergic Reactions: Skin rash, joint and muscle discomfort, fever.
Headache, dizziness.
Irritation of tongue, nausea, vomiting, diarrhea.
Water retention, weight gain.

Serious Adverse Effects
Allergic Reactions: Hepatitis with jaundice (see Glossary).
Idiosyncratic Reaction: Episodes of high fever (not due to infection), 1% of users.
Bone marrow depression (see Glossary): fatigue, weakness, fever, sore throat, abnormal bleeding or bruising.
Inflammation of the pancreas: abdominal pain, fever, nausea, vomiting.
Parkinson-like disorders (see Glossary).
Behavioral changes: depression, confusion, nightmares.

▷ **Possible Effects on Sexual Function:** Decreased male and female libido (14%), impotence (24% to 80%), inhibited ejaculation (rare), inhibited female orgasm (related to higher doses), male breast enlargement and tenderness, female breast enlargement with milk production (26%), loss of menstruation.

▷ **Adverse Effects That May Mimic Natural Diseases or Disorders**
Liver toxicity may suggest viral hepatitis.
Idiosyncratic fever may suggest a viral flulike infection.
Abnormal involuntary movements of extremities may suggest Huntington's disease.

Natural Diseases or Disorders That May Be Activated by This Drug
Porphyria, latent coronary artery insufficiency, lupus erythematosus–like syndrome.

CAUTION
1. If this drug is used as the sole agent, the blood pressure may be very erratic. Observe for the development of tolerance and loss of effectiveness.
2. This drug is most effective when combined with a diuretic.
3. Avoid concurrent use with other drugs known to depress bone marrow function.
4. Report the development of any tendency to emotional depression.

Precautions for Use
By Infants and Children: Observe for the development of hemolytic anemia, abnormal liver function, excessive sedation and nightmares.
By Those over 60 Years of Age: The basic rule in treating hypertension after 60 is to proceed cautiously. Unacceptably high blood pressure should be reduced without creating risks associated with excessively low blood pressure. Sudden, rapid and excessive reduction of blood pressure can predispose to stroke or heart attack. Adverse effects are common: drowsiness (50%), depression (10%), forgetfulness, reduced

mental acuity, nasal congestion, dry mouth, hallucinations. This drug can cause parkinsonism or intensify existing parkinsonism.

▷ **Advisability of Use During Pregnancy**
Pregnancy Category: B (tentative). See Pregnancy Code inside back cover.
Animal studies: No birth defects reported in mice, rats or rabbits.
Human studies: Information from adequate studies of pregnant women is not available.
Use this drug only if clearly needed. Use the minimal effective dose.

Advisability of Use if Breast-Feeding
Presence of this drug in breast milk: Yes.
If drug is necessary, monitor infant for drowsiness and inadequate feeding.

Habit-Forming Potential: None.

Effects of Overdosage: Marked drowsiness, weakness, confusion, nausea, vomiting, stupor progressing to coma.

Possible Effects of Long-Term Use: Water retention (if not taken with a diuretic). Development of hemolytic anemia (see Glossary).

Suggested Periodic Examinations While Taking This Drug (at physician's discretion)
Complete blood cell counts, liver function tests.

▷ **While Taking This Drug, Observe the Following**
Foods: Avoid excessive salt. When possible, avoid high-protein foods at the time this drug is taken; this drug competes with proteins for absorption.
Beverages: No restrictions. May be taken with milk.
▷ *Alcohol:* Use with extreme caution until the combined effects have been determined. This combination can cause marked sedation and exaggerated drop in blood pressure.
Tobacco Smoking: No interactions expected.
▷ *Other Drugs*
Methyldopa may ***increase*** the effects of
• tolbutamide (Orinase), and cause excessive hypoglycemia.
• other drugs with sedative effects, and cause excessive sedation.
Methyldopa ***taken concurrently*** with
• beta blocker drugs may rarely cause hypertensive reactions (see Drug Class, Section Four).
• haloperidol (Haldol) may cause dementia, disorientation and abnormal behavior.
• monoamine oxidase (MAO) type A inhibitor drugs may cause hallucinations and hypertension (see Drug Class, Section Four).
• phenothiazines may cause hypertension (see Drug Class, Section Four).
The following drugs may ***decrease*** the effects of methyldopa
• tricyclic antidepressants (see Drug Class, Section Four).

▷ *Driving, Hazardous Activities:* This drug may cause drowsiness and fatigue. Restrict activities as necessary.

Aviation Note: The use of this drug **may be a disqualification** for piloting. Consult a designated Aviation Medical Examiner.

Exposure to Sun: No restrictions.

Heavy Exercise or Exertion: Use caution. Excessive physical activity may increase the possibility of orthostatic hypotension. Isometric exercises—the "overload" technique for strengthening individual muscles—can raise blood pressure significantly. Ask your physician for guidance.

Discontinuation: It may be advisable to discontinue this drug 5 to 7 days before surgery under general anesthesia. Consult your surgeon and/or anesthesiologist regarding dosage adjustment or withdrawal of this drug prior to surgery.

METHYLPHENIDATE
(meth il FEN i dayt)

Introduced: 1956

Class: Stimulant, amphetaminelike drugs

Prescription: USA: Yes
Canada: Yes

Controlled Drug: USA: C-II*
Canada: <C>

Available as Generic: USA: Yes
Canada: No

Brand Names: Ritalin, Ritalin-SR

BENEFITS versus RISKS	
Possible Benefits	*Possible Risks*
EFFECTIVE CONTROL OF NARCOLEPSY	POTENTIAL FOR SERIOUS PSYCHOLOGICAL DEPENDENCE
USEFUL AS ADJUNCTIVE TREATMENT IN THE ATTENTION DEFICIT DISORDERS OF CHILDHOOD	SUPPRESSION OF GROWTH IN CHILDHOOD
Useful in treatment of mild to moderate depression	Abnormal behavior
Useful in some cases of emotional withdrawal in the elderly	Rare blood cell disorders

*See Schedules of Controlled Drugs inside back cover.

▷ **Principal Uses**

As a Single Drug Product: Used primarily to treat (1) narcolepsy, recurrent spells of uncontrollable drowsiness and sleep; and (2) attention-deficit disorders of childhood, formerly known as the hyperactive child syndrome, minimal brain damage and minimal brain dysfunction. Additional uses include the treatment of mild to moderate depression, and the management of apathetic and withdrawal states in the elderly.

How This Drug Works: Not completely established. It is thought that this drug may increase the release of the nerve impulse transmitter norepinephrine. The resulting stimulation of brain function improves alertness and concentration, and increases learning ability and attention span. The primary action that calms the overactive child is not known.

Available Dosage Forms and Strengths
                    Tablets — 5 mg, 10 mg, 20 mg
        Tablets, prolonged-action — 20 mg

▷ **Usual Adult Dosage Range:**   5 to 20 mg 2 or 3 times/day. **Note: Actual dosage and administration schedule must be determined by the physician for each patient individually.**

▷ **Dosing Instructions:**   Take tablet 30 to 45 minutes before meals. The regular tablet may be crushed for administration; the prolonged-action tablet should be taken whole, not crushed.

Usual Duration of Use: Continual use on a regular schedule for 3 to 4 weeks is usually necessary to determine this drug's effectiveness in controlling the symptoms of narcolepsy or improving the behavior of attention-deficit children. Long-term use (months to years) requires supervision and periodic evaluation by your physician. Consult your physician on a regular basis.

▷ **This Drug Should Not Be Taken If**
  • you have had an allergic reaction to it previously.
  • you have glaucoma (inadequately treated).
  • you are experiencing a period of severe anxiety, nervous tension or emotional depression.

▷ **Inform Your Physician Before Taking This Drug If**
  • you have high blood pressure, angina or epilepsy.
  • you are taking, or have taken within the past 14 days, any monoamine oxidase (MAO) type A inhibitor drug (see Drug Class, Section Four).

Possible Side-Effects (natural, expected and unavoidable drug actions)
  Nervousness, insomnia.

▷ **Possible Adverse Effects** (unusual, unexpected and infrequent reactions)
  If any of the following develop, consult your physician promptly for guidance.

Mild Adverse Effects
  Allergic Reactions: Skin rash, hives, drug fever, joint pains.
  Headache, dizziness, rapid and forceful heart palpitation.
  Reduced appetite, nausea, abdominal discomfort.
Serious Adverse Effects
  Allergic Reactions: Severe skin reactions, extensive bruising due to allergic destruction of blood platelets (see Glossary).
  Idiosyncratic Reaction: Abnormal patterns of behavior.
  Abnormally low red blood cell and white blood cell counts.

▷ **Possible Effects on Sexual Function:**   None reported.

Natural Diseases or Disorders That May Be Activated by This Drug
  Latent epilepsy.

CAUTION
  1. Careful dosage adjustments on an individual basis are mandatory.
  2. Paradoxical reactions (see Glossary) can occur, causing aggravation of initial symptoms for which this drug was prescribed.

Precautions for Use
  By Infants and Children: Safety and effectiveness for use by those under 6 years of age have not been established. If this drug is not benefical in managing an attention deficit disorder after a trial of one month, it should be discontinued. During long-term use, monitor the child for normal growth and development.
  By Those over 60 Years of Age: Start with small doses to determine your tolerance for this drug. You may be more susceptible to the development of nervousness, agitation, insomnia, high blood pressure, angina or disturbance of heart rhythm.

▷ **Advisability of Use During Pregnancy**
  Pregnancy Category: B (tentative). See Pregnancy Code inside back cover.
  Animal studies: No birth defects found in mouse studies.
  Human studies: Information from adequate studies of pregnant women is not available.
  Use this drug only if clearly needed. Ask physician for guidance.

Advisability of Use if Breast-Feeding
  Presence of this drug in breast milk: Unknown.
  Avoid drug or refrain from nursing.

Habit-Forming Potential: This drug can produce tolerance and cause serious psychological dependence (see Glossary), a potentially dangerous characteristic of amphetaminelike drugs (see Drug Class, Section Four).

Effects of Overdosage: Headache, vomiting, agitation, tremors, muscle twitching, dry mouth, sweating, fever, confusion, hallucinations, seizures, coma.

Possible Effects of Long-Term Use: Suppression of growth (in weight and/ or height) has been reported in children during long-term use of this drug.

Suggested Periodic Examinations While Taking This Drug (at physician's discretion)
Complete blood cell counts, blood pressure measurements.

▷ **While Taking This Drug, Observe the Following**
Foods: Avoid foods rich in tyramine (see Glossary); this drug in combination with tyramine may cause an excessive rise in blood pressure.
Beverages: Avoid beverages prepared from meat or meat extracts. This drug may be taken with milk.
▷ *Alcohol:* Avoid beer, Chianti wines and vermouth.
Tobacco Smoking: No interactions expected.
▷ *Other Drugs*
Methylphenidate may *increase* the effects of
- tricyclic antidepressants, and enhance their toxic effects (see Drug Class, Section Four).

Methylphenidate may *decrease* the effects of
- guanethidine (Ismelin), and impair its ability to lower blood pressure.

Methylphenidate *taken concurrently* with
- anticonvulsants may cause a significant change in the pattern of epileptic seizures; dosage adjustments may be necessary for proper control.
- monoamine oxidase (MAO) type A inhibitor drugs (see Drug Class, Section Four) may cause a significant rise in blood pressure. Avoid the concurrent use of these drugs.

▷ *Driving, Hazardous Activities:* This drug may cause dizziness or drowsiness. Restrict activities as necessary.
Aviation Note: The use of this drug *is a disqualification* for piloting. Consult a designated Aviation Medical Examiner.
Exposure to Sun: No restrictions.
Discontinuation: If it has been necessary to use this drug for an extended period of time, do not discontinue it abruptly. Careful supervision is necessary during withdrawal to prevent severe depression and erratic behavior.

METHYLPREDNISOLONE
(meth il pred NIS oh lohn)

Introduced: 1957

Class: Cortisonelike drugs

Prescription: USA: Yes
Canada: Yes

Controlled Drug: USA: No
Canada: No

Available as Generic: USA: Yes
        Canada: No

Brand Names: Medrol, Medrol Enpak

BENEFITS versus RISKS	
Possible Benefits	*Possible Risks*
EFFECTIVE RELIEF OF SYMPTOMS IN A WIDE VARIETY OF INFLAMMATORY AND ALLERGIC DISORDERS	Short-term use (up to 10 days) is usually well tolerated
EFFECTIVE IMMUNO-SUPPRESSION in selected benign and malignant disorders	Long-term use (exceeding 2 weeks) is associated with many possible adverse effects: ALTERED MOOD AND PERSONALITY CATARACTS, GLAUCOMA HYPERTENSION OSTEOPOROSIS ASEPTIC BONE NECROSIS INCREASED SUSCEPTIBILITY TO INFECTIONS (See Possible Adverse Effects and Possible Effects of Long-Term Use)

▷ **Principal Uses**

As a Single Drug Product: This potent drug of the cortisone class is used in the treatment of a wide variety of allergic and inflammatory conditions. It is used most commonly in the management of serious skin disorders, asthma, regional enteritis, ulcerative colitis and all types of major rheumatic disorders including bursitis, tendinitis and most forms of arthritis.

How This Drug Works: Not fully established. It is thought that this drug's anti-inflammatory effect is due to its ability to inhibit the normal defensive functions of certain white blood cells. Its immunosuppressant effect is attributed to a reduced production of lymphocytes and antibodies.

Available Dosage Forms and Strengths
        Ointment — 0.25%, 1%
    Retention enema — 40 mg/bottle
        Tablets — 2 mg, 4 mg, 8 mg, 16 mg, 24 mg, 32 mg

▷ **Usual Adult Dosage Range:**   4 to 48 mg daily as a single dose or in divided doses. **Note: Actual dosage and administration schedule must be determined by the physician for each patient individually.**

▷ **Dosing Instructions:**   Take with or following food to prevent stomach irritation, preferably in the morning. The tablet may be crushed for administration.

Usual Duration of Use: For acute disorders: 4 to 10 days. For chronic disorders: according to individual requirements. The duration of use should not exceed the time necessary to obtain adequate symptomatic relief in acute self-limiting conditions, or the time required to stabilize a chronic condition and permit gradual withdrawal. Because of its intermediate duration of action, this drug is appropriate for alternate-day administration. Consult your physician on a regular basis.

▷ **This Drug Should Not Be Taken If**
  • you have had an allergic reaction to any dosage form of it previously.
  • you have active peptic ulcer disease.
  • you have an active infection of the eye caused by the herpes simplex virus.
  • you have active tuberculosis.

▷ **Inform Your Physician Before Taking This Drug If**
  • you have had an unfavorable reaction to any cortisonelike drug in the past.
  • you have a history of peptic ulcer disease, thrombophlebitis or tuberculosis.
  • you have any of the following: diabetes, glaucoma, high blood pressure, deficient thyroid function or myasthenia gravis.
  • you plan to have surgery of any kind in the near future.

Possible Side-Effects (natural, expected and unavoidable drug actions)
Increased appetite, weight gain, retention of salt and water, excretion of potassium, increased susceptibility to infection.

▷ **Possible Adverse Effects** (unusual, unexpected and infrequent reactions)
If any of the following develop, consult your physician promptly for guidance.
Mild Adverse Effects
Allergic Reaction: Skin rash.
Headache, dizziness, insomnia.
Acid indigestion, abdominal distension.
Muscle cramping and weakness.
Acne, excessive growth of facial hair.
Serious Adverse Effects
Mental and emotional disturbances of serious magnitude.
Reactivation of latent tuberculosis.
Development of peptic ulcer.
Increased blood pressure.
Development of inflammation of the pancreas.

Thrombophlebitis (inflammation of a vein with the formation of blood clot)—pain or tenderness in thigh or leg, with or without swelling of the foot, ankle or leg.

Pulmonary embolism (movement of a blood clot to the lung)—sudden shortness of breath, pain in the chest, coughing, bloody sputum.

▷ **Possible Effects on Sexual Function:**   Altered timing and pattern of menstruation.

▷ **Adverse Effects That May Mimic Natural Diseases or Disorders**
Pattern of symptoms and signs resembling Cushing's syndrome.

Natural Diseases or Disorders That May Be Activated by This Drug
Latent diabetes, glaucoma, peptic ulcer disease, tuberculosis.

CAUTION
1. It is advisable to carry a card of personal identification with a notation that you are taking this drug, if your course of treatment is to exceed 1 week.
2. Do not discontinue this drug abruptly if you are using it for long-term treatment.
3. If vaccination against measles, rabies, smallpox or yellow fever is required, discontinue this drug 72 hours before vaccination and do not resume it for at least 14 days after vaccination.

Precautions for Use
By Infants and Children: Avoid prolonged use if possible. During long-term use, observe for suppression of normal growth and the possibility of increased intracranial pressure. Following long-term use, the child may be at risk for adrenal gland deficiency during stress for as long as 18 months after cessation of this drug.

By Those over 60 Years of Age: Cortisonelike drugs should be used very sparingly after 60 and only when the disorder under treatment is unresponsive to adequate trials of unrelated drugs. Avoid prolonged use of this drug. Continual use (even in small doses) can increase the severity of diabetes, enhance fluid retention, raise blood pressure, weaken resistance to infection, induce stomach ulcer and accelerate the development of cataract and osteoporosis.

▷ **Advisability of Use During Pregnancy**
Pregnancy Category: C (tentative). See Pregnancy Code inside back cover.
Animal studies: Birth defects reported in mice, rats and rabbits.
Human studies: Information from adequate studies of pregnant women is not available.
Avoid completely during the first 3 months. Limit use during the last 6 months as much as possible. If used, examine infant for possible deficiency of adrenal gland function.

Advisability of Use if Breast-Feeding
Presence of this drug in breast milk: Yes.
Avoid drug or refrain from nursing.

Habit-Forming Potential: Use of this drug to suppress symptoms over an extended period of time may produce a state of functional dependence (see Glossary). In the treatment of conditions like asthma and rheumatoid arthritis, it is advisable to keep the dose as small as possible and to attempt drug withdrawal after periods of reasonable improvement. Such procedures may reduce the degree of "steroid rebound"— the return of symptoms as the drug is withdrawn.

Effects of Overdosage: Fatigue, muscle weakness, stomach irritation, acid indigestion, excessive sweating, facial flushing, fluid retention, swelling of extremities, increased blood pressure.

Possible Effects of Long-Term Use: Increased blood sugar (possible diabetes), increased fat deposits on the trunk of the body ("buffalo hump"), rounding of the face ("moon face"), thinning and fragility of skin, loss of texture and strength of bones (osteoporosis, aseptic necrosis), cataracts, glaucoma, retarded growth and development in children.

Suggested Periodic Examinations While Taking This Drug (at physician's discretion)
   Measurements of blood pressure, blood sugar and potassium levels.
   Complete eye examinations at regular intervals.
   Chest X-ray if history of tuberculosis.
   Determination of the rate of development of the growing child to detect retardation of normal growth.

▷ **While Taking This Drug, Observe the Following**
   Foods: No interactions expected. Ask physician regarding need to restrict salt intake or to eat potassium-rich foods. During long-term use of this drug, it is advisable to eat a high-protein diet.
   Nutritional Support: During long-term use, take a vitamin D supplement. During wound repair, take a zinc supplement.
   Beverages: No restrictions. Drink all forms of milk liberally.
▷   *Alcohol:* No interactions expected. Use caution if you are prone to peptic ulcer disease.
   Tobacco Smoking: Nicotine increases the blood levels of naturally produced cortisone and related hormones. Heavy smoking may add to the expected actions of this drug and requires close observation for excessive effects.
   Marijuana Smoking: May cause additional impairment of immunity.
▷   *Other Drugs*
   Methylprednisolone may **decrease** the effects of
   • isoniazid (INH, Niconyl, etc.).
   • salicylates (aspirin, sodium salicylate, etc.).
   Methylprednisolone **taken concurrently** with
   • oral anticoagulants may either increase or decrease their effectiveness; consult physician regarding the need for prothrombin time testing and dosage adjustment.

The following drugs may *decrease* the effects of methylprednisolone

- antacids may reduce its absorption.
- barbiturates (Amytal, Butisol, phenobarbital, etc.).
- phenytoin (Dilantin, etc.).
- rifampin (Rifadin, Rimactane, etc.).

▷ *Driving, Hazardous Activities:* Usually no restrictions. Be alert to the rare occurrence of dizziness.

Aviation Note: The use of this drug *may be a disqualification* for piloting. Consult a designated Aviation Medical Examiner.

Exposure to Sun: No restrictions.

Occurrence of Unrelated Illness: This drug may decrease natural resistance to infection. Inform your physician if you develop an infection of any kind. It may also reduce your body's ability to respond to the stress of acute illness, injury or surgery. Keep your physician fully informed of any significant changes in your state of health.

Discontinuation: If you have been taking this drug for an extended period of time, do not discontinue it abruptly. Ask physician for guidance regarding gradual withdrawal. For a period of 2 years after discontinuing this drug, it is essential in the event of illness, injury or surgery that you inform attending medical personnel that you have used this drug in the past. The period of impaired response to stress following the use of cortisonelike drugs may last for 1 to 2 years.

METOCLOPRAMIDE
(met oh kloh PRA mide)

Introduced: 1973

Class: Gastrointestinal stimulant, antivomiting agent

Prescription: USA: Yes
Canada: Yes

Controlled Drug: USA: No
Canada: No

Available as Generic: No

Brand Names: ✦Emex, ✦Maxeran, Maxolon, Reglan

BENEFITS versus RISKS

Possible Benefits	*Possible Risks*
EFFECTIVE STOMACH STIMULANT FOR CORRECTING DELAYED EMPTYING	Sedation and fatigue (10%)
	Parkinson-like reactions (see Glossary), 1 in 500
Symptomatic relief in reflux esophagitis	Tardive dyskinesia (see Glossary), rare
Relief of nausea and vomiting associated with migraine headache	

▷ **Principal Uses**

As a Single Drug Product: Used primarily to stimulate contractions of the stomach and thereby facilitate timely emptying of the stomach in disorders such as (1) the stomach retention (gastroparesis) associated with diabetes; (2) acid reflux from the stomach into the esophagus (esophagitis); (3) the nausea and vomiting associated with migraine headaches; and (4) the nausea and vomiting induced by anticancer drugs.

How This Drug Works: Not completely established. It is thought that this drug inhibits relaxation of the stomach muscles and enhances the stimulation of the parasympathetic nervous system that is responsible for stomach muscle contractions. This action accelerates emptying of the stomach into the intestine.

Available Dosage Forms and Strengths
Injection — 5 mg per ml, 10 mg per ml
  Syrup — 5 mg per 5-ml teaspoonful
Tablets — 5 mg, 10 mg

▷ **Usual Adult Dosage Range:**   10 to 15 mg 4 times/day. The total daily dose should not exceed 0.5 mg per kilogram of body weight. **Note: Actual dosage and administration schedule must be determined by the physician for each patient individually.**

▷ **Dosing Instructions:**   Take tablet or syrup 30 minutes before each meal and at bedtime. The tablet may be crushed for administration.

Usual Duration of Use: Continual use on a regular schedule for 5 to 7 days is usually necessary to determine this drug's effectiveness in accelerating stomach emptying and relieving symptoms of heartburn, fullness and belching. Long-term use (months to years) requires supervision and periodic evaluation by your physician. Consult your physician on a regular basis.

▷ **This Drug Should Not Be Taken If**
• you have had an allergic reaction to it previously.
• you have a seizure disorder of any kind.
• you have active gastrointestinal bleeding.
• you have a pheochromocytoma (adrenaline-producing tumor).

▷ **Inform Your Physician Before Taking This Drug If**
• you are allergic or overly sensitive to procaine or procainamide.
• you have impaired liver or kidney function.
• you have Parkinson's disease.
• you are taking any atropinelike drugs, antipsychotic drugs or opioid analgesics (see Drug Classes, Section Four).

Possible Side-Effects (natural, expected and unavoidable drug actions)
Drowsiness and lethargy (10%), breast tenderness and swelling, milk production.

▷ **Possible Adverse Effects** (unusual, unexpected and infrequent reactions)
If any of the following develop, consult your physician promptly for guidance.
Mild Adverse Effects
Allergic Reaction: Skin rash.
Headache, dizziness, restlessness, depression, insomnia.
Dry mouth, nausea, diarrhea, constipation.
Serious Adverse Effects
Parkinson-like reactions (see Glossary).
Tardive dyskinesia (see Glossary).

▷ **Possible Effects on Sexual Function**
Decreased libido (80%), impaired erection (60%), decreased sperm count.
Altered timing and pattern of menstruation.

Precautions for Use
By Infants and Children: Observe for the early development of Parkinson-like reactions soon after starting treatment. Use the smallest effective dose to minimize such reactions.
By Those over 60 Years of Age: Parkinson-like reactions and tardive dyskinesias are more likely to occur with the use of high doses over an extended period of time. Determine the smallest effective dose and use this only when clearly needed.

▷ **Advisability of Use During Pregnancy**
Pregnancy Category: B (tentative). See Pregnancy Code inside back cover.
Animal studies: No birth defects found due to this drug.
Human studies: Information from adequate studies of pregnant women is not available.
Use this drug only if clearly needed.

Advisability of Use if Breast-Feeding
Presence of this drug in breast milk: Yes.
Avoid drug or refrain from nursing.

Habit-Forming Potential: None.

Effects of Overdosage: Marked drowsiness, confusion, muscle spasms, jerking movements of head and face, tremors, shuffling gait.

Possible Effects of Long-Term Use: Parkinson-like reactions may appear within several months of use. Tardive dyskinesias usually occur after a year of continual use; they may persist after this drug is discontinued.

Suggested Periodic Examinations While Taking This Drug (at physician's discretion)
During long-term use, observe for the development of fine, wormlike movements on the surface of the tongue; these may be the first indications of an emerging tardive dyskinesia.

▷ **While Taking This Drug, Observe the Following**
Foods: No restrictions.
Beverages: No restrictions. May be taken with milk.
▷ *Alcohol:* Use with extreme caution. Combined effects can result in excessive sedation and marked intoxication. Alcohol is best avoided.
Tobacco Smoking: No interactions expected.
▷ *Other Drugs*
Metoclopramide may **decrease** the effects of
- cimetidine (Tagamet).
- digoxin (slow-dissolving dosage forms), and reduce its effectiveness.

Metoclopramide **taken concurrently** with
- major antipsychotic drugs (phenothiazines, thiothixenes, haloperidol, etc.) may increase the risk of developing Parkinson-like reactions.

The following drugs may **decrease** the effects of metoclopramide
- atropinelike drugs.
- opioid analgesics (see Drug Class, Section Four).
▷ *Driving, Hazardous Activities:* This drug may cause drowsiness and dizziness. Restrict activities as necessary.
Aviation Note: The use of this drug **may be a disqualification** for piloting. Consult a designated Aviation Medical Examiner.
Exposure to Sun: No restrictions.

METOLAZONE
(me TOHL a zohn)

Introduced: 1974

Class: Antihypertensive, diuretic, sulfonamides

Prescription: USA: Yes
Canada: Yes

Controlled Drug: USA: No
Canada: No

Available as Generic: USA: No
Canada: No

Brand Names: Diulo, Microx, Zaroxolyn

BENEFITS versus RISKS	
Possible Benefits	*Possible Risks*
EFFECTIVE, WELL-TOLERATED DIURETIC	Loss of body potassium
	Increased blood sugar
POSSIBLY EFFECTIVE IN MILD HYPERTENSION	Increased blood uric acid
	Rare liver damage, jaundice
ENHANCES EFFECTIVENESS OF OTHER ANTIHYPERTENSIVES	Rare blood cell disorder: abnormally low white blood cell count

▷ **Principal Uses**

   As a Single Drug Product: Diuretics of this class are used to primarily to (1) increase the volume of urine (diuresis) to correct the excessive fluid retention associated with congestive heart failure and certain types of liver and kidney disease; and (2) initiate treatment for high blood pressure (hypertension). They are often the first drugs tried ("step 1") in treating mild to moderate hypertension.

   How This Drug Works: By increasing the elimination of salt and water from the body (through increased urine production), this drug reduces the volume of fluid in the blood and body tissues and lowers the sodium content throughout the body. By relaxing the walls of smaller arteries and allowing them to expand, this drug increases the total capacity of the arterial system. The combined effect of these two actions (reduced blood volume in expanded space) results in lowering of blood pressure.

Available Dosage Forms and Strengths

   Tablets — 0.5 mg, 2.5 mg, 5 mg, 10 mg

▷ **Usual Adult Dosage Range:** As antihypertensive: 2.5 to 5 mg/day initially; 2.5 to 10 mg/day for maintenance. As diuretic: 2.5 to 10 mg/day initially; the smallest effective dose should be determined. The total daily dose should not exceed 20 mg. **Note: Actual dosage and administration schedule must be determined by the physician for each patient individually.**

▷ **Dosing Instructions:** May be taken with or following food to reduce stomach irritation. Best taken as one dose in the morning to avoid nighttime urination. The tablet may be crushed for administration.

   Usual Duration of Use: Continual use on a regular schedule for 2 to 3 weeks is usually necessary to determine this drug's effectiveness in lowering high blood pressure. Long-term use (months to years) requires periodic evaluation of response and possible dosage adjustment. Use as a diuretic should be intermittent with "drug holidays" (no drug taken) to reduce the risk of sodium and potassium imbalance. Consult your physician on a regular basis.

▷ **This Drug Should Not Be Taken If**
   • you have had an allergic reaction to it previously.

▷ **Inform Your Physician Before Taking This Drug If**
   • you are allergic to any form of "sulfa" drug.
   • you are pregnant or planning pregnancy.
   • you have a history of kidney or liver disease.
   • you have diabetes, gout or lupus erythematosus.
   • you are taking any form of cortisone, digitalis, oral antidiabetic drug or insulin.
   • you plan to have surgery under general anesthesia in the near future.

Possible Side-Effects (natural, expected and unavoidable drug actions)
Light-headedness on arising from sitting or lying position (see Orthostatic Hypotension in Glossary).
Increase in blood sugar level, affecting control of diabetes.
Increase in blood uric acid level, affecting control of gout.
Decrease in blood potassium level, causing muscle weakness and cramping.

▷ **Possible Adverse Effects** (unusual, unexpected and infrequent reactions)
If any of the following develop, consult your physician promptly for guidance.
Mild Adverse Effects
Allergic Reactions: Skin rashes, hives.
Headache, dizziness, blurred vision.
Reduced appetite, indigestion, nausea, vomiting, diarrhea.
Serious Adverse Effects
Allergic Reactions: Hepatitis with jaundice (see Glossary).
Idiosyncratic Reactions: Muscle pains and cramping, seizures, collapse.
Acute gout attacks (in susceptible individuals).
Acute to chronic muscle disorders (due to potassium loss).
Abnormally low white blood cell count: fever, sore throat, infections.

▷ **Possible Effects on Sexual Function:** None reported.

▷ **Adverse Effects That May Mimic Natural Diseases or Disorders**
Liver reaction may suggest viral hepatitis.

Natural Diseases or Disorders That May Be Activated by This Drug
Diabetes, gout, systemic lupus erythematosus (questionable).

CAUTION
1. Do not exceed recommended doses. Increased dosage can cause excessive loss of sodium and potassium, with resultant loss of appetite, nausea, fatigue, weakness, confusion and tingling in the extremities.
2. If you are also taking a digitalis preparation (digitoxin, digoxin), ensure an adequate intake of high-potassium foods to prevent potassium deficiency—a potential cause of digitalis toxicity. (See Table of High Potassium Foods in Section Six).

Precautions for Use
By Infants and Children: Safety and effectiveness for use by those under 12 years of age have not been established. Avoid overdosage that could cause serious dehydration. Significant potassium loss can occur within the first 2 weeks of drug use.
By Those over 60 Years of Age: Small doses are advisable until your individual response has been determined. You may be more susceptible to the development of impaired thinking, orthostatic hypotension, potassium loss and blood sugar increase. Overdosage and extended use of this drug can cause excessive loss of body water, thickening (in-

creased viscosity) of the blood and an increased tendency for the blood to clot—predisposing to stroke, heart attack or thrombophlebitis (vein inflammation with blood clot).

▷ **Advisability of Use During Pregnancy**
Pregnancy Category: B (tentative). See Pregnancy Code inside back cover.
Animal studies: No birth defects reported in mouse, rat or rabbit studies.
Human studies: Information from adequate studies of pregnant women is not available.
This drug should not be used during pregnancy unless a very serious complication occurs for which this drug is significantly beneficial. Ask physician for guidance.

Advisability of Use if Breast-Feeding
Presence of this drug in breast milk: Yes.
Avoid drug if possible. If use is necessary, monitor nursing infant closely and discontinue drug or nursing if adverse effects develop.

Habit-Forming Potential: None.

Effects of Overdosage: Dry mouth, thirst, lethargy, weakness, muscle cramping, nausea, vomiting, drowsiness progressing to stupor or coma.

Possible Effects of Long-Term Use: Impaired balance of water, salt and potassium in blood and body tissues. Development of diabetes in predisposed individuals. Pathological changes in the parathyroid glands (with increased blood calcium levels and decreased blood phosphate levels) have been reported with long-term use of thiazide diuretics, a class chemically related to this diuretic.

Suggested Periodic Examinations While Taking This Drug (at physician's discretion)
Complete blood cell counts, measurements of blood levels of sodium, potassium, chloride, sugar and uric acid.
Kidney and liver function tests.

▷ **While Taking This Drug, Observe the Following**
Foods: Consult your physician regarding the advisability of eating foods rich in potassium. If so advised, see the Table of High Potassium Foods in Section Six. Follow physician's advice regarding the use of salt.
Beverages: No restrictions. This drug may be taken with milk.
▷ *Alcohol:* Use with caution until the combined effects have been determined. Alcohol may exaggerate the blood-pressure-lowering effects of this drug and cause orthostatic hypotension.
Tobacco Smoking: No interactions expected. Follow physician's advice.
▷ *Other Drugs*
Metolazone may ***increase*** the effects of
  • other antihypertensive drugs; dosage adjustments may be necessary

to prevent excessive lowering of blood pressure.
- lithium, and cause lithium toxicity.

Metolazone may *decrease* the effects of
- oral antidiabetic drugs (sulfonylureas); dosage adjustments may be necessary for proper control of blood sugar.

Metolazone *taken concurrently* with
- digitalis preparations (digitoxin, digoxin) requires very careful monitoring and dosage adjustments to prevent fluctuations of blood potassium levels and serious disturbances of heart rhythm.

The following drugs may *decrease* the effects of metolazone
- cholestyramine (Cuemid, Questran) may interfere with its absorption.
- colestipol (Colestid) may interfere with its absorption.

Take cholestyramine and colestipol 1 hour before any oral diuretic.

▷ *Driving, Hazardous Activities:* Use caution until the possible occurrence of orthostatic hypotension, dizziness or impaired vision has been determined.

Aviation Note: The use of this drug *may be a disqualification* for piloting. Consult a designated Aviation Medical Examiner.

Exposure to Sun: Use caution until sensitivity has been determined. This drug may cause photosensitivity (see Glossary).

Exposure to Heat: Avoid excessive perspiring, which could cause additional loss of salt and water from the body.

Heavy Exercise or Exertion: Avoid exertion that produces light-headedness, excessive fatigue or muscle cramping. Isometric exercises—the "overload" technique for strengthening individual muscles—can raise blood pressure significantly. Ask physician for guidance regarding participation in this form of exercise.

Occurrence of Unrelated Illness: Illnesses that cause vomiting or diarrhea can produce a serious imbalance of important body chemistry. Consult your physician for guidance.

Discontinuation: This drug should not be stopped abruptly following long-term use; serious diuretic-withdrawal fluid retention (edema) can develop after sudden discontinuation. The dose should be reduced gradually. It may be advisable to discontinue this drug 5 to 7 days before major surgery. Ask your physician, surgeon and/or anesthesiologist for guidance regarding dosage adjustment or drug withdrawal.

METOPROLOL
(me TOH proh lohl)

Introduced: 1974

Class: Antihypertensive, beta-adrenergic blocker

Prescription: USA: Yes
Canada: Yes

Controlled Drug: USA: No
Canada: No

Available as Generic: No

Brand Names: ✦Apo-Metoprolol, ✦Betaloc, ✦Co-Betaloc [CD], Lopressor, Lopressor HCT [CD], ✦Novometoprol

---

BENEFITS versus RISKS

Possible Benefits	*Possible Risks*
EFFECTIVE, WELL-TOLERATED ANTIHYPERTENSIVE in mild to moderate high blood pressure	CONGESTIVE HEART FAILURE in advanced heart disease Worsening of angina in coronary heart disease (abrupt withdrawal) Masking of low blood sugar (hypoglycemia) in drug-treated diabetes Provocation of asthma (with high doses)

▷ **Principal Uses**

As a Single Drug Product: The treatment of mild to moderately severe high blood pressure. May be used alone or concurrently with other anti-hypertensive drugs, such as diuretics. Also used to reduce the risk of recurrent heart attack.

How This Drug Works: By blocking certain actions of the sympathetic nervous system, this drug
- reduces the rate the contraction force of the heart, thus lowering the ejection pressure of the blood leaving the heart.
- reduces the degree of contraction of blood vessel walls, resulting in their relaxation and expansion and consequent lowering of blood pressure.
- prolongs the conduction time of nerve impulses through the heart, of benefit in the management of certain heart rhythm disorders.

Available Dosage Forms and Strengths
Injection — 1 mg per ml
Tablets — 50 mg, 100 mg

▷ **Usual Adult Dosage Range:**   Initially, 50 mg twice daily (12 hours apart). The dose may be increased gradually at intervals of 7 to 10 days as needed and tolerated, up to 300 mg/day. For maintenance, 100 mg twice/day. The total daily dose should not exceed 450 mg. **Note: Actual dosage and administration schedule must be determined by the physician for each patient individually.**

▷ **Dosing Instructions:**   May be taken without regard to eating. The tablet may be crushed for administration. Do not discontinue this drug abruptly.

Usual Duration of Use: Continual use on a regular schedule for 10 to 14 days is usually necessary to determine this drug's effectiveness in lowering blood pressure. The long-term use of this drug (months to years) will be determined by the course of your blood pressure over time and your response to the overall treatment program (weight reduction, salt restriction, smoking cessation, etc.). Consult your physician on a regular basis.

Currently a "Drug of Choice" for initiating treatment of hypertension with a single drug, especially for those subject to bronchial asthma or diabetes.

▷ **This Drug Should Not Be Taken If**
- you have had an allergic reaction to it previously.
- you have congestive heart failure.
- you have an abnormally slow heart rate or a serious form of heart block.
- you are taking, or have taken within the past 14 days, any monoamine oxidase (MAO) type A inhibitor drug (see Drug Class, Section Four).

▷ **Inform Your Physician Before Taking This Drug If**
- you have had an adverse reaction to any beta blocker drug in the past (see Drug Class, Section Four).
- you have a history of serious heart disease, with or without episodes of heart failure.
- you have a history of hay fever (allergic rhinitis), asthma, chronic bronchitis or emphysema.
- you have a history of overactive thyroid function (hyperthyroidism).
- you have a history of low blood sugar (hypoglycemia).
- you have impaired liver or kidney function.
- you have diabetes or myasthenia gravis.
- you are currently taking any form of digitalis, quinidine or reserpine, or any calcium blocker drug (see Drug Class, Section Four).
- you plan to have surgery under general anesthesia in the near future.

Possible Side-Effects (natural, expected and unavoidable drug actions)
Lethargy and fatigability (10%), cold extremities, slow heart rate (15%), light-headedness in upright position (see Orthostatic Hypotension in Glossary).

▷ **Possible Adverse Effects** (unusual, unexpected and infrequent reactions)
If any of the following develop, consult your physician promptly for guidance.
Mild Adverse Effects
Allergic Reactions: Skin rash, itching.
Headache, dizziness (10%), insomnia, abnormal dreams.
Indigestion, nausea, vomiting, constipation, diarrhea.
Joint and muscle discomfort, fluid retention (edema).

Serious Adverse Effects
Mental depression (5%), anxiety.
Chest pain, shortness of breath, precipitation of congestive heart failure.
Induction of bronchial asthma (in asthmatic individuals).

▷ **Possible Effects on Sexual Function:** Decreased libido (4 times more common in men); impaired erection (less common with this drug than with most other beta blockers); Peyronie's disease (see Glossary).

CAUTION
1. **Do not discontinue this drug suddenly** without the knowledge and guidance of your physician. Carry a notation on your person that you are taking this drug.
2. Consult your physician or pharmacist before using nasal decongestants usually present in over-the-counter cold preparations and nose drops. These can cause sudden increases in blood pressure when taken concurrently with beta blocker drugs.
3. Report the development of any tendency to emotional depression.

Precautions for Use
By Infants and Children: Safety and effectiveness for use by those under 12 years of age have not been established. However, if this drug is used, observe for the development of low blood sugar (hypoglycemia) during periods of reduced food intake.
By Those over 60 Years of Age: Proceed **cautiously** with all antihypertensive drugs. Unacceptably high blood pressure should be reduced without creating the risks associated with excessively low blood pressure. Start treatment with small doses, and monitor the blood pressure response frequently. Sudden, rapid and excessive reduction of blood pressure can predispose to stroke or heart attack. Observe for dizziness, unsteadiness, tendency to fall, confusion, hallucinations, depression or urinary frequency.

▷ **Advisability of Use During Pregnancy**
Pregnancy Category: B (tentative). See Pregnancy Code inside back cover.
Animal studies: No significant increase in birth defects due to this drug.
Human studies: Information from adequate studies of pregnant women is not available.
Use this drug only if clearly needed. Ask physician for guidance.

Advisability of Use if Breast-Feeding
Presence of this drug in breast milk: Yes, in large amounts.
Avoid drug or refrain from nursing.

Habit-Forming Potential: None.

Effects of Overdosage: Weakness, slow pulse, low blood pressure, fainting, cold and sweaty skin, congestive heart failure, possible coma and convulsions.

Possible Effects of Long-Term Use: Reduced heart reserve and eventual heart failure in susceptible individuals with advanced heart disease.

Suggested Periodic Examinations While Taking This Drug (at physician's discretion)
Measurements of blood pressure, evaluation of heart function.

▷ **While Taking This Drug, Observe the Following**
Foods: No restrictions. Avoid excessive salt intake.
Beverages: No restrictions. May be taken with milk.
▷ *Alcohol:* Use with caution until the combined effect has been determined. Alcohol may exaggerate this drug's ability to lower the blood pressure and may increase its mild sedative effect.
Tobacco Smoking: Nicotine may reduce this drug's effectiveness in treating high blood pressure. In addition, high doses of this drug may potentiate the constriction of the bronchial tubes caused by regular smoking.
▷ *Other Drugs*
Metoprolol may ***increase*** the effects of
- other antihypertensive drugs, and cause excessive lowering of the blood pressure. Dosage adjustments may be necessary.
- reserpine (Ser-Ap-Es, etc.), and cause sedation, depression, slowing of the heart rate and lowering of the blood pressure.
- verapamil (Calan, Isoptin), and cause excessive depression of heart function; monitor this combination closely.
Metoprolol ***taken concurrently*** with
- clonidine (Catapres) requires close monitoring for rebound high blood pressure if clonidine is withdrawn while metoprolol is still being taken.
- insulin requires close monitoring to avoid undetected hypoglycemia (see Glossary).
The following drugs may ***increase*** the effects of metoprolol
- cimetidine (Tagamet).
- methimazole (Tapazole).
- oral contraceptives.
- propylthiouracil (Propacil).
The following drugs may ***decrease*** the effects of metoprolol
- barbiturates (phenobarbital, etc.).
- indomethacin (Indocin), and possibly other "aspirin substitutes," may impair metoprolol's antihypertensive effect.
- rifampin (Rifadin, Rimactane).
▷ *Driving, Hazardous Activities:* Use caution until the full extent of drowsiness, lethargy and blood pressure change has been determined.
Aviation Note: The use of this drug ***is a disqualification*** for piloting. Consult a designated Aviation Medical Examiner.
Exposure to Sun: No restrictions.
Exposure to Heat: Caution advised. Hot environments can lower the blood pressure and exaggerate the effects of this drug.

Exposure to Cold: Caution advised. Cold environments can enhance the circulatory deficiency in the extremities that may occur with this drug. The elderly should take precautions to prevent hypothermia (see Glossary).

Heavy Exercise or Exertion: It is advisable to avoid exertion that produces light-headedness, excessive fatigue or muscle cramping. The use of this drug may intensify the hypertensive response to isometric exercise.

Occurrence of Unrelated Illness: The fever that accompanies systemic infections can lower the blood pressure and require adjustment of dosage. Illnesses that cause nausea or vomiting may interrupt the regular dosage schedule. Ask your physician for guidance.

Discontinuation: It is advisable to avoid sudden discontinuation of this drug in all situations. If possible, gradual reduction of dose over a period of 2 to 3 weeks is recommended. Ask your physician for specific guidance.

METRONIDAZOLE
(me troh NI da zohl)

Introduced: 1960

Class: Anti-infective

Prescription: USA: Yes
Canada: Yes

Controlled Drug: USA: No
Canada: No

Available as Generic: Yes

Brand Names: ✦Apo-Metronidazole, Flagyl, Metizol, MetroGel, Metryl, ✦Neo-Tric, ✦Novonidazole, ✦PMS-Metronidazole, Protostat

BENEFITS versus RISKS	
Possible Benefits	*Possible Risks*
EFFECTIVE TREATMENT FOR TRICHOMONAS INFECTIONS, AMEBIC DYSENTERY AND GIARDIASIS	Superinfection with yeast organisms
Effective treatment for some anaerobic bacterial infections	Peripheral neuropathy (see Glossary)
Effective local treatment for rosacea	Abnormally low white blood cell count (transient)
	Aggravation of epilepsy

▷ **Principal Uses**

As a Single Drug Product: Used primarily to treat trichomonas infections of the vaginal canal and cervix and of the male urethra. It is also used to treat amebic dysentery, giardia infections of the intestine and serious infections caused by certain strains of anaerobic bacteria. A more recent use is the treatment of rosacea with local application of a gel dosage form.

How This Drug Works: By interacting with DNA, this drug destroys essential components of the nucleus that are necessary for the cell life and growth of infecting organisms.

Available Dosage Forms and Strengths
Gel — 0.75%
Injection — 500 mg per 100 ml
Tablets — 250 mg, 500 mg

▷ **Usual Adult Dosage Range:** Varies with infection to be treated.
For trichomoniasis: One-day course—2 grams as a single dose; or 1 gram for 2 doses 12 hours apart. Seven-day course—250 mg 3 times/day for 7 consecutive days. (The 7-day course is preferred.)
For amebiasis: 500 to 750 mg 3 times/day for 5 to 10 consecutive days.
For giardiasis: 2 grams once/day for 3 days; or 250 to 500 mg 3 times/day for 5 to 7 days.
The total daily dosage should not exceed 4 grams (4000 mg).
Note: Actual dosage and administration schedule must be determined by the physician for each patient individually.

▷ **Dosing Instructions:** May be taken with or following food to reduce stomach irritation. The tablet may be crushed for administration.

Usual Duration of Use: Continual use on a regular schedule as outlined is necessary to ensure this drug's effectiveness. Do not repeat the course of treatment without your physician's approval.

▷ **This Drug Should Not Be Taken If**
• you have had an allergic reaction to it previously.
• you currently have a bone marrow or blood cell disorder.
• you have any type of central nervous system disorder, including epilepsy.

▷ **Inform Your Physician Before Taking This Drug If**
• you have a history of any type of blood cell disorder, especially one induced by drugs.
• you have impaired liver or kidney function.
• you are pregnant or breast-feeding.

Possible Side-Effects (natural, expected and unavoidable drug actions)
A sharp, metallic, unpleasant taste.
Dark discoloration of the urine (of no significance).
Superinfection (see Glossary) by yeast organisms in the mouth or vagina.

▷ **Possible Adverse Effects** (unusual, unexpected and infrequent reactions)
If any of the following develop, consult your physician promptly for guidance.

Mild Adverse Effects
 Allergic Reactions: Skin rash, hives, flushing, itching.
 Headache, dizziness, incoordination, unsteadiness.
 Loss of appetite, nausea, vomiting, abdominal cramps, diarrhea.
 Irritation of mouth and tongue, possibly due to yeast infection.
Serious Adverse Effects
 Idiosyncratic Reactions: Abnormal behavior, confusion, depression.
 Peripheral neuropathy (see Glossary).
 Abnormally low white blood cell count (transient): fever, sore throat, infections.

▷ **Possible Effects on Sexual Function:** Decreased libido; decreased vaginal secretions (difficult or painful intercourse).

Possible Delayed Adverse Effects: Studies have shown that this drug can cause cancer in mice and possibly in rats. There is no evidence to date that this drug causes cancer in man when used in the dosages specified earlier. Follow your physician's instructions exactly. Avoid unnecessary or prolonged use.

▷ **Adverse Effects That May Mimic Natural Diseases or Disorders**
 Behavioral changes may suggest spontaneous psychosis.

Natural Diseases or Disorders That May Be Activated by This Drug
 Latent yeast infections.

CAUTION
 1. Troublesome and persistent diarrhea can develop in sensitive individuals. If diarrhea persists for more than 24 hours, discontinue this drug and consult with your physician.
 2. Discontinue this drug immediately if you develop any indications of toxic effects on the brain or nervous system: confusion, irritability, dizziness, incoordination, unsteady stance or gait, muscle jerking or twitching, numbness or weakness in the extremities.

Precautions for Use
 By Infants and Children: Avoid use in those with a history of bone marrow or blood cell disorders.
 By Those over 60 Years of Age: Natural changes in the skin may predispose to yeast infections in the genital and anal regions. Report the development of rashes and itching promptly.

▷ **Advisability of Use During Pregnancy**
 Pregnancy Category: X (tentative). See Pregnancy Code inside back cover.
 Animal studies: No birth defects reported in rat studies. However, this drug is known to cause cancer in mice and possibly in rats.
 Human studies: No increase in birth defects reported in 206 exposures to this drug during the first 3 months. However, information from adequate studies of pregnant women is not available.

The manufacturer advises against the use of this drug during the first 3 months. Use during the last 6 months is not advised unless it is absolutely essential to the mother's health.

Advisability of Use if Breast-Feeding
Presence of this drug in breast milk: Yes.
Avoid drug or refrain from nursing.

Habit-Forming Potential: None.

Effects of Overdosage: Weakness, stomach irritation, nausea, vomiting, confusion, disorientation.

Possible Effects of Long-Term Use: None reported. Avoid long-term use.

Suggested Periodic Examinations While Taking This Drug (at physician's discretion)
Complete blood cell counts.

▷ **While Taking This Drug, Observe the Following**
Foods: No restrictions.
Beverages: No restrictions. May be taken with milk.
▷ *Alcohol:* Use caution until combined effects have been determined. A disulfiramlike reaction has been reported (see Glossary).
Tobacco Smoking: No interactions expected.
▷ *Other Drugs*
Metronidazole may *increase* the effects of
• warfarin (Coumadin, etc.), and cause abnormal bleeding. The prothrombin time should be monitored closely, especially during the first 10 days of concurrent use.
Metronidazole *taken concurrently* with
• disulfiram (Antabuse) may cause severe emotional and behavioral disturbances.
▷ *Driving, Hazardous Activities:* This drug may cause dizziness or incoordination. Restrict activities as necessary.
Aviation Note: The use of this drug *may be a disqualification* for piloting. Consult a designated Aviation Medical Examiner.
Exposure to Sun: No restrictions.

MEXILETINE
(mex IL e teen)

Introduced: 1973

Class: Antiarrhythmic

Prescription: USA: Yes
Canada: Yes

Controlled Drug: USA: No
Canada: No

Available as Generic: No

Brand Name: Mexitil

```
┌─────────────────────────────────────────────────────────────┐
│                    BENEFITS versus RISKS                     │
│                                                              │
│      Possible Benefits              Possible Risks           │
│   EFFECTIVE TREATMENT IN      NARROW TREATMENT RANGE         │
│   30% OF SELECTED HEART       FREQUENT ADVERSE EFFECTS       │
│   RHYTHM DISORDERS              (up to 40% of users)         │
│                               WORSENING OF SOME             │
│                                 ARRHYTHMIAS                  │
│                               Rare seizures, liver injury and│
│                                 reduced white blood cell count│
└─────────────────────────────────────────────────────────────┘
```

▷ **Principal Uses**

As a Single Drug Product: This drug is classified as a Class 1B agent, similar to lidocaine in its actions. It is used primarily to correct and prevent the recurrence of (1) abnormally rapid heart rates (tachycardia) that arise in the ventricles (lower heart chambers); and (2) premature beats arising in the ventricles.

How This Drug Works: By slowing the transmission of electrical impulses throughout the conduction system of the heart, this drug assists in restoring normal heart rate and rhythm in selected types of arrhythmia.

Available Dosage Forms and Strengths
Capsules — 150 mg, 200 mg, 250 mg

▷ **Usual Adult Dosage Range:** Initiate treatment with 200 mg/8 hours. At intervals of 2 to 3 days, increase dose by 50 to 100 mg as needed and tolerated. The total daily dosage should not exceed 1200 mg. Measurement of drug blood levels is advised (when available) to determine the optimal dose and schedule. **Note: Actual dosage and administration schedule must be determined by the physician for each patient individually.**

▷ **Dosing Instructions:** Take with food or antacid to reduce stomach irritation. Take at same times each day to obtain uniform results. The capsule may be opened for administration.

Usual Duration of Use: Continual use on a regular schedule for 1 to 2 weeks is usually necessary to determine this drug's effectiveness in correcting or preventing responsive rhythm disorders. Long-term use requires supervision and periodic evaluation by your physician. Consult your physician on a regular basis.

▷ **This Drug Should Not Be Taken If**
  • you have had an allergic reaction to it previously.
  • you have second-degree or third-degree heart block (determined by electrocardiogram), uncorrected by a pacemaker.

▷ **Inform Your Physician Before Taking This Drug If**
- you have had any unfavorable reactions to other antiarrhythmic drugs in the past.
- you have a history of heart disease of any kind, especially "heart block" or heart failure.
- you have impaired liver function.
- you have a seizure disorder of any kind.
- you are taking any form of digitalis, a potassium supplement or any diuretic drug that can cause excessive loss of body potassium (ask physician).

Possible Side-Effects (natural, expected and unavoidable drug actions)
Nervousness (11%), light-headedness (10%).

▷ **Possible Adverse Effects** (unusual, unexpected and infrequent reactions)
If any of the following develop, consult your physician promptly for guidance.
Mild Adverse Effects
Allergic Reaction: Skin rash (4%).
Headache (7%), dizziness (26%), visual disturbance (7%), fatigue (3%), weakness (5%), tremor (13%).
Loss of appetite, indigestion, nausea (39%), vomiting, constipation (4%), diarrhea (5%), abdominal pain (1%).
Serious Adverse Effects
Idiosyncratic Reactions: Depression, confusion, amnesia, hallucinations, seizures (all rare).
Drug-induced heart rhythm disorders (1%), shortness of breath (5%), palpitations (7%), chest pain (7%), swelling of feet.
Urinary retention.
Liver damage with jaundice (see Glossary).
Abnormally low white blood cell and blood platelet counts (rare): fever, sore throat, abnormal bleeding or bruising.

▷ **Possible Effects on Sexual Function:**   Decreased libido, impotence (rare).

▷ **Adverse Effects That May Mimic Natural Diseases or Disorders**
Liver toxicity may suggest viral hepatitis.

Natural Diseases or Disorders That May Be Activated by This Drug
Latent epilepsy.

CAUTION
1. Thorough evaluation of your heart function (including electrocardiograms) is necessary prior to using this drug.
2. Periodic evaluation of your heart function is necessary to determine your response to this drug. Some individuals may experience worsening of their heart rhythm disorder and/or deterioration of heart function. Close monitoring of heart rate, rhythm and overall performance is essential.

3. Dosage must be adjusted carefully for each individual. Do not change your dosage without the knowledge and supervision of your physician.
4. Do not take any other antiarrhythmic drug while taking this drug unless you are directed to do so by your physician.
5. Carry a card of personal identification with the notation that you are taking this drug. Inform all attending medical personnel that you are taking this drug, especially if you require surgery of any kind.

Precautions for Use

By Infants and Children: Safety and effectiveness for use by those under 12 years of age have not been established. Initial use of this drug requires hospitalization and supervision by a qualified cardiologist.

By Those over 60 Years of Age: Reduced liver function may require reduction in dosage. Observe carefully for light-headedness, dizziness, unsteadiness and tendency to fall.

▷ Advisability of Use During Pregnancy

Pregnancy Category: C (tentative). See Pregnancy Code inside back cover.

Animal studies: No birth defects reported in mice, rats or rabbits. However, an increased rate of fetal resorption was found.

Human studies: Information from adequate studies of pregnant women is not available.

Avoid during first 3 months. Use this drug only if clearly needed. Ask physician for guidance.

Advisability of Use if Breast-Feeding

Presence of this drug in breast milk: Yes.

Avoid drug or refrain from nursing.

Habit-Forming Potential: None.

Effects of Overdosage: Impaired urination, constipation, marked drop in blood pressure, abnormal heart rhythms, congestive heart failure, dizziness, incoordination, seizures.

Possible Effects of Long-Term Use: None reported.

Suggested Periodic Examinations While Taking This Drug (at physician's discretion)

Electrocardiograms, complete blood cell counts, liver function tests.

▷ While Taking This Drug, Observe the Following

Foods: No restrictions. Ask physician regarding need for salt restriction.

Beverages: No restrictions. May be taken with milk.

▷ *Alcohol:* Use caution until the combined effects have been determined. Alcohol can increase the blood-pressure-lowering effects of this drug.

Tobacco Smoking: Nicotine can cause irritability of the heart and reduce the effectiveness of this drug. Follow physician's advice regarding smoking.

▷ *Other Drugs*

Mexiletine may *increase* the effects of
- antihypertensive drugs, and cause excessive lowering of blood pressure.
- beta blocker drugs (see Drug Class, Section Four).

The following drugs may *decrease* the effects of mexiletine
- phenytoin (Dilantin, etc.).
- rifampin (Rifadin, Rimactane).

▷ *Driving, Hazardous Activities:* This drug may cause weakness, dizziness or blurred vision. Restrict activities as necessary.

Aviation Note: The use of this drug *may be a disqualification* for piloting. Consult a designated Aviation Medical Examiner.

Exposure to Sun: No restrictions.

Occurrence of Unrelated Illness: Disorders that cause vomiting, diarrhea or dehydration can affect this drug's action adversely. Report such developments promptly.

Discontinuation: This drug should not be discontinued abruptly following long-term use. Ask your physician for guidance regarding gradual dose reduction.

MINOCYCLINE
(min oh SI kleen)

Introduced: 1970

Class: Antibiotic, tetracyclines

Prescription: USA: Yes
Canada: Yes

Controlled Drug: USA: No
Canada: No

Available as Generic: No

Brand Name: Minocin

BENEFITS versus RISKS

Possible Benefits	*Possible Risks*
EFFECTIVE TREATMENT OF INFECTIONS due to susceptible microorganisms	Allergic reactions
	Drug-induced colitis
	Drug-induced dizziness and unsteadiness
	Fungal superinfections

▷ **Principal Uses**

As a Single Drug Product: This member of the tetracycline drug class is used primarily to treat (1) a broad range of infections caused by susceptible bacteria and protozoa, and (2) severe, resistant pustular acne.

How This Drug Works: This drug prevents the growth and multiplication of susceptible bacteria by interfering with their formation of essential proteins.

Available Dosage Forms and Strengths
　　　　　Capsules — 50 mg, 100 mg
　　　Oral suspension — 50 mg per 5-ml teaspoonful (5% alcohol)
　　Tablets, film-coated — 50 mg, 100 mg

▷ **Usual Adult Dosage Range:**   Initially, 200 mg; then 100 mg/12 hours or 50 mg/6 hours. The total daily dosage should not exceed 350 mg the first day or 200 mg thereafter. **Note: Actual dosage and administration schedule must be determined by the physician for each patient individually.**

▷ **Dosing Instructions:**   May be taken without regard to food. Take at same time each day, with a full glass of water or milk. Take the full course prescribed. The tablet may be crushed and the capsule may be opened for administration.

Usual Duration of Use: The time required to control the infection and be free of fever and symptoms for 48 hours. This varies with the nature of the infection.

▷ **This Drug Should Not Be Taken If**
  • you are allergic to any tetracycline drug (see Drug Class, Section Four).
  • you are pregnant or breast-feeding.

▷ **Inform Your Physician Before Taking This Drug If**
  • it is prescribed for a child under 8 years of age.
  • you have a history of liver or kidney disease.
  • you have systemic lupus erythematosus.
  • you are taking any penicillin drug.
  • you are taking any anticoagulant drug.
  • you plan to have surgery under general anesthesia in the near future.

Possible Side-Effects (natural, expected and unavoidable drug actions)
　　Superinfections (see Glossary), often due to yeast organisms. These can occur in the mouth, intestinal tract, rectum and/or vagina, resulting in rectal and vaginal itching.

▷ **Possible Adverse Effects** (unusual, unexpected and infrequent reactions)
　　If any of the following develop, consult your physician promptly for guidance.
　　Mild Adverse Effects
　　Allergic Reactions: Skin rash, hives, itching of hands and feet, swelling of face or extremities.
　　Marked dizziness, unsteadiness, incoordination (usually occurs during the first 3 days).

Pigmentation of skin.

Loss of appetite, stomach irritation, nausea, vomiting, diarrhea.

Irritation of mouth or tongue, "black tongue," sore throat, abdominal cramping or pain.

Serious Adverse Effects

Allergic Reactions: Anaphylactic reaction (see Glossary), asthma, fever, swollen joints, abnormal bleeding or bruising.

Permanent discoloration and/or malformation of teeth when taken under 8 years of age, including unborn child and infant.

▷ **Possible Effects on Sexual Function:**   None reported.

Natural Diseases or Disorders That May Be Activated by This Drug
Systemic lupus erythematosus.

CAUTION
1. Antacids, dairy products and preparations containing aluminum, bismuth, calcium, iron, magnesium or zinc can prevent adequate absorption of this drug and reduce its effectiveness significantly.
2. Troublesome and persistent diarrhea can develop in sensitive individuals. If diarrhea persists for more than 24 hours, discontinue this drug and consult your physician.
3. If surgery under general anesthesia is required while taking this drug, the choice of anesthetic agent must be considered carefully to prevent serious kidney damage.

Precautions for Use
By Infants and Children: If possible, tetracyclines should not be given to children under 8 years of age because of the risk of permanent discoloration and deformity of the teeth. Rarely, young infants may develop increased intracranial pressure within the first 4 days of receiving this drug. Tetracyclines may inhibit normal bone growth and development.

By Those over 60 Years of Age: Dosage must be carefully individualized and based upon determinations of kidney function. Natural skin changes may predispose to severe and prolonged itching reactions in the genital and anal regions.

▷ **Advisability of Use During Pregnancy**
Pregnancy Category: D (tentative). See Pregnancy Code inside back cover.
Animal studies: Tetracycline causes limb defects in rats, rabbits and chickens.
Human studies: Information from studies of pregnant women indicates that this drug can cause impaired development and discoloration of teeth and other developmental defects.
It is advisable to avoid this drug completely during entire pregnancy.

Advisability of Use if Breast-Feeding
Presence of this drug in breast milk: Yes.
Avoid drug or refrain from nursing.

Habit-Forming Potential: None.

Effects of Overdosage: Dizziness, nausea, vomiting, diarrhea.

Possible Effects of Long-Term Use: Superinfections; rarely, impairment of bone marrow, liver or kidney function.

Suggested Periodic Examinations While Taking This Drug (at physician's discretion)
>   Complete blood cell counts, liver and kidney function tests.
>   During extended use, sputum and stool examinations may detect early superinfection due to yeast organisms.

▷ **While Taking This Drug, Observe the Following**
   Foods: No restrictions.
   Beverages: No restrictions.
▷   *Alcohol:* No interactions expected. However, it is best avoided if you have active liver disease.
   Tobacco Smoking: No interactions expected.
▷   *Other Drugs*
   Tetracyclines may *increase* the effects of
   • oral anticoagulants, and make it necessary to reduce their dosage.
   • digoxin (Lanoxin), and cause digitalis toxicity.
   • lithium (Eskalith, Lithane, etc.), and increase the risk of lithium toxicity.
   Tetracyclines may *decrease* the effects of
   • oral contraceptives, and impair their effectiveness in preventing pregnancy.
   • penicillins, and impair their effectiveness in treating infections.
   Tetracyclines *taken concurrently* with
   • methoxyflurane anesthesia may impair kidney function.
   The following drugs may *decrease* the effects of tetracyclines
   • antacids (aluminum and magnesium preparations, sodium bicarbonate, etc.) may reduce drug absorption.
   • iron and mineral preparations may reduce drug absorption.
▷   *Driving, Hazardous Activities:* This drug may cause marked dizziness or incoordination. Restrict activities as necessary.
   Aviation Note: The use of this drug *may be a disqualification* for piloting. Consult a designated Aviation Medical Examiner.
   Exposure to Sun: Use caution until sensitivity has been determined. Some tetracyclines can cause photosensitivity (see Glossary).

MINOXIDIL
(min OX i dil)

Introduced: 1972

Class: Antihypertensive, hair growth stimulant

Prescription: USA: Yes
   Canada: Yes

Controlled Drug: USA: No
   Canada: No

Available as Generic: Yes

Brand Names: Loniten, Minodyl, Rogaine

```
┌─────────────────────────────────────────────────────────────┐
│                    BENEFITS versus RISKS                      │
│                                                               │
│      Possible Benefits              Possible Risks            │
│   A POTENT, LONG-ACTING          EXCESSIVE BODY HAIR          │
│      ANTIHYPERTENSIVE               GROWTH (in 80% of users)  │
│   EFFECTIVE IN 75% OF CASES      SALT AND WATER RETENTION     │
│      OF SEVERE HYPERTENSION      Excessively rapid heart rate │
│   EFFECTIVE IN ACCELERATED       Aggravation of angina        │
│      AND MALIGNANT               Local scalp irritation (topical use) │
│      HYPERTENSION                                             │
│   Moderately effective in treating                            │
│      male-pattern baldness in 39% of                          │
│      users                                                    │
└─────────────────────────────────────────────────────────────┘
```

▷ **Principal Uses**

As a Single Drug Product: Principal uses include (1) the treatment of severe high blood pressure that cannot be controlled by conventional therapy; (2) the treatment of male-pattern baldness, using a topical solution applied to the scalp.

How This Drug Works: (1) By causing direct relaxation of the constricted muscles within the walls of small arteries throughout the body, this drug permits expansion of the arteries with resultant lowering of blood pressure. (2) The exact mechanism by which this drug stimulates hair growth is not completely known. It is thought that it may increase the size of previously closed small blood vessels in the scalp (improve blood flow) and restore small hair follicles to normal size and activity.

Available Dosage Forms and Strengths
Tablets — 2.5 mg, 10 mg
Topical solution — 2%

▷ **Usual Adult Dosage Range:** For hypertension: Initially, 5 mg/24 hours in one dose. Gradually increase dose to 10 mg, 20 mg, then 40 mg/24 hours, taken in 1 or 2 divided doses daily, as needed and tolerated. The usual maintenance dose is 10 to 40 mg/24 hours. The total daily dosage should not exceed 50 mg. For male-pattern baldness: Apply thinly 1 ml of topical solution to the balding area of the scalp twice daily. The total daily dosage should not exceed 2 ml. **Note: Actual dosage and administration schedule must be determined by the physician for each patient individually.**

▷ **Dosing Instructions:** For hypertension: Tablets may be taken with or following food to prevent nausea. Take at the same time each day. The tablet may be crushed for administration. For baldness: *The topical solution is for external, local use only; it is not to be swallowed.* Begin application at the center of the bald area; apply thinly to cover the entire area. The scalp and hair must be dry at the time of application. Follow carefully the instructions that accompany the applicator you have purchased.

Usual Duration of Use: Continual use on a regular schedule for 3 to 7 days is usually necessary to determine this drug's effectiveness in controlling severe hypertension. Continual use of the topical solution for at least 4 months is necessary to determine its ability to promote hair growth. Long-term use (months to years) of both dosage forms requires supervision and periodic evaluation by your physician. Consult your physician on a regular basis.

▷ **This Drug Should Not Be Taken If**
- you have had an allergic reaction to it previously.
- you are known to have a pheochromocytoma (an adrenaline-producing tumor).
- you have pulmonary hypertension due to mitral valve stenosis.

▷ **Inform Your Physician Before Taking This Drug If**
- you are pregnant or planning pregnancy.
- you have a history of coronary artery disease or impaired heart function.
- you have a history of stroke or impaired brain circulation.
- you have impaired liver or kidney function.

Possible Side-Effects (natural, expected and unavoidable drug actions)
Increased heart rate, fluid retention with weight gain (7%), excessive hair growth on face, arms, legs and back (80%).

▷ **Possible Adverse Effects** (unusual, unexpected and infrequent reactions)
If any of the following develop, consult your physician promptly for guidance.
Mild Adverse Effects
Allergic Reactions: Skin rash (less than 1%). Localized dermatitis at site of application of topical solution.
Headache, dizziness, fainting (1% to 2%).
Nausea, increased thirst.
Serious Adverse Effects
Idiosyncratic Reaction: Fluid formation around the heart (pericardial effusion) (3%).
Development of angina pectoris; development of high blood pressure in the lung circulation (pulmonary hypertension).

▷ **Possible Effects on Sexual Function:**   Breast tenderness (less than 1%).

Natural Diseases or Disorders That May Be Activated by This Drug
Latent coronary artery disease with symptomatic angina.

CAUTION

1. The long-term use of this drug for hypertension usually requires the concurrent use of an effective diuretic to counteract salt and water retention.
2. The long-term use of this drug for hypertension often requires the concurrent use of a beta blocker drug to control excessive acceleration of the heart rate.
3. It is best to avoid the concurrent use of this drug and guanethidine; the combination can cause severe orthostatic hypotension (see Glossary).
4. Consult your physician regarding the advisability of using a "no salt added" diet.
5. Only very small amounts of this drug are absorbed into the general circulation when the topical solution is applied to the scalp. However, some systemic effects have been reported. Inform your physician promptly if you experience any unusual symptoms while using the topical solution.

Precautions for Use

By Infants and Children: Dosage schedules should be determined by a qualified pediatrician. Monitor closely for salt and water retention.

By Those over 60 Years of Age: This drug must be used very cautiously by this age group. Start treatment with small doses and limit the total daily dose to 75 mg. Headache, palpitation and rapid heart rate due to this drug are more common in this age group and can mimic acute anxiety states. Observe for dizziness, unsteadiness, fainting and falling.

▷ **Advisability of Use During Pregnancy**

Pregnancy Category: C (tentative). See Pregnancy Code inside back cover.

Animal studies: No birth defects reported in rats or rabbits. However, studies did reveal decreased fertility and increased fetal deaths.

Human studies: Information from adequate studies of pregnant women is not available.

Avoid during the first 3 months. Use only if clearly needed during the last 6 months.

Advisability of Use if Breast-Feeding

Presence of this drug in breast milk: Yes.

Avoid drug or refrain from nursing.

Habit-Forming Potential: None.

Effects of Overdosage: Headache, dizziness, weakness, nausea, marked low blood pressure, weak and rapid pulse, loss of consciousness.

Possible Effects of Long-Term Use: Excessive growth of body hair occurs in 80% of users after 1 to 2 months of continual treatment for hypertension. Close to 100% of users will experience this effect after 1 year of continual treatment. This may be accompanied by darkening of the skin and coarsening of facial features.

Suggested Periodic Examinations While Taking This Drug (at physician's discretion)

Body weight measurement for insidious gain due to water retention. Electrocardiographic and echocardiographic heart examinations.

▷ **While Taking This Drug, Observe the Following**

Foods: Avoid excessive salt and heavily salted foods.

Beverages: No restrictions. May be taken with milk.

▷ *Alcohol:* Use with extreme caution until combined effects have been determined. Alcohol can exaggerate the blood-pressure-lowering effects of this drug.

Tobacco Smoking: Best avoided. Nicotine can contribute significantly to the development of angina in susceptible individuals.

▷ *Other Drugs*

Minoxidil may *increase* the effects of

• all other antihypertensive drugs; careful dosage adjustments are mandatory.

Minoxidil *taken concurrently* with

• guanethidine (Ismelin, Esimil) may cause severe orthostatic hypotension; avoid this combination.

▷ *Driving, Hazardous Activities:* This drug may cause dizziness and fatigue. Restrict activities as necessary.

Aviation Note: The use of this drug *is a disqualification* for piloting. Consult a designated Aviation Medical Examiner.

Exposure to Sun: No restrictions.

Discontinuation: This drug should not be stopped abruptly. If it is to be discontinued, consult your physician regarding gradual reduction in dosage and appropriate replacement with other drugs for the management of hypertension. Following discontinuation of the topical solution, the pretreatment pattern of baldness may return within 3 to 4 months.

MISOPROSTOL
(mi soh PROH stohl)

Introduced: 1987

Class: Stomach ulcer preventive, antiulcer

Prescription: USA: Yes
Canada: Yes

Controlled Drug: USA: No
Canada: No

Available as Generic: USA: No
Canada: No

Brand Name: Cytotec

+--+
| **BENEFITS versus RISKS** |
| |
| *Possible Benefits*   *Possible Risks* |
| EFFECTIVE PREVENTION OF   ABORTION (11%) |
| STOMACH ULCERATION   Diarrhea (14% to 40%), transient |
| WHILE TAKING ANTI- |
| INFLAMMATORY DRUGS (93% |
| reduction of ulcer development) |
| Effective treatment of duodenal |
| ulcer |
+--+

▷ **Principal Uses**

> *As a Single Drug Product:* Used primarily to prevent development of stom-
> ach ulcers during long-term use of anti-inflammatory drugs as ther-
> apy for arthritis and related conditions. Also used (in Canada and
> other countries) for treatment of active duodenal ulcer unrelated to
> use of anti-inflammatory drugs.

How This Drug Works: This drug protects the lining tissues of the stomach
and duodenum and prevents ulceration due to anti-inflammatory
drugs by using several mechanisms: (1) replacing tissue prostaglandins that are depleted by anti-inflammatory drugs; (2) inhibiting the
secretion of stomach acid; (3) increasing the local production of bicarbonate (to neutralize acids) and of mucus (to protect stomach and
duodenal tissues). The combined effects prevent new ulcer formation
and promote healing of existing ulcer(s).

Available Dosage Forms and Strengths
Tablets — 200 mcg

▷ **Usual Adult Dosage Range**

> For prevention of stomach ulcer—100 to 200 mcg 4 times daily, taken
> concurrently during the use of any anti-inflammatory drug (see An-
> tiarthritic/Anti-inflammatory Drug Class, Section Four).
> For treatment of duodenal ulcer—200 mcg 4 times daily for 4 to 8
> weeks.
> **Note: Actual dosage and administration schedule must be determined
> by the physician for each patient individually.**

▷ **Dosing Instructions:**   Take the prescribed dose with each of 3 daily meals;
take the last (fourth) dose of the day with food at bedtime. The tablet
may be crushed for administration.

Usual Duration of Use: For prevention of stomach ulcer, continual use on
a regular schedule is recommended for the entire period of anti-
inflammatory drug use. For treatment of duodenal ulcer, continual
use on a regular schedule for 4 weeks is recommended; if ulcer heal-

ing is not complete, a second course of 4 weeks is advised. Long-term use (months to years) requires periodic evaluation of response and dosage adjustment. Consult your physician on a regular basis.

Possible Advantages of This Drug: Significantly more effective than histamine (H-2)-blocking drugs (cimetidine, famotidine, nizatidine, ranitidine) or sucralfate in preventing the development of stomach ulcers.

Currently a "Drug of Choice" for the routine prevention of stomach ulcers induced by long-term use of antiarthritic/anti-inflammatory drugs.

▷ **This Drug Should Not Be Taken If**
- you have had an allergic reaction to it previously.
- you are allergic to any type of prostaglandin.
- you are pregnant or breast-feeding.
- you are not able or willing to use effective contraception (oral contraceptives or intrauterine device) while taking this drug.

▷ **Inform Your Physician Before Taking This Drug If**
- you have a history of peptic ulcer disease or Crohn's disease.
- you have impaired kidney function.
- you have a seizure disorder.

Possible Side-Effects (natural, expected and unavoidable drug actions)
Diarrhea (14% to 40% of users), usually beginning after 13 days of use and subsiding spontaneously after 8 days.
Abortion (miscarriage) of pregnancy (11% of users); this is often incomplete and accompanied by serious uterine bleeding that may require hospitalization and urgent treatment.

▷ **Possible Adverse Effects** (unusual, unexpected and infrequent reactions)
If any of the following develop, consult your physician promptly for guidance.
Mild Adverse Effects
Allergic Reaction: Skin rash.
Headache (2.4%), dizziness.
Abdominal pain (12.8%), indigestion (2%), nausea (3.2%), vomiting (1.3%), flatulence (2.9%), constipation (1.1%).
Menstrual irregularity (0.3%), menstrual cramps (0.6%), heavy menstrual flow (0.5%), spotting between periods (0.7%).
Serious Adverse Effects
Allergic Reactions: None reported.
Post-menopausal vaginal bleeding; this may require further evaluation.

▷ **Possible Effects on Sexual Function:** Reduced libido and impotence reported rarely, but causal relationship not established.

▷ **Natural Diseases or Disorders That May Be Activated by This Drug**
Latent epilepsy.

CAUTION
1. Do not take this drug if you are pregnant. It can cause abortion.
2. Do not make this drug available to others who may be pregnant or who may become pregnant.
3. If your physician prescribes this drug for you, it is advisable that you have a negative serum pregnancy test within 2 weeks before starting treatment.
4. Start taking this drug only on the second or third day of your next normal menstrual period.
5. Also initiate effective contraceptive measures when you begin to take this drug. Discuss the use of oral contraceptives or intrauterine devices with your physician.
6. Should pregnancy occur while you are taking this drug, discontinue it immediately and inform your physician.

Precautions for Use
By Infants and Children: Safety and effectiveness for use by those under 18 years of age have not been established.

By Those over 60 Years of Age: This drug is usually well tolerated by this age group. However, some forms of prostaglandins can cause drops in blood pressure; observe for periods of light-headedness or faintness that may indicate low blood pressure. Report any such development to your physician.

▷ **Advisability of Use During Pregnancy**
Pregnancy Category: X. See Pregnancy Code inside back cover.
Animal studies: No birth defects due to this drug found in rat or rabbit studies.
Human studies: Information from studies of pregnant women confirms that this drug can cause abortion, sometimes incomplete; unpassed products of conception can cause life-threatening complications.
Avoid this drug completely.

Advisability of Use if Breast-Feeding
Presence of this drug in breast milk: Unknown.
Avoid drug or refrain from nursing.

Habit-Forming Potential: None.

Effects of Overdosage: Abdominal pain, diarrhea, fever, drowsiness, weakness, tremor, convulsions, difficult breathing.

Possible Effects of Long-Term Use: Unknown at this time.

Suggested Periodic Examinations While Taking This Drug (at physician's discretion)
Monitoring for accidental pregnancy.

▷ **While Taking This Drug, Observe the Following**
Foods: No restrictions.
Beverages: No restrictions. May be taken with milk.

▷   *Alcohol:* No interactions expected. However, use sparingly if at all; alcohol can promote the development of stomach ulcer and reduce the effectiveness of this drug.

Tobacco Smoking: No interactions expected. However, nicotine is conducive to the development of stomach ulcer. Smoking should be avoided.

▷   *Other Drugs*

Misoprostol *taken concurrently* with

• antacids that contain magnesium may increase the risk of diarrhea; avoid this combination.

▷   *Driving, Hazardous Activities:* This drug may cause dizziness, light-headedness, stomach pain or diarrhea. Restrict activities as necessary.

Aviation Note: The use of this drug *may be a disqualification* for piloting. Consult a designated Aviation Medical Examiner.

Exposure to Sun: No restrictions.

Discontinuation: This drug should be taken concurrently while you are taking antiarthritic/anti-inflammatory drugs that can induce stomach ulceration. Consult your physician if you have reason to discontinue it prematurely.

MOLINDONE
(moh LIN dohn)

Introduced: 1971

Class: Strong tranquilizer, antipsychotic

Prescription: USA: Yes

Controlled Drug: USA: No

Available as Generic: No

Brand Name: Moban

BENEFITS versus RISKS

Possible Benefits	*Possible Risks*
EFFECTIVE TREATMENT OF SOME CASES OF ACUTE AND CHRONIC SCHIZOPHRENIA	NARROW TREATMENT MARGIN SERIOUS TOXIC EFFECTS ON BRAIN:
May be effective in schizophrenia that has not responded to other drugs	PARKINSON-LIKE REACTIONS
	SEVERE RESTLESSNESS
	ABNORMAL INVOLUNTARY MOVEMENTS
	TARDIVE DYSKINESIAS (see Glossary)
	Liver toxicity, jaundice
	Atropinelike side-effects

▷ **Principal Uses**

As a Single Drug Product: Used primarily in the management of acute and chronic schizophrenia to control thought disorder, disorientation, hallucinations, perceptual distortions and hostility. It is sometimes effective in chronic schizophrenic individuals who have not responded to other antipsychotic drugs.

How This Drug Works: Not completely established. It is thought that by decreasing dopamine activity in the reticular activating system of the brain, this drug improves distorted patterns of thinking and behavior.

Available Dosage Forms and Strengths
Concentrate — 20 mg per ml
Tablets — 5 mg, 10 mg, 25 mg, 50 mg, 100 mg

▷ **Usual Adult Dosage Range:** Initially, 50 to 75 mg/day in 3 or 4 divided doses; dose may be increased gradually in 3 to 4 days to 100 mg/day as needed and tolerated. For maintenance: mild psychosis—5 to 15 mg, 3 or 4 times/day; moderate psychosis—10 to 25 mg, 3 or 4 times/day; severe psychosis—up to 225 mg/day, in 3 or 4 divided doses. The total daily dosage should not exceed 225 mg. **Note: Actual dosage and administration schedule must be determined by the physician for each patient individually.**

▷ **Dosing Instructions:** Take with food or milk to reduce stomach irritation. The liquid concentrate may be diluted with water, milk, fruit juice or carbonated beverages. The tablet may be crushed for administration.

Usual Duration of Use: Continual use on a regular schedule for 3 to 6 weeks is usually necessary to determine this drug's effectiveness in controlling the features of schizophrenia. Long-term use (months to years) requires supervision and periodic evaluation by your physician. Consult your physician on a regular basis.

▷ **This Drug Should Not Be Taken If**
 • you have had an allergic reaction to it previously.
 • you have acute alcoholic intoxication.

▷ **Inform Your Physician Before Taking This Drug If**
 • you are taking any drugs that have sedative effects.
 • you use alcohol excessively.
 • you have any type of seizure disorder.
 • you have any type of glaucoma.
 • you have Parkinson's disease or an enlarged prostate gland.
 • you have impaired liver or kidney function.
 • you have a history of breast cancer.

Possible Side-Effects (natural, expected and unavoidable drug actions)
Drowsiness, dry mouth, nasal congestion, constipation, impaired urination.
Parkinson-like reactions (see Glossary).

▷ **Possible Adverse Effects** (unusual, unexpected and infrequent reactions)
If any of the following develop, consult your physician promptly for guidance.

Mild Adverse Effects

Allergic Reaction: Skin rash.

Headache, dizziness, blurred vision, lethargy, unsteadiness, insomnia, depression, euphoria, ringing in ears.

Rapid heartbeat, low blood pressure, fainting.

Loss of appetite, indigestion, nausea.

Serious Adverse Effects

Allergic Reactions: Liver reaction with jaundice.

Spasms of face and neck muscles, abnormal involuntary movements of extremities, severe restlessness.

Development of tardive dyskinesias (see Glossary).

Neuroleptic malignant syndrome: high fever, fast heart rate, difficult breathing, severe muscle rigidity, loss of bladder control, seizures.

▷ **Possible Effects on Sexual Function**

Increased libido; male breast enlargement and tenderness; female breast enlargement with milk formation.

Altered timing and pattern of menstruation.

▷ **Adverse Effects That May Mimic Natural Diseases or Disorders**

Parkinson-like reactions may be mistaken for naturally occurring Parkinson's disease.

Liver reactions may suggest viral hepatitis.

CAUTION

1. This drug may alter the pattern of epileptic seizures and require dosage adjustments of anticonvulsant drugs.
2. Obtain prompt evaluation of any change or disturbance of vision.
3. There is a very narrow margin between the effective therapeutic dose and the dose that can cause Parkinson-like reactions. Inform your physician promptly if suggestive symptoms develop.

Precautions for Use

By Infants and Children: Safety and effectiveness for use by those under 12 years of age have not been established.

By Those over 60 Years of Age: Start treatment with small doses. This drug can aggravate an existing prostatism (see Glossary). You may be more susceptible to the development of Parkinson-like reactions or tardive dyskinesia. Report any suggestive symptoms promptly.

▷ **Advisability of Use During Pregnancy**

Pregnancy Category: B (tentative). See Pregnancy Code inside back cover.

Animal studies: No birth defects reported in mice, rats or rabbits.

Human studies: Information from adequate studies of pregnant women is not available.

Because of its inherent toxicity for brain tissue, avoid use during pregnancy if possible.

Advisability of Use if Breast-Feeding
Presence of this drug in breast milk: Unknown.
Avoid drug or refrain from nursing.

Habit-Forming Potential: None.

Effects of Overdosage: Marked drowsiness, weakness, tremor, agitation, impaired stance and gait, stupor progressing to coma, possible seizures.

Possible Effects of Long-Term Use: Development of tardive dyskinesias.

Suggested Periodic Examinations While Taking This Drug (at physician's discretion)
Complete blood cell counts, liver function tests.

▷ **While Taking This Drug, Observe the Following**
Foods: No restrictions.
Beverages: No restrictions. May be taken with milk.
▷ *Alcohol:* Avoid completely. Alcohol can increase the sedative action of this drug and enhance its depressant effects on brain function. Also, this drug can increase the intoxicating effects of alcohol.
Tobacco Smoking: No interactions expected.
▷ *Other Drugs*
Molindone may *increase* the effects of
• all drugs containing atropine or having atropinelike effects (see Drug Class, Section Four).
• all drugs with sedative effects, and cause excessive sedation.
Molindone *taken concurrently* with
• antiepileptic drugs (anticonvulsants) may require close monitoring for changes in seizure patterns and need for dosage adjustments.
▷ *Driving, Hazardous Activities:* This drug may cause dizziness and drowsiness. Restrict activities as necessary.
Aviation Note: The use of this drug *is a disqualification* for piloting. Consult a designated Aviation Medical Examiner.
Exposure to Sun: No restrictions.
Exposure to Heat: Use caution and avoid excessive heat as much as possible. This drug may impair the regulation of body temperature and increase the risk of heat stroke.
Discontinuation: Do not stop taking this drug suddenly after long-term use. Ask your physician for guidance regarding gradual dosage reduction and withdrawal.

NADOLOL
(nay DOH lohl)

Introduced: 1976

Class: Antianginal, anti-hypertensive, beta-adrenergic blocker

Prescription: USA: Yes
Canada: Yes

Controlled Drug: USA: No
Canada: No

Available as Generic: No

Brand Names: Corgard, Corzide [CD]

BENEFITS versus RISKS

Possible Benefits	*Possible Risks*
EFFECTIVE, WELL-TOLERATED ANTIHYPERTENSIVE in mild to moderate high blood pressure	CONGESTIVE HEART FAILURE in advanced heart disease
EFFECTIVE ANTIANGINAL DRUG IN CLASSICAL CORONARY ARTERY DISEASE with moderate to severe angina	Provocation of asthma (in predisposed individuals)
	Masking of hypoglycemia in drug-dependent diabetes
	Worsening of angina following abrupt withdrawal

▷ **Principal Uses**

As a Single Drug Product: This beta blocker drug is used primarily to (1) treat moderately high blood pressure, and (2) contribute to the management of coronary artery disease by preventing attacks of effort-induced angina. (This drug is contraindicated in Prinzmetal's vasospastic angina.)

As a Combination Drug Product [CD]: This drug is available in combination with bendroflumethiazide, a mild diuretic "step 1" antihypertensive drug. This combination product is more effective and more convenient for long-term use.

How This Drug Works: By blocking certain actions of the sympathetic nervous system, this drug

- reduces the rate and contraction force of the heart, thus lowering the oxygen requirement of the heart muscle and reducing the ejection pressure of the blood leaving the heart; these actions reduce the frequency of angina and lower blood pressure.
- reduces the degree of contraction of blood vessel walls, resulting in their relaxation and expansion and consequent lowering of blood pressure.
- prolongs the conduction time of nerve impulses through the heart, of benefit in the management of certain heart rhythm disorders.

Available Dosage Forms and Strengths
Tablets — 40 mg, 80 mg, 120 mg, 160 mg

▷ **Usual Adult Dosage Range:** For hypertension: Initially, 40 mg daily in one dose; this may be increased gradually as needed and tolerated, up to 640 mg/24 hours. The usual maintenance dose is 80 to 320 mg/24 hours. The total daily dosage should not exceed 640 mg. For angina: Initially, 40 mg daily in one dose; increase gradually at intervals of 3 to 7 days up to 240 mg/24 hours. The usual maintenance dose is 80 to 240 mg/24 hours. The total daily dose should not exceed 240 mg. **Note: Actual dosage and administration schedule must be determined by the physician for each patient individually.**

▷ **Dosing Instructions:** May be taken without regard to eating. The tablet may be crushed for administration. Do not discontinue this drug abruptly.

Usual Duration of Use: Continual use on a regular schedule for 10 to 14 days is usually necessary to determine this drug's effectiveness in lowering blood pressure and preventing effort-induced angina. The long-term use of this drug (months to years) will be determined by the course of your blood pressure and angina over time and your response to the overall treatment program (weight reduction, salt restriction, smoking cessation, etc.). Consult your physician on a regular basis.

Possible Advantages of This Drug
Does not reduce blood flow to the kidney.
Can be used concurrently with other drugs that may reduce blood flow to the kidney (such as most anti-inflammatory aspirin substitutes).

Currently a "Drug of Choice" for initiating treatment of hypertension with a single drug.

▷ **This Drug Should Not Be Taken If**
- you have had an allergic reaction to it previously.
- you have congestive heart failure.
- you have an abnormally slow heart rate or a serious form of heart block.
- you are subject to bronchial asthma.
- you are presently experiencing seasonal hay fever.
- you are taking, or have taken within the past 14 days, any monoamine oxidase (MAO) type A inhibitor drug (see Drug Class, Section Four).

▷ **Inform Your Physician Before Taking This Drug If**
- you have had an adverse reaction to any beta blocker drug in the past (see Drug Class, Section Four).
- you have a history of serious heart disease, with or without episodes of heart failure.
- you have a history of hay fever (allergic rhinitis), asthma, chronic bronchitis or emphysema.

- you have a history of overactive thyroid function (hyperthyroidism).
- you have a history of low blood sugar (hypoglycemia).
- you have impaired liver or kidney function.
- you have diabetes or myasthenia gravis.
- you are currently taking any form of digitalis, quinidine or reserpine, or any calcium blocker drug (see Drug Class, Section Four).
- you plan to have surgery under general anesthesia in the near future.

Possible Side-Effects (natural, expected and unavoidable drug actions)
Lethargy and fatigability, cold extremities, slow heart rate, light-headedness in upright position (see Orthostatic Hypotension in Glossary).

▷ **Possible Adverse Effects** (unusual, unexpected and infrequent reactions)
If any of the following develop, consult your physician promptly for guidance.
Mild Adverse Effects
Allergic Reactions: Skin rash, itching, drug fever.
Headache, dizziness, insomnia, vivid dreaming, visual disturbances, ringing in ears, slurred speech.
Indigestion, nausea, vomiting, diarrhea, abdominal pain.
Numbness and tingling of extremities.
Serious Adverse Effects
Allergic Reaction: Facial swelling.
Chest pain, shortness of breath, precipitation of congestive heart failure.
Intensification of heart block.
Induction of bronchial asthma (in asthmatic individuals).
Masking of warning indications of acute hypoglycemia in drug-treated diabetes.

▷ **Possible Effects on Sexual Function:** Decreased libido, impotence (4%), impaired erection (36%).

▷ **Adverse Effects That May Mimic Natural Diseases or Disorders**
Impaired circulation to the extremities may resemble Raynaud's phenomenon.

Natural Diseases or Disorders That May Be Activated by This Drug
Bronchial asthma, Prinzmetal's variant (vasospastic) angina, latent Raynaud's disease, myasthenia gravis (questionable).

CAUTION
1. *Do not discontinue this drug suddenly* without the knowledge and guidance of your physician. Carry a notation on your person that you are taking this drug.
2. Consult your physician or pharmacist before using nasal decongestants usually present in over-the-counter cold preparations and nose drops. These can cause sudden increases in blood pressure when taken concurrently with beta blocker drugs.
3. Report the development of any tendency to emotional depression.

Precautions for Use

By Infants and Children: Safety and effectiveness for use by those under 12 years of age have not been established. However, if this drug is used, observe for the development of low blood sugar (hypoglycemia) during periods of reduced food intake.

By Those over 60 Years of Age: Proceed **cautiously** with all antihypertensive drugs. Unacceptably high blood pressure should be reduced without creating the risks associated with excessively low blood pressure. Start treatment with small doses, and monitor the blood pressure response frequently. Sudden, rapid and excessive reduction of blood pressure can predispose to stroke or heart attack. Observe for dizziness, unsteadiness, tendency to fall, confusion, hallucinations, depression or urinary frequency.

▷ **Advisability of Use During Pregnancy**

Pregnancy Category: C (tentative). See Pregnancy Code inside back cover.

Animal studies: No significant increase in birth defects due to this drug, but embryotoxicity reported in rabbits.

Human studies: Information from adequate studies of pregnant women is not available.

Avoid use during the first 3 months if possible. Use this drug only if clearly needed. Ask physician for guidance.

Advisability of Use if Breast-Feeding

Presence of this drug in breast milk: Yes, in large amounts.

Avoid drug or refrain from nursing.

Habit-Forming Potential: None.

Effects of Overdosage: Weakness, slow pulse, low blood pressure, fainting, cold and sweaty skin, congestive heart failure, possible coma and convulsions.

Possible Effects of Long-Term Use: Reduced heart reserve and eventual heart failure in susceptible individuals with advanced heart disease.

Suggested Periodic Examinations While Taking This Drug (at physician's discretion)

Measurements of blood pressure, evaluation of heart function.

▷ **While Taking This Drug, Observe the Following**

Foods: No restrictions. Avoid excessive salt intake.

Beverages: No restrictions. May be taken with milk.

▷ *Alcohol:* Use with caution until the combined effect has been determined. Alcohol may exaggerate this drug's ability to lower blood pressure and may increase its mild sedative effect.

Tobacco Smoking: Nicotine may reduce this drug's effectiveness in treating high blood pressure and angina. In addition, high doses of this drug may potentiate the constriction of the bronchial tubes caused by regular smoking.

▷   *Other Drugs*

Nadolol may *increase* the effects of

- other antihypertensive drugs, and cause excessive lowering of blood pressure. Dosage adjustments may be necessary.
- reserpine (Ser-Ap-Es, etc.), and cause sedation, depression, slowing of the heart rate and lowering of blood pressure.
- verapamil (Calan, Isoptin), and cause excessive depression of heart function; monitor this combination closely.

Nadolol may *decrease* the effects of

- theophyllines (Aminophyllin, Theo-Dur, etc.), and reduce their effectiveness in treating asthma.

Nadolol *taken concurrently* with

- clonidine (Catapres) requires close monitoring for rebound high blood pressure if clonidine is withdrawn while nadolol is still being taken.
- insulin requires close monitoring to avoid undetected hypoglycemia (see Glossary).

The following drugs may *decrease* the effects of nadolol

- indomethacin (Indocin), and possibly other "aspirin substitutes," may impair nadolol's antihypertensive effect.

▷   *Driving, Hazardous Activities:* Use caution until the full extent of drowsiness, lethargy and blood pressure change has been determined.

Aviation Note: The use of this drug *is a disqualification* for piloting. Consult a designated Aviation Medical Examiner.

Exposure to Sun: No restrictions.

Exposure to Heat: Caution advised. Hot environments can lower the blood pressure and exaggerate the effects of this drug.

Exposure to Cold: Caution advised. Cold environments can enhance the circulatory deficiency in the extremities that may occur with this drug. The elderly should take precautions to prevent hypothermia (see Glossary).

Heavy Exercise or Exertion: It is advisable to avoid exertion that produces light-headedness, excessive fatigue or muscle cramping. The use of this drug may intensify the hypertensive response to isometric exercise.

Occurrence of Unrelated Illness: The fever that accompanies systemic infections can lower the blood pressure and require adjustment of dosage. Illnesses that cause nausea or vomiting may interrupt the regular dosage schedule. Ask your physician for guidance.

Discontinuation: It is advisable to avoid sudden discontinuation of this drug in all situations. If possible, gradual reduction of dose over a period of 2 to 3 weeks is recommended. Ask your physician for specific guidance.

NAPROXEN
(na PROX en)

Introduced: 1974

Class: Mild analgesic, anti-inflammatory

Prescription: USA: Yes
Canada: Yes

Controlled Drug: USA: No
Canada: No

Available as Generic: No

Brand Names: Anaprox, Anaprox DS, ✦Apo-Naproxen, Naprosyn, ✦Naxen, ✦Novoanaprox

---

BENEFITS versus RISKS

Possible Benefits	*Possible Risks*
EFFECTIVE RELIEF OF MILD TO MODERATE PAIN AND INFLAMMATION	Gastrointestinal pain, ulceration, bleeding (rare)
	Drug-induced hepatitis with jaundice (rare)
	Rare kidney damage
	Mild fluid retention
	Reduced white blood cell and platelet counts

▷ **Principal Uses**

As a Single Drug Product: Used primarily to relieve mild to moderately severe pain associated with (1) musculoskeletal injuries; (2) acute and chronic gout, rheumatoid arthritis and osteoarthritis; (3) dental, obstetrical and orthopedic surgery; and (4) menstrual cramps. It is also used to prevent and relieve migrainelike headaches.

How This Drug Works: Not completely established. It is thought that this drug reduces the tissue concentrations of prostaglandins (and related compounds), chemicals involved in the production of inflammation and pain.

Available Dosage Forms and Strengths

Oral suspension — 125 mg per 5-ml teaspoonful
Tablets — 250 mg, 275 mg, 375 mg, 500 mg, 550 mg

▷ **Usual Adult Dosage Range**

As analgesic: initially, 500 mg; then 250 mg every 6 to 8 hours as needed.
As antiarthritic: 250, 375 or 500 mg twice/day, 12 hours apart.
As antigout: initially, 750 mg; then 250 mg/8 hours until acute attack is relieved.
For menstrual pain: initially, 500 mg; then 250 mg every 6 to 8 hours as needed.

The total daily dosage should not exceed 1650 mg.

Note: Actual dosage and administration schedule must be determined by the physician for each patient individually.

▷ **Dosing Instructions:**   Take either on an empty stomach or with food or milk to prevent stomach irritation. Take with a full glass of water and remain upright (do not lie down) for 30 minutes. The tablet may be crushed for administration.

Usual Duration of Use: Continual use on a regular schedule for 1 to 2 weeks is usually necessary to determine this drug's effectiveness in relieving the discomfort of arthritis. Long-term use requires supervision and periodic evaluation by the physician. Consult your physician on a regular basis.

▷ **This Drug Should Not Be Taken If**
- you have had an allergic reaction to it previously.
- you are subject to asthma or nasal polyps caused by aspirin.
- you have active peptic ulcer disease or any form of gastrointestinal bleeding.
- you have a bleeding disorder or a blood cell disorder.
- you have active liver disease.
- you have severe impairment of kidney function.

▷ **Inform Your Physician Before Taking This Drug If**
- you are allergic to aspirin or to other aspirin substitutes.
- you have a history of peptic ulcer disease or any type of bleeding disorder.
- you have impaired liver or kidney function.
- you have high blood pressure or a history of heart failure.
- you are taking any of the following: acetaminophen, aspirin or other aspirin substitutes, anticoagulants, oral antidiabetic drugs.

Possible Side-Effects (natural, expected and unavoidable drug actions)
Fluid retention (weight gain), prolongation of bleeding time.

▷ **Possible Adverse Effects** (unusual, unexpected and infrequent reactions)
If any of the following develop, consult your physician promptly for guidance.
Mild Adverse Effects
Allergic Reactions: Skin rash, hives, itching, localized swellings, spontaneous bruising.
Headache, dizziness, altered or blurred vision, ringing in the ears, drowsiness, fatigue, inability to concentrate.
Mouth sores, indigestion, nausea, vomiting, abdominal pain, diarrhea.
Serious Adverse Effects
Active peptic ulcer, stomach or intestinal bleeding, diverticulitis.
Liver damage with jaundice (see Glossary).
Kidney damage with painful urination, bloody urine, reduced urine formation.

Visual disturbances due to corneal changes, lens opacities, retinal changes.

Impaired hearing.

Reduction of white blood cell and/or platelet counts.

▷ **Possible Effects on Sexual Function**
Inhibited ejaculation (1 report).
Altered timing and pattern of menstruation.

Possible Delayed Adverse Effects: Mild anemia due to "silent" blood loss from the stomach (less than that caused by aspirin).

▷ **Adverse Effects That May Mimic Natural Diseases or Disorders**
Liver reaction may suggest viral hepatitis.

Natural Diseases or Disorders That May Be Activated by This Drug
Peptic ulcer disease, ulcerative colitis.

CAUTION
1. Dosage should always be limited to the smallest amount that produces reasonable improvement.
2. This drug may mask early indications of infection. Inform your physician if you think you are developing an infection of any kind.

Precautions for Use
By Infants and Children: Indications and dosage recommendations for use by those under 12 years of age have not been established.
By Those over 60 Years of Age: Small doses are advisable until tolerance is determined. Observe for any indications of liver or kidney toxicity, fluid retention, dizziness, confusion, impaired memory, stomach bleeding or constipation.

▷ **Advisability of Use During Pregnancy**
Pregnancy Category: B (tentative). See Pregnancy Code inside back cover.
Animal studies: No birth defects reported in mice, rats or rabbits.
Human studies: Information from adequate studies of pregnant women is not available.
Avoid this drug during the last 3 months. Use it during the first 6 months only if clearly needed. Ask physician for guidance.

Advisability of Use if Breast-Feeding
Presence of this drug in breast milk: Yes, in minute amounts.
Avoid drug or refrain from nursing.

Habit-Forming Potential: None.

Effects of Overdosage: Possible drowsiness, dizziness, ringing in the ears, nausea, vomiting, indigestion.

Possible Effects of Long-Term Use: Eye changes such as opacities in the cornea or lens, retinal changes in the macular area. Kidney damage.

Suggested Periodic Examinations While Taking This Drug (at physician's discretion)

Complete blood cell counts, liver and kidney function tests.

Complete eye examinations if vision is altered in any way.

Hearing examinations if ringing in the ears or hearing loss develops.

▷ **While Taking This Drug, Observe the Following**

Foods: No restrictions.

Beverages: No restrictions. May be taken with milk.

▷ *Alcohol:* Use with caution. The irritant action of alcohol on the stomach lining, added to the irritant action of this drug in sensitive individuals, can increase the risk of stomach ulceration and/or bleeding.

Tobacco Smoking: No interactions expected.

▷ *Other Drugs*

Naproxen may *increase* the effects of

- acetaminophen (Tylenol, etc.), and increase the risk of kidney damage; avoid prolonged use of this combination.
- anticoagulants (Coumadin, etc.), and increase the risk of bleeding; monitor prothrombin time and adjust dose accordingly.

Naproxen *taken concurrently* with the following drugs may increase the risk of bleeding; avoid these combinations:

- aspirin.
- dipyridamole (Persantine).
- indomethacin (Indocin).
- sulfinpyrazone (Anturane).
- valproic acid (Depakene).

▷ *Driving, Hazardous Activities:* This drug may cause drowsiness or dizziness. Restrict activities as necessary.

Aviation Note: The use of this drug *may be a disqualification* for piloting. Consult a designated Aviation Medical Examiner.

Exposure to Sun: No restrictions.

NEOSTIGMINE
(nee oh STIG meen)

Introduced: 1931

Class: Antimyasthenic

Prescription: USA: Yes
Canada: No

Controlled Drug: USA: No
Canada: No

Available as Generic: USA: Yes
Canada: No

Brand Name: Prostigmin

BENEFITS versus RISKS

Possible Benefits	*Possible Risks*
MODERATELY EFFECTIVE TREATMENT OF OCULAR AND MILD FORMS OF MYASTHENIA GRAVIS (symptomatic relief of muscle weakness)	Cholinergic crisis (overdose): excessive salivation, nausea, vomiting, stomach cramps, diarrhea, shortness of breath (asthmalike wheezing), excessive weakness

---

▷ **Principal Uses**

As a Single Drug Product: Used primarily to treat the ocular and milder forms of myasthenia gravis by providing temporary relief of muscle weakness and fatigability. It is most useful in long-term treatment when there is little or no difficulty in swallowing.

How This Drug Works: This drug inhibits cholinesterase, the enzyme that destroys acetylcholine. This results in higher levels of acetylcholine, the nerve transmitter that facilitates the stimulation of muscular activity. The net effects are increased muscle strength and endurance.

Available Dosage Forms and Strengths

Injection — 0.25, 0.5, 1.0 mg per ml

Tablets — 15 mg

▷ **Usual Adult Dosage Range:**   Initially: 15 mg/3 to 4 hours; adjust dosage as needed and tolerated. Maintenance: up to 300 mg/24 hours; the average dose is 75 to 150 mg/24 hours. **Note: Actual dosage and administration schedule must be determined by the physician for each patient individually.**

▷ **Dosing Instructions:**   Take with food or milk to reduce the intensity of side-effects. Larger portions of the daily maintenance dosage should be timed according to the pattern of fatigue and weakness. The tablet may be crushed for administration.

Usual Duration of Use: Continual use on a regular schedule (with dosage adjustment) for 10 to 14 days is usually necessary to determine this drug's effectiveness in relieving the symptoms of myasthenia gravis. Long-term use (months to years) requires periodic evaluation of response and dosage adjustment. Consult your physician on a regular basis.

▷ **This Drug Should Not Be Taken If**
- you have had an allergic reaction to it previously.
- you are known to be allergic to bromide compounds.

▷ **Inform Your Physician Before Taking This Drug If**
- you have any type of seizure disorder.
- you are subject to heart rhythm disorders or bronchial asthma.

- you have recurrent urinary tract infections.
- you have prostatism (see Glossary).
- you plan to have surgery under general anesthesia in the near future.

Possible Side-Effects (natural, expected and unavoidable drug actions)
Small pupils, watering of eyes, slow pulse, excessive salivation, nausea, vomiting, stomach cramps, diarrhea, urge to urinate, increased sweating.

▷ **Possible Adverse Effects** (unusual, unexpected and infrequent reactions)
If any of the following develop, consult your physician promptly for guidance.
Mild Adverse Effects
Allergic Reaction: Skin rash.
Nervousness, anxiety, unsteadiness, muscle cramps or twitching.
Serious Adverse Effects
Confusion, slurred speech, seizures, difficult breathing (asthmatic wheezing).
Increased muscle weakness or paralysis.
Excessive vomiting or diarrhea may induce abnormally low blood potassium levels (hypokalemia). This will accentuate muscle weakness.

▷ **Possible Effects on Sexual Function:** None reported.

▷ **Adverse Effects That May Mimic Natural Diseases or Disorders**
Seizures may suggest the possibility of epilepsy.

Natural Diseases or Disorders That May Be Activated by This Drug
Latent bronchial asthma.

CAUTION
1. Certain drugs can block the action of this drug and reduce its effectiveness in treating myasthenia gravis. (See *Other Drugs* below.) Consult your physician before starting any new drug, prescription or over-the-counter.
2. The dosage schedule of this drug must be carefully individualized for each patient. Variations in response may occur from time to time. Because generalized muscle weakness is a major symptom of both myasthenia crisis (underdosage) and cholinergic crisis (overdosage), it may be difficult to recognize the correct cause. As a rule, weakness that begins within 1 hour after taking this drug probably represents overdosage; weakness that begins 3 or more hours after taking this drug is probably due to underdosage. Observe these time relationships and inform your physician.
3. During long-term use of this drug, observe for the possible development of resistance to the drug's therapeutic action (loss of effectiveness). Consult your physician regarding the advisability of discontinuing this drug for a few days to see if responsiveness can be restored.

Precautions for Use
By Infants and Children: Dosage and administration schedule must be modified if kidney function is severely impaired.

By Those over 60 Years of Age: The natural decline of kidney function with aging may require smaller doses to prevent accumulation of this drug to toxic levels.

▷ **Advisability of Use During Pregnancy**
Pregnancy Category: C (tentative). See Pregnancy Code inside back cover.

Animal studies: No information available.

Human studies: Information from adequate studies of pregnant women is not available.

There are no reports of birth defects due to the use of this drug during pregnancy. However, there are reports of significant muscular weakness in 20% of newborn infants whose mothers had taken this drug during pregnancy. Ask your physician for guidance.

Advisability of Use if Breast-Feeding
Presence of this drug in breast milk: Probably not.

Monitor nursing infant closely and discontinue drug or nursing if adverse effects develop.

Habit-Forming Potential: None.

Effects of Overdosage: Generalized muscular weakness, blurred vision, very small pupils, slow heart rate, difficult breathing (wheezing), excessive salivation, nausea, vomiting, stomach cramps, diarrhea, muscle cramps or twitching. This syndrome constitutes the cholinergic crisis.

Possible Effects of Long-Term Use: Development of tolerance (see Glossary) with loss of therapeutic effectiveness.

Suggested Periodic Examinations While Taking This Drug (at physician's discretion)
Assessment of drug effectiveness and dosage schedule for optimal therapeutic results.

▷ **While Taking This Drug, Observe the Following**
Foods: No restrictions.

Beverages: No restrictions. May be taken with milk.

▷   *Alcohol:* Use caution until the combined effects are determined. Weakness and unsteadiness may be accentuated.

Tobacco Smoking: No interactions expected.

▷   *Other Drugs*
The following drugs may *decrease* the effects of neostigmine
- atropine (belladonna).
- clindamycin (Cleocin).
- guanadrel (Hylorel).
- guanethidine (Esimil, Ismelin).

- procainamide (Procan SR, Pronestyl).
- quinidine (Cardioquin, Duraquin, etc.).
- quinine (Quinamm).

▷ *Driving, Hazardous Activities:* This drug may cause blurred vision, confusion or generalized weakness. Restrict activities as necessary.

Aviation Note: The use of this drug *is a disqualification* for piloting. Consult a designated Aviation Medical Examiner.

Exposure to Sun: No restrictions.

Exposure to Heat: Use caution. This may cause excessive sweating and increased weakness.

Exposure to Environmental Chemicals: Avoid excessive exposure (inhalation, skin contamination) to the insecticides Baygon, Diazinon and Sevin. These can accentuate the potential toxicity of this drug.

Discontinuation: Do not discontinue this drug abruptly without your physician's knowledge and guidance.

NIACIN
(NI a sin)

Other Names: Nicotinic acid, vitamin B-3

Introduced: 1937

Class: Anticholesterol, vasodilator, vitamins

Prescription: USA: Tablets and liquid—no; capsules—yes
Canada: No

Controlled Drug: USA: No
Canada: No

Available as Generic: USA: Yes
Canada: Yes

Brand Names: ✦Antivert [CD], Niac, Nicobid, Nico-400, Nicolar, Nicotinex, ✦Novoniacin, Slo-Niacin, Span-Niacin-150

BENEFITS versus RISKS

Possible Benefits	*Possible Risks*
EFFECTIVE REDUCTION OF TOTAL CHOLESTEROL, LOW DENSITY CHOLESTEROL AND TRIGLYCERIDES IN TYPES II, III, IV AND V CHOLESTEROL DISORDERS (25% reduction of total cholesterol, 35% reduction of LDL cholesterol, and 20% elevation of HDL cholesterol, a beneficial effect) Specific prevention and treatment of pellagra (niacin-deficiency disease)	Activation of peptic ulcer Drug-induced hepatitis Aggravation of diabetes or gout

---

▷ **Principal Uses**

As a Single Drug Product: This drug is used to treat three unrelated disorders: (1) certain patterns of abnormally high blood levels of cholesterol and triglycerides in individuals considered to be at high risk for the development of coronary artery heart disease; (2) pellagra, a niacin (vitamin B-3) deficiency disorder characterized by dementia, dermatitis and diarrhea; and (3) certain types of vertigo and tinnitus (ringing in the ears).

As a Combination Drug Product [CD]: In Canada this drug is combined with meclizine to enhance its effectiveness in the treatment of motion sickness and vertigo.

How This Drug Works

The mechanism by which this drug reduces cholesterol and triglyceride blood levels is not completely known. It is thought that it may inhibit the initial production of triglycerides and impair the conversion of fatty tissue to cholesterol and triglycerides.

This drug corrects the specific deficiency of vitamin B-3 that is responsible for the symptoms of pellagra.

This drug causes direct dilation of peripheral blood vessels in the skin of the face and neck; for this reason it has been used to increase the blood flow to the inner ear in an attempt to relieve some types of vertigo and ringing in the ears. The effectiveness of this application is questionable.

Available Dosage Forms and Strengths

Capsules, prolonged-action — 125 mg, 250 mg, 300 mg, 400 mg, 500 mg

Oral solution — 50 mg per 5-ml teaspoonful

Tablets — 20 mg, 25 mg, 50 mg, 100 mg, 500 mg
Tablets, prolonged-action — 150 mg, 250 mg, 500 mg, 750 mg

▷ **Usual Adult Dosage Range**
For cholesterol disorders: Initially 100 mg 3 times daily. Dose may be increased in increments of 300 mg daily at intervals of 4 to 7 days as needed and tolerated. The usual maintenance dose is 1 to 2 grams 3 times daily. The total daily dosage should not exceed 6 grams.
For prevention of pellagra: 10 to 20 mg daily.
For treatment of pellagra: 50 mg 3 to 10 times daily.
Note: Actual dosage and administration schedule must be determined by the physician for each patient individually.

▷ **Dosing Instructions:**   Take with or immediately following meals to prevent stomach irritation. Also take one-half of an adult's aspirin tablet or 1 children's aspirin tablet with each dose of niacin to prevent facial flushing and itching. Dosage should be increased very slowly over 2 to 3 months as needed. The prolonged-action form of niacin is preferable to improve tolerance. The regular tablet may be crushed for administration, but the prolonged-action capsules and tablets should not be altered.

Usual Duration of Use: Continual use on a regular schedule for 3 to 5 weeks is usually necessary to determine this drug's effectiveness in reducing elevated levels of cholesterol and triglycerides. Long-term use (months to years) requires periodic evaluation of response and dosage adjustment. Consult your physician on a regular basis.

Currently a "Drug of Choice" for initiating treatment of elevated LDL cholesterol and VLDL triglycerides. See Cholesterol Disorders in Section Two.

▷ **This Drug Should Not Be Taken If**
• you have had an allergic reaction to it previously.
• you have active peptic ulcer disease or inflammatory bowel disease.
• you have active liver disease.

▷ **Inform Your Physician Before Taking This Drug If**
• you are prone to low blood pressure.
• you have a heart rhythm disorder of any kind.
• you have a history of peptic ulcer disease, inflammatory bowel disease, liver disease, jaundice or gallbladder disease (with or without gallstones).
• you have diabetes or gout.

Possible Side-Effects (natural, expected and unavoidable drug actions)
Flushing, itching, tingling and feeling of warmth usually in the face and neck. Sensitive individuals may experience orthostatic hypotension (see Glossary).

▷ **Possible Adverse Effects** (unusual, unexpected and infrequent reactions)
   If any of the following develop, consult your physician promptly for guidance.
   Mild Adverse Effects
     Allergic Reactions: Skin rash, itching, hives.
     Headache, dizziness, faintness, impaired vision.
     Indigestion, nausea, vomiting, diarrhea.
     Dryness of skin, grayish-black pigmentation of skin folds.
   Serious Adverse Effects
     Drug-induced hepatitis with jaundice (see Glossary): yellow eyes and skin, dark-colored urine, light-colored stools.
     Worsening of diabetes and gout.
     Development of heart rhythm disorders.

▷ **Possible Effects on Sexual Function:** None reported.

▷ **Adverse Effects That May Mimic Natural Diseases or Disorders**
   Liver reactions may suggest viral hepatitis.

Natural Diseases or Disorders That May Be Activated by This Drug
   Latent diabetes, gout, inflammatory bowel disease or peptic ulcer.

CAUTION
   1. Large doses may cause significant increases in blood levels of sugar and uric acid. Those who have diabetes or gout should monitor their status regularly.
   2. Comply fully with all recommendations for periodic measurements of blood cholesterol and triglyceride levels. These are essential to monitoring your response to treatment and determining the need for changes in dosage or medication.

Precautions for Use
   By Infants and Children: Safety and effectiveness for use of large doses by those under 12 years of age have not been established.
   By Those over 60 Years of Age: Observe for the possible development of low blood pressure (light-headedness, dizziness, faintness) and heart rhythm disorders.

▷ **Advisability of Use During Pregnancy**
   Pregnancy Category: C (tentative). See Pregnancy Code inside back cover.
   Animal studies: Significant birth defects due to this drug were found in chicks.
   Human studies: Information from adequate studies of pregnant women is not available.
   Use this drug only if clearly needed. Avoid completely during the first 3 months.

Advisability of Use if Breast-Feeding
   Presence of this drug in breast milk: Unknown.
   Avoid drug or refrain from nursing.

Habit-Forming Potential: None.

Effects of Overdosage: Generalized flushing, nausea, vomiting, stomach cramps, diarrhea, weakness, fainting.

Possible Effects of Long-Term Use: Increased blood levels of sugar and uric acid; liver damage.

Suggested Periodic Examinations While Taking This Drug (at physician's discretion)
Measurements of blood levels of total cholesterol, HDL and LDL cholesterol fractions, triglycerides, sugar and uric acid.
Liver function tests.

▷ **While Taking This Drug, Observe the Following**
Foods: Follow the low-cholesterol diet prescribed by your physician.
Beverages: No restrictions. May be taken with milk.
▷ *Alcohol:* Use with caution until the combined effects have been determined. Alcohol used with large doses of this drug may cause excessive lowering of blood pressure.
Tobacco Smoking: No interactions expected.
▷ *Other Drugs*
Niacin may *increase* the effects of
• some antihypertensive drugs, and cause excessive lowering of blood pressure.
Niacin may *decrease* the effects of
• antidiabetic drugs (insulin and sulfonylureas), by raising the level of blood sugar.
• probenecid (Benemid) and sulfinpyrazone (Anturane), by raising the level of blood uric acid.
▷ *Driving, Hazardous Activities:* This drug may cause dizziness and faintness. Restrict activities as necessary.
Aviation Note: The use of this drug *may be a disqualification* for piloting. Consult a designated Aviation Medical Examiner.
Exposure to Sun: No restrictions.
Discontinuation: Do not discontinue this drug without your physician's knowledge and guidance. Abrupt withdrawal may be followed by excessive increase in blood cholesterol and triglyceride levels.

NICARDIPINE
(ni KAR de peen)

Introduced: 1984

Class: Antianginal, antihypertensive, calcium channel blocker

Prescription: USA: Yes

Controlled Drug: USA: No

Available as Generic: USA: No

Brand Name: Cardene

BENEFITS versus RISKS	
Possible Benefits	*Possible Risks*
EFFECTIVE PREVENTION OF CLASSICAL ANGINA-OF-EFFORT	Increase in angina upon starting treatment (7%)
EFFECTIVE TREATMENT OF HYPERTENSION	Water retention, ankle swelling (8%)

▷ **Principal Uses**

As a Single Drug Product: Used primarily to treat (1) classical angina-of-effort (due to atherosclerotic disease of the coronary arteries) in individuals who have not responded to or cannot tolerate the nitrates and beta blocker drugs customarily used to treat this disorder; (2) mild to moderately severe hypertension.

How This Drug Works: Not completely established. It is thought that by blocking the normal passage of calcium through certain cell walls (which is necessary for the function of nerve and muscle tissue), this drug inhibits the contraction of coronary arteries and peripheral arterioles. As a result of these effects, this drug

• promotes dilation of the coronary arteries (antianginal effect).
• reduces the degree of contraction of peripheral arterial walls, resulting in their relaxation and consequent lowering of blood pressure. This further reduces the workload of the heart during exertion and contributes to the prevention of angina.

Available Dosage Forms and Strengths

Capsules — 20 mg, 30 mg

▷ **Usual Adult Dosage Range:**   Initially 20 mg 3 times daily, 6 to 8 hours apart. Dose may be increased gradually at 3-day intervals (as needed and tolerated) up to 40 mg 3 times daily. The total daily dosage should not exceed 120 mg. **Note: Actual dosage and administration schedule must be determined by the physician for each patient individually.**

▷ **Dosing Instructions:**   May be taken with or following food to reduce stomach irritation. However, if taken after a high-fat meal, total absorption of this drug may be reduced by 20% to 30%. The capsule should be swallowed whole (not altered).

Usual Duration of Use: Continual use on a regular schedule for 2 to 4 weeks is usually necessary to determine this drug's effectiveness in reducing the frequency and severity of angina or controlling hypertension. For long-term use (months to years), determine the smallest effective dose. Supervision and periodic evaluation are essential. Consult your physician on a regular basis.

▷ **This Drug Should Not Be Taken If**
- you have had an allergic reaction to it previously.
- you have advanced aortic stenosis.

▷ **Inform Your Physician Before Taking This Drug If**
- you have had an unfavorable response to any calcium blocker drug in the past (see Drug Class, Section Four).
- you are currently taking any form of digitalis or a beta blocker drug (see Drug Class, Section Four).
- you are taking any drugs that lower blood pressure.
- you are taking cimetidine (Tagamet) or cyclosporine (Sandimmune).
- you have a history of congestive heart failure, heart attack or stroke.
- you are subject to disturbances of heart rhythm.
- you have impaired liver or kidney function.

Possible Side-Effects (natural, expected and unavoidable drug actions)
Rapid heart rate (3.4%), swelling of the feet and ankles (8%), flushing and sensation of warmth (9.7%).

▷ **Possible Adverse Effects** (unusual, unexpected and infrequent reactions)
If any of the following develop, consult your physician promptly for guidance.
Mild Adverse Effects
Allergic Reaction: Skin rash (0.4% to 1.2%).
Headache (6.4% to 8.2%), dizziness (4% to 6.9%), weakness (4.2% to 5.8%), nervousness (0.6%), blurred vision, confusion.
Palpitation (3.3% to 4.1%), shortness of breath (0.6%).
Indigestion (0.8% to 1.5%), nausea (1.9% to 2.2%), vomiting (0.4%), constipation (0.6%).
Serious Adverse Effects
Allergic Reactions: None reported.
Increased frequency or severity of angina on initiation of treatment or following an increase in dose (7%).
Marked drop in blood pressure with fainting (0.8%).

▷ **Possible Effects on Sexual Function:** Rare impotence (less than 1%).

▷ **Adverse Effects That May Mimic Natural Diseases or Disorders**
Flushing and warmth may resemble menopausal "hot flushes."

CAUTION
1. If you are monitoring your own blood pressure, make your measurements just before each dose and 1–2 hours after each dose to obtain an accurate picture of this drug's effect. This will detect excessive fluctuations between high and low readings.
2. Be sure to inform all physicians and dentists you consult that you are taking this drug. Note the use of this drug on your card of personal identification.

3. You may use nitroglycerin and other nitrate drugs as needed to relieve acute episodes of angina pain. However, if you detect that your angina attacks are becoming more frequent or intense, notify your physician promptly.

Precautions for Use

By Infants and Children: Safety and effectiveness for use by those under 18 years of age have not been established.

By Those over 60 Years of Age: Usually well tolerated by this age group. However, observe for the development of weakness, dizziness, fainting and falling. Take necessary precautions to prevent injury. Report promptly any changes in your pattern of thirst and urination.

▷ **Advisability of Use During Pregnancy**

Pregnancy Category: C (tentative). See Pregnancy Code inside back cover.

Animal studies: Embryo and fetal toxicity reported in small animals, but no birth defects due to this drug.

Human studies: Information from adequate studies of pregnant women is not available.

Avoid this drug during the first 3 months. Use during the last 6 months only if clearly needed. Ask physician for guidance.

Advisability of Use if Breast-Feeding

Presence of this drug in breast milk: Probably yes.

Avoid drug or refrain from nursing.

Habit-Forming Potential: None.

Effects of Overdosage: Weakness, light-headedness, fainting, fast pulse, low blood pressure, shortness of breath, flushed and warm skin, tremors.

Possible Effects of Long-Term Use: None reported.

Suggested Periodic Examinations While Taking This Drug (at physician's discretion)

Evaluations of heart function, including electrocardiograms; measurements of blood pressure in supine, sitting and standing positions.

▷ **While Taking This Drug, Observe the Following**

Foods: No restrictions. Avoid excessive salt intake.

Beverages: No restrictions. May be taken with milk.

▷   *Alcohol:* Use with caution until combined effects have been determined. Alcohol may exaggerate the drop in blood pressure experienced by some individuals.

Tobacco Smoking: Nicotine may reduce the effectiveness of this drug. Follow your physician's advice regarding smoking.

Marijuana Smoking: Possible reduced effectiveness of this drug; mild to moderate increase in angina; possible changes in electrocardiogram, confusing interpretation.

▷ *Other Drugs*
Nicardipine may *increase* the effects of
- cyclosporine (Sandimmune), and cause kidney toxicity.

Nicardipine *taken concurrently* with
- beta blocker drugs or digitalis preparations (see Drug Classes, Section Four) may affect heart rate and rhythm adversely. Careful monitoring by your physician is necessary if these drugs are taken concurrently.

The following drugs may *increase* the effects of nicardipine
- cimetidine (Tagamet).

▷ *Driving, Hazardous Activities:* Usually no restrictions. This drug may cause drowsiness or dizziness. Restrict activities as necessary.

Aviation Note: Coronary artery disease and hypertension *are disqualifications* for piloting. Consult a designated Aviation Medical Examiner.

Exposure to Sun: No restrictions.

Exposure to Heat: Caution advised. Hot environments can exaggerate the blood-pressure-lowering effects of this drug. Observe for light-headedness or weakness.

Heavy Exercise or Exertion: This drug may improve your ability to be more active without resulting angina pain. Use caution and avoid excessive exercise that could impair heart function in the absence of warning pain.

Discontinuation: Do not discontinue this drug abruptly. Consult your physician regarding gradual withdrawal. Observe for the possible development of rebound angina.

NIFEDIPINE
(ni FED i peen)

Introduced: 1972

Class: Antianginal, calcium channel blocker

Prescription: USA: Yes
Canada: Yes

Controlled Drug: USA: No
Canada: No

Available as Generic: No

Brand Names: Adalat, Procardia

BENEFITS versus RISKS	
Possible Benefits	*Possible Risks*
EFFECTIVE PREVENTION OF BOTH MAJOR TYPES OF ANGINA	Rare increase in angina upon starting treatment
	Rare precipitation of congestive heart failure
	Very rare drug-induced hepatitis

▷ **Principal Uses**

As a Single Drug Product: Used primarily to treat (1) angina pectoris due to coronary artery spasm (Prinzmetal's variant angina) that occurs spontaneously and is not associated with exertion; and (2) classical angina-of-effort (due to atherosclerotic disease of the coronary arteries) in individuals who have not responded to or cannot tolerate the nitrates and beta blocker drugs customarily used to treat this disorder.

How This Drug Works: Not completely established. It is thought that by blocking the normal passage of calcium through certain cell walls (which is necessary for the function of nerve and muscle tissue), this drug slows the spread of electrical activity through the conduction system of the heart and inhibits the contraction of coronary arteries and peripheral arterioles. As a result of these combined effects, this drug

- prevents spontaneous spasm of the coronary arteries (Prinzmetal's type of angina).
- reduces the rate and contraction force of the heart during exertion, thus lowering the oxygen requirement of the heart muscle; this reduces the occurrence of effort-induced angina (classical angina pectoris).
- reduces the degree of contraction of peripheral arterial walls, resulting in their relaxation and consequent lowering of blood pressure. This further reduces the workload of the heart during exertion and contributes to the prevention of angina.

Available Dosage Forms and Strengths
Capsules — 10 mg, 20 mg

▷ **Usual Adult Dosage Range:**   Initially, 10 mg 3 times daily. Dose may be increased gradually at 7- to 14-day intervals (as needed and tolerated) up to 30 mg 3 or 4 times/day. The usual maintenance dose is 10 to 20 mg 3 times/day. The total daily dosage should not exceed 180 mg. **Note: Actual dosage and administration schedule must be determined by the physician for each patient individually.**

▷ **Dosing Instructions:**   May be taken with or following food to reduce stomach irritation. The capsule should be swallowed whole (not altered).

Usual Duration of Use: Continual use on a regular schedule for 2 to 4 weeks is usually necessary to determine this drug's effectiveness in reducing the frequency and severity of angina. For long-term use (months to years), determine the smallest effective dose. Supervision and periodic evaluation by your physician are essential. Consult your physician on a regular basis.

▷ **This Drug Should Not Be Taken If**
- you have had an allergic reaction to it previously.
- you have active liver disease.
- you have low blood pressure—systolic pressure below 90.

▷ **Inform Your Physician Before Taking This Drug If**
- you have had an unfavorable response to any calcium blocker drug in the past.
- you are currently taking any form of digitalis or a beta blocker drug (see Drug Class, Section Four).
- you are taking any drugs that lower blood pressure.
- you have a history of congestive heart failure, heart attack or stroke.
- you are subject to disturbances of heart rhythm.
- you have impaired liver or kidney function.
- you have diabetes.
- you have a history of drug-induced liver damage.

Possible Side-Effects (natural, expected and unavoidable drug actions)
Low blood pressure, rapid heart rate, swelling of the feet and ankles (7%), flushing and sensation of warmth (25%), sweating.

▷ **Possible Adverse Effects** (unusual, unexpected and infrequent reactions)
If any of the following develop, consult your physician promptly for guidance.
Mild Adverse Effects
Allergic Reactions: Skin rash, hives, itching, fever.
Headache (23%), dizziness (27%), weakness (12%), nervousness (7%), blurred vision.
Palpitation (7%), shortness of breath, wheezing (6%), cough.
Heartburn (11%), nausea, cramps, diarrhea (2%).
Tremors, muscle cramps (8%).
Serious Adverse Effects
Allergic Reaction: Drug-induced hepatitis (very rare).
Idiosyncratic Reactions: Joint stiffness and inflammation.
Increased frequency or severity of angina on initiation of treatment or following an increase in dose.
Marked drop in blood pressure with fainting.

▷ **Possible Effects on Sexual Function:** Altered timing and pattern of menstruation; excessive menstrual bleeding.

▷ **Adverse Effects That May Mimic Natural Diseases or Disorders**
An allergic rash and swelling of the legs may resemble erysipelas.
Drug-induced hepatitis may suggest viral hepatitis.

CAUTION
1. Be sure to inform all physicians and dentists you consult that you are taking this drug. Note the use of this drug on your card of personal identification.
2. You may use nitroglycerin and other nitrate drugs as needed to relieve acute episodes of angina pain. However, if you detect that your angina attacks are becoming more frequent or intense, notify your physician promptly.

Precautions for Use
By Infants and Children: Safety and effectiveness for use by those under 12 years of age have not been established.
By Those over 60 Years of Age: You may be more susceptible to the development of weakness, dizziness, fainting and falling. Take necessary precautions to prevent injury. Report promptly any changes in your pattern of thirst and urination.

▷ **Advisability of Use During Pregnancy**
Pregnancy Category: C (tentative). See Pregnancy Code inside back cover.
Animal studies: Embryo and fetal deaths reported in mice, rats and rabbits; birth defects reported in rats.
Human studies: Information from adequate studies of pregnant women is not available.
Avoid this drug during the first 3 months. Use during the last 6 months only if clearly needed. Ask physician for guidance.

Advisability of Use if Breast-Feeding
Presence of this drug in breast milk: Unknown.
Avoid drug or refrain from nursing.

Habit-Forming Potential: None.

Effects of Overdosage: Weakness, light-headedness, fainting, fast pulse, low blood pressure, shortness of breath, flushed and warm skin, tremors.

Possible Effects of Long-Term Use: None reported.

Suggested Periodic Examinations While Taking This Drug (at physician's discretion)
Evaluations of heart function, including electrocardiograms; measurements of blood pressure in supine, sitting and standing positions.

▷ **While Taking This Drug, Observe the Following**
Foods: No restrictions. Avoid excessive salt intake.
Beverages: No restrictions. May be taken with milk.
▷ *Alcohol:* Use with caution until combined effects have been determined. Alcohol may exaggerate the drop in blood pressure experienced by some individuals.
Tobacco Smoking: Nicotine may reduce the effectiveness of this drug. Follow your physician's advice regarding smoking.
Marijuana Smoking: Possible reduced effectiveness of this drug; mild to moderate increase in angina; possible changes in electrocardiogram, confusing interpretation.
▷ *Other Drugs*
Nifedipine **taken concurrently** with
• beta blocker drugs or digitalis preparations (see Drug Classes, Section Four) may affect heart rate and rhythm adversely. Careful monitoring by your physician is necessary if these drugs are taken concurrently.

The following drugs may *increase* the effects of nifedipine
- cimetidine (Tagamet).

▷ *Driving, Hazardous Activities:* Usually no restrictions. This drug may cause drowsiness or dizziness. Restrict activities as necessary.

Aviation Note: Coronary artery disease *is a disqualification* for piloting. Consult a designated Aviation Medical Examiner.

Exposure to Sun: No restrictions.

Exposure to Heat: Caution advised. Hot environments can exaggerate the blood-pressure-lowering effects of this drug. Observe for light-headedness or weakness.

Heavy Exercise or Exertion: This drug may improve your ability to be more active without resulting angina pain. Use caution and avoid excessive exercise that could impair heart function in the absence of warning pain.

Discontinuation: Do not discontinue this drug abruptly. Consult your physician regarding gradual withdrawal. Observe for the possible development of rebound angina.

NITROFURANTOIN
(ni troh fyur AN toin)

Introduced: 1953   **Class:** Urinary anti-infective

Prescription: USA: Yes   **Controlled Drug:** USA: No
Canada: Yes   Canada: No

Available as Generic: Yes

Brand Names: ✦Apo-Nitrofurantoin, Furadantin, Furalan, Macrodantin, Macrodantin MACPAC, ✦Nephronex, ✦Novofuran

---

BENEFITS versus RISKS

Possible Benefits	*Possible Risks*
EFFECTIVE TREATMENT OF SOME URINARY TRACT INFECTIONS	ALLERGIC REACTIONS: Anaphylaxis Rashes, hives Repetitive asthma Lung inflammation Drug-induced hepatitis Peripheral neuropathy (see Glossary) Blood cell disorders: hemolytic anemia (see Glossary) Reduced white blood cell count Superinfections

▷ **Principal Uses**

> *As a Single Drug Product:* Because this drug is concentrated in the urine and attains only low levels in the blood, its use is limited to the prevention or treatment of infections in the urinary tract.

How This Drug Works: Not completely established. It is thought that by interfering with some bacterial enzyme systems, this drug is bacteriostatic (growth retarding) in low to moderate concentrations and bactericidal (killing) in high concentrations.

Available Dosage Forms and Strengths
> Capsules — 25 mg, 50 mg, 100 mg
> Oral suspension — 25 mg per 5-ml teaspoonful
> Tablets — 50 mg, 100 mg

▷ **Usual Adult Dosage Range:** For treatment of active infections: 50 to 100 mg/6 hours. For prevention: 50 to 100 mg once/day at bedtime. The total daily dosage should not exceed 600 mg. **Note: Actual dosage and administration schedule must be determined by the physician for each patient individually.**

▷ **Dosing Instructions:** Preferably taken with or following food to facilitate absorption and reduce stomach irritation. The tablet may be crushed and the capsule opened for administration, but this drug can stain the teeth yellow on contact.

Usual Duration of Use: Continual use on a regular schedule for 7 to 10 days is usually necessary to determine this drug's effectiveness in curing urinary tract infections. Long-term use for prevention (months to years) requires supervision and periodic evaluation by your physician. Consult your physician on a regular basis.

▷ **This Drug Should Not Be Taken If**
- you have had an allergic reaction to it previously.
- you have severely impaired kidney function.
- you have active liver disease.
- you are in the last month of pregnancy.

▷ **Inform Your Physician Before Taking This Drug If**
- you are allergic to any nitrofuran drug.
- you have impaired liver or kidney function.
- you have a deficiency of glucose-6-phosphate dehydrogenase in your red blood cells.
- you have chronic anemia or diabetes.

Possible Side-Effects (natural, expected and unavoidable drug actions)
Superinfections (see Glossary) in the urinary tract.
Brown discoloration of the urine, of no significance.

▷ **Possible Adverse Effects** (unusual, unexpected and infrequent reactions)
If any of the following develop, consult your physician promptly for guidance.

Mild Adverse Effects
 Allergic Reactions: Skin rashes, hives, localized swellings, itching, fever.
 Headache, dizziness, drowsiness, burning and tearing of eyes, impaired color vision, muscle aching, loss of hair.
 Loss of appetite, nausea, vomiting, diarrhea, abdominal cramping.
Serious Adverse Effects
 Allergic Reactions: Anaphylaxis (see Glossary), interstitial pneumonitis (lung inflammation), asthma, hepatitis.
 Idiosyncratic Reaction: Hemolytic anemia (see Glossary).
 Peripheral neuropathy (see Glossary).
 Blood cell disorders: reduced red and white blood cell counts.

▷ **Possible Effects on Sexual Function:**   None reported.

▷ **Adverse Effects That May Mimic Natural Diseases or Disorders**
 Allergic pneumonitis may suggest an infectious pneumonia.
 Allergic hepatitis may suggest viral hepatitis.

Natural Diseases or Disorders That May Be Activated by This Drug
 Latent asthma.

CAUTION
 Troublesome and persistent diarrhea can develop in sensitive individuals. If diarrhea persists for more than 24 hours, discontinue this drug and consult your physician.

Precautions for Use
 By Infants and Children: This drug should not be used in infants under 1 month of age. Observe closely for the possible development of increased intracranial pressure.
 By Those over 60 Years of Age: Dosage must be carefully individualized on the basis of kidney function. This age group is more susceptible to skin rashes, nausea, vomiting and constipation.

▷ **Advisability of Use During Pregnancy**
 Pregnancy Category: C (tentative). See Pregnancy Code inside back cover.
 Animal studies: No information available.
 Human studies: No significant increase in birth defects reported in 590 exposures. Information from adequate studies of pregnant women is not available.
 Avoid use of drug during the last few weeks of pregnancy. Use otherwise only if clearly needed. Ask your physician for guidance.

Advisability of Use if Breast-Feeding
 Presence of this drug in breast milk: Yes, in small amounts.
 Avoid drug or refrain from nursing.

Habit-Forming Potential: None.

Effects of Overdosage: Nausea, vomiting, diarrhea.

Possible Effects of Long-Term Use: Allergic reactions in lungs or liver, peripheral neuropathy, superinfections within the urinary tract.

Suggested Periodic Examinations While Taking This Drug (at physician's discretion)
Complete blood cell counts, liver function tests, X-ray examinations of lungs during long-term use.

▷ **While Taking This Drug, Observe the Following**
Foods: No restrictions. Eat liberally of the following foods: beef, chicken, lamb and pork liver, asparagus, navy beans (good sources of folic acid).
Beverages: No restrictions. May be taken with milk.
▷ *Alcohol:* Use with extreme caution until the combined effects have been determined. This drug, in combination with alcohol, may cause a disulfiramlike reaction (see Glossary) in sensitive individuals.
Tobacco Smoking: No interactions expected.
▷ *Other Drugs*
The following drugs may **decrease** the effects of nitrofurantoin
• antacids that contain magnesium can prevent the absorption of nitrofurantoin and reduce its effectiveness.
▷ *Driving, Hazardous Activities:* This drug may cause dizziness. Restrict activities as necessary.
Aviation Note: The use of this drug **may be a disqualification** for piloting. Consult a designated Aviation Medical Examiner.
Exposure to Sun: No restrictions.

NITROGLYCERIN
(ni troh GLIS er in)

Introduced: 1847   **Class:** Antianginal, nitrates

Prescription: USA: Yes   **Controlled Drug:** USA: No
    Canada: No   Canada: No

Available as Generic: Yes

Brand Names: Deponit, Minitran Transdermal Delivery System, Nitro-Bid, Nitrodisc, Nitro-Dur, Nitro-Dur II, Nitrogard, ✦Nitrogard-SR, Nitroglyn, Nitrol, Nitrolingual Spray, Nitrong, ✦Nitrong SR, Nitrospan, ✦Nitrostabilin, Nitrostat, Transderm-Nitro, ✦Tridil

BENEFITS versus RISKS	
Possible Benefits	*Possible Risks*
EFFECTIVE RELIEF AND PREVENTION OF ANGINA EFFECTIVE ADJUNCTIVE TREATMENT IN SELECTED CASES OF CONGESTIVE HEART FAILURE	Orthostatic hypotension (see Glossary) with and without fainting Skin rash (rare) Altered hemoglobin with large doses (very rare)

▷ **Principal Uses**

As a Single Drug Product: Used primarily in the treatment of symptomatic coronary artery disease. The rapid-action forms are used to relieve acute attacks of anginal pain at their onset. The sustained-action forms are used to prevent the development of angina.

How This Drug Works: By direct action on the muscles in blood vessel walls, this drug relaxes and dilates both arteries and veins. Its beneficial effects in the management of angina are due to two mechanisms of action: (1) dilation of narrowed coronary arteries; (2) dilation of veins in the general circulation, with consequent reduction of the volume and pressure of blood entering the heart. The net effects are improved blood supply to the heart muscle and reduced workload for the heart. Both actions reduce the frequency and severity of angina.

Available Dosage Forms and Strengths

Canisters, translingual spray — 13.8 grams (200 doses), 0.4 mg per metered dose
Capsules, prolonged-action — 2.5 mg, 2.6 mg, 6.5 mg, 9 mg
Ointment — 2%
Tablets, buccal — 1 mg, 2 mg, 3 mg
Tablets, prolonged-action — 2.6 mg, 6.5 mg, 9 mg
Tablets, sublingual — 0.15 mg, 0.3 mg, 0.4 mg, 0.6 mg
Transdermal systems — 2.5 mg, 5 mg, 7.5 mg, 10 mg, 15 mg

▷ **Usual Adult Dosage Range:** According to dosage form:

Sublingual spray—1 metered spray (0.4 mg) under tongue/3 to 5 minutes, up to 3 doses within 15 minutes, to relieve acute angina. To prevent angina, 1 spray taken 5 to 10 minutes before exertion.

Sublingual tablets—0.15 to 0.6 mg dissolved under tongue at 5-minute intervals to relieve acute angina.

Prolonged-action tablets—1.3 to 6.5 mg at 8- to 12-hour intervals to prevent angina.

Prolonged-action capsules—2.5 to 9 mg at 8- to 12-hour intervals to prevent angina.

Ointment—2.5 to 5 cm (1 to 2 inches, 15 to 30 mg) applied in a thin, even layer of uniform size to hairless skin at 3- to 4-hour intervals to prevent angina.

Buccal tablets—1 to 2 mg/4 to 5 hours placed between cheek and gum.

Transdermal patches—5-sq.-cm to 30-sq.-cm patch applied to hairless skin once/24 hours to prevent angina.

Note: Actual dosage and administration schedule must be determined by the physician for each patient individually.

▷ **Dosing Instructions:** Dosage forms to be swallowed are best taken when stomach is empty (1 hour before or 2 hours after eating) to obtain maximal blood levels. Tablets should not be crushed for administration. Capsules may be opened, but the contents should not be crushed or chewed before swallowing.

Usual Duration of Use: Continual use on a regular schedule for 3 to 5 days is usually necessary to determine this drug's effectiveness in preventing and relieving acute anginal attacks. Individual dosage adjustments will be necessary for optimal results. Long-term use (months to years) requires supervision and periodic evaluation by your physician. Consult your physician on a regular basis.

▷ **This Drug Should Not Be Taken If**
- you have had an allergic reaction to it previously.
- you are severely anemic.
- you have closed-angle glaucoma (inadequately treated).

▷ **Inform Your Physician Before Taking This Drug If**
- you have had an unfavorable response to other nitrate drugs in the past.
- you have low blood pressure.
- you have any form of glaucoma.

Possible Side-Effects (natural, expected and unavoidable drug actions)
Flushing of face, headaches (50%), orthostatic hypotension (see Glossary), rapid heart rate, palpitation.

▷ **Possible Adverse Effects** (unusual, unexpected and infrequent reactions)
If any of the following develop, consult your physician promptly for guidance.
Mild Adverse Effects
Allergic Reaction: Skin rash.
Throbbing headaches (may be severe and persistent), dizziness, fainting.
Nausea, vomiting.
Serious Adverse Effects
Allergic Reactions: Severe skin reactions with peeling.
Idiosyncratic Reaction: Methemoglobinemia (very rare).

▷ **Possible Effects on Sexual Function**
Correction of impotence (1 report following sublingual use).
The preventive use of nitroglycerin prior to sexual activity has been recommended to eliminate or reduce the risk of angina. Consult your physician for guidance.

▷ **Adverse Effects That May Mimic Natural Diseases or Disorders**

Hypotensive spells (sudden drops in blood pressure) due to this drug may be mistaken for late-onset epilepsy.

CAUTION

1. This drug can provoke migraine headaches in susceptible individuals.
2. In the presence of impaired brain circulation (cerebral arteriosclerosis), this drug can cause transient ischemic attacks—periods of temporary speech impairment, paralysis, numbness, etc.
3. The development of tolerance to long-acting forms of nitrates will render the sublingual tablets ineffective for the relief of acute angina. Sensitivity to the drug's antianginal effect is restored after one week of abstinence from the long-acting forms.
4. Many over-the-counter (OTC) drug products for allergies, colds and coughs contain drugs that may counteract the desired effects of this drug. Ask your physician or pharmacist for guidance before using any such medications.

Precautions for Use

By Infants and Children: Limited usefulness and experience in this age group. Dosage schedules not established.

By Those over 60 Years of Age: Begin treatment with small doses and increase dose cautiously as needed and tolerated. You may be more susceptible to the development of flushing, throbbing headache, dizziness, "blackout" spells, fainting and falling.

▷ **Advisability of Use During Pregnancy**

Pregnancy Category: C (tentative). See Pregnancy Code inside back cover.

Animal studies: No information available.

Human studies: Information from adequate studies of pregnant women is not available.

Use this drug only if clearly needed. Ask physician for guidance.

Advisability of Use if Breast-Feeding

Presence of this drug in breast milk: Unknown.

Monitor nursing infant closely and discontinue drug or nursing if adverse effects develop.

Habit-Forming Potential: None.

Effects of Overdosage: Throbbing headache, dizziness, marked flushing, nausea, vomiting, abdominal cramps, confusion, delirium, paralysis, seizures, circulatory collapse.

Possible Effects of Long-Term Use: The development of tolerance (see Glossary) and the temporary loss of effectiveness.

Suggested Periodic Examinations While Taking This Drug (at physician's discretion)

Measurements of blood pressure and internal eye pressures.

Evaluation of hemoglobin.

▷ **While Taking This Drug, Observe the Following**

Foods: No restrictions.

Beverages: No restrictions. May be taken with milk.

▷   *Alcohol:* Use extreme caution until the combined effects have been determined. Avoid alcohol completely in the presence of any side-effects or adverse effects from nitroglycerin. Never use alcohol in the presence of a nitroglycerin headache.

Tobacco Smoking: Nicotine can reduce the effectiveness of this drug. Follow your physician's advice regarding smoking.

Marijuana Smoking: Possible reduced effectiveness of this drug; mild to moderate increase in angina; possible changes in the electrocardiogram, confusing interpretation.

▷   *Other Drugs*

Nitroglycerin *taken concurrently* with

- antihypertensive drugs may cause excessive lowering of blood pressure. Careful dosage adjustments may be necessary.

The following drugs may *increase* the effects of nitroglycerin

- aspirin, in analgesic doses (500 mg or more).

▷   *Driving, Hazardous Activities:* Usually no restrictions. This drug may cause dizziness or faintness. Restrict activities as necessary.

Aviation Note: Coronary artery disease *is a disqualification* for piloting. Consult a designated Aviation Medical Examiner.

Exposure to Sun: No restrictions.

Exposure to Heat: Use caution. Hot environments can cause significant lowering of blood pressure.

Exposure to Cold: Cold environments can increase the need for this drug and limit its effectiveness.

Heavy Exercise or Exertion: This drug can increase your tolerance for exercise. Use good judgment regarding excessive exertion in the absence of anginal pain.

Discontinuation: Do not stop this drug abruptly after long-term use. It is advisable to reduce the dose (of the prolonged-action dosage forms) gradually over a period of 4 to 6 weeks. Observe for rebound angina.

Special Storage Instructions: For sublingual tablets, to prevent loss of strength

- keep tablets in the original glass container.
- do not transfer tablets to a plastic or metallic container (such as a pillbox).
- do not place absorbent cotton, paper (such as the prescription label), or other material inside the container.
- do not store other drugs in the same container.
- close the container tightly immediately after each use.
- store at room temperature.

NIZATIDINE
(ni ZA te deen)

Introduced: 1986

Class: Antiulcer, H-2 receptor blocker

Prescription: USA: Yes

Controlled Drug: USA: No

Available as Generic: No

Brand Name: Axid

BENEFITS versus RISKS

Possible Benefits	*Possible Risks*
EFFECTIVE TREATMENT OF PEPTIC ULCER DISEASE: relief of symptoms, acceleration of healing (in 80% to 90% of cases), prevention of recurrence (in 65% to 80% of cases) CONTROL OF HYPERSECRETORY STOMACH DISORDERS Beneficial in treatment of reflux esophagitis	Drug-induced liver damage (rare) Abnormally low blood platelet count (rare)

▷ **Principal Uses**

As a Single Drug Product: Used primarily in the treatment of peptic ulcer disease, both benign stomach (gastric) ulcer and duodenal ulcer. It is used specifically to hasten the healing of ulcer and to prevent recurrence. Also used to control the excessive production of stomach acid in the Zollinger-Ellison syndrome. Though its effectiveness has not been fully established, this drug is also used in the management of esophagitis (as with hiatal hernia) and upper gastrointestinal bleeding.

How This Drug Works: By blocking the action of histamine, this drug effectively inhibits the secretion of stomach acid and thus creates a more favorable environment for the healing of peptic ulcers.

Available Dosage Forms and Strengths
Capsules — 150 mg, 300 mg

▷ **Usual Adult Dosage Range:** For active peptic ulcer: 150 mg 2 times daily, 12 hours apart; or 300 mg once daily at bedtime. For prevention of recurrent ulcer: 150 mg at bedtime. **Note: Actual dosage and administration schedule must be determined by the physician for each patient individually.**

▷ **Dosing Instructions:** To obtain the longest period of stomach acid reduction, this drug should be taken with or immediately following food. The capsule may be opened for administration.

Usual Duration of Use: Continual use on a regular schedule for 4 to 6 weeks is usually necessary to determine this drug's effectiveness in healing active peptic ulcer. Long-term use (months to years) for prevention of ulcer recurrence requires individual consideration by your physician.

Possible Advantages of This Drug
Effective ulcer treatment with once-a-day dosage.
Minimal adverse effects.
Does not cause confusion; does not reduce sperm count or sexual potency.
No significant drug interactions.

▷ **This Drug Should Not Be Taken If**
- you have had an allergic reaction to any dosage form of it previously.

▷ **Inform Your Physician Before Taking This Drug If**
- you are allergic to other H-2 receptor blockers: cimetidine (Tagamet), famotidine (Pepcid), ranitidine (Zantac).
- you have impaired liver or kidney function.
- you are taking large doses of aspirin.

Possible Side-Effects (natural, expected and unavoidable drug actions)
None reported.

▷ **Possible Adverse Effects** (unusual, unexpected and infrequent reactions)
If any of the following develop, consult your physician promptly for guidance.
Mild Adverse Effects
Allergic Reaction: Skin rash, hives (0.5%).
Drowsiness (2.4%), sweating (1.0%).
Serious Adverse Effects
Allergic Reaction: Exfoliative dermatitis.
Drug-induced liver injury (without jaundice), reversible.
Reduced blood platelet count: abnormal bleeding or bruising (rare).

▷ **Possible Effects on Sexual Function:** Male breast enlargement (rare).

CAUTION
1. Do not discontinue this drug abruptly. (Ulcer activation and perforation have occurred following abrupt cessation of cimetidine, a closely related drug.)
2. After discontinuation of this drug, inform your physician promptly if you experience a return of symptoms indicative of ulcer reactivation.

Precautions for Use

By Infants and Children: Safety and effectiveness for use by those under 12 years of age have not been established.

By Those over 60 Years of Age: This drug may contribute to the formation of stomach phytobezoars (masses of undigested vegetable fibers). Individuals with poor chewing ability (missing teeth) and those who have had partial gastrectomy or vagotomy (stomach surgery) are most susceptible. Observe for loss of appetite, stomach fullness, nausea and vomiting.

▷ **Advisability of Use During Pregnancy**

Pregnancy Category: C (tentative). See Pregnancy Code inside back cover.
  Animal studies: Rabbit studies revealed significant birth defects of the heart, brain and spinal cord.
  Human studies: Information from adequate studies of pregnant women is not available.
  Avoid drug during the first 3 months if possible. Use this drug only if clearly needed. Ask physician for guidance.

Advisability of Use if Breast-Feeding

Presence of this drug in breast milk: Probably yes.
Avoid drug or refrain from nursing.

Habit-Forming Potential: None.

Effects of Overdosage: Based on animal studies: excessive tearing, salivation, vomiting, diarrhea.

Possible Effects of Long-Term Use: None reported.

Suggested Periodic Examinations While Taking This Drug (at physician's discretion)
  Complete blood cell counts, liver function tests.

▷ **While Taking This Drug, Observe the Following**

Foods: Protein-rich foods produce maximal stomach acid secretion. Follow the diet prescribed to derive optimal benefit from this drug.
Beverages: No restrictions. May be taken with milk.
▷ *Alcohol:* No interactions with drug. However, alcoholic beverages increase stomach acidity and can reduce the effectiveness of this drug.
▷ *Other Drugs*
  Nizatidine may *increase* the effects of
  • aspirin (when aspirin is taken in large doses—3900 mg/day).
  The following drugs may *decrease* the effects of nizatidine
  • antacids containing aluminum and magnesium hydroxide can reduce absorption of nizatidine by 10%. Avoid antacids for 2 hours before and after taking nizatidine.
▷ *Driving, Hazardous Activities:* This drug may cause drowsiness. Restrict activities as necessary.
Aviation Note: The use of this drug *may be a disqualification* for piloting. Consult a designated Aviation Medical Examiner.

Exposure to Sun: No restrictions.

Discontinuation: Do not discontinue this drug suddenly if taken for peptic ulcer disease. Consult physician for withdrawal instructions. This drug does not provide an extended protective effect. Be alert to the possibility of ulcer recurrence anytime after discontinuation.

NORFLOXACIN
(nor FLOX a sin)

Introduced: 1986

Class: Anti-infectives

Prescription: USA: Yes
Canada: Yes

Controlled Drug: USA: No
Canada: No

Available as Generic: USA: No
Canada: No

Brand Name: Noroxin

BENEFITS versus RISKS

Possible Benefits	*Possible Risks*
HIGH CURE RATE (95%) IN TREATMENT OF URINARY TRACT INFECTIONS	Infrequent nausea, indigestion
	Rare impairment of vision
	Rare seizure
Effective treatment of bacterial gastroenteritis and gonorrhea	

▷ **Principal Uses**

As a Single Drug Product: Used primarily to treat urinary tract infections (in adults) caused by a wide variety of bacteria sensitive to the action of this drug. It is also used to treat acute gastroenteritis caused by certain bacteria, to prevent traveler's diarrhea and to treat gonorrhea.

How This Drug Works: By inhibiting essential enzyme systems of bacterial nucleic acids (DNA), this drug prevents bacterial reproduction (with low doses) and destroys bacteria (with higher doses).

Available Dosage Forms and Strengths
Tablets — 400 mg

▷ **Usual Adult Dosage Range:** Uncomplicated urinary tract infections—400 mg/12 hours for 3 days. Complicated urinary tract infections—400 mg/12 hours for 10 to 21 days. Total daily dosage should not exceed 800 mg. **Note: Actual dosage and administration schedule must be determined by the physician for each patient individually.**

▷ **Dosing Instructions:** Preferably taken with a full glass of water 1 hour before or 2 hours after eating. Avoid antacids for 2 hours after taking this drug. The tablet may be crushed for administration. Take the full course prescribed.

Usual Duration of Use: Continual use on a regular schedule for 3 to 21 days (depending upon the nature of the infection) is usually necessary to determine this drug's effectiveness in eradicating the infection.

Possible Advantages of This Drug: Highly effective in treating adults with urinary tract infections due to virtually all varieties of causative bacteria. This drug kills bacteria rapidly, preventing the development of bacterial resistance to the action of the drug.

Currently a "Drug of Choice" for starting anti-infective treatment prior to obtaining the results of urine bacterial culture and sensitivity tests.

▷ **This Drug Should Not Be Taken If**
- you have had an allergic reaction to any dosage form of it previously.
- you are pregnant or breast-feeding.
- it is prescribed for a child under 18 years of age.

▷ **Inform Your Physician Before Taking This Drug If**
- you are allergic to cinoxacin (Cinobac) or nalidixic acid (NegGram).
- you have a seizure disorder.
- you have impaired liver or kidney function.

Possible Side-Effects (natural, expected and unavoidable drug actions)
None reported.

▷ **Possible Adverse Effects** (unusual, unexpected and infrequent reactions)
If any of the following develop, consult your physician promptly for guidance.
Mild Adverse Effects
Allergic Reactions: Skin rash (0.4%), hives (0.1%), localized swelling, itching (0.1%).
Headache (1.6%), dizziness (1.2%), mental depression (4 reports), seizures (3 reports).
Drowsiness, mood alterations, nervousness, insomnia, hallucinations (all less than 1%).
Visual disturbances: blurred or double vision, altered color vision, increased sensitivity to light (all less than 0.1%).
Dry mouth, decreased appetite (0.1%), nausea (2%), indigestion (0.3%), vomiting, (0.2%), diarrhea (0.2%).
Swollen or painful tendons and joints (0.1%).
Serious Adverse Effects
Allergic Reactions: Exfoliative dermatitis (1 report), anaphylactic reaction (see Glossary; 1 report).

▷ **Possible Effects on Sexual Function:** None reported.

Natural Diseases or Disorders That May Be Activated by This Drug
Latent epilepsy.

CAUTION
1. With high doses or prolonged use, crystal formation in the kidney can occur. This can be prevented by drinking copious amounts of water, up to 2 quarts/24 hours.
2. This drug may decrease the formation of saliva and predispose to the formation of dental cavities or gum disease. Consult your dentist if mouth dryness persists.

Precautions for Use
By Infants and Children: Safety for use by those who have not attained complete bone growth has not been established. This drug can impair normal bone growth and development in test animals. Avoid its use in children until complete bone development is assured.
By Those over 60 Years of Age: Impaired kidney function may require dosage reduction. Consult your physician.

▷ **Advisability of Use During Pregnancy**
Pregnancy Category: C (tentative). See Pregnancy Code inside back cover.
Animal studies: Mouse, rat, rabbit and monkey studies reveal no birth defects due to this drug. However, this drug can cause impaired bone development in immature dogs.
Human studies: Information from adequate studies of pregnant women is not available.
This drug should be avoided during entire pregnancy.

Advisability of Use if Breast-Feeding
Presence of this drug in breast milk: Unknown.
Avoid drug or refrain from nursing.

Habit-Forming Potential: None.

Effects of Overdosage: No information available.

Possible Effects of Long-Term Use: Crystal formation in kidneys with high doses and inadequate fluid intake.

Suggested Periodic Examinations While Taking This Drug (at physician's discretion)
Liver function tests, urine analysis.

▷ **While Taking This Drug, Observe the Following**
Foods: No restrictions.
Beverages: No restrictions.
▷ *Alcohol:* No interactions expected.
Tobacco Smoking: No interactions expected.
▷ *Other Drugs*
Nitrofurantoin (Macrodantin, etc.) **taken concurrently** with norfloxacin may antagonize the antibacterial action of norfloxacin in the urinary tract. Avoid this combination.

The following drug may **increase** the effects of norfloxacin
- probenecid (Benemid).

The following drugs may **decrease** the effects of norfloxacin
- antacids may reduce its absorption.

▷ *Driving, Hazardous Activities:* This drug may cause dizziness or impaired vision. Restrict activities as necessary.

Aviation Note: The use of this drug **may be a disqualification** for piloting. Consult a designated Aviation Medical Examiner.

Exposure to Sun: Sunglasses advised if eyes are overly sensitive to bright light.

Discontinuation: If you experience no adverse effects from this drug, take the full course prescribed for maximal results. Consult your physician regarding termination of treatment.

NORTRIPTYLINE
(nor TRIP ti leen)

Introduced: 1963

Class: Antidepressant

Prescription: USA: Yes
Canada: Yes

Controlled Drug: USA: No
Canada: No

Available as Generic: USA: No
Canada: No

Brand Names: Aventyl, Pamelor

BENEFITS versus RISKS	
Possible Benefits	*Possible Risks*
EFFECTIVE RELIEF OF ENDOGENOUS DEPRESSION	ADVERSE BEHAVIORAL EFFECTS: confusion, disorientation, hallucinations, delusions
Possibly beneficial in other depressive disorders	
Possibly beneficial in the management of some types of chronic, severe pain	CONVERSION OF DEPRESSION TO MANIA in manic-depressive disorders
	Aggravation of schizophrenia
	Irregular heart rhythms
	Rare blood cell abnormalities

▷ **Principal Uses**

As a Single Drug Product

Used primarily to relieve the symptoms associated with spontaneous (endogenous) depression, and to initiate the restoration of normal mood. This drug should be used only when a diagnosis of a true, primary depression of significant degree has been established. It should not be used to treat the symptoms of mild and transient (reactive) depression that may be associated with many life situations in the absence of a bona fide affective illness.

It is also used in conjunction with other drugs to manage chronic, severe pain associated with such conditions as cancer, migraine headache, severe arthritis, peripheral neuropathy, AIDS, etc.

How This Drug Works: It is thought that this drug relieves depression by slowly restoring to normal levels certain constituents of brain tissue (norepinephrine and serotonin) that transmit nerve impulses.

Available Dosage Forms and Strengths
>   Capsules — 10 mg, 25 mg, 50 mg, 75 mg
> Oral solution — 10 mg per 5-ml teaspoonful (alcohol 4%)

▷ **Usual Adult Dosage Range:**   Initially 25 mg 3 or 4 times daily. Dose may be increased cautiously as needed and tolerated by 10 to 25 mg daily at intervals of 1 week. Usual maintenance dose is 50 to 100 mg/24 hours. Total dose should not exceed 150 mg/24 hours. When the optimal requirement is determined, it may be taken at bedtime as one dose. **Note: Actual dosage and administration schedule must be determined by the physician for each patient individually.**

▷ **Dosing Instructions:**   May be taken without regard to meals. The capsule may be opened for administration.

Usual Duration of Use: Some benefit may be apparent within 1 to 2 weeks, but adequate response may require continual use for 3 months or longer. Long-term use should not exceed 6 months without evaluation regarding the need for continuation of the drug. Consult your physician on a regular basis.

▷ **This Drug Should Not Be Taken If**
- you have had an allergic reaction to it previously.
- you are taking or have taken within the past 14 days any monoamine oxidase (MAO) type A inhibitor drug (see Drug Class, Section Four).
- you are recovering from a recent heart attack.
- you have narrow-angle glaucoma.

▷ **Inform Your Physician Before Taking This Drug If**
- you are allergic or sensitive to any other tricyclic antidepressant (see Drug Class, Section Four).
- you have a history of any of the following: diabetes, epilepsy, glaucoma, heart disease, prostate gland enlargement or overactive thyroid function.
- you plan to have surgery under general anesthesia in the near future.

Possible Side-Effects (natural, expected and unavoidable drug actions)
Light-headedness, drowsiness, blurred vision, dry mouth, constipation, impaired urination (see Prostatism in Glossary).

▷ **Possible Adverse Effects** (unusual, unexpected and infrequent reactions)
If any of the following develop, consult your physician promptly for guidance.

Mild Adverse Effects

Allergic Reactions: Skin rash, hives, swelling of face or tongue, drug fever (see Glossary).

Headache, dizziness, weakness, fainting, unsteady gait, tremors.

Peculiar taste, irritation of tongue or mouth, nausea, indigestion.

Fluctuation of blood sugar levels.

Serious Adverse Effects

Allergic Reactions: Hepatitis, with or without jaundice (see Glossary).

Confusion, disorientation, hallucinations, delusions.

Aggravation of paranoid psychoses and schizophrenia; seizures.

Heart palpitation and irregular rhythm.

Bone marrow depression (see Glossary)—fatigue, weakness, fever, sore throat, abnormal bleeding or bruising.

Peripheral neuritis (see Glossary)—numbness, tingling, pain, loss of strength in arms and legs.

Parkinson-like disorders (see Glossary)—usually mild and infrequent; more likely to occur in the elderly.

▷ **Possible Effects on Sexual Function:** Decreased libido, increased libido (antidepressant effect), male impotence, inhibited female orgasm, male and female breast enlargement, milk production, swelling of testicles.

▷ **Adverse Effects That May Mimic Natural Diseases or Disorders**
Liver toxicity may suggest viral hepatitis.

Natural Diseases or Disorders That May Be Activated by This Drug
Latent diabetes, epilepsy, glaucoma, prostatism.

CAUTION
1. Dosage must be adjusted for each person individually. Report for follow-up evaluation and laboratory tests as directed by your physician.
2. It is advisable to withhold this drug if electroconvulsive therapy (ECT, "shock" treatment) is to be used to treat your depression.

Precautions for Use

By Infants and Children: Safety and effectiveness for use by those under 6 years of age have not been established.

By Those over 60 Years of Age: Usual dosage is 30 to 50 mg daily in divided doses. During the first 2 weeks of treatment, observe for the development of confusion, agitation, forgetfulness, disorientation, delusions and hallucinations. Reduction of dosage or discontinuation may be necessary. Unsteadiness may predispose to falling and injury. This drug can increase the degree of impaired urination associated with prostate gland enlargement (prostatism).

▷ **Advisability of Use During Pregnancy**

Pregnancy Category: C (tentative). See Pregnancy Code inside back cover.

Animal studies: Results are inconclusive.

Human studies: No defects reported in 21 exposures to amitriptyline, a closely related drug. Information from adequate studies of pregnant women is not available for this drug.

Avoid use of drug during first 3 months. Use during last 6 months only if clearly needed. Ask your physician for guidance.

Advisability of Use if Breast-Feeding

Presence of this drug in breast milk: Yes, in small amounts.

Monitor nursing infant closely and discontinue drug or nursing if adverse effects develop: excessive drowsiness and failure to feed.

Habit-Forming Potential: Psychological or physical dependence is rare and unexpected.

Effects of Overdosage: Confusion, hallucinations, marked drowsiness, heart palpitations, dilated pupils, tremors, stupor, deep sleep, coma, convulsions.

Suggested Periodic Examinations While Taking This Drug (at physician's discretion)

Complete blood cell counts, liver function tests, serial blood pressure readings and electrocardiograms.

▷ **While Taking This Drug, Observe the Following**

Foods: No restrictions. This drug may increase the appetite and cause excessive weight gain.

Beverages: No restrictions. May be taken with milk.

▷ *Alcohol:* Avoid completely. This drug can markedly increase the intoxicating effects of alcohol and accentuate its depressant action on brain function.

Tobacco Smoking: May hasten the elimination of this drug. Higher doses may be necessary.

▷ *Other Drugs*

Nortriptyline may *increase* the effects of

- atropinelike drugs (see Drug Class, Section Four).
- dicoumarol, and increase the risk of bleeding.
- epinephrine (Adrenalin).

Nortriptyline may *decrease* the effects of

- clonidine (Catapres).
- ephedrine (Primatene tablets).
- guanethidine (Ismelin).

Nortriptyline *taken concurrently* with

- disulfiram (Antabuse) may cause acute dementia: confusion, disorientation, hallucinations.
- monoamine oxidase (MAO) type A inhibitor drugs may cause high fever, delirium and convulsions (see Drug Class, Section Four).

- thyroid preparations may impair heart rhythm and function. Ask physician for guidance regarding adjustment of thyroid dose.

The following drugs may *increase* the effects of nortriptyline

- cimetidine (Tagamet), and cause nortriptyline toxicity.
- quinidine (Quinaglute, etc,), and cause nortriptyline toxicity.

The following drugs may *decrease* the effects of nortriptyline

- barbiturates (see Drug Class, Section Four), and reduce its effectiveness.

▷ *Driving, Hazardous Activities:* This drug may impair mental alertness, judgment, physical coordination and reaction time. Avoid hazardous activities.

Aviation Note: The use of this drug *is a disqualification* for piloting. Consult a designated Aviation Medical Examiner.

Exposure to Sun: Use caution until sensitivity to sun has been determined. This drug may cause photosensitivity (see Glossary).

Exposure to Heat: This drug can inhibit sweating and impair the body's adaptation to hot environments, increasing the risk of heat stroke. Avoid saunas.

Exposure to Cold: The elderly should use caution and avoid conditions conducive to hypothermia (see Glossary).

Discontinuation: It is advisable to discontinue this drug gradually. Abrupt withdrawal after long-term use can cause headache, malaise and nausea.

ORAL CONTRACEPTIVES
(or al kon tra SEP tivs)

Other Names: Estrogens/progestins

Introduced: 1956   **Class:** Female sex hormones

Prescription: USA: Yes   **Controlled Drug:** USA: No
Canada: Yes   Canada: No

Available as Generic: USA: No
Canada: No

Brand Names: Brevicon, Demulen, Enovid, Levlen, Loestrin, Lo/Ovral, Micronor*, ✦Minestrin 1/20, Modicon, Nelova, Nelova 10/11, Nordette, Norethin 1/35E, Norethin 1/50M, Norinyl, Norlestrin, Nor-Q.D.*, Ortho-Novum, Ovcon, Ovral, Ovrette*, ✦Synphasic, Tri-Levlen, Tri-Norinyl, Triphasil

*"Mini-Pill" type, contains progestin only.

```
┌─────────────────────────────────────────────────────────────────────┐
│                    BENEFITS versus RISKS                              │
│                                                                       │
│        Possible Benefits                    Possible Risks            │
│   HIGHLY EFFECTIVE FOR              SERIOUS, LIFE-THREATENING          │
│     CONTRACEPTIVE                     THROMBOEMBOLIC                   │
│     PROTECTION                        DISORDERS in susceptible         │
│   Moderately effective as adjunctive    individuals                   │
│     treatment in management of      Hypertension                      │
│     excessive menses and            Fluid retention                   │
│     endometriosis                   Intensification of migrainelike    │
│                                        headaches                       │
│                                     Intensification of fibrocystic     │
│                                        breast changes                  │
│                                     Accelerated growth of uterine      │
│                                        fibroid tumors                  │
│                                     Drug-induced hepatitis with        │
│                                        jaundice                        │
│                                     Benign liver tumors (rare)         │
└─────────────────────────────────────────────────────────────────────┘
```

▷ **Principal Uses**

As a Single Drug Product: The "Mini-Pill" contains only one component—a progestin. This has been shown to be slightly less effective than the combination of estrogen and progestin in preventing pregnancy.

As a Combination Drug Product [CD]: Most oral contraceptives consist of a combination of a type of estrogen and a type of progestin. These products are the most effective form of contraception available. While used primarily to prevent pregnancy, they are sometimes used to treat menstrual irregularity, excessively heavy menstrual flow and endometriosis.

How This Drug Works: When the combination of an estrogen and a progestin is taken in sufficient dosage and on a regular basis, the blood and tissue levels of these hormones increase to resemble those that occur during pregnancy. This results in suppression of the two pituitary gland hormones that normally produce ovulation (the formation and release of an egg by the ovary). In addition, these drugs may (1) alter the cervical mucus so that it resists the passage of sperm, and (2) alter the lining of the uterus so that it resists implantation of the egg (if ovulation occurs).

Available Dosage Forms and Strengths

Tablets — several combinations of synthetic estrogens and progestins in varying strengths; see the package label of the brand prescribed.

▷ **Usual Adult Dosage Range:**   Initiate treatment with the first tablet on the fifth day after the onset of menstruation. Follow with 1 tablet daily (taken at the same time each day) for 21 consecutive days. Resume treatment on the eighth day following the last tablet taken during

the preceding cycle. The schedule is to take the drug daily for 3 weeks
and to omit it for 1 week. For the Mini-Pill (progestin only), initiate
treatment on the first day of menstruation and take 1 tablet daily,
every day, throughout the year (no interruption). **Note: Actual dosage
and administration schedule must be determined by the physician
for each patient individually.**

▷ **Dosing Instructions:**   May be taken with or after food to reduce stomach
   irritation. To ensure regular (every day) use and uniform blood levels,
   it is advisable to take the tablet at the same time daily. The tablets
   may be crushed for administration.

Usual Duration of Use: According to individual needs and circumstances.
   Long-term use (months to years) requires supervision and periodic
   evaluation by your physician every 6 months.

▷ **This Drug Should Not Be Taken If**
   • you have had a significant allergic reaction to any dosage form of it
     previously.
   • you have a history of thrombophlebitis, embolism, heart attack or
     stroke.
   • you have breast cancer.
   • you have active liver disease, seriously impaired liver function or a
     history of liver tumor.
   • you have abnormal and unexplained vaginal bleeding.
   • you have sickle cell disease.
   • you are pregnant.

▷ **Inform Your Physician Before Taking This Drug If**
   • you have had an unfavorable reaction to any oral contraceptive pre-
     viously.
   • you have a history of cancer of the breast or reproductive organs.
   • you have any of the following conditions: fibrocystic breast changes,
     fibroid tumors of the uterus, endometriosis, migrainelike headaches,
     epilepsy, asthma, heart disease, high blood pressure, gallbladder dis-
     ease, diabetes or porphyria.
   • you smoke tobacco on a regular basis.
   • you plan to have surgery in the near future.

Possible Side-Effects (natural, expected and unavoidable drug actions)
   Fluid retention, weight gain, "breakthrough" bleeding (spotting in middle of menstrual cycle), altered menstrual pattern, lack of menstruation (during and following cessation of drug), increased susceptibility
   to yeast infection of the genital tissues.

▷ **Possible Adverse Effects** (unusual, unexpected and infrequent reactions)
   **If any of the following develop, consult your physician promptly for
   guidance.**

Mild Adverse Effects

Allergic Reactions: Skin rash, hives, itching.

Headache, nervous tension, irritability, accentuation of migraine headaches.

Nausea, vomiting, bloating, diarrhea.

Tannish pigmentation of the face.

Reduced tolerance to contact lenses.

Impaired color vision: blue tinge to objects, blue halo around lights.

Serious Adverse Effects

Allergic Reactions: Erythema multiforme and nodosum (skin reactions), loss of scalp hair.

Idiosyncratic Reactions: Joint and muscle pains.

Emotional depression, rise in blood pressure (in susceptible individuals).

Eye changes: optic neuritis, retinal thrombosis, altered curvature of the cornea, cataracts.

Gallbladder disease, benign liver tumors, jaundice, rise in blood sugar.

Erosion of uterine cervix, enlargement of uterine fibroid tumors, cystitislike syndrome.

Thrombophlebitis (inflammation of a vein with formation of blood clot)—pain or tenderness in thigh or leg, with or without swelling of foot or leg.

Pulmonary embolism (movement of blood clot to lung)—sudden shortness of breath, pain in chest, coughing, bloody sputum.

Stroke (blood clot in brain)—headaches, blackout, sudden weakness or paralysis of any part of the body, severe dizziness, altered vision, slurred speech, inability to speak.

Heart attack (blood clot in coronary artery)—sudden pain in chest, neck, jaw or arm; weakness; sweating; nausea.

Mesenteric thrombosis—blood clot in abdominal artery.

▷ **Possible Effects on Sexual Function**

Decreased libido (14% to 50%).

Altered character of menstruation; midcycle spotting.

Breast enlargement and tenderness with milk production.

Absent menstruation and infertility (temporary) after discontinuation of drug.

Possible Delayed Adverse Effects: Estrogens taken during pregnancy can predispose the female child to the later development of cancer of the vagina or cervix following puberty.

▷ **Adverse Effects That May Mimic Natural Diseases or Disorders**

Liver reactions may suggest viral hepatitis.

Natural Diseases or Disorders That May Be Activated by This Drug

Latent hypertension, diabetes mellitus, acute intermittent porphyria, lupus erythematosus–like syndrome.

CAUTION

1. The incidence of serious adverse effects due to the use of these drugs is very low. However, any unusual development should be reported and evaluated promptly.
2. Studies indicate that women over 30 years of age who smoke and use oral contraceptives are at significantly greater risk of having a serious cardiovascular event than are nonusers.
3. The risk of thromboembolism increases with the amount of estrogen in the product and with the age of the user. Low-estrogen combinations are advised.
4. It is advisable to discontinue these drugs 1 month prior to elective surgery to reduce the risk of postsurgical thromboembolism.
5. Investigate promptly any alteration or disturbance of vision that occurs during the use of these drugs.
6. Investigate promptly the nature of recurrent, persistent or severe headaches that develop while taking these drugs.
7. Observe for significant change of mood. Discontinue this drug if depression develops.
8. Certain commonly used drugs may reduce the effectiveness of oral contraceptives. Some of these are listed in the category of *Other Drugs*.
9. Diarrhea lasting more than a few hours (and occurring during the days the drug is taken) can prevent adequate absorption of these drugs and impair their effectiveness as contraceptives.
10. If 2 consecutive menstrual periods are missed, consult your physician regarding the advisability of performing a pregnancy test. Do not continue to use these drugs until your pregnancy status is determined.

▷ **Advisability of Use During Pregnancy**

Pregnancy Category: X. See Pregnancy Code inside back cover.

Animal studies: Genital defects reported in mice and guinea pigs; cleft palate reported in rodents.

Human studies: Information from studies of pregnant women indicates that estrogens can masculinize the female fetus. In addition, limb defects and heart malformations have been reported.

It is now known that estrogens taken during pregnancy can predispose the female child to the development of cancer of the vagina or cervix following puberty. *Avoid these drugs completely during entire pregnancy.*

Advisability of Use if Breast-Feeding

Presence of these drugs in breast milk: Yes, in minute amounts.

These drugs may suppress milk formation if started early following delivery.

Breast-feeding is considered to be safe during the use of oral contraceptives.

Habit-Forming Potential: None.

Effects of Overdosage: Headache, drowsiness, nausea, vomiting, fluid retention, abnormal vaginal bleeding, breast enlargement and discomfort.

Possible Effects of Long-Term Use: High blood pressure, gallbladder disease with stones, accelerated growth of uterine fibroid tumors, absent menstruation and impaired fertility after discontinuation of drug.

Suggested Periodic Examinations While Taking This Drug (at physician's discretion)

Regular (every 6 months) evaluation of the breasts and pelvic organs, including Pap smears. Liver function tests as indicated.

▷ **While Taking This Drug, Observe the Following**

Foods: Avoid excessive use of salt if fluid retention occurs.

Beverages: No restrictions. May be taken with milk.

▷   *Alcohol:* No interactions expected.

Tobacco Smoking: Recent studies indicate that heavy smoking (15 or more cigarettes daily) in association with the use of oral contraceptives significantly increases the risk of heart attack (coronary thrombosis). Heavy smoking should be considered a contraindication to the use of oral contraceptives.

▷   *Other Drugs*

Oral contraceptives may ***increase*** the effects of

- some benzodiazepines, and cause excessive sedation.
- metoprolol (Lopressor), and cause excessive beta blocker effects.
- prednisolone and prednisone, and cause excessive cortisonelike effects.
- theophyllines, and increase the risk of toxic effects.

Oral contraceptives ***taken concurrently*** with

- antidiabetic drugs may cause unpredictable fluctuations of blood sugar.
- tricyclic antidepressants (Elavil, Sinequan, etc.) may enhance their adverse effects and reduce their antidepressant effectiveness.
- troleandomycin (TAO) may increase the incidence of liver toxicity and jaundice.
- warfarin (Coumadin) may cause unpredictable alterations of prothrombin activity.

The following drugs may ***decrease*** the effects of oral contraceptives (and impair their effectiveness)

- barbiturates (phenobarbital, etc.; see Drug Class, Section Four).
- carbamazepine (Tegretol).
- griseofulvin (Fulvicin, etc.).
- penicillins (ampicillin, penicillin V).
- phenytoin (Dilantin).
- primidone (Mysoline).
- rifampin (Rifadin, Rimactane).
- tetracyclines (see Drug Class, Section Four).

▷ *Driving, Hazardous Activities:* Usually no restrictions. Consult your physician for assessment of individual risk and for guidance regarding specific restrictions.

Aviation Note: Usually no restrictions. However, it is advisable to observe for the rare occurrence of disturbed vision and to restrict activities accordingly. Consult a designated Aviation Medical Examiner.

Exposure to Sun: Use caution until full effect is known. These drugs can cause photosensitivity (see Glossary).

Discontinuation: Do not discontinue this drug if "breakthrough" bleeding occurs. If spotting or bleeding continues, consult your physician. A preparation with a higher estrogen content may be required. Remember: Omitting this drug for only 1 day may allow pregnancy to occur. It is advisable to avoid pregnancy for 3 to 6 months after discontinuing these drugs; aborted fetuses from women who became pregnant within 6 months after discontinuation reveal significantly increased chromosome abnormalities.

OXAZEPAM
(ox AZ e pam)

Introduced: 1965

Class: Mild tranquilizer, benzodiazepines

Prescription: USA: Yes
Canada: Yes

Controlled Drug: USA: C-IV*
Canada: No

Available as Generic: USA: Yes
Canada: Yes

Brand Names: ✦Apo-Oxazepam, ✦Novoxapam, ✦Oxpam, Serax, ✦Zapex, Zaxopam

BENEFITS versus RISKS	
Possible Benefits	*Possible Risks*
RELIEF OF ANXIETY AND NERVOUS TENSION in 70% to 80% of users	Habit-forming potential with prolonged use
Wide margin of safety with therapeutic doses	Minor impairment of mental functions
Very few drug interactions	Very rare jaundice
	Very rare blood cell disorders

▷ **Principal Uses**

As a Single Drug Product: Used primarily to (1) provide short-term relief of mild to moderate anxiety; (2) relieve the symptoms of acute alcohol

*See Schedules of Controlled Drugs inside back cover.

withdrawal: agitation, tremors, hallucinations, incipient delirium tremens.

How This Drug Works: It is thought that this drug produces a calming effect by enhancing the action of the nerve transmitter gamma-aminobutyric acid (GABA), which in turn blocks the arousal of higher brain centers.

Available Dosage Forms and Strengths
Capsules — 10 mg, 15 mg, 30 mg
Tablets — 15 mg

▷ **Usual Adult Dosage Range:** 30 to 120 mg/24 hours, in 3 or 4 divided doses. The total daily dosage should not exceed 180 mg. **Note: Actual dosage and administration schedule must be determined by the physician for each patient individually.**

▷ **Dosing Instructions:** May be taken on empty stomach or with food or milk as needed to prevent stomach irritation. The tablet may be crushed and the capsule may be opened for administration. Do not discontinue this drug abruptly if taken for more than 4 weeks.

Usual Duration of Use: Continual use on a regular schedule for 3 to 5 days is usually necessary to determine this drug's effectiveness in relieving moderate anxiety. Limit continual use to 1 to 3 weeks. Avoid uninterrupted and prolonged use.

▷ **This Drug Should Not Be Taken If**
- you have had an allergic reaction to any dosage form of it previously.
- you have acute narrow-angle glaucoma.
- it is prescribed for a child under 6 years of age.

▷ **Inform Your Physician Before Taking This Drug If**
- you are allergic to any benzodiazepine drug (see Drug Class, Section Four).
- you have a history of alcoholism or drug abuse.
- you are pregnant or planning pregnancy.
- you have impaired liver or kidney function.
- you have a history of serious depression or mental disorder.
- you have any of the following: asthma, emphysema, epilepsy, myasthenia gravis.
- you are taking any drugs with sedative effects.

Possible Side-Effects (natural, expected and unavoidable drug actions)
Drowsiness, lethargy, unsteadiness, "hangover" effects on the day following bedtime use.

▷ **Possible Adverse Effects** (unusual, unexpected and infrequent reactions)
If any of the following develop, consult your physician promptly for guidance.

Mild Adverse Effects
Allergic Reactions: Skin rashes, hives.
Dizziness, fainting, blurred vision, double vision, slurred speech, sweating, nausea.
Serious Adverse Effects
Allergic Reactions: Liver reaction with jaundice (see Glossary).
Abnormally low white blood cell count: fever, sore throat, infections.
Paradoxical responses of excitement, agitation, anger, rage.

▷ **Possible Effects on Sexual Function:**   Altered timing and pattern of menstruation.

▷ **Adverse Effects That May Mimic Natural Diseases or Disorders**
Liver reaction with jaundice may suggest viral hepatitis.

CAUTION
1. This drug should not be discontinued abruptly if it has been taken continually for more than 4 weeks.
2. The concurrent use of some over-the-counter drug products that contain antihistamines (allergy and cold preparations, sleep aids) can cause excessive sedation in sensitive individuals.

Precautions for Use
By Infants and Children: Safety and effectiveness for use by those under 6 years of age have not been established. This drug should not be used in the hyperactive or psychotic child of any age. Observe for excessive sedation and incoordination.
By Those over 60 Years of Age: It is advisable to use smaller doses at longer intervals to avoid overdosage. Observe for the possible development of lethargy, indifference, fatigue, weakness, unsteadiness, disturbing dreams, nightmares and paradoxical reactions of excitement, agitation, anger, hostility and rage.

▷ **Advisability of Use During Pregnancy**
Pregnancy Category: C (tentative). See Pregnancy Code inside back cover.
Animal studies: No birth defects found in mice, rats or rabbits.
Human studies: Information from adequate studies of pregnant women is not available. No birth defects have been reported with the use of this drug. However, available information regarding the use of other drugs of this class (benzodiazepines) is conflicting and inconclusive. Some studies found an increase in serious birth defects associated with the use of 2 benzodiazepines. Other studies have found no significant increase in birth defects.
Frequent use in late pregnancy can cause the "floppy infant" syndrome in the newborn: weakness, lethargy, unresponsiveness, depressed breathing, low body temperature. Avoid use during entire pregnancy if possible.

Advisability of Use if Breast-Feeding
Presence of this drug in breast milk: Yes.
Avoid drug or refrain from nursing.

Habit-Forming Potential: This drug can produce psychological and/or physical dependence (see Glossary) if used in large doses for an extended period of time.

Effects of Overdosage: Marked drowsiness, weakness, feeling of drunkenness, staggering gait, tremor, stupor progressing to deep sleep or coma.

Possible Effects of Long-Term Use: Psychological and/or physical dependence, rare blood cell disorders.

Suggested Periodic Examinations While Taking This Drug (at physician's discretion)

Complete blood cell counts during long-term use.
Liver function tests.

▷ **While Taking This Drug, Observe the Following**

Foods: No restrictions.

Beverages: Avoid excessive intake of caffeine-containing beverages: coffee, tea, cola. May be taken with milk.

▷ *Alcohol:* Use with extreme caution until the combined effect is determined. Alcohol may increase the depressant effects of this drug on the brain. It is advisable to avoid alcohol completely—throughout the day and night—if it is necessary to drive or to engage in any hazardous activity.

Tobacco Smoking: Heavy smoking may reduce the calming action of this drug.

Marijuana Smoking: Increased sedation and significant impairment of intellectual and physical performance.

▷ *Other Drugs*

Oxazepam may ***increase*** the effects of
- digoxin (Lanoxin), and cause digoxin toxicity.
- phenytoin (Dilantin), and cause phenytoin toxicity.

Oxazepam may ***decrease*** the effects of
- levodopa (Sinemet, etc.), and reduce its effectiveness in treating Parkinson's disease.

The following drugs may ***decrease*** the effects of oxazepam
- oral contraceptives.
- theophylline (Aminophylline, Theo-Dur, etc.).

▷ *Driving, Hazardous Activities:* This drug can impair mental alertness, judgment, physical coordination and reaction time. Avoid hazardous activities accordingly.

Aviation Note: The use of this drug ***is a disqualification*** for piloting. Consult a designated Aviation Medical Examiner.

Exposure to Sun: No restrictions.

Exposure to Heat: Use caution until the effect of excessive perspiration is determined. Because of reduced urine volume, this drug may accumulate in the body and produce effects of overdosage.

Discontinuation: Avoid sudden discontinuation if this drug has been taken for over 4 weeks without interruption. Dosage should be tapered gradually to prevent a withdrawal syndrome that could include depression, confusion, hallucinations, tremor, seizures, muscle cramping, sweating and vomiting.

OXYCODONE
(ox ee KOH dohn)

Introduced: 1950

Prescription: USA: Yes
Canada: Yes

Available as Generic: USA: Yes
Canada: No

Class: Analgesic, narcotic

Controlled Drug: USA: C-II*
Canada: <N>

Brand Names: ✦Oxycocet [CD], ✦Oxycodan [CD], Percocet [CD], ✦Percocet-Demi [CD], Percodan [CD], Percodan-Demi [CD], Roxicodone, ✦Supeudol, Tylox [CD]

BENEFITS versus RISKS

Possible Benefits	*Possible Risks*
EFFECTIVE RELIEF OF MODERATE TO SEVERE PAIN	POTENTIAL FOR HABIT FORMATION (DEPENDENCE) Sedative effects Mild allergic reactions (infrequent) Nausea, constipation

---

▷ **Principal Uses**

As a Single Drug Product: Used primarily in tablet and suppository form (Canada) to relieve moderate to severe pain.

As a Combination Drug Product [CD]: Oxycodone is available in combinations with acetaminophen and with aspirin. These milder pain relievers are added to enhance the analgesic effect and to reduce fever when present.

How This Drug Works: Acting primarily as a depressant of certain brain functions, this drug suppresses the perception of pain and calms the emotional response to pain.

Available Dosage Forms and Strengths
Solution — 5 mg per 5-ml teaspoonful
Suppositories — 10 mg, 20 mg (Canada)
Tablets — 5 mg, 10 mg (Canada)

*See Schedules of Controlled Drugs inside back cover.

Tablets — 2.44 mg, 4.88 mg (in combination drugs)

▷ **Usual Adult Dosage Range:** 5 mg/3 to 6 hours as needed. May be increased to 10 mg/4 hours if needed for severe pain. The total daily dosage should not exceed 60 mg. **Note: Actual dosage and administration schedule must be determined by the physician for each patient individually.**

▷ **Dosing Instructions:** May be taken with or following food to reduce stomach irritation or nausea. The tablet may be crushed for administration.

Usual Duration of Use: As required to control pain. Continual use should not exceed 5 to 7 days without interruption and reassessment of need.

▷ **This Drug Should Not Be Taken If**
  • you have had an allergic reaction to any dosage form of it previously.
  • you are having an acute attack of asthma.

▷ **Inform Your Physician Before Taking This Drug If**
  • you have had an unfavorable reaction to any narcotic drug in the past.
  • you have a history of drug abuse or alcoholism.
  • you have chronic lung disease with impaired breathing.
  • you have impaired liver or kidney function.
  • you have gallbladder disease, a seizure disorder or an underactive thyroid gland.
  • you have difficulty emptying the urinary bladder.
  • you are taking any other drugs that have a sedative effect.
  • you plan to have surgery under general anesthesia in the near future.

Possible Side-Effects (natural, expected and unavoidable drug actions)
  Drowsiness, light-headedness, dry mouth, urinary retention, constipation.

▷ **Possible Adverse Effects** (unusual, unexpected and infrequent reactions)
  If any of the following develop, consult your physician promptly for guidance.
  Mild Adverse Effects
  Allergic Reactions: Skin rash, hives, itching.
  Idiosyncratic Reactions: Skin rash and itching when combined with dairy products (milk or cheese).
  Dizziness, impaired concentration, sensation of drunkenness, confusion, depression, blurred or double vision.
  Nausea, vomiting.
  Serious Adverse Effects
  Impaired breathing: use with caution in chronic lung disease.

▷ **Possible Effects on Sexual Function:** None reported.

CAUTION
1. If you have asthma, chronic bronchitis or emphysema, the excessive use of this drug may cause significant respiratory difficulty, thickening of bronchial secretions and suppression of coughing.
2. The concurrent use of this drug with atropinelike drugs can increase the risk of urinary retention and reduced intestinal function.
3. Do not take this drug following acute head injury.

Precautions for Use
By Infants and Children: Do not use this drug in children under 2 years of age because of their vulnerability to life-threatening respiratory depression.

By Those over 60 Years of Age: Use small doses initially and increase dosage as needed and tolerated. Limit use to short-term treatment only. There may be increased susceptibility to the development of drowsiness, dizziness, unsteadiness, falling, urinary retention and constipation (often leading to fecal impaction).

▷ **Advisability of Use During Pregnancy**
Pregnancy Category: C (tentative). See Pregnancy Code inside back cover.
Animal studies: No information available.
Human studies: Information from adequate studies of pregnant women is not available. Oxycodone taken repeatedly during the last few weeks before delivery may cause withdrawal symptoms in the newborn infant.
Use this drug only if clearly needed and in small, infrequent doses.

Advisability of Use if Breast-Feeding
Presence of this drug in breast milk: Unknown.
Avoid drug or refrain from nursing.

Habit-Forming Potential: Psychological and/or physical dependence can develop with use of large doses for an extended period of time.

Effects of Overdosage: Drowsiness, restlessness, agitation, nausea, vomiting, dry mouth, vertigo, weakness, lethargy, stupor, coma, seizures.

Possible Effects of Long-Term Use: Psychological and physical dependence, chronic constipation.

Suggested Periodic Examinations While Taking This Drug (at physician's discretion)
None.

▷ **While Taking This Drug, Observe the Following**
Foods: No restrictions.
Beverages: No restrictions. May be taken with milk.
▷ *Alcohol:* Use extreme caution until the combined effects have been determined. Oxycodone can intensify the intoxicating effects of alcohol, and alcohol can intensify the depressant effects of oxycodone on brain function, breathing and circulation.

Tobacco Smoking: No interactions expected.

Marijuana Smoking: Increase in drowsiness and pain relief; impairment of mental and physical performance.

▷ *Other Drugs*

Oxycodone may **increase** the effects of
- other drugs with sedative effects.
- atropinelike drugs, and increase the risk of constipation and urinary retention.

▷ *Driving, Hazardous Activities:* This drug can impair mental alertness, judgment, reaction time and physical coordination. Avoid hazardous activities accordingly.

Aviation Note: The use of this drug **is a disqualification** for piloting. Consult a designated Aviation Medical Examiner.

Exposure to Sun: No restrictions.

Discontinuation: It is advisable to limit this drug to short-term use. If it is necessary to use it for extended periods of time, discontinuation should be gradual to minimize possible effects of withdrawal.

OXYMETAZOLINE
(ox ee met AZ oh leen)

Introduced: 1964

Class: Decongestant

Prescription: USA: No
Canada: No

Controlled Drug: USA: No
Canada: No

Available as Generic: USA: Yes
Canada: No

Brand Names: Afrin, Allerest 12 Hour Nasal, Coricidin Nasal Mist, Dristan Long Lasting, Duramist Plus, Duration, 4-Way Long Acting Nasal Spray, ◆Nafrine, Neo-Synephrine 12 Hour, Nostrilla, NTZ Long Acting Nasal, Ocuclear, Sinarest 12-Hour Nasal Spray, Sinex Long Acting

---

BENEFITS versus RISKS

Possible Benefits	*Possible Risks*
EFFECTIVE, LONG-LASTING DECONGESTION OF NASAL AND SINUS TISSUES EFFECTIVE DECONGESTION OF INFLAMED EYES	"REBOUND" CONGESTION WITH EXCESSIVE USE Mild irritation of ocular or nasal tissues Systemic effects (via absorption with excessive use): nervousness, insomnia, hypertension

---

▷ **Principal Uses**

As a Single Drug Product: Used primarily as a decongestant nose drop or spray to relieve swelling and congestion of the nasal membranes due to colds or allergy. It is also used as an eye drop to relieve inflammation and swelling of the conjunctival membranes ("red eyes") due to allergy or chemical irritation.

How This Drug Works: By contracting the walls of arterioles and thus reducing their size, this drug decreases the volume of blood in the tissues, resulting in shrinkage of tissue mass (decongestion). This expands the nasal airway and enlarges the openings into the sinuses and eustachian tubes. The same action on the conjunctival vessels in the eye results in clearing of the capillary congestion (redness) and swelling.

Available Dosage Forms and Strengths

Eye drops — 0.025%

Nasal spray — 0.05%

Nose drops — 0.05%

Pediatric nose drops — 0.025%

▷ **Usual Adult Dosage Range:** Eye drops: 1 or 2 drops in affected eye/6 to 8 hours. Nose drops and spray: 2 or 3 drops or sprays into each nostril twice/day, morning and evening, 12 hours apart. For long-term use, consult your physician.

▷ **Dosing Instructions:** Do not exceed the recommended doses. The nasal spray is more effective than the drops and is less likely to cause systemic absorption.

Usual Duration of Use: Continual use on a regular schedule for 3 to 5 days is usually necessary to determine this drug's effectiveness in relieving eye and nasal congestion. If there is no significant improvement after 1 week of use, consult your physician for further evaluation.

▷ **This Drug Should Not Be Taken If**
- you have had an allergic reaction to it previously.
- for the eye drops: you have untreated narrow-angle glaucoma or an active eye infection.

▷ **Inform Your Physician Before Taking This Drug If**
- you have high blood pressure or heart disease.
- you have diabetes or an overactive thyroid gland (hyperthyroidism).
- you are taking any beta blocker drug (see Drug Class, Section Four).
- you are taking, or have taken within the past 14 days, any monoamine oxidase (MAO) type A inhibitor drug (see Drug Class, Section Four).

Possible Side-Effects (natural, expected and unavoidable drug actions)
Dryness or irritation of the nose, nervousness, insomnia.

▷ **Possible Adverse Effects** (unusual, unexpected and infrequent reactions)
   If any of the following develop, consult your physician promptly for guidance.
   Mild Adverse Effects
   Headache, light-headedness, burning or stinging of the nose, heart palpitation, tremors.
   Serious Adverse Effects
   None reported.

▷ **Possible Effects on Sexual Function:**   None reported.

   CAUTION
   1. Too frequent use, or extended use, of nose drops or sprays containing this drug may cause a secondary rebound congestion resulting in a form of functional dependence (see Glossary).
   2. Many over-the-counter drug products for allergies, colds and coughs contain drugs that may interact unfavorably with this drug. Ask your physician or pharmacist for guidance before using such medications.

   Precautions for Use
   By Infants and Children: Children may be especially susceptible to systemic absorption of this drug. Avoid excessive use.
   By Those over 60 Years of Age: Use small doses until your tolerance has been determined. Observe for possible nervousness, insomnia or palpitation.

▷ **Advisability of Use During Pregnancy**
   Pregnancy Category: C (tentative). See Pregnancy Code inside back cover.
   Animal studies: No information available.
   Human studies: Information from adequate studies of pregnant women is not available.
   Limit use to small, infrequent doses.

   Advisability of Use if Breast-Feeding
   Presence of this drug in breast milk: Unknown.
   Monitor nursing infant closely and discontinue drug or nursing if adverse effects develop.

   Habit-Forming Potential: Frequent or excessive use may cause functional dependence (see Glossary).

   Effects of Overdosage: Headache, restlessness, anxiety, agitation, palpitation, sweating.

   Possible Effects of Long-Term Use: Secondary rebound congestion and chemical irritation of nasal tissues.

   Suggested Periodic Examinations While Taking This Drug (at physician's discretion)
   None required.

▷ **While Taking This Drug, Observe the Following**
  Foods: No restrictions.
  Beverages: Heavy use of coffee or tea may add to the nervousness or in-
    somnia experienced by sensitive individuals.
▷ *Alcohol:* No interactions expected.
  Tobacco Smoking: No interactions expected.
▷ *Other Drugs*
  Oxymetazoline **taken concurrently** with
  • beta blocker drugs or monoamine oxidase (MAO) type A inhibitor
    drugs may cause dangerous elevations of blood pressure. Observe for
    headache or palpitation.
▷ *Driving, Hazardous Activities:* No restrictions.
  Aviation Note: The use of this drug **may be a disqualification** for piloting.
    Consult a designated Aviation Medical Examiner.
  Exposure to Sun: No restrictions.

PENBUTOLOL
(pen BYU toh lohl)

Introduced: 1976

Class: Antihypertensive, beta-
adrenergic blocker

Prescription: USA: Yes

Controlled Drug: USA: No

Available as Generic: No

Brand Name: Levatol

BENEFITS versus RISKS	
Possible Benefits	*Possible Risks*
EFFECTIVE, WELL-TOLERATED ANTIHYPERTENSIVE in mild to moderate high blood pressure	CONGESTIVE HEART FAILURE in advanced heart disease
	Worsening of angina in coronary heart disease (abrupt withdrawal)
	Masking of low blood sugar (hypoglycemia) in drug-treated diabetes
	Provocation of asthma

▷ **Principal Uses**
  As a Single Drug Product: The treatment of mild to moderately severe high
    blood pressure. May be used alone or concurrently with other anti-
    hypertensive drugs, such as diuretics.

How This Drug Works: By blocking certain actions of the sympathetic nervous system, this drug
- reduces the rate and contraction force of the heart, thus lowering the ejection pressure of the blood leaving the heart.
- reduces the degree of contraction of blood vessel walls, resulting in their relaxation and expansion and consequent lowering of blood pressure.

Available Dosage Forms and Strengths
Tablets — 20 mg

▷ **Usual Adult Dosage Range:** Initially 20 mg once daily. The dose may be increased gradually by 10 mg/day at intervals of 2 weeks as needed and tolerated up to 80 mg/day. For maintenance, 20 to 40 mg once daily is usually adequate. The total daily dose should not exceed 80 mg. **Note: Actual dosage and administration schedule must be determined by the physician for each patient individually.**

▷ **Dosing Instructions:** May be taken without regard to eating. The tablet may be crushed for administration. Do not discontinue this drug abruptly.

Usual Duration of Use: Continual use on a regular schedule for 2 to 3 weeks is usually necessary to determine this drug's effectiveness in lowering blood pressure. The long-term use of this drug (months to years) will be determined by the course of your blood pressure over time and your response to the overall treatment program (weight reduction, salt restriction, smoking cessation, etc.). Consult your physician on a regular basis.

Possible Advantages of This Drug
Adequate control of blood pressure with a single daily dose.
Causes less slowing of the heart rate than most other beta blocker drugs.

Currently a "Drug of Choice" for initiating treatment of hypertension with a single drug.

▷ **This Drug Should Not Be Taken If**
- you have had an allergic reaction to it previously.
- you have congestive heart failure.
- you have an abnormally slow heart rate or a serious form of heart block.
- you are subject to bronchial asthma.

▷ **Inform Your Physician Before Taking This Drug If**
- you have had an adverse reaction to any beta blocker drug in the past (see Drug Class, Section Four).
- you have a history of serious heart disease, with or without episodes of heart failure.
- you have a history of hay fever (allergic rhinitis), asthma, chronic bronchitis or emphysema.

- you have a history of overactive thyroid function (hyperthyroidism).
- you have a history of low blood sugar (hypoglycemia).
- you have impaired liver or kidney function.
- you have diabetes or myasthenia gravis.
- you have impaired circulation in the extremities (Raynaud's disorder, claudication pains in legs).
- you are currently taking any form of digitalis, quinidine or reserpine, or any calcium blocker drug (see Drug Class, Section Four).
- you plan to have surgery under general anesthesia in the near future.

Possible Side-Effects (natural, expected and unavoidable drug actions)
Lethargy and fatigability, cold extremities, slow heart rate, light-headedness in upright position (see Orthostatic Hypotension in Glossary).

▷ **Possible Adverse Effects** (unusual, unexpected and infrequent reactions)
If any of the following develop, consult your physician promptly for guidance.
Mild Adverse Effects
Allergic Reactions: Skin rash, itching, reversible hair loss.
Headache, dizziness, blurred vision, insomnia, abnormal dreams.
Indigestion, nausea, vomiting, constipation, diarrhea.
Joint and muscle discomfort.
Serious Adverse Effects
Allergic Reactions: Anaphylactoid reaction (see Glossary).
Mental depression, anxiety, disorientation, short-term memory loss, hallucinations.
Chest pain, shortness of breath, precipitation of congestive heart failure.
Induction of bronchial asthma (in asthmatic individuals).
Aggravation of myasthenia gravis.
Abnormally low white blood cell and platelet counts: fever, sore throat, abnormal bleeding or bruising.

▷ **Possible Effects on Sexual Function:**   Decreased libido and impotence, rare but more common with higher doses; Peyronie's disease (see Glossary).

▷ **Adverse Effects That May Mimic Natural Diseases or Disorders**
Reduced blood flow to extremities may resemble Raynaud's phenomenon (see Glossary).

Natural Diseases or Disorders That May Be Activated by This Drug
Raynaud's disease, intermittent claudication, myasthenia gravis.

CAUTION
1. *Do not discontinue this drug suddenly* without the knowledge and guidance of your physician. Carry a notation on your person that you are taking this drug.
2. Consult your physician or pharmacist before using nasal decongestants usually present in over-the-counter cold preparations and

nose drops. These can cause sudden increases in blood pressure when taken concurrently with beta blocker drugs.
3. Report the development of any tendency to emotional depression.

Precautions for Use

By Infants and Children: Safety and effectiveness for use by those under 12 years of age have not been established. However, if this drug is used, observe for the development of low blood sugar (hypoglycemia) during periods of reduced food intake.

By Those over 60 Years of Age: Proceed **cautiously** with all antihypertensive drugs. Unacceptably high blood pressure should be reduced without creating the risks associated with excessively low blood pressure. Start treatment with small doses, and monitor the blood pressure response frequently. Sudden, rapid and excessive reduction of blood pressure can predispose to stroke or heart attack. Observe for dizziness, unsteadiness, tendency to fall, confusion, hallucinations, depression or urinary frequency.

▷ **Advisability of Use During Pregnancy**

Pregnancy Category: C (tentative). See Pregnancy Code inside back cover.
Animal studies: No birth defects due to this drug found in rat or rabbit studies.
Human studies: Information from adequate studies of pregnant women is not available.
Use this drug only if clearly needed. Ask physician for guidance.

Advisability of Use if Breast-Feeding

Presence of this drug in breast milk: Unknown.
Avoid drug or refrain from nursing.

Habit-Forming Potential: None.

Effects of Overdosage: Weakness, slow pulse, low blood pressure, fainting, cold and sweaty skin, congestive heart failure, possible coma and convulsions.

Possible Effects of Long-Term Use: Reduced heart reserve and eventual heart failure in susceptible individuals with advanced heart disease.

Suggested Periodic Examinations While Taking This Drug (at physician's discretion)
Measurements of blood pressure, evaluation of heart function.
Complete blood cell counts.

▷ **While Taking This Drug, Observe the Following**

Foods: No restrictions. Avoid excessive salt intake.
Beverages: No restrictions. May be taken with milk.
▷ *Alcohol:* Use with caution until the combined effect has been determined. Alcohol may exaggerate this drug's ability to lower the blood pressure and may increase its mild sedative effect.

Tobacco Smoking: Nicotine may reduce this drug's effectiveness in treating high blood pressure. In addition, high doses of this drug may potentiate the constriction of the bronchial tubes caused by regular smoking.

▷ *Other Drugs*

Penbutolol may *increase* the effects of

- other antihypertensive drugs, and cause excessive lowering of the blood pressure. Dosage adjustments may be necessary.
- reserpine (Ser-Ap-Es, etc.), and cause sedation, depression, slowing of the heart rate and lowering of the blood pressure. This combination is best avoided.
- verapamil (Calan, Isoptin), and cause excessive depression of heart function; monitor this combination closely.

Penbutolol *taken concurrently* with

- clonidine (Catapres) requires close monitoring for rebound high blood pressure if clonidine is withdrawn while penbutolol is still being taken.
- insulin requires close monitoring to avoid undetected hypoglycemia (see Glossary).

The following drugs may *increase* the effects of penbutolol

- methimazole (Tapazole).
- oral contraceptives.
- propylthiouracil (Propacil).

The following drugs may *decrease* the effects of penbutolol

- barbiturates (phenobarbital, etc.).
- indomethacin (Indocin), and possibly other "aspirin substitutes," may impair pindolol's antihypertensive effect.
- rifampin (Rifadin, Rimactane).

▷ *Driving, Hazardous Activities:* Use caution until the full extent of fatigue, dizziness and blood pressure change have been determined.

Aviation Note: The use of this drug *is a disqualification* for piloting. Consult a designated Aviation Medical Examiner.

Exposure to Sun: No restrictions.

Exposure to Heat: Caution advised. Hot environments can lower the blood pressure and exaggerate the effects of this drug.

Exposure to Cold: Caution advised. Cold environments can enhance the circulatory deficiency in the extremities that may occur with this drug. The elderly should take precautions to prevent hypothermia (see Glossary).

Heavy Exercise or Exertion: It is advisable to avoid exertion that produces light-headedness, excessive fatigue or muscle cramping. The use of this drug may intensify the hypertensive response to isometric exercise.

Occurrence of Unrelated Illness: The fever that accompanies systemic infections can lower the blood pressure and require adjustment of dosage. Illnesses that cause nausea or vomiting may interrupt the regular dosage schedule. Ask your physician for guidance.

Discontinuation: It is advisable to avoid sudden discontinuation of this drug in all situations. If possible, gradual reduction of dose over a period of 2 to 3 weeks is recommended. Ask your physician for specific guidance.

PENICILLIN V
(pen i SIL in VEE)

Introduced: 1953

Class: Antibiotic, penicillins

Prescription: USA: Yes
Canada: Yes

Controlled Drug: USA: No
Canada: No

Available as Generic: USA: Yes
Canada: Yes

Brand Names: ✦Apo-Penicillin VK, Beepen VK, Betapen-VK, Ledercillin VK, ✦Nadopen-V, ✦Novopen-VK, Penapar VK, ✦Pen-Vee, Pen-Vee K, ✦PVF, ✦PVF K, Robicillin VK, Uticillin VK, V-Cillin K, ✦VC-K 500, Veetids

---

BENEFITS versus RISKS

Possible Benefits	*Possible Risks*
EFFECTIVE TREATMENT OF INFECTIONS due to susceptible microorganisms	ALLERGIC REACTIONS, mild to severe, in 3% of the general population and 15% of allergic individuals Superinfections (yeast) Drug-induced colitis

---

▷ **Principal Uses**

As a Single Drug Product: This type of penicillin is used primarily to treat responsive infections of the upper and lower respiratory tract, the middle ear and the skin. Equally important uses are the prevention of rheumatic fever and the prevention of bacterial endocarditis in individuals with valvular heart disease.

How This Drug Works: This drug destroys susceptible infecting bacteria by interfering with their ability to produce new protective cell walls as they multiply and grow.

Available Dosage Forms and Strengths
Oral solution — 125 mg, 250 mg per 5-ml teaspoonful
Tablets — 125 mg, 250 mg, 500 mg

▷ **Usual Adult Dosage Range:**   Dosage is based upon the results of sensitivity testing of the causative organism, the severity of the infection and the response of the patient. Depending upon the specific infection, the dosage range is 125 to 500 mg/6 to 8 hours. For the prevention of bacterial endocarditis: 2 grams (2000 mg) taken 1 hour before the procedure, followed by 1 gram 6 hours later. The total daily dosage should not exceed 7 grams (7000 mg). **Note: Actual dosage and administration schedule must be determined by the physician for each patient individually.**

▷ **Dosing Instructions:**   May be taken on an empty stomach or with food or milk. Absorption may be slightly faster if taken when stomach is empty. The tablet may be crushed for administration.

Usual Duration of Use: For all streptococcal infections—not less than 10 consecutive days (without interruption) to reduce the possibility of developing rheumatic fever or glomerulonephritis. For all other infections—as long as necessary to eradicate the infection.

▷ **This Drug Should Not Be Taken If**
  • you have had an allergic reaction to any dosage form of it previously.
  • you are certain you are allergic to *any* form of penicillin.

▷ **Inform Your Physician Before Taking This Drug If**
  • you suspect you may be allergic to penicillin or you have a history of a previous "reaction" of any type to penicillin.
  • you are allergic to any cephalosporin antibiotic (Ancef, Anspor, Ceclor, Ceporan, Ceporex, Kafocin, Keflex, Keflin, Kefzol, Loridine, Ultracef, Velosef; see Drug Class, Section Four).
  • you are allergic by nature (hay fever, asthma, hives, eczema).

Possible Side-Effects (natural, expected and unavoidable drug actions)
Superinfections (see Glossary), often due to yeast organisms.

▷ **Possible Adverse Effects** (unusual, unexpected and infrequent reactions)
  If any of the following develop, consult your physician promptly for guidance.
  Mild Adverse Effects
  Allergic Reactions: Skin rashes, hives, itching.
  Irritations of mouth and tongue, "black tongue," nausea, vomiting, mild diarrhea, dizziness (rare).
  Serious Adverse Effects
  Allergic Reactions: Anaphylactic reaction (see Glossary), severe skin reactions, drug fever, swollen painful joints, sore throat, abnormal bleeding or bruising.
  Drug-induced colitis.

▷ **Possible Effects on Sexual Function:**   None reported.

CAUTION
1. Take the exact dose and the full course prescribed.
2. This drug should not be used concurrently with antibiotics like erythromycin or tetracycline.

Precautions for Use

By Infants and Children: Observe the allergic child closely for evidence of a developing allergy to penicillin. This drug may cause diarrhea, which sometimes necessitates discontinuation.

By Those over 60 Years of Age: Natural changes in the skin may predispose to prolonged itching reactions in the genital and anal regions. Report such reactions promptly.

▷ **Advisability of Use During Pregnancy**

Pregnancy Category: B (tentative). See Pregnancy Code inside back cover.
Animal studies: Birth defects of the limbs reported in mice. (Not confirmed in other studies.)
Human studies: Information from adequate studies of pregnant women indicates no increased risk of birth defects in 3546 pregnancies exposed to penicillin derivatives.
This drug is considered safe for use during any period of pregnancy.

Advisability of Use if Breast-Feeding

Presence of this drug in breast milk: Yes.
The nursing infant may be sensitized to penicillin and be at risk for developing diarrhea or yeast infections.
Avoid drug if possible or refrain from nursing.

Habit-Forming Potential: None.

Effects of Overdosage: Possible nausea, vomiting and/or diarrhea.

Possible Effects of Long-Term Use: Superinfections, often due to yeast organisms.

Suggested Periodic Examinations While Taking This Drug (at physician's discretion)
Complete blood cell counts, kidney function tests.

▷ **While Taking This Drug, Observe the Following**

Foods: No restrictions.
Beverages: No restrictions. May be taken with milk.
▷ *Alcohol:* No interactions expected.
Tobacco Smoking: No interactions expected.
▷ *Other Drugs*

Penicillin V may *decrease* the effects of
• oral contraceptives in some women, and impair their effectiveness in preventing pregnancy.
The following drugs may *decrease* the effects of penicillin V
• antacids may reduce the absorption of penicillin V.

- chloramphenicol (Chloromycetin).
- erythromycin (Erythrocin, E-Mycin, etc.).
- tetracyclines (Achromycin, Declomycin, Minocin, etc.). (See Drug Class, Section Four.)

▷ *Driving, Hazardous Activities:* Usually no restrictions. Be alert to the rare occurrence of dizziness and/or nausea, and restrict activities accordingly.

Aviation Note: The use of this drug *may be a disqualification* for piloting. Consult a designated Aviation Medical Examiner.

Exposure to Sun: No restrictions.

Special Storage Instructions: Oral solutions should be refrigerated.

Observe the Following Expiration Times: Do not take the oral solution of this drug if older than 7 days when kept at room temperature or 14 days when kept refrigerated.

PENTAZOCINE
(pen TAZ oh seen)

Introduced: 1967

Class: Analgesic, narcotic

Prescription: USA: Yes
Canada: Yes

Controlled Drug: USA: C-IV*
Canada: <N>

Available as Generic: USA: No
Canada: No

Brand Names: Talacen [CD], Talwin, Talwin Compound [CD], ✦Talwin Compound-50 [CD], Talwin Nx [CD]

BENEFITS versus RISKS	
Possible Benefits	*Possible Risks*
EFFECTIVE RELIEF OF MODERATE TO SEVERE PAIN	POTENTIAL FOR HABIT FORMATION (DEPENDENCE)
	Sedative effects
	Mental and behavioral disturbances
	Low blood pressure, fainting
	Nausea, constipation

▷ **Principal Uses**

As a Single Drug Product: Used exclusively to relieve acute or chronic pain of moderate to severe degree from any cause.

*See Schedules of Controlled Drugs inside back cover.

As a Combination Drug Product [CD]: Pentazocine is available in combinations with acetaminophen and with aspirin. These milder pain relievers are added to enhance the analgesic effect and to reduce fever when present. In the USA the tablet form of pentazocine also contains naloxone (Talwin Nx), a narcotic antagonist that renders the drug ineffective if abused.

How This Drug Works: Acting primarily as a depressant of certain brain functions, this drug suppresses the perception of pain and calms the emotional response to pain.

Available Dosage Forms and Strengths
Injection — 30 mg per ml
Tablets — 50 mg (Canada)
Tablets — 50 mg with 0.5 mg of naloxone (USA)

▷ **Usual Adult Dosage Range:** 50 mg/3 to 4 hours as needed. May be increased to 100 mg/4 hours if needed for severe pain. The total daily dosage should not exceed 600 mg. **Note: Actual dosage and administration schedule must be determined by the physician for each patient individually.**

▷ **Dosing Instructions:** May be taken with or following food to reduce stomach irritation or nausea. The tablet may be crushed for administration.

Usual Duration of Use: As required to control pain. Continual use should not exceed 5 to 7 days without interruption and reassessment of need.

▷ **This Drug Should Not Be Taken If**
- you have had an allergic reaction to any dosage form of it previously.
- you are having an acute attack of asthma.

▷ **Inform Your Physician Before Taking This Drug If**
- you have had an unfavorable reaction to any narcotic drug in the past.
- you have a history of drug abuse or alcoholism.
- you have chronic lung disease with impaired breathing.
- you have impaired liver or kidney function.
- you have gallbladder disease, a seizure disorder or an underactive thyroid gland.
- you have difficulty emptying the urinary bladder.
- you are taking any other drugs that have a sedative effect.
- you plan to have surgery under general anesthesia in the near future.

Possible Side-Effects (natural, expected and unavoidable drug actions)
Drowsiness, light-headedness, weakness, urinary retention, constipation.

▷ **Possible Adverse Effects** (unusual, unexpected and infrequent reactions)
If any of the following develop, consult your physician promptly for guidance.

Mild Adverse Effects
  Allergic Reactions: Skin rash, hives, itching, swelling of face.
  Headache, dizziness, impaired concentration, sensation of drunkenness, blurred or double vision, flushing, sweating.
  Nausea, vomiting, indigestion, diarrhea.
Serious Adverse Effects
  Marked drop in blood pressure, possible fainting.
  Impaired breathing: use with caution in chronic lung disease.
  Mental and behavioral disturbances, hallucinations, tremor.
  Bone marrow depression (see Glossary) of a mild and reversible nature (rare).
  Aggravation of prostatism (see Glossary).

▷ **Possible Effects on Sexual Function:**   None reported.

CAUTION
  1. The use of this drug with atropinelike drugs may increase the risk of urinary retention and reduced intestinal function.
  2. Do not take this drug following acute head injury.

Precautions for Use
  By Infants and Children: Safety and effectiveness for use by those under 12 years of age have not been established.
  By Those over 60 Years of Age: Use small doses initially and increase dosage as needed and tolerated. Limit use to short-term treatment only. There may be increased susceptibility to the development of drowsiness, dizziness, unsteadiness, falling, urinary retention and constipation.

▷ **Advisability of Use During Pregnancy**
  Pregnancy Category: C (tentative). See Pregnancy Code inside back cover.
  Animal studies: Significant birth defects reported in hamsters.
  Human studies: Information from adequate studies of pregnant women is not available. Pentazocine taken repeatedly during the last few weeks before delivery may cause withdrawal symptoms in the newborn infant.
  Avoid this drug during the first 3 months. Use only if clearly needed and in small, infrequent doses during the last 6 months.

Advisability of Use if Breast-Feeding
  Presence of this drug in breast milk: Unknown.
  Avoid drug or refrain from nursing.

Habit-Forming Potential: Psychological and/or physical dependence can develop with use of large doses for an extended period of time.

Effects of Overdosage: Anxiety, disturbed thoughts, hallucinations, progressive drowsiness, stupor, depressed breathing.

Possible Effects of Long-Term Use: Psychological and physical dependence, chronic constipation.

Suggested Periodic Examinations While Taking This Drug (at physician's discretion)

Complete blood cell counts, if used for an extended period of time.

▷ **While Taking This Drug, Observe the Following**

Foods: No restrictions.

Beverages: No restrictions. May be taken with milk.

▷ *Alcohol:* Use extreme caution until the combined effects have been determined. Pentazocine can intensify the intoxicating effects of alcohol, and alcohol can intensify the depressant effects of pentazocine on brain function, breathing and circulation.

Tobacco Smoking: Heavy smoking may reduce the effectiveness of pentazocine and make larger doses necessary.

Marijuana Smoking: Increase in drowsiness and pain relief; impairment of mental and physical performance.

▷ *Other Drugs*

Pentazocine may *increase* the effects of

• other drugs with sedative effects.

• atropinelike drugs, and increase the risk of constipation and urinary retention.

▷ *Driving, Hazardous Activities:* This drug can impair mental alertness, judgment, reaction time and physical coordination. Avoid hazardous activities accordingly.

Aviation Note: The use of this drug *is a disqualification* for piloting. Consult a designated Aviation Medical Examiner.

Exposure to Sun: No restrictions.

Discontinuation: It is advisable to limit this drug to short-term use. If it is necessary to use it for extended periods of time, discontinuation should be gradual to minimize possible effects of withdrawal.

PENTOXIFYLLINE
(pen tox I fi leen)

Other Name: Oxpentifylline

Introduced: 1972

Class: Blood flow agent, xanthines

Prescription: USA: Yes
Canada: Yes

Controlled Drug: USA: No
Canada: No

Available as Generic: No

Brand Name: Trental

```
┌─────────────────────────────────────────────────────────────────┐
│                      BENEFITS versus RISKS                        │
│                                                                   │
│        Possible Benefits              Possible Risks              │
│   IMPROVED BLOOD FLOW IN        Reduced blood pressure, angina,   │
│     PERIPHERAL ARTERIAL           abnormal heart rhythms (in      │
│     DISEASE                       susceptible individuals)        │
│   REDUCTION OF                  Indigestion, nausea, vomiting     │
│     INTERMITTENT                Dizziness, flushing               │
│     CLAUDICATION PAIN                                             │
└─────────────────────────────────────────────────────────────────┘
```

▷ **Principal Uses**

As a Single Drug Product: Used primarily (as adjunctive treatment) in the management of peripheral obstructive arterial disease to improve arterial blood flow and reduce the frequency and severity of muscle pain due to intermittent claudication.

How This Drug Works: This drug is thought to improve blood flow through the microcirculation and to increase the oxygen supply to working muscles by way of three mechanisms: (1) reduction of blood viscosity due to decreased levels of fibrinogen in the blood; (2) increased flexibility of the red blood cells (carrying oxygen) due to an increase in cyclic AMP (enzyme) within red blood cells; this permits easier passage through the minute blood vessels of the microcirculation; and (3) prevention of red blood cell and platelet aggregation.

Available Dosage Forms and Strengths

Tablets, prolonged-action — 400 mg

▷ **Usual Adult Dosage Range:** 400 mg 3 times/day. If adverse nervous system or gastrointestinal effects occur, reduce the dose to 400 mg twice/day. **Note: Actual dosage and administration schedule must be determined by the physician for each patient individually.**

▷ **Dosing Instructions:** Take with or following food to reduce stomach irritation. Swallow the tablet whole without breaking, crushing or chewing.

Usual Duration of Use: Continual use on a regular schedule for 2 to 4 weeks is usually necessary to determine this drug's effectiveness in preventing or delaying the pains of intermittent claudication associated with walking. Treatment for 2 to 3 months is recommended to determine full effectiveness. Long-term use (months to years) requires supervision and periodic evaluation by your physician. Consult your physician on a regular basis.

Possible Advantages of This Drug

Reduces blood viscosity and thereby improves blood flow through small vessels.

Increases supply of oxygen to working muscles.

Currently a "Drug of Choice" for treating peripheral arterial disease and reducing the frequency and severity of intermittent claudication pain.

▷ **This Drug Should Not Be Taken If**
 • you have had an allergic reaction to it previously.

▷ **Inform Your Physician Before Taking This Drug If**
 • you are allergic to other xanthine drugs: caffeine, theophylline, theobromine.
 • you have impaired kidney function.
 • you have low blood pressure, impaired brain circulation or coronary artery disease.
 • you smoke tobacco.
 • you are taking any antihypertensive drugs.

Possible Side-Effects (natural, expected and unavoidable drug actions)
Usually none with recommended doses.

▷ **Possible Adverse Effects** (unusual, unexpected and infrequent reactions)
If any of the following develop, consult your physician promptly for guidance.
Mild Adverse Effects
Allergic Reaction: Skin rash.
Headache (1.2%), dizziness (1.9%), tremor.
Indigestion (2.8%), nausea (2.2%), vomiting (1.2%).
Serious Adverse Effects
Development of angina or heart rhythm disorders in the presence of coronary artery disease.

▷ **Possible Effects on Sexual Function:**   None reported.

CAUTION
Use this drug with caution in the presence of impaired circulation within the brain (cerebral arteriosclerosis) or coronary artery disease. If any related symptoms develop, consult your physician for prompt evaluation.

Precautions for Use
By Infants and Children: Safety and effectiveness for use by those under 18 years of age have not been established. Use by this age group is not anticipated.
By Those over 60 Years of Age: You may be more susceptible to the adverse effects listed. Observe closely for any indications of dizziness or chest pain and report these promptly.

▷ **Advisability of Use During Pregnancy**
Pregnancy Category: C (tentative). See Pregnancy Code inside back cover.
Animal studies: Increased fetal resorptions reported in rats, but no birth defects found in rats or rabbits.
Human studies: Information from adequate studies of pregnant women is not available.

Avoid use during the first 3 months. Use otherwise only if clearly needed.

Advisability of Use if Breast-Feeding
Presence of this drug in breast milk: Yes.
Avoid drug or refrain from nursing.

Habit-Forming Potential: None.

Effects of Overdosage: Drowsiness, flushing, faintness, excitement, seizures.

Possible Effects of Long-Term Use: None reported.

Suggested Periodic Examinations While Taking This Drug (at physician's discretion)
Blood pressure measurements, evaluation of heart status.

▷ **While Taking This Drug, Observe the Following**
Foods: No restrictions.
Beverages: No restrictions. May be taken with milk.
▷ *Alcohol:* Use caution until the combined effects have been determined. Alcohol may increase the blood-pressure-lowering effect of this drug.
Tobacco Smoking: Nicotine constricts arteries and will impair the effectiveness of this drug significantly. Avoid all use of tobacco.
▷ *Other Drugs*
Pentoxifylline may *increase* the effects of
- antihypertensive drugs, and cause excessive lowering of blood pressure.
- warfarin (Coumadin, etc.), and increase the possibility of unwanted bleeding; monitor prothrombin times as appropriate.
▷ *Driving, Hazardous Activities:* This drug may cause drowsiness or dizziness. Restrict activities as necessary.
Aviation Note: The use of this drug *may be a disqualification* for piloting. Consult a designated Aviation Medical Examiner.
Exposure to Sun: No restrictions.

PERGOLIDE
(PER go lide)

Introduced: 1980

Class: Antiparkinsonism, dopamine agonist, ergot derivative

Prescription: USA: Yes (Expected to become available in 1989)

Controlled Drug: USA: No

Available as Generic: USA: No

Brand Name: Permax

```
┌─────────────────────────────────────────────────────────────┐
│                   BENEFITS versus RISKS                      │
│                                                              │
│      Possible Benefits              Possible Risks           │
│  ADDITIVE RELIEF OF             ABNORMAL INVOLUNTARY         │
│    SYMPTOMS OF PARKINSON'S         MOVEMENTS (62%)           │
│    DISEASE when used            HALLUCINATIONS (14%)         │
│    concurrently with levodopa/  INITIAL FALL IN BLOOD        │
│    carbidopa (Sinemet)            PRESSURE/ORTHOSTATIC       │
│  PERMITS A 5% TO 30%              HYPOTENSION (10%)          │
│    REDUCTION IN SINEMET                                      │
│    DOSAGE                                                    │
└─────────────────────────────────────────────────────────────┘
```

▷ **Principal Uses**

As a Single Drug Product: Used solely as an adjunct to levodopa/carbidopa treatment of Parkinson's disease for those individuals who experience intolerable abnormal movements (dyskinesia) and/or increasing "on-off" episodes due to levodopa. The addition of pergolide (1) permits reduction of the daily dose of levodopa with consequent lessening of dyskinesia and erratic drug response, and (2) provides additional relief of parkinsonian symptoms.

How This Drug Works: By directly stimulating the dopamine receptor sites in the corpus striatum of the brain, this drug helps to compensate for the deficiency of dopamine that is responsible for the rigidity, tremor and sluggish movement characteristic of Parkinson's disease.

Available Dosage Forms and Strengths

Tablets — 0.05 mg, 0.25 mg, 1 mg

▷ **Usual Adult Dosage Range**

Initially 0.05 mg daily for the first 2 days; gradually increase the daily dose by 0.1 mg or 0.15 mg every third day over the next 12 days. If needed and tolerated, the daily dose may be increased further by 0.25 mg every third day until an optimal respose is achieved. The total daily dosage should be divided into 3 equal portions and given at 6 to 8 hour intervals. The usual maintenance dose is 3 mg/24 hours; do not exceed 5 mg/24 hours.

During the gradual introduction of pergolide, the concurrent dose of levodopa/carbidopa (Sinemet) may be cautiously decreased in accord with your physician's instructions.

Note: Actual dosage and administration schedule must be determined by the physician for each patient individually.

▷ **Dosing Instructions:**   Take with food or milk to reduce stomach irritation. The tablet may be crushed for administration.

Usual Duration of Use: Continual use on a regular schedule for 4 to 6 weeks is usually necessary to determine this drug's effectiveness in

controlling the symptoms of Parkinson's disease and permitting reduction of levodopa/carbidopa dosage. Long-term use (months to years) requires periodic evaluation of response and dosage adjustment. Consult your physician on a regular basis.

Possible Advantages of This Drug: It may provide a more effective and uniform control of parkinsonian symptoms and a significant reduction of some adverse effects of long-term levodopa therapy.

▷ **This Drug Should Not Be Taken If**
- you have had an allergic reaction to it previously.
- you have had a serious adverse effect from any ergot preparation in the past.
- you have severe coronary artery disease or peripheral vascular disease.

▷ **Inform Your Physician Before Taking This Drug If**
- you have constitutionally low blood pressure.
- you are pregnant or breast-feeding.
- you are taking any antihypertensive drugs or antipsychotic drugs (see Drug Classes, Section Four).
- you have any degree of coronary artery disease, especially angina or a history of heart attack.
- you have any type of heart rhythm disorder.
- you have impaired liver or kidney function.
- you have a seizure disorder.

Possible Side-Effects (natural, expected and unavoidable drug actions)
Weakness (4.2%), chest pain—possibly anginal (3.7%), peripheral edema (7.4%), orthostatic hypotension (see Glossary) (10%).

▷ **Possible Adverse Effects** (unusual, unexpected and infrequent reactions)
If any of the following develop, consult your physician promptly for guidance.
Mild Adverse Effects
Allergic Reactions: Skin rash (3.2%), facial swelling (1.1%).
Headache (5.3%), dizziness (19%), hallucinations (14%), confusion (11%), drowsiness (10%), insomnia (8%), anxiety (6%), double vision (2%).
Nasal congestion (12%), shortness of breath (5%), palpitation (2%), fainting (2%).
Altered taste (1.6%), loss of appetite (4.8%), dry mouth (3.7%), indigestion (6.4%), nausea (24%), vomiting (2.7%), constipation (10%), diarrhea (6.4%).
Serious Adverse Effects
Allergic Reactions: None reported.
Idiosyncratic Reactions: "Flulike" symptoms (3%).
Abnormal involuntary movements (dyskinesia) (62%), psychotic behavior (2%).

▷ **Possible Effects on Sexual Function:** Infrequent reports of altered libido (both increased and decreased), impotence, breast pain, priapism (see Glossary).

▷ **Adverse Effects That May Mimic Natural Diseases or Disorders**
Effects on mental function and behavior may resemble psychotic disorders.

▷ **Natural Diseases or Disorders That May Be Activated by This Drug**
Coronary artery disease with anginal syndrome, heart rhythm disorders, Raynaud's syndrome (see Glossary), seizure disorders.

CAUTION
1. This drug can initiate dyskinesias and can intensify existing dyskinesias. Observe carefully for the development of tremors, twitching or abnormal, involuntary movements of any kind. Report these promptly.
2. Begin treatment with low doses to prevent the possibility of excessive drop in blood pressure. See dosage routine outlined above.
3. Inform your physician promptly if you become pregnant or plan pregnancy. This drug has been reported (rarely) to cause abortion and birth defects.

Precautions for Use
By Infants and Children: This drug is not utilized by this age group.
By Those over 60 Years of Age: Small initial doses are mandatory. Observe closely for any tendency to light-headedness or faintness, especially on arising from a lying or sitting position. You may be more susceptible to the development of impaired thinking, confusion, agitation, nightmares or hallucinations.

▷ **Advisability of Use During Pregnancy**
Pregnancy Category: B (tentative). See Pregnancy Code inside back cover.
Animal studies: No birth defects due to this drug were found in mouse or rabbit studies.
Human studies: Information from adequate studies of pregnant women is not available. However, there are four reports of birth defects associated with the use of this drug and infrequent reports of abortion. Causal relationships have not been established, but prudence advises against the use of this drug during pregnancy. Consult your physician for guidance.

Advisability of Use if Breast-Feeding
Presence of this drug in breast milk: Unknown.
Avoid drug or refrain from nursing.

Habit-Forming Potential: None.

Effects of Overdosage: Nausea, vomiting, palpitations, low blood pressure, agitation, severe involuntary movements, hallucinations, seizures.

Possible Effects of Long-Term Use: Increased risk of developing dyskinesias.

Suggested Periodic Examinations While Taking This Drug (at physician's discretion)
Regular evaluation of drug response, heart function and blood pressure status.

▷ **While Taking This Drug, Observe the Following**
Foods: No restrictions.
Beverages: No restrictions. May be taken with milk.
▷ *Alcohol:* Use caution until the combined effects have been determined. Alcohol can exaggerate the blood-pressure-lowering and sedative effects of this drug.
Tobacco Smoking: No interactions expected.
▷ *Other Drugs*
Pergolide *taken concurrently* with
- antihypertensive drugs (and other drugs that can lower blood pressure) requires careful monitoring for excessive drops in pressure. Dosage adjustments may be necessary.

The following drugs may *decrease* the effects of pergolide and diminish its effectiveness
- chlorprothixene (Taractan).
- haloperidol (Haldol).
- metoclopramide (Reglan).
- phenothiazines (see Drug Class, Section Four).
- thiothixene (Navane).
▷ *Driving, Hazardous Activities:* This drug may cause dizziness, drowsiness, impaired coordination or fainting. Restrict activities as necessary.
Aviation Note: The use of this drug *is a disqualification* for piloting. Consult a designated Aviation Medical Examiner.
Exposure to Sun: No restrictions.
Exposure to Heat: Use caution until the combined effects have been determined. Hot environments can cause lowering of blood pressure.
Discontinuation: Do not discontinue this drug abruptly. Sudden withdrawal can cause confusion, paranoid thinking and severe hallucinations. Consult your physician regarding a schedule for gradual withdrawal.

PERPHENAZINE
(per FEN a zeen)

Introduced: 1957

Class: Strong tranquilizer, phenothiazines

Prescription: USA: Yes
Canada: Yes

Controlled Drug: USA: No
Canada: No

Available as Generic: USA: No
Canada: Yes

Brand Names: ✦Apo-Perphenazine, ✦Elavil Plus [CD], Etrafon [CD], Etrafon-A [CD], Etrafon Forte [CD], ✦Phenazine, ✦PMS Levazine, Triavil [CD], Trilafon

BENEFITS versus RISKS	
Possible Benefits	*Possible Risks*
EFFECTIVE CONTROL OF ACUTE MENTAL DISORDERS in the majority of patients	SERIOUS TOXIC EFFECTS ON BRAIN with long-term use
Beneficial effects on thinking, mood and behavior	Liver damage with jaundice (infrequent)
Relief of anxiety and tension	Rare blood cell disorders:
Moderately effective control of nausea and vomiting	hemolytic anemia, abnormally low white blood cell and platelet counts

▷ **Principal Uses**

As a Single Drug Product: This antipsychotic drug is used primarily to treat acute and chronic psychotic disorders such as agitated depression, schizophrenia and similar states of mental dysfunction. It may be used as a tranquilizer in the management of agitated and disruptive behavior in the absence of true psychosis. Less frequently, it may be used to relieve severe nausea or vomiting.

As a Combination Drug Product [CD]: This drug is available in combination with amitriptyline, an effective antidepressant. In some cases of severe agitated depression, the combination of a specific antipsychotic drug and a specific antidepressant drug will be more effective than either drug used alone.

How This Drug Works: Not completely established. Present theory is that by inhibiting the action of dopamine, this drug acts to correct an imbalance of nerve impulse transmissions that is thought to be responsible for certain mental disorders.

Available Dosage Forms and Strengths

Concentrate — 16 mg per 5-ml teaspoonful
Injection — 5 mg per ml
Tablets — 2 mg, 4 mg, 8 mg, 16 mg
Tablets, prolonged-action — 8 mg

▷ **Usual Adult Dosage Range:** Initially 2 to 16 mg 2 to 4 times daily. Dose may be increased by 4 mg at 3- to 4-day intervals as needed and tolerated. Usual dosage range is 8 to 24 mg daily. The total daily dosage should not exceed 64 mg. **Note: Actual dosage and administration schedule must be determined by the physician for each patient individually.**

▷ **Dosing Instructions:**   May be taken with or following meals to reduce stomach irritation. The regular tablets may be crushed for administration; the prolonged-action tablets should be taken whole, not broken, crushed or chewed.

Usual Duration of Use: Continual use on a regular schedule for several weeks is usually necessary to determine this drug's effectiveness in controlling psychotic disorders. If it is not significantly beneficial within 6 weeks, it should be discontinued. Long-term use (months to years) requires periodic evaluation of response, appropriate dosage adjustment and consideration of continued need. Consult your physician on a regular basis.

▷ **This Drug Should Not Be Taken If**
   • you are allergic to any of the drugs bearing the brand names listed.
   • you have active liver disease.
   • you have cancer of the breast.
   • you have a current blood cell or bone marrow disorder.

▷ **Inform Your Physician Before Taking This Drug If**
   • you are allergic or abnormally sensitive to any phenothiazine drug (see Drug Class, Section Four).
   • you have impaired liver or kidney function.
   • you have any type of seizure disorder.
   • you have diabetes, glaucoma or heart disease.
   • you have a history of lupus erythematosus.
   • you are taking any drug with sedative effects.
   • you plan to have surgery under general or spinal anesthesia in the near future.

Possible Side-Effects (natural, expected and unavoidable drug actions)
   Drowsiness (usually during the first 2 weeks), orthostatic hypotension (see Glossary), blurred vision, dry mouth, nasal congestion, constipation, impaired urination.
   Pink or purple coloration of urine, of no significance.

▷ **Possible Adverse Effects** (unusual, unexpected and infrequent reactions)
   If any of the following develop, consult your physician promptly for guidance.
   Mild Adverse Effects
   Allergic Reactions: Skin rash, hives, low-grade fever.
   Lowering of body temperature, especially in the elderly. (See Hypothermia in Glossary).
   Increased appetite and weight gain.
   Dizziness, weakness, agitation, insomnia, impaired day and night vision.
   Chronic constipation, fecal impaction.
   Serious Adverse Effects
   Allergic Reactions: Hepatitis with jaundice (see Glossary), severe skin reactions, anaphylactic reaction (see Glossary).

Idiosyncratic Reaction: High fever.

Depression, disorientation, seizures, deposits in cornea, lens and retina.

Rapid heart rate, heart rhythm disorders.

Blood cell disorders: hemolytic anemia, reduced white blood cell and blood platelet counts.

Nervous system reactions: Parkinson-like disorders (see Glossary), severe restlessness, muscle spasms involving the face and neck, tardive dyskinesia (see Glossary).

▷ **Possible Effects on Sexual Function**

Altered timing and pattern of menstruation.

Female breast enlargement with milk production.

Male breast enlargement and tenderness.

Inhibited ejaculation.

False positive pregnancy test results.

▷ **Adverse Effects That May Mimic Natural Diseases or Disorders**

Nervous system reactions may suggest true Parkinson's disease.

Liver reactions may suggest viral hepatitis.

Reactions resembling systemic lupus erythematosus can occur.

Natural Diseases or Disorders That May Be Activated by This Drug

Latent epilepsy, glaucoma, diabetes mellitus, prostatism (see Glossary).

CAUTION

1. Many over-the-counter medications (see OTC Drugs in Glossary) for allergies, colds and coughs contain drugs that can interact unfavorably with this drug. Ask your physician or pharmacist for guidance before using any such medications.

2. Antacids that contain aluminum and/or magnesium can prevent the absorption of this drug and reduce its effectiveness.

3. Obtain prompt evaluation of any change or disturbance of vision.

Precautions for Use

By Infants and Children: Use of this drug is not recommended in children under 12 years of age. Do not use this drug in the presence of symptoms suggestive of Reye syndrome (see Glossary). Children with acute infectious diseases (flulike infections, chicken pox, measles, etc.) are more prone to develop muscular spasms of the face, back and extremities when this drug is given to control nausea or vomiting.

By Those over 60 Years of Age: Small doses are advisable until individual response has been determined. You may be more susceptible to the development of drowsiness, lethargy, constipation, lowering of body temperature (hypothermia) and orthostatic hypotension (see Glossary). This drug can enhance existing prostatism (see Glossary). You may also be more susceptible to the development of Parkinson-like reactions and/or tardive dyskinesia (see discussion of these terms in Glossary). These reactions must be recognized early since they may become unresponsive to treatment and irreversible.

▷ **Advisability of Use During Pregnancy**
Pregnancy Category: C (tentative). See Pregnancy Code inside back cover.
Animal studies: Cleft palate reported in mouse and rat studies.
Human studies: No increase in birth defects reported in 166 exposures. Information from adequate studies of pregnant women is not available.
Avoid drug during the first 3 months; avoid during the last month because of possible effects on the newborn infant.

Advisability of Use if Breast-Feeding
Presence of this drug in breast milk: Yes, in minute amounts.
Monitor nursing infant closely and discontinue drug or nursing if adverse effects develop.

Habit-Forming Potential: None.

Effects of Overdosage: Marked drowsiness, weakness, tremor, agitation, unsteadiness, deep sleep, coma, convulsions.

Possible Effects of Long-Term Use
Opacities in the cornea or lens of the eye, pigmentation of the retina.
Tardive dyskinesia (see Glossary).

Suggested Periodic Examinations While Taking This Drug (at physician's discretion)
Complete blood cell counts, especially between the fourth and tenth weeks of treatment.
Liver function tests, electrocardiograms.
Complete eye examinations—eye structures and vision.
Careful inspection of the tongue for early evidence of fine, involuntary, wavelike movements that could indicate the beginning of tardive dyskinesia.

▷ **While Taking This Drug, Observe the Following**
Foods: No restrictions.
Nutritional Support: A riboflavin (vitamin B-2) supplement should be taken with long-term use.
Beverages: No restrictions. May be taken with milk.
▷ *Alcohol:* Avoid completely. Alcohol can increase the sedative action of phenothiazines and accentuate their depressant effects on brain function and blood pressure. Phenothiazines can increase the intoxicating effects of alcohol.
Tobacco Smoking: Possible reduction of drowsiness from drug.
Marijuana Smoking: Moderate increase in drowsiness; accentuation of orthostatic hypotension; increased risk of precipitating latent psychoses, confusing the interpretation of mental status and drug responses.
▷ *Other Drugs*
Perphenazine may *increase* the effects of

- all sedative drugs, especially meperidine (Demerol), and cause excessive sedation.
- all atropinelike drugs, and cause nervous system toxicity.

Perphenazine may *decrease* the effects of

- guanethidine (Ismelin, Esimil), and reduce its effectiveness in lowering blood pressure.

Perphenazine *taken concurrently* with

- lithium (Lithobid, Lithotabs) may impair the effectiveness of lithium and cause nervous system toxicity.

The following drugs may *decrease* the effects of perphenazine

- antacids containing aluminum and/or magnesium.
- barbiturates (see Drug Class, Section Four).
- benztropine (Cogentin).
- disulfiram (Antabuse).
- trihexyphenidyl (Artane).

▷ *Driving, Hazardous Activities:* This drug can impair mental alertness, judgment and physical coordination. Avoid hazardous activities.

Aviation Note: The use of this drug *is a disqualification* for piloting. Consult a designated Aviation Medical Examiner.

Exposure to Sun: Use caution until sensitivity has been determined. Some phenothiazines can cause photosensitivity (see Glossary).

Exposure to Heat: Use caution and avoid excessive heat as much as possible. This drug may impair the regulation of body temperature and increase the risk of heat stroke.

Exposure to Cold: Use caution and dress warmly. This drug can increase the risk of hypothermia in the elderly.

Discontinuation: After a period of long-term use, do not discontinue this drug suddenly. Gradual withdrawal over 2 to 3 weeks under physician supervision is recommended. Do not discontinue this drug without your physician's knowledge and approval. The relapse rate of schizophrenia after discontinuation is 50% to 60%.

PHENAZOPYRIDINE
(fen az oh PEER i deen)

Introduced: 1927

Class: Urinary analgesic

Prescription: USA: Varies
Canada: No

Controlled Drug: USA: No
Canada: No

Available as Generic: USA: Yes
Canada: No

Brand Names: Azo Gantanol [CD], Azo Gantrisin [CD], Azo-Standard, Baridium, Di-Azo, ✦Phenazo, Pyridium, Pyridium Plus [CD], ✦Pyronium, Thiosulfil-A [CD], Urobiotic-250 [CD], ✦Uro Gantanol [CD]

BENEFITS versus RISKS	
Possible Benefits	*Possible Risks*
EFFECTIVE RELIEF OF URINARY URGENCY AND DISCOMFORT	DRUG-INDUCED HEPATITIS (rare) Hemolytic anemia (rare)

▷ **Principal Uses**

As a Single Drug Product: Used exclusively in the treatment of lower urinary tract infections and irritations to relieve the urgency to urinate and the discomfort that accompanies the passage of urine (as in cystitis, urethritis and prostatitis).

As a Combination Drug Product [CD]: This drug is available in combinations with several anti-infective drugs that are commonly used to treat urinary tract infections. Each combination product provides a drug to eradicate the infection and a drug to relieve the discomfort during the early period of treatment.

How This Drug Works: Not completely established. By its direct local anesthetic effect on the tissues lining the lower urinary tract, this drug provides symptomatic relief of pain, burning, pressure and the sense of urgency to void.

Available Dosage Forms and Strengths
Tablets — 100 mg, 200 mg

▷ **Usual Adult Dosage Range:**   100 to 200 mg 3 or 4 times/day, as needed and tolerated. **Note: Actual dosage and administration schedule must be determined by the physician for each patient individually.**

▷ **Dosing Instructions:**   Take with or after food to reduce stomach irritation. The tablet should be taken whole, not broken or crushed for administration.

Usual Duration of Use: Continual use on a regular schedule for 12 to 24 hours is usually necessary to determine this drug's effectiveness in relieving urinary urgency and discomfort. This drug is intended for short-term use; do not continue to take it after the bladder disorder has been corrected.

▷ **This Drug Should Not Be Taken If**
  • you have had an allergic reaction to it previously.
  • you have active liver disease.

▷ **Inform Your Physician Before Taking This Drug If**
  • you have a history of liver or kidney disease.
  • you have had a drug-induced blood cell disorder in the past.

Possible Side-Effects (natural, expected and unavoidable drug actions)
Reddish-orange discoloration of the urine (of no significance).

▷ **Possible Adverse Effects** (unusual, unexpected and infrequent reactions)
If any of the following develop, consult your physician promptly for guidance.
Mild Adverse Effects
Allergic Reaction: Skin rash.
Headache, dizziness, indigestion, abdominal cramping.
Serious Adverse Effects
Allergic Reactions: Drug-induced hepatitis, with or without jaundice (see Glossary).
Idiosyncratic Reaction: Hemolytic anemia (see Glossary) in sensitive individuals; this is more likely to occur in the presence of impaired kidney function.

▷ **Possible Effects on Sexual Function:**   None reported.

▷ **Adverse Effects That May Mimic Natural Diseases or Disorders**
Liver reaction may suggest viral hepatitis.

CAUTION
It is important to understand that this drug is only an analgesic, and that its action is limited to the relief of symptoms. It has no curative effect on the underlying condition that is responsible for the symptoms. Consult your physician regarding the need for specific anti-infective therapy.

Precautions for Use
By Infants and Children: Consult your physician regarding appropriate dosage. Limit use to the time required for adequate relief of symptoms.
By Those over 60 Years of Age: The natural decline in kidney function that occurs after 60 may require that you use smaller doses. Observe for the development of a yellowish coloration of the eyes or skin—an indication of excessive drug accumulation. If this occurs, consult your physician.

▷ **Advisability of Use During Pregnancy**
Pregnancy Category: B (tentative). See Pregnancy Code inside back cover.
Animal studies: No birth defects found.
Human studies: Information from studies of pregnant women indicates no increase in birth defects in 1109 exposures to this drug.
Limit use to small doses for short periods of time. Ask your physician for guidance.

Advisability of Use if Breast-Feeding
Presence of this drug in breast milk: Unknown.
Avoid drug or refrain from nursing.

Habit-Forming Potential: None.

Effects of Overdosage: Nausea, vomiting, abdominal discomfort, skin discoloration, hemolytic anemia (in susceptible individuals), altered hemoglobin resulting in weakness and shortness of breath.

Possible Effects of Long-Term Use: Orange-yellow discoloration of the skin; hemolytic anemia.

Suggested Periodic Examinations While Taking This Drug (at physician's discretion)
None for short-term use; red blood cell counts and liver-function tests during long-term use.

▷ **While Taking This Drug, Observe the Following**
Foods: No restrictions.
Beverages: No restrictions.
▷ *Alcohol:* No interactions expected.
Tobacco Smoking: No interactions expected.
▷ *Other Drugs:* No significant interactions with other drugs have been reported.
▷ *Driving, Hazardous Activities:* Usually no restrictions. This drug may cause dizziness. Restrict activities as necessary.
Aviation Note: The use of this drug **may be a disqualification** for piloting. Consult a designated Aviation Medical Examiner.
Exposure to Sun: No restrictions.

PHENELZINE
(FEN el zeen)

Introduced: 1961

Class: Antidepressant, MAO type A inhibitor

Prescription: USA: Yes
Canada: Yes

Controlled Drug: USA: No
Canada: No

Available as Generic: No

Brand Name: Nardil

BENEFITS versus RISKS

Possible Benefits	*Possible Risks*
EFFECTIVE RELIEF OF REACTIVE, NEUROTIC, ATYPICAL DEPRESSIONS with associated anxiety or phobia Beneficial in some depressions that are not responsive to other treatments	DANGEROUS INTERACTIONS WITH MANY DRUGS AND FOODS CONDUCIVE TO HYPERTENSIVE CRISIS DISORDERED HEART RATE AND RHYTHM Drug-induced hepatitis (rare) Mental changes: agitation, confusion, impaired memory, hypomania

---

▷ **Principal Uses**

As a Single Drug Product: This potent MAO type A inhibitor drug is used exclusively to treat severe situational (reactive or neurotic) depression, atypical depression, and (though less effective) severe endogenous depression. Because of the supervision required during its use and its potential for serious adverse effects, this drug is usually reserved to treat depressions that have not responded satisfactorily to other antidepressant therapy.

How This Drug Works: Not completely established. It is thought that by inhibiting the action of a certain enzyme (monoamine oxidase type A) in brain tissue, this drug produces an increase of those nerve impulse transmitters that maintain normal mood and emotional stability.

Available Dosage Forms and Strengths
Tablets — 15 mg

▷ **Usual Adult Dosage Range:** Initially, 15 mg 3 times/day; increase rapidly up to 60 mg/day, as needed and tolerated, until improvement is apparent. For maintenance, reduce dose gradually over several weeks to the smallest dose that will maintain optimal improvement; this may be as low as 15 mg daily or every other day. The total daily dosage should not exceed 90 mg. **Note: Actual dosage and administration schedule must be determined by the physician for each patient individually.**

▷ **Dosing Instructions:** May be taken on an empty stomach or with food. Do not take this drug in the late evening; it can interfere with sleep. The tablet may be crushed for administration.

Usual Duration of Use: Continual use on a regular schedule for 3 to 4 weeks is usually necessary to determine this drug's effectiveness in relieving depression. Once the optimal maintenance dose has been determined, it may be continued indefinitely. Long-term use (months to years) requires supervision and periodic evaluation by your physician. Consult your physician on a regular basis.

▷ **This Drug Should Not Be Taken If**
- you have had an allergic reaction to it previously.
- you have advanced heart disease.
- you have active liver disease or impaired liver function.
- you have an adrenaline-producing tumor (pheochromocytoma).
- you are taking any of the following drugs: another MAO type A inhibitor, a tricyclic antidepressant, carbamazepine (see Drug Classes, Section Four).

▷ **Inform Your Physician Before Taking This Drug If**
- you have high blood pressure.
- you have had a stroke, or you have impaired circulation to the brain.

- you have coronary heart disease.
- you have frequent or severe headaches.
- you have diabetes, epilepsy, schizophrenia or an overactive thyroid gland (hyperthyroidism).
- you have impaired kidney function.
- you plan to have surgery under general or spinal anesthesia in the near future.

Possible Side-Effects (natural, expected and unavoidable drug actions)
Insomnia if taken in the evening.
Orthostatic hypotension (see Glossary).
Fluid retention (swelling of feet and ankles).

▷ **Possible Adverse Effects** (unusual, unexpected and infrequent reactions)
If any of the following develop, consult your physician promptly for guidance.
Mild Adverse Effects
Allergic Reaction: Skin rash.
Headache, dizziness, drowsiness, weakness, agitation, confusion, impaired memory, tremors, muscle twitching, blurred vision, impaired red-green color vision.
Dry mouth, increased appetite, indigestion, constipation.
Serious Adverse Effects
Drug-induced hepatitis with jaundice (see Glossary).
Hypertensive crisis: rapid and extreme rise in blood pressure, severe throbbing headache, palpitation, nausea, vomiting, sweating, risk of brain hemorrhage.
Unusual excitement or nervousness.
Disturbances of heart rate and rhythm.

▷ **Possible Effects on Sexual Function**
Decreased libido (30% of males, 28% of females).
Impaired erection (50%); inhibited ejaculation (60%).
Inhibited orgasm (30% of males, 35% of females).

▷ **Adverse Effects That May Mimic Natural Diseases or Disorders**
Drug-induced hepatitis may suggest viral hepatitis.

Natural Diseases or Disorders That May Be Activated by This Drug
Latent epilepsy, schizophrenia.
This drug may convert a depression into the manic phase of a manic-depressive disorder.

CAUTION
1. Careful dosage adjustment is mandatory. Determine the lowest effective dose and do not exceed it.
2. The development of a severe headache or palpitation may indicate a dangerous elevation of blood pressure. Discontinue this drug immediately and consult your physician.

3. This drug may suppress anginal pain that would normally serve as a warning of excessive demand on the heart.

4. This drug may increase the possibility of hypoglycemic reactions if used concurrently with insulin or oral antidiabetic drugs (sulfonylureas; see Drug Class, Section Four). It may also delay recovery from hypoglycemia.

5. This drug can alter the threshold for convulsions in anyone with epilepsy or a seizure disorder. Dosages of anticonvulsant drugs may require adjustment.

6. This drug should be discontinued 2 weeks before elective surgery under general or spinal anesthesia. Consult your surgeon or anesthesiologist.

7. Many over-the-counter drug products contain ingredients that can cause serious interactions if taken concurrently with this drug. Avoid use of the following: cold and sinus medications, nasal decongestants, hay fever preparations, asthma inhalants, appetite and weight control products, "pep" pills. Consult your physician or pharmacist regarding their safe use with this drug.

8. It is advisable to carry a card of personal identification with the notation that you are taking this drug. Notify all medical personnel that may attend you that you are taking this drug.

Precautions for Use

By Infants and Children: Safety and effectiveness for use by those under 16 years of age have not been established.

By Those over 60 Years of Age: This drug is not recommended for use by anyone over 60. However, if poor response to other treatment justifies consideration of a trial of this drug, it is inadvisable to use it in the presence of high blood pressure, hardening of the arteries, impaired circulation within the brain or coronary artery disease. This drug will intensify existing prostatism (see Glossary). Fluid retention is more prominent in this age group.

▷ Advisability of Use During Pregnancy

Pregnancy Category: C (tentative). See Pregnancy Code inside back cover.
Animal studies: No information available.
Human studies: Information from adequate studies of pregnant women is not available. Birth defects have been reported with the use of this drug.
Avoid this drug completely if possible. Ask your physician for guidance.

Advisability of Use if Breast-Feeding

Presence of this drug in breast milk: Probably yes.
Avoid drug or refrain from nursing.

Habit-Forming Potential: None.

Effects of Overdosage: Overstimulation, agitation, anxiety, restlessness, insomnia, confusion, delirium, hallucinations, seizures, high fever, circulatory collapse, coma.

Possible Effects of Long-Term Use: The conversion of mental depression into a state of hypomania: excessive mental and physical activity, excitement, agitation, loud and rapid talking, delusional thinking.

Suggested Periodic Examinations While Taking This Drug (at physician's discretion)
Blood pressure measurements in lying, sitting and standing positions. Complete blood cell counts, liver function tests.

▷ **While Taking This Drug, Observe the Following**
Foods: ***All tyramine-rich foods should be avoided completely.*** See Tyramine in the Glossary for a compete list of foods and beverages to avoid while taking this drug.
Beverages: Limit coffee, tea and cola beverages to one serving daily. See Tyramine in the Glossary.
▷ *Alcohol:* Use extreme caution until the combined effects have been determined. Alcohol can increase the depressant effects of this drug on brain function.
Tobacco Smoking: No interactions expected.
▷ *Other Drugs*
Phenelzine may ***increase*** the effects of
- amphetamine and related drugs.
- appetite suppressants.
- all drugs with stimulant effects on the nervous system, and cause excessive rise in blood pressure.
- all drugs with sedative effects, and cause excessive sedation.
- insulin.
- sulfonylureas (see Drug Class, Section Four).

Phenelzine ***taken concurrently*** with
- carbamazepine (Tegretol) may cause severe toxic reactions.
- levodopa (Dopar, Sinemet) may cause a dangerous rise in blood pressure.
- meperidine (Demerol) may cause high fever, seizures and coma.
- methyldopa (Aldomet) may cause a dangerous rise in blood pressure.
- methylphenidate (Ritalin) may cause severe headache, weakness and numbness in the extremities.
- tricyclic antidepressants may cause severe toxic reactions including high fever, delirium, tremor, seizures and coma.

Note: Consult your physician before taking ***any other drugs*** while taking phenelzine.
▷ *Driving, Hazardous Activities:* This drug may cause dizziness, drowsiness and blurred vision. Restrict activities as necessary.
Aviation Note: The use of this drug ***is a disqualification*** for piloting. Consult a designated Aviation Medical Examiner.
Exposure to Sun: No restrictions.
Occurrence of Unrelated Illness: Because of the very serious and life-threatening interactions that can occur between this drug and many others, it is mandatory that you inform each physician and dentist you consult that you are taking this drug.

Discontinuation: If this drug is not effective after 4 weeks of continual use, it should be discontinued. If it is effective, continue to take it in proper dosage until advised to stop. Do not discontinue it abruptly. If another antidepressant is to be tried, a drug-free waiting period of 14 days must elapse between the discontinuation of this drug and initiation of the new one. All precautions regarding the avoidance of tyramine-rich foods and other drugs must be observed during this 14-day period.

PHENOBARBITAL
(fee noh BAR bi tawl)

Other Name: Phenobarbitone

Introduced: 1912

Class: Sedative, anticonvulsant, barbiturates

Prescription: USA: Yes
Canada: Yes

Controlled Drug: USA: C-IV*
Canada: <C>

Available as Generic: Yes

Brand Names: Barbidonna [CD], Barbidonna Elixir [CD], Barbita, Belladenal [CD], Belladenal-S [CD], ✦Belladenal Spacetabs [CD], ✦Bellergal [CD], Bellergal-S [CD], ✦Bellergal Spacetabs [CD], Bronchotabs [CD], Bronkolixir [CD], Chardonna-2 [CD], ✦Diclophen [CD], Dilantin w/Phenobarbital [CD], Donnatal [CD], Donnazyme [CD], ✦Gardenal, Kinesed [CD], Luminal, Mudrane GG Elixir & Tablets [CD], Mudrane Tablets [CD], ✦Neuro-Spasex [CD], ✦Neuro-Trasentin [CD], ✦Neuro-Trasentin Forte [CD], ✦Phenaphen Capsules [CD], ✦Phenaphen No. 2, 3, 4 [CD], Quadrinal [CD], Solfoton, Tedral Preparations [CD]

BENEFITS versus RISKS	
Possible Benefits	*Possible Risks*
EFFECTIVE CONTROL OF TONIC-CLONIC SEIZURES AND ALL TYPES OF PARTIAL SEIZURES	POTENTIAL FOR DEPENDENCE LIFE-THREATENING TOXICITY WITH OVERDOSAGE
EFFECTIVE CONTROL OF FEBRILE SEIZURES OF CHILDHOOD	Drug-induced hepatitis Rare blood cell disorders: abnormally low red cell, white cell and platelet counts
Effective relief of anxiety and nervous tension	

*See Schedules of Controlled Drugs inside back cover.

▷ **Principal Uses**

As a Single Drug Product: This barbiturate drug has two primary uses: (1) as a mild sedative to relieve anxiety, nervous tension and insomnia; and (2) as an anticonvulsant to control grand mal epilepsy and all types of partial seizures. It is also used to control febrile seizures of childhood.

As a Combination Drug Product [CD]: This drug is available in many combinations with derivatives of belladonna, an antispasmodic commonly used to treat functional disorders of the gastrointestinal tract. It is also available in combination with bronchodilators for the treatment of asthma, and with ergotamine for the treatment of headaches.

How This Drug Works: Not completely established. It is thought that by impeding the transfer of sodium and potassium across cell membranes, this drug selectively blocks the transmission of nerve impulses. This could serve to produce a sedative effect and to suppress the spread of nerve impulses that are responsible for epileptic seizures.

Available Dosage Forms and Strengths
Capsules — 16 mg
Elixir — 15 mg, 20 mg per 5-ml teaspoonful
Tablets — 8 mg, 16 mg, 32 mg, 65 mg, 100 mg

▷ **Usual Adult Dosage Range:** As sedative: 15 to 30 mg 2 to 4 times/day. As hypnotic: 100 to 200 mg at bedtime. As anticonvulsant: 100 to 200 mg given as a single dose at bedtime. The total daily dosage should not exceed 600 mg. **Note: Actual dosage and administration schedule must be determined by the physician for each patient individually.**

▷ **Dosing Instructions:** May be taken with or after food to reduce stomach irritation. Regular tablets may be crushed and capsules opened for administration. Prolonged-action dosage forms should be swallowed whole without alteration.

Usual Duration of Use: Continual use on a regular schedule for 3 to 5 days is usually necessary to determine this drug's effectiveness in relieving anxiety and tension, and for 4 to 6 weeks to determine its ability to control seizures. If used to treat anxiety-tension states, its use should not exceed 4 weeks without reappraisal of continued need. Long-term use for seizure control (months to years) requires supervision and periodic evaluation by your physician. Consult your physician on a regular basis.

▷ **This Drug Should Not Be Taken If**
• you have had an allergic reaction to it previously.
• you are subject to acute intermittent porphyria (see Glossary).

▷ **Inform Your Physician Before Taking This Drug If**
• you are allergic or overly sensitive to any barbiturate drug (see Drug Class, Section Four).

- you are pregnant or planning pregnancy.
- you have a history of alcohol or drug abuse.
- you are taking any drugs with sedative effects.
- you have any type of seizure disorder.
- you have myasthenia gravis.
- you have impaired liver, kidney or thyroid gland function.
- you plan to have surgery under general anesthesia in the near future.

Possible Side-Effects (natural, expected and unavoidable drug actions)
Drowsiness, impaired concentration, mental and physical sluggishness.

▷ **Possible Adverse Effects** (unusual, unexpected and infrequent reactions)
If any of the following develop, consult your physician promptly for guidance.
Mild Adverse Effects
Allergic Reactions: Skin rashes, hives, localized swellings of face, drug fever (see Glossary).
Dizziness, unsteadiness, impaired vision, double vision.
Nausea, vomiting, diarrhea.
Shoulder-hand syndrome: pain and stiffness in the shoulder, pain and swelling in the hand.
Serious Adverse Effects
Allergic Reactions: Drug-induced hepatitis with jaundice (see Glossary).
Idiosyncratic Reactions: Paradoxical excitement and delirium (instead of sedation).
Mental depression, abnormal involuntary movements.
Blood cell disorders: deficiencies of all blood cell types causing fatigue, weakness, fever, sore throat, abnormal bleeding or bruising.

▷ **Possible Effects on Sexual Function**
Decreased libido and/or impotence (16%).
Decreased effectiveness of oral contraceptives taken concurrently (71%).

▷ **Adverse Effects That May Mimic Natural Diseases or Disorders**
Liver reactions may suggest viral hepatitis.

Natural Diseases or Disorders That May Be Activated by This Drug
Acute intermittent and/or cutaneous porphyria, systemic lupus erythematosus.

CAUTION
1. Anticonvulsant drug therapy must be carefully individualized. Accurate diagnosis and classification of the seizure pattern are essential to the correct selection of the most appropriate drug for seizure control.
2. Emotional stress or physical trauma (including surgery) may require increased anticonvulsant dosage to control seizures.
3. Prolonged-action dosage forms of this drug are not appropriate for the treatment of seizures and should not be used.

Precautions for Use

By Infants and Children: This drug should not be given to the hyperkinetic child. Observe for possible paradoxical stimulation and hyperactivity; this can occur in 10% to 40% of children. Changes associated with puberty characteristically slow the metabolism of this drug and permit its gradual accumulation. Blood levels of this drug in young adolescents should be monitored every 3 months to detect rising concentrations and early toxicity. Adjust dosage as necessary.

By Those over 60 Years of Age: It is advisable to avoid all barbiturates in the elderly. If use of this drug is attempted, start with small doses until tolerance has been determined. Observe for confusion, delirium, agitation and excitement. Do not use this drug concurrently with other drugs for mental disorders. This drug is conducive to the development of hypothermia (see Glossary).

▷ **Advisability of Use During Pregnancy**

Pregnancy Category: D (tentative). See Pregnancy Code inside back cover.

Animal studies: Conflicting reports of cleft palate and skeletal defects in mouse, rat and rabbit studies.

Human studies: Information from studies of pregnant women indicates no increase in birth defects in 8037 exposures to this drug. However, it is reported that barbiturates can cause fetal damage when taken during pregnancy.

Avoid use of drug during entire pregnancy if possible. If it is clearly needed to control seizures, the mother should receive vitamin K prior to delivery and the infant should receive it at birth.

Advisability of Use if Breast-Feeding

Presence of this drug in breast milk: Yes, in small amounts.

Monitor nursing infant closely and discontinue drug or nursing if adverse effects develop.

Habit-Forming Potential: Psychological and physical dependence can occur with prolonged use of excessive doses—300 to 700 mg/day for 1 to 2 months. Dependence is not likely to occur with usual sedative or anticonvulsant doses.

Effects of Overdosage: Behavior similar to alcoholic intoxication: confusion, slurred speech, physical incoordination, staggering gait, drowsiness, stupor progressing to coma.

Possible Effects of Long-Term Use: Psychological and/or physical dependence; syndrome of chronic intoxication: headache, depression, impaired vision, dizziness, slurred speech, incoordination. Megaloblastic anemia due to folic acid deficiency. Rickets or osteomalacia due to deficiencies of vitamin D and calcium.

Suggested Periodic Examinations While Taking This Drug (at physician's discretion)

Complete blood cell counts, liver function tests.

During long-term use: blood levels of folic acid, vitamin B-12, calcium and phosphorus; skeletal X-ray studies for demineralization of bone.

▷ **While Taking This Drug, Observe the Following**

> *Foods:* No restrictions. Eat liberally of foods rich in folic acid: fortified breakfast cereals, liver, legumes, green leafy vegetables.

> *Beverages:* No restrictions. May be taken with milk or fruit juices.

▷ *Alcohol:* Avoid completely. Alcohol can increase greatly the sedative and depressant actions of this drug on brain functions.

> *Tobacco Smoking:* May enhance the sedative effects of this drug and increase drowsiness.

> *Marijuana Smoking:* Increased drowsiness, unsteadiness; significantly impaired mental and physical performance.

▷ *Other Drugs*

> Phenobarbital may *increase* the effects of
> - all other drugs with sedative effects, and cause excessive sedation.

> Phenobarbital may *decrease* the effects of
> - anticoagulants (Coumadin, etc.), and require dosage adjustments.
> - certain beta blockers (Inderal, Lopressor), and reduce their effectiveness.
> - cortisonelike drugs.
> - doxycycline (Vibramycin), and reduce its effectiveness.
> - griseofulvin (Fulvicin, etc.), and reduce its effectiveness.
> - oral contraceptives, and reduce their effectiveness in preventing pregnancy.
> - quinidine (Quinaglute, etc.), and reduce its effectiveness.
> - theophyllines (Aminophyllin, Theo-Dur, etc.), and reduce their antiasthmatic effectiveness.

> Phenobarbital *taken concurrently* with
> - phenytoin (Dilantin) may alter phenytoin blood levels: a high phenobarbital level will increase the phenytoin level; a low phenobarbital level will decrease the phenytoin level. Periodic determination of blood levels of both drugs is advised.

> The following drugs may *increase* the effects of phenobarbital
> - valproic acid (Depakene).

▷ *Driving, Hazardous Activities:* This drug may cause drowsiness and may impair mental alertness, judgment, physical coordination and reaction time. Restrict activities as necessary.

> *Aviation Note:* The use of this drug **is a disqualification** for piloting. Consult a designated Aviation Medical Examiner.

> *Exposure to Sun:* Use caution until sensitivity has been determined. This drug may cause photosensitivity.

> *Exposure to Cold:* Observe the elderly for possible hypothermia (see Glossary) while taking this drug.

> *Discontinuation:* If used as an anticonvulsant, this drug must not be discontinued abruptly. Sudden withdrawal can precipitate status epilepticus (repetitive seizures). Gradual reduction in dosage should be made over a period of 3 months. Total drug withdrawal may be attempted after a period of 3 to 5 years without a seizure. However, seizures are likely to recur in 40% of adults and in 20% to 30% of children.

PHENYLBUTAZONE
(fen il BYU ta zohn)

Introduced: 1949

Class: Mild analgesic, anti-inflammatory

Prescription: USA: Yes
Canada: Yes

Controlled Drug: USA: No
Canada: No

Available as Generic: Yes

Brand Names: ♦Apo-Phenylbutazone, Azolid, Butazolidin, ♦Butone [CD], ♦Intrabutazone, ♦Neo-Zoline-M [CD], ♦Novobutazone, ♦Phenbuff

BENEFITS versus RISKS	
Possible Benefits	*Possible Risks*
PROMPT, EFFECTIVE RELIEF OF INFLAMMATION AND PAIN IN MODERATELY SEVERE ARTHRITIS, GOUT, BURSITIS AND SUPERFICIAL PHLEBITIS (FOR SHORT-TERM USE)	BONE MARROW DEPRESSION MAY BE SEVERE
	DRUG-INDUCED HEPATITIS
	KIDNEY DAMAGE, IMPAIRED FUNCTION
	GASTROINTESTINAL ULCER FORMATION AND BLEEDING
	HYPERTENSION
	HEART MUSCLE DAMAGE
	EYE DAMAGE: OPTIC NEURITIS
	EAR DAMAGE: HEARING LOSS

▷ **Principal Uses**

As a Single Drug Product: This potent anti-inflammatory drug is used primarily for the short-term relief of pain and inflammation associated with moderately severe arthritis, gout, bursitis, tendinitis and superficial phlebitis. Because of its potential for severe toxicity, it is not considered to be an "aspirin substitute." Its use should be limited to those conditions that do not respond to less toxic drugs.

How This Drug Works: Not completely established. It is thought that this drug acts somewhat like aspirin, by suppressing the formation of prostaglandins and related substances that are involved in the production of inflammation.

Available Dosage Forms and Strengths
Capsules — 100 mg
Tablets — 100 mg

▷ **Usual Adult Dosage Range:** For arthritis: Initially, 100 to 200 mg 3 times/day; for maintenance, 100 mg 1 to 4 times/day. For acute gout: Initially, 400 mg as a single dose; then 100 mg/4 hours for 4 days or until the acute attack is relieved; continual use should not exceed 1 week. Alternate course for gout: 200 mg/4 hours for 4 days or until acute attack is relieved; continual use should not exceed 2 weeks. **Note: Actual dosage and administration schedule must be determined by the physician for each patient individually.**

▷ **Dosing Instructions:** Take with or following food to reduce stomach irritation. The tablet may be crushed and the capsule may be opened for administration.

Usual Duration of Use: Continual use on a regular schedule for 2 to 5 days is usually necessary to determine this drug's effectiveness in relieving acute pain in arthritis, gout and related conditions. This drug should be limited to short-term use only. If significant improvement does not occur within 1 week, this drug should be discontinued. The maximal period of continual use should not exceed 10 to 14 days.

▷ **This Drug Should Not Be Taken If**
- you have had an allergic reaction to it previously, or to oxyphenbutazone (Tandearil), a closely related drug.
- you have a history of serious adverse effects from drugs.
- you have a history of a blood cell or bone marrow disorder.
- you have a history of stomach or intestinal ulceration or bleeding.
- you have a history of disease or impaired function of the thyroid, heart, liver or kidneys.
- you have high blood pressure.

▷ **Inform Your Physician Before Taking This Drug If**
- you are allergic to aspirin or aspirin substitutes (anti-inflammatory analgesics).
- you are taking any other drugs at this time, either prescription or over-the-counter drugs.
- you are taking anticoagulants.
- you have glaucoma.

Possible Side-Effects (natural, expected and unavoidable drug actions)
Salt and water retention, reduced urine output.

▷ **Possible Adverse Effects** (unusual, unexpected and infrequent reactions)
If any of the following develop, consult your physician promptly for guidance.
Mild Adverse Effects
Allergic Reactions: Skin rashes, hives, itching, drug fever (see Glossary).
Headache, drowsiness, lethargy, nervousness, confusion, tremors.
Indigestion, stomach pain, nausea, vomiting, diarrhea.
Progressive gain in weight and rise in blood pressure; these are indications to discontinue this drug.
Serious Adverse Effects
Allergic Reactions: Severe skin reactions, high fever, swollen and painful joints, salivary gland enlargement, anaphylactic reaction (see Glossary).

Bone marrow depression (see Glossary): fatigue, weakness, fever, sore throat, abnormal bleeding or bruising.

Drug-induced hepatitis, with or without jaundice (see Glossary).

Kidney damage, impaired kidney function, kidney failure.

Stomach and intestinal ulceration and/or bleeding.

Damage to heart muscle (myocarditis) and heart covering (pericarditis).

Eye damage: injuries to optic nerve and retina, impaired vision.

Ear damage: loss of hearing.

▷ **Possible Effects on Sexual Function:** None reported.

Possible Delayed Adverse Effects: The development of leukemia following the use of this drug has been reported. A cause-and-effect relationship (see Glossary) has not been established.

▷ **Adverse Effects That May Mimic Natural Diseases or Disorders**
Liver reactions may suggest viral hepatitis.

Natural Diseases or Disorders That May Be Activated by This Drug
Latent hypertension, peptic ulcer disease, ulcerative colitis.

CAUTION
1. This drug should never be used for mild and trivial conditions. It has high potential for serious and life-threatening adverse effects.
2. Follow your physician's instructions fully regarding periodic examinations while taking this drug. These are essential for the early detection of possible adverse effects.

Precautions for Use
By Infants and Children: Safety and effectiveness for use by those under 15 years of age have not been established.

By Those over 60 Years of Age: Many authorities advise that this drug should not be used by this age group. More than 60% of users over 61 years of age experience adverse effects from this drug. The elderly and the debilitated are clearly more vulnerable to the toxic effects of this drug. Its use is not recommended.

▷ **Advisability of Use During Pregnancy**
Pregnancy Category: D (tentative). See Pregnancy Code inside back cover.

Animal studies: Evidence of embryo toxicity reported.

Human studies: Information from adequate studies of pregnant women is not available. Two cases of birth defects following use of this drug have been reported. A causal relationship has not been established.

One manufacturer of this drug recommends that it not be used during pregnancy.

Advisability of Use if Breast-Feeding
Presence of this drug in breast milk: Yes.

Avoid drug or refrain from nursing.

Habit-Forming Potential: None.

Effects of Overdosage: Headache, dizziness, insomnia, mental and behavioral disturbances, hallucinations, seizures, coma.

Possible Effects of Long-Term Use: Bone marrow depression. Development of thyroid gland enlargement (goiter), with or without altered function.

Suggested Periodic Examinations While Taking This Drug (at physician's discretion)
Complete blood cell counts and urine analysis should be made before the drug is taken and during the course of treatment at intervals of 1 to 2 weeks.
Liver function tests.

▷ **While Taking This Drug, Observe the Following**
Foods: No restrictions. Avoid excessive salt.
Beverages: No restrictions. May be taken with milk.
▷ *Alcohol:* Avoid completely because of its irritant effect on the stomach, increasing the risk of ulceration and bleeding.
Tobacco Smoking: No interactions expected.
▷ *Other Drugs*
Phenylbutazone may *increase* the effects of
• anticoagulants (Coumadin, etc.), and cause bleeding.
• lithium (Lithane, Lithotabs, etc.), and increase the risk of lithium toxicity.
• phenytoin (Dilantin), and cause phenytoin toxicity.
• sulfonylureas (see Drug Class, Section Four), and increase the risk of hypoglycemia.
▷ *Driving, Hazardous Activities:* This drug may cause dizziness, confusion and impaired vision or hearing. Restrict activities as necessary.
Aviation Note: The use of this drug *may be a disqualification* for piloting. Consult a designated Aviation Medical Examiner.
Exposure to Sun: Use caution until sensitivity has been determined. This drug may cause photosensitivity (see Glossary).

PHENYTOIN
(FEN i toh in)

Other Name: Diphenylhydantoin

Introduced: 1938

Class: Anticonvulsant, hydantoins

Prescription: USA: Yes
Canada: Yes

Controlled Drug: USA: No
Canada: No

Available as Generic: USA: Yes
Canada: No

Brand Names: Dilantin, Dilantin w/Phenobarbital [CD], Diphenylan, ✦Mebroin [CD]

BENEFITS versus RISKS

Possible Benefits	*Possible Risks*
EFFECTIVE CONTROL OF TONIC-CLONIC (GRAND MAL), PSYCHOMOTOR (TEMPORAL LOBE), MYOCLONIC AND FOCAL SEIZURES IN 80% OF USERS	VERY NARROW TREATMENT MARGIN POSSIBLE BIRTH DEFECTS Overgrowth of gums Excessive hair growth Rare blood cell disorders: impaired production of all blood cells Drug-induced hepatitis Drug-induced nephritis

---

▷ **Principal Uses**

As a Single Drug Product: Used primarily as an antiepileptic drug to control grand mal, psychomotor, myoclonic and focal seizures. Though not officially approved, this drug is also used to initiate treatment of trigeminal neuralgia; it is sometimes effective in relieving the severe facial pain of this disorder.

As a Combination Drug Product [CD]: This drug is available in combination with phenobarbital, another effective anticonvulsant. Some seizure disorders require the combined actions of these two drugs for effective control.

How This Drug Works: Not completely established. It is thought that by promoting the loss of sodium from nerve fibers, this drug lowers and stabilizes their excitability and thereby inhibits the repetitious spread of electrical impulses along nerve pathways. This action may prevent seizures altogether, or it may reduce their frequency and severity.

Available Dosage Forms and Strengths

Capsules (extended) — 30 mg, 100 mg
Capsules (prompt) — 30 mg, 100 mg
Injection — 50 mg per ml
Oral suspension — 30 mg, 125 mg per 5-ml teaspoonful
Tablets, chewable — 50 mg

▷ **Usual Adult Dosage Range:** Initially, 100 mg 3 times/day. Dose may be increased cautiously by 100 mg/week as needed and tolerated. After the optimal maintenance dose has been determined, the total daily dose may be taken as a single dose every 24 hours if Dilantin capsules are used. No other formulation is approved for once-a-day use. The total daily dosage should not exceed 600 mg. **Note: Actual dosage and administration schedule must be determined by the physician for each patient individually.**

▷ **Dosing Instructions:** May be taken with or after food to reduce stomach irritation. The capsule may be opened and the tablet may be crushed for administration.

Usual Duration of Use: Continual use on a regular schedule for 2 to 3 weeks is usually necessary to determine this drug's effectiveness in reducing the frequency and severity of seizures. Optimal control will require careful dosage adjustments over a period of several months. Long-term use (months to years) requires ongoing supervision and periodic evaluation by your physician. Consult your physician on a regular basis.

▷ **This Drug Should Not Be Taken If**
- you have had an allergic reaction to this drug or to other hydantoin drugs previously.

▷ **Inform Your Physician Before Taking This Drug If**
- you are taking any other drugs at this time.
- you have a history of liver disease or impaired liver function.
- you have low blood pressure, diabetes or any type of heart disease.
- you plan to have surgery under general anesthesia in the near future.

Possible Side-Effects (natural, expected and unavoidable drug actions)
Mild fatigue, sluggishness and drowsiness (in sensitive individuals).
Pink to red to brown coloration of urine (of no significance).

▷ **Possible Adverse Effects** (unusual, unexpected and infrequent reactions)
If any of the following develop, consult your physician promptly for guidance.
Mild Adverse Effects
Allergic Reactions: Skin rashes (5% to 10%), hives, drug fever (see Glossary).
Headache, dizziness, nervousness, insomnia, muscle twitching.
Nausea, vomiting, constipation.
Overgrowth of gum tissues (most common in children).
Excessive growth of body hair (most common in young girls).
Serious Adverse Effects
Allergic Reactions: Drug-induced hepatitis, with or without jaundice (see Glossary). Drug-induced nephritis, with acute kidney failure. Severe skin reactions. Generalized enlargement of lymph glands (pseudolymphoma).
Idiosyncratic Reaction: Hemolytic anemia (see Glossary).
Acute psychotic episodes (rare).
Bone marrow depression (see Glossary): fatigue, weakness, fever, sore throat, abnormal bleeding or bruising.
Mental confusion, unsteadiness, double vision, jerky eye movements, slurred speech.
Joint pain and swelling.
Elevated blood sugar, due to inhibition of insulin release.

▷ **Possible Effects on Sexual Function**
Decreased libido and/or impotence (11%).
Peyronie's disease (see Glossary).
Decreased effectiveness of oral contraceptives taken concurrently (24%).

▷ **Adverse Effects That May Mimic Natural Diseases or Disorders**
Drug-induced hepatitis may suggest viral hepatitis.
Skin reactions may resemble lupus erythematosus.

Natural Diseases or Disorders That May Be Activated by This Drug
Latent diabetes, porphyria, systemic lupus erythematosus.

CAUTION

1. Some brand name capsules of this drug have a significantly longer duration of action than generic name capsules of the same strength. To assure a correct dosing schedule, it is necessary to distinguish between "prompt" action and "extended" action capsules. Do not substitute one for the other without your physician's knowledge and guidance.
2. When used for the treatment of epilepsy, *this drug must not be stopped abruptly.*
3. The wide variation of this drug's action from person to person requires careful individualization of dosage schedules. Periodic measurements of blood levels of this drug can be very helpful in determining appropriate dosage. (See Therapeutic Drug Monitoring in Section One.)
4. Regularity of drug use is essential for successful management of seizure disorders. Take this drug at the same time each day.
5. Shake the suspension form of this drug thoroughly before measuring the dose. Use a standard measuring device to assure that the dose is based upon a 5-ml teaspoon.
6. Side-effects and mild adverse effects are usually most apparent during the first several days of treatment, and often subside with continued use.
7. It may be necessary to take folic acid to prevent anemia while taking this drug. Consult your physician regarding this.
8. It is advisable to carry a card of personal identification with a notation that you are taking this drug.

Precautions for Use
By Infants and Children: Elimination of this drug varies widely with age. Careful monitoring by periodic measurement of blood levels is essential for all ages. Some children will require more than one dose daily for good control. Observe for early indications of drug toxicity: jerky eye movements, unsteadiness in stance and gait, slurred speech, abnormal involuntary movements of the extremities and odd behavior.
By Those over 60 Years of Age: You may be more sensitive to all of the actions of this drug and require smaller doses. Observe closely for any indications of early toxicity: drowsiness, fatigue, confusion, unsteadiness, disturbances of vision, slurred speech, muscle twitching.

▷ **Advisability of Use During Pregnancy**

Pregnancy Category: D (tentative). See Pregnancy Code inside back cover.

Animal studies: Cleft lip and palate, skeletal and visceral defects in mice; skeletal and visceral defects in rats.

Human studies: Available information is conflicting. Some studies suggest a small but significant increase in the occurrence of birth defects associated with the use of phenytoin during pregnancy. The incidence of birth defects in children of epileptics not taking anticonvulsant drugs is 3.2%; the incidence with the use of anticonvulsant drugs during pregnancy increases to 6.4%. The "fetal hydantoin syndrome" in the newborn infant exposed to phenytoin during pregnancy consists of birth defects of the skull, face and limbs, deficient growth and development, and subnormal intelligence and performance. Other effects on the infant include reduction in blood clotting factors that predispose it to severe bruising and hemorrhage.

Discuss with your physician the advantages and possible disadvantages of using this drug during pregnancy. It is advisable to use the smallest maintenance dose that will control seizures. In addition, you should be given vitamin K during the last month of pregnancy to prevent a deficiency of blood clotting factors in the fetus.

Advisability of Use if Breast-Feeding

Presence of this drug in breast milk: Yes, in trace amounts.

Monitor nursing infant closely and discontinue drug or nursing if adverse effects develop.

Habit-Forming Potential: None.

Effects of Overdosage: Drowsiness, jerky eye movements, hand tremor, unsteadiness, slurred speech, hallucinations, delusions, nausea, vomiting, stupor progressing to coma.

Possible Effects of Long-Term Use: Low blood calcium resulting in rickets or osteomalacia; megaloblastic anemia; peripheral neuropathy (see Glossary); schizophreniclike psychosis. Lymphosarcoma, malignant lymphoma and leukemia have been associated with long-term use; a cause-and-effect relationship (see Glossary) has not been established.

Suggested Periodic Examinations While Taking This Drug (at physician's discretion)

Monitoring of blood phenytoin levels to guide dosage.

Complete blood cell counts, liver function tests.

Measurements of the following blood levels: glucose, calcium, phosphorus, folic acid, vitamin B-12.

Skeletal X-ray studies for demineralization of bone.

▷ **While Taking This Drug, Observe the Following**

Foods: No restrictions.

Nutritional Support: Supplements of folic acid, calcium, vitamin D and vitamin K may be necessary.

Beverages: No restrictions. May be taken with milk.

▷ *Alcohol:* Use extreme caution until the combined effects have been determined. Alcohol (in large quantities or with continual use) may reduce this drug's effectiveness in preventing seizures.

Tobacco Smoking: No interactions expected.

▷ *Other Drugs*

Phenytoin may *decrease* the effects of
- cortisonelike drugs (see Drug Class, Section Four).
- cyclosporine.
- doxycycline (Vibramycin, etc.).
- levodopa (Larodopa, Sinemet).
- methadone (Dolophine).
- mexiletine (Mexitil).
- oral contraceptives.
- quinidine (Quinaglute, etc.).

Phenytoin *taken concurrently* with
- oral anticoagulants (Coumadin, etc.) can either increase or decrease the anticoagulant effect; monitor this combination very closely with serial prothrombin testing.
- primidone (Mysoline) may alter primidone actions and enhance its toxicity.
- theophyllines (Aminophyllin, Theo-Dur, etc.) may cause a decrease in the effectiveness of both drugs.

The following drugs may *increase* the effects of phenytoin
- chloramphenicol (Chloromycetin).
- cimetidine (Tagamet).
- disulfiram (Antabuse).
- isoniazid (INH, Niconyl, etc.).
- phenacemide (Phenurone).
- phenylbutazone (Butazolidin).
- sulfonamides (see Drug Class, Section Four).
- trimethoprim (Proloprim, Trimpex).
- valproic acid (Depakene).

The following drugs may *decrease* the effects of phenytoin
- bleomycin.
- carmustine.
- cisplatin.
- diazoxide.
- folic acid.
- methotrexate.
- rifampin.
- vinblastine.

▷ *Driving, Hazardous Activities:* This drug may impair mental alertness, vision and coordination. Restrict activities as necessary.

Aviation Note: The use of this drug *is a disqualification* for piloting. Consult a designated Aviation Medical Examiner.

Exposure to Sun: Use caution. This drug may cause photosensitivity (see Glossary).

Occurrence of Unrelated Illness: Intercurrent infections may slow the elimination of this drug and increase the risk of toxicity due to higher blood levels.

Discontinuation: **This drug must not be discontinued abruptly.** Sudden withdrawal can precipitate severe and repeated seizures. If this drug is to be discontinued, gradual reduction in dosage should be made over a period of 3 months. Total drug withdrawal may be attempted after a period of 3 to 4 years without a seizure. However, seizures are likely to recur in 40% of adults and in 20% to 30% of children.

PILOCARPINE
(pi loh KAR peen)

Introduced: 1875

Class: Antiglaucoma

Prescription: USA: Yes
Canada: No

Controlled Drug: USA: No
Canada: No

Available as Generic: Yes

Brand Names: Almocarpine, E-Pilo Preparations [CD], Isopto Carpine, ✦Minims, ✦Miocarpine, Ocusert Pilo-20,-40, PE Preparations [CD], Pilagan, Pilocar, ✦Pilopine HS

BENEFITS versus RISKS

Possible Benefits	*Possible Risks*
EFFECTIVE REDUCTION OF INTERNAL EYE PRESSURE FOR CONTROL OF ACUTE AND CHRONIC GLAUCOMA	Mild side-effects with systemic absorption Minor eye discomfort Altered vision

---

▷ **Principal Uses**

As a Single Drug Product: This drug is used exclusively for the management of all types of glaucoma. Selection of the appropriate dosage form and strength must be carefully individualized.

As a Combination Drug Product [CD]: This drug is combined with epinephrine (in eye drop solutions) to utilize the actions of both drugs in lowering internal eye pressure. The opposite effects of these two drugs on the size of the pupil (pilocarpine constricts, epinephrine dilates) provides a balance that prevents excessive constriction or dilation.

How This Drug Works: By directly stimulating constriction of the pupil, this drug enlarges the outflow canal in the anterior chamber of the eye and promotes the drainage of excess fluid (aqueous humor), thus lowering the internal eye pressure.

Available Dosage Forms and Strengths
> Eye drop solutions — 0.25%, 0.5%, 1%, 2%, 3%, 4%, 5%, 6%, 8%, 10%
> Gel — 4%
> Ocuserts — 20 mcg, 40 mcg

▷ **Usual Adult Dosage Range:**   For chronic glaucoma: Eye drop solutions—1 drop of a 0.5% to 4% solution 4 times/day. Eye gel—apply 0.5 inch strip of gel into the eye once daily at bedtime. Ocusert—insert one into affected eye and replace every 7 days with a new one. **Note: Actual dosage and administration schedule must be determined by the physician for each patient individually.**

▷ **Dosing Instructions:**   To avoid excessive absorption into the body, press finger against inner corner of the eye (to close off the tear duct) during and for 2 minutes following instillation of the eye drop. Place the gel and the Ocusert in the eye at bedtime.

Usual Duration of Use: Continual use on a regular schedule for 1 to 2 weeks is usually necessary to determine this drug's effectiveness in controlling internal eye pressure. Long-term use (months to years) requires supervision and periodic evaluation by your physician. Consult your physician on a regular basis.

▷ **This Drug Should Not Be Taken If**
  • you have had an allergic reaction to it previously.
  • you have active bronchial asthma.

▷ **Inform Your Physician Before Taking This Drug If**
  • you have a history of bronchial asthma.
  • you have a history acute iritis.

Possible Side-Effects (natural, expected and unavoidable drug actions)
Temporary impairment of vision, usually lasting 2 to 3 hours following instillation of drops.

▷ **Possible Adverse Effects** (unusual, unexpected and infrequent reactions)
  If any of the following develop, consult your physician promptly for guidance.
  Mild Adverse Effects
  Allergic Reactions: Itching of the eyes, itching and/or swelling of the eyelids.
  Headache, heart palpitation, tremors.
  Serious Adverse Effects
  Provocation of acute asthma in susceptible individuals.

▷ **Possible Effects on Sexual Function:**   None reported.

Precautions for Use
  By Those over 60 Years of Age: Maintain personal cleanliness to prevent eye infections. Report promptly any indication of possible infection involving the eyes.

▷ **Advisability of Use During Pregnancy**

Pregnancy Category: C (tentative). See Pregnancy Code inside back cover.
Animal studies: Significant birth defects due to this drug reported in rats.
Human studies: Information from adequate studies of pregnant women is not available.
Limit use to the smallest effective dose. Minimize systemic absorption (see Dosing Instructions).

Advisability of Use if Breast-Feeding

Presence of this drug in breast milk: May be present in small amounts.
Monitor nursing infant closely and discontinue drug or nursing if adverse effects develop.

Habit-Forming Potential: None.

Effects of Overdosage: Flushing of face, increased flow of saliva, sweating.
If solution is swallowed: nausea, vomiting, diarrhea, profuse sweating, rapid pulse, difficult breathing, loss of consciousness.

Possible Effects of Long-Term Use: Development of tolerance (see Glossary), temporary loss of effectiveness.

Suggested Periodic Examinations While Taking This Drug (at physician's discretion)

Measurement of internal eye pressure on a regular basis.
Examination of eyes for development of cataracts.

▷ **While Taking This Drug, Observe the Following**

Foods: No restrictions.
Beverages: No restrictions.
▷ *Alcohol:* Use caution until the combined effect has been determined. If this drug is absorbed, it may prolong the effect of alcohol on the brain.
Tobacco Smoking: No interactions expected.
Marijuana Smoking: Sustained additional decrease in internal eye pressure.
▷ *Other Drugs*
The following drugs may **decrease** the effects of pilocarpine
  • atropine and drugs with atropinelike actions (see Drug Class, Section Four).
▷ *Driving, Hazardous Activities:* This drug may impair your ability to focus your vision properly. Restrict activities as necessary.
Aviation Note: The use of this drug **may be a disqualification** for piloting. Consult a designated Aviation Medical Examiner.
Exposure to Sun: No restrictions.
Discontinuation: Do not discontinue the regular use of this drug without consulting your physician. Periodic discontinuation and temporary substitution of another drug may be necessary to preserve its effectiveness in treating glaucoma.

PINDOLOL
(PIN doh lohl)

Introduced: 1972

Class: Antihypertensive, beta-adrenergic blocker

Prescription: USA: Yes
Canada: Yes

Controlled Drug: USA: No
Canada: No

Available as Generic: No

Brand Names: ✦Viskazide [CD], Visken

BENEFITS versus RISKS

Possible Benefits	*Possible Risks*
EFFECTIVE, WELL-TOLERATED ANTIHYPERTENSIVE in mild to moderate high blood pressure	CONGESTIVE HEART FAILURE in advanced heart disease Worsening of angina in coronary heart disease (abrupt withdrawal) Masking of low blood sugar (hypoglycemia) in drug-treated diabetes Provocation of asthma (with high doses)

▷ **Principal Uses**

As a Single Drug Product: The treatment of mild to moderately severe high blood pressure. May be used alone or concurrently with other anti-hypertensive drugs, such as diuretics.

As a Combination Drug Product [CD]: This drug is available in combination with hydrochlorothiazide (in Canada). The addition of a thiazide diuretic to this beta blocker drug enhances its effectiveness as an antihypertensive.

How This Drug Works: By blocking certain actions of the sympathetic nervous system, this drug
* reduces the rate and contraction force of the heart, thus lowering the ejection pressure of the blood leaving the heart.
* reduces the degree of contraction of blood vessel walls, resulting in their relaxation and expansion and consequent lowering of blood pressure.

Available Dosage Forms and Strengths
Tablets — 5 mg, 10 mg

▷ **Usual Adult Dosage Range:** Initially, 5 mg twice daily (12 hours apart). The dose may be increased gradually by 10 mg/day at intervals of 2 to 3 weeks as needed and tolerated up to 60 mg/day. For maintenance,

5 to 10 mg 2 or 3 times/day. The total daily dose should not exceed 60 mg. **Note: Actual dosage and administration schedule must be determined by the physician for each patient individually.**

▷ **Dosing Instructions:** May be taken without regard to eating. The tablet may be crushed for administration. Do not discontinue this drug abruptly.

Usual Duration of Use: Continual use on a regular schedule for 2 to 3 weeks is usually necessary to determine this drug's effectiveness in lowering blood pressure. The long-term use of this drug (months to years) will be determined by the course of your blood pressure over time and your response to the overall treatment program (weight reduction, salt restriction, smoking cessation, etc.). Consult your physician on a regular basis.

Possible Advantages of This Drug: Causes less slowing of the heart rate than most other beta blocker drugs.

Currently a "Drug of Choice" for initiating treatment of hypertension with a single drug.

▷ **This Drug Should Not Be Taken If**
- you have had an allergic reaction to it previously.
- you have congestive heart failure.
- you have an abnormally slow heart rate or a serious form of heart block.
- you are taking, or have taken within the past 14 days, any monoamine oxidase (MAO) type A inhibitor drug (see Drug Class, Section Four).

▷ **Inform Your Physician Before Taking This Drug If**
- you have had an adverse reaction to any beta blocker drug in the past (see Drug Class, Section Four).
- you have a history of serious heart disease, with or without episodes of heart failure.
- you have a history of hay fever (allergic rhinitis), asthma, chronic bronchitis or emphysema.
- you have a history of overactive thyroid function (hyperthyroidism).
- you have a history of low blood sugar (hypoglycemia).
- you have impaired liver or kidney function.
- you have diabetes or myasthenia gravis.
- you are currently taking any form of digitalis, quinidine or reserpine, or any calcium blocker drug (see Drug Class, Section Four).
- you plan to have surgery under general anesthesia in the near future.

Possible Side-Effects (natural, expected and unavoidable drug actions)
Lethargy and fatigability (15%), cold extremities, slow heart rate, lightheadedness in upright position (see Orthostatic Hypotension in Glossary).

▷ **Possible Adverse Effects** (unusual, unexpected and infrequent reactions)
If any of the following develop, consult your physician promptly for guidance.
Mild Adverse Effects
Allergic Reactions: Skin rash, itching.
Headache (5%), dizziness (17%), insomnia (19%), abnormal dreams.
Indigestion, nausea (7%), vomiting, constipation, diarrhea.
Joint and muscle discomfort (11%), fluid retention (edema) (11%).
Serious Adverse Effects
Mental depression, anxiety.
Chest pain, shortness of breath, precipitation of congestive heart failure.
Induction of bronchial asthma (in asthmatic individuals).

▷ **Possible Effects on Sexual Function:**   Decreased libido, impaired erection (rare).

CAUTION
1. *Do not discontinue this drug suddenly* without the knowledge and guidance of your physician. Carry a notation on your person that you are taking this drug.
2. Consult your physician or pharmacist before using nasal decongestants usually present in over-the-counter cold preparations and nose drops. These can cause sudden increases in blood pressure when taken concurrently with beta blocker drugs.
3. Report the development of any tendency to emotional depression.

Precautions for Use
By Infants and Children: Safety and effectiveness for use by those under 12 years of age have not been established. However, if this drug is used, observe for the development of low blood sugar (hypoglycemia) during periods of reduced food intake.
By Those over 60 Years of Age: Proceed *cautiously* with all antihypertensive drugs. Unacceptably high blood pressure should be reduced without creating the risks associated with excessively low blood pressure. Start treatment with small doses, and monitor the blood pressure response frequently. Sudden, rapid and excessive reduction of blood pressure can predispose to stroke or heart attack. Observe for dizziness, unsteadiness, tendency to fall, confusion, hallucinations, depression or urinary frequency.

▷ **Advisability of Use During Pregnancy**
Pregnancy Category: B (tentative). See Pregnancy Code inside back cover.
Animal studies: No significant increase in birth defects due to this drug.
Human studies: Information from adequate studies of pregnant women is not available.
Use this drug only if clearly needed. Ask physician for guidance.

Advisability of Use if Breast-Feeding
Presence of this drug in breast milk: Yes.
Avoid drug or refrain from nursing.

Habit-Forming Potential: None.

Effects of Overdosage: Weakness, slow pulse, low blood pressure, fainting, cold and sweaty skin, congestive heart failure, possible coma and convulsions.

Possible Effects of Long-Term Use: Reduced heart reserve and eventual heart failure in susceptible individuals with advanced heart disease.

Suggested Periodic Examinations While Taking This Drug (at physician's discretion)
Measurements of blood pressure, evaluation of heart function.

▷ **While Taking This Drug, Observe the Following**
Foods: No restrictions. Avoid excessive salt intake.
Beverages: No restrictions. May be taken with milk.
▷ *Alcohol:* Use with caution until the combined effect has been determined. Alcohol may exaggerate this drug's ability to lower the blood pressure and may increase its mild sedative effect.
Tobacco Smoking: Nicotine may reduce this drug's effectiveness in treating high blood pressure. In addition, high doses of this drug may potentiate the constriction of the bronchial tubes caused by regular smoking.
▷ *Other Drugs*
Pindolol may *increase* the effects of
- other antihypertensive drugs, and cause excessive lowering of the blood pressure. Dosage adjustments may be necessary.
- reserpine (Ser-Ap-Es, etc.), and cause sedation, depression, slowing of the heart rate and lowering of the blood pressure.
- verapamil (Calan, Isoptin), and cause excessive depression of heart function; monitor this combination closely.

Pindolol *taken concurrently* with
- clonidine (Catapres) requires close monitoring for rebound high blood pressure if clonidine is withdrawn while pindolol is still being taken.
- insulin requires close monitoring to avoid undetected hypoglycemia (see Glossary).

The following drugs may *increase* the effects of pindolol
- cimetidine (Tagamet).
- methimazole (Tapazole).
- oral contraceptives.
- propylthiouracil (Propacil).

The following drugs may *decrease* the effects of pindolol
- barbiturates (phenobarbital, etc.).
- indomethacin (Indocin), and possibly other "aspirin substitutes," may impair pindolol's antihypertensive effect.
- rifampin (Rifadin, Rimactane).

▷ *Driving, Hazardous Activities:* Use caution until the full extent of fatigue, dizziness and blood pressure change have been determined.

Aviation Note: The use of this drug *is a disqualification* for piloting. Consult a designated Aviation Medical Examiner.

Exposure to Sun: No restrictions.

Exposure to Heat: Caution advised. Hot environments can lower the blood pressure and exaggerate the effects of this drug.

Exposure to Cold: Caution advised. Cold environments can enhance the circulatory deficiency in the extremities that may occur with this drug. The elderly should take precautions to prevent hypothermia (see Glossary).

Heavy Exercise or Exertion: It is advisable to avoid exertion that produces light-headedness, excessive fatigue or muscle cramping. The use of this drug may intensify the hypertensive response to isometric exercise.

Occurrence of Unrelated Illness: The fever that accompanies systemic infections can lower the blood pressure and require adjustment of dosage. Illnesses that cause nausea or vomiting may interrupt the regular dosage schedule. Ask your physician for guidance.

Discontinuation: It is advisable to avoid sudden discontinuation of this drug in all situations. If possible, gradual reduction of dose over a period of 2 to 3 weeks is recommended. Ask your physician for specific guidance.

PIROXICAM
(peer OX i kam)

Introduced: 1978

Class: Mild analgesic, anti-inflammatory

Prescription: USA: Yes
Canada: Yes

Controlled Drug: USA: No
Canada: No

Available as Generic: No

Brand Names: ✦Apo-Piroxicam, Feldene, ✦Novopirocam

BENEFITS versus RISKS	
Possible Benefits	*Possible Risks*
EFFECTIVE RELIEF OF MILD TO MODERATE PAIN AND INFLAMMATION	Gastrointestinal pain, ulceration, bleeding (rare)
	Drug-induced hepatitis (rare)
	Rare kidney damage
	Mild fluid retention
	Reduced white blood cell and platelet counts

▷ **Principal Uses**

As a Single Drug Product: Used primarily to relieve mild to moderately severe pain and inflammation associated with (1) rheumatoid arthritis, (2) osteoarthritis and (3) acute and chronic gout.

How This Drug Works: Not completely established. It is thought that this drug suppresses the formation of prostaglandins (and related compounds), chemicals involved in the production of inflammation and pain.

Available Dosage Forms and Strengths
Capsules — 10 mg, 20 mg

▷ **Usual Adult Dosage Range:**   As antiarthritic: 10 mg twice daily, 12 hours apart; or 20 mg once daily. The total daily dosage should not exceed 40 mg, and then for no more than 5 days. **Note: Actual dosage and administration schedule must be determined by the physician for each patient individually.**

▷ **Dosing Instructions:**   Take with or following food to prevent stomach irritation. Take with a full glass of water and remain upright (do not lie down) for 30 minutes. The capsule may be opened for administration.

Usual Duration of Use: Continual use on a regular schedule for 2 weeks is usually necessary to determine this drug's effectiveness in relieving the discomfort of arthritis. Long-term use (months to years) requires supervision and periodic evaluation by your physician. Consult your physician on a regular basis.

▷ **This Drug Should Not Be Taken If**
- you have had an allergic reaction to it previously.
- you are subject to asthma or nasal polyps caused by aspirin.
- you have active peptic ulcer disease or any form of gastrointestinal bleeding.
- you have a bleeding disorder or a blood cell disorder.
- you have active liver disease.
- you have severe impairment of kidney function.

▷ **Inform Your Physician Before Taking This Drug If**
- you are allergic to aspirin or to other aspirin substitutes.
- you have a history of peptic ulcer disease, regional enteritis or ulcerative colitis.
- you have a history of any type of bleeding disorder.
- you have impaired liver or kidney function.
- you have high blood pressure or a history of heart failure.
- you are taking any of the following: acetaminophen, aspirin or other aspirin substitutes, anticoagulants, oral antidiabetic drugs.
- you plan to have surgery of any type in the near future.

Possible Side-Effects (natural, expected and unavoidable drug actions)
Fluid retention (weight gain), prolongation of bleeding time.

▷ **Possible Adverse Effects** (unusual, unexpected and infrequent reactions)
If any of the following develop, consult your physician promptly for guidance.
Mild Adverse Effects
Allergic Reactions: Skin rash, itching, spontaneous bruising.
Headache, dizziness, altered or blurred vision, ringing in the ears, drowsiness, fatigue, inability to concentrate.
Indigestion, nausea, vomiting, abdominal pain, diarrhea.
Serious Adverse Effects
Active peptic ulcer, stomach or intestinal bleeding.
Drug-induced liver damage.
Kidney damage with painful urination, bloody urine, reduced urine formation.
Rare bone marrow depression (see Glossary): fatigue, weakness, fever, sore throat, abnormal bleeding or bruising.

▷ **Possible Effects on Sexual Function:**   None reported.

Possible Delayed Adverse Effects: Mild anemia due to "silent" blood loss from the stomach (less than that caused by aspirin).

▷ **Adverse Effects That May Mimic Natural Diseases or Disorders**
Liver reaction may suggest viral hepatitis.

Natural Diseases or Disorders That May Be Activated by This Drug
Peptic ulcer disease, ulcerative colitis.

CAUTION
1. Dosage should always be limited to the smallest amount that produces reasonable improvement.
2. This drug may mask early indications of infection. Inform your physician if you think you are developing an infection of any kind.

Precautions for Use
By Infants and Children: Indications and dosage recommendations for use by those under 12 years of age have not been established.
By Those over 60 Years of Age: Small doses are advisable until tolerance is determined. Observe for any indications of liver or kidney toxicity, fluid retention, dizziness, confusion, impaired memory, stomach bleeding or constipation.

▷ **Advisability of Use During Pregnancy**
Pregnancy Category: B (tentative). See Pregnancy Code inside back cover.
Animal studies: No birth defects reported due to this drug.
Human studies: Information from adequate studies of pregnant women is not available.
The manufacturer does not recommend the use of this drug during pregnancy.

Advisability of Use if Breast-Feeding
Presence of this drug in breast milk: Unknown.
Avoid drug or refrain from nursing.

Habit-Forming Potential: None.

Effects of Overdosage: Possible drowsiness, dizziness, ringing in the ears, nausea, vomiting, indigestion.

Possible Effects of Long-Term Use: Development of anemia due to "silent" bleeding from the gastrointestinal tract.

Suggested Periodic Examinations While Taking This Drug (at physician's discretion)
Complete blood cell counts, liver and kidney function tests.
Complete eye examinations if vision is altered in any way.
Hearing examinations if ringing in the ears or hearing loss develops.

▷ **While Taking This Drug, Observe the Following**
Foods: No restrictions.
Beverages: No restrictions. May be taken with milk.
▷ *Alcohol:* Use with caution. The irritant action of alcohol on the stomach lining, added to the irritant action of this drug in sensitive individuals, can increase the risk of stomach ulceration and/or bleeding.
Tobacco Smoking: No interactions expected.
▷ *Other Drugs*
Piroxicam may *increase* the effects of
• acetaminophen (Tylenol, etc.), and increase the risk of kidney damage; avoid prolonged use of this combination.
• anticoagulants (Coumadin, etc.), and increase the risk of bleeding; monitor prothrombin time, adjust dose accordingly.
Piroxicam *taken concurrently* with the following drugs may increase the risk of bleeding; avoid these combinations:
• aspirin.
• dipyridamole (Persantine).
• indomethacin (Indocin).
• sulfinpyrazone (Anturane).
• valproic acid (Depakene).
▷ *Driving, Hazardous Activities:* This drug may cause drowsiness or dizziness. Restrict activities as necessary.
Aviation Note: The use of this drug *may be a disqualification* for piloting. Consult a designated Aviation Medical Examiner.
Exposure to Sun: No restrictions.

POTASSIUM
(poh TAS ee um)

Introduced: 1939   **Class:** Potassium preparations
Prescription: USA: Yes   **Controlled Drug:** USA: No
Canada: No   Canada: No

Available as Generic: Yes

Brand Names: ✦Apo-K, Kaochlor, Kaochlor-Eff, Kaon, Kaon-Cl, Kay Ciel, K-Lor, Klorvess, Klotrix, K-Lyte, K-Lyte/Cl, K-Lyte DS, K+10, K-Tab, Micro-K, Micro-K Extencaps, Micro-K LS, ✦Neo-K, Slow-K, Ten-K, Trikates

---

BENEFITS versus RISKS

Possible Benefits	*Possible Risks*
EFFECTIVE PREVENTION AND TREATMENT OF POTASSIUM DEFICIENCY (HYPOKALEMIA)	DEVELOPMENT OF EXCESSIVE POTASSIUM (HYPERKALEMIA) Ulceration and perforation of stomach or intestine with use of slow-release or enteric-coated tablets (these forms no longer recommended)

▷ **Principal Uses**

As a Single Drug Product: This drug is used primarily in conjunction with those diuretics that cause excessive loss of potassium from the body. Potassium preparations are usually given to stabilize the blood level within the normal range. Dosage adjustments may be necessary from time to time.

How This Drug Works: By maintaining or replenishing the normal potassium content of cells, this drug preserves or restores such normal cellular functions as the transmission of nerve impulses, the contraction of muscle fibers, the regulation of kidney function and the secretion of stomach juices.

Available Dosage Forms and Strengths

Capsules, prolonged-action —	8 mEq, 10 mEq
Liquids —	10 mEq, 15 mEq, 20 mEq, 30 mEq, 40 mEq, 45 mEq per 15-ml tablespoonful
Powders —	15 mEq, 20 mEq, 25 mEq per packet
Suspension, prolonged-action —	20 mEq per packet
Tablets —	2 mEq, 2.5 mEq, 5 mEq
Tablets, chewable —	1 mEq, 2.5 mEq
Tablets, effervescent —	20 mEq, 25 mEq, 50 mEq
Tablets, enteric-coated —	4 mEq
Tablets, prolonged-action —	6.7 mEq, 8 mEq, 10 mEq
Tablets, wax matrix —	6.7 mEq, 8 mEq, 10 mEq

▷ **Usual Adult Dosage Range:** Depends upon the dosage form prescribed. Follow your physician's prescribed dose exactly. **Note: Actual dosage and administration schedule must be determined by the physician for each patient individually.**

▷ **Dosing Instructions:**   Take each dose with food or immediately following a meal to reduce stomach irritation. Regular tablets should be swallowed whole. Soluble tablets and powders should be dissolved completely in 4 ounces of cold water or juice and sipped slowly over a period of 5 to 10 minutes. Liquid forms should be diluted in 4 ounces of water or juice. The prolonged-action capsules should be swallowed whole and not opened for administration. Wax matrix and enteric-coated tablets are not recommended because of their potential for causing localized erosion and ulceration of gastrointestinal tissues.

Usual Duration of Use: This must be determined by your physician. Periods of use will depend upon your concurrent use of diuretics, the potassium content of your diet and periodic measurement of your blood potassium level. Consult your physician on a regular basis.

▷ **This Drug Should Not Be Taken If**
  • you have had an allergic reaction to it previously.
  • you have severe impairment of kidney function.
  • you are taking any drug that contains amiloride, spironolactone or triamterene.

▷ **Inform Your Physician Before Taking This Drug If**
  • you are taking any of the following: a cortisonelike drug, a digitalis preparation, a diuretic (see Drug Classes, Section Four).
  • you have Addison's disease (adrenal gland deficiency).
  • you have diabetes or any form of heart disease.
  • you have a history of kidney disease or impaired kidney function.
  • you have a history of familial periodic paralysis.

Possible Side-Effects (natural, expected and unavoidable drug actions)
A mild laxative effect for some individuals.

▷ **Possible Adverse Effects** (unusual, unexpected and infrequent reactions)
If any of the following develop, consult your physician promptly for guidance.
Mild Adverse Effects
Nausea, vomiting, abdominal discomfort, diarrhea. (These usually occur if potassium is taken undiluted or on an empty stomach.)
Serious Adverse Effects
Potassium accumulation, resulting in abnormally high blood levels. Immediate treatment is mandatory.
Potassium in enteric-coated tablets or slow-release (wax matrix) tablets can cause ulceration of the stomach or intestine with risk of bleeding and/or perforation.

▷ **Possible Effects on Sexual Function:**   None reported.

CAUTION
  1. Dosage must be carefully individualized. Periodic evaluation of overall condition and blood potassium levels is essential to safe and

effective management. Excessively high blood levels of potassium can occur without warning. Do not exceed the prescribed dose.

2. Inform your physician promptly if you are taking a tablet form of this drug and you become aware of any difficulty in swallowing.
3. If you have chronic constipation, it is advisable that you avoid potassium in tablet form.
4. Some salt substitutes contain a large amount of potassium. If you are using a salt substitute, consult your physician regarding its continued use or any necessary adjustment in the dosage of your potassium preparation.

Precautions for Use
By Those over 60 Years of Age: Your potassium balance must be maintained within strict limitations. Serious adverse effects can occur when the potassium level is either above or below the normal range. Adhere to your dosage schedule exactly.

▷ **Advisability of Use During Pregnancy**
Pregnancy Category: A (tentative). See Pregnancy Code inside back cover.
Animal studies: No information available.
Human studies: Information from adequate studies of pregnant women is not available.
Potassium is a normal and essential constituent of body tissues. Potassium preparations can be used safely during pregnancy. Adhere strictly to prescribed dosage schedules.

Advisability of Use if Breast-Feeding
Presence of this drug in breast milk: Yes.
Monitor nursing infant closely and discontinue drug or nursing if adverse effects develop.

Habit-Forming Potential: None.

Effects of Overdosage: Lethargy, weakness and heaviness of legs, numbness and tingling in the extremities, confusion, irregular heart rhythm, drop in blood pressure, seizures, coma, heart arrest.

Possible Effects of Long-Term Use: Reduced absorption of vitamin B-12, resulting in anemia in some individuals.

Suggested Periodic Examinations While Taking This Drug (at physician's discretion)
Measurement of blood potassium levels.

▷ **While Taking This Drug, Observe the Following**
Foods: No restrictions. Consult your physician regarding any special modifications of your diet.
Beverages: No restrictions.
▷   *Alcohol:* No interactions expected.
Tobacco Smoking: No interactions expected.

▷ *Other Drugs*
Potassium *taken concurrently* with
- amiloride, spironolactone or triamterene may cause an excessive rise in blood potassium levels. This can be extremely dangerous; avoid the concurrent use of these diuretics and any form of potassium.
- digitalis preparations requires very careful monitoring of dosage and heart status.

▷ *Driving, Hazardous Activities:* No restrictions.
Aviation Note: The use of this drug *may be a disqualification* for piloting. Consult a designated Aviation Medical Examiner.
Exposure to Sun: No restrictions.
Discontinuation: Do not discontinue this drug suddenly if you are taking digitalis. Ask your physician for guidance if you find it necessary to discontinue potassium medication for any reason.

PRAZEPAM
(PRA ze pam)

Introduced: 1969

Class: Mild tranquilizer, benzodiazepines

Prescription: USA: Yes

Controlled Drug: USA: C-IV*

Available as Generic: USA: No

Brand Name: Centrax

BENEFITS versus RISKS	
Possible Benefits	*Possible Risks*
RELIEF OF ANXIETY AND NERVOUS TENSION in 70% to 80% of users	Habit-forming potential with prolonged use
Wide margin of safety with therapeutic doses	Minor impairment of mental functions
Very few drug interactions	

▷ **Principal Uses**
As a Single Drug Product: Used primarily to (1) provide short-term relief of mild to moderate anxiety; (2) relieve the symptoms of acute alcohol withdrawal: agitation, tremors, hallucinations, incipient delirium tremens.

How This Drug Works: It is thought that this drug produces a calming effect by enhancing the action of the nerve transmitter gamma-ami-

*See Schedules of Controlled Drugs inside back cover.

nobutyric acid (GABA), which in turn blocks the arousal of higher brain centers.

Available Dosage Forms and Strengths
Capsules — 5 mg, 10 mg, 20 mg
Tablets — 10 mg

▷ **Usual Adult Dosage Range:**   20 to 60 mg/24 hours, in 3 or 4 divided doses. The total daily dosage should not exceed 60 mg. **Note: Actual dosage and administration schedule must be determined by the physician for each patient individually.**

▷ **Dosing Instructions:**   May be taken on empty stomach or with food or milk as needed to prevent stomach irritation. The tablet may be crushed and the capsule may be opened for administration. Do not discontinue this drug abruptly if taken for more than 4 weeks.

Usual Duration of Use: Continual use on a regular schedule for 3 to 5 days is usually necessary to determine this drug's effectiveness in relieving moderate anxiety. Limit continual use to 1 to 3 weeks. Avoid uninterrupted and prolonged use.

▷ **This Drug Should Not Be Taken If**
  • you have had an allergic reaction to any dosage form of it previously.
  • you have acute narrow-angle glaucoma.
  • it is prescribed for a child under 18 years of age.

▷ **Inform Your Physician Before Taking This Drug If**
  • you are allergic to any benzodiazepine drug (see Drug Class, Section Four).
  • you have a history of alcoholism or drug abuse.
  • you are pregnant or planning pregnancy.
  • you have impaired liver or kidney function.
  • you have a history of serious depression or mental disorder.
  • you have any of the following: asthma, emphysema, epilepsy, myasthenia gravis.
  • you are taking any drugs with sedative effects.

Possible Side-Effects (natural, expected and unavoidable drug actions)
Drowsiness (6%), lethargy (11%), unsteadiness (5%), "hangover" effects on the day following bedtime use.

▷ **Possible Adverse Effects** (unusual, unexpected and infrequent reactions)
If any of the following develop, consult your physician promptly for guidance.
Mild Adverse Effects
Allergic Reactions: Skin rashes, hives, itching.
Dizziness (8%), fainting, weakness (7%), confusion, blurred vision, double vision, slurred speech, sweating, nausea.

Serious Adverse Effects
Paradoxical responses of excitement, agitation, anger, rage.

▷ **Possible Effects on Sexual Function:** None reported.

CAUTION
1. This drug should not be discontinued abruptly if it has been taken continually for more than 4 weeks.
2. The concurrent use of some over-the-counter drug products that contain antihistamines (allergy and cold preparations, sleep aids) can cause excessive sedation in sensitive individuals.

Precautions for Use
By Infants and Children: Safety and effectiveness for use by those under 18 years of age have not been established. This drug should not be used in the hyperactive or psychotic child of any age. Observe for excessive sedation and incoordination.
By Those over 60 Years of Age: It is advisable to use smaller doses at longer intervals to avoid overdosage. Observe for the possible development of lethargy, indifference, fatigue, weakness, unsteadiness, disturbing dreams, nightmares and paradoxical reactions of excitement, agitation, anger, hostility and rage.

▷ **Advisability of Use During Pregnancy**
Pregnancy Category: C (tentative). See Pregnancy Code inside back cover.
Animal studies: No information available.
Human studies: Information from adequate studies of pregnant women is not available. No birth defects have been reported with the use of this drug. However, available information regarding the use of other drugs of this class (benzodiazepines) is conflicting and inconclusive. Some studies found an increase in serious birth defects associated with the use of 2 benzodiazepines. Other studies have found no significant increase in birth defects.
Frequent use in late pregnancy can cause the "floppy infant" syndrome in the newborn: weakness, lethargy, unresponsiveness, depressed breathing, low body temperature.
Avoid use during entire pregnancy if possible.

Advisability of Use if Breast-Feeding
Presence of this drug in breast milk: Probably yes.
Avoid drug or refrain from nursing.

Habit-Forming Potential: This drug can produce psychological and/or physical dependence (see Glossary) if used in large doses for an extended period of time.

Effects of Overdosage: Marked drowsiness, weakness, feeling of drunkenness, staggering gait, tremor, stupor progressing to deep sleep or coma.

Possible Effects of Long-Term Use: Psychological and/or physical dependence.

Suggested Periodic Examinations While Taking This Drug (at physician's discretion)
Complete blood cell counts during long-term use.

▷ **While Taking This Drug, Observe the Following**
Foods: No restrictions.
Beverages: Avoid excessive intake of caffeine-containing beverages: coffee, tea, cola. May be taken with milk.

▷ *Alcohol:* Use with extreme caution until the combined effect has been determined. Alcohol may increase the depressant effects of this drug on the brain. It is advisable to avoid alcohol completely—throughout the day and night—if it is necessary to drive or to engage in any hazardous activity.

Tobacco Smoking: Heavy smoking may reduce the calming action of this drug.

Marijuana Smoking: Increased sedation and significant impairment of intellectual and physical performance.

▷ *Other Drugs*
The following drugs may *increase* the effects of prazepam
- cimetidine (Tagamet).
- disulfiram (Antabuse).
- oral contraceptives.

▷ *Driving, Hazardous Activities:* This drug can impair mental alertness, judgment, physical coordination and reaction time. Avoid hazardous activities accordingly.

Aviation Note: The use of this drug *is a disqualification* for piloting. Consult a designated Aviation Medical Examiner.

Exposure to Sun: No restrictions.

Exposure to Heat: Use caution until the effect of excessive perspiration is determined. Because of reduced urine volume, this drug may accumulate in the body and produce effects of overdosage.

Exposure to Cold: The elderly should dress warmly and avoid situations and environments conducive to hypothermia (see Glossary).

Discontinuation: Avoid sudden discontinuation if this drug has been taken for over 4 weeks without interruption. Dosage should be tapered gradually to prevent a withdrawal syndrome that could include depression, confusion, hallucinations, tremor, seizures, muscle cramping, sweating and vomiting.

PRAZOSIN
(PRA zoh sin)

Introduced: 1970   **Class:** Antihypertensive
Prescription: USA: Yes   **Controlled Drug:** USA: No
           Canada: Yes   Canada: No

Available as Generic: Yes

Brand Names: Minipress, Minizide [CD]

BENEFITS versus RISKS

Possible Benefits	*Possible Risks*
EFFECTIVE INITIAL THERAPY FOR MILD TO MODERATE HYPERTENSION	"First dose" drop in blood pressure with fainting (0.15%)
EFFECTIVE "STEP 2 OR 3" ANTIHYPERTENSIVE IN 60% TO 70% OF CASES OF MODERATE TO SEVERE HYPERTENSION when used adjunctively with other antihypertensive drugs	Induction of paroxysmal tachycardia (rare)
EFFECTIVE CONTROL OF HYPERTENSION IN PHEOCHROMOCYTOMA	
Effective in presence of impaired kidney function	

▷ **Principal Uses**

As a Single Drug Product: Used primarily to initiate treatment in mild to moderate hypertension. Also used as a "step 2" or "step 3" antihypertensive drug, in conjunction with other drugs, to treat moderate to severe hypertension.

As a Combination Drug Product [CD]: This drug is available in combination with polythiazide, a diuretic of the thiazide class of drugs that are usually used as "step 1" medications to initiate treatment for hypertension. By utilizing two different methods of drug action, this combination product is more effective and more convenient for long-term use.

How This Drug Works: It is thought that by blocking certain actions of the sympathetic nervous system, this drug causes direct relaxation and expansion of blood vessel walls, thus lowering the pressure of the blood within the vessels.

Available Dosage Forms and Strengths

Capsules — 1 mg, 2 mg, 5 mg

▷ **Usual Adult Dosage Range:** Initiate treatment with a "test dose" of 1 mg to determine the patient's response within the first 2 hours. If tolerated satisfactorily, increase dose cautiously up to 15 mg/24 hours in 2 or 3 divided doses. The total daily dosage should not exceed 20 mg. **Note: Actual dosage and administration schedule must be determined by the physician for each patient individually.**

▷ **Dosing Instructions:** May be taken without regard to food. The capsule may be opened for administration.

Usual Duration of Use: Continual use on a regular schedule for 4 to 6 weeks is usually necessary to determine this drug's effectiveness in controlling hypertension. Long-term use (months to years) requires supervision and periodic evaluation by your physician. Consult your physician on a regular basis.

Possible Advantages of This Drug
Effective initial treatment of hypertension.
Does not alter blood cholesterol, potassium or sugar levels.

▷ **This Drug Should Not Be Taken If**
- you have had an allergic reaction to it previously.
- you are experiencing mental depression.
- you have angina (active coronary artery disease) and you are not taking a beta-blocking drug. (Consult your physician.)

▷ **Inform Your Physician Before Taking This Drug If**
- you have experienced orthostatic hypotension (see Glossary) when using other antihypertensive drugs.
- you have a history of mental depression.
- you have impaired circulation to the brain, or a history of stroke.
- you have coronary artery disease.
- you have active liver disease or impaired liver function.
- you plan to have surgery under general anesthesia in the near future.

Possible Side-Effects (natural, expected and unavoidable drug actions)
Orthostatic hypotension, drowsiness (7%), salt and water retention, dry mouth, nasal congestion, constipation.

▷ **Possible Adverse Effects** (unusual, unexpected and infrequent reactions)
If any of the following develop, consult your physician promptly for guidance.
Mild Adverse Effects
Allergic Reactions: Skin rash, itching.
Headache (7.8%), dizziness (10.3%), fatigue (6.9%), weakness (6.5%), nervousness, sweating, numbness and tingling, blurred vision, reddened eyes, ringing in the ears.
Palpitation (5.3%), rapid heart rate, shortness of breath.
Nausea (4.9%), vomiting, diarrhea, abdominal pain.
Urinary frequency and incontinence.
Serious Adverse Effects
Mental depression, sleep disturbance.
Paroxysmal tachycardia (heart rates of 120 to 160).

▷ **Possible Effects on Sexual Function**
Decreased libido (14%); impotence (less than 1%).
Priapism (see Glossary).

Natural Diseases or Disorders That May Be Activated by This Drug
Latent coronary artery insufficiency.

CAUTION
1. Observe for the possible "first dose" response of precipitous drop in blood pressue, with or without fainting; this usually occurs within 30 to 90 minutes. Limit initial doses to 1 mg taken at bedtime for the first 3 days; remain supine after taking these trial doses.
2. Impaired kidney function may increase your sensitivity to this drug and require smaller than usual doses.

Precautions for Use
By Infants and Children: Safety and effectiveness for use by those under 12 years of age have not been established.
By Those over 60 Years of Age: Begin treatment with no more than 1 mg/ day for the first 3 days. Subsequent increases in dose must be very gradual and carefully supervised by your physician. The occurrence of orthostatic hypotension can cause unexpected falls and injury; sit or lie down promptly if you feel light-headed or dizzy. Report any indications of dizziness or chest pain promptly.

▷ **Advisability of Use During Pregnancy**
Pregnancy Category: C (tentative). See Pregnancy Code inside back cover.
Animal studies: No birth defects found.
Human studies: Information from adequate studies of pregnant women is not available.
Use this drug only if clearly needed. Ask your physician for guidance.

Advisability of Use if Breast-Feeding
Presence of this drug in breast milk: Yes, in small amounts.
Monitor nursing infant closely and discontinue drug or nursing if adverse effects develop.

Habit-Forming Potential: None.

Effects of Overdosage: Orthostatic hypotension, headache, generalized flushing, rapid heart rate, extreme weakness, irregular heart rhythm, circulatory collapse.

Possible Effects of Long-Term Use: None reported.

Suggested Periodic Examinations While Taking This Drug (at physician's discretion)
Measurements of blood pressure in lying, sitting and standing positions.
Measurements of body weight to detect fluid retention.

▷ **While Taking This Drug, Observe the Following**

Foods: No restrictions. Avoid excessive salt intake.

Beverages: No restrictions. May be taken with milk.

▷   *Alcohol:* Use with extreme caution until the combined effects have been determined. Alcohol can exaggerate the blood-pressure-lowering actions of this drug and cause excessive reduction.

Tobacco Smoking: Nicotine can contribute significantly to this drug's ability to intensify coronary insufficiency in susceptible individuals. All forms of tobacco should be avoided.

▷   *Other Drugs*

The following drugs may *increase* the effects of prazosin

• beta-adrenergic-blocking drugs (see Drug Class, Section Four); the severity and duration of the "first dose" hypotensive response may be increased.

▷   *Driving, Hazardous Activities:* This drug may cause dizziness or drowsiness. Restrict activities as necessary.

Aviation Note: The use of this drug *is a disqualification* for piloting. Consult a designated Aviation Medical Examiner.

Exposure to Sun: No restrictions.

Exposure to Cold: Use caution until combined effect has been determined. Cold environments may increase this drug's ability to cause coronary insufficiency (angina) in susceptible individuals.

Heavy Exercise or Exertion: Excessive exertion can augment this drug's ability to induce angina. See Profile of Angina in Section Two.

Discontinuation: If you are taking this drug as part of your treatment program for congestive heart failure, do not discontinue it abruptly. Ask your physician for guidance.

PREDNISOLONE
(pred NIS oh lohn)

Introduced: 1955

Class: Cortisonelike drugs

Prescription: USA: Yes
Canada: Yes

Controlled Drug: USA: No
Canada: No

Available as Generic: USA: Yes
Canada: Yes

Brand Names: ✦Ak-Cide [CD], ✦Ak-Tate, Delta-Cortef, ✦Inflamase, ✦Inflamase Forte, ✦Nova-Pred, ✦Novoprednisolone, ✦Pred Forte, ✦Pred Mild, Prelone

```
┌─────────────────────────────────────────────────────────────────────┐
│                      BENEFITS versus RISKS                          │
│                                                                     │
│      Possible Benefits                    Possible Risks            │
│  EFFECTIVE RELIEF OF            Short-term use (up to 10 days) is    │
│    SYMPTOMS IN A WIDE            usually well tolerated              │
│    VARIETY OF INFLAMMATORY     Long-term use (exceeding 2           │
│    AND ALLERGIC DISORDERS       weeks) is associated with many      │
│  EFFECTIVE IMMUNO-              possible adverse effects:            │
│    SUPPRESSION in selected       ALTERED MOOD AND                   │
│    benign and malignant disorders    PERSONALITY                   │
│  Prevention of rejection in organ   CATARACTS, GLAUCOMA            │
│    transplantation               HYPERTENSION                      │
│                                  OSTEOPOROSIS                      │
│                                  ASEPTIC BONE NECROSIS             │
│                                  INCREASED SUSCEPTIBILITY          │
│                                    TO INFECTIONS                    │
│                                (See Possible Adverse Effects and    │
│                                  Possible Effects of Long-Term      │
│                                  Use below)                         │
└─────────────────────────────────────────────────────────────────────┘
```

▷ **Principal Uses**

As a Single Drug Product: This potent drug of the cortisone class is used in the treatment of a wide variety of allergic and inflammatory conditions. It is used most commonly in the management of serious skin disorders, asthma, regional enteritis, ulcerative colitis and all types of major rheumatic disorders including bursitis, tendinitis and most forms of arthritis.

How This Drug Works: Not fully established. It is thought that this drug's anti-inflammatory effect is due to its ability to inhibit the normal defensive functions of certain white blood cells. Its immunosuppressant effect is attributed to a reduced production of lymphocytes and antibodies.

Available Dosage Forms and Strengths
   Syrup — 15 mg per 5-ml teaspoonful
   Tablets — 5 mg

▷ **Usual Adult Dosage Range:** 5 to 60 mg daily as a single dose or in divided doses. The total daily dosage should not exceed 250 mg. **Note: Actual dosage and administration schedule must be determined by the physician for each patient individually.**

▷ **Dosing Instructions:** Take with or following food to prevent stomach irritation, preferably in the morning. The tablet may be crushed for administration.

Usual Duration of Use: For acute disorders: 4 to 10 days. For chronic disorders: according to individual requirements. The duration of use should not exceed the time necessary to obtain adequate symptomatic relief in acute self-limiting conditions; or the time required to stabilize a chronic condition and permit gradual withdrawal. Because of its intermediate duration of action, this drug is appropriate for alternate day administration. Consult your physician on a regular basis.

▷ **This Drug Should Not Be Taken If**
- you have had an allergic reaction to any dosage form of it previously.
- you have active peptic ulcer disease.
- you have an active infection of the eye caused by the herpes simplex virus.
- you have active tuberculosis.

▷ **Inform Your Physician Before Taking This Drug If**
- you have had an unfavorable reaction to any cortisonelike drug in the past.
- you have a history of peptic ulcer disease, thrombophlebitis or tuberculosis.
- you have any of the following: diabetes, glaucoma, high blood pressure, deficient thyroid function or myasthenia gravis.
- you plan to have surgery of any kind in the near future.

Possible Side-Effects (natural, expected and unavoidable drug actions)
Increased appetite, weight gain, retention of salt and water, excretion of potassium, increased susceptibility to infection.

▷ **Possible Adverse Effects** (unusual, unexpected and infrequent reactions)
If any of the following develop, consult your physician promptly for guidance.
Mild Adverse Effects
Allergic Reaction: Skin rash.
Headache, dizziness, insomnia.
Acid indigestion, abdominal distention.
Muscle cramping and weakness.
Acne, excessive growth of facial hair.
Serious Adverse Effects
Mental and emotional disturbances of serious magnitude.
Reactivation of latent tuberculosis.
Development of peptic ulcer.
Increased blood pressure.
Development of inflammation of the pancreas.
Thrombophlebitis (inflammation of a vein with the formation of blood clot)—pain or tenderness in thigh or leg, with or without swelling of the foot, ankle or leg.
Pulmonary embolism (movement of a blood clot to the lung)—sudden shortness of breath, pain in the chest, coughing, bloody sputum.

▷ **Adverse Effects That May Mimic Natural Diseases or Disorders**
Pattern of symptoms and signs resembling Cushing's syndrome.

▷ **Possible Effects on Sexual Function**

> Altered timing and pattern of menstruation.
> Correction of male infertility when due to autoantibodies that suppress sperm activity.

Natural Diseases or Disorders That May Be Activated by This Drug
Latent diabetes, glaucoma, peptic ulcer disease, tuberculosis.

CAUTION
> 1. It is advisable to carry a card of personal identification with a notation that you are taking this drug, if your course of treatment is to exceed 1 week.
> 2. Do not discontinue this drug abruptly if you are using it for long-term treatment.
> 3. If vaccination against measles, rabies, smallpox or yellow fever is required, discontinue this drug 72 hours before vaccination and do not resume it for at least 14 days after vaccination.

Precautions for Use
> *By Infants and Children:* Avoid prolonged use if possible. During long-term use, observe for suppression of normal growth and the possibility of increased intracranial pressure. Following long-term use, the child may be at risk for adrenal gland deficiency during stress for as long as 18 months after cessation of this drug.
> *By Those over 60 Years of Age:* Cortisonelike drugs should be used very sparingly after 60 and only when the disorder under treatment is unresponsive to adequate trials of unrelated drugs. Avoid prolonged use of this drug. Continual use (even in small doses) can increase the severity of diabetes, enhance fluid retention, raise blood pressure, weaken resistance to infection, induce stomach ulcer and accelerate the development of cataract and osteoporosis.

▷ **Advisability of Use During Pregnancy**
> *Pregnancy Category:* C (tentative). See Pregnancy Code inside back cover.
> Animal studies: Birth defects reported in mice, rats and rabbits.
> Human studies: Information from adequate studies of pregnant women is not available.
> Avoid completely during the first 3 months. Limit use during the last 6 months as much as possible. If used, examine infant for possible deficiency of adrenal gland function.

Advisability of Use if Breast-Feeding
> Presence of this drug in breast milk: Yes.
> Avoid drug or refrain from nursing.

Habit-Forming Potential: Use of this drug to suppress symptoms over an extended period of time may produce a state of functional dependence (see Glossary). In the treatment of conditions like asthma and rheumatoid arthritis, it is advisable to keep the dose as small as possible and to attempt drug withdrawal after periods of reasonable improvement. Such procedures may reduce the degree of "steroid rebound"—the return of symptoms as the drug is withdrawn.

Effects of Overdosage: Fatigue, muscle weakness, stomach irritation, acid indigestion, excessive sweating, facial flushing, fluid retention, swelling of extremities, increased blood pressure.

Possible Effects of Long-Term Use: Increased blood sugar (possible diabetes), increased fat deposits on the trunk of the body ("buffalo hump"), rounding of the face ("moon face"), thinning and fragility of skin, loss of texture and strength of bones (osteoporosis, aseptic necrosis), cataracts, glaucoma, retarded growth and development in children.

Suggested Periodic Examinations While Taking This Drug (at physician's discretion)

Measurements of blood pressure, blood sugar and potassium levels.

Complete eye examinations at regular intervals.

Chest X-ray if history of tuberculosis.

Determination of the rate of development of the growing child to detect retardation of normal growth.

▷ **While Taking This Drug, Observe the Following**

Foods: No interactions expected. Ask physician regarding need to restrict salt intake or to eat potassium-rich foods. During long-term use of this drug, it is advisable to eat a high-protein diet.

Nutritional Support: During long-term use, take a vitamin D supplement. During wound repair, take a zinc supplement.

Beverages: No restrictions. Drink all forms of milk liberally.

▷   *Alcohol:* No interactions expected. Use caution if you are prone to peptic ulcer disease.

Tobacco Smoking: Nicotine increases the blood levels of naturally produced cortisone and related hormones. Heavy smoking may add to the expected actions of this drug and requires close observation for excessive effects.

Marijuana Smoking: May cause additional impairment of immunity.

▷   *Other Drugs*

Prednisolone may *decrease* the effects of

• isoniazid (INH, Niconyl, etc.).

• salicylates (aspirin, sodium salicylate, etc.).

Prednisolone *taken concurrently* with

• oral anticoagulants may either increase or decrease their effectiveness; consult physician regarding the need for prothrombin time testing and dosage adjustment.

The following drugs may *decrease* the effects of prednisolone

• antacids may reduce its absorption.

• barbiturates (Amytal, Butisol, phenobarbital, etc.).

• phenytoin (Dilantin, etc.).

• rifampin (Rifadin, Rimactane, etc.).

▷ *Driving, Hazardous Activities:* Usually no restrictions. Be alert to the rare occurrence of dizziness.

Aviation Note: The use of this drug **may be a disqualification** for piloting. Consult a designated Aviation Medical Examiner.

Exposure to Sun: No restrictions.

Occurrence of Unrelated Illness: This drug may decrease natural resistance to infection. Inform your physician if you develop an infection of any kind. It may also reduce your body's ability to respond to the stress of acute illness, injury or surgery. Keep your physician fully informed of any significant changes in your state of health.

Discontinuation: If you have been taking this drug for an extended period of time, do not discontinue it abruptly. Ask physician for guidance regarding gradual withdrawal. For a period of 2 years after discontinuing this drug, it is essential in the event of illness, injury or surgery that you inform attending medical personnel that you have used this drug in the past. The period of impaired response to stress following the use of cortisonelike drugs may last for 1 to 2 years.

PREDNISONE
(PRED ni sohn)

Introduced: 1955

Class: Cortisonelike drugs

Prescription: USA: Yes
  Canada: Yes

Controlled Drug: USA: No
  Canada: No

Available as Generic: USA: Yes
  Canada: Yes

Brand Names: ✦Apo-Prednisone, Deltasone, Meticorten, ✦Novoprednisone, Orasone, ✦Winpred

BENEFITS versus RISKS	
Possible Benefits	**Possible Risks**
EFFECTIVE RELIEF OF SYMPTOMS IN A WIDE VARIETY OF INFLAMMATORY AND ALLERGIC DISORDERS EFFECTIVE IMMUNOSUPPRESSION in selected benign and malignant disorders Prevention of rejection in organ transplantation	Short-term use (up to 10 days) is usually well tolerated Long-term use (exceeding 2 weeks) is associated with many possible adverse effects: ALTERED MOOD AND PERSONALITY CATARACTS, GLAUCOMA HYPERTENSION OSTEOPOROSIS ASEPTIC BONE NECROSIS INCREASED SUSCEPTIBILITY TO INFECTIONS (See Possible Adverse Effects and Possible Effects of Long-Term Use below)

▷ **Principal Uses**

As a Single Drug Product: This potent drug of the cortisone class is used in the treatment of a wide variety of allergic and inflammatory conditions. It is used most commonly in the management of serious skin disorders, asthma, regional enteritis, ulcerative colitis and all types of major rheumatic disorders including bursitis, tendinitis and most forms of arthritis.

How This Drug Works: Not fully established. It is thought that this drug's anti-inflammatory effect is due to its ability to inhibit the normal defensive functions of certain white blood cells. Its immunosuppressant effect is attributed to a reduced production of lymphocytes and antibodies.

Available Dosage Forms and Strengths

Oral solution — 5 mg per 5-ml teaspoonful
Syrup — 5 mg per 5-ml teaspoonful (alcohol 5%)
Tablets — 1 mg, 2.5 mg, 5 mg, 10 mg, 20 mg, 25 mg, 50 mg

▷ **Usual Adult Dosage Range:**   5 to 60 mg daily as a single dose or in divided doses. The total daily dosage should not exceed 250 mg. **Note: Actual dosage and administration schedule must be determined by the physician for each patient individually.**

▷ **Dosing Instructions:**   Take with or following food to prevent stomach irritation, preferably in the morning. The tablet may be crushed for administration.

Usual Duration of Use: For acute disorders: 4 to 10 days. For chronic disorders: according to individual requirements. The duration of use should not exceed the time necessary to obtain adequate symptomatic relief in acute self-limiting conditions; or the time required to stabilize a chronic condition and permit gradual withdrawal. Because of its intermediate duration of action, this drug is appropriate for alternate day administration. Consult your physician on a regular basis.

▷ **This Drug Should Not Be Taken If**
- you have had an allergic reaction to any dosage form of it previously.
- you have active peptic ulcer disease.
- you have an active infection of the eye caused by the herpes simplex virus.
- you have active tuberculosis.

▷ **Inform Your Physician Before Taking This Drug If**
- you have had an unfavorable reaction to any cortisonelike drug in the past.
- you have a history of peptic ulcer disease, thrombophlebitis or tuberculosis.
- you have any of the following: diabetes, glaucoma, high blood pressure, deficient thyroid function or myasthenia gravis.
- you plan to have surgery of any kind in the near future.

Possible Side-Effects (natural, expected and unavoidable drug actions)
Increased appetite, weight gain, retention of salt and water, excretion of potassium, increased susceptibility to infection.

▷ **Possible Adverse Effects** (unusual, unexpected and infrequent reactions)
If any of the following develop, consult your physician promptly for guidance.
Mild Adverse Effects
Allergic Reaction: Skin rash.
Headache, dizziness, insomnia.
Acid indigestion, abdominal distention.
Muscle cramping and weakness.
Acne, excessive growth of facial hair.
Serious Adverse Effects
Mental and emotional disturbances of serious magnitude.
Reactivation of latent tuberculosis.
Development of peptic ulcer.
Increased blood pressure.
Development of inflammation of the pancreas.
Thrombophlebitis (inflammation of a vein with the formation of blood clot)—pain or tenderness in thigh or leg, with or without swelling of the foot, ankle or leg.
Pulmonary embolism (movement of a blood clot to the lung)—sudden shortness of breath, pain in the chest, coughing, bloody sputum.

▷ **Possible Effects on Sexual Function**
Altered timing and pattern of menstruation.
Correction of male infertility when due to autoantibodies that suppress sperm activity.

▷ **Adverse Effects That May Mimic Natural Diseases or Disorders**
Pattern of symptoms and signs resembling Cushing's syndrome.

Natural Diseases or Disorders That May Be Activated by This Drug
Latent diabetes, glaucoma, peptic ulcer disease, tuberculosis.

CAUTION
1. It is advisable to carry a card of personal identification with a notation that you are taking this drug, if your course of treatment is to exceed 1 week.
2. Do not discontinue this drug abruptly if you are using it for long-term treatment.
3. If vaccination against measles, rabies, smallpox or yellow fever is required, discontinue this drug 72 hours before vaccination and do not resume it for at least 14 days after vaccination.

Precautions for Use
By Infants and Children: Avoid prolonged use if possible. During long-term use, observe for suppression of normal growth and the possibility of increased intracranial pressure. Following long-term use, the child may be at risk for adrenal gland deficiency during stress for as long as 18 months after cessation of this drug.
By Those over 60 Years of Age: Cortisonelike drugs should be used very sparingly after 60 and only when the disorder under treatment is unresponsive to adequate trials of unrelated drugs. Avoid the prolonged use of this drug. Continual use (even in small doses) can increase the severity of diabetes, enhance fluid retention, raise blood pressure, weaken resistance to infection, induce stomach ulcer and accelerate development of cataract and osteoporosis.

▷ **Advisability of Use During Pregnancy**
Pregnancy Category: C (tentative). See Pregnancy Code inside back cover.
Animal studies: Birth defects reported in mice, rats and rabbits.
Human studies: Information from adequate studies of pregnant women is not available.
Avoid completely during the first 3 months. Limit use during the last 6 months as much as possible. If used, examine infant for possible deficiency of adrenal gland function.

Advisability of Use if Breast-Feeding
Presence of this drug in breast milk: Yes.
Avoid drug or refrain from nursing.

Habit-Forming Potential: Use of this drug to suppress symptoms over an extended period of time may produce a state of functional dependence (see Glossary). In the treatment of conditions like asthma and rheumatoid arthritis, it is advisable to keep the dose as small as possible and to attempt drug withdrawal after periods of reasonable improvement. Such procedures may reduce the degree of "steroid rebound"—the return of symptoms as the drug is withdrawn.

Effects of Overdosage: Fatigue, muscle weakness, stomach irritation, acid indigestion, excessive sweating, facial flushing, fluid retention, swelling of extremities, increased blood pressure.

Possible Effects of Long-Term Use: Increased blood sugar (possible diabetes), increased fat deposits on the trunk of the body ("buffalo hump"), rounding of the face ("moon face"), thinning and fragility of skin, loss of texture and strength of bones (osteoporosis, aseptic necrosis), cataracts, glaucoma, retarded growth and development in children.

Suggested Periodic Examinations While Taking This Drug (at physician's discretion)
Measurements of blood pressure, blood sugar and potassium levels.
Complete eye examinations at regular intervals.
Chest X-ray if history of tuberculosis.
Determination of the rate of development of the growing child to detect retardation of normal growth.

▷ **While Taking This Drug, Observe the Following**
Foods: No interactions expected. Ask physician regarding need to restrict salt intake or to eat potassium-rich foods. During long-term use of this drug, it is advisable to eat a high-protein diet.
Nutritional Support: During long-term use, take a vitamin D supplement. During wound repair, take a zinc supplement.
Beverages: No restrictions. Drink all forms of milk liberally.
▷ *Alcohol:* No interactions expected. Use caution if you are prone to peptic ulcer disease.
Tobacco Smoking: Nicotine increases the blood levels of naturally produced cortisone and related hormones. Heavy smoking may add to the expected actions of this drug and requires close observation for excessive effects.
Marijuana Smoking: May cause additional impairment of immunity.
▷ *Other Drugs*
Prednisone may *decrease* the effects of
• isoniazid (INH, Niconyl, etc.).
• salicylates (aspirin, sodium salicylate, etc.).
Prednisone *taken concurrently* with
• oral anticoagulants may either increase or decrease their effectiveness; consult physician regarding the need for prothrombin time testing and dosage adjustment.
The following drugs may *decrease* the effects of prednisone
• antacids may reduce its absorption.

- barbiturates (Amytal, Butisol, phenobarbital, etc.).
- phenytoin (Dilantin, etc.).
- rifampin (Rifadin, Rimactane, etc.).

▷ *Driving, Hazardous Activities:* Usually no restrictions. Be alert to the rare occurrence of dizziness.

Aviation Note: The use of this drug **may be a disqualification** for piloting. Consult a designated Aviation Medical Examiner.

Exposure to Sun: No restrictions.

Occurrence of Unrelated Illness: This drug may decrease natural resistance to infection. Inform your physician if you develop an infection of any kind. It may also reduce your body's ability to respond to the stress of acute illness, injury or surgery. Keep your physician fully informed of any significant changes in your state of health.

Discontinuation: If you have been taking this drug for an extended period of time, do not discontinue it abruptly. Ask physician for guidance regarding gradual withdrawal. For a period of 2 years after discontinuing this drug, it is essential in the event of illness, injury or surgery that you inform attending medical personnel that you have used this drug in the past. The period of impaired response to stress following the use of cortisonelike drugs may last for 1 to 2 years.

PRIMIDONE
(PRI mi dohn)

Introduced: 1953

Class: Anticonvulsant

Prescription: USA: Yes
  Canada: Yes

Controlled Drug: USA: No
  Canada: No

Available as Generic: USA: Yes
  Canada: Yes

Brand Names: ✦Apo-Primidone, Myidone, Mysoline, ✦Sertan

BENEFITS versus RISKS	
Possible Benefits	*Possible Risks*
EFFECTIVE CONTROL OF TONIC-CLONIC (GRAND MAL) AND ALL TYPES OF PARTIAL SEIZURES	Allergic skin reactions Rare blood cell disorders: megaloblastic anemia, deficient white blood cells and platelets

▷ **Principal Uses**

As a Single Drug Product: This drug is used exclusively to control generalized grand mal seizures and all types of partial seizures. It can be used to supplement the anticonvulsant action of phenytoin.

How This Drug Works: Not completely established. This drug reduces and stabilizes the excitability of nerve fibers and inhibits the repetitious spread of electrical impulses along nerve pathways. This action may prevent seizures altogether, or it may reduce their frequency and severity. (Part of this drug's action is attributable to phenobarbital, one of its conversion products in the body.)

Available Dosage Forms and Strengths
Oral suspensions — 250 mg per 5-ml teaspoonful
Tablets — 50 mg, 250 mg

▷ **Usual Adult Dosage Range:**   Initially, 250 mg/24 hours as a single dose at bedtime for 1 week; 2nd week, 250 mg/12 hours; 3rd week, 250 mg 3 times/day, 6 to 8 hours apart; 4th week, 250 mg 4 times/day, 4 to 6 hours apart. The total daily dosage should not exceed 2000 mg. **Note: Actual dosage and administration schedule must be determined by the physician for each patient individually.**

▷ **Dosing Instructions:**   May be taken with or following food to reduce stomach irritation. The tablet may be crushed for administration. Shake the suspension well before measuring the dose.

Usual Duration of Use: Continual use on a regular schedule for 2 to 4 weeks is usually necessary to determine this drug's effectiveness in reducing the frequency and severity of seizures. Long-term use (months to years) requires supervision and periodic evaluation by your physician. Consult your physician on a regular basis.

▷ **This Drug Should Not Be Taken If**
- you have had an allergic reaction to it previously.
- you are allergic to phenobarbital.
- you have a history of porphyria.

▷ **Inform Your Physician Before Taking This Drug If**
- you have had an allergic or idiosyncratic reaction to any barbiturate drug in the past.
- you have a family history of intermittent porphyria.
- you have impaired liver, kidney or thyroid gland function.
- you have asthma, emphysema or myasthenia gravis.
- you are pregnant or planning pregnancy.
- you plan to have surgery under general anesthesia in the near future.

Possible Side-Effects (natural, expected and unavoidable drug actions)
Drowsiness, impaired concentration, mental and physical sluggishness.

▷ **Possible Adverse Effects** (unusual, unexpected and infrequent reactions)
If any of the following develop, consult your physician promptly for guidance.
Mild Adverse Effects
Allergic Reactions: Skin rashes, hives, localized swellings.
"Hangover" effect, dizziness, unsteadiness, impaired vision, double vision, fatigue, emotional disturbances.

Low blood pressure, faintness.

Nausea, vomiting, thirst, increased urine volume.

Serious Adverse Effects

Allergic Reaction: Swelling of lymph glands.

Idiosyncratic Reactions: Paradoxical anxiety, agitation, restlessness, rage.

Visual hallucinations.

Blood cell disorders: megaloblastic anemia due to folic acid depletion; deficient production of white blood cells and blood platelets.

▷ **Possible Effects on Sexual Function**

Decreased libido and/or impotence (22%).

Decreased effectiveness of oral contraceptives taken concurrently.

▷ **Adverse Effects That May Mimic Natural Diseases or Disorders**

Allergic swelling of lymph glands may suggest a naturally occurring lymphoma.

Natural Diseases or Disorders That May Be Activated by This Drug

Acute intermittent and/or cutaneous porphyria (see Glossary).

Systemic lupus erythematosus.

CAUTION

1. This drug must not be stopped abruptly.
2. The wide variation of this drug's action from person to person requires careful individualization of dosage schedules.
3. Regularity of drug use is essential for the successful management of seizure disorders. Take your medication at the same time each day.
4. Side-effects and mild adverse effects are usually most apparent during the first several weeks of treatment and often subside with continued use.
5. It may be necessary to take folic acid to prevent anemia while taking this drug. Consult your physician.
6. It is advisable to carry a card of personal identification with a notation that you are taking this drug.

Precautions for Use

By Infants and Children: This drug should be used with caution in the hyperkinetic (overactive) child. Observe for possible paradoxical hyperactivity. Changes associated with puberty characteristically slow the metabolism of phenobarbital and permit its gradual accumulation. Measurements of blood levels in young adolescents can detect rising concentrations of this drug that could lead to toxicity. (See Therapeutic Drug Monitoring in Section One.)

By Those over 60 Years of Age: It is advisable to avoid all barbiturates in the elderly. If use of this drug is attempted, start with small doses until tolerance has been determined. Observe for confusion, delirium, agitation or paradoxical excitement. This drug may be conducive to hypothermia (see Glossary).

▷ **Advisability of Use During Pregnancy**

Pregnancy Category: D (tentative). See Pregnancy Code inside back cover.

Animal studies: Birth defects due to this drug reported in mice.

Human studies: Information from adequate studies of pregnant women is not available. However, recent reports suggest a possible association between the use of this drug during the first 3 months of pregnancy and the development of birth defects in the fetus. Discuss with your physician the advantages and possible disadvantages of using this drug during pregnancy. If it is used, determine the smallest maintenance dose that will prevent seizures.

The newborn infants of mothers who take this drug during pregnancy may develop abnormal bleeding or bruising due to the deficiency of certain blood clotting factors in the blood. Consult your physician regarding the need to take vitamin K during the last month of pregnancy.

Advisability of Use if Breast-Feeding

Presence of this drug in breast milk: Yes.

Monitor nursing infant closely and discontinue drug or nursing if adverse effects develop.

Habit-Forming Potential: None.

Effects of Overdosage: Drowsiness, jerky eye movements, blurred vision, staggering gait, incoordination, slurred speech, stupor progressing to coma.

Possible Effects of Long-Term Use: Enlargement of lymph glands; enlargement of thyroid gland. Megaloblastic anemia due to folic acid deficiency. Reduced blood levels of calcium and phosphorus, leading to rickets in children and loss of bone texture (osteomalacia) in adults.

Suggested Periodic Examinations While Taking This Drug (at physician's discretion)

Complete blood cell counts. Measurements of blood levels of calcium and phosphorus. Evaluation of lymph and thyroid glands. Skeletal X-ray examinations for bone demineralization during long-term use.

▷ **While Taking This Drug, Observe the Following**

Foods: No restrictions.

Nutritional Support: Consult your physician regarding the need for supplements of calcium, vitamin D, folic acid and vitamin K.

Beverages: No restrictions. May be taken with milk or fruit juice.

▷ *Alcohol:* Avoid completely. Alcohol can increase greatly the sedative and depressant effects of this drug on brain function.

Tobacco Smoking: May enhance the sedative effects of this drug and increase drowsiness.

▷ *Other Drugs*

Note: 15% of primidone is converted to phenobarbital in the body. See the Drug Profile of Phenobarbital for possible interactions with other drugs.

▷ *Driving, Hazardous Activities:* This drug may cause drowsiness and dizziness; it can also impair mental alertness, vision and physical coordination. Restrict activities as necessary.

Aviation Note: The use of this drug *is a disqualification* for piloting. Consult a designated Aviation Medical Examiner.

Exposure to Sun: No restrictions.

Occurrence of Unrelated Illness: Notify your physician of any illness or injury that prevents the use of this drug according to your regular dosage schedule.

Discontinuation: Do not discontinue this drug without your physician's knowledge and approval. Sudden withdrawal of any anticonvulsant drug can cause severe and repeated seizures.

PROBENECID
(proh BEN e sid)

Introduced: 1951

Class: Antigout

Prescription: USA: Yes
  Canada: No

Controlled Drug: USA: No
  Canada: No

Available as Generic: USA: Yes
  Canada: No

Brand Names: ✦Ampicin PRB [CD], Benemid, ✦Benuryl, ColBenemid [CD], Polycillin-PRB [CD], Probalan, ✦Pro-Biosan 500 Kit [CD]

BENEFITS versus RISKS	
Possible Benefits	*Possible Risks*
EFFECTIVE LONG-TERM PREVENTION OF ACUTE ATTACKS OF GOUT	Formation of uric acid kidney stones
Useful adjunct to penicillin therapy (to achieve high blood and tissue levels of penicillin)	Bone marrow depression (aplastic anemia) (rare)
	Drug-induced liver and kidney damage (both rare)

▷ **Principal Uses**

As a Single Drug Product: Used primarily in the long-term management of gout to prevent acute attacks. While effective for prevention, it has no beneficial effects in relieving the joint inflammation and pain of the acute episode. In fact, it may aggravate and prolong the symptoms of acute gout.

As a Combination Drug Product [CD]: This drug is available in combination with colchicine, a drug often used for the treatment of acute gout. Each drug has a different mechanism of action; when used in combination they provide both relief of the acute manifestations of gout and some measure of protection from recurrence of acute attacks.

How This Drug Works: By acting on the tubular systems of the kidney to increase the amount of uric acid excreted in the urine, this drug reduces the levels of uric acid in the blood and body tissues. By acting on the tubular systems of the kidney to decrease the amount of penicillin excreted in the urine, this drug prolongs the presence of penicillin in the blood and helps achieve higher concentrations in body tissues.

Available Dosage Forms and Strengths
Tablets — 500 mg

▷ **Usual Adult Dosage Range:** Antigout: Initially, 250 mg twice/day for 1 week; then 500 mg twice/day. Adjunct to penicillin therapy: 500 mg 4 times/day. **Note: Actual dosage and administration schedule must be determined by the physician for each patient individually.**

▷ **Dosing Instructions:** Take with or following food to reduce stomach irritation. Drink 2.5 to 3 quarts of liquids daily. The tablet may be crushed for administration.

Usual Duration of Use: Continual use on a regular schedule for several months is usually necessary to determine this drug's effectiveness in preventing acute attacks of gout. Long-term use (months to years) requires supervision and periodic evaluation by your physician. Consult your physician on a regular basis.

▷ **This Drug Should Not Be Taken If**
- you have had an allergic reaction to it previously.
- you have active liver disease.
- you have an active blood cell or bone marrow disorder.
- you are experiencing an attack of acute gout at the present time.

▷ **Inform Your Physician Before Taking This Drug If**
- you have a history of kidney disease or kidney stones.
- you have a history of liver disease or impaired liver function.
- you have a history of peptic ulcer disease.
- you have a history of a blood cell or bone marrow disorder.
- you are taking any drug product that contains aspirin or aspirinlike drugs.

Possible Side-Effects (natural, expected and unavoidable drug actions)
Development of kidney stones (composed of uric acid); this is preventable. Consult your physician regarding the use of sodium bicarbonate (or other urine alkalizer) to prevent stone formation.

▷ **Possible Adverse Effects** (unusual, unexpected and infrequent reactions)
  If any of the following develop, consult your physician promptly for guidance.
  Mild Adverse Effects
  Allergic Reactions: Skin rash, itching, drug fever (see Glossary).
  Headache, dizziness, flushing of face.
  Reduced appetite, sore gums, nausea, vomiting.
  Serious Adverse Effects
  Allergic Reaction: Anaphylactic reaction (see Glossary).
  Idiosyncratic Reaction: Hemolytic anemia (see Glossary).
  Bone marrow depression (see Glossary): fatigue, weakness, fever, sore throat, abnormal bleeding or bruising.
  Drug-induced liver damage with jaundice (see Glossary).
  Drug-induced kidney damage: marked fluid retention, reduced urine formation.

▷ **Possible Effects on Sexual Function:**   None reported.

▷ **Adverse Effects That May Mimic Natural Diseases or Disorders**
  Liver reactions may suggest viral hepatitis.
  Kidney reactions may suggest nephrosis.

  CAUTION
  1. This drug should not be started until 2 to 3 weeks after an acute attack of gout has subsided.
  2. This drug may increase the frequency of acute attacks of gout during the first few months of treatment. Concurrent use of colchicine is advised to prevent acute attacks. See the Profile of Gout in Section Two.
  3. Aspirin (and aspirin-containing drug products) can reduce the effectiveness of this drug. Use acetaminophen or a nonaspirin analgesic for pain relief as needed.

  Precautions for Use
  By Infants and Children: Safety and effectiveness for use by those under 2 years of age have not been established.
  By Those over 60 Years of Age: The natural decline in kidney function that occurs after 60 may require adjustment of your dosage. You may be more susceptible to the serious adverse effects of this drug. Report any unusual symptoms promptly for evaluation.

▷ **Advisability of Use During Pregnancy**
  Pregnancy Category: C (tentative). See Pregnancy Code inside back cover.
  Animal studies: No information available.
  Human studies: Information from adequate studies of pregnant women is not available.
  This drug has been used during pregnancy with no reports of birth defects or adverse effects on the fetus. Ask your physician for guidance.

Advisability of Use if Breast-Feeding
Presence of this drug in breast milk: Unknown.
Avoid drug or refrain from nursing.

Habit-Forming Potential: None.

Effects of Overdosage: Stomach irritation, nausea, vomiting, nervous agitation, delirium, seizures, coma.

Possible Effects of Long-Term Use: Formation of kidney stones. Kidney damage in sensitive individuals.

Suggested Periodic Examinations While Taking This Drug (at physician's discretion)
Complete blood cell counts, measurements of blood uric acid, liver and kidney function tests.

▷ **While Taking This Drug, Observe the Following**
Foods: Follow physician's advice regarding the need for a low-purine diet.
Beverages: A large intake of coffee, tea or cola beverages may reduce the effectiveness of treatment.
▷ *Alcohol:* No interactions expected. However, large amounts of alcohol can raise the blood uric acid level and reduce the effectiveness of treatment.
Tobacco Smoking: No interactions expected.
▷ *Other Drugs*
Probenecid may *increase* the effects of
- clofibrate (Atromid S).
- dyphylline (Neothylline).
- methotrexate (Mexate), and increase its toxicity.
- thiopental (Pentothal), and prolong its anesthetic effect.
Probenecid *taken concurrently* with
- penicillins may cause a threefold to fivefold increase in penicillin blood levels, greatly increasing the effectiveness of each penicillin dose.
The following drugs may *decrease* the effects of probenecid
- aspirin and other salicylates may reduce its effectiveness in promoting the excretion of uric acid.
▷ *Driving, Hazardous Activities:* This drug may cause dizziness. Restrict activities as necessary.
Aviation Note: The use of this drug *may be a disqualification* for piloting. Consult a designated Aviation Medical Examiner.
Exposure to Sun: No restrictions.
Discontinuation: Do not discontinue this drug without consulting your physician.

PROBUCOL
(PROH byu kohl)

Introduced: 1971

Prescription: USA: Yes
Canada: Yes

Available as Generic: USA: No
Canada: No

Brand Name: Lorelco

Class: Anticholesterol

Controlled Drug: USA: No
Canada: No

BENEFITS versus RISKS	
Possible Benefits	*Possible Risks*
EFFECTIVE REDUCTION OF TOTAL CHOLESTEROL AND LOW DENSITY CHOLESTEROL IN TYPE IIa CHOLESTEROL DISORDERS (15% to 20% reduction of total cholesterol, 10% to 15% reduction of LDL cholesterol when used in conjunction with a low-cholesterol diet)	CONCURRENT REDUCTION (22% to 25%) OF HIGH DENSITY (HDL) CHOLESTEROL (This is thought to be undesirable in the prevention and treatment of atherosclerosis.) Diarrhea, indigestion (10%)

▷ **Principal Uses**

As a Single Drug Product: Used for the reduction of abnormally high blood levels of cholesterol (type IIa) that have not responded to adequate control of diet, weight, diabetes and hypothyroidism.

How This Drug Works: Not completely known. It is thought that this drug may inhibit the absorption of dietary cholesterol, may inhibit the early stages of cholesterol production in the liver and may increase the rate of LDL cholesterol destruction and elimination.

Available Dosage Forms and Strengths
Tablets — 250 mg, 500 mg

▷ **Usual Adult Dosage Range:** 250 mg to 500 mg twice daily. **Note: Actual dosage and administration schedule must be determined by the physician for each patient individually.**

▷ **Dosing Instructions:** Take with the morning and evening meals. The tablet may be crushed for administration.

Usual Duration of Use: Continual use on a regular schedule for 3 to 6 months is usually necessary to determine this drug's effectiveness in lowering cholesterol blood levels. Long-term use (months to years) requires periodic evaluation of response and dosage adjustment. Consult your physician on a regular basis.

▷ **This Drug Should Not Be Taken If**
- you have had an allergic reaction to it previously.
- you have had a heart attack (myocardial infarction) recently.

▷ **Inform Your Physician Before Taking This Drug If**
- you are pregnant.
- you have a history of heart disease, heart rhythm disorder or abnormal electrocardiogram.
- you have impaired liver function or gallstones.

Possible Side-Effects (natural, expected and unavoidable drug actions)
None.

▷ **Possible Adverse Effects** (unusual, unexpected and infrequent reactions)
If any of the following develop, consult your physician promptly for guidance.
Mild Adverse Effects
Allergic Reactions: Rash, itching, swelling (angioedema) of face, mouth, hands or feet.
Headache, dizziness, numbness or tingling in extremities.
Indigestion, excessive gas, abdominal discomfort, nausea, vomiting, diarrhea.
Serious Adverse Effects
Idiosyncratic Reactions: Dizziness, fainting, chest pain, heart palpitations.
Altered electrocardiogram in some individuals.

▷ **Possible Effects on Sexual Function**
Altered timing and pattern of menstruation.
Impotence (rare).

CAUTION
1. Report promptly the development of chest pain, heart palpitations, dizziness or faintness.
2. Comply fully with all recommendations for periodic measurements of blood cholesterol and triglyceride levels. These are essential to monitoring your response to treatment and determining the need for changes in dosage or medication.

Precautions for Use
By Infants and Children: Safety and effectiveness for use by those under 12 years of age have not been established.
By Those over 60 Years of Age: It is advisable to have an electrocardiogram before starting this drug and at intervals of 6 months until it is determined that there is no drug-induced alteration of heart function.

▷ **Advisability of Use During Pregnancy**
Pregnancy Category: B (tentative). See Pregnancy Code inside back cover.
Animal studies: No drug-induced birth defects found in rodents.

Human studies: Information from adequate studies of pregnant women is not available.

Use this drug only if clearly needed. Because of the long persistence of this drug in body tissues, it is recommended that the drug be discontinued and that birth control be used for 6 months before attempting to establish pregnancy.

The manufacturer does not recommend the use of this drug during pregnancy.

Advisability of Use if Breast-Feeding
Presence of this drug in breast milk: Unknown.
Avoid drug or refrain from nursing.

Habit-Forming Potential: None.

Effects of Overdosage: Abdominal distress, nausea, vomiting, diarrhea.

Possible Effects of Long-Term Use: Decrease in high density (HDL) cholesterol blood levels; increase in triglyceride blood levels.

Suggested Periodic Examinations While Taking This Drug (at physician's discretion)
Measurements of blood levels of total cholesterol, HDL and LDL cholesterol fractions and triglycerides.
Electrocardiograms (selectively).

▷ **While Taking This Drug, Observe the Following**
Foods: Follow the low-cholesterol diet prescribed by your physician.
Beverages: No restrictions.
▷ *Alcohol:* No interactions expected.
Tobacco Smoking: No interactions expected.
▷ *Other Drugs*
Probucol may *decrease* the effects of
  • chenodiol (Chenix), and impair its effectiveness in the treatment of gallstones.
▷ *Driving, Hazardous Activities:* This drug may cause dizziness or faintness in sensitive individuals. Restrict activities as necessary.
Aviation Note: The use of this drug *is usually not a disqualification* for piloting. Consult a designated Aviation Medical Examiner.
Exposure to Sun: No restrictions.
Discontinuation: Do not discontinue this drug without your physician's knowledge and guidance. Abrupt withdrawal may be followed by prompt and excessive increase in blood cholesterol levels.

PROCAINAMIDE
(proh kayn A mide)

Introduced: 1950

Class: Antiarrhythmic

Prescription: USA: Yes
Canada: Yes

Controlled Drug: USA: No
Canada: No

Available as Generic: USA: Yes
      Canada: No

Brand Names: Procamide SR, Procan SR, Pronestyl, Pronestyl-SR

BENEFITS versus RISKS	
Possible Benefits	*Possible Risks*
EFFECTIVE TREATMENT OF SELECTED HEART RHYTHM DISORDERS	NARROW TREATMENT RANGE INDUCTION OF SYSTEMIC LUPUS ERYTHEMATOSUS SYNDROME in 20% of long-term users Provocation of abnormal heart rhythms Blood cell disorders: insufficient white blood cells and platelets

▷ **Principal Uses**

As a Single Drug Product: This drug is classified as a Type 1 anti-arrhythmic agent, similar to disopyramide and quinidine in its actions. It is used primarily to abolish and prevent the recurrence of premature beats arising in the atria (upper chambers) and the ventricles (lower chambers) of the heart. It is also useful in the treatment and prevention of atrial fibrillation, atrial flutter and abnormally rapid heart rates (tachycardia) that originate in the atria or the ventricles.

How This Drug Works: By slowing the activity of the pacemaker and delaying the transmission of electrical impulses through the conduction system and muscle of the heart, this drug assists in restoring normal heart rate and rhythm.

Available Dosage Forms and Strengths

      Capsules — 250 mg, 375 mg, 500 mg
      Injections — 100 mg per ml, 500 mg per ml
      Tablets — 250 mg, 375 mg, 500 mg
Tablets, prolonged-action — 250 mg, 500 mg, 750 mg, 1000 mg

▷ **Usual Adult Dosage Range:**   Dose varies according to indication for use. Premature atrial or ventricular contractions: 250 to 500 mg/3 hours. Paroxysmal atrial tachycardia: initially, 1250 mg, followed in 1 hour by 750 mg; then 500 to 1000 mg/2 hours as needed and tolerated. Atrial fibrillation and flutter: the heart should be digitalized first; then initiate procainamide with 1250 mg, followed in 1 hour by 750 mg; follow with 500 to 1000 mg/2 hours as needed and tolerated. For maintenance: 500 to 1000 mg/4 to 6 hours. The total daily dosage should not exceed 6000 mg. **Note: Actual dosage and administration schedule must be determined by the physician for each patient individually.**

▷ **Dosing Instructions:** Preferably taken on an empty stomach, 1 hour before or 2 hours after eating. However, it may be taken with or following food to reduce stomach irritation. The regular capsules may be opened and the regular tablets may be crushed for administration; however, the prolonged-action tablets should be swallowed whole without alteration.

Usual Duration of Use: Continual use on a regular schedule for 24 to 48 hours is usually necessary to determine this drug's effectiveness in correcting or preventing responsive rhythm disorders. Long-term use requires supervision and periodic evaluation by your physician. Consult your physician on a regular basis.

▷ **This Drug Should Not Be Taken If**
- you have had an allergic reaction to it previously.
- you have second-degree or third-degree heart block (determined by electrocardiogram).

▷ **Inform Your Physician Before Taking This Drug If**
- you are allergic to procaine (Novocain) or to other local anesthetics of the "-caine" drug class, such as those commonly used for glaucoma testing and for dental procedures.
- you have had any unfavorable reactions to other antiarrhythmic drugs in the past.
- you have a history of heart disease of any kind, especially "heart block."
- you have a history of low blood pressure.
- you have a history of lupus erythematosus.
- you have a history of abnormally low blood platelet counts from any cause.
- you have impaired liver or kidney function.
- you have myasthenia gravis.
- you have an enlarged prostate gland.
- you are taking any form of digitalis or any diuretic drug that can cause excessive loss of body potassium (ask physician).
- you plan to have surgery under general anesthesia in the near future.

Possible Side-Effects (natural, expected and unavoidable drug actions)
Drop in blood pressure in susceptible individuals.

▷ **Possible Adverse Effects** (unusual, unexpected and infrequent reactions)
If any of the following develop, consult your physician promptly for guidance.
Mild Adverse Effects
Allergic Reactions: Skin rash, hives, itching, drug fever (see Glossary). Weakness, light-headedness.
Loss of appetite, bitter taste, indigestion, nausea, vomiting, diarrhea.
Serious Adverse Effects
Allergic Reactions: Systemic lupus erythematosuslike syndrome: fever, skin eruptions, joint and muscle pains, pleurisy. (This is reported to occur in at least 20% of users.)

Idiosyncratic Reactions: Mental depression, hallucinations, psychotic behavior, hemolytic anemia (see Glossary).

Severe drop in blood pressure, fainting.

Asthmalike breathing difficulties.

Induction of new heart rhythm disturbances.

Inability to empty urinary bladder, prostatism (see Glossary).

Blood cell disorders: abnormally low white blood cell count, causing fever, sore throat, infections; abnormally low blood platelet count, causing abnormal bleeding or bruising.

▷ **Possible Effects on Sexual Function:**   None reported.

▷ **Adverse Effects That May Mimic Natural Diseases or Disorders**
Rare liver reaction may suggest viral hepatitis.

Natural Diseases or Disorders That May Be Activated by This Drug
Systemic lupus erythematosus, myasthenia gravis.

CAUTION
1. Thorough evaluation of your heart function (including electrocardiograms) is necessary prior to using this drug.
2. Periodic evaluation of your heart function is necessary to determine your response to this drug. Some individuals may experience worsening of their heart rhythm disorder and/or deterioration of heart function. Close monitoring of heart rate, rhythm and overall performance is essential.
3. Dosage must be adjusted carefully for each individual. Do not change your dosage without the knowledge and supervision of your physician.
4. Do not take any other antiarrhythmic drug while taking this drug unless directed to do so by your physician.

Precautions for Use
By Infants and Children: Blood cell counts should be monitored for loss of white blood cells.
By Those over 60 Years of Age: Reduced kidney function may require reduction in dosage. Observe carefully for light-headedness, dizziness, unsteadiness and tendency to fall.

▷ **Advisability of Use During Pregnancy**
Pregnancy Category: C (tentative). See Pregnancy Code inside back cover.
Animal studies: No information available.
Human studies: Information from adequate studies of pregnant women is not available.
Use this drug only if clearly needed.

Advisability of Use if Breast-Feeding
Presence of this drug in breast milk: Unknown.
Avoid drug or refrain from nursing.

Habit-Forming Potential: None.

Effects of Overdosage: Loss of appetite, nausea, vomiting, weakness, faintness, irregular heart rhythm, stupor, circulatory collapse, heart arrest.

Possible Effects of Long-Term Use: Lupus erythematosus–like syndrome (see above).

Suggested Periodic Examinations While Taking This Drug (at physician's discretion)
Complete blood cell counts.
Blood tests for the development of lupus erythematosus (LE) cells and antinuclear antibodies.
Electrocardiograms to monitor the full effect of this drug on the mechanisms that influence heart rate and rhythm.

▷ **While Taking This Drug, Observe the Following**
Foods: No restrictions.
Beverages: Avoid excessive intake of coffee, tea and cola beverages. Avoid iced drinks. May be taken with milk.
▷   *Alcohol:* Use caution until the combined effects have been determined. Alcohol can increase the blood-pressure-lowering effects of this drug.
Tobacco Smoking: Nicotine can cause irritability of the heart and reduce the effectiveness of this drug. Follow physician's advice regarding smoking.
▷   *Other Drugs*
Procainamide may *increase* the effects of
 • antihypertensive drugs, and cause excessive lowering of blood pressure.
The following drugs may *increase* the effects of procainamide
 • amiodirone.
 • cimetidine (Tagamet).
▷   *Driving, Hazardous Activities:* This drug may cause dizziness or weakness. Restrict activities as necessary.
Aviation Note: The use of this drug *may be a disqualification* for piloting. Consult a designated Aviation Medical Examiner.
Exposure to Sun: No restrictions.
Exposure to Heat: Use caution. Hot environments are conducive to lower blood pressure.
Occurrence of Unrelated Illness: Disorders that cause vomiting, diarrhea or dehydration can affect this drug's action adversely. Report such developments promptly.
Discontinuation: This drug should not be discontinued abruptly following long-term use. Ask your physician for guidance regarding gradual dose reduction.

PROCHLORPERAZINE
(proh klor PER a zeen)

Introduced: 1956

Class: Strong tranquilizer, antiemetic, phenothiazines

Prescription: USA: Yes
Canada: Yes

Controlled Drug: USA: No
Canada: No

Available as Generic: USA: Yes
Canada: No

Brand Names: ✦Combid [CD], Compazine, ✦Stemetil

BENEFITS versus RISKS

Possible Benefits	*Possible Risks*
EFFECTIVE CONTROL OF ACUTE MENTAL DISORDERS in the majority of patients: beneficial effects on thinking, mood and behavior	SERIOUS TOXIC EFFECTS ON BRAIN with long-term use
EFFECTIVE CONTROL OF NAUSEA AND VOMITING	Liver damage with jaundice (infrequent)
Relief of anxiety and nervous tension	Rare blood cell disorders: abnormally low white cell and platelet counts

---

▷ **Principal Uses**

As a Single Drug Product: This member of the phenothiazine class is used primarily to relieve severe nausea and vomiting. Although it has sedative and antipsychotic effects characteristic of this class, it is used less often as a major tranquilizer.

How This Drug Works: Not completely established. Present theory is that by inhibiting the action of dopamine, this drug acts to correct an imbalance of nerve impulse transmissions that is thought to be responsible for certain mental disorders. By blocking the action of dopamine in the chemoreceptor trigger zone of the brain, this drug prevents excessive stimulation of the vomiting center.

Available Dosage Forms and Strengths

Capsules, prolonged-action — 10 mg, 15 mg, 30 mg
Injection — 5 mg per ml
Suppositories — 2.5 mg, 5 mg, 25 mg
Syrup — 5 mg per 5-ml teaspoonful
Tablets — 5 mg, 10 mg, 25 mg

▷ **Usual Adult Dosage Range:** Initially, 5 mg/6 to 8 hours. If needed and tolerated, dose may be increased by 5 mg at intervals of 3 to 4 days. Usual range is 35 to 60 mg/24 hours. The total daily dosage should not exceed 150 mg. **Note: Actual dosage and administration schedule must be determined by the physician for each patient individually.**

▷ **Dosing Instructions:**   May be taken with or following food to reduce stomach irritation. The tablets may be crushed for administration. Prolonged-action capsules should be swallowed whole without alteration.

Duration of Use: Continual use on a regular schedule for 12 to 24 hours is usually necessary to determine this drug's effectiveness in controlling nausea and vomiting. If used for severe anxiety-tension states or acute psychotic behavior, a trial of several weeks is usually necessary to determine effectiveness. If not significantly beneficial within 6 weeks, it should be discontinued. Consult your physician on a regular basis.

▷ **This Drug Should Not Be Taken If**
- you have had an allergic reaction to it previously.
- you have active liver disease.
- you have cancer of the breast.
- you have a current blood cell or bone marrow disorder.

▷ **Inform Your Physician Before Taking This Drug If**
- you are allergic or abnormally sensitive to any phenothiazine drug (see Drug Class, Section Four).
- you have impaired liver or kidney function.
- you have any type of seizure disorder.
- you have diabetes, glaucoma or heart disease.
- you have a history of lupus erythematosus.
- you are taking any drug with sedative effects.
- you plan to have surgery under general or spinal anesthesia in the near future.

Possible Side-Effects (natural, expected and unavoidable drug actions)
Drowsiness (usually during the first 2 weeks), orthostatic hypotension (see Glossary), blurred vision, dry mouth, nasal congestion, constipation, impaired urination.
Pink or purple coloration of urine, of no significance.

▷ **Possible Adverse Effects** (unusual, unexpected and infrequent reactions)
If any of the following develop, consult your physician promptly for guidance.
Mild Adverse Effects
Allergic Reactions: Skin rash, hives, low-grade fever.
Lowering of body temperature, especially in the elderly. (See Hypothermia in Glossary.)
Increased appetite and weight gain.
Dizziness, weakness, agitation, insomnia, impaired day and night vision.
Chronic constipation, fecal impaction.

Serious Adverse Effects

Allergic Reactions: Hepatitis with jaundice (see Glossary), usually between second and fourth week; high fever; asthma; anaphylactic reaction (see Glossary).

Idiosyncratic Reaction: Toxic dermatitis.

Depression, disorientation, seizures.

Disturbances of heart rhythm, rapid heart rate.

Bone marrow depression (see Glossary): fever, sore throat, abnormal bleeding or bruising.

Parkinson-like disorders (see Glossary); muscle spasms of face, jaw, neck, back, extremities; extreme restlessness; slowed movements, muscle rigidity, tremors; tardive dyskinesias (see Glossary).

▷ **Possible Effects on Sexual Function**

Altered timing and pattern of menstruation.

Female breast enlargement with milk production.

Male breast enlargement and tenderness.

Inhibited ejaculation; priapism (see Glossary).

Causes false positive pregnancy test result.

▷ **Adverse Effects That May Mimic Natural Diseases or Disorders**

Nervous system reactions may suggest Parkinson's disease.

Liver reactions may suggest viral hepatitis.

Reactions resembling systemic lupus erythematosus can occur.

Natural Diseases or Disorders That May Be Activated by This Drug

Latent epilepsy, glaucoma, diabetes mellitus, prostatism (see Glossary).

CAUTION

1. Many over-the-counter medications (see OTC Drugs in Glossary) for allergies, colds and coughs contain drugs that can interact unfavorably with this drug. Ask your physician or pharmacist for guidance before using any such medications.
2. Antacids that contain aluminum and/or magnesium can prevent the absorption of this drug and reduce its effectiveness.
3. Obtain prompt evaluation of any change or disturbance of vision.

Precautions for Use

By Infants and Children: Do not use this drug in infants under 2 years of age, or in children of any age with symptoms suggestive of Reye syndrome (see Glossary). Children with acute illnesses ("flulike" infections, measles, chicken pox, etc.) are very susceptible to adverse effects when this drug is given to control nausea and vomiting.

By Those over 60 Years of Age: Small doses are advisable until individual response has been determined. You may be more susceptible to the development of drowsiness, lethargy, constipation, lowering of body temperature (hypothermia) and orthostatic hypotension (see Glossary). This drug can enhance existing prostatism (see Glossary). You may also be more susceptible to the development of Parkinson-like reactions and/or tardive dyskinesia (see discussion of these terms in

Glossary). These reactions must be recognized early since they may become unresponsive to treatment and irreversible.

▷ **Advisability of Use During Pregnancy**
Pregnancy Category: C (tentative). See Pregnancy Code inside back cover.
Animal studies: Cleft palate reported in mouse and rat studies.
Human studies: No increase in birth defects reported in 2023 exposures. Information from adequate studies of pregnant women is not available.
Limit use to small and infrequent doses. Avoid drug during the last month because of possible effects on the newborn infant.

Advisability of Use if Breast-Feeding
Presence of this drug in breast milk: Yes, in small amounts.
Monitor nursing infant closely and discontinue drug or nursing if adverse effects develop.

Habit-Forming Potential: None.

Effects of Overdosage: Marked drowsiness, weakness, tremor, agitation, unsteadiness, deep sleep, coma, convulsions.

Possible Effects of Long-Term Use: Tardive dyskinesias. Eye changes: opacities in cornea or lens, retinal pigmentation.

Suggested Periodic Examinations While Taking This Drug (at physician's discretion)
Complete blood cell counts, especially between the fourth and tenth weeks of treatment.
Liver function tests, electrocardiograms.
Complete eye examinations—eye structures and vision.
Careful inspection of the tongue for early evidence of fine, involuntary, wavelike movements that could indicate the beginning of tardive dyskinesia.

▷ **While Taking This Drug, Observe the Following**
Foods: No restrictions.
Nutritional Support: A riboflavin (vitamin B-2) supplement should be taken with long-term use.
Beverages: No restrictions. May be taken with milk.
▷ *Alcohol:* Avoid completely. Alcohol can increase the sedative action of phenothiazines and accentuate their depressant effects on brain function and blood pressure. Phenothiazines can increase the intoxicating effects of alcohol.
Tobacco Smoking: Possible reduction of drowsiness from drug.
Marijuana Smoking: Moderate increase in drowsiness; accentuation of orthostatic hypotension; increased risk of precipitating latent psychoses, confusing the interpretation of mental status and drug responses.

▷ *Other Drugs*

Prochlorperazine may *increase* the effects of
- all sedative drugs, especially meperidine (Demerol), and cause excessive sedation.
- all atropinelike drugs, and cause nervous system toxicity.

Prochlorperazine may *decrease* the effects of
- guanethidine (Ismelin, Esimil), and reduce its effectiveness in lowering blood pressure.

Prochlorperazine *taken concurrently* with
- propranolol (Inderal) may cause increased effects of both drugs; monitor drug effects closely and adjust dosages as necessary.

The following drugs may *decrease* the effects of prochlorperazine
- antacids containing aluminum and/or magnesium.
- benztropine (Cogentin).
- trihexyphenidyl (Artane).

▷ *Driving, Hazardous Activities:* This drug can impair mental alertness, judgment and physical coordination. Avoid hazardous activities.

Aviation Note: The use of this drug *is a disqualification* for piloting. Consult a designated Aviation Medical Examiner.

Exposure to Sun: Use caution until sensitivity has been determined. Some phenothiazines can cause photosensitivity (see Glossary).

Exposure to Heat: Use caution and avoid excessive heat as much as possible. This drug may impair the regulation of body temperature and increase the risk of heat stroke.

Exposure to Cold: Use caution and dress warmly. This drug can increase the risk of hypothermia in the elderly.

Discontinuation: After a period of long-term use, do not discontinue this drug suddenly. Gradual withdrawal over 2 to 3 weeks under physician supervision is recommended.

PROMETHAZINE
(proh METH a zeen)

Introduced: 1945

Class: Antiemetic, antihistamines, phenothiazines

Prescription: USA: Yes
Canada: No

Controlled Drug: USA: No
Canada: No

Available as Generic: USA: Yes
Canada: Yes

Brand Names: ✦Histanil, K-Phen, Pentazine, Phenergan, Phenergan-D [CD], Phenergan w/Codeine [CD], ✦PMS Promethazine, Prorex

---

BENEFITS versus RISKS

Possible Benefits	*Possible Risks*
EFFECTIVE SYMPTOMATIC RELIEF OF ALLERGIC RHINITIS AND DERMATOSIS	EXCESSIVE SEDATION in sensitive individuals
Moderately effective prevention and treatment of motion sickness, nausea and vomiting	Atropinelike effects
	Rare blood cell disorders: abnormally low white cell and platelet counts
Effective as mild sedative and hypnotic	

▷ **Principal Uses**

As a Single Drug Product: This versatile drug shares the characteristics of two major drug classes, the antihistamines and the phenothiazines. It is used to provide symptomatic relief in allergic disorders (hay fever, hives, etc.), to control nausea and vomiting and to produce mild sedation.

As a Combination Drug Product [CD]: This drug is often combined with analgesics such as aspirin or codeine to enhance their pain-relieving action by producing mild sedation. It is also used in cough mixtures for its drying (antihistaminic) effect.

How This Drug Works: Not completely established. This drug reduces the intensity of the allergic response by blocking the action of histamine after it has been released from sensitized tissue cells. It reduces the sensitivity of the nerve endings in the labyrinth (inner ear) and blocks the transmission of excessive nerve impulses to the vomiting center in the brain. The way this drug produces sedation and light sleep is not known.

Available Dosage Forms and Strengths

        Injections — 25 mg per ml, 50 mg per ml
    Suppositories — 12.5 mg, 25 mg, 50 mg
          Syrups — 6.25 mg per 5-ml teaspoonful (alcohol 7%), 25 mg per 5-ml teaspoonful (alcohol 1.5%)
        Tablets — 12.5 mg, 25 mg, 50 mg

▷ **Usual Adult Dosage Range:**   12.5 to 25 mg/4 to 6 hours as needed. The total daily dosage should not exceed 150 mg. **Note: Actual dosage and administration schedule must be determined by the physician for each patient individually.**

▷ **Dosing Instructions:**   Preferably taken with or following food to reduce stomach irritation. The tablets may be crushed for administration.

Usual Duration of Use: Continual use on a regular schedule for 3 to 5 days is usually necessary to determine this drug's effectiveness in relieving allergic symptoms or controlling vomiting. If not effective within 5 days, it should be discontinued.

▷ **This Drug Should Not Be Taken If**
- you have had an allergic reaction to it previously.
- you have a blood cell or bone marrow disorder.
- you have narrow-angle glaucoma (not adequately treated).

▷ **Inform Your Physician Before Taking This Drug If**
- you are allergic or overly sensitive to any phenothiazine drug (see Drug Class, Section Four).
- you are taking any drugs with sedative effects.
- you have a seizure disorder or bronchial asthma.
- you have impaired liver function.
- you have a history of peptic ulcer disease.
- you have an enlarged prostate gland or prostatism (see Glossary).

Possible Side-Effects (natural, expected and unavoidable drug actions)
Drowsiness (25% of users), lethargy, impaired concentration, dry mouth, constipation, impaired urination, reduced tolerance for contact lenses.

▷ **Possible Adverse Effects** (unusual, unexpected and infrequent reactions)
If any of the following develop, consult your physician promptly for guidance.
Mild Adverse Effects
Allergic Reactions: Skin rash, hives.
Headache, dizziness, unsteadiness, confusion, nervousness, excitation, irritability, tremor, insomnia, numbness and tingling, blurred vision, double vision, ringing in ears.
Loss of appetite, stomach irritation, nausea, vomiting, diarrhea.
Rapid heart rate, palpitation, low blood pressure.
Chest tightness, asthmatic wheezing, thickening of bronchial secretions.
Serious Adverse Effects
Allergic Reactions: Drug-induced hepatitis with jaundice (see Glossary).
Idiosyncratic Reactions: Euphoria, hysteria.
Nervous system reactions: Muscle spasms of the face, neck, back and extremities: rolling of the eyes, twisting of the neck, arching of the back, spasms of the hands and feet.
Blood cell disorders: abnormally low white blood cell and blood platelet counts, causing fever, sore throat, infections, abnormal bleeding or bruising (all very rare).

▷ **Possible Effects on Sexual Function:** None reported.

▷ **Adverse Effects That May Mimic Natural Diseases or Disorders**
Drug-induced hepatitis may suggest viral hepatitis.

Natural Diseases or Disorders That May Be Activated by This Drug
Latent epilepsy, glaucoma, prostatism (see Glossary).

CAUTION
1. This drug should not be used alone to treat symptoms of lower respiratory tract disease, including asthma.

2. Avoid this drug for at least 5 days before skin testing for possible allergens.

Precautions for Use

By Infants and Children: This drug should not be used in premature or full-term newborn infants. The young child is especially sensitive to the nervous system effects of antihistamines and phenothiazines. Children with acute illnesses ("flulike" infections, measles, chicken pox, etc.) are very susceptible to muscular spasms of the face, neck, back or extremities when this drug is used to control nausea and vomiting. Avoid this drug completely during such infections; there is evidence to suggest that it may contribute to the development of Reye syndrome (see Glossary).

By Those over 60 Years of Age: You may be more susceptible to the development of drowsiness, dizziness and lethargy and to impaired thinking, judgment and memory. The sedative effect of this drug can cause a hypoactive syndrome that may be misinterpreted as senility or emotional depression. This drug can increase the symptoms of prostatism (see Glossary).

▷ Advisability of Use During Pregnancy

Pregnancy Category: B (tentative). See Pregnancy Code inside back cover.

Animal studies: No birth defects reported in rats.

Human studies: No significant increase in birth defects reported in 746 exposures to this drug.

Avoid use of this drug during the last 3 months; it can reduce certain blood clotting factors in the fetus and cause bleeding in the newborn infant.

Advisability of Use if Breast-Feeding

Presence of this drug in breast milk: Yes.

Avoid drug or refrain from nursing.

Habit-Forming Potential: None.

Effects of Overdosage: Marked drowsiness, weakness, unsteadiness, agitation, delirium, deep sleep, coma, seizures.

Possible Effects of Long-Term Use: The development of tolerance and loss of effectiveness.

Suggested Periodic Examinations While Taking This Drug (at physician's discretion)

Complete blood cell counts.

▷ While Taking This Drug, Observe the Following

Foods: No restrictions.

Beverages: No restrictions. May be taken with milk.

▷   *Alcohol:* Use extreme caution until the combined effects have been determined. The combination of alcohol and antihistamines can cause rapid and marked sedation.

Tobacco Smoking: No interactions expected.
▷ *Other Drugs*
    Promethazine may *increase* the effects of
    • all sedative drugs, and cause excessive sedation.
    • atropine and atropinelike drugs (see Drug Class, Section Four).
▷ *Driving, Hazardous Activities:* This drug may cause dizziness or drowsiness. Restrict activities as necessary.
    Aviation Note: The use of this drug *is a disqualification* for piloting. Consult a designated Aviation Medical Examiner.
    Exposure to Sun: Use caution until sensitivity has been determined. This drug may cause photosensitivity (see Glossary).

PROPOXYPHENE
(proh POX i feen)

Introduced: 1955   **Class:** Analgesic, narcotic

Prescription: USA: Yes   **Controlled Drug:** USA: C-IV*
    Canada: Yes   Canada: <N>

Available as Generic: Yes

Brand Names: Darvocet-N 50/100 [CD], Darvon, Darvon-N, Darvon w/ASA [CD], Darvon Compound [CD], Darvon Compound-65 [CD], Darvon-N w/ASA [CD], ✦Darvon-N Compound [CD], Dolene, Dolene AP-65 [CD], Dolene Compound-65 [CD], ✦Novopropoxyn, ✦Novopropoxyn Compound [CD], ✦642, Wygesic [CD]

BENEFITS versus RISKS

Possible Benefits	*Possible Risks*
EFFECTIVE RELIEF OF MILD TO MODERATE PAIN	POTENTIAL FOR HABIT FORMATION (DEPENDENCE)
	Sedative effects
	Drug-induced hepatitis (very rare)

▷ **Principal Uses**
    As a Single Drug Product: This drug is used exclusively as an analgesic to relieve mild to moderate pain.
    As a Combination Drug Product [CD]: It is available in combinations with acetaminophen and with aspirin. These milder pain relievers are added to enhance the analgesic effect and to reduce fever when present. Some combinations also contain caffeine to counteract the sedative effects of the analgesics.

*See Schedules of Controlled Drugs inside back cover.

How This Drug Works: Acting primarily as a depressant of certain brain functions, this drug suppresses the perception of pain and calms the emotional response to pain.

Available Dosage Forms and Strengths
  Capsules — 32 mg, 65 mg
  Oral suspension — 50 mg per 5-ml teaspoonful
  Tablets — 100 mg

▷ **Usual Adult Dosage Range:** For propoxyphene: 65 mg/4 hours as needed. The total daily dosage should not exceed 390 mg. For propoxyphene napsylate (Darvon-N): 100 mg/4 hours as needed. The total daily dose should not exceed 600 mg. **Note: Actual dosage and administration schedule must be determined by the physician for each patient individually.**

▷ **Dosing Instructions:** May be taken with or following food to reduce stomach irritation or nausea. The tablet may be crushed and the capsule may be opened for administration.

Usual Duration of Use: As required to control pain. Continual use should not exceed 5 to 7 days without interruption and reassessment of need.

▷ **This Drug Should Not Be Taken If**
  • you have had an allergic reaction to any dosage form of it previously.
  • you are having an acute attack of asthma.

▷ **Inform Your Physician Before Taking This Drug If**
  • you have had an unfavorable reaction to any narcotic drug in the past.
  • you have a history of drug abuse or alcoholism.
  • you have chronic lung disease with impaired breathing.
  • you have impaired liver or kidney function.
  • you are taking any other drugs that have a sedative effect.

Possible Side-Effects (natural, expected and unavoidable drug actions)
  Drowsiness, light-headedness, constipation.

▷ **Possible Adverse Effects** (unusual, unexpected and infrequent reactions)
  If any of the following develop, consult your physician promptly for guidance.
  Mild Adverse Effects
  Allergic Reactions: Skin rash, itching.
  Headache, dizziness, weakness, confusion, blurred vision.
  Nausea, vomiting, abdominal discomfort.
  Serious Adverse Effects
  Allergic Reactions: Hepatitis with jaundice (see Glossary).
  Paradoxical excitement, agitation, insomnia.

▷ **Possible Effects on Sexual Function:** None reported.

▷ **Precautions for Use**
By Infants and Children: Safety and effectiveness for use by those under 12 years of age have not been established.
By Those over 60 Years of Age: Use small doses initially and increase dosage as needed and tolerated. Limit use to short-term treatment only. There may be increased susceptibility to the development of drowsiness, dizziness, unsteadiness, falling and constipation (possibly leading to fecal impaction).

▷ **Advisability of Use During Pregnancy**
Pregnancy Category: C (tentative). See Pregnancy Code inside back cover.
Animal studies: No birth defects due to this drug were found.
Human studies: Information from studies of pregnant women indicates no significant increase in birth defects in 2914 exposures to this drug.
Use this drug only if clearly needed and in small, infrequent doses.

Advisability of Use if Breast-Feeding
Presence of this drug in breast milk: Yes, in small amounts.
Monitor nursing infant closely and discontinue drug or nursing if adverse effects develop.

Habit-Forming Potential: Psychological and/or physical dependence can develop with use of large doses for an extended period of time.

Effects of Overdosage: Drowsiness, restlessness, agitation, nausea, vomiting, dry mouth, vertigo, weakness, lethargy, stupor, coma, seizures.

Possible Effects of Long-Term Use: Psychological and physical dependence, chronic constipation.

Suggested Periodic Examinations While Taking This Drug (at physician's discretion)
None.

▷ **While Taking This Drug, Observe the Following**
Foods: No restrictions.
Beverages: No restrictions. May be taken with milk.
▷ *Alcohol:* Use extreme caution until the combined effects have been determined. Propoxyphene can intensify the intoxicating effects of alcohol, and alcohol can intensify the depressant effects of propoxyphene on brain function.
Tobacco Smoking: Heavy smoking may reduce the effectiveness of this drug.
Marijuana Smoking: Increase in drowsiness and pain relief; impairment of mental and physical performance.
▷ *Other Drugs*
Propoxyphene may ***increase*** the effects of
• other drugs with sedative effects.
• oral anticoagulants (Coumadin, etc.), and increase the risk of bleeding.

- carbamazepine (Tegretol), and increase its toxicity.
- doxepin (Sinequan), and increase its toxicity.

▷ *Driving, Hazardous Activities:* This drug can impair mental alertness, judgment, reaction time and physical coordination. Avoid hazardous activities accordingly.

Aviation Note: The use of this drug **is a disqualification** for piloting. Consult a designated Aviation Medical Examiner.

Exposure to Sun: No restrictions.

Discontinuation: It is advisable to limit this drug to short-term use. If it is necessary to use it for extended periods of time, discontinuation should be gradual to minimize possible effects of withdrawal.

PROPRANOLOL
(proh PRAN oh lohl)

Introduced: 1966

Class: Antianginal, antiarrhythmic, antihypertensive, migraine preventive, beta-adrenergic blocker

Prescription: USA: Yes
Canada: Yes

Controlled Drug: USA: No
Canada: No

Available as Generic: Yes

Brand Names: ✦Apo-Propranolol, ✦Detensol, Inderal, Inderal-LA, Inderide [CD], Inderide LA [CD], Ipran, ✦Novopranol, ✦PMS Propranolol

---

BENEFITS versus RISKS

Possible Benefits	*Possible Risks*
EFFECTIVE, WELL-TOLERATED AS: ANTIANGINAL DRUG in effort-induced angina; ANTIARRHYTHMIC DRUG in certain heart rhythm disorders; ANTIHYPERTENSIVE DRUG in mild to moderate hypertension	CONGESTIVE HEART FAILURE in advanced heart disease
	Worsening of angina in coronary heart disease (if drug is abruptly withdrawn)
EFFECTIVE PREVENTION OF MIGRAINE HEADACHES	Masking of low blood sugar (hypoglycemia) in drug-treated diabetes
Effective adjunct in the prevention of recurrent heart attack (myocardial infarction)	Provocation of asthma
Effective adjunct in the management of pheochromocytoma	Rare blood cell disorders: low white cell and platelet counts

▷ **Principal Uses**

As a Single Drug Product: This first beta blocker drug is used primarily to treat several serious cardiovascular disorders: classical effort-induced angina, certain types of heart rhythm disturbance and high blood pressure. It is also beneficial in preventing the recurrence of heart attacks (myocardial infarction). In addition, it is used to reduce the frequency and severity of migraine headaches. Other uses (not "officially approved" at this time) include the control of physical manifestations of anxiety and nervous tension (as in stage fright), the control of familial tremors and the control of symptoms associated with markedly overactive thyroid gland function (thyrotoxicosis).

As a Combination Drug Product [CD]: This drug is available in combination with hydrochlorothiazide for the treatment of hypertension. This combination product includes two "step 1" drugs with different mechanisms of action; it is intended to provide greater effectiveness and convenience for long-term use.

How This Drug Works: By blocking certain actions of the sympathetic nervous system, this drug

- reduces the rate and contraction force of the heart, thus lowering the ejection pressure of the blood leaving the heart and reducing the oxygen requirement for heart function.
- reduces the degree of contraction of blood vessel walls, resulting in their relaxation and expansion and consequent lowering of blood pressure.
- prolongs the conduction time of nerve impulses through the heart, of benefit in the management of certain heart rhythm disorders.

Available Dosage Forms and Strengths

Capsules, prolonged-action — 80 mg, 120 mg, 160 mg
Concentrate — 80 mg/ml
Injection — 1 mg per ml
Oral solution — 4 mg/ml, 8 mg/ml
Tablets — 10 mg, 20 mg, 40 mg, 60 mg, 80 mg, 90 mg

▷ **Usual Adult Dosage Range:** Varies with indication.

Antianginal: Initially, 10 to 20 mg 3 or 4 times/day; increase dose gradually every 3 to 7 days as needed and tolerated. The total daily dosage should not exceed 320 mg.

Antiarrhythmic: 10 to 30 mg 3 or 4 times/day as needed and tolerated.

Antihypertensive: Initially, 40 mg twice/day; increase dose gradually as needed and tolerated. The total daily dosage should not exceed 640 mg.

Migraine headache prevention: Initially, 20 mg 4 times/day; increase dose gradually as needed and tolerated. The total daily dosage should not exceed 240 mg.

Note: Actual dosage and administration schedule must be determined by the physician for each patient individually.

▷ **Dosing Instructions:**   Preferably taken 1 hour before eating to maximize absorption. The tablet may be crushed for administration; to prevent a possible numbing effect (harmless), mix with soft food and swallow promptly. The prolonged-action capsules should be swallowed whole without alteration. Do not discontinue this drug abruptly.

Usual Duration of Use: Continual use on a regular schedule for 10 to 14 days is usually necessary to determine this drug's effectiveness in preventing angina, controlling heart rhythm disorders and lowering blood pressure. Maximal effectiveness may require continual use for 6 to 8 weeks. The long-term use of this drug (months to years) will be determined by the course of your symptoms over time and your response to the overall treatment program (weight reduction, salt restriction, smoking cessation, etc.). Consult your physician on a regular basis.

▷ **This Drug Should Not Be Taken If**
  • you have had an allergic reaction to it previously.
  • you have Prinzmetal's variant angina (coronary artery spasm).
  • you have congestive heart failure.
  • you have an abnormally slow heart rate or a serious form of heart block.
  • you are taking, or have taken within the past 14 days, any monoamine oxidase (MAO) type A inhibitor drug (see Drug Class, Section Four).

▷ **Inform Your Physician Before Taking This Drug If**
  • you have had an adverse reaction to any beta blocker drug in the past (see Drug Class, Section Four).
  • you have a history of serious heart disease, with or without episodes of heart failure.
  • you have a history of hay fever (allergic rhinitis), asthma, chronic bronchitis or emphysema.
  • you have a history of overactive thyroid function (hyperthyroidism).
  • you have a history of low blood sugar (hypoglycemia).
  • you have impaired liver or kidney function.
  • you have diabetes or myasthenia gravis.
  • you are currently taking any form of digitalis, quinidine or reserpine, or any calcium blocker drug (see Drug Class, Section Four).
  • you plan to have surgery under general anesthesia in the near future.

Possible Side-Effects (natural, expected and unavoidable drug actions)
Lethargy and fatigability, cold extremities, slow heart rate, light-headedness in upright position (see orthostatic hypotension in Glossary).

▷ **Possible Adverse Effects** (unusual, unexpected and infrequent reactions)
If any of the following develop, consult your physician promptly for guidance.
Mild Adverse Effects
Allergic Reactions: Skin rash, temporary loss of hair, drug fever (see Glossary).

Headache, dizziness, insomnia, vivid dreams.

Indigestion, nausea, vomiting, diarrhea.

Serious Adverse Effects

Idiosyncratic Reactions: Acute behavioral disturbances: disorientation, confusion, hallucinations, amnesia.

Mental depression, anxiety.

Chest pain, shortness of breath, precipitation of congestive heart failure.

Induction of bronchial asthma (in asthmatic individuals).

Rare blood cell disorders: abnormally low white blood cell count, causing fever and sore throat; abnormally low blood platelet count, causing abnormal bleeding or bruising.

▷ **Possible Effects on Sexual Function**

Decreased libido; impaired erection (28%); impotence (15%).

This drug has been found to have the highest incidence of libido reduction and erectile impairment of all beta blocker drugs.

Male infertility (inhibited sperm motility); Peyronie's disease (see Glossary).

▷ **Adverse Effects That May Mimic Natural Diseases or Disorders**

Reduced blood flow to extremities may resemble Raynaud's phenomenon (see Glossary).

Natural Diseases or Disorders That May Be Activated by This Drug

Prinzmetal's variant angina, Raynaud's disease, intermittent claudication, myasthenia gravis (questionable).

CAUTION

1. *Do not discontinue this drug suddenly* without the knowledge and guidance of your physician. Carry a notation on your person that you are taking this drug.
2. Consult your physician or pharmacist before using nasal decongestants usually present in over-the-counter cold preparations and nose drops. These can cause sudden increases in blood pressure when taken concurrently with beta blocker drugs.
3. Report the development of any tendency to emotional depression.

Precautions for Use

By Infants and Children: Safety and effectiveness for use by those under 12 years of age have not been established. However, if this drug is used, observe for the development of low blood sugar (hypoglycemia) during periods of reduced food intake.

By Those over 60 Years of Age: Proceed *cautiously* with all antihypertensive drugs. Unacceptably high blood pressure should be reduced without creating the risks associated with excessively low blood pressure. Start treatment with small doses, and monitor the blood pressure response frequently. Sudden, rapid and excessive reduction of blood pressure can predispose to stroke or heart attack. Observe for dizziness, unsteadiness, tendency to fall, confusion, hallucinations, depression or urinary frequency.

▷ **Advisability of Use During Pregnancy**
   Pregnancy Category: C (tentative). See Pregnancy Code inside back cover.
      Animal studies: No significant increase in birth defects due to this drug.
      Some toxic effects on embryo reported.
      Human studies: Information from adequate studies of pregnant women
      is not available.
      Avoid use of drug during the first 3 months if possible. Use this drug
      only if clearly needed. Ask your physician for guidance.

Advisability of Use if Breast-Feeding
   Presence of this drug in breast milk: Yes.
   Monitor nursing infant closely and discontinue drug or nursing if ad-
   verse effects develop.

Habit-Forming Potential: None.

Effects of Overdosage: Weakness, slow pulse, low blood pressure, fainting,
   cold and sweaty skin, congestive heart failure, possible coma and convulsions.

Possible Effects of Long-Term Use: Reduced heart reserve and eventual
   heart failure in susceptible individuals with advanced heart disease.

Suggested Periodic Examinations While Taking This Drug (at physician's
   discretion)
   Complete blood cell counts.
   Measurements of blood pressure, evaluation of heart function.

▷ **While Taking This Drug, Observe the Following**
   Foods: No restrictions. Avoid excessive salt intake.
   Beverages: No restrictions. May be taken with milk.
▷ *Alcohol:* Use with caution until the combined effect has been determined.
      Alcohol may exaggerate this drug's ability to lower the blood pressure
      and may increase its mild sedative effect.
   Tobacco Smoking: Nicotine may reduce this drug's effectiveness in treat-
      ing angina, heart rhythm disorders and high blood pressure. Smoking
      increases the rate of elimination of this drug and decreases its blood
      levels, especially in younger individuals. In addition, high doses of
      this drug may potentiate the constriction of the bronchial tubes
      caused by regular smoking.
▷ *Other Drugs*
   Propranolol may **increase** the effects of
   • other antihypertensive drugs, and cause excessive lowering of blood
     pressure. Dosage adjustments may be necessary.
   • lidocaine (Xylocaine, etc.).
   • reserpine (Ser-Ap-Es, etc.), and cause sedation, depression, slowing
     of the heart rate and lowering of the blood pressure.
   • verapamil (Calan, Isoptin), and cause excessive depression of heart
     function; monitor this combination closely.
   Propranolol may **decrease** the effects of

- theophyllines (Aminophyllin, Theo-Dur, etc.), and reduce their antiasthmatic effectiveness.

Propranolol *taken concurrently* with

- clonidine (Catapres) requires close monitoring for rebound high blood pressure if clonidine is withdrawn while propranolol is still being taken.
- epinephrine (Adrenalin, etc.) may cause marked rise in blood pressure and slowing of the heart rate.
- insulin requires close monitoring to avoid undetected hypoglycemia (see Glossary).

The following drugs may *increase* the effects of propranolol

- chlorpromazine (Thorazine, etc.).
- cimetidine (Tagamet).
- methimazole (Tapazole).
- propylthiouracil (Propacil).

The following drugs may *decrease* the effects of propranolol

- barbiturates (phenobarbital, etc.).
- indomethacin (Indocin), and possibly other "aspirin substitutes," may impair propranolol's antihypertensive effect.
- rifampin (Rifadin, Rimactane).

▷ *Driving, Hazardous Activities:* Use caution until the full extent of drowsiness, lethargy and blood pressure change have been determined.

Aviation Note: The use of this drug *may be a disqualification* for piloting. Consult a designated Aviation Medical Examiner.

Exposure to Sun: No restrictions.

Exposure to Heat: Caution advised. Hot environments can lower blood pressure and exaggerate the effects of this drug.

Exposure to Cold: Caution advised. Cold environments can enhance the circulatory deficiency in the extremities that may occur with this drug. The elderly should take precautions to prevent hypothermia (see Glossary).

Heavy Exercise or Exertion: It is advisable to avoid exertion that produces light-headedness, excessive fatigue or muscle cramping. The use of this drug may intensify the hypertensive response to isometric exercise.

Occurrence of Unrelated Illness: The fever that accompanies systemic infections can lower blood pressure and require adjustment of dosage. Illnesses that cause nausea or vomiting may interrupt the regular dosage schedule. Ask your physician for guidance.

Discontinuation: It is advisable to avoid sudden discontinuation of this drug in all situations; this is especially true in the presence of coronary artery disease. If possible, gradual reduction of dose over a period of 2 to 3 weeks is recommended. Ask your physician for specific guidance.

PYRIDOSTIGMINE
(peer id oh STIG meen)

Introduced: 1962

Class: Antimyasthenic

Prescription: USA: Yes
Canada: No

Controlled Drug: USA: No
Canada: No

Available as Generic: USA: No
Canada: No

Brand Names: Mestinon, Mestinon Timespan, Regonol

BENEFITS versus RISKS

Possible Benefits	*Possible Risks*
MODERATELY EFFECTIVE TREATMENT OF OCULAR AND MILD FORMS OF MYASTHENIA GRAVIS (symptomatic relief of muscle weakness)	Cholinergic crisis (overdose): excessive salivation, nausea, vomiting, stomach cramps, diarrhea, shortness of breath (asthmalike wheezing), excessive weakness

---

▷ **Principal Uses**

As a Single Drug Product: Used primarily to treat the ocular and milder forms of myasthenia gravis by providing temporary relief of muscle weakness and fatigability. It is most useful in long-term treatment when there is little or no difficulty in swallowing.

How This Drug Works: This drug inhibits cholinesterase, the enzyme that destroys acetylcholine. This results in higher levels of acetylcholine, the nerve transmitter that facilitates the stimulation of muscular activity. The net effects are increased muscle strength and endurance.

Available Dosage Forms and Strengths
Syrup — 60 mg per 5-ml teaspoonful (5% alcohol)
Tablets — 60 mg
Tablets, prolonged-action — 180 mg

▷ **Usual Adult Dosage Range:** Initially: 60 to 120 mg/3 to 4 hours; adjust dosage as needed and tolerated. Maintenance: 60 to 1500 mg/24 hours; the average dose is 600 mg/24 hours. Prolonged-action tablets: 180 to 540 mg once or twice a day, at least 6 hours apart. **Note: Actual dosage and administration schedule must be determined by the physician for each patient individually.**

▷ **Dosing Instructions:** Take with food or milk to reduce the intensity of side-effects. Larger portions of the daily maintenance dosage should be timed according to the pattern of fatigue and weakness. The syrup will permit a finer adjustment of dosage. The regular tablet may be crushed for administration. The prolonged-action tablet should be taken whole (not altered).

Usual Duration of Use: Continual use on a regular schedule (with dosage adjustment) for 10 to 14 days is usually necessary to determine this drug's effectiveness in relieving the symptoms of myasthenia gravis. Long-term use (months to years) requires periodic evaluation of response and dosage adjustment. Consult your physician on a regular basis.

▷ **This Drug Should Not Be Taken If**
  • you are known to be allergic to bromide compounds.

▷ **Inform Your Physician Before Taking This Drug If**
  • you are subject to heart rhythm disorders or bronchial asthma.
  • you have recurrent urinary tract infections.
  • you have prostatism (see Glossary).
  • you plan to have surgery under general anesthesia in the near future.

Possible Side-Effects (natural, expected and unavoidable drug actions)
  Small pupils, watering of eyes, slow pulse, excessive salivation, nausea, vomiting, stomach cramps, diarrhea, urge to urinate, increased sweating.

▷ **Possible Adverse Effects** (unusual, unexpected and infrequent reactions)
  If any of the following develop, consult your physician promptly for guidance.
  Mild Adverse Effects
  Allergic Reaction: Skin rash.
  Nervousness, anxiety, unsteadiness, muscle cramps or twitching.
  Loss of scalp hair.
  Serious Adverse Effects
  Confusion, slurred speech, seizures, difficult breathing (asthmatic wheezing).
  Increased muscle weakness or paralysis.
  Excessive vomiting or diarrhea may induce abnormally low blood potassium levels (hypokalemia). This will accentuate muscle weakness.

▷ **Possible Effects on Sexual Function:** None reported.

▷ **Adverse Effects That May Mimic Natural Diseases or Disorders**
  Seizures may suggest the possibility of epilepsy.

Natural Diseases or Disorders That May Be Activated by This Drug
  Latent bronchial asthma.

CAUTION
  1. Certain drugs can block the action of this drug and reduce its effectiveness in treating myasthenia gravis. (See *Other Drugs* below.) Consult your physician before starting any new drug, prescription or over-the-counter.

2. The dosage schedule of this drug must be carefully individualized for each patient. Variations in response may occur from time to time. Because generalized muscle weakness is a major symptom of both myasthenia crisis (underdosage) and cholinergic crisis (overdosage), it may be difficult to recognize the correct cause. As a rule, weakness that begins within 1 hour after taking this drug probably represents overdosage; weakness that begins 3 or more hours after taking this drug is probably due to underdosage. Observe these time relationships and inform your physician.

3. During long-term use of this drug, observe for the possible development of resistance to the drug's therapeutic action (loss of effectiveness). Consult your physician regarding the advisability of discontinuing this drug for a few days to see if responsiveness can be restored.

Precautions for Use

By Infants and Children: The syrup form of this drug permits greater precision of dosage adjustment and ease of administration in this age group.

By Those over 60 Years of Age: The natural decline of kidney function with aging may require smaller doses to prevent accumulation of this drug to toxic levels.

▷ **Advisability of Use During Pregnancy**

Pregnancy Category: C (tentative). See Pregnancy Code inside back cover.

Animal studies: No information available.

Human studies: Information from adequate studies of pregnant women is not available.

There are no reports of birth defects due to the use of this drug during pregnancy. However, there are reports of significant muscular weakness in newborn infants whose mothers had taken this drug during pregnancy. Ask your physician for guidance.

Advisability of Use if Breast-Feeding

Presence of this drug in breast milk: Probably not.

Monitor nursing infant closely and discontinue drug or nursing if adverse effects develop.

Habit-Forming Potential: None.

Effects of Overdosage: Generalized muscular weakness, blurred vision, very small pupils, slow heart rate, difficult breathing (wheezing), excessive salivation, nausea, vomiting, stomach cramps, diarrhea, muscle cramps or twitching. This syndrome constitutes the cholinergic crisis.

Possible Effects of Long-Term Use: Development of tolerance (see Glossary) with loss of therapeutic effectiveness.

Suggested Periodic Examinations While Taking This Drug (at physician's discretion)

Assessment of drug effectiveness and dosage schedule for optimal therapeutic results.

▷ **While Taking This Drug, Observe the Following**

Foods: No restrictions.

Beverages: No restrictions. May be taken with milk.

▷ *Alcohol:* Use caution until the combined effects are determined. Weakness and unsteadiness may be accentuated.

Tobacco Smoking: No interactions expected.

▷ *Other Drugs*

The following drugs may *decrease* the effects of pyridostigmine

• atropine (belladonna).

• clindamycin (Cleocin).

• guanadrel (Hylorel).

• guanethidine (Esimil, Ismelin).

• procainamide (Procan SR, Pronestyl).

• quinidine (Cardioquin, Duraquin, etc.).

• quinine (Quinamm).

▷ *Driving, Hazardous Activities:* This drug may cause blurred vision, confusion or generalized weakness. Restrict activities as necessary.

Aviation Note: The use of this drug *is a disqualification* for piloting. Consult a designated Aviation Medical Examiner.

Exposure to Sun: No restrictions.

Exposure to Heat: Use caution. This may cause excessive sweating and increased weakness.

Exposure to Environmental Chemicals: Avoid excessive exposure (inhalation, skin contamination) to the insecticides Baygon, Diazinon and Sevin. These can accentuate the potential toxicity of this drug.

Discontinuation: Do not discontinue this drug abruptly without your physician's knowledge and guidance.

QUINIDINE
(KWIN i deen)

Introduced: 1918

Class: Antiarrhythmic

Prescription: USA: Yes
Canada: No

Controlled Drug: USA: No
Canada: No

Available as Generic: Yes

Brand Names: ✦Apo-Quinidine, ✦Biquin Durules, Cardioquin, Cin-Quin, Duraquin, ✦Novoquinidine, Quinaglute Dura-Tabs, ✦Quinate, Quinidex Extentabs, ✦Quinobarb [CD]*, Quinora

*Quinobarb contains phenylethylbarbiturate, a sedative of the barbiturate class.

```
┌─────────────────────────────────────────────────────────────────────┐
│                      BENEFITS versus RISKS                          │
│                                                                       │
│      Possible Benefits                    Possible Risks             │
│   EFFECTIVE TREATMENT OF          NARROW TREATMENT RANGE             │
│   SELECTED HEART RHYTHM           FREQUENT ADVERSE EFFECTS           │
│   DISORDERS                         (30% of users)                   │
│                                   NUMEROUS ALLERGIC AND              │
│                                     IDIOSYNCRATIC REACTIONS          │
│                                   Dose-related toxicity              │
│                                   Provocation of abnormal heart      │
│                                     rhythms                          │
│                                   Abnormally low blood platelet      │
│                                     count (rare)                     │
└─────────────────────────────────────────────────────────────────────┘
```

▷ **Principal Uses**

As a Single Drug Product: Used primarily to control the following types of abnormal heart rhythm: atrial fibrillation and flutter, paroxysmal atrial tachycardia, paroxysmal ventricular tachycardia, premature atrial and ventricular contractions.

As a Combination Drug Product [CD]: This drug is available (in Canada) in combination with a barbiturate, a mild sedative that is added to allay the anxiety and nervous tension that often accompany heart rhythm disorders.

How This Drug Works: By slowing the activity of the pacemaker and delaying the transmission of electrical impulses through the conduction system and muscle of the heart, this drug assists in restoring normal heart rate and rhythm.

Available Dosage Forms and Strengths

Capsules — 200 mg, 300 mg

Injections — 80 mg, 200 mg per ml

Tablets — 100 mg, 200 mg, 275 mg, 300 mg

Tablets, prolonged-action — 300 mg, 324 mg, 330 mg

▷ **Usual Adult Dosage Range:** Test dose: 200 mg, then observe for 2 hours for evidence of idiosyncrasy.

Dose varies with indication:

Premature atrial or ventricular contractions: 200 to 300 mg 3 or 4 times/day.

Paroxysmal atrial tachycardia: 400 to 600 mg/2 to 3 hours until paroxysm is terminated.

Atrial flutter: digitalize first; then individualize dosage schedule as appropriate.

Atrial fibrillation: digitalize first; then try 200 mg/2 to 3 hours for 5 to 8 doses; increase dose daily until normal rhythm is restored or toxic effects develop.

Maintenance schedule: 200 to 300 mg 3 or 4 times/day. The total daily dosage should not exceed 4000 mg.

Note: Actual dosage and administration schedule must be determined by the physician for each patient individually.

▷ **Dosing Instructions:** Preferably taken on an empty stomach to achieve high blood levels rapidly. However, it may be taken with or following food to reduce stomach irritation. The regular tablets may be crushed and the capsules opened for administration. The prolonged-action forms should be swallowed whole without alteration.

Usual Duration of Use: Continual use on a regular schedule for 2 to 4 days is usually necessary to determine this drug's effectiveness in correcting or preventing responsive abnormal rhythms. Long-term use (months to years) requires supervision and periodic evaluation by your physician. Consult your physician on a regular basis.

▷ **This Drug Should Not Be Taken If**
- you have had an allergic or idiosyncratic reaction to any dosage form of it previously.
- you currently have an acute infection of any kind.

▷ **Inform Your Physician Before Taking This Drug If**
- you have coronary artery disease or myasthenia gravis.
- you have a history of hyperthyroidism.
- you have had a deficiency of blood platelets in the past from any cause.
- you are now taking, or have taken recently, any digitalis preparation (digitoxin, digoxin, etc.).
- you plan to have surgery under general anesthesia in the near future.

Possible Side-Effects (natural, expected and unavoidable drug actions)
Drop in blood pressure, may be marked in sensitive individuals.

▷ **Possible Adverse Effects** (unusual, unexpected and infrequent reactions)
If any of the following develop, consult your physician promptly for guidance.
Mild Adverse Effects
Allergic Reactions: Skin rash, hives, itching, drug fever (rare).
Dose-related toxicity (cinchonism): blurred vision, ringing in the ears, loss of hearing, dizziness.
Nausea, vomiting, diarrhea (20% to 30% of users).
Serious Adverse Effects
Allergic Reactions: Severe skin reactions, hemolytic anemia (see Glossary), joint and muscle pains, anaphylactic reaction (see Glossary), reduced blood platelet count, drug-induced hepatitis (see Glossary).
Idiosyncratic Reactions: Skin rash, rapid heart rate, acute delirium and combative behavior, difficult breathing.
Heart conduction abnormalities.
Optic neuritis, impaired vision.
Abnormally low white blood cell count: fever, sore throat, infections.

▷ **Possible Effects on Sexual Function:** None reported.

▷ **Adverse Effects That May Mimic Natural Diseases or Disorders**
Drug-induced hepatitis may suggest viral hepatitis.

Natural Diseases or Disorders That May Be Activated by This Drug
Systemic lupus erythematosus, myasthenia gravis, psoriasis (in sensitive individuals).

CAUTION
1. The effects of this drug are very unpredictable because of the wide variation in response from person to person. Dosage adjustments must be based upon individual reaction. Notify your physician of any events that you suspect may be drug related.
2. It is advisable to carry a card of personal identification that includes a notation that you are taking this drug.

Precautions for Use
By Infants and Children: A test for drug idiosyncrasy should be made before starting treatment with this drug. If there is no beneficial response after 3 days of adequate dosage, this drug should be discontinued.
By Those over 60 Years of Age: Small doses are mandatory until your individual response has been determined. Observe for the development of light-headedness, dizziness, weakness or sense of impending faint. Use caution to prevent falls.

▷ **Advisability of Use During Pregnancy**
Pregnancy Category: C (tentative). See Pregnancy Code inside back cover.
Animal studies: No information available.
Human studies: Information from adequate studies of pregnant women is not available. No birth defects have been reported following use of this drug during pregnancy.
Use this drug only if clearly needed.

Advisability of Use if Breast-Feeding
Presence of this drug in breast milk: Yes.
Avoid drug or refrain from nursing.

Habit-Forming Potential: None.

Effects of Overdosage: Nausea, vomiting, ringing in the ears, headache, jerky eye movements, double vision, altered color vision, confusion, delirium, hot skin, seizures, coma.

Possible Effects of Long-Term Use: None reported.

Suggested Periodic Examinations While Taking This Drug (at physician's discretion)
Complete blood cell counts, electrocardiograms.

▷ **While Taking This Drug, Observe the Following**
Foods: No restrictions.
Beverages: No restrictions. May be taken with milk.

▷ *Alcohol:* Use caution until the combined effects have been determined. Alcohol may enhance the blood-pressure-lowering effects of this drug.

Tobacco Smoking: Nicotine can increase irritability of the heart and aggravate rhythm disorders. Avoid all forms of tobacco.

▷ *Other Drugs*

Quinidine may *increase* the effects of
- anticoagulants (Coumadin, etc.), and increase the risk of bleeding.
- digitoxin and digoxin (Lanoxin), and cause digitalis toxicity.

The following drugs may *increase* the effects of quinidine
- amiodarone.
- cimetidine (Tagamet).

The following drugs may *decrease* the effects of quinidine
- barbiturates (phenobarbital, etc.).
- phenytoin (Dilantin).
- rifampin (Rifadin, Rimactane).

▷ *Driving, Hazardous Activities:* This drug may cause dizziness and alter vision. Restrict activities as necessary.

Aviation Note: The use of this drug *may be a disqualification* for piloting. Consult a designated Aviation Medical Examiner.

Exposure to Sun: No restrictions.

RANITIDINE
(ra NI te deen)

Introduced: 1981

Class: Antiulcer, H-2 receptor blocker

Prescription: USA: Yes
Canada: Yes

Controlled Drug: USA: No
Canada: No

Available as Generic: No

Brand Name: Zantac

BENEFITS versus RISKS

Possible Benefits	*Possible Risks*
EFFECTIVE TREATMENT OF PEPTIC ULCER DISEASE: relief of symptoms, acceleration of healing, prevention of recurrence	Drug-induced hepatitis (rare)
	Confusion (in severely ill elderly patients)
CONTROL OF HYPERSECRETORY STOMACH DISORDERS	Rare blood cell disorders
Beneficial in treatment of reflux esophagitis	

▷ **Principal Uses**

As a Single Drug Product: Used primarily in the treatment of peptic ulcer disease, both benign stomach (gastric) ulcer and duodenal ulcer. It is used specifically to hasten the healing of ulcer and to prevent recurrence. Also used to control the excessive production of stomach acid in the Zollinger-Ellison syndrome. Though its effectiveness has not been fully established, this drug is also widely used in the management of esophagitis (as with hiatal hernia) and upper gastrointestinal bleeding.

How This Drug Works: By blocking the action of histamine, this drug effectively inhibits the secretion of stomach acid and thus creates a more favorable environment for the healing of peptic ulcers.

Available Dosage Forms and Strengths
Injection — 0.5 mg per ml, 25 mg per ml
Syrup — 15 mg per ml (7.5% alcohol)
Tablets — 150 mg, 300 mg

▷ **Usual Adult Dosage Range:** For active peptic ulcer and hypersecretory states: 150 mg 2 times daily, 12 hours apart. For prevention of recurrent ulcer: 150 mg at bedtime. **Note: Actual dosage and administration schedule must be determined by the physician for each patient individually.**

▷ **Dosing Instructions:** To obtain the longest period of stomach acid reduction, this drug should be taken with or immediately following meals. The tablet may be crushed for administration.

Usual Duration of Use: Continual use on a regular schedule for 4 to 6 weeks is usually necessary to determine this drug's effectiveness in healing active peptic ulcer. Long-term use (months to years) for prevention of ulcer recurrence requires individual consideration by your physician.

▷ **This Drug Should Not Be Taken If**
• you have had an allergic reaction to any dosage form of it previously.

▷ **Inform Your Physician Before Taking This Drug If**
• you are allergic to any other histamine (H-2)-blocking drug (see Drug Class, Section Four).
• you have impaired liver or kidney function.
• you are taking an oral anticoagulant.

Possible Side-Effects (natural, expected and unavoidable drug actions)
None reported.

▷ **Possible Adverse Effects** (unusual, unexpected and infrequent reactions)
If any of the following develop, consult your physician promptly for guidance.

Mild Adverse Effects
Allergic Reaction: Skin rash.
Headache, malaise, dizziness.
Nausea, constipation, diarrhea.
Serious Adverse Effects
Idiosyncratic Reaction: Confusion in the elderly and debilitated.
Drug-induced hepatitis (see Glossary).
Bone marrow depression (see Glossary)—weakness, fever, sore throat, abnormal bleeding or bruising.

▷ **Possible Effects on Sexual Function:** Decreased libido, impotence, male breast enlargement and tenderness (all rare).

▷ **Adverse Effects That May Mimic Natural Diseases or Disorders**
Liver reactions may suggest viral hepatitis.

CAUTION
1. Do not discontinue this drug abruptly. (Ulcer activation and perforation have occurred following abrupt cessation of cimetidine, a closely related drug.)
2. After discontinuation of this drug, inform your physician promptly if you experience a return of symptoms indicative of ulcer reactivation.

Precautions for Use
By Infants and Children: Safety and effectiveness for use by those under 12 years of age have not been established.
By Those over 60 Years of Age: Observe for the development of nervous agitation or confusion. This drug may contribute to the formation of stomach phytobezoars (masses of undigested vegetable fibers). Individuals with poor chewing ability (missing teeth) and those who have had partial gastrectomy or vagotomy (stomach surgery) are most susceptible. Observe for loss of appetite, stomach fullness, nausea and vomiting.

▷ **Advisability of Use During Pregnancy**
Pregnancy Category: B (tentative). See Pregnancy Code inside back cover.
Animal studies: No birth defects reported.
Human studies: Information from adequate studies of pregnant women is not available.
Use this drug only if clearly needed. Ask physician for guidance.

Advisability of Use if Breast-Feeding
Presence of this drug in breast milk: Yes.
Avoid drug or refrain from nursing.

Habit-Forming Potential: None.

Effects of Overdosage: Confusion, delirium, slurred speech, flushing, sweating, drowsiness, muscle twitching, seizures, coma.

Possible Effects of Long-Term Use: None reported.

Suggested Periodic Examinations While Taking This Drug (at physician's discretion)
  Complete blood cell counts, liver function tests.

▷ **While Taking This Drug, Observe the Following**
  Foods: Protein-rich foods produce maximal stomach acid secretion. Follow the diet prescribed to derive optimal benefit from this drug.
  Beverages: No restrictions. May be taken with milk.
▷ *Alcohol:* No interactions with drug. However, alcoholic beverages increase stomach acidity and can reduce the effectiveness of this drug.
▷ *Other Drugs*
    Ranitidine may *increase* the effects of
    • oral anticoagulants, and increase the risk of bleeding.
▷ *Driving, Hazardous Activities:* This drug may cause dizziness. Restrict activities as necessary.
  Aviation Note: The use of this drug *may be a disqualification* for piloting. Consult a designated Aviation Medical Examiner.
  Exposure to Sun: No restrictions.
  Discontinuation: Do not discontinue this drug suddenly if taken for peptic ulcer disease. Consult physician for withdrawal instructions. This drug does not provide an extended protective effect. Be alert to the possibility of ulcer recurrence anytime after discontinuation.

RESERPINE
(re SER peen)

Other Names: Deserpidine, rauwolfia

Introduced: 1953   **Class:** Antihypertensive

Prescription: USA: Yes   **Controlled Drug:** USA: No
          Canada: Yes   Canada: No

Available as Generic: Yes

Brand Names: Demi-Regroton [CD], Diupres [CD], Diutensin-R [CD], Dureticyl [CD], Enduronyl [CD], Enduronyl Forte [CD], Esidrix [CD], Hydropres [CD], ✦Hygroton-Reserpine [CD], ✦Novoreserpine, Oreticyl [CD], Rauzide [CD], Regroton [CD], ✦Reserfia, Ser-Ap-Es [CD], Serpalan, Serpasil, Serpasil-Apresoline [CD], Unipres [CD]

BENEFITS versus RISKS

Possible Benefits	*Possible Risks*
Moderately effective "step 2" antihypertensive in mild to moderate hypertension when used concurrently with a diuretic	INDUCTION OF MENTAL DEPRESSION (can be severe and prolonged)
	ACTIVATION OF PEPTIC ULCER, GASTROINTESTINAL BLEEDING
	Frequent nasal congestion and diarrhea
	Reduced libido, sexual impotence
	Mental disturbances

▷ **Principal Uses**

As a Single Drug Product: Used primarily as a "step 2" antihypertensive drug in the treatment of mild to moderate hypertension. Originally introduced as a tranquilizer for the treatment of schizophrenia, it is seldom used for this purpose currently.

As a Combination Drug Product [CD]: This drug is available in combination with most of the thiazide diuretics, the conventional "step 1" antihypertensive medication. One popular product combines reserpine, hydrochlorothiazide and hydralazine, a "step 2 or 3" antihypertensive. These combinations are more effective for treating moderate to severe hypertension.

How This Drug Works: By depleting the nerve impulse transmitter norepinephrine from nerve terminals, this drug reduces the ability of the sympathetic nervous system to maintain the degree of blood vessel constriction that is responsible for high blood pressure. The reduced availability of norepinephrine results in relaxation of blood vessel walls and lowering of blood pressure.

Available Dosage Forms and Strengths
Tablets — 0.1 mg, 0.25 mg, 1 mg

▷ **Usual Adult Dosage Range:** As antihypertensive: Initially, 0.1 to 0.5 mg/24 hours for 1 to 2 weeks. Adjust dose as needed and tolerated. The usual maintenance dose is 0.1 to 0.25 mg/24 hours. The total daily dosage should not exceed 1.0 mg/24 hours. **Note: Actual dosage and administration schedule must be determined by the physician for each patient individually.**

▷ **Dosing Instructions:** Take with or following food to reduce stomach irritation. The tablet may be crushed for administration. The prolonged-action capsule should be swallowed whole without alteration.

Usual Duration of Use: Continual use on a regular schedule for 3 to 6 weeks is usually necessary to determine this drug's full effectiveness in controlling hypertension. Long-term use (months to years) requires supervision and periodic evaluation by your physician. Consult your physician on a regular basis.

▷ **This Drug Should Not Be Taken If**
- you have had an allergic reaction to any form of reserpine previously.
- you are mentally depressed, or you have had a depression in the past.
- you have an active peptic ulcer, or a history of peptic ulcer disease.
- you have active regional enteritis, ulcerative colitis or a history of ulcerative bowel disease.

▷ **Inform Your Physician Before Taking This Drug If**
- you have a seizure disorder.
- you are subject to migraine headaches.
- you have any form of heart disease.
- you have gallbladder disease.
- you are taking any of the following drugs: anticoagulants, a digitalis preparation, quinidine, levodopa, antidepressants, sedatives or a monoamine oxidase (MAO) type A inhibitor (see Drug Classes, Section Four).
- you plan to have surgery under general anesthesia in the near future.

Possible Side-Effects (natural, expected and unavoidable drug actions)
Drowsiness and lethargy (especially during the first few weeks), reddening of the eyes, nasal stuffiness (frequent), dry mouth, increased hunger contractions, acid indigestion, intestinal cramping, diarrhea, water retention.

▷ **Possible Adverse Effects** (unusual, unexpected and infrequent reactions)
If any of the following develop, consult your physician promptly for guidance.
Mild Adverse Effects
Allergic Reactions: Skin rashes, itching.
Headache, dizziness, nosebleeds.
Nausea, vomiting, persistent diarrhea.
Serious Adverse Effects
Allergic Reactions: Reduction of blood platelet count, with or without spontaneous bruising.
Idiosyncratic Reactions: Paradoxical nervousness, agitation, confusion, nightmares, hallucinations.
Bronchospasm, asthmatic wheezing.
Mental depression, may be severe.
Peptic ulcer activation, with or without bleeding.

▷ **Possible Effects on Sexual Function**
Decreased libido and/or impotence (33%); inhibited ejaculation (14%).
Male breast enlargement and tenderness.
Female breast enlargement with milk production.

▷ **Adverse Effects That May Mimic Natural Diseases or Disorders**
Parkinson-like muscle rigidity and lethargic behavior may suggest true Parkinson's disease.

Natural Diseases or Disorders That May Be Activated by This Drug
Migraine headaches, mental depression, peptic ulcer disease, systemic lupus erythematosus.

CAUTION
1. Discontinue this drug at the first indication of despondency, loss of appetite, early morning awakening (insomnia), or impaired sex drive or performance.
2. Avoid concurrent use of drugs with strong sedative effects, antidepressants, levodopa and monoamine oxidase (MAO) type A inhibitors.
3. If surgery is planned, consult your surgeon and/or anesthesiologist regarding the need to discontinue this drug prior to surgery.

Precautions for Use
By Infants and Children: Continual use for a minimum of 7 to 14 days is necessary to determine this drug's effectiveness as an antihypertensive. Observe carefully for excessive drowsiness, emotional instability or gastrointestinal disturbances.

By Those over 60 Years of Age: Start treatment with small doses and proceed cautiously. Unacceptably high blood pressure should be reduced without creating the risks associated with excessively low blood pressure. Sudden, rapid and excessive reduction of blood pressure can predispose to stroke or heart attack. This age group is more susceptible to the development of impaired thinking, depression (6%), confusion, nightmares and orthostatic hypotension (see Glossary).

▷ **Advisability of Use During Pregnancy**
Pregnancy Category: D (tentative). See Pregnancy Code inside back cover.
Animal studies: Significant eye defects reported in rats.
Human studies: Information from adequate studies of pregnant women is not available. Significant birth defects have been reported with the use of this drug during the first 3 months.
Use of this drug during the last month of pregnancy can cause lethargy, nasal congestion, breathing difficulties and poor feeding in the newborn infant.
Avoid this drug during the first 3 months and the last month. Use it otherwise only if clearly needed.

Advisability of Use if Breast-Feeding
Presence of this drug in breast milk: Yes.
Avoid drug or refrain from nursing.

Habit-Forming Potential: None.

Effects of Overdosage: Marked drowsiness, flushed skin, incoordination, tremors, slow and weak pulse, slow and shallow breathing, diarrhea, stupor progressing to coma.

Possible Effects of Long-Term Use: None reported.

Suggested Periodic Examinations While Taking This Drug (at physician's discretion)

Complete blood cell counts.

Assessment of emotional status for unrecognized depression.

▷ **While Taking This Drug, Observe the Following**

Foods: No restrictions. Avoid excessive salt intake.

Beverages: No restrictions. May be taken with milk.

▷   *Alcohol:* Use with extreme caution until the combined effects have been determined. This drug can increase the intoxicating effects of alcohol. Both of these drugs depress brain function.

Tobacco Smoking: No interactions expected.

Marijuana Smoking: Significant increase in drowsiness; possible accentuation of hypotension; possible precipitation of depression.

▷   *Other Drugs*

Reserpine may **decrease** the effects of

- levodopa (Dopar, Sinemet), and reduce its effectiveness in treating Parkinson's disease.

Reserpine **taken concurrently** with

- anticonvulsants may lower the convulsive threshold in susceptible individuals and alter seizure patterns.
- digitalis preparations may cause rhythm disorders in susceptible individuals.
- monoamine oxidase (MAO) type A inhibitors may cause excessive stimulation of the nervous system (theoretical).
- quinidine may cause rhythm disorders in susceptible individuals.
- warfarin (Coumadin, etc.) may cause decreased anticoagulant effect with short-term use and increased anticoagulant effect with long-term use.

▷   *Driving, Hazardous Activities:* This drug may impair mental alertness, judgment, physical coordination and reaction time. Restrict activities as necessary.

Aviation Note: The use of this drug **is a disqualification** for piloting. Consult a designated Aviation Medical Examiner.

Exposure to Sun: No restrictions.

Exposure to Cold: Use caution. Monitor the elderly for excessive hypotension and other changes conducive to hypothermia (see Glossary).

RIFAMPIN
(RIF am pin)

Other Name: Rifampicin

Introduced: 1967

Class: Antibiotic, rifamycins

Prescription: USA: Yes
Canada: Yes

Controlled Drug: USA: No
Canada: No

Available as Generic: No

Brand Names: Rifadin, Rifamate [CD], Rimactane, Rimactane/INH Dual
Pack [CD], ✦Rofact

BENEFITS versus RISKS

Possible Benefits	*Possible Risks*
EFFECTIVE TREATMENT OF TUBERCULOSIS in combination with other drugs	DRUG-INDUCED HEPATITIS DRUG-INDUCED NEPHRITIS Flulike syndrome
EFFECTIVE PREVENTION OF MENINGITIS by the elimination of meningococcus from the throat of carriers	Rare blood cell disorder: abnormally low blood platelet count

---

▷ **Principal Uses**

As a Single Drug Product: This antibiotic drug is used primarily to treat active tuberculosis. It is usually given concurrently with other antitubercular drugs to enhance its effectiveness. It is also used to eliminate the meningitis germ (meningococcus) from the throats of healthy carriers so it cannot be spread to others. It is not effective in the treatment of active meningitis.

As a Combination Drug Product [CD]: This drug is available in combination with isoniazid, another antitubercular drug that delays the development of drug-resistant strains of the tuberculosis germ.

How This Drug Works: This drug prevents the growth and multiplication of susceptible tuberculosis organisms by blocking specific enzyme systems that are involved in the formation of essential proteins.

Available Dosage Forms and Strengths

Capsules — 150 mg, 300 mg

▷ **Usual Adult Dosage Range:** For tuberculosis: 600 mg once/day. For meningococcus carriers: 600 mg once/day for 4 days. The total daily dosage should not exceed 600 mg. **Note: Actual dosage and administration schedule must be determined by the physician for each patient individually.**

▷ **Dosing Instructions:** Preferably taken with 8 ounces of water on an empty stomach (1 hour before or 2 hours after eating). However, it may be taken with food if necessary to reduce stomach irritation. The capsule may be opened and the contents mixed with applesauce or jelly for administration.

Usual Duration of Use: Continual use on a regular schedule for several months is usually necessary to determine this drug's effectiveness in promoting recovery from tuberculosis. Long-term use (possibly 1 to

2 years) requires ongoing supervision and periodic evaluation by your physician. Consult your physician on a regular basis.

▷ **This Drug Should Not Be Taken If**
- you have had an allergic reaction to it previously.
- you have active liver disease.

▷ **Inform Your Physician Before Taking This Drug If**
- you are pregnant.
- you have a history of liver disease or impaired liver function.
- you consume alcohol daily.
- you are taking an oral contraceptive. (An alternate method of contraception is advised.)
- you are taking an anticoagulant.

Possible Side-Effects (natural, expected and unavoidable drug actions)
Red, orange or brown discoloration of tears, sweat, saliva, sputum, urine or stool. Yellow discoloration of the skin (not jaundice). Note: In the absence of symptoms indicating illness, any discoloration is a harmless drug effect and does not indicate toxicity.
Possible fungal superinfections (see Glossary).

▷ **Possible Adverse Effects** (unusual, unexpected and infrequent reactions)
If any of the following develop, consult your physician promptly for guidance.
Mild Adverse Effects
Allergic Reactions: Skin rash, hives, itching, drug fever (see Glossary).
Headache, drowsiness, dizziness, blurred vision, impaired hearing, vague numbness and tingling.
Loss of appetite, heartburn, nausea, vomiting, abdominal cramps, diarrhea.
Serious Adverse Effects
Flulike syndrome: fever, chills, headache, dizziness, musculoskeletal pain, difficult breathing.
Drug-induced liver damage, with or without jaundice.
Drug-induced kidney damage: impaired urine production, bloody or cloudy urine.
Excessively low blood platelet count: abnormal bleeding or bruising.

▷ **Possible Effects on Sexual Function**
Altered timing and pattern of menstruation.
Decreased effectiveness of oral contraceptives taken concurrently.

▷ **Adverse Effects That May Mimic Natural Diseases or Disorders**
Liver reactions may suggest viral hepatitis.
Kidney reactions may suggest an infectious nephritis.

CAUTION
1. This drug may permanently discolor soft contact lenses.
2. This drug may reduce the effectiveness of oral contraceptives; unplanned pregnancy could occur; an alternate method of contraception is advised.

3. When this drug is used alone in the treatment of tuberculosis, bacterial strains that are resistant to this drug can develop rapidly. This drug should only be used in conjunction with other antitubercular drugs.

4. To ensure the best possible response to treatment, take the full course of medication prescribed; this may be for several months or years.

Precautions for Use

By Infants and Children: Monitor closely for possible liver toxicity or deficiency of blood platelets.

By Those over 60 Years of Age: Natural changes in body composition and function make you more susceptible to the adverse effects of this drug. Report promptly any indications of possible drug toxicity.

▷ **Advisability of Use During Pregnancy**

Pregnancy Category: C (tentative). See Pregnancy Code inside back cover.

Animal studies: Cleft palate and spinal defects reported in rodent studies.

Human studies: Information from adequate studies of pregnant women is not available.

If possible, avoid use of drug during the first 3 months.

Advisability of Use if Breast-Feeding

Presence of this drug in breast milk: Yes.

Avoid drug or refrain from nursing.

Habit-Forming Potential: None.

Effects of Overdosage: Nausea, vomiting, drowsiness, unconsciousness, severe liver damage, jaundice.

Possible Effects of Long-Term Use: Superinfections, fungal overgrowth of mouth or tongue.

Suggested Periodic Examinations While Taking This Drug (at physician's discretion)

Complete blood cell counts, liver and kidney function tests.

Hearing acuity tests if hearing loss is suspected.

▷ **While Taking This Drug, Observe the Following**

Foods: No restrictions.

Beverages: No restrictions.

▷ *Alcohol:* It is best to avoid alcohol completely to reduce the risk of potential liver toxicity.

Tobacco Smoking: No interactions expected.

▷ *Other Drugs*

Rifampin may *decrease* the effects of

• anticoagulants (Coumadin, etc.), and reduce their effectiveness.

• beta blockers (see Drug Class, Section Four).

• cortisonelike drugs (see Drug Class, Section Four).

- cyclosporine.
- digitoxin.
- methadone (Dolophine).
- mexiletine (Mexitil).
- oral contraceptives.
- phenytoin (Dilantin).
- progestins.
- quinidine.
- sulfonylureas (see Drug Class, Section Four).
- theophyllines (Aminophyllin, Theo-Dur, etc.).

The following drug may *decrease* the effects of rifampin
- aminosalicylic acid (PAS), and reduce its antitubercular effectiveness.

▷ *Driving, Hazardous Activities:* This drug may cause dizziness, drowsiness, impaired vision and impaired hearing. Restrict activities as necessary.

Aviation Note: The use of this drug *may be a disqualification* for piloting. Consult a designated Aviation Medical Examiner.

Exposure to Sun: No restrictions.

Discontinuation: It is advisable not to interrupt or discontinue this drug without consulting your physician. Intermittent administration can increase the possibility of developing allergic reactions.

SELEGILINE
(se LEDGE i leen)

Other Name: Deprenyl

Introduced: 1981

Class: Antiparkinsonism, monoamine oxidase (MAO) type B inhibitor

Prescription: USA: Yes (Expected to become available in 1989)

Controlled Drug: USA: No

Available as Generic: USA: No

Brand Name: Eldepryl

BENEFITS versus RISKS	
Possible Benefits	*Possible Risks*
ADDITIVE RELIEF OF SYMPTOMS OF PARKINSON'S DISEASE when used concurrently with levodopa/ carbidopa (Sinemet) PERMITS UP TO 30% REDUCTION IN SINEMET DOSAGE with resultant decrease in adverse effects	ABNORMAL INVOLUNTARY MOVEMENTS (12%) HALLUCINATIONS (5.4%) INITIAL FALL IN BLOOD PRESSURE/ORTHOSTATIC HYPOTENSION (1.8%)

▷ **Principal Uses**

As a Single Drug Product: Used solely as an adjunct to levodopa/carbidopa treatment of Parkinson's disease for those individuals who experience intolerable abnormal movements (dyskinesia) and/or increasing "on-off" episodes due to loss of effectiveness of levodopa. The addition of selegiline (1) permits reduction of the daily dose of levodopa (by 25% to 30%) with consequent lessening of dyskinesia and erratic drug response, and (2) provides additional relief of parkinsonian symptoms.

How This Drug Works: By (1) inhibiting monoamine oxidase type B, the enzyme that inactivates dopamine in the brain, and by (2) slowing the restorage of released dopamine at nerve terminals, this drug helps to correct the deficiency of dopamine that is responsible for the rigidity, tremor and sluggish movement characteristic of Parkinson's disease.

Available Dosage Forms and Strengths
Tablets — 5 mg

▷ **Usual Adult Dosage Range**

5 mg once or twice daily. The usual maintenance dose is 5 mg after breakfast and 5 mg after lunch. A total daily dose of 10 mg is adequate to achieve optimal benefit from this drug. Higher doses do not result in further improvement and are not advised.

During the gradual introduction of selegiline, the concurrent dose of levodopa/carbidopa (Sinemet) may be cautiously decreased in accord with your physician's instructions. Concurrent Sinemet dosage should be reduced by 10% to 20% when selegiline is started.

Note: Actual dosage and administration schedule must be determined by the physician for each patient individually.

▷ **Dosing Instructions:** Take with food or milk to reduce stomach irritation. The tablet may be crushed for administration.

Usual Duration of Use: Continual use on a regular schedule for 4 to 6 weeks is usually necessary to determine this drug's effectiveness in controlling the symptoms of Parkinson's disease and permitting reduction of levodopa/carbidopa dosage. Long-term use (months to years) requires periodic evaluation of response and dosage adjustment. Consult your physician on a regular basis.

Possible Advantages of This Drug

It may provide a more effective and uniform control of parkinsonian symptoms and a significant reduction of some adverse effects associated with long-term levodopa therapy. Fifty to 60% of users show improvement.

It does not lose its effectiveness with long-term use.

It does not require avoidance of foods containing tyramine, as is necessary with monoamine oxidase (MAO) type A inhibitors.

It causes no life-threatening or irreversible adverse effects.

▷ **This Drug Should Not Be Taken If**
- you have had an allergic reaction to it previously.
- you have Huntington's disease, hereditary (essential) tremor or tardive dyskinesia (see Glossary).
- you are pregnant or breast-feeding.

▷ **Inform Your Physician Before Taking This Drug If**
- you have constitutionally low blood pressure.
- you have peptic ulcer disease.
- you have a history of heart rhythm disorder.
- you are taking any antihypertensive drugs or antipsychotic drugs (see Drug Classes, Section Four).

Possible Side-Effects (natural, expected and unavoidable drug actions)
Weakness (0.3%), orthostatic hypotension (see Glossary) (1.8%), dry mouth (2%), insomnia (1.5%).

▷ **Possible Adverse Effects** (unusual, unexpected and infrequent reactions)
If any of the following develop, consult your physician promptly for guidance.
Mild Adverse Effects
Headache (0.3%), dizziness (2.2%), agitation (2.5%).
Palpitations (0.2%), fainting (0.1%).
Altered taste (0.1%), nausea and vomiting (7%), stomach pain (0.1%).
Serious Adverse Effects
Dyskinesias: abnormal involuntary movements (12%).
Confusion and hallucinations (5.4%), depression (0.4%), psychosis (0.2%).
Aggravation of peptic ulcer (0.2%), gastrointestinal bleeding (0.2%).

▷ **Possible Effects on Sexual Function:**   None reported.

▷ **Adverse Effects That May Mimic Natural Diseases or Disorders**
Effects on mental function and behavior may resemble psychotic disorders.

▷ **Natural Diseases or Disorders That May Be Activated by This Drug**
Peptic ulcer disease.

CAUTION
1. This drug can initiate dyskinesias and can intensify existing dyskinesias. Observe carefully for the development of tremors, twitching or abnormal, involuntary movements of any kind. Report these promptly.
2. This drug potentiates the effects of levodopa. When this drug is added to current levodopa treatment, adverse effects of levodopa may develop or be intensified. It is necessary to reduce the dose of levodopa by 10% to 20% when treatment with selegiline begins.
3. Inform your physician promptly if you become pregnant or plan pregnancy. The manufacturer does not recommend the use of this drug during pregnancy.

Precautions for Use

By Infants and Children: This drug is not utilized by this age group.

By Those over 60 Years of Age: This drug is well tolerated by the elderly. Observe closely for any tendency to light-headedness or faintness, especially on arising from a lying or sitting position.

▷ **Advisability of Use During Pregnancy**

Pregnancy Category: B (tentative). See Pregnancy Code inside back cover.

Animal studies: No birth defects due to this drug were found in rat studies.

Human studies: Information from adequate studies of pregnant women is not available. The manufacturer advises that this drug should not be taken during pregnancy.

Advisability of Use if Breast-Feeding

Presence of this drug in breast milk: Unknown.

Avoid drug or refrain from nursing.

Habit-Forming Potential: None.

Effects of Overdosage: Nausea, vomiting, palpitations, low blood pressure, agitation, severe involuntary movements, hallucinations.

Possible Effects of Long-Term Use: None reported.

Suggested Periodic Examinations While Taking This Drug (at physician's discretion)

Regular evaluation of drug response, heart function and blood pressure status.

▷ **While Taking This Drug, Observe the Following**

Foods: No restrictions.

Beverages: No restrictions. May be taken with milk.

▷ *Alcohol:* Use caution until the combined effects have been determined. Alcohol may exaggerate the blood-pressure-lowering and sedative effects of this drug.

Tobacco Smoking: No interactions expected.

▷ *Other Drugs*

Selegiline **taken concurrently** with

- antihypertensive drugs (and other drugs that can lower blood pressure) requires careful monitoring for excessive drops in pressure. Dosage adjustments may be necessary.

The following drugs may **decrease** the effects of selegiline and diminish its effectiveness

- chlorprothixene (Taractan).
- haloperidol (Haldol).
- metoclopramide (Reglan).
- phenothiazines (see Drug Class, Section Four).
- reserpine (Ser-Ap-Es, etc.), in high doses.
- thiothixene (Navane).

▷ *Driving, Hazardous Activities:* This drug may cause dizziness, drowsiness, impaired coordination or fainting. Restrict activities as necessary.

Aviation Note: The use of this drug **is a disqualification** for piloting. Consult a designated Aviation Medical Examiner.

Exposure to Sun: No restrictions.

Exposure to Heat: Use caution until the combined effects have been determined. Hot environments can cause lowering of blood pressure.

Discontinuation: Do not discontinue this drug abruptly. Sudden withdrawal can cause prompt increase in parkinsonian symptoms and deterioration of control. Consult your physician regarding a schedule for gradual withdrawal and concurrent adjustment of Sinemet or other appropriate drugs.

SPIRONOLACTONE
(speer on oh LAK tohn)

Introduced: 1959

Class: Diuretic

Prescription: USA: Yes
Canada: Yes

Controlled Drug: USA: No
Canada: No

Available as Generic: USA: Yes
Canada: No

Brand Names: Aldactone, Aldactazide [CD], Alatone, ◆Novospiroton, ◆Novospirozine [CD], ◆Sincomen

---

BENEFITS versus RISKS

Possible Benefits	*Possible Risks*
EFFECTIVE PREVENTION OF POTASSIUM LOSS when used adjunctively with other diuretics	ABNORMALLY HIGH BLOOD POTASSIUM LEVEL with excessive use
EFFECTIVE DIURETIC IN REFRACTORY CASES OF FLUID RETENTION when used adjunctively with other diuretics	Enlargement of male breast tissue Masculinization effects in women: excessive hair growth, deepening of the voice

---

▷ **Principal Uses**

As a Single Drug Product: This mild diuretic is used as part of the treatment program for the management of congestive heart failure and disorders of the liver and kidney that are accompanied by excessive fluid retention (edema). It is also used in conjunction with other measures to treat high blood pressure. It is used primarily in situations where it is advisable to prevent loss of potassium from the body.

As a Combination Drug Product [CD]: This drug is available in combination with hydrochlorothiazide, a different kind of diuretic that promotes the loss of potassium from the body. Spironolactone is used in this combination to counteract the potassium-wasting effect of the thiazide diuretic.

How This Drug Works: Not completely established. It is thought that by inhibiting the action of aldosterone (an adrenal gland hormone), this drug prevents the reabsorption of sodium and the excretion of potassium by the kidney. Thus the drug promotes the excretion of sodium (and water with it) and the retention of potassium.

Available Dosage Forms and Strengths
Tablets — 25 mg, 50 mg, 100 mg

▷ **Usual Adult Dosage Range:**   Initially, 25 to 100 mg/day for 5 days. The dose is then adjusted according to individual response. The usual maintenance dose is 50 to 200 mg/day, divided into 2 to 4 doses. The total daily dosage should not exceed 400 mg. **Note: Actual dosage and administration schedule must be determined by the physician for each patient individually.**

▷ **Dosing Instructions:**   May be taken with or following meals to promote absorption of the drug and to reduce stomach irritation. The tablet may be crushed for administration. Intermittent or alternate day use is recommended to minimize the possibility of sodium and potassium imbalance.

Usual Duration of Use: Continual use on a regular schedule for 5 to 10 days is usually necessary to determine this drug's effectiveness in clearing edema, and for 2 to 3 weeks to determine its effect on hypertension. Long-term use (months to years) requires supervision and periodic evaluation by your physician. Consult your physician on a regular basis.

▷ **This Drug Should Not Be Taken If**
  • you have had an allergic reaction to it previously.
  • you have severely impaired liver or kidney function.

▷ **Inform Your Physician Before Taking This Drug If**
  • you have a history of liver or kidney disease.
  • you have diabetes.
  • you are taking any of the following: an anticoagulant, antihypertensives, a digitalis preparation, another diuretic, lithium or a potassium preparation.
  • you plan to have surgery under general anesthesia in the near future.

Possible Side-Effects (natural, expected and unavoidable drug actions)
Abnormally high blood potassium levels (42%), abnormally low blood sodium levels (12%), dehydration (17%).

▷ **Possible Adverse Effects** (unusual, unexpected and infrequent reactions)
   If any of the following develop, consult your physician promptly for guidance.
   Mild Adverse Effects
   Allergic Reactions: Skin rash, hives, itching, drug fever (see Glossary).
   Headache, dizziness, unsteadiness, weakness, drowsiness, lethargy, confusion.
   Dry mouth, nausea, vomiting, diarrhea.
   Serious Adverse Effects
   Allergic Reaction: Abnormally low blood platelet count (rare).
   Symptomatic potassium excess: confusion, numbness and tingling in lips and extremities, fatigue, weakness, shortness of breath, slow heart rate, low blood pressure.
   Masculine pattern of hair growth and deepening of the voice in women.
   Stomach ulceration with bleeding (rare).

▷ **Possible Effects on Sexual Function**
   Decreased libido (close to 100%); impaired erection or impotence (30%).
   Male breast enlargement and tenderness (close to 100% with high doses).
   Female breast enlargement (100% with high doses); altered timing and pattern of menstruation; postmenopausal bleeding.
   Decreased vaginal secretion.

   CAUTION
   1. Do not take potassium supplements or increase your intake of potassium-rich foods while taking this drug.
   2. Do not discontinue this drug abruptly unless abnormally high blood levels of potassium develop.
   3. Ordinary doses of aspirin (600 mg) may reverse the diuretic effect of this drug. Observe response to this drug combination.
   4. Avoid the excessive use of salt substitutes that contain potassium; these are a potential cause of potassium excess.

Precautions for Use
   By Infants and Children: Limit the continual use of this drug in children to 1 month. Observe closely for indications of potassium accumulation.
   By Those over 60 Years of Age: The natural decline in kidney function may predispose to potassium retention in the body. Limit continual use of this drug to periods of 2 to 3 weeks. Observe for indications of potassium excess: slow heart rate, irregular heart rhythms, low blood pressure, confusion, drowsiness. The excessive use of diuretics can cause harmful loss of body water (dehydration), increased viscosity of the blood and an increased tendency of the blood to clot, predisposing to stroke, heart attack or thrombophlebitis.

▷ **Advisability of Use During Pregnancy**
   Pregnancy Category: D (tentative). See Pregnancy Code inside back cover.
   Animal studies: This drug causes feminization of male rat fetuses.

Human studies: Information from adequate studies of pregnant women is not available.

This drug should not be used during pregnancy unless a very serious complication of pregnancy occurs for which this drug is significantly beneficial.

Advisability of Use if Breast-Feeding

Presence of this drug in breast milk: A metabolic by-product (canrenone) is present.

Avoid drug or refrain from nursing.

Habit-Forming Potential: None.

Effects of Overdosage: Thirst, drowsiness, fatigue, weakness, nausea, vomiting, confusion, irregular heart rhythm, low blood pressure.

Possible Effects of Long-Term Use: Potassium accumulation to abnormally high blood levels. Male breast enlargement.

Suggested Periodic Examinations While Taking This Drug (at physician's discretion)

Measurements of blood sodium, potassium and chloride levels.

Kidney function tests.

▷ **While Taking This Drug, Observe the Following**

Foods: No restrictions. Avoid excessive restriction of salt.

Beverages: No restrictions. May be taken with milk.

▷   *Alcohol:* Use with caution until the combined effects have been determined. Alcohol may enhance the drowsiness and the blood-pressure-lowering effect of this drug.

Tobacco Smoking: No interactions expected.

▷   *Other Drugs*

Spironolactone may *increase* the effects of
- digoxin (Lanoxin).

Spironolactone may *decrease* the effects of
- anticoagulants (Coumadin, etc.).

Spironolactone *taken concurrently* with
- captopril (Capoten) may cause excessively high blood potassium levels.
- digitoxin (Crystodigin) may cause either increased or decreased digitoxin effects (unpredictable).
- lithium may cause accumulation of lithium to toxic levels.
- potassium preparations may cause excessively high blood potassium levels.

The following drugs may *decrease* the effects of spironolactone
- aspirin may reduce its diuretic effectiveness.

▷   *Driving, Hazardous Activities:* This drug may cause dizziness and drowsiness. Restrict activities as necessary.

Aviation Note: The use of this drug *may be a disqualification* for piloting. Consult a designated Aviation Medical Examiner.

Exposure to Sun: No restrictions.

Discontinuation: With high dosage or prolonged use, it is advisable to withdraw this drug gradually. Ask your physician for guidance.

SUCRALFATE
(soo KRAL fayt)

Introduced: 1978

Class: Antiulcer

Prescription: USA: Yes
   Canada: Yes

Controlled Drug: USA: No
   Canada: No

Available as Generic: No

Brand Names: Carafate, ✦Sulcrate

BENEFITS versus RISKS	
Possible Benefits	*Possible Risks*
EFFECTIVE TREATMENT IN PEPTIC ULCER DISEASE	Constipation
No serious adverse effects	Skin rash, hives, itching
No significant drug interactions	

▷ **Principal Uses**

As a Single Drug Product: Used exclusively in the management of peptic ulcer disease to promote healing of both stomach (gastric) and duodenal ulcer. It is effective when used alone, but may be used in conjunction with antacids when these are needed for pain relief.

How This Drug Works: Not completely established. It is thought that this drug promotes ulcer healing by several mechanisms: (1) the formation of a protective coating over the ulcer site to prevent further erosion by stomach acid; (2) the inhibition of the digestive action of pepsin; (3) the protection of injured tissue at the ulcer margins; (4) the stimulation of active healing (tissue repair).

Available Dosage Forms and Strengths
   Tablets — 0.5 gram, 1 gram

▷ **Usual Adult Dosage Range:** 1 gram 4 times/day. **Note: Actual dosage and administration schedule must be determined by the physician for each patient individually.**

▷ **Dosing Instructions:** Take with water on an empty stomach at least 1 hour before or 2 hours after each meal and at bedtime. Swallow the tablets whole; do not alter or chew. Take the full course prescribed.

Usual Duration of Use: Continual use on a regular schedule for 6 to 8 weeks is usually necessary to determine this drug's effectiveness in promoting the healing of peptic ulcers. Use beyond 8 weeks must be determined by your physician.

▷ **This Drug Should Not Be Taken If**
   • you have had an allergic reaction to it previously.

▷ **Inform Your Physician Before Taking This Drug If**
   • you have chronic constipation.
   • you are taking any other drugs at this time.

Possible Side-Effects (natural, expected and unavoidable drug actions)
   Constipation (2.2%).

▷ **Possible Adverse Effects** (unusual, unexpected and infrequent reactions)
   If any of the following develop, consult your physician promptly for guidance.
   Mild Adverse Effects
   Allergic Reactions: Skin rash, hives, itching.
   Dizziness, light-headedness, drowsiness.
   Dry mouth, indigestion, nausea, cramping, diarrhea.
   Serious Adverse Effects
   None reported.

▷ **Possible Effects on Sexual Function:**   None reported.

   CAUTION
   1. If antacids are needed to relieve ulcer pain, do not take them within half an hour before or 1 hour after the dose of sucralfate.
   2. This drug may impair the absorption of other drugs if they are taken close together. It is advisable to avoid taking any other drugs within 2 hours of taking sucralfate. This applies especially to cimetidine (Tagamet), phenytoin (Dilantin) and tetracyclines.

▷ **Advisability of Use During Pregnancy**
   Pregnancy Category: B (tentative). See Pregnancy Code inside back cover.
   Animal studies: No birth defects due to this drug reported in mouse, rat and rabbit studies.
   Human studies: Information from adequate studies of pregnant women is not available.
   Because only very small amounts of this drug are absorbed, it is probably safe for use at any time during pregnancy. However, it should be used only if clearly needed. Ask your physician for guidance.

Advisability of Use if Breast-Feeding
   Presence of this drug in breast milk: Unknown.
   Monitor nursing infant closely and discontinue drug or nursing if adverse effects develop.

Habit-Forming Potential: None.

Effects of Overdosage: Nausea, stomach cramping, possible diarrhea.

Possible Effects of Long-Term Use: Deficiencies of vitamins A, D, E and K due to impaired absorption from the intestine.

Suggested Periodic Examinations While Taking This Drug (at physician's discretion)
None required.

▷ **While Taking This Drug, Observe the Following**
Foods: No restrictions. Follow diet prescribed by your physician.
Beverages: No restrictions. This drug is preferably taken with water.
▷ *Alcohol:* No interactions with drug expected. However, alcohol is best avoided because of its irritant effect on the stomach.
Tobacco Smoking: No interactions expected. However, nicotine can delay ulcer healing and reduce the effectiveness of this drug. Avoid all forms of tobacco.
▷ *Other Drugs*
Sucralfate may *decrease* the effects of
- cimetidine (Tagamet).
- digoxin (Lanoxin).
- phenytoin (Dilantin, etc.).
- tetracycline (Achromycin, Tetracyn, etc.).
- warfarin (Coumadin, etc.), and reduce its effectiveness as an anti-coagulant.
▷ *Driving, Hazardous Activities:* This drug may cause dizziness or drowsiness. Restrict activities as necessary.
Aviation Note: The use of this drug *may be a disqualification* for piloting. Consult a designated Aviation Medical Examiner.
Exposure to Sun: No restrictions.

SULFAMETHOXAZOLE
(sul fa meth OX a zohl)

Introduced: 1961   **Class:** Anti-infective, sulfonamides

Prescription: USA: Yes   **Controlled Drug:** USA: No
Canada: Yes   Canada: No

Available as Generic: Yes

Brand Names: ✦Apo-Sulfamethoxazole, ✦Apo-Sulfatrim [CD], ✦Apo-Sulfatrim DS [CD], Azo Gantanol [CD], Bactrim [CD], Bactrim DS [CD], Bethaprim [CD], Comoxol [CD], Cotrim [CD], Gantanol, ✦Novotrimel [CD], ✦Novotrimel DS [CD], ✦Protrin [CD], ✦Protrin DF [CD], ✦Roubac [CD], Septra [CD], Septra DS [CD], ✦Uro Gantanol [CD], Uroplus DS [CD], Uroplus SS [CD]

BENEFITS versus RISKS

Possible Benefits	*Possible Risks*
EFFECTIVE ANTIMICROBIAL ACTION against susceptible bacteria and protozoa	Allergic reactions: mild to severe skin reactions, anaphylaxis, myocarditis
	Rare blood cell disorders: aplastic anemia, hemolytic anemia, abnormally low white cell and platelet counts
	Drug-induced liver damage
	Drug-induced kidney damage

▷ **Principal Uses**

As a Single Drug Product: This member of the sulfonamide class is used to treat a variety of bacterial and protozoal infections. It is most commonly used to treat certain infections of the urinary tract.

As a Combination Drug Product [CD]: This drug is available in combination with phenazopyridine, an analgesic drug that relieves the discomfort associated with acute infections of the urinary bladder and urethra. This combination provides early symptomatic relief while the underlying infection is being eradicated. This drug is also available in combination with another antibacterial drug—trimethoprim. This combination is quite effective in the treatment of certain types of middle ear infection, bronchitis, pneumonia and certain infections of the intestinal tract and the urinary tract.

How This Drug Works: This drug prevents the growth and multiplication of susceptible bacteria by interfering with their formation of folic acid, an essential nutrient.

Available Dosage Forms and Strengths

Oral suspension — 500 mg per 5-ml teaspoonful

Tablets — 500 mg, 1 gram

▷ **Usual Adult Dosage Range:** Initially, 2 grams; then 1 gram every 8 to 12 hours, depending upon the severity of the infection. The total daily dosage should not exceed 3 grams. **Note: Actual dosage and administration schedule must be determined by the physician for each patient individually.**

▷ **Dosing Instructions:** Preferably taken on an empty stomach, 1 hour before or 2 hours after eating. However, it may be taken with or following food to reduce stomach irritation. The tablet may be crushed for administration.

Usual Duration of Use: Continual use on a regular schedule for 4 to 7 days is usually necessary to determine this drug's effectiveness in controlling responsive infections. Treatment should be continued until the patient is free of symptoms for 48 hours. Limit treatment to no more than 14 days if possible.

Currently a "Drug of Choice" (when combined with trimethoprim) for preventing pneumonia (due to pneumocystis carinii) in patients with AIDS.

▷ **This Drug Should Not Be Taken If**
- you are allergic to *any* sulfonamide drug (see Drug Class, Section Four).
- you are in the last month of pregnancy.
- you are breast-feeding.

▷ **Inform Your Physician Before Taking This Drug If**
- you are allergic to any sulfonamide derivative: acetazolamide, thiazide diuretics, sulfonylurea antidiabetic drugs (see Drug Classes, Section Four).
- you are allergic by nature: history of hay fever, asthma, hives, eczema.
- you have impaired liver or kidney function.
- you have a personal or family history of porphyria.
- you have had a drug-induced blood cell or bone marrow disorder in the past.
- you are currently taking any oral anticoagulant, antidiabetic drug or phenytoin.
- you plan to have surgery under pentothal anesthesia while taking this drug.

Possible Side-Effects (natural, expected and unavoidable drug actions)
Brownish coloration of the urine, of no significance.
Superinfections, bacterial or fungal (see Glossary).

▷ **Possible Adverse Effects** (unusual, unexpected and infrequent reactions)
If any of the following develop, consult your physician promptly for guidance.
Mild Adverse Effects
Allergic Reactions: Skin rashes, hives, itching, localized swellings, reddened eyes.
Headache, dizziness, unsteadiness, ringing in the ears.
Loss of appetite, irritation of the mouth and tongue, nausea, vomiting, abdominal pain, diarrhea.
Serious Adverse Effects
Allergic Reactions: Drug fever (see Glossary), swollen glands, painful joints, anaphylaxis (see Glossary). Allergic reaction in the heart muscle (myocarditis), allergic pneumonitis, allergic hepatitis. Severe skin reactions.
Idiosyncratic Reaction: Hemolytic anemia (see Glossary).
Bone marrow depression (see Glossary): fatigue, weakness, fever, sore throat, abnormal bleeding or bruising.

Pancreatitis; kidney damage: bloody or cloudy urine, reduced urine volume.

Psychotic reactions, hallucinations, seizures, hearing loss, peripheral neuropathy (see Glossary).

▷ **Possible Effects on Sexual Function:** None reported.

▷ **Adverse Effects That May Mimic Natural Diseases or Disorders**

Liver reactions may suggest viral hepatitis.

Lung reactions may suggest an infectious pneumonia.

Natural Diseases or Disorders That May Be Activated by This Drug

Goiter, acute intermittent porphyria, polyarteritis nodosa, systemic lupus erythematosus (questionable).

CAUTION

1. A large intake of water (up to 2 quarts daily) is necessary to ensure an adequate volume of urine.
2. Shake liquid dosage forms thoroughly before measuring each dose.

Precautions for Use

By Infants and Children: This drug should not be used in infants under 2 months of age.

By Those over 60 Years of Age: Small doses taken at longer intervals often achieve adequate blood and tissue drug levels. Observe for the development of reduced urine volume, fever, sore throat, abnormal bleeding or bruising or skin irritation with itching, particularly in the anal or genital regions.

▷ **Advisability of Use During Pregnancy**

Pregnancy Category: C (tentative). See Pregnancy Code inside back cover.

Animal studies: Cleft palate and skeletal birth defects reported in mice and rats.

Human studies: No increase in birth defects reported in 4584 exposures to various sulfonamides during pregnancy.

Avoid use of drug during the last month of pregnancy because of possible adverse effects on the newborn infant.

Advisability of Use if Breast-Feeding

Presence of this drug in breast milk: Yes.

Avoid drug or refrain from nursing.

Habit-Forming Potential: None.

Effects of Overdosage: Headache, dizziness, nausea, vomiting, abdominal cramping, toxic fever, coma, jaundice, kidney failure.

Possible Effects of Long-Term Use: Superinfections, bacterial or fungal. Development of goiter, with or without hypothyroidism. Excessive loss of vitamin C via urine.

Suggested Periodic Examinations While Taking This Drug (at physician's discretion)

Complete blood cell counts, weekly for the first 8 weeks.

Urine analysis weekly.

Liver and kidney function tests.

▷ **While Taking This Drug, Observe the Following**

Foods: No restrictions.

Beverages: No restrictions. May be taken with milk.

▷ *Alcohol:* Use caution until the combined effect has been determined. Sulfonamide drugs can increase the intoxicating effects of alcohol.

Tobacco Smoking: No interactions expected.

▷ *Other Drugs*

Sulfamethoxazole may *increase* the effects of

• anticoagulants (Coumadin, etc.), and increase the risk of bleeding.

• sulfonylureas (see Drug Class, Section Four), and increase the risk of hypoglycemia.

Sulfamethoxazole may *decrease* the effects of

• cyclosporine, and reduce its immunosuppressive effect.

• penicillins.

▷ *Driving, Hazardous Activities:* This drug may cause dizziness. Restrict activities as necessary.

Aviation Note: The use of this drug **may be a disqualification** for piloting. Consult a designated Aviation Medical Examiner.

Exposure to Sun: Use caution until sensitivity has been determined. Some sulfonamide drugs can cause photosensitivity (see Glossary).

SULFASALAZINE
(sul fa SAL a zeen)

Introduced: 1949

Class: Bowel anti-inflammatory, sulfonamides

Prescription: USA: Yes
Canada: Yes

Controlled Drug: USA: No
Canada: No

Available as Generic: USA: Yes
Canada: No

Brand Names: Azaline, Azulfidine, Azulfidine EN-tabs, ✦PMS Sulfasalazine, ✦PMS Sulfasalazine E.C., ✦Salazopyrin, ✦SAS-Enema, ✦SAS Enteric-500, SAS-500

```
+----------------------------------------------------------------------+
|                      BENEFITS versus RISKS                           |
|                                                                      |
|       Possible Benefits                  Possible Risks              |
|   EFFECTIVE SUPPRESSION OF       Allergic reactions: mild to severe   |
|      INFLAMMATORY BOWEL             skin reactions                   |
|      DISEASE                     Rare blood cell disorders: aplastic  |
|   SYMPTOMATIC RELIEF IN             anemia, hemolytic anemia,         |
|      TREATMENT OF REGIONAL          abnormally low white cell and     |
|      ENTERITIS AND ULCERATIVE       platelet counts                  |
|      COLITIS                     Drug-induced liver damage            |
|                                  Drug-induced kidney damage           |
+----------------------------------------------------------------------+
```

▷ **Principal Uses**

As a Single Drug Product: This member of the sulfonamide class is used exclusively to treat inflammatory disease of the lower intestinal tract: regional enteritis (Crohn's disease) and ulcerative colitis. It is usually taken by mouth, but may also be used in retention enemas.

How This Drug Works: Not completely established. Possible methods of this drug's action include

- an anti-inflammatory action that suppresses the formation of prostaglandins (and related compounds), tissue substances that induce inflammation, tissue destruction and diarrhea.
- an anti-infective action that may prevent the growth and multiplication of certain infective agents in the intestine and colon. (This method of action is questionable.)

Available Dosage Forms and Strengths

Oral suspension — 250 mg per 5-ml teaspoonful

Tablets — 500 mg

Tablets, enteric-coated — 500 mg

▷ **Usual Adult Dosage Range:** Initially, 1 to 2 grams every 6 to 8 hours until symptoms are adequately controlled. For maintenance, 500 mg/6 hours. The total daily dosage should not exceed 12 grams. **Note: Actual dosage and administration schedule must be determined by the physician for each patient individually.**

▷ **Dosing Instructions:** Preferably taken with 8 ounces of water on an empty stomach, 1 hour before or 2 hours after eating. However, it may be taken with or following food to reduce stomach irritation. Intervals between doses (day and night) should be no longer than 8 hours. The regular tablet may be crushed for administration; the enteric-coated tablet should be swallowed whole without alteration.

Usual Duration of Use: Continual use on a regular schedule for 1 to 3 weeks is usually necessary to determine this drug's effectiveness in controlling the symptoms of regional enteritis or ulcerative colitis. Long-term use (months to years) requires supervision and periodic evaluation by your physician. Consult your physician on a regular basis.

▷ **This Drug Should Not Be Taken If**
- you are allergic to *any* sulfonamide drug (see Drug Class, Section Four), or to aspirin (or other salicylates).
- you are in the last month of pregnancy.
- you are breast-feeding.

▷ **Inform Your Physician Before Taking This Drug If**
- you are allergic to any sulfonamide derivative: acetazolamide, thiazide diuretics, sulfonylurea antidiabetic drugs (see Drug Classes, Section Four).
- you are allergic by nature: history of hay fever, asthma, hives, eczema.
- you have impaired liver or kidney function.
- you have a personal or family history of porphyria.
- you have had a drug-induced blood cell or bone marrow disorder in the past.
- you are currently taking any oral anticoagulant, antidiabetic drug or phenytoin.
- you plan to have surgery under pentothal anesthesia while taking this drug.

Possible Side-Effects (natural, expected and unavoidable drug actions)
Brownish coloration of the urine, of no significance.
Superinfections, bacterial or fungal (see Glossary).

▷ **Possible Adverse Effects** (unusual, unexpected and infrequent reactions)
If any of the following develop, consult your physician promptly for guidance.
Mild Adverse Effects
Allergic Reactions: Skin rashes, hives, itching.
Headache, dizziness.
Loss of appetite, irritation of the mouth and tongue, nausea, vomiting, abdominal pain, diarrhea.
Serious Adverse Effects
Allergic Reactions: Drug fever (see Glossary), swollen glands, painful joints, anaphylaxis (see Glossary). Allergic pneumonitis, allergic hepatitis. Severe skin reactions.
Idiosyncratic Reaction: Hemolytic anemia (see Glossary).
Bone marrow depression (see Glossary): fatigue, weakness, fever, sore throat, abnormal bleeding or bruising.
Pancreatitis; kidney damage: bloody or cloudy urine, reduced urine volume.
Peripheral neuropathy (see Glossary).

▷ **Possible Effects on Sexual Function:**   Decreased production of sperm, reversible infertility.

▷ **Adverse Effects That May Mimic Natural Diseases or Disorders**
Liver reactions may suggest viral hepatitis.
Lung reactions may suggest an infectious pneumonia.

Natural Diseases or Disorders That May Be Activated by This Drug
Goiter, acute intermittent porphyria.

CAUTION
1. A large intake of water (up to 2 quarts daily) is necessary to ensure an adequate volume of urine.
2. Shake liquid dosage forms thoroughly before measuring each dose.

Precautions for Use
By Infants and Children: Safety and effectiveness for use by those under 2 years of age have not been established.
By Those over 60 Years of Age: Observe for the development of reduced urine volume, fever, sore throat, abnormal bleeding or bruising or skin irritation with itching, particularly in the anal or genital regions.

▷ **Advisability of Use During Pregnancy**
Pregnancy Category: C (tentative). See Pregnancy Code inside back cover.
Animal studies: Cleft palate and skeletal birth defects due to sulfonamides reported in mice and rats.
Human studies: No increase in birth defects reported in 4584 exposures to various sulfonamides during pregnancy.
Avoid use of drug during the last month of pregnancy because of possible adverse effects on the newborn infant.

Advisability of Use if Breast-Feeding
Presence of this drug in breast milk: Yes.
Avoid drug or refrain from nursing.

Habit-Forming Potential: None.

Effects of Overdosage: Headache, dizziness, nausea, vomiting, abdominal cramping, toxic fever, coma, jaundice, kidney failure.

Possible Effects of Long-Term Use: Development of goiter, with or without hypothyroidism. An orange-yellow discoloration of the skin has been reported. This is not jaundice.

Suggested Periodic Examinations While Taking This Drug (at physician's discretion)
Complete blood cell counts, weekly for the first 8 weeks.
Urine analysis weekly.
Liver and kidney function tests.

▷ **While Taking This Drug, Observe the Following**
Foods: No restrictions. Follow prescribed diet.
Beverages: No restrictions. May be taken with milk.
▷ *Alcohol:* Use caution until the combined effect has been determined. Sulfonamide drugs can increase the intoxicating effects of alcohol.

Tobacco Smoking: No interactions expected.

▷ *Other Drugs*

Sulfasalazine may ***increase*** the effects of
- anticoagulants (Coumadin, etc.), and increase the risk of bleeding.
- sulfonylureas (see Drug Class, Section Four), and increase the risk of hypoglycemia.

Sulfasalazine may ***decrease*** the effects of
- digoxin (Lanoxin).

▷ *Driving, Hazardous Activities:* This drug may cause dizziness. Restrict activities as necessary.

Aviation Note: The use of this drug ***may be a disqualification*** for piloting. Consult a designated Aviation Medical Examiner.

Exposure to Sun: Use caution until sensitivity has been determined. Some sulfonamide drugs can cause photosensitivity (see Glossary).

SULFISOXAZOLE
(sul fi SOX a zohl)

Introduced: 1949

Class: Anti-infective, sulfonamides

Prescription: USA: Yes
   Canada: Yes

Controlled Drug: USA: No
   Canada: No

Available as Generic: Yes

Brand Names: ✦Apo-Sulfisoxazole, Azo Gantrisin [CD], Gantrisin, Lipo Gantrisin, ✦Novosoxazole, Pediazole [CD]

BENEFITS versus RISKS

Possible Benefits	*Possible Risks*
EFFECTIVE ANTIMICROBIAL ACTION against susceptible bacteria and protozoa	Allergic reactions: mild to severe skin reactions, anaphylaxis
	Rare blood cell disorders: aplastic anemia, hemolytic anemia, abnormally low white cell and platelet counts
	Drug-induced liver damage
	Drug-induced kidney damage

▷ **Principal Uses**

As a Single Drug Product: This member of the sulfonamide class is used to treat a variety of bacterial and protozoal infections. It is most commonly used to treat certain infections of the urinary tract.

As a Combination Drug Product [CD]: This drug is available in combination with phenazopyridine, an analgesic drug that relieves the discomfort associated with acute infections of the urinary bladder and urethra. This combination provides early symptomatic relief while the underlying infection is being eradicated.

How This Drug Works: This drug prevents the growth and multiplication of susceptible bacteria by interfering with their formation of folic acid, an essential nutrient.

Available Dosage Forms and Strengths

Emulsion, prolonged-action — 1 gram per 5-ml teaspoonful
Eye drops — 4%
Eye ointment — 4%
Injection — 400 mg per ml
Pediatric suspension — 500 mg per 5-ml teaspoonful
Syrup — 500 mg per 5-ml teaspoonful
Tablets — 500 mg

▷ **Usual Adult Dosage Range:**   Initially, 2 to 4 grams; then 750 to 1500 mg (1.5 grams) every 4 hours, or 1 to 2 grams every 6 hours, depending upon the severity of the infection. The total daily dosage should not exceed 12 grams. **Note: Actual dosage and administration schedule must be determined by the physician for each patient individually.**

▷ **Dosing Instructions:**   Preferably taken with 8 ounces of water on an empty stomach, 1 hour before or 2 hours after eating. However, it may be taken with or following food to reduce stomach irritation. The tablet may be crushed for administration.

Usual Duration of Use: Continual use on a regular schedule for 7 to 10 days is usually necessary to determine this drug's effectiveness in controlling responsive infections. Treatment should be continued until the patient is free of symptoms for 48 hours. Limit treatment to no more than 14 days if possible.

▷ **This Drug Should Not Be Taken If**
- you are allergic to *any* sulfonamide drug (see Drug Class, Section Four).
- you are in the last month of pregnancy.
- you are breast-feeding.

▷ **Inform Your Physician Before Taking This Drug If**
- you are allergic to any sulfonamide derivative: acetazolamide, thiazide diuretics, sulfonylurea antidiabetic drugs (see Drug Classes, Section Four).
- you are allergic by nature: history of hay fever, asthma, hives, eczema.
- you have impaired liver or kidney function.
- you have a personal or family history of porphyria.

- you have had a drug-induced blood cell or bone marrow disorder in the past.
- you are currently taking any oral anticoagulant, antidiabetic drug or phenytoin.
- you plan to have surgery under pentothal anesthesia while taking this drug.

Possible Side-Effects (natural, expected and unavoidable drug actions)
Brownish coloration of the urine, of no significance.
Superinfections, bacterial or fungal (see Glossary).

▷ **Possible Adverse Effects** (unusual, unexpected and infrequent reactions)
If any of the following develop, consult your physician promptly for guidance.
Mild Adverse Effects
Allergic Reactions: Skin rashes, hives, itching, localized swellings, reddened eyes.
Headache, dizziness, unsteadiness, ringing in the ears.
Loss of appetite, irritation of the mouth and tongue, nausea, vomiting, abdominal pain, diarrhea.
Serious Adverse Effects
Allergic Reactions: Drug fever (see Glossary), swollen glands, painful joints, anaphylaxis (see Glossary). Allergic hepatitis. Severe skin reactions.
Idiosyncratic Reaction: Hemolytic anemia (see Glossary).
Bone marrow depression (see Glossary): fatigue, weakness, fever, sore throat, abnormal bleeding or bruising.
Kidney damage: bloody or cloudy urine, reduced urine volume.
Peripheral neuropathy (see Glossary).

▷ **Possible Effects on Sexual Function:**   None reported.

▷ **Adverse Effects That May Mimic Natural Diseases or Disorders**
Liver reactions may suggest viral hepatitis.

Natural Diseases or Disorders That May Be Activated by This Drug
Goiter, acute intermittent porphyria.

CAUTION
1. A large intake of water (up to 2 quarts daily) is necessary to ensure an adequate volume of urine.
2. Shake liquid dosage forms thoroughly before measuring each dose.

Precautions for Use
By Infants and Children: This drug should not be used in infants under 2 months of age.
By Those over 60 Years of Age: Small doses taken at longer intervals often achieve adequate blood and tissue drug levels. Observe for the development of reduced urine volume, fever, sore throat, abnormal bleeding or bruising or skin irritation with itching, particularly in the anal or genital regions.

▷ **Advisability of Use During Pregnancy**
  Pregnancy Category: C (tentative). See Pregnancy Code inside back cover.
    Animal studies: Cleft palate and skeletal birth defects due to sulfonamides reported in mice and rats.
    Human studies: No increase in birth defects reported in 4287 exposures
      to this drug during pregnancy.
    Avoid use of drug during the last month of pregnancy because of possible adverse effects on the newborn infant.

Advisability of Use if Breast-Feeding
  Presence of this drug in breast milk: Yes.
  Avoid drug or refrain from nursing.

Habit-Forming Potential: None.

Effects of Overdosage: Headache, dizziness, nausea, vomiting, abdominal
  cramping, toxic fever, coma, jaundice, kidney failure.

Possible Effects of Long-Term Use: Superinfections, bacterial or fungal.
  Development of goiter, with or without hypothyroidism. Excessive
  loss of vitamin C via urine.

Suggested Periodic Examinations While Taking This Drug (at physician's
  discretion)
  Complete blood cell counts, weekly for the first 8 weeks.
  Urine analysis weekly.
  Liver and kidney function tests.

▷ **While Taking This Drug, Observe the Following**
  Foods: No restrictions.
  Beverages: No restrictions. May be taken with milk.
▷ *Alcohol:* Use caution until the combined effect has been determined. Sulfonamide drugs can increase the intoxicating effects of alcohol.
  Tobacco Smoking: No interactions expected.
▷ *Other Drugs*
    Sulfisoxazole may *increase* the effects of
    • anticoagulants (Coumadin, etc.), and increase the risk of bleeding.
    • sulfonylureas (see Drug Class, Section Four), and increase the risk of
      hypoglycemia.
    Sulfisoxazole may *decrease* the effects of
    • penicillins.
▷ *Driving, Hazardous Activities:* This drug may cause dizziness. Restrict activities as necessary.
  Aviation Note: The use of this drug *may be a disqualification* for piloting.
      Consult a designated Aviation Medical Examiner.
  Exposure to Sun: Use caution until sensitivity has been determined. Some
      sulfonamide drugs can cause photosensitivity (see Glossary).

SULINDAC
(sul IN dak)

Introduced: 1976

Class: Mild analgesic, anti-
inflammatory

Prescription: USA: Yes
Canada: Yes

Controlled Drug: USA: No
Canada: No

Available as Generic: No

Brand Name: Clinoril

BENEFITS versus RISKS

Possible Benefits	*Possible Risks*
EFFECTIVE RELIEF OF MILD TO MODERATE PAIN AND INFLAMMATION	Gastrointestinal pain, ulceration, bleeding (rare) Rare liver damage Rare kidney damage Rare bone marrow depression (aplastic anemia)

▷ **Principal Uses**

As a Single Drug Product: Used primarily to relieve mild to moderately severe pain associated with (1) rheumatoid arthritis and osteoarthritis; (2) acute and chronic gout; and (3) bursitis, tendinitis and related disorders.

How This Drug Works: Not completely established. It is thought that this drug reduces the tissue concentrations of prostaglandins (and related compounds), substances involved in the production of inflammation and pain.

Available Dosage Forms and Strengths
Tablets — 150 mg, 200 mg

▷ **Usual Adult Dosage Range:** 150 to 200 mg twice/day, 12 hours apart. The total daily dosage should not exceed 400 mg. **Note: Actual dosage and administration schedule must be determined by the physician for each patient individually.**

▷ **Dosing Instructions:** Preferably taken on an empty stomach, 1 hour before or 2 hours after eating. However, it may be taken with or after food if necessary to reduce stomach irritation. Take with a full glass of water and remain upright (do not lie down) for 30 minutes. The tablet may be crushed for administration.

Usual Duration of Use: Continual use on a regular schedule for 2 to 3 weeks is usually necessary to determine this drug's effectiveness in

relieving the discomfort of arthritis. Acute gout usually responds within 7 days. Shoulder bursitis or tendinitis usually responds within 7 to 14 days. Long-term use (months to years) requires supervision and periodic evaluation by your physician. Consult your physician on a regular basis.

▷ **This Drug Should Not Be Taken If**
- you have had an allergic reaction to it previously.
- you are subject to asthma or nasal polyps caused by aspirin.
- you have active peptic ulcer disease or any form of gastrointestinal bleeding.
- you have a bleeding disorder or a blood cell disorder.
- you have severe impairment of liver or kidney function.

▷ **Inform Your Physician Before Taking This Drug If**
- you are allergic to aspirin or to other aspirin substitutes.
- you have a history of peptic ulcer disease or any type of bleeding disorder.
- you have impaired liver or kidney function.
- you have high blood pressure or a history of heart failure.
- you are taking any of the following: acetaminophen, aspirin or other aspirin substitutes, anticoagulants, oral antidiabetic drugs.

Possible Side-Effects (natural, expected and unavoidable drug actions)
Fluid retention (edema).
Drowsiness in sensitive individuals.

▷ **Possible Adverse Effects** (unusual, unexpected and infrequent reactions)
If any of the following develop, consult your physician promptly for guidance.
Mild Adverse Effects
Allergic Reactions: Skin rash, hives, itching.
Headache, dizziness, mild numbness and tingling, blurred vision, ringing in the ears.
Mouth sores, indigestion, nausea, vomiting, constipation, diarrhea.
Serious Adverse Effects
Allergic Reactions: Anaphylactic reaction (see Glossary), severe skin reactions.
Idiosyncratic Reactions: Drug-induced pneumonitis with fever.
Active peptic ulcer, with or without bleeding.
Liver damage with jaundice (see Glossary).
Kidney damage with painful urination, bloody urine, reduced urine formation.
Rare bone marrow depression (see Glossary): fatigue, weakness, fever, sore throat, abnormal bleeding or bruising.

▷ **Possible Effects on Sexual Function**
Vaginal bleeding (less than 1%).
Male breast enlargement (causal relationship not established).

Possible Delayed Adverse Effects: Mild anemia due to "silent" blood loss from the stomach (less than that caused by aspirin).

▷ **Adverse Effects That May Mimic Natural Diseases or Disorders**
Liver reaction may suggest viral hepatitis.

Natural Diseases or Disorders That May Be Activated by This Drug
Peptic ulcer disease, ulcerative colitis.

CAUTION
1. Dosage should always be limited to the smallest amount that produces reasonable improvement.
2. This drug may mask early indications of infection. Inform your physician if you think you are developing an infection of any kind.

Precautions for Use
By Infants and Children: Safety and effectiveness for use by those under 12 years of age have not been established.
By Those over 60 Years of Age: Small doses are advisable until tolerance is determined. Observe for any indications of liver or kidney toxicity, fluid retention, dizziness, confusion, impaired memory, stomach bleeding or constipation.

▷ **Advisability of Use During Pregnancy**
Pregnancy Category: C (tentative). See Pregnancy Code inside back cover.
  Animal studies: A low incidence of birth defects has been reported but not confirmed.
  Human studies: Information from adequate studies of pregnant women is not available.
  The manufacturer does not recommend the use of this drug during pregnancy.

Advisability of Use if Breast-Feeding
Presence of this drug in breast milk: Unknown.
Avoid drug or refrain from nursing.

Habit-Forming Potential: None.

Effects of Overdosage: Stomach irritation, nausea, vomiting, diarrhea.

Possible Effects of Long-Term Use: Fluid retention.

Suggested Periodic Examinations While Taking This Drug (at physician's discretion)
  Complete blood cell counts, liver and kidney function tests, complete eye examinations if vision is altered in any way.

▷ **While Taking This Drug, Observe the Following**
Foods: No restrictions.
Beverages: No restrictions. May be taken with milk.

▷ *Alcohol:* Use with caution. The irritant action of alcohol on the stomach lining, added to the irritant action of this drug in sensitive individuals, can increase the risk of stomach ulceration and/or bleeding.

Tobacco Smoking: No interactions expected.

▷ *Other Drugs*

Sulindac may **increase** the effects of

- acetaminophen (Tylenol, etc.), and increase the risk of kidney damage; avoid prolonged use of this combination.
- anticoagulants (Coumadin, etc.), and increase the risk of bleeding; monitor prothrombin time, adjust dose accordingly.

Sulindac **taken concurrently** with the following drugs may increase the risk of bleeding; avoid these combinations:

- aspirin.
- dipyridamole (Persantine).
- indomethacin (Indocin).
- sulfinpyrazone (Anturane).
- valproic acid (Depakene).

▷ *Driving, Hazardous Activities:* This drug may cause drowsiness or dizziness. Restrict activities as necessary.

Aviation Note: The use of this drug **may be a disqualification** for piloting. Consult a designated Aviation Medical Examiner.

Exposure to Sun: No restrictions.

TAMOXIFEN
(ta MOX i fen)

Introduced: 1973

Class: Antiestrogen, anticancer

Prescription: USA: Yes
Canada: Yes

Controlled Drug: USA: No
Canada: No

Available as Generic: No

Brand Names: Nolvadex, ◆Nolvadex-D, ◆Tamofen

BENEFITS versus RISKS	
Possible Benefits	*Possible Risks*
EFFECTIVE ADJUNCTIVE TREATMENT IN ADVANCED BREAST CANCER in 30% to 40% of cases	Severe increase in tumor or bone pain, transient
	Thromophlebitis, pulmonary embolism
	Abnormally high blood calcium levels
	Eye changes: corneal opacities, retinal injury

▷ **Principal Uses**

As a Single Drug Product: Used primarily as an alternative to estrogens and androgens (male sex hormones) to treat advanced breast cancer in postmenopausal women. It is also used to stimulate ovulation in premenopausal women with infertility.

How This Drug Works: Not completely established. It is thought that by blocking the uptake of estradiol (estrogen), this drug removes or reduces a stimulus to breast cancer cells.

Available Dosage Forms and Strengths
Tablets — 10 mg, 20 mg (in Canada)

▷ **Usual Adult Dosage Range:** 10 to 20 mg twice/day, morning and evening. **Note: Actual dosage and administration schedule must be determined by the physician for each patient individually.**

▷ **Dosing Instructions:** May be taken either on an empty stomach or with food. The tablet may be crushed for administration.

Usual Duration of Use: Continual use on a regular schedule for 4 to 10 weeks is usually necessary to determine this drug's effectiveness in controlling the growth and spread of advanced breast cancer. In the presence of bone involvement, treatment for several months may be required to evaluate effectiveness. Long-term use (months to years) requires supervision and periodic evaluation by your physician. Consult your physician on a regular basis.

▷ **This Drug Should Not Be Taken If**
• you have had a serious allergic or adverse reaction to it previously.
• you have active phlebitis.
• you have a significant deficiency of white blood cells or blood platelets.

▷ **Inform Your Physician Before Taking This Drug If**
• you have a history of thrombophlebitis or pulmonary embolism.
• you have a history of abnormally high blood calcium levels.
• you have a history of any type of blood cell or bone marrow disorder.
• you have cataracts or other visual impairment.
• you have impaired liver function.
• you plan to have surgery in the near future.

Possible Side-Effects (natural, expected and unavoidable drug actions)
Hot flashes, fluid retention, weight gain.

▷ **Possible Adverse Effects** (unusual, unexpected and infrequent reactions)
If any of the following develop, consult your physician promptly for guidance.
Mild Adverse Effects
Allergic Reaction: Skin rash.
Headache, dizziness, drowsiness, depression, fatigue, confusion.
Nausea, vomiting, itching in genital area, loss of hair.

Serious Adverse Effects
Initial "flare" of severe pain in tumor or involved bone.
Development of thrombophlebitis, risk of pulmonary embolism.
Eye changes: corneal opacities, retinal injury.
Development of abnormally high blood calcium levels.
Transient decreases in white blood cells and blood platelets.

▷ **Possible Effects on Sexual Function**
Premenopausal: altered timing and pattern of menstruation.
Postmenopausal: vaginal bleeding.
This drug may be effective in treating the following conditions:
- male infertility due to abnormally low sperm counts.
- male breast enlargement and tenderness.
- chronic female breast pain (mastalgia).

CAUTION
1. If this drug is used prior to your menopause, it may induce ovulation and predispose to pregnancy. Since this drug should not be
   used during pregnancy, some method of contraception (other than
   oral contraceptives) is advised.
2. Do not take any form of estrogen while taking this drug; estrogens
   can inhibit tamoxifen's effectiveness.

▷ **Advisability of Use During Pregnancy**
Pregnancy Category: X (tentative). See Pregnancy Code inside back cover.
Animal studies: No birth defects due to this drug reported.
Human studies: Information from adequate studies of pregnant women
   is not available.
This drug can have estrogenic effects. It should not be used during preg-
   nancy.

Advisability of Use if Breast-Feeding
Presence of this drug in breast milk: Unknown.
Avoid drug or refrain from nursing.

Habit-Forming Potential: None.

Effects of Overdosage: No information available.

Possible Effects of Long-Term Use: Development of abnormally high blood
   calcium levels.

Suggested Periodic Examinations While Taking This Drug (at physician's
   discretion)
Complete blood cell counts, measurements of blood calcium levels.
Complete eye examinations if impaired vision occurs.

▷ **While Taking This Drug, Observe the Following**
Foods: No restrictions.
Beverages: No restrictions. May be taken with milk.
▷ *Alcohol:* No interactions expected.

Tobacco Smoking: No interactions expected.

▷ *Other Drugs*
The following drugs may **decrease** the effects of tamoxifen
- estrogens.
- oral contraceptives (those that contain estrogens).

▷ *Driving, Hazardous Activities:* This drug may cause dizziness or drowsiness. Restrict activities as necessary.

Aviation Note: The use of this drug **may be a disqualification** for piloting. Consult a designated Aviation Medical Examiner.

Exposure to Sun: No restrictions.

TEMAZEPAM
(tem AZ e pam)

Introduced: 1978

Class: Hypnotic, benzodiazepines

Prescription: USA: Yes
Canada: Yes

Controlled Drug: USA: C-IV*
Canada: No

Available as Generic: USA: Yes
Canada: No

Brand Names: Razepam, Restoril, Temaz

BENEFITS versus RISKS

Possible Benefits	*Possible Risks*
EFFECTIVE HYPNOTIC after 4 weeks of continual use	Habit-forming potential with long-term use
Wide margin of safety with therapeutic doses	Minor impairment of mental functions ("hangover" effect)

▷ **Principal Uses**

As a Single Drug Product: This member of the benzodiazepine class of "minor tranquilizers" is used exclusively as a bedtime sedative to induce sleep.

How This Drug Works: It is thought that this drug produces a calming effect by enhancing the action of the nerve transmitter gamma-aminobutyric acid (GABA), which in turn blocks the arousal of higher brain centers and helps to induce sleep.

Available Dosage Forms and Strengths
Capsules — 15 mg, 30 mg

▷ **Usual Adult Dosage Range:** 15 to 30 mg at bedtime. Total daily dosage should not exceed 90 mg. **Note: Actual dosage and administration**

*See Schedules of Controlled Drugs inside back cover.

schedule must be determined by the physician for each patient individually.

▷ **Dosing Instructions:** Preferably taken on an empty stomach to hasten absorption and induce sleep rapidly. The capsule may be opened for administration. Do not discontinue this drug abruptly if taken for more than 4 weeks.

Usual Duration of Use: Periods of 3 to 5 nights intermittently, repeated as needed with appropriate dosage adjustment. Avoid uninterrupted and prolonged use. The duration of use should not exceed 2 weeks without reappraisal of continued need.

▷ **This Drug Should Not Be Taken If**
- you have had an allergic reaction to it previously.
- you have acute narrow-angle glaucoma, inadequately treated.

▷ **Inform Your Physician Before Taking This Drug If**
- you are allergic to any benzodiazepine drug (see Drug Class, Section Four).
- you have a history of alcoholism or drug abuse.
- you are pregnant or planning pregnancy.
- you have impaired liver or kidney function.
- you have a history of serious depression or mental disorder.
- you are taking other drugs with sedative effects.
- you have any of the following: asthma, emphysema, epilepsy, myasthenia gravis.

Possible Side-Effects (natural, expected and unavoidable drug actions)
"Hangover" effects on arising: drowsiness, lethargy and unsteadiness.

▷ **Possible Adverse Effects** (unusual, unexpected and infrequent reactions)
If any of the following develop, consult your physician promptly for guidance.
Mild Adverse Effects
Allergic Reactions: Skin rash, hives.
Dizziness, fainting, slurred speech, nausea, indigestion.
Serious Adverse Effects
Idiosyncratic Reactions: Nervousness, talkativeness, irritability, apprehension, euphoria, excitement, hallucinations.

▷ **Possible Effects on Sexual Function:** None reported.

CAUTION
1. This drug should not be discontinued abruptly if it has been taken continually for more than 4 weeks.
2. The concurrent use of some over-the-counter drug products that contain antihistamines (allergy and cold preparations, sleep aids) can cause excessive sedation in sensitive individuals.
3. Regular nightly use of any hypnotic drug should be avoided.

4. If you experience a "hangover" effect, avoid hazardous activities (driving, etc.) and the use of alcohol.

Precautions for Use

By Infants and Children: Safety and effectiveness for use by those under 18 years of age have not been established.

By Those over 60 Years of Age: It is advisable to use smaller doses (15 mg) at first to determine your response. Observe for the possible development of lethargy, indifference, fatigue, weakness, unsteadiness, disturbing dreams, nightmares and paradoxical reactions of excitement, agitation, anger, hostility and rage.

▷ ### Advisability of Use During Pregnancy

Pregnancy Category: X (tentative). See Pregnancy Code inside back cover.

Animal studies: Rib defects reported in rats; skull and rib defects reported in rabbits.

Human studies: Information from adequate studies of pregnant women is not available.

Avoid use during entire pregnancy.

Advisability of Use if Breast-Feeding

Presence of this drug in breast milk: Probably yes.

Avoid drug or refrain from nursing.

Habit-Forming Potential: This drug can produce psychological and/or physical dependence (see Glossary) if used in large doses for an extended period of time. Avoid continual use.

Effects of Overdosage: Marked drowsiness, weakness, feeling of drunkenness, staggering gait, tremor, stupor progressing to deep sleep or coma.

Possible Effects of Long-Term Use: Psychological and/or physical dependence.

Suggested Periodic Examinations While Taking This Drug (at physician's discretion)

Complete blood cell counts during long-term use.

▷ ### While Taking This Drug, Observe the Following

Foods: No restrictions.

Beverages: Avoid excessive intake of caffeine-containing beverages (coffee, tea, cola) within 4 hours of taking this drug. May be taken with milk.

▷ *Alcohol:* Use with extreme caution until the combined effect has been determined. Alcohol may increase the absorption of this drug and add to its depressant effects on the brain. It is advisable to avoid alcohol completely throughout the day and night if it is necessary to drive or to engage in any hazardous activity.

Tobacco Smoking: Heavy smoking may reduce the hypnotic action of this drug.

Marijuana Smoking: Increased sedation and significant impairment of intellectual and physical performance.

▷ *Other Drugs*

Temazepam may ***increase*** the effects of
- digoxin (Lanoxin), and cause digoxin toxicity.
- phenytoin (Dilantin), and cause phenytoin toxicity.

Temazepam may ***decrease*** the effects of
- levodopa (Sinemet, etc.), and reduce its effectiveness in treating Parkinson's disease.

The following drugs may ***increase*** the effects of temazepam
- cimetidine (Tagamet).
- disulfiram (Antabuse).
- isoniazid (INH, Rifamate, etc.).
- oral contraceptives.
- valproic acid (Depakene).

The following drugs may ***decrease*** the effects of temazepam
- rifampin (Rimactane, etc.).
- theophylline (Aminophylline, Theo-Dur, etc.).

▷ *Driving, Hazardous Activities:* This drug can impair mental alertness, judgment, physical coordination and reaction time. Avoid hazardous activities accordingly.

Aviation Note: The use of this drug ***is a disqualification*** for piloting. Consult a designated Aviation Medical Examiner.

Exposure to Sun: No restrictions.

Exposure to Heat: Use caution until the effect of excessive perspiration is determined. Because of reduced urine volume, this drug may accumulate in the body and produce effects of overdosage.

Discontinuation: Avoid sudden discontinuation if this drug has been taken for over 4 weeks without interruption. Dosage should be tapered gradually to prevent a withdrawal syndrome that could include depression, confusion, hallucinations, tremor, seizures, muscle cramping, sweating and vomiting.

TERAZOSIN
(ter AY zoh sin)

Introduced: 1987   **Class:** Antihypertensive

Prescription: USA: Yes   **Controlled Drug:** USA: No

Available as Generic: No

Brand Name: Hytrin

```
┌─────────────────────────────────────────────────────────────┐
│                   BENEFITS versus RISKS                       │
│                                                               │
│      Possible Benefits            Possible Risks              │
│   EFFECTIVE TREATMENT OF      "First dose" drop in blood      │
│     MILD TO MODERATE            pressure with fainting (1%)   │
│   HYPERTENSION when used      Fluid retention (5.5%)          │
│   alone or in combination     Rapid heart rate (1.9%)         │
│   with other antihypertensive                                 │
│   drugs                                                       │
└─────────────────────────────────────────────────────────────┘
```

▷ **Principal Uses**

As a Single Drug Product: Used primarily as a "step 1" antihypertensive drug to initiate treatment of mild to moderate hypertension. Also used in conjunction with other drugs to treat moderate to severe hypertension.

How This Drug Works: It is thought that by blocking certain actions of the sympathetic nervous system, this drug causes direct relaxation and expansion of blood vessel walls, thus lowering the pressure of the blood within the vessels.

Available Dosage Forms and Strengths

Tablets — 1 mg, 2 mg, 5 mg

▷ **Usual Adult Dosage Range:** Initiate treatment with a "test dose" of 1 mg to determine the patient's response within the first 2 hours. If tolerated satisfactorily, increase dose cautiously (as needed and tolerated) up to 5 mg/24 hours taken as a single dose at bedtime. Total daily dosage should not exceed 20 mg. **Note: Actual dosage and administration schedule must be determined by the physician for each patient individually.**

▷ **Dosing Instructions:** Preferably taken at bedtime to avoid orthostatic hypotension (see Glossary). May be taken without regard to food. The tablet may be crushed for administration.

Usual Duration of Use: Continual use on a regular schedule for 6 to 8 weeks is usually necessary to determine this drug's effectiveness in controlling hypertension. Long-term use (months to years) requires supervision and periodic evaluation by your physician. Consult your physician on a regular basis.

Possible Advantages of This Drug

May be used to initiate treatment.
Usually effective with once-a-day dosage.
Rarely causes depression or impotence.
Does not alter blood cholesterol, potassium or sugar.

▷ **This Drug Should Not Be Taken If**
- you have had an allergic reaction to it previously.
- you are experiencing mental depression.

- you have angina (active coronary artery disease) and you are not taking a beta-blocking drug. (Consult your physician.)

▷ **Inform Your Physician Before Taking This Drug If**
- you have experienced orthostatic hypotension (see Glossary) when using other antihypertensive drugs.
- you have a history of mental depression.
- you have impaired circulation to the brain, or a history of stroke.
- you have coronary artery disease.
- you have active liver disease or impaired liver function.
- you have impaired kidney function.
- you plan to have surgery under general anesthesia in the near future.

Possible Side-Effects (natural, expected and unavoidable drug actions)
Orthostatic hypotension (1.3%), drowsiness (5.4%), salt and water retention (5.5%), dry mouth, nasal congestion (5.9%), constipation.

▷ **Possible Adverse Effects** (unusual, unexpected and infrequent reactions)
If any of the following develop, consult your physician promptly for guidance.
Mild Adverse Effects
Allergic Reaction: Skin rash.
Headache (16.2%), dizziness (19.3%), fatigue (6.9%), weakness (11.3%), nervousness (2.3%), sweating, numbness and tingling (2.9%), blurred vision (1.6%).
Palpitation (4.3%), rapid heart rate (1.9%), shortness of breath (3.1%).
Nausea (4.4%), vomiting, diarrhea, abdominal pain.
Serious Adverse Effects
Mental depression (0.3%).

▷ **Possible Effects on Sexual Function:** Impotence (1.2%).

Natural Diseases or Disorders That May Be Activated by This Drug
Latent coronary artery insufficiency.

CAUTION
1. Observe for the possible "first dose" response of precipitous drop in blood pressue, with or without fainting; this usually occurs within 30 to 90 minutes. Limit initial doses to 1 mg taken at bedtime for the first 3 days; remain supine after taking these trial doses.
2. Impaired kidney function may increase your sensitivity to this drug and require smaller than usual doses.
3. Consult your physician if you plan to use over-the-counter remedies for allergic rhinitis or head colds; these preparations contain drugs that may interact with terazosin.

Precautions for Use
By Infants and Children: Safety and effectiveness for use by those under 12 years of age have not been established.
By Those over 60 Years of Age: Begin treatment with no more than 1 mg/day for the first 3 days. Subsequent increases in dose must be very

gradual and carefully supervised by your physician. The occurrence of orthostatic hypotension can cause unexpected falls and injury; sit or lie down promptly if you feel light-headed or dizzy. Report any indications of dizziness or chest pain promptly.

▷ **Advisability of Use During Pregnancy**
Pregnancy Category: C (tentative). See Pregnancy Code inside back cover.
   Animal studies: No birth defects found in rat or rabbit studies.
   Human studies: Information from adequate studies of pregnant women is not available.
   Use this drug only if clearly needed. Ask your physician for guidance.

Advisability of Use if Breast-Feeding
   Presence of this drug in breast milk: Unknown.
   Monitor nursing infant closely and discontinue drug or nursing if adverse effects develop.

Habit-Forming Potential: None.

Effects of Overdosage: Orthostatic hypotension, headache, generalized flushing, rapid heart rate, extreme weakness, irregular heart rhythm, circulatory collapse.

Possible Effects of Long-Term Use: None reported.

Suggested Periodic Examinations While Taking This Drug (at physician's discretion)
   Measurements of blood pressure in lying, sitting and standing positions.
   Measurements of body weight to detect fluid retention.

▷ **While Taking This Drug, Observe the Following**
Foods: No restrictions. Avoid excessive salt intake.
Beverages: No restrictions. May be taken with milk.
▷ *Alcohol:* Use with extreme caution until the combined effects have been determined. Alcohol can exaggerate the blood-pressure-lowering actions of this drug and cause excessive reduction.
Tobacco Smoking: Nicotine can contribute significantly to this drug's ability to intensify coronary insufficiency in susceptible individuals. All forms of tobacco should be avoided.
▷ *Other Drugs*
   The following drugs may **increase** the effects of terazosin
   • beta-adrenergic-blocking drugs (see Drug Class, Section Four); the severity and duration of the "first dose" hypotensive response may be increased.
   The following drugs may **decrease** the effects of terazosin
   • estrogens.
   • indomethacin (Indocin).
▷ *Driving, Hazardous Activities:* This drug may cause dizziness or drowsiness. Restrict activities as necessary.
Aviation Note: The use of this drug **is a disqualification** for piloting. Consult a designated Aviation Medical Examiner.

Exposure to Sun: No restrictions.

Exposure to Cold: Use caution until combined effect has been determined. Cold environments may increase this drug's ability to cause coronary insufficiency (angina) and hypothermia (see Glossary) in susceptible individuals.

Heavy Exercise or Exertion: Excessive exertion can augment this drug's ability to induce angina. See Angina in Section Two.

Discontinuation: If you are taking this drug as part of your treatment program for congestive heart failure, do not discontinue it abruptly. Ask your physician for guidance.

TERBUTALINE
(ter BYU ta leen)

Introduced: 1974

Class: Antiasthmatic, bronchodilator

Prescription: USA: Yes
Canada: Yes

Controlled Drug: USA: No
Canada: No

Available as Generic: No

Brand Names: Brethaire, Brethine, Bricanyl, ✦Bricanyl Spacer

BENEFITS versus RISKS	
Possible Benefits	*Possible Risks*
VERY EFFECTIVE RELIEF OF BRONCHOSPASM	Increased blood pressure
	Fine hand tremor
	Irregular heart rhythm (with excessive use)

▷ **Principal Uses**

As a Single Drug Product: To relieve acute bronchial asthma and to reduce the frequency and severity of chronic, recurrent asthmatic attacks; also used to relieve reversible bronchospasm associated with chronic bronchitis and emphysema.

How This Drug Works: By stimulating certain sympathetic nerve terminals, this drug acts to dilate those bronchial tubes that are in sustained constriction, thereby increasing the size of the airway and improving the ability to breathe.

Available Dosage Forms and Strengths
Aerosol — 0.2 mg/actuation, 0.25 mg/actuation (Canada)
Injection — 1 mg per ml
Tablets — 2.5 mg, 5 mg

▷ **Usual Adult Dosage Range:**   Aerosol: 0.4 mg taken in 2 separate inhalations 1 minute apart; repeat every 4 to 6 hours as needed. Tablets: 2.5 to 5 mg taken 3 times/day, 6 hours apart. The total daily dosage should not exceed 15 mg. **Note: Actual dosage and administration schedule must be determined by the physician for each patient individually.**

▷ **Dosing Instructions:**   May be taken on empty stomach or with food or milk. Tablets may be crushed for administration. For aerosol, follow the written instructions carefully. Do not overuse.

Usual Duration of Use: According to individual requirements. Do not use beyond the time necessary to terminate episodes of asthma.

Possible Advantages of This Drug
Rapid onset of action.
Long duration of action.
Highly effective relief of asthma.

▷ **This Drug Should Not Be Taken If**
- you have had an allergic reaction to any dosage form of it previously.
- you currently have an irregular heart rhythm.
- you are taking, or have taken within the past 2 weeks, any monoamine oxidase (MAO) type A inhibitor drug (see Drug Class, Section Four).

▷ **Inform Your Physician Before Taking This Drug If**
- you are overly sensitive to other drugs that stimulate the sympathetic nervous system.
- you are currently using epinephrine (Adrenalin, Primatene Mist, etc.) to relieve asthmatic breathing.
- you have a seizure disorder.
- you have any type of heart or circulatory disorder, especially high blood pressure or coronary heart disease.
- you have diabetes or an overactive thyroid gland (hyperthyroidism).
- you are taking any form of digitalis or any stimulant drug.

Possible Side-Effects (natural, expected and unavoidable drug actions)
Aerosol: dryness or irritation of mouth or throat, altered taste. Tablet: nervousness, tremor, palpitation.

▷ **Possible Adverse Effects** (unusual, unexpected and infrequent reactions)
If any of the following develop, consult your physician promptly for guidance.
Mild Adverse Effects
Headache, dizziness, drowsiness, restlessness, insomnia.
Rapid, pounding heartbeat; increased sweating; muscle cramps in arms and legs.
Nausea, heartburn, vomiting.

Serious Adverse Effects
Rapid or irregular heart rhythm, intensification of angina, increased blood pressure.

▷ **Possible Effects on Sexual Function:** None reported.

Natural Diseases or Disorders That May Be Activated By This Drug
Latent coronary artery disease, diabetes or high blood pressure.

CAUTION
1. Concurrent use of this drug by aerosol inhalation with beclomethasone aerosol (Beclovent, Vanceril) may increase the risk of toxicity due to fluorocarbon propellants. It is advisable to use this aerosol 20 to 30 minutes *before* beclomethasone aerosol. This will reduce the risk of toxicity and will enhance the penetration of beclomethasone.
2. *Avoid excessive use of aerosol inhalation.* The excessive or prolonged use of this drug by inhalation can reduce its effectiveness and cause serious heart rhythm disturbances, including cardiac arrest.
3. Do not use this drug concurrently with epinephrine. These two drugs may be used alternately if an interval of 4 hours is allowed between doses.
4. If you do not respond to your usually effective dose, ask your physician for guidance. Do not increase the size or frequency of the dose without your physician's approval.

Precautions for Use
By Infants and Children: Safety and effectiveness for use by those under 12 years of age have not been established.
By Those over 60 Years of Age: Avoid excessive and continual use. If acute asthma is not relieved promptly, other drugs will have to be tried. Observe for the development of nervousness, palpitations, irregular heart rhythm and muscle tremors. Use with extreme caution if you have hardening of the arteries, heart disease or high blood pressure.

▷ **Advisability of Use During Pregnancy**
Pregnancy Category: B (tentative). See Pregnancy Code inside back cover.
Animal studies: No significant birth defects reported in mouse and rat studies.
Human studies: Information from adequate studies of pregnant women is not available.
Use only if clearly needed. Ask your physician for guidance.

Advisability of Use if Breast-Feeding
Presence of this drug in breast milk: Yes.
Monitor nursing infant closely and discontinue drug or nursing if adverse effects develop.

Habit-Forming Potential: None.

Effects of Overdosage: Nervousness, palpitation, rapid heart rate, sweating, headache, tremor, vomiting, chest pain.

Possible Effects of Long-Term Use: Loss of effectiveness. See *CAUTION* category above.

Suggested Periodic Examinations While Taking This Drug (at physician's discretion)
Blood pressure measurements, evaluation of heart status.

▷ **While Taking This Drug, Observe the Following**
Foods: No restrictions.
Beverages: Avoid excessive use of caffeine-containing beverages: coffee, tea, cola, chocolate.
▷ *Alcohol:* No interactions expected.
Tobacco Smoking: No interactions expected.
▷ *Other Drugs*
Terbutaline *taken concurrently* with
  • monoamine oxidase (MAO) type A inhibitor drugs may cause excessive increase in blood pressure and undesirable heart stimulation (see Drug Class, Section Four).
The following drugs may *decrease* the effects of terbutaline
  • beta blocker drugs may impair its effectiveness (see Drug Class, Section Four).
▷ *Driving, Hazardous Activities:* Usually no restrictions. Use caution if excessive nervousness or dizziness occurs.
Aviation Note: The use of this drug *is a disqualification* for piloting. Consult a designated Aviation Medical Examiner.
Exposure to Sun: No restrictions.
Heavy Exercise or Exertion: Use caution. Excessive exercise can induce asthma in sensitive individuals.

TERFENADINE
(ter FEN a deen)

Introduced: 1977   **Class:** Antihistamines

Prescription: USA: Yes   **Controlled Drug:** USA: No
     Canada: No   Canada: No

Available as Generic: No

Brand Names: Seldane, Seldane-D

BENEFITS versus RISKS

Possible Benefits	*Possible Risks*
EFFECTIVE RELIEF OF ALLERGIC RHINITIS AND ALLERGIC SKIN DISORDERS	Infrequent headache Mild fatigue Minor digestive disturbances Slight atropinelike effects

---

▷ **Principal Uses**

As a Single Drug Product: Used primarily to provide symptomatic relief in allergic and related disorders: seasonal and perennial allergic rhinitis (hay fever), allergic conjunctivitis and vasomotor rhinitis; also in hives and localized swellings (angioedema) of allergic origin.

How This Drug Works: Antihistamines reduce the intensity of the allergic response by blocking the action of histamine after it has been released from sensitized tissue cells in the eyes, nose and skin.

Available Dosage Forms and Strengths

Suspension — 30 mg per 5-ml teaspoonful (Canada)

Tablets — 60 mg

▷ **Usual Adult Dosage Range:** 60 mg every 8 to 12 hours as needed. The total daily dosage should not exceed 360 mg. **Note: Actual dosage and administration schedule must be determined by the physician for each patient individually.**

▷ **Dosing Instructions:** May be taken with food or milk to prevent stomach irritation. The tablet may be crushed for administration.

Usual Duration of Use: Continual use on a regular schedule for 2 to 3 days is usually necessary to determine this drug's effectiveness in relieving the symptoms of allergic rhinitis and dermatosis. It may be necessary to take this drug throughout the entire pollen season, depending upon individual sensitivity. However, antihistamines should not be taken continually (without interruption) for long-term use. Limit their use to periods that require symptomatic relief. Consult your physician on a regular basis.

Possible Advantages of This Drug

Fast onset of action, relief within one hour.

No loss of effectiveness with continual use.

No drowsiness or impaired mental function that is so characteristic of other antihistamines.

▷ **This Drug Should Not Be Taken If**

- you have had an allergic reaction to any dosage form of it previously.
- you are currently undergoing allergy skin tests.

▷ **Inform Your Physician Before Taking This Drug If**

- you have had any allergic reactions or unfavorable responses to the previous use of antihistamines.

Possible Side-Effects (natural, expected and unavoidable drug actions)
Dry nose, mouth or throat.

▷ **Possible Adverse Effects** (unusual, unexpected and infrequent reactions)
If any of the following develop, consult your physician promptly for guidance.
Mild Adverse Effects
Allergic Reactions: Skin rash, itching.
Headache, nervousness, fatigue.
Increased appetite, indigestion, nausea, vomiting.
Serious Adverse Effects
None reported.

▷ **Possible Effects on Sexual Function**
Altered timing and pattern of menstruation.
Female breast enlargement with milk production.

CAUTION
1. Discontinue this drug 4 days before diagnostic skin testing procedures in order to prevent false negative test results.
2. Do not use this drug if you have active bronchial asthma, bronchitis or pneumonia. It may thicken bronchial mucus and make it more difficult to remove (by absorption or coughing).

Precautions for Use
By Infants and Children: Safety and effectiveness for use by those under 12 years of age have not been established.
By Those over 60 Years of Age: You may be more susceptible to the development of headache and fatigue. Use smaller doses at longer intervals if necessary.

▷ **Advisability of Use During Pregnancy**
Pregnancy Category: C (tentative). See Pregnancy Code inside back cover.
Animal studies: No birth defects due to this drug reported.
Human studies: Information from adequate studies of pregnant women is not available.
Use this drug only if clearly needed. Ask your physician for guidance.

Advisability of Use if Breast-Feeding
Presence of this drug in breast milk: Unknown.
Avoid drug or refrain from nursing.

Habit-Forming Potential: None.

Effects of Overdosage: No information available. No serious or threatening effects expected.

Possible Effects of Long-Term Use: None reported.

Suggested Periodic Examinations While Taking This Drug (at physician's discretion)
None required.

▷ **While Taking This Drug, Observe the Following**

Foods: No restrictions.

Beverages: No restrictions. May be taken with milk.

▷ *Alcohol:* No interactions expected.

Tobacco Smoking: No interactions expected.

▷ *Other Drugs:* No significant interactions reported to date.

Hazardous Activities: No restrictions.

Aviation Note: The use of this drug *is probably not a disqualification* for piloting. Consult a designated Aviation Medical Examiner.

Exposure to Sun: No restrictions.

TETRACYCLINE
(te trah SI kleen)

Introduced: 1953

Class: Antibiotic, tetracyclines

Prescription: USA: Yes
Canada: Yes

Controlled Drug: USA: No
Canada: No

Available as Generic: Yes

Brand Names: Achromycin, Achromycin V, ✦Apo-Tetra, Cyclopar, ✦Medicycline, Mysteclin-F [CD], ✦Neo-Tetrine, Nor-Tet, ✦Novotetra, Panmycin, Retet, Robitet, Sumycin, Tetra-C, Tetracyn, Tetralan, Tetram, Tropicycline

---

BENEFITS versus RISKS

Possible Benefits	*Possible Risks*
EFFECTIVE TREATMENT OF INFECTIONS due to susceptible bacteria and protozoa	ALLERGIC REACTIONS, mild to severe: ANAPHYLAXIS, DRUG-INDUCED HEPATITIS (rare) Drug-induced colitis Superinfections (bacterial or fungal) Rare blood cell disorders: hemolytic anemia, abnormally low white cell and platelet counts

---

▷ **Principal Uses**

As a Single Drug Product: This member of the tetracycline drug class is used primarily to (1) treat a broad range of infections caused by susceptible bacteria and protozoa (short-term use); and (2) treat severe, resistant pustular acne (long-term use).

As a Combination Drug Product [CD]: This drug is available in combination with amphotericin B, an antifungal antibiotic that is provided to reduce the risk of developing an overgrowth of yeast organisms (superinfection) of the gastrointestinal tract.

How This Drug Works: This drug prevents the growth and multiplication of susceptible bacteria by interfering with their formation of essential proteins.

Available Dosage Forms and Strengths

Capsules — 100 mg, 250 mg, 500 mg
Ointment — 3%
Ointment, ophthalmic — 10 mg per gram
Solution, topical — 2.2 mg per ml
Suspension, ophthalmic — 10 mg per ml
Suspension, oral — 125 mg per 5-ml teaspoonful
Tablets — 250 mg, 500 mg

▷ **Usual Adult Dosage Range:** 250 to 500 mg/6 hours, or 500 to 1000 mg/12 hours. The total daily dosage should not exceed 4000 mg (4 grams). **Note: Actual dosage and administration schedule must be determined by the physician for each patient individually.**

▷ **Dosing Instructions:** Preferably taken on an empty stomach, 1 hour before or 2 hours after eating. However, to reduce stomach irritation it may be taken with crackers that contain insignificant amounts of iron, calcium, magnesium or zinc. Avoid all dairy products for 2 hours before and after taking this drug. Take at the same time each day, with a full glass of water. Take the full course prescribed. The tablet may be crushed and the capsule may be opened for administration.

Usual Duration of Use: The time required to control the acute infection and be free of fever and symptoms for 48 hours. This varies with the nature of the infection. Long-term use (months to years, as for treatment of acne) requires supervision and periodic evaluation. Consult your physician on a regular basis.

▷ **This Drug Should Not Be Taken If**
• you are allergic to any tetracycline drug (see Drug Class, Section Four).
• you are pregnant or breast-feeding.

▷ **Inform Your Physician Before Taking This Drug If**
• it is prescribed for a child under 8 years of age.
• you have a history of liver or kidney disease.
• you have systemic lupus erythematosus.
• you are taking any penicillin drug.
• you are taking any anticoagulant drug.
• you plan to have surgery under general anesthesia in the near future.

Possible Side-Effects (natural, expected and unavoidable drug actions)

> Superinfections (see Glossary), often due to yeast organisms. These can occur in the mouth, intestinal tract, rectum and/or vagina, resulting in rectal and vaginal itching.

▷ **Possible Adverse Effects** (unusual, unexpected and infrequent reactions)

If any of the following develop, consult your physician promptly for guidance.

Mild Adverse Effects

> Allergic Reactions: Skin rash, hives, itching of hands and feet, swelling of face or extremities.
>
> Loss of appetite, stomach irritation, nausea, vomiting, diarrhea.
>
> Irritation of mouth or tongue, "black tongue," sore throat, abdominal cramping or pain.

Serious Adverse Effects

> Allergic Reactions: Anaphylactic reaction (see Glossary), asthma, fever, swollen joints and lymph glands.
>
> Drug-induced hepatitis with jaundice.
>
> Permanent discoloration and/or malformation of teeth when taken under 8 years of age, including unborn child and infant.
>
> Impaired vision, increased intracranial pressure.
>
> Drug-induced colitis.
>
> Rare blood cell disorders: hemolytic anemia (see Glossary); abnormally low white blood cell count, causing fever, sore throat and infections; abnormally low blood platelet count, causing abnormal bleeding or bruising.

▷ **Possible Effects on Sexual Function:**   Decreased effectiveness of oral contraceptives taken concurrently (several case reports of pregnancy).

▷ **Adverse Effects That May Mimic Natural Diseases or Disorders**

> Drug-induced hepatitis may suggest viral hepatitis.

Natural Diseases or Disorders That May Be Activated by This Drug

> Systemic lupus erythematosus.

CAUTION

1. Antacids, dairy products and preparations containing aluminum, bismuth, calcium, iron, magnesium or zinc can prevent adequate absorption of this drug and reduce its effectiveness significantly.
2. Troublesome and persistent diarrhea can develop in sensitive individuals. If diarrhea persists for more than 24 hours, discontinue this drug and consult your physician.
3. If surgery under general anesthesia is required while taking this drug, the choice of anesthetic agent must be considered carefully to prevent serious kidney damage.

Precautions for Use

> *By Infants and Children:* If possible, tetracyclines should not be given to children under 8 years of age because of the risk of permanent dis-

coloration and deformity of the teeth. Rarely, young infants may develop increased intracranial pressure within the first 4 days of receiving this drug. Tetracyclines may inhibit normal bone growth and development.

By Those over 60 Years of Age: Dosage must be carefully individualized and based upon determinations of kidney function. Natural skin changes may predispose to severe and prolonged itching reactions in the genital and anal regions.

▷ **Advisability of Use During Pregnancy**

Pregnancy Category: D (tentative). See Pregnancy Code inside back cover.

Animal studies: Tetracycline causes limb defects in rats, rabbits and chickens.

Human studies: Information from studies of pregnant women indicates that this drug can cause impaired development and discoloration of teeth and other developmental defects.

It is advisable to avoid this drug completely during entire pregnancy.

Advisability of Use if Breast-Feeding

Presence of this drug in breast milk: Yes.

Avoid drug or refrain from nursing.

Habit-Forming Potential: None.

Effects of Overdosage: Stomach burning, nausea, vomiting, diarrhea.

Possible Effects of Long-Term Use: Superinfections; rarely, impairment of bone marrow, liver or kidney function.

Suggested Periodic Examinations While Taking This Drug (at physician's discretion)

Complete blood cell counts, liver and kidney function tests.

During extended use, sputum and stool examinations may detect early superinfection due to yeast organisms.

▷ **While Taking This Drug, Observe the Following**

Foods: Avoid cheeses, yogurt, ice cream, iron-fortified cereals and supplements and meats for 2 hours before and after taking this drug. Calcium and iron can combine with this drug and reduce its absorption significantly.

Beverages: Avoid all forms of milk for 2 hours before and after taking this drug.

▷ *Alcohol:* No interactions expected. However, it is best avoided if you have active liver disease.

Tobacco Smoking: No interactions expected.

▷ *Other Drugs*

Tetracyclines may ***increase*** the effects of

- oral anticoagulants, and make it necessary to reduce their dosage.
- digoxin (Lanoxin), and cause digitalis toxicity.
- lithium (Eskalith, Lithane, etc.), and increase the risk of lithium toxicity.

Tetracyclines may *decrease* the effects of
- oral contraceptives, and impair their effectiveness in preventing pregnancy.
- penicillins, and impair their effectiveness in treating infections.

Tetracyclines *taken concurrently* with
- methoxyflurane anesthesia may impair kidney function.

The following drugs may *decrease* the effects of tetracyclines
- antacids (aluminum and magnesium preparations, sodium bicarbonate, etc.) may reduce drug absorption.
- iron and mineral preparations may reduce drug absorption.

▷ *Driving, Hazardous Activities:* Usually no restrictions. However, this drug may cause nausea or diarrhea. Restrict activities as necessary.

Aviation Note: The use of this drug *may be a disqualification* for piloting. Consult a designated Aviation Medical Examiner.

Exposure to Sun: Use caution until sensitivity has been determined. Some tetracyclines can cause photosensitivity (see Glossary).

THEOPHYLLINE
(thee OFF i lin)

Other Names: Aminophylline, oxtriphylline

Introduced: 1929

Class: Antiasthmatic, bronchodilator, xanthines

Prescription: USA: Yes
Canada: No

Controlled Drug: USA: No
Canada: No

Available as Generic: Yes

Brand Names: Accurbron, Amesec [CD], Brondecon [CD], Bronkaid Tablets [CD], Bronkodyl, Bronkolixir [CD], Bronkotabs [CD], Choledyl, Constant-T, Elixicon, Elixophyllin, LaBID, Lodrane, Marax [CD], Marax DF [CD], Mudrane GG Elixir & Tablets [CD], Mudrane Tablets [CD], ✦PMS Theophylline, ✦Pulmophylline, Quadrinal [CD], Quibron [CD], Quibron Plus [CD], Quibron-T Dividose, ✦Quibron-T/SR, Respbid, Slo-bid, Slo-Phyllin, Slo-Phyllin GG [CD], Slo-Phyllin Gyrocaps, Somophyllin-CRT, Somophyllin-DF, Somophyllin-T, ✦Somophyllin-12, Sustaire, ✦Tedral Preparations [CD], Theobid Duracaps, Theo-Dur, Theolair, Theophyl-SR, Theo-24, Theovent

```
┌─────────────────────────────────────────────────────────────┐
│                    BENEFITS versus RISKS                    │
│      Possible Benefits              Possible Risks          │
│  EFFECTIVE RELIEF OF ACUTE    NARROW TREATMENT RANGE        │
│    BRONCHIAL ASTHMA           FREQUENT STOMACH              │
│  MODERATELY EFFECTIVE           DISTRESS                     │
│    CONTROL OF CHRONIC,        Gastrointestinal bleeding     │
│    RECURRENT BRONCHIAL        Central nervous system toxicity,│
│    ASTHMA                       seizures                     │
│  Moderately effective symptomatic  Heart rhythm disturbances │
│    relief in chronic bronchitis and                         │
│    emphysema                                                │
└─────────────────────────────────────────────────────────────┘
```

▷ **Principal Uses**

As a Single Drug Product: Used primarily to relieve the shortness of breath and wheezing characteristic of acute bronchial asthma, and to prevent the recurrence of asthmatic episodes. It is also useful in relieving the asthmaticlike symptoms that are associated with some types of chronic bronchitis and emphysema.

As a Combination Drug Product [CD]: This drug is available in combination with several other drugs that are beneficial in the overall management of bronchial asthma and related conditions. Ephedrine is added to enhance the bronchodilator effects; guaifenesin is added to provide an expectorant effect that thins the mucus secretions in the bronchial tubes; mild sedatives such as phenobarbital are added to allay the anxiety that often accompanies acute attacks of asthma.

How This Drug Works: By inhibiting the enzyme phosphodiesterase, this drug produces an increase in the tissue chemical cyclic AMP. This causes relaxation of the muscles in the bronchial tubes and blood vessels of the lung, resulting in relief of bronchospasm, expanded lung capacity and improved lung circulation.

Available Dosage Forms and Strengths

Capsules — 100 mg, 200 mg, 250 mg

Capsules, prolonged-action — 50 mg, 60 mg, 75 mg, 100 mg, 125 mg, 130 mg, 200 mg, 250 mg, 260 mg, 300 mg

Elixir — 80 mg, 150 mg per 15-ml tablespoonful

Oral solution — 80 mg, 160 mg per 15-ml tablespoonful

Oral suspension — 300 mg per 15-ml tablespoonful

Syrup — 80 mg, 150 mg per 15-ml tablespoonful

Tablets — 100 mg, 125 mg, 200 mg, 250 mg, 300 mg

Tablets, prolonged-action — 100 mg, 200 mg, 250 mg, 300 mg, 400 mg, 450 mg, 500 mg

▷ **Usual Adult Dosage Range:**   Because of its potential toxicity, this drug is given according to body weight. For acute asthma: Initially, 6 mg/kg as the first dose; then 3 mg/kg every 6 hours for 12 hours; then 3 mg/kg every 8 hours as needed. For maintenance: 16 mg/kg/24 hours, or 400 mg/24 hours, whichever is less, taken in 3 or 4 divided doses at intervals of 6 to 8 hours. The total daily dosage should not exceed 900 mg. **Note: Actual dosage and administration schedule must be determined by the physician for each patient individually.**

▷ **Dosing Instructions:**   May be taken with or following food to reduce stomach irritation. The regular capsules may be opened and the regular tablets may be crushed for administration. The prolonged action dosage forms should be swallowed whole and not altered.

Usual Duration of Use: Continual use on a regular schedule for 48 to 72 hours is usually necessary to determine this drug's effectiveness in controlling the breathing impairment associated with bronchial asthma and chronic lung disease. Long-term use (months to years) requires supervision and periodic evaluation by your physician. Consult your physician on a regular basis.

▷ **This Drug Should Not Be Taken If**
- you have had an allergic reaction to it previously.
- you have active peptic ulcer disease.

▷ **Inform Your Physician Before Taking This Drug If**
- you have had an unfavorable reaction to any xanthine drug previously (see Drug Class, Section Four).
- you have a history of peptic ulcer disease.
- you have impaired liver or kidney function.
- you have hypertension, heart disease or any type of heart rhythm disorder.

Possible Side-Effects (natural, expected and unavoidable drug actions)
Nervousness, insomnia, rapid heart rate, increased urine volume.

▷ **Possible Adverse Effects** (unusual, unexpected and infrequent reactions)
If any of the following develop, consult your physician promptly for guidance.
Mild Adverse Effects
Allergic Reactions: Skin rash, hives.
Headache, dizziness, irritability, tremor, fatigue, weakness.
Loss of appetite, nausea, vomiting, abdominal pain, diarrhea, excessive thirst.
Flushing of face.
Serious Adverse Effects
Idiosyncratic Reactions: Marked anxiety, confusion, behavioral disturbances.
Central nervous system toxicity: muscle twitching, seizures.
Heart rhythm abnormalities, rapid breathing, low blood pressure.

Gastrointestinal bleeding.

▷ **Possible Effects on Sexual Function:**   None reported.

Natural Diseases or Disorders That May Be Activated by This Drug
Latent peptic ulcer disease.

CAUTION
1. This drug should not be taken concurrently with other antiasthmatic drugs unless you are directed to do so by your physician. Serious overdosage could result.
2. It has been reported that influenza vaccine may delay the elimination of this drug and cause accumulation to toxic levels.

Precautions for Use
By Infants and Children: Observe for indications of toxicity: irritability, agitation, tremors, lethargy, fever, vomiting, rapid heart rate and breathing, seizures.
By Those over 60 Years of Age: Start treatment with small doses until your tolerance has been determined. You may be more susceptible to the development of stomach irritation, nausea, vomiting or diarrhea. When used concurrently with coffee (caffeine) or with nasal decongestants, this drug may cause excessive stimulation and a hyperactivity syndrome.

▷ **Advisability of Use During Pregnancy**
Pregnancy Category: C (tentative). See Pregnancy Code inside back cover.
Animal studies: Significant birth defects due to this drug reported in mice.
Human studies: Information from adequate studies of pregnant women is not available. No increase in birth defects reported in 394 exposures to this drug.
Avoid this drug during the first 3 months. Use it otherwise only if clearly needed. Ask your physician for guidance.

Advisability of Use if Breast-Feeding
Presence of this drug in breast milk: Yes.
Avoid drug or refrain from nursing.

Habit-Forming Potential: None.

Effects of Overdosage: Nausea, vomiting, restlessness, irritability, confusion, delirium, seizures, high fever, weak pulse, coma.

Possible Effects of Long-Term Use: Gastrointestinal irritation.

Suggested Periodic Examinations While Taking This Drug (at physician's discretion)
Measurement of blood theophylline levels, especially with high dosage or long-term use. (See Therapeutic Drug Monitoring in Section One.)

▷ **While Taking This Drug, Observe the Following**

Foods: No restrictions.

Beverages: Avoid excessive use of caffeine-containing beverages: coffee, tea, cola; this combination could cause nervousness and insomnia.

▷ *Alcohol:* No interactions expected. May have additive effect on stomach irritation.

Tobacco Smoking: May hasten the elimination of this drug and reduce its effectiveness. Higher doses may be necessary to maintain a therapeutic blood level.

▷ *Other Drugs*

Theophylline may *decrease* the effects of
- lithium (Lithane, Lithobid, etc.), and reduce its effectiveness.

Theophylline *taken concurrently* with
- halothane (anesthesia) may cause heart rhythm abnormalities.
- phenytoin (Dilantin) may cause decreased effects of both drugs.

The following drugs may *increase* the effects of theophylline
- cimetidine (Tagamet) may cause theophylline toxicity.
- erythromycin (E-Mycin, Erythrocin, etc.) may cause theophylline toxicity.
- oral contraceptives.
- troleandomycin (TAO).

The following drugs may *decrease* the effects of theophylline
- barbiturates (phenobarbital, etc.).
- beta blocker drugs (see Drug Class, Section Four).
- rifampin (Rifadin, Rimactane, etc.).

▷ *Driving, Hazardous Activities:* This drug may cause dizziness. Restrict activities as necessary.

Aviation Note: The use of this drug *may be a disqualification* for piloting. Consult a designated Aviation Medical Examiner.

Exposure to Sun: No restrictions.

Occurrence of Unrelated Illness: Acute viral respiratory infections can delay the elimination of this drug significantly. Observe closely for indications of toxicity and the need to reduce dosage or lengthen the dosage interval.

Discontinuation: Avoid prolonged and unnecessary use of this drug. When you have achieved an asthma-free state, withdraw this drug gradually over several days.

THIORIDAZINE
(thi oh RID a zeen)

Introduced: 1959

Class: Strong tranquilizer, phenothiazines

Prescription: USA: Yes
Canada: Yes

Controlled Drug: USA: No
Canada: No

Available as Generic: USA: Yes
        Canada: Yes

Brand Names: ✦Apo-Thioridazine, Mellaril, Mellaril-S, Millazine, ✦Novo-ridazine, ✦PMS Thioridazine

---

BENEFITS versus RISKS

Possible Benefits	*Possible Risks*
EFFECTIVE CONTROL OF ACUTE MENTAL DISORDERS in the majority of patients: beneficial effects on thinking, mood and behavior Relief of anxiety, agitation and tension Possibly effective in the management of the hyperactivity syndrome in children	SERIOUS TOXIC EFFECTS ON BRAIN with long-term use Liver damage with jaundice (infrequent) Rare blood cell disorders: abnormally low white blood cell count

---

▷ **Principal Uses**

As a Single Drug Product: This antipsychotic drug is used primarily in the management of the following conditions: moderate to marked depression with significant anxiety and nervous tension; agitation, anxiety, depression and exaggerated fears in the elderly; severe behavioral problems in children characterized by hyperexcitability, combativeness, short attention span and rapid swings in mood.

How This Drug Works: Not completely established. Present theory is that by inhibiting the action of dopamine in certain brain centers, this drug acts to correct an imbalance of nerve impulse transmissions that is thought to be responsible for certain mental disorders.

Available Dosage Forms and Strengths
        Concentrate — 30 mg, 100 mg per ml
     Oral suspension — 25 mg, 100 mg per 5-ml teaspoonful
          Tablets — 10 mg, 15 mg, 25 mg, 50 mg, 100 mg, 150 mg, 200 mg

▷ **Usual Adult Dosage Range:**   Initially, 25 to 100 mg 3 times/day. Dose may be increased by 25 to 50 mg at 3- to 4-day intervals as needed and tolerated. Usual dosage range is 200 to 800 mg daily, divided into 2 to 4 doses. The total daily dosage should not exceed 800 mg. **Note: Actual dosage and administration schedule must be determined by the physician for each patient individually.**

▷ **Dosing Instructions:**   May be taken with or following meals to reduce stomach irritation. The tablets may be crushed for administration.

Usual Duration of Use: Continual use on a regular schedule for 3 to 4 weeks is usually necessary to determine this drug's effectiveness in controlling psychotic disorders. If not significantly beneficial within 6 weeks, it should be discontinued. Long-term use (months to years) requires periodic evaluation of response, appropriate dosage adjustment and consideration of continued need. Consult your physician on a regular basis.

▷ **This Drug Should Not Be Taken If**
- you are allergic to any of the drugs bearing the brand names listed above.
- you have active liver disease.
- you have cancer of the breast.
- you have a current blood cell or bone marrow disorder.

▷ **Inform Your Physician Before Taking This Drug If**
- you are allergic or abnormally sensitive to any phenothiazine drug (see Drug Class, Section Four).
- you have impaired liver or kidney function.
- you have any type of seizure disorder.
- you have diabetes, glaucoma or heart disease.
- you have a history of lupus erythematosus.
- you are taking any drug with sedative effects.
- you plan to have surgery under general or spinal anesthesia in the near future.

Possible Side-Effects (natural, expected and unavoidable drug actions)
Drowsiness (usually during the first 2 weeks), orthostatic hypotension (see Glossary), blurred vision, dry mouth, nasal congestion, constipation, impaired urination.
Pink or purple coloration of urine, of no significance.

▷ **Possible Adverse Effects** (unusual, unexpected and infrequent reactions)
If any of the following develop, consult your physician promptly for guidance.
Mild Adverse Effects
Allergic Reactions: Skin rash, hives, low-grade fever.
Lowering of body temperature, especially in the elderly. (See Hypothermia in Glossary.)
Increased appetite and weight gain.
Weakness, agitation, insomnia, impaired day and night vision.
Chronic constipation, fecal impaction.
Serious Adverse Effects
Allergic Reactions: Hepatitis with jaundice (see Glossary), severe skin reactions.
Depression, disorientation, seizures, loss of peripheral vision.
Rapid heart rate, heart rhythm disorders.
Blood cell disorders: reduced white blood cell count (more common in the elderly).

Nervous system reactions: Parkinson-like disorders (see Glossary), severe restlessness, muscle spasms involving the face and neck, tardive dyskinesia (see Glossary).

▷ **Possible Effects on Sexual Function**

Decreased male and female libido; inhibited ejaculation (49% to 60%); impotence (54%); impaired female orgasm; priapism (see Glossary).
Male breast enlargement and tenderness.
Female breast enlargement with milk production.
Altered timing and pattern of menstruation.
False positive pregnancy test results.

▷ **Adverse Effects That May Mimic Natural Diseases or Disorders**

Nervous system reactions may suggest true Parkinson's disease.
Liver reactions may suggest viral hepatitis.
Reactions resembling systemic lupus erythematosus can occur.

Natural Diseases or Disorders That May Be Activated by This Drug

Latent epilepsy, glaucoma, diabetes mellitus, prostatism (see Glossary).

CAUTION

1. Many over-the-counter medications (see OTC Drugs in Glossary) for allergies, colds and coughs contain drugs that can interact unfavorably with this drug. Ask your physician or pharmacist for guidance before using any such medications.
2. Antacids that contain aluminum and/or magnesium can prevent the absorption of this drug and reduce its effectiveness.
3. Obtain prompt evaluation of any change or disturbance of vision.

Precautions for Use

By Infants and Children: Use of this drug is not recommended in children under 2 years of age. Do not use this drug in the presence of symptoms suggestive of Reye syndrome (see Glossary). Children with acute infectious diseases ("flulike" infections, chicken pox, measles, etc.) are more prone to develop muscular spasms of the face, back and extremities when this drug is given for any reason.

By Those over 60 Years of Age: Small doses are advisable until individual response has been determined. You may be more susceptible to the development of drowsiness, lethargy, constipation, lowering of body temperature (hypothermia) and orthostatic hypotension (see Glossary). This drug can enhance existing prostatism (see Glossary). You may also be more susceptible to the development of Parkinson-like reactions and/or tardive dyskinesia (see discussion of these terms in Glossary). These reactions must be recognized early since they may become unresponsive to treatment and irreversible.

▷ **Advisability of Use During Pregnancy**

Pregnancy Category: C (tentative). See Pregnancy Code inside back cover.
Animal studies: The results of rodent studies are conflicting.

Human studies: No increase in birth defects reported in 23 exposures. Information from adequate studies of pregnant women is not available.

Avoid drug during the first 3 months. Use it otherwise only if clearly needed. Ask your physician for guidance.

Advisability of Use if Breast-Feeding
Presence of this drug in breast milk: Yes, in minute amounts.
Monitor nursing infant closely and discontinue drug or nursing if adverse effects develop.

Habit-Forming Potential: None.

Effects of Overdosage: Marked drowsiness, weakness, tremor, agitation, unsteadiness, deep sleep, coma, convulsions.

Possible Effects of Long-Term Use: Opacities in the cornea or lens of the eye, pigmentation of the retina. Tardive dyskinesia (see Glossary).

Suggested Periodic Examinations While Taking This Drug (at physician's discretion)
Complete blood cell counts, especially between the fourth and tenth weeks of treatment.
Liver function tests, electrocardiograms.
Complete eye examinations—eye structures and vision.
Careful inspection of the tongue for early evidence of fine, involuntary, wavelike movements that could indicate the beginning of tardive dyskinesia.

▷ **While Taking This Drug, Observe the Following**
Foods: No restrictions.
Nutritional Support: A riboflavin (vitamin B-2) supplement should be taken with long-term use.
Beverages: No restrictions. May be taken with milk.
▷ *Alcohol:* Avoid completely. Alcohol can increase the sedative action of phenothiazines and accentuate their depressant effects on brain function and blood pressure. Phenothiazines can increase the intoxicating effects of alcohol.
Tobacco Smoking: Possible reduction of drowsiness from drug.
Marijuana Smoking: Moderate increase in drowsiness; accentuation of orthostatic hypotension; increased risk of precipitating latent psychoses, confusing the interpretation of mental status and drug responses.
▷ *Other Drugs*
Thioridazine may *increase* the effects of
• all sedative drugs, especially meperidine (Demerol), and cause excessive sedation.
• all atropinelike drugs, and cause nervous system toxicity.
Thioridazine may *decrease* the effects of

- guanethidine (Ismelin, Esimil), and reduce its effectiveness in lowering blood pressure.

Thioridazine *taken concurrently* with

- lithium (Lithobid, Lithotabs) may impair the effectiveness of lithium and cause nervous system toxicity.

The following drugs may *decrease* the effects of thioridazine

- antacids containing aluminum and/or magnesium.
- barbiturates (see Drug Class, Section Four).
- benztropine (Cogentin).
- disulfiram (Antabuse).
- trihexyphenidyl (Artane).

▷ *Driving, Hazardous Activities:* This drug can impair mental alertness, judgment and physical coordination. Avoid hazardous activities.

Aviation Note: The use of this drug *is a disqualification* for piloting. Consult a designated Aviation Medical Examiner.

Exposure to Sun: Use caution until sensitivity has been determined. Some phenothiazines can cause photosensitivity (see Glossary).

Exposure to Heat: Use caution and avoid excessive heat as much as possible. This drug may impair the regulation of body temperature and increase the risk of heat stroke.

Exposure to Cold: Use caution and dress warmly. This drug can increase the risk of hypothermia in the elderly.

Discontinuation: After a period of long-term use, do not discontinue this drug suddenly. Gradual withdrawal over 2 to 3 weeks under physician supervision is recommended. Do not discontinue this drug without your physician's knowledge and approval.

THIOTHIXENE
(thi oh THIX een)

Introduced: 1967

Class: Strong tranquilizer, thioxanthenes

Prescription: USA: Yes
Canada: Yes

Controlled Drug: USA: No
Canada: No

Available as Generic: USA: Yes
Canada: No

Brand Name: Navane

BENEFITS versus RISKS

Possible Benefits	*Possible Risks*
EFFECTIVE CONTROL OF ACUTE MENTAL DISORDERS in the majority of patients: beneficial effects on thinking, mood and behavior	SERIOUS TOXIC EFFECTS ON BRAIN with long-term use
	Liver damage with jaundice (rare)
	Rare blood cell disorders: abnormally low white blood cell count

▷ **Principal Uses**

As a Single Drug Product: This antipsychotic drug is used to ameliorate the psychotic thinking and behavior associated with acute psychoses of unknown nature, episodes of mania and paranoia, and acute schizophrenia.

How This Drug Works: Not completely established. Present theory is that, by inhibiting the action of dopamine, this drug acts to correct an imbalance of nerve impulse transmissions that is thought to be responsible for certain mental disorders.

Available Dosage Forms and Strengths

Capsules — 1 mg, 2 mg, 5 mg, 10 mg, 20 mg
Concentrate — 5 mg per ml
Injections — 2 mg, 5 mg per ml

▷ **Usual Adult Dosage Range:**   Initially, 2 to 5 mg 2 or 3 times daily. Dose may be increased by 2 mg at 3- to 4-day intervals as needed and tolerated. Usual dosage range is 20 to 30 mg daily. The total daily dosage should not exceed 60 mg. **Note: Actual dosage and administration schedule must be determined by the physician for each patient individually.**

▷ **Dosing Instructions:**   May be taken with or following meals to reduce stomach irritation. The capsules may be opened for administration. The liquid concentrate must be diluted just before administration by adding it to 8 ounces of water, milk, fruit juice or carbonated beverage.

Usual Duration of Use: Continual use on a regular schedule for several weeks is usually necessary to determine this drug's effectiveness in controlling psychotic disorders. If not significantly beneficial within 6 weeks, it should be discontinued. Long-term use (months to years) requires periodic evaluation of response, appropriate dosage adjustment and consideration of continued need. Consult your physician on a regular basis.

▷ **This Drug Should Not Be Taken If**
- you have had an allergic reaction to it previously.
- you have active liver disease.
- you have cancer of the breast.
- you have a current blood cell or bone marrow disorder.

▷ **Inform Your Physician Before Taking This Drug If**
- you are allergic or abnormally sensitive to other thioxanthene drugs or any phenothiazine drug (see Drug Classes, Section Four).
- you have impaired liver or kidney function.
- you have any type of seizure disorder.
- you have diabetes, glaucoma or heart disease.
- you have a history of lupus erythematosus.
- you are taking any drug with sedative effects.

- you drink alcohol daily.
- you plan to have surgery under general or spinal anesthesia in the near future.

Possible Side-Effects (natural, expected and unavoidable drug actions)
Mild drowsiness (usually during the first 2 weeks), orthostatic hypotension (see Glossary), blurred vision, dry mouth, nasal congestion, constipation, impaired urination.

▷ **Possible Adverse Effects** (unusual, unexpected and infrequent reactions)
If any of the following develop, consult your physician promptly for guidance.
Mild Adverse Effects
Allergic Reactions: Skin rash, hives, itching.
Lowering of body temperature, especially in the elderly. (See Hypothermia in Glossary.)
Fluid retention, weight gain.
Dizziness, weakness, agitation, insomnia, impaired vision.
Nausea, vomiting.
Serious Adverse Effects
Allergic Reactions: Rare hepatitis with jaundice (see Glossary), anaphylactic reaction (see Glossary).
Idiosyncratic Reactions: Paradoxical worsening of psychotic symptoms. Development of the neuroleptic malignant syndrome: high fever, high (or low) blood pressure, severe muscle rigidity, impaired breathing, rapid heart rate, seizures.
Depression, disorientation, seizures, deposits in cornea and lens.
Rapid heart rate, heart rhythm disorders.
Blood cell disorders: reduced white blood cell count.
Nervous system reactions: Parkinson-like disorders (see Glossary), severe restlessness, muscle spasms involving the face and neck, tardive dyskinesia (see Glossary).

▷ **Possible Effects on Sexual Function**
Altered timing and pattern of menstruation.
Impotence (rare).
Male breast enlargement and tenderness.
Female breast enlargement with milk production.

▷ **Adverse Effects That May Mimic Natural Diseases or Disorders**
Nervous system reactions may suggest true Parkinson's disease or Reye syndrome (see Glossary).
Liver reactions may suggest viral hepatitis.

Natural Diseases or Disorders That May Be Activated by This Drug
Latent epilepsy, glaucoma, prostatism (see Glossary).

CAUTION
1. Many over-the-counter medications (see OTC Drugs in Glossary) for allergies, colds and coughs contain drugs that can interact unfa-

vorably with this drug. Ask your physician or pharmacist for guidance before using any such medications.

2. Antacids that contain aluminum and/or magnesium may prevent the absorption of this drug and reduce its effectiveness.
3. Obtain prompt evaluation of any change or disturbance of vision.

Precautions for Use

By Infants and Children: Use of this drug is not recommended in children under 12 years of age. Do not use this drug in the presence of symptoms suggestive of Reye syndrome (see Glossary). Children with acute infectious diseases ("flulike" infections, chicken pox, measles, etc.) are more prone to develop muscular spasms of the face, back and extremities when this drug is given.

By Those over 60 Years of Age: Small doses are advisable until individual response has been determined. You may be more susceptible to the development of drowsiness, lethargy, constipation, lowering of body temperature (hypothermia) and orthostatic hypotension (see Glossary). This drug can enhance existing prostatism (see Glossary). You may also be more susceptible to the development of Parkinson-like reactions and/or tardive dyskinesia (see discussion of these terms in Glossary). These reactions must be recognized early since they may become unresponsive to treatment and irreversible.

▷ **Advisability of Use During Pregnancy**
Pregnancy Category: B (tentative). See Pregnancy Code inside back cover.
Animal studies: No birth defects reported in rats, rabbits or monkeys.
Human studies: Information from adequate studies of pregnant women is not available.
Avoid drug during the first 3 months if possible. Avoid during the last month because of possible effects on the newborn infant.

Advisability of Use if Breast-Feeding
Presence of this drug in breast milk: Unknown.
Avoid drug or refrain from nursing.

Habit-Forming Potential: None.

Effects of Overdosage: Marked drowsiness, weakness, tremor, agitation, unsteadiness, deep sleep, coma, convulsions.

Possible Effects of Long-Term Use: Opacities in the cornea or lens of the eye, pigmentation of the retina. Tardive dyskinesia (see Glossary).

Suggested Periodic Examinations While Taking This Drug (at physician's discretion)
Complete blood cell counts, especially between the fourth and tenth weeks of treatment.
Liver function tests, electrocardiograms.
Complete eye examinations—eye structures and vision.

Careful inspection of the tongue for early evidence of fine, involuntary, wavelike movements that could indicate the beginning of tardive dyskinesia.

▷ **While Taking This Drug, Observe the Following**
Foods: No restrictions.
Beverages: No restrictions. May be taken with milk.
▷ *Alcohol:* Avoid completely. Alcohol can increase the sedative action of thiothixene and accentuate its depressant effects on brain function and blood pressure. Thiothixene can increase the intoxicating effects of alcohol.
Tobacco Smoking: No interactions expected.
Marijuana Smoking: Moderate increase in drowsiness; accentuation of orthostatic hypotension; increased risk of precipitating latent psychoses, confusing the interpretation of mental status and drug responses.
▷ *Other Drugs*
Thiothixene may *increase* the effects of
• all sedative drugs, especially barbiturates and narcotic analgesics, and cause excessive sedation.
• all atropinelike drugs, and cause nervous system toxicity.
Thiothixene may *decrease* the effects of
• guanethidine (Ismelin, Esimil), and reduce its effectiveness in lowering blood pressure.
The following drugs may *decrease* the effects of thiothixene
• antacids containing aluminum and/or magnesium.
• barbiturates (see Drug Class, Section Four).
• benztropine (Cogentin).
• trihexyphenidyl (Artane).
▷ *Driving, Hazardous Activities:* This drug can impair mental alertness, judgment and physical coordination. Avoid hazardous activities.
Aviation Note: The use of this drug *is a disqualification* for piloting. Consult a designated Aviation Medical Examiner.
Exposure to Sun: Use caution until sensitivity has been determined. This drug can cause photosensitivity (see Glossary).
Exposure to Heat: Use caution and avoid excessive heat as much as possible. This drug may impair the regulation of body temperature and increase the risk of heat stroke.
Exposure to Cold: Use caution and dress warmly. This drug can increase the risk of hypothermia in the elderly.
Discontinuation: After a period of long-term use, do not discontinue this drug suddenly. Gradual withdrawal over 2 to 3 weeks under physician supervision is recommended. Do not discontinue this drug without your physician's knowledge and approval. The relapse rate of schizophrenia after discontinuation is 50% to 60%.

THYROID
(THI royd)

Introduced: 1896

Class: Thyroid hormones

Prescription: USA: Yes
Canada: Yes

Controlled Drug: USA: No
Canada: No

Available as Generic: Yes

Brand Names: Armour Thyroid, Proloid, S-P-T, Thyrar, Thyroid Strong, Thyroid USP Enseals

---

BENEFITS versus RISKS

Possible Benefits	*Possible Risks*
EFFECTIVE REPLACEMENT THERAPY IN STATES OF THYROID HORMONE DEFICIENCY (HYPOTHYROIDISM) EFFECTIVE TREATMENT OF SIMPLE GOITER AND CHRONIC THYROIDITIS EFFECTIVE TREATMENT OF THYROID GLAND CANCER	Intensification of angina in presence of coronary artery disease

---

▷ **Principal Uses**

As a Single Drug Product: This natural form of thyroid hormones (derived from animal thyroid glands) is used primarily to correct a deficiency of these hormones (hypothyroidism). In the absence of true thyroid deficiency, the use of this drug to treat nonspecific fatigue, obesity, infertility or slow growth is inappropriate and possibly harmful.

How This Drug Works: Not completely established. By altering the processes of cellular chemistry that store energy in an inactive (reserve) form, this drug makes more energy available for biochemical activity and increases the rate of cellular metabolism of all tissues throughout the body.

Available Dosage Forms and Strengths

Capsules — 65 mg, 130 mg, 195 mg, 325 mg
Tablets — 16 mg, 32 mg, 65 mg, 98 mg, 100 mg, 130 mg, 195 mg, 200 mg, 260 mg, 325 mg
Tablets, enteric-coated — 32 mg, 65 mg, 130 mg
Tablets, sugar-coated — 32 mg, 65 mg, 130 mg, 195 mg

▷ **Usual Adult Dosage Range:**   Initially, 60 mg/day; increase dose by 60 mg at intervals of 1 month as needed and tolerated. The usual maintenance dose is 60 to 180 mg/day. **Note: Actual dosage and administration schedule must be determined by the physician for each patient individually.**

▷ **Dosing Instructions:**   Preferably taken in the morning on an empty stomach to ensure maximal absorption and uniform results. The capsules may be opened and the uncoated tablets may be crushed for administration.

Usual Duration of Use: Continual use on a regular schedule for 4 to 6 weeks is usually necessary to determine this drug's effectiveness in correcting the symptoms of thyroid deficiency. Long-term use (months to years, possibly for life) requires supervision and periodic evaluation by your physician. Consult your physician on a regular basis.

▷ **This Drug Should Not Be Taken If**
- you have had an allergic reaction to it previously.
- you are recovering from a recent heart attack; ask your physician for guidance.
- you are using it to lose weight and your thyroid function is normal (no deficiency).

▷ **Inform Your Physician Before Taking This Drug If**
- you have high blood pressure, any form of heart disease or diabetes.
- you have a history of Addison's disease or adrenal gland deficiency.
- you are taking any antiasthmatic medications.
- you are taking an anticoagulant.

Possible Side-Effects (natural, expected and unavoidable drug actions)
None if dosage is adjusted correctly.

▷ **Possible Adverse Effects** (unusual, unexpected and infrequent reactions)
If any of the following develop, consult your physician promptly for guidance.
Mild Adverse Effects
Allergic Reactions: Skin rash, hives.
Headache in sensitive individuals, even with proper dosage adjustment.
Serious Adverse Effects
Increased frequency or intensity of angina in the presence of coronary artery disease.

▷ **Possible Effects on Sexual Function**
Altered menstrual pattern during dosage adjustments.
Possibly beneficial in treating impaired sexual function that is associated with true hypothyroidism.

Natural Diseases or Disorders That May Be Activated by This Drug
Latent coronary artery disease.

CAUTION
1. The need for and response to thyroid hormone treatment varies greatly from person to person. Careful supervision of individual response is necessary to determine correct dosage. Do not change your dosage schedule without consulting your physician.
2. Thyroid hormonal content of drug products may vary significantly among commercial brands. To ensure consistent results from your medication, it is advisable to continue using the same brand throughout your treatment program.

Precautions for Use
By Infants and Children: This drug is not appropriate for treating hypothyroidism in infants and young children. The drug of choice for this purpose is thyroxine. (See the Drug Profile of Thyroxine that follows.)
By Those over 60 Years of Age: This drug must be used cautiously by this age group. Usually the requirements for thyroid hormone replacement are about 25% lower than in younger adults. Observe closely for any indications that suggest possible overdosage.

▷ **Advisability of Use During Pregnancy**
Pregnancy Category: A (tentative). See Pregnancy Code inside back cover.
Animal studies: No information available.
Human studies: Thyroid hormones do not reach the fetus (cross the placenta) in significant amounts. Clinical experience has shown that appropriate use of thyroid hormones causes no adverse effects on the fetus.
Use this drug only if clearly needed and with carefully adjusted dosage.

Advisability of Use if Breast-Feeding
Presence of this drug in breast milk: Yes.
Breast-feeding is considered safe with correctly adjusted dosage.

Habit-Forming Potential: None.

Effects of Overdosage: Headache, sense of increased body heat, nervousness, increased sweating, hand tremors, insomnia, rapid and irregular heart action, diarrhea, muscle cramping, weight loss.

Possible Effects of Long-Term Use: Bone loss (osteoporosis) in the lumbar vertebrae (spine).

Suggested Periodic Examinations While Taking This Drug (at physician's discretion)
Measurement of thyroid hormone levels in blood.

▷ **While Taking This Drug, Observe the Following**
Foods: No restrictions.
Beverages: No restrictions.
▷ *Alcohol:* No interactions expected.
Tobacco Smoking: No interactions expected.

▷   *Other Drugs*
Thyroid may *increase* the effects of
- warfarin (Coumadin), and increase the risk of bleeding; reduction in the dosage of anticoagulant is usually necessary.

Thyroid may *decrease* the effects of
- digoxin (Lanoxin), when correcting hypothyroidism; a larger dose of digoxin may be needed.

Thyroid *taken concurrently* with
- all antidiabetic drugs (insulin and sulfonylureas) may require an increase in the dosage of the antidiabetic agent to obtain proper control of blood sugar levels. After correct doses of both drugs have been determined, a reduction in the dose of thyroid may require a simultaneous reduction in the dose of the antidiabetic drug to prevent hypoglycemia.
- tricyclic antidepressants (see Drug Class, Section Four) may cause an increase in the activity of both drugs; monitor for indications of overdosage of each drug.

The following drugs may *decrease* the effects of thyroid
- cholestyramine (Cuemid, Questran) may reduce its absorption; intake of the two drugs should be separated by 5 hours.

▷   *Driving, Hazardous Activities:* No restrictions.
Aviation Note: The use of this drug *is probably not a disqualification* for piloting. Consult a designated Aviation Medical Examiner.
Exposure to Sun: No restrictions.
Exposure to Heat: This drug may decrease individual tolerance to warm environments, increasing discomfort due to heat. Consult your physician if you develop symptoms of overdosage during the warm months of the year.
Heavy Exercise or Exertion: Use caution if you have angina (coronary artery disease). This drug may increase the frequency or severity of angina during physical activity.
Discontinuation: This drug must be taken continually on a regular schedule to correct thyroid deficiency. Do not discontinue it without consulting your physician.

THYROXINE
(thi ROX een)

Other Names: Levothyroxine, L-thyroxine, T-4

Introduced: 1953   **Class:** Thyroid hormones

Prescription: USA: Yes   **Controlled Drug:** USA: No
　　　　Canada: Yes   　　　　Canada: No

Available as Generic: USA: Yes
　　　　Canada: No

Brand Names: ◆Eltroxin, Euthroid [CD], Levothroid, Levoxine, Synthroid, Thyrolar [CD]

BENEFITS versus RISKS

Possible Benefits	*Possible Risks*
EFFECTIVE REPLACEMENT THERAPY IN STATES OF THYROID HORMONE DEFICIENCY (HYPOTHYROIDISM)	Intensification of angina in presence of coronary artery disease
EFFECTIVE TREATMENT OF SIMPLE GOITER AND CHRONIC THYROIDITIS	Drug-induced hyperthyroidism (with excessive dosage)
EFFECTIVE TREATMENT OF THYROID GLAND CANCER	

▷ **Principal Uses**

As a Single Drug Product: This synthetic thyroid hormone is used primarily to correct thyroid deficiency (hypothyroidism). In addition, it is used to suppress thyroid function in the treatment of simple goiter and the management of Hashimoto's thyroiditis. It is also of value as adjunctive therapy in the management of thyroid gland cancer.

As a Combination Drug Product [CD]: This thyroid hormone is available in combination with the other principal thyroid hormone, liothyronine, in a preparation that resembles the natural hormone material produced by the thyroid gland.

How This Drug Works: Not completely established. By altering the processes of cellular chemistry that store energy in an inactive (reserve) form, this drug makes more energy available for biochemical activity and increases the rate of cellular metabolism of all tissues throughout the body.

Available Dosage Forms and Strengths

Injections — 100 mcg per ml, 200 mcg per vial

Tablets — 0.0125 mg, 0.025 mg, 0.05 mg, 0.075 mg, 0.1 mg, 0.112 mg, 0.125 mg, 0.15 mg, 0.175 mg, 0.2 mg, 0.3 mg

▷ **Usual Adult Dosage Range:** Initially, 0.05 to 0.10 mg/day. The dose may be increased at intervals of 2 to 3 weeks as needed and tolerated. The usual maintenance dose is 0.025 to 0.3 mg/day. The total daily dosage should not exceed 0.4 mg. **Note: Actual dosage and administration schedule must be determined by the physician for each patient individually.**

▷ **Dosing Instructions:** Preferably taken in the morning on an empty stomach to ensure maximal absorption and uniform results. The tablets may be crushed for administration.

Usual Duration of Use: Continual use on a regular schedule for 4 to 6 weeks is usually necessary to determine this drug's effectiveness in correcting the symptoms of thyroid deficiency. Long-term use (months to years, possibly for life) requires supervision and periodic evaluation by your physician. Consult your physician on a regular basis.

▷ **This Drug Should Not Be Taken If**
- you have had an allergic reaction to it previously.
- you are recovering from a recent heart attack; ask your physician for guidance.
- you are using it to lose weight and your thyroid function is normal (no deficiency).

▷ **Inform Your Physician Before Taking This Drug If**
- you have high blood pressure, any form of heart disease or diabetes.
- you have a history of Addison's disease or adrenal gland deficiency.
- you are taking any antiasthmatic medications.
- you are taking an anticoagulant.

Possible Side-Effects (natural, expected and unavoidable drug actions)
None if dosage is adjusted correctly.

▷ **Possible Adverse Effects** (unusual, unexpected and infrequent reactions)
If any of the following develop, consult your physician promptly for guidance.
Mild Adverse Effects
Allergic Reactions: Skin rash, hives.
Headache in sensitive individuals, even with proper dosage adjustment.
Serious Adverse Effects
Increased frequency or intensity of angina in the presence of coronary artery disease.
Note: Other adverse effects are manifestations of excessive dosage. See Effects of Overdosage category.

▷ **Possible Effects on Sexual Function**
Altered menstrual pattern during dosage adjustments.
Possibly beneficial in treating impaired sexual function that is associated with true hypothyroidism.

Natural Diseases or Disorders That May Be Activated by This Drug
Latent coronary artery insufficiency (angina), diabetes.

CAUTION
1. The need for and response to thyroid hormone treatment varies greatly from person to person. Careful supervision of individual response is necessary to determine correct dosage. Do not change your dosage schedule without consulting your physician.
2. In the absence of verified thyroid deficiency, this drug should not be used to treat nonspecific fatigue, obesity, infertility or slow growth. Such use is inappropriate and could be harmful.

Precautions for Use
By Infants and Children: To facilitate normal growth and development, the thyroid-deficient child often requires higher dosage than the

adult. A transient loss of hair may occur during the early months of treatment.

By Those over 60 Years of Age: This drug must be used cautiously by this age group. Usually the requirements for thyroid hormone replacement are about 25% lower than in younger adults. Observe closely for any indications that suggest possible overdosage.

▷ **Advisability of Use During Pregnancy**

Pregnancy Category: A (tentative). See Pregnancy Code inside back cover.

Animal studies: Cataract formation reported in rat studies. Other defects reported in rabbit and guinea pig studies.

Human studies: Thyroid hormones do not reach the fetus (cross the placenta) in significant amounts. Clinical experience has shown that appropriate use of thyroid hormones causes no adverse effects on the fetus.

Use this drug only if clearly needed and with carefully adjusted dosage.

Advisability of Use if Breast-Feeding

Presence of this drug in breast milk: Yes, in minimal amounts.

Breast-feeding is considered safe with correctly adjusted dosage.

Habit-Forming Potential: None.

Effects of Overdosage: Headache, sense of increased body heat, nervousness, increased sweating, hand tremors, insomnia, rapid and irregular heart action, diarrhea, muscle cramping, weight loss.

Possible Effects of Long-Term Use: Bone loss (osteoporosis) in the lumbar vertebrae (spine).

Suggested Periodic Examinations While Taking This Drug (at physician's discretion)

Measurement of thyroid hormone levels in blood.

▷ **While Taking This Drug, Observe the Following**

Foods: No restrictions.

Beverages: No restrictions.

▷   *Alcohol:* No interactions expected.

Tobacco Smoking: No interactions expected.

▷   *Other Drugs*

Thyroxine may ***increase*** the effects of

- warfarin (Coumadin), and increase the risk of bleeding; reduction in the dosage of anticoagulant is usually necessary.

Thyroxine may ***decrease*** the effects of

- digoxin (Lanoxin), when correcting hypothyroidism; a larger dose of digoxin may be needed.

Thyroxine ***taken concurrently*** with

- all antidiabetic drugs (insulin and sulfonylureas) may require an increase in the dosage of the antidiabetic agent to obtain proper control of blood sugar levels. After correct doses of both drugs have been determined, a reduction in the dose of thyroid may require a simultaneous reduction in the dose of the antidiabetic drug to prevent hypoglycemia.

- tricyclic antidepressants (see Drug Class, Section Four) may cause an increase in the activity of both drugs; monitor for indications of overdosage of each drug.

The following drugs may *decrease* the effects of thyroxine

- cholestyramine (Cuemid, Questran) may reduce its absorption; intake of the two drugs should be separated by 5 hours.

▷ *Driving, Hazardous Activities:* No restrictions.

Aviation Note: The use of this drug *is probably not a disqualification* for piloting. Consult a designated Aviation Medical Examiner.

Exposure to Sun: No restrictions.

Exposure to Heat: This drug may decrease individual tolerance to warm environments, increasing discomfort due to heat. Consult your physician if you develop symptoms of overdosage during the warm months of the year.

Heavy Exercise or Exertion: Use caution if you have angina (coronary artery disease). This drug may increase the frequency or severity of angina during physical activity.

Discontinuation: This drug must be taken continually on a regular schedule to correct thyroid deficiency. Do not discontinue it without consulting your physician.

TIMOLOL
(TI moh lohl)

Introduced: 1972

Class: Antianginal, antiglaucoma, antihypertensive, migraine preventive, beta-adrenergic blocker

Prescription: USA: Yes
  Canada: Yes

Controlled Drug: USA: No
  Canada: No

Available as Generic: USA: No
  Canada: No

Brand Names: Blocadren, Timolide [CD], Timoptic

```
┌─────────────────────────────────────────────────────────────┐
│                   BENEFITS versus RISKS                      │
│        Possible Benefits              Possible Risks         │
│  EFFECTIVE, WELL-TOLERATED      CONGESTIVE HEART FAILURE      │
│  AS: ANTIANGINAL DRUG in          in advanced heart disease  │
│  effort-induced angina;         Worsening of angina in coronary│
│  ANTIGLAUCOMA DRUG in             heart disease (if drug is  │
│  open-angle glaucoma;             abruptly withdrawn)        │
│  ANTIHYPERTENSIVE DRUG          Masking of low blood sugar   │
│  in mild to moderate              (hypoglycemia) in drug-treated│
│  hypertension                     diabetes                  │
│  EFFECTIVE PREVENTION OF        Provocation of asthma        │
│  MIGRAINE HEADACHES                                          │
│  Effective adjunct in the                                   │
│  prevention of recurrent heart                              │
│  attack (myocardial infarction)                             │
└─────────────────────────────────────────────────────────────┘
```

▷ **Principal Uses**

As a Single Drug Product: This member of the beta blocker drug class is used primarily to treat (1) classical effort-induced angina, certain types of heart rhythm disturbance and high blood pressure; (2) increased internal eye pressure and chronic open-angle glaucoma. It is also beneficial in preventing the recurrence of heart attacks (myocardial infarction). In addition, it is used to reduce the frequency and severity of migraine headaches.

As a Combination Drug Product [CD]: This drug is available in combination with hydrochlorothiazide for the treatment of hypertension. This combination product includes two "step 1" drugs with different mechanisms of action; it is intended to provide greater effectiveness and convenience for long-term use.

How This Drug Works: By blocking certain actions of the sympathetic nervous system, this drug
- reduces the rate and contraction force of the heart, thus lowering the ejection pressure of the blood leaving the heart and reducing the oxygen requirement for heart function.
- reduces the degree of contraction of blood vessel walls, resulting in their relaxation and expansion and consequent lowering of blood pressure.
- prolongs the conduction time of nerve impulses through the heart, of benefit in the management of certain heart rhythm disorders.
- slows the formation of fluid (aqueous humor) in the anterior chamber of the eye and improves its drainage from the eye, thus lowering the internal eye pressure.

Available Dosage Forms and Strengths
Eye solutions — 0.25%, 0.5%
Tablets — 5 mg, 10 mg, 20 mg

▷ **Usual Adult Dosage Range:** Varies with indication.

Antianginal and antihypertensive: Initially, 10 mg 2 times/day; increase dose gradually every 7 days as needed and tolerated. Usual maintenance dose is 10 to 20 mg twice/day. The total daily dosage should not exceed 60 mg.

Migraine headache prevention: Initially, 10 mg 2 times/day; increase dose as needed to 10 mg in the morning and 20 mg at night.

Recurrent heart attack prevention: 10 mg twice/day.

Antiglaucoma: 1 drop in affected eye every 12 to 24 hours.

Note: Actual dosage and administration schedule must be determined by the physician for each patient individually.

▷ **Dosing Instructions:** Preferably taken 1 hour before eating to maximize absorption. The tablet may be crushed for administration. Do not discontinue this drug abruptly.

Usual Duration of Use: Continual use on a regular schedule for 10 to 14 days is usually necessary to determine this drug's effectiveness in preventing angina, controlling heart rhythm disorders and lowering blood pressure. Maximal effectiveness may require continual use for 6 to 8 weeks. The long-term use of this drug (months to years) will be determined by the course of your symptoms over time and your response to the overall treatment program (weight reduction, salt restriction, smoking cessation, etc.). Consult your physician on a regular basis.

Currently a "Drug of Choice" for initiating treatment of hypertension with a single drug.

▷ **This Drug Should Not Be Taken If**
- you have had an allergic reaction to it previously.
- you have Prinzmetal's variant angina (coronary artery spasm).
- you have congestive heart failure.
- you have an abnormally slow heart rate or a serious form of heart block.
- you are taking, or have taken within the past 14 days, any monoamine oxidase (MAO) type A inhibitor drug (see Drug Class, Section Four).

▷ **Inform Your Physician Before Taking This Drug If**
- you have had an adverse reaction to any beta blocker drug in the past (see Drug Class, Section Four).
- you have a history of serious heart disease, with or without episodes of heart failure.
- you have a history of hay fever (allergic rhinitis), asthma, chronic bronchitis or emphysema.
- you have a history of overactive thyroid function (hyperthyroidism).
- you have a history of low blood sugar (hypoglycemia).
- you have impaired liver or kidney function.
- you have diabetes or myasthenia gravis.

- you are currently taking any form of digitalis, quinidine or reserpine, or any calcium blocker drug (see Drug Class, Section Four).
- you plan to have surgery under general anesthesia in the near future.

Possible Side-Effects (natural, expected and unavoidable drug actions)
Lethargy and fatigability, cold extremities, slow heart rate, light-headedness in upright position (see Orthostatic Hypotension in Glossary).

▷ **Possible Adverse Effects** (unusual, unexpected and infrequent reactions)
If any of the following develop, consult your physician promptly for guidance.

Mild Adverse Effects
Allergic Reactions: Skin rash, itching.
Headache, dizziness, visual disturbances, vivid dreams.
Indigestion, nausea, vomiting, diarrhea.
Numbness and tingling in extremities.

Serious Adverse Effects
Allergic Reactions: Laryngospasm, severe dermatitis.
Idiosyncratic Reactions: Acute behavioral disturbances: depression, hallucinations.
Chest pain, shortness of breath, precipitation of congestive heart failure.
Induction of bronchial asthma (in asthmatic individuals).
Masking of warning signs of impending low blood sugar (hypoglycemia) in drug-treated diabetes.

▷ **Possible Effects on Sexual Function**
Decreased libido, impaired erection, impotence.
Note: All of these effects can occur with the use of timolol eye drops at recommended dosage.

▷ **Adverse Effects That May Mimic Natural Diseases or Disorders**
Reduced blood flow to extremities may resemble Raynaud's phenomenon (see Glossary).

Natural Diseases or Disorders That May Be Activated by This Drug
Prinzmetal's variant angina, Raynaud's disease, intermittent claudication, myasthenia gravis (questionable).

CAUTION
1. ***Do not discontinue this drug suddenly*** without the knowledge and guidance of your physician. Carry a notation on your person that you are taking this drug.
2. Consult your physician or pharmacist before using nasal decongestants usually present in over-the-counter cold preparations and nose drops. These can cause sudden increases in blood pressure when taken concurrently with beta blocker drugs.
3. Report the development of any tendency to emotional depression (rare with this drug).

Precautions for Use

By Infants and Children: Safety and effectiveness for use by those under 12 years of age have not been established. However, if this drug is used, observe for the development of low blood sugar (hypoglycemia) during periods of reduced food intake.

By Those over 60 Years of Age: Proceed **cautiously** with all antihypertensive drugs. Unacceptably high blood pressure should be reduced without creating the risks associated with excessively low blood pressure. Start treatment with small doses, and monitor the blood pressure response frequently. Sudden, rapid and excessive reduction of blood pressure can predispose to stroke or heart attack. Observe for dizziness, unsteadiness, tendency to fall, confusion, hallucinations, depression or urinary frequency.

▷ **Advisability of Use During Pregnancy**

Pregnancy Category: C (tentative). See Pregnancy Code inside back cover.
Animal studies: No significant increase in birth defects due to this drug.
Human studies: Information from adequate studies of pregnant women is not available.
Avoid use of drug during the first 3 months if possible. Use this drug only if clearly needed. Ask your physician for guidance.

Advisability of Use if Breast-Feeding

Presence of this drug in breast milk: Probably yes.
Monitor nursing infant closely and discontinue drug or nursing if adverse effects develop.

Habit-Forming Potential: None.

Effects of Overdosage: Weakness, slow pulse, low blood pressure, fainting, cold and sweaty skin, congestive heart failure, possible coma and convulsions.

Possible Effects of Long-Term Use: Reduced heart reserve and eventual heart failure in susceptible individuals with advanced heart disease.

Suggested Periodic Examinations While Taking This Drug (at physician's discretion)

Complete blood cell counts (because of adverse effects of other drugs of this class).
Measurements of blood pressure, evaluation of heart function.

▷ **While Taking This Drug, Observe the Following**

Foods: No restrictions. Avoid excessive salt intake.
Beverages: No restrictions. May be taken with milk.
▷ *Alcohol:* Use with caution until the combined effect has been determined. Alcohol may exaggerate this drug's ability to lower the blood pressure and may increase its mild sedative effect.
Tobacco Smoking: Nicotine may reduce this drug's effectiveness in treating angina, heart rhythm disorders and high blood pressure. In ad-

dition, high doses of this drug may potentiate the constriction of the bronchial tubes caused by regular smoking.

▷ *Other Drugs*

Timolol may *increase* the effects of

- other antihypertensive drugs, and cause excessive lowering of blood pressure. Dosage adjustments may be necessary.
- lidocaine (Xylocaine, etc.).
- reserpine (Ser-Ap-Es, etc.), and cause sedation, depression, slowing of the heart rate and lowering of the blood pressure.
- verapamil (Calan, Isoptin), and cause excessive depression of heart function; monitor this combination closely.

Timolol may *decrease* the effects of

- theophyllines (Aminophyllin, Theo-Dur, etc.), and reduce their antiasthmatic effectiveness.

Timolol *taken concurrently* with

- clonidine (Catapres) requires close monitoring for rebound high blood pressure if clonidine is withdrawn while timolol is still being taken.
- epinephrine (Adrenalin, etc.) may cause marked rise in blood pressure and slowing of the heart rate.
- insulin requires close monitoring to avoid undetected hypoglycemia (see Glossary).

The following drugs may *increase* the effects of timolol

- chlorpromazine (Thorazine, etc.)
- cimetidine (Tagamet).
- methimazole (Tapazole).
- propylthiouracil (Propacil).

The following drugs may *decrease* the effects of timolol

- barbiturates (phenobarbital, etc.).
- indomethacin (Indocin), and possibly other "aspirin substitutes," may impair timolol's antihypertensive effect.
- rifampin (Rifadin, Rimactane).

▷ *Driving, Hazardous Activities:* Use caution until the full extent of dizziness, lethargy and blood pressure change have been determined.

Aviation Note: The use of this drug *may be a disqualification* for piloting. Consult a designated Aviation Medical Examiner.

Exposure to Sun: No restrictions.

Exposure to Heat: Caution advised. Hot environments can lower blood pressure and exaggerate the effects of this drug.

Exposure to Cold: Caution advised. Cold environments can enhance the circulatory deficiency in the extremities that may occur with this drug. The elderly should take precautions to prevent hypothermia (see Glossary).

Heavy Exercise or Exertion: It is advisable to avoid exertion that produces light-headedness, excessive fatigue or muscle cramping. The use of this drug may intensify the hypertensive response to isometric exercise.

Occurrence of Unrelated Illness: The fever that accompanies systemic infections can lower blood pressure and require adjustment of dosage. Illnesses that cause nausea or vomiting may interrupt the regular dosage schedule. Ask your physician for guidance.

Discontinuation: It is advisable to avoid sudden discontinuation of this drug in all situations; this is especially true in the presence of coronary artery disease. If possible, gradual reduction of dose over a period of 2 to 3 weeks is recommended. Ask your physician for specific guidance.

TOCAINIDE
(toh KAY nide)

Introduced: 1976

Prescription: USA: Yes
Canada: Yes

Available as Generic: USA: No
Canada: No

Brand Name: Tonocard

Class: Antiarrhythmic

Controlled Drug: USA: No
Canada: No

BENEFITS versus RISKS

Possible Benefits	*Possible Risks*
EFFECTIVE TREATMENT OF SELECTED HEART RHYTHM DISORDERS (ventricular)	DRUG-INDUCED HEART RHYTHM DISORDERS (10.9%) CONGESTIVE HEART FAILURE (4%) Rare blood cell disorders: aplastic anemia, abnormally low white blood cell and platelet counts Drug-induced lung damage

---

▷ **Principal Uses**

As a Single Drug Product: This drug is classified as a Type 1 antiarrhythmic agent, similar to procainamide and quinidine in its actions. It is used primarily to correct and prevent the recurrence of (1) abnormally rapid heart rates (tachycardia) that arise in the ventricles (lower heart chambers); and (2) premature beats arising in the ventricles.

How This Drug Works: By slowing the transmission of electrical impulses throughout the conduction system of the heart, this drug assists in restoring normal heart rate and rhythm.

Available Dosage Forms and Strengths
Tablets — 400 mg, 600 mg

▷ **Usual Adult Dosage Range:**   Do not take a loading dose. Initiate treatment with 400 mg/8 hours. If needed and tolerated, the dose may be increased gradually to 600 mg/8 hours. The total daily dosage should not exceed 2400 mg. **Note: Actual dosage and administration schedule must be determined by the physician for each patient individually.**

▷ **Dosing Instructions:**   May be taken without regard to meals, but may be taken with or following food if desired to reduce stomach irritation. Take at same time each day to obtain uniform results. The tablet may be crushed for administration.

Usual Duration of Use: Continual use on a regular schedule for 1 to 2 weeks is usually necessary to determine this drug's effectiveness in correcting or preventing responsive rhythm disorders. Long-term use requires supervision and periodic evaluation by your physician. Consult your physician on a regular basis.

▷ **This Drug Should Not Be Taken If**
  • you have had an allergic reaction to it previously.
  • you are allergic to local anesthetics of the Novocain type.
  • you have second-degree or third-degree heart block (with no pacemaker).

▷ **Inform Your Physician Before Taking This Drug If**
  • you have had any unfavorable reactions to other antiarrhythmic drugs in the past.
  • you have a history of heart disease of any kind, especially heart block.
  • you have impaired liver or kidney function.
  • you are taking any form of digitalis, a potassium supplement or any diuretic drug that can cause excessive loss of body potassium (ask physician).

Possible Side-Effects (natural, expected and unavoidable drug actions)
Flushing, increased sweating, light-headedness.
The onset of tremors indicates that the dose is reaching the maximum that can be tolerated.

▷ **Possible Adverse Effects** (unusual, unexpected and infrequent reactions)
If any of the following develop, consult your physician promptly for guidance.
Mild Adverse Effects
Allergic Reactions: Skin rash (8%), hives, itching.
Headache (4%), dizziness (15%), visual disturbance (1.5%), fatigue (0.8%), tremor (8%), numbness (9%).
Loss of appetite, indigestion, nausea (14%), vomiting (4%), diarrhea (4%).

Serious Adverse Effects

Idiosyncratic Reactions: Confusion, disorientation, hallucinations (2.7%).

Drug-induced heart rhythm disorders (10%), congestive heart failure (4%), shortness of breath, palpitations, chest pain.

Drug-induced lung damage: pneumonitis and fibrosis, causing cough and breathing difficulty. (Usually occurs after 3 to 18 weeks of drug use.)

Bone marrow depression (see Glossary): fatigue, weakness, fever, sore throat, abnormal bleeding or bruising. (Usually occurs after 2 to 12 weeks of drug use.)

▷ **Possible Effects on Sexual Function:** None reported.

▷ **Adverse Effects That May Mimic Natural Diseases or Disorders**
Lung reactions may suggest an infectious bronchitis or pneumonia.

CAUTION

1. Thorough evaluation of your heart function (including electrocardiograms) is necessary prior to using this drug.
2. Periodic evaluation of your heart function is necessary to determine your response to this drug. Some individuals may experience worsening of their heart rhythm disorder and/or deterioration of heart function. Close monitoring of heart rate, rhythm and overall performance is essential.
3. Dosage must be adjusted carefully for each individual. Do not change your dosage without the knowledge and supervision of your physician.
4. Do not take any other antiarrhythmic drug while taking this drug unless directed to do so by your physician.

Precautions for Use

By Infants and Children: Safety and effectiveness for use by those under 12 years of age have not been established. Initial use of this drug requires hospitalization and supervision by a qualified cardiologist.

By Those over 60 Years of Age: Reduced kidney function may require reduction in dosage. Observe carefully for light-headedness, dizziness, unsteadiness and tendency to fall.

▷ **Advisability of Use During Pregnancy**

Pregnancy Category: C (tentative). See Pregnancy Code inside back cover.

Animal studies: No birth defects reported in rat or rabbit studies; however, an increase in fetal resorptions, stillbirths and abortions was reported.

Human studies: Information from adequate studies of pregnant women is not available.

Avoid this drug during first 3 months. Use this drug only if clearly needed. Ask your physician for guidance.

Advisability of Use if Breast-Feeding
Presence of this drug in breast milk: Unknown.
Avoid drug or refrain from nursing.

Habit-Forming Potential: None.

Effects of Overdosage: Impaired urination, constipation, marked drop in blood pressure, abnormal heart rhythms, slow heart rate, congestive heart failure, seizures.

Possible Effects of Long-Term Use: None reported.

Suggested Periodic Examinations While Taking This Drug (at physician's discretion)
Electrocardiograms, complete blood cell counts, measurements of potassium blood levels.

▷ **While Taking This Drug, Observe the Following**
Foods: No restrictions. Ask physician regarding need for salt restriction and advisability of eating potassium-rich foods.
Beverages: No restrictions. May be taken with milk.
▷ *Alcohol:* Use caution until the combined effects have been determined. Alcohol can increase the blood-pressure-lowering effects of this drug.
Tobacco Smoking: Nicotine can cause irritability of the heart and reduce the effectiveness of this drug. Follow physician's advice regarding smoking.
▷ *Other Drugs*
Tocainide may *increase* the effects of
• antihypertensive drugs, and cause excessive lowering of blood pressure.
• beta blocker drugs (see Drug Class, Section Four).
The following drugs may *decrease* the effects of tocainide
• diuretics that promote potassium loss.
▷ *Driving, Hazardous Activities:* This drug may cause dizziness or blurred vision. Restrict activities as necessary.
Aviation Note: The use of this drug *may be a disqualification* for piloting. Consult a designated Aviation Medical Examiner.
Exposure to Sun: No restrictions.
Occurrence of Unrelated Illness: Disorders that cause vomiting, diarrhea or dehydration can affect this drug's action adversely. Report such developments promptly.
Discontinuation: This drug should not be discontinued abruptly following long-term use. Ask your physician for guidance regarding gradual dose reduction.

TOLAZAMIDE
(tohl AZ a mide)

Introduced: 1966   **Class:** Antidiabetic, sulfonylureas
Prescription: USA: Yes   **Controlled Drug:** USA: No

Available as Generic: Yes

Brand Names: Ronase, Tolamide, Tolinase

BENEFITS versus RISKS

Possible Benefits	*Possible Risks*
Assistance in regulating blood sugar in noninsulin-dependent diabetes (adjunctive to appropriate diet and weight control)	HYPOGLYCEMIA, severe and prolonged Drug-induced liver damage Rare bone marrow depression (see Glossary) Hemolytic anemia (see Glossary)

▷ **Principal Uses**

As a Single Drug Product: To assist in the control of mild to moderately severe type II diabetes mellitus (adult, maturity-onset) that does not require insulin, but that cannot be adequately controlled by diet alone.

How This Drug Works: It is thought that this drug (1) stimulates the release of insulin (by a pancreas that is capable of responding to stimulation), and (2) enhances the utilization of insulin by appropriate tissues.

Available Dosage Forms and Strengths

Tablets — 100 mg, 250 mg, 500 mg

▷ **Usual Adult Dosage Range:**   Initially, 100 to 250 mg daily with breakfast. At 7-day intervals, the dose may be increased by increments of 100 to 250 mg daily as needed and tolerated. The total daily dosage should not exceed 1000 mg (1 gram). A "loading" or priming dose is not necessary and should not be given. **Note: Actual dosage and administration schedule must be determined by the physician for each patient individually.**

▷ **Dosing Instructions:**   If the daily maintenance dose is found to be more than 500 mg, the total dose should be divided into 2 equal doses: the first taken with the morning meal, the second with the evening meal. The tablet may be crushed for administration.

Usual Duration of Use: Continual use on a regular schedule for several weeks is usually necessary to determine this drug's effectiveness in controlling diabetes. Failure to respond to maximal doses within 1 month constitutes a primary failure. Up to 10% of those who respond initially may develop secondary failure of the drug later. The duration of effective use can only be determined by periodic measurement of the blood sugar. Consult your physician on a regular basis.

▷ **This Drug Should Not Be Taken If**
- you have had an allergic reaction to it previously.
- you have severe impairment of liver or kidney function.
- you are pregnant.

▷ **Inform Your Physician Before Taking This Drug If**
- you are allergic to other sulfonylurea drugs or to "sulfa" drugs. (See Drug Classes, Section Four).
- your diabetes has been unstable or "brittle" in the past.
- you do not know how to recognize or treat hypoglycemia (see Glossary).
- you have a history of congestive heart failure, peptic ulcer disease, cirrhosis of the liver, hypothyroidism or porphyria.

Possible Side-Effects (natural, expected and unavoidable drug actions)
If drug dosage is excessive or food intake is delayed or inadequate, abnormally low blood sugar (hypoglycemia) will occur as a predictable drug effect.

▷ **Possible Adverse Effects** (unusual, unexpected and infrequent reactions)
If any of the following develop, consult your physician promptly for guidance.
Mild Adverse Effects
Allergic Reactions: Skin rash, hives, itching, drug fever.
Headache, ringing in the ears.
Indigestion, heartburn, nausea, vomiting, diarrhea.
Serious Adverse Effects
Allergic Reactions: Hepatitis with jaundice (see Glossary).
Idiosyncratic Reactions: Hemolytic anemia (see Glossary); disulfiram-like reaction with concurrent use of alcohol (see Glossary), infrequent with this drug.
Bone marrow depression (see Glossary): fatigue, weakness, fever, sore throat, abnormal bleeding or bruising.

▷ **Possible Effects on Sexual Function**   None reported.

▷ **Adverse Effects That May Mimic Natural Diseases or Disorders**
Liver reactions may suggest viral hepatitis.

CAUTION
1. This drug must be regarded as only one part of the total program for the management of your diabetes. It is not a substitute for a properly prescribed diet and regular exercise.
2. Over a period of time (usually several months), this drug may lose its effectiveness in controlling blood sugar levels. Periodic follow-up examinations are necessary to monitor all aspects of response to drug treatment.

Precautions for Use
By Infants and Children: This drug is not effective in type I (juvenile, growth-onset) insulin-dependent diabetes.

By Those over 60 Years of Age: This drug should be used with caution in this age group. Start treatment with 100 mg/day; increase dosage cautiously and monitor closely to prevent hypoglycemic reactions. Repeated episodes of hypoglycemia in the elderly can cause brain damage.

▷ **Advisability of Use During Pregnancy**
Pregnancy Category: C (tentative). See Pregnancy Code inside back cover.
Animal studies: No birth defects due to this drug reported in rats.
Human studies: Information from adequate studies of pregnant women is not available.
Because uncontrolled blood sugar levels during pregnancy are associated with a higher incidence of birth defects, many experts recommend that insulin (instead of an oral agent) be used as necessary to control diabetes during the entire pregnancy.
Use during pregnancy is not recommended by the manufacturer.

Advisability of Use if Breast-Feeding
Presence of this drug in breast milk: Probably yes.
Avoid drug or refrain from nursing.

Habit-Forming Potential: None.

Effects of Overdosage: Symptoms of mild to severe hypoglycemia: headache, light-headedness, faintness, nervousness, confusion, tremor, sweating, heart palpitation, weakness, hunger, nausea, vomiting, stupor progressing to coma.

Possible Effects of Long-Term Use: Reduced function of the thyroid gland (hypothyroidism). Reports of increased frequency and severity of heart and blood vessel diseases associated with long-term use of this class of drugs are highly controversial and inconclusive. A direct cause-and-effect relationship (see Glossary) is tenuous. Ask your physician for guidance.

Suggested Periodic Examinations While Taking This Drug (at physician's discretion)
Complete blood cell counts, liver function tests, thyroid function tests, periodic evaluation of heart and circulatory system.

▷ **While Taking This Drug, Observe the Following**
Foods: Follow the diabetic diet prescribed by your physician.
Beverages: As directed in the diabetic diet. May be taken with milk.
▷   *Alcohol:* Use with extreme caution until the combined effect has been determined. Alcohol can exaggerate this drug's hypoglycemic effect. This drug infrequently causes a marked intolerance of alcohol resulting in a disulfiramlike reaction (see Glossary): facial flushing, sweating, palpitation.
Tobacco Smoking: No interactions expected.

▷ *Other Drugs*

The following drugs may *increase* the effects of tolazamide
- aspirin, and other salicylates.
- cimetidine (Tagamet).
- clofibrate (Atromid S).
- fenfluramine (Pondimin).
- monoamine oxidase (MAO) type A inhibitor drugs (see Drug Class, Section Four).
- phenylbutazone (Butazolidin).
- ranitidine (Zantac).

The following drugs may *decrease* the effects of tolazamide
- beta blocker drugs (see Drug Class, Section Four).
- bumetanide (Bumex).
- diazoxide (Proglycem).
- ethacrynic acid (Edecrin).
- furosemide (Lasix).
- phenytoin (Dilantin).
- thiazide diuretics (see Drug Class, Section Four).

▷ *Driving, Hazardous Activities:* Regulate your dosage schedule, eating schedule and physical activities very carefully to prevent hypoglycemia. Be able to recognize the early symptoms of hypoglycemia so you can avoid hazardous activities and take corrective measures.

Aviation Note: Diabetes *is a disqualification* for piloting. Consult a designated Aviation Medical Examiner.

Exposure to Sun: Use caution until sensitivity has been determined. Some drugs of this class can cause photosensitivity (see Glossary).

Occurrence of Unrelated Illness: Acute infections, illnesses causing vomiting or diarrhea, serious injuries and surgical procedures can interfere with diabetic control and may require the use of insulin. If any of these conditions occur, consult your physician promptly.

Discontinuation: Because of the possibility of secondary failure, it is advisable to evaluate the continued benefit of this drug every 6 months.

TOLBUTAMIDE
(tohl BYU ta mide)

Introduced: 1956   **Class:** Antidiabetic, sulfonylureas

Prescription: USA: Yes   **Controlled Drug:** USA: No
Canada: Yes   Canada: No

Available as Generic: Yes

Brand Names: ✦Apo-Tolbutamide, ✦Mobenol, ✦Novobutamide, Oramide, Orinase

---

BENEFITS versus RISKS

Possible Benefits	*Possible Risks*
Assistance in regulating blood sugar in noninsulin-dependent diabetes (adjunctive to appropriate diet and weight control)	HYPOGLYCEMIA, severe and prolonged Drug-induced liver damage Rare bone marrow depression (See Glossary) Hemolytic anemia (See Glossary)

▷ **Principal Uses**

As a Single Drug Product: To assist in the control of mild to moderately severe type II diabetes mellitus (adult, maturity-onset) that does not require insulin, but that cannot be adequately controlled by diet alone.

How This Drug Works: It is thought that this drug (1) stimulates the release of insulin (by a pancreas that is capable of responding to stimulation), and (2) enhances the utilization of insulin by appropriate tissues.

Available Dosage Forms and Strengths

Tablets — 250 mg, 500 mg

▷ **Usual Adult Dosage Range:** Initially, 500 mg twice a day. The dose may be increased or decreased every 48 to 72 hours until the minimal amount required for satisfactory control is determined. The usual range is 500 to 2000 mg/24 hours. The total daily dosage should not exceed 3000 mg (3 grams). A "loading" or priming dose is not necessary and should not be given. **Note: Actual dosage and administration schedule must be determined by the physician for each patient individually.**

▷ **Dosing Instructions:** May be taken with food (morning and evening meals) to reduce stomach irritation. The tablet may be crushed for administration.

Usual Duration of Use: Continual use on a regular schedule for several weeks is usually necessary to determine this drug's effectiveness in controlling diabetes. Failure to respond to maximal doses within 1 month constitutes a primary failure. Up to 15% of those who respond initially may develop secondary failure of the drug within the first year. The duration of effective use can only be determined by periodic measurement of the blood sugar. Consult your physician on a regular basis.

▷ **This Drug Should Not Be Taken If**
- you have had an allergic reaction to it previously.
- you have severe impairment of liver or kidney function.
- you are pregnant.

▷ **Inform Your Physician Before Taking This Drug If**
- you are allergic to other sulfonylurea drugs or to "sulfa" drugs. (See Drug Classes, Section Four).
- your diabetes has been unstable or "brittle" in the past.
- you do not know how to recognize or treat hypoglycemia (see Glossary).
- you have a history of congestive heart failure, peptic ulcer disease, cirrhosis of the liver, hypothyroidism or porphyria.

Possible Side-Effects (natural, expected and unavoidable drug actions)
If drug dosage is excessive or food intake is delayed or inadequate, abnormally low blood sugar (hypoglycemia) will occur as a predictable drug effect.

▷ **Possible Adverse Effects** (unusual, unexpected and infrequent reactions)
If any of the following develop, consult your physician promptly for guidance.
Mild Adverse Effects
Allergic Reactions: Skin rash, hives, itching, drug fever.
Headache, ringing in the ears, weakness.
Indigestion, heartburn, nausea, vomiting.
Serious Adverse Effects
Allergic Reactions: Hepatitis with jaundice (see Glossary).
Idiosyncratic Reactions: Hemolytic anemia (see Glossary); disulfiram-like reaction with concurrent use of alcohol (see Glossary), infrequent with this drug.
Bone marrow depression (see Glossary): fatigue, weakness, fever, sore throat, abnormal bleeding or bruising.

▷ **Possible Effects on Sexual Function**   None reported.

▷ **Adverse Effects That May Mimic Natural Diseases or Disorders**
Liver reactions may suggest viral hepatitis.

Natural Diseases or Disorders That May Be Activated by This Drug
Acute intermittent porphyria (see Glossary).

CAUTION
1. This drug must be regarded as only one part of the total program for the management of your diabetes. It is not a substitute for a properly prescribed diet and regular exercise.
2. Over a period of time (usually several months), this drug may lose its effectiveness in controlling blood sugar levels. Periodic follow-up examinations are necessary to monitor all aspects of response to drug treatment.

Precautions for Use
By Infants and Children: This drug is not effective in type I (juvenile, growth-onset) insulin-dependent diabetes.
By Those over 60 Years of Age: This drug should be used with caution in this age group. Start treatment with 500 mg/day; increase dosage

cautiously and monitor closely to prevent hypoglycemic reactions. Repeated episodes of hypoglycemia in the elderly can cause brain damage.

▷ **Advisability of Use During Pregnancy**
   Pregnancy Category: C (tentative). See Pregnancy Code inside back cover.
   Animal studies: Ocular and bone birth defects reported in rat studies.
   Human studies: Information from adequate studies of pregnant women is not available.
   Because uncontrolled blood sugar levels during pregnancy are associated with a higher incidence of birth defects, many experts recommend that insulin (instead of an oral agent) be used as necessary to control diabetes during the entire pregnancy.
   Use during pregnancy is not recommended by the manufacturer.

Advisability of Use if Breast-Feeding
   Presence of this drug in breast milk: Yes.
   Avoid drug or refrain from nursing.

Habit-Forming Potential: None.

Effects of Overdosage: Symptoms of mild to severe hypoglycemia: headache, light-headedness, faintness, nervousness, confusion, tremor, sweating, heart palpitation, weakness, hunger, nausea, vomiting, stupor progressing to coma.

Possible Effects of Long-Term Use: Reduced function of the thyroid gland (hypothyroidism). Reports of increased frequency and severity of heart and blood vessel diseases associated with long-term use of this class of drugs are highly controversial and inconclusive. A direct cause-and-effect relationship (see Glossary) is tenuous. Ask your physician for guidance.

Suggested Periodic Examinations While Taking This Drug (at physician's discretion)
   Complete blood cell counts, liver function tests, thyroid function tests, periodic evaluation of heart and circulatory system.

▷ **While Taking This Drug, Observe the Following**
   Foods: Follow the diabetic diet prescribed by your physician.
   Beverages: As directed in the diabetic diet. May be taken with milk.
▷ *Alcohol:* Use with extreme caution until the combined effect has been determined. Alcohol can exaggerate this drug's hypoglycemic effect. This drug infrequently causes a marked intolerance of alcohol resulting in a disulfiramlike reaction (see Glossary): facial flushing, sweating, palpitation.
   Tobacco Smoking: No interactions expected.
▷ *Other Drugs*
   The following drugs may *increase* the effects of tolbutamide
   • aspirin, and other salicylates.

- chloramphenicol (Chloromycetin).
- cimetidine (Tagamet).
- clofibrate (Atromid S).
- fenfluramine (Pondimin).
- monoamine oxidase (MAO) type A inhibitor drugs (see Drug Class, Section Four).
- phenylbutazone (Butazolidin).
- ranitidine (Zantac).
- sulfonamide drugs (see Drug Class, Section Four).

The following drugs may *decrease* the effects of tolbutamide

- beta blocker drugs (see Drug Class, Section Four).
- bumetanide (Bumex).
- diazoxide (Proglycem).
- ethacrynic acid (Edecrin).
- furosemide (Lasix).
- phenytoin (Dilantin).
- rifampin (Rifadin, Rimactane).
- thiazide diuretics (see Drug Class, Section Four).

▷ *Driving, Hazardous Activities:* Regulate your dosage schedule, eating schedule and physical activities very carefully to prevent hypoglycemia. Be able to recognize the early symptoms of hypoglycemia so you can avoid hazardous activities and take corrective measures.

Aviation Note: Diabetes *is a disqualification* for piloting. Consult a designated Aviation Medical Examiner.

Exposure to Sun: Use caution until sensitivity has been determined. Some drugs of this class can cause photosensitivity (see Glossary).

Occurrence of Unrelated Illness: Acute infections, illnesses causing vomiting or diarrhea, serious injuries and surgical procedures can interfere with diabetic control and may require the use of insulin. If any of these conditions occur, consult your physician promptly.

Discontinuation: Because of the possibility of secondary failure, it is advisable to evaluate the continued benefit of this drug every 6 months.

TOLMETIN
(TOHL met in)

Introduced: 1976

Class: Mild analgesic, anti-inflammatory

Prescription: USA: Yes
Canada: Yes

Controlled Drug: USA: No
Canada: No

Available as Generic: No

Brand Names: Tolectin, Tolectin DS

BENEFITS versus RISKS

Possible Benefits	*Possible Risks*
EFFECTIVE RELIEF OF MILD TO MODERATE PAIN AND INFLAMMATION	Gastrointestinal pain, ulceration, bleeding (rare)
	Rare liver damage
	Rare kidney damage
	Rare blood cell disorders: hemolytic anemia, abnormally low white blood cell and platelet counts

---

▷ **Principal Uses**

As a Single Drug Product: Used primarily to relieve mild to moderately severe pain and inflammation associated with (1) acute and chronic rheumatoid arthritis; (2) osteoarthritis; and (3) juvenile rheumatoid arthritis.

How This Drug Works: Not completely established. It is thought that this drug reduces the tissue concentrations of prostaglandins (and related compounds), substances involved in the production of inflammation and pain.

Available Dosage Forms and Strengths
    Capsules — 400 mg
    Tablets — 200 mg

▷ **Usual Adult Dosage Range:**   Initially, 400 mg 3 times/day. For maintenance: adjust dosage from 600 mg to 1600 mg daily as needed, taken in 3 or 4 divided doses. The total daily dosage should not exceed 2000 mg (2.0 grams) for rheumatoid arthritis, or 1600 mg (1.6 grams) for osteoarthritis. **Note: Actual dosage and administration schedule must be determined by the physician for each patient individually.**

▷ **Dosing Instructions:**   Preferably taken on an empty stomach, 1 hour before or 2 hours after eating. However, it may be taken with or after food if necessary to reduce stomach irritation. Take with a full glass of water and remain upright (do not lie down) for 30 minutes. Schedule dosing to include one in the morning and one at bedtime. The capsule may be opened and the tablet may be crushed for administration.

Usual Duration of Use: Continual use on a regular schedule for 1 to 2 weeks is usually necessary to determine this drug's effectiveness in relieving the discomfort of arthritis. Long-term use (months to years) requires supervision and periodic evaluation by your physician. Consult your physician on a regular basis.

▷ **This Drug Should Not Be Taken If**
    • you have had an allergic reaction to it previously.
    • you are subject to asthma or nasal polyps caused by aspirin.

- you have active peptic ulcer disease or any form of gastrointestinal bleeding.
- you have a bleeding disorder or a blood cell disorder.
- you have severe impairment of liver or kidney function.

▷ **Inform Your Physician Before Taking This Drug If**
- you are allergic to aspirin or to other aspirin substitutes.
- you have a history of peptic ulcer disease or any type of bleeding disorder.
- you have impaired liver or kidney function.
- you have high blood pressure or a history of heart failure.
- you are taking any of the following: acetaminophen, aspirin or other aspirin substitutes, anticoagulants, oral antidiabetic drugs.

Possible Side-Effects (natural, expected and unavoidable drug actions)
Fluid retention (edema).
Drowsiness in sensitive individuals.

▷ **Possible Adverse Effects** (unusual, unexpected and infrequent reactions)
If any of the following develop, consult your physician promptly for guidance.
Mild Adverse Effects
Allergic Reactions: Skin rash, hives, itching.
Headache, dizziness, blurred vision, ringing in the ears.
Mouth sores, indigestion, nausea, vomiting, constipation, diarrhea.
Serious Adverse Effects
Allergic Reactions: Anaphylactic reaction (see Glossary), severe skin reactions.
Active peptic ulcer, with or without bleeding.
Liver damage with jaundice (see Glossary).
Kidney damage with painful urination, bloody urine, reduced urine formation.
Abnormally low white blood cell count: fever, sore throat.
Abnormally low blood platelet count: abnormal bleeding or bruising.

▷ **Possible Effects on Sexual Function:**   None reported.

Possible Delayed Adverse Effects: Mild anemia due to "silent" blood loss from the stomach (less than that caused by aspirin).

▷ **Adverse Effects That May Mimic Natural Diseases or Disorders**
Liver reaction may suggest viral hepatitis.

Natural Diseases or Disorders That May Be Activated by This Drug
Peptic ulcer disease, ulcerative colitis.

CAUTION
1. Dosage should always be limited to the smallest amount that produces reasonable improvement.
2. This drug may mask early indications of infection. Inform your physician if you think you are developing an infection of any kind.

Precautions for Use

By Infants and Children: Safety and effectiveness for use by those under 2 years of age have not been established.

By Those over 60 Years of Age: Small doses are advisable until tolerance is determined. Observe for any indications of liver or kidney toxicity, fluid retention, dizziness, confusion, impaired memory, stomach bleeding or constipation.

▷ Advisability of Use During Pregnancy

Pregnancy Category: B (tentative). See Pregnancy Code inside back cover.

Animal studies: No birth defects due to this drug reported.

Human studies: Information from adequate studies of pregnant women is not available.

The manufacturer does not recommend the use of this drug during pregnancy.

Advisability of Use if Breast-Feeding

Presence of this drug in breast milk: Unknown.

Avoid drug or refrain from nursing.

Habit-Forming Potential: None.

Effects of Overdosage: Stomach irritation, nausea, vomiting, diarrhea.

Possible Effects of Long-Term Use: Fluid retention.

Suggested Periodic Examinations While Taking This Drug (at physician's discretion)

Complete blood cell counts, liver and kidney function tests, complete eye examinations if vision is altered in any way.

▷ While Taking This Drug, Observe the Following

Foods: No restrictions.

Beverages: No restrictions. May be taken with milk.

▷   *Alcohol:* Use with caution. The irritant action of alcohol on the stomach lining, added to the irritant action of this drug in sensitive individuals, can increase the risk of stomach ulceration and/or bleeding.

Tobacco Smoking: No interactions expected.

▷   *Other Drugs*

Tolmetin may *increase* the effects of

- acetaminophen (Tylenol, etc.), and increase the risk of kidney damage; avoid prolonged use of this combination.
- anticoagulants (Coumadin, etc.), and increase the risk of bleeding; monitor prothrombin time, adjust dose accordingly.

Tolmetin *taken concurrently* with the following drugs may increase the risk of bleeding; avoid these combinations:

- aspirin.
- dipyridamole (Persantine).
- indomethacin (Indocin).
- sulfinpyrazone (Anturane).

- valproic acid (Depakene).

▷ *Driving, Hazardous Activities:* This drug may cause drowsiness or dizziness. Restrict activities as necessary.

Aviation Note: The use of this drug **may be a disqualification** for piloting. Consult a designated Aviation Medical Examiner.

Exposure to Sun: No restrictions.

TRAZODONE
(TRAZ oh dohn)

Introduced: 1967

Class: Antidepressants

Prescription: USA: Yes
Canada: Yes

Controlled Drug: USA: No
Canada: No

Available as Generic: USA: Yes
Canada: No

Brand Name: Desyrel, Trialodine

BENEFITS versus RISKS

Possible Benefits	*Possible Risks*
EFFECTIVE TREATMENT IN ALL TYPES OF DEPRESSIVE ILLNESS, with or without anxiety	Adverse behavioral effects: confusion, disorientation, delusions, hallucinations (all infrequent)
	Potential for inducing heart rhythm disorders (in individuals with heart disease)

▷ **Principal Uses**

As a Single Drug Product: Used to provide symptomatic relief in all types of depression, with or without anxiety or agitation. The primary intent is to initiate restoration of normal mood with a minimum of adverse drug effects.

How This Drug Works: Not completely established. It is thought that this drug increases the availability of the nerve impulse transmitter serotonin within certain brain centers and thereby relieves the symptoms of emotional depression.

Available Dosage Forms and Strengths

Tablets — 50 mg, 100 mg, 150 mg, 300 mg

▷ **Usual Adult Dosage Range:** Initially, 50 mg 3 times/day. The dose may be increased by 50 mg daily at intervals of 3 or 4 days as needed and tolerated. The total daily dosage should not exceed 400 mg. **Note: Actual dosage and administration schedule must be determined by the physician for each patient individually.**

▷ **Dosing Instructions:**   Best taken with food to improve absorption. The tablet may be crushed for administration. If excessive drowsiness or dizziness occurs, it is advisable to take a larger portion of the total daily dose at bedtime and to divide the remaining amount into 2 or 3 smaller doses to be taken during the day.

Usual Duration of Use: Continual use on a regular schedule for 2 to 4 weeks is usually necessary to determine this drug's effectiveness in relieving the symptoms of depression. Long-term use (weeks to months) requires supervision and periodic evaluation by your physician. Consult your physician on a regular basis.

▷ **This Drug Should Not Be Taken If**
- you have had an allergic reaction to it previously.
- you are recovering from a recent heart attack (myocardial infarction).
- you are taking, or have taken within the past 14 days, any monoamine oxidase (MAO) type A inhibitor drug (see Drug Class, Section Four).

▷ **Inform Your Physician Before Taking This Drug If**
- you have a history of any of the following: alcoholism, epilepsy, heart disease (especially heart rhythm disorders).
- you have impaired liver or kidney function.
- you are taking any antihypertensive drugs.
- you plan to have surgery under general anesthesia in the near future.

Possible Side-Effects (natural, expected and unavoidable drug actions)
Drowsiness, light-headedness, blurred vision, dry mouth, constipation.

▷ **Possible Adverse Effects** (unusual, unexpected and infrequent reactions)
If any of the following develop, consult your physician promptly for guidance.
Mild Adverse Effects
Allergic Reaction: Skin rash.
Headache, dizziness, fatigue, impaired concentration, nervousness, tremors.
Rapid heart rate, palpitations.
Peculiar taste, stomach discomfort, nausea, vomiting, diarrhea.
Muscular aches and pains.
Serious Adverse Effects
Behavioral effects: Confusion, anger, hostility, disorientation, impaired memory, delusions, hallucinations, nightmares.
Irregular heart rhythms, low blood pressure, fainting.

▷ **Possible Effects on Sexual Function**
Decreased male libido; increased female libido.
Inhibited ejaculation, impotence, priapism (see Glossary).
Altered timing and pattern of menstruation.

CAUTION

1. If you experience a significant degree of mouth dryness while using this drug, consult your dentist regarding the risk of gum erosion or tooth decay. Ask for his guidance in ways to keep the mouth comfortably moist.
2. It is advisable to withhold this drug if electroconvulsive therapy (ECT) is to be used.

Precautions for Use

By Infants and Children: Safety and effectiveness for use by those under 18 years of age have not been established.

By Those over 60 Years of Age: During the first two weeks of treatment, observe for the development of restlessness, agitation, excitement, forgetfulness, confusion or disorientation. Be aware of possible unsteadiness and incoordination that may predispose to falling. This drug may enhance prostatism (see Glossary).

▷ **Advisability of Use During Pregnancy**

Pregnancy Category: C (tentative). See Pregnancy Code inside back cover.
Animal studies: Fetal deaths and birth defects reported.
Human studies: Information from adequate studies of pregnant women is not available.
Avoid this drug completely during the first 3 months. Use otherwise only if clearly needed. Ask your physician for guidance.

Advisability of Use if Breast-Feeding

Presence of this drug in breast milk: Yes.
Avoid drug or refrain from nursing.

Habit-Forming Potential: None.

Effects of Overdosage: Marked drowsiness, weakness, confusion, tremors, low blood pressure, rapid heart rate, stupor, coma, possible seizures.

Possible Effects of Long-Term Use: None reported.

Suggested Periodic Examinations While Taking This Drug (at physician's discretion)

Complete blood cell counts. (This drug may cause slight reductions in white blood cell counts. This should be monitored closely if infection, sore throat or fever develops.)
Serial blood pressure readings and electrocardiograms.

▷ **While Taking This Drug, Observe the Following**

Foods: No restrictions.
Beverages: No restrictions. May be taken with milk.
▷ *Alcohol:* Avoid completely. This drug can increase markedly the intoxicating effects of alcohol and accentuate its depressant action on brain functions.
Tobacco Smoking: No interactions expected.

▷ *Other Drugs*

Trazodone may **increase** the effects of

- antihypertensive drugs, and cause excessive lowering of blood pressure; dosage adjustments may be necessary.
- drugs with sedative effects, and cause excessive sedation.
- phenytoin (Dilantin), by raising its blood level; observe for phenytoin toxicity.

▷ *Driving, Hazardous Activities:* This drug may cause dizziness or drowsiness. Restrict activities as necessary.

Aviation Note: The use of this drug **is a disqualification** for piloting. Consult a designated Aviation Medical Examiner.

Exposure to Sun: No restrictions.

Discontinuation: It is advisable to discontinue this drug gradually. Ask your physician for guidance in dosage reduction over an appropriate period of time.

TRIAMTERENE
(tri AM ter een)

Introduced: 1964

Class: Diuretic

Prescription: USA: Yes
Canada: Yes

Controlled Drug: USA: No
Canada: No

Available as Generic: No

Brand Names: ✦Apo-Triazide [CD], Dyazide [CD], Dyrenium, Maxzide [CD], Maxzide-25 [CD], ✦Novotriamzide [CD]

BENEFITS versus RISKS

Possible Benefits	*Possible Risks*
EFFECTIVE PREVENTION OF POTASSIUM LOSS when used adjunctively with other diuretics	ABNORMALLY HIGH BLOOD POTASSIUM LEVEL with excessive use
EFFECTIVE DIURETIC IN REFRACTORY CASES OF FLUID RETENTION when used adjunctively with other diuretics	Rare blood cell disorders: megaloblastic anemia, abnormally low white blood cell and platelet counts

---

▷ **Principal Uses**

As a Single Drug Product: This mild diuretic is used as part of the treatment program for the management of congestive heart failure and disorders of the liver and kidney that are accompanied by excessive fluid retention (edema). It is also used in conjunction with other measures to treat high blood pressure. It is used primarily in situations where it is advisable to prevent loss of potassium from the body.

As a Combination Drug Product [CD]: This drug is available in combination with hydrochlorothiazide, a different kind of diuretic that promotes the loss of potassium from the body. Triamterene is used in this combination to counteract the potassium-wasting effect of the thiazide diuretic.

How This Drug Works: Not completely established. It is thought that by inhibiting the enzyme system that initiates the sodium-potassium exchange process, this drug prevents the reabsorption of sodium and the excretion of potassium by the kidney. Thus the drug promotes the excretion of sodium (and water with it) and the retention of potassium.

Available Dosage Forms and Strengths
  Capsules — 50 mg, 100 mg

▷ **Usual Adult Dosage Range:** Initially, 100 mg twice daily. The dose is then adjusted according to individual response. The usual maintenance dose is 100 to 200 mg/day, divided into 2 doses. The total daily dosage should not exceed 300 mg. **Note: Actual dosage and administration schedule must be determined by the physician for each patient individually.**

▷ **Dosing Instructions:** May be taken with or following meals to promote absorption of the drug and to reduce stomach irritation. The capsule may be opened for administration. Intermittent or alternate-day use is recommended to minimize the possibility of sodium and potassium imbalance.

Usual Duration of Use: Continual use on a regular schedule for 3 to 5 days is usually necessary to determine this drug's effectiveness in clearing edema, and for 2 to 3 weeks to determine its effect on hypertension. Long-term use (months to years) requires supervision and periodic evaluation by your physician. Consult your physician on a regular basis.

▷ **This Drug Should Not Be Taken If**
  • you have had an allergic reaction to it previously.
  • you have severely impaired liver or kidney function.

▷ **Inform Your Physician Before Taking This Drug If**
  • you have a history of liver or kidney disease.
  • you have diabetes or gout.
  • you are taking any of the following: antihypertensives, a digitalis preparation, another diuretic, lithium or a potassium preparation.
  • you plan to have surgery under general anesthesia in the near future.

Possible Side-Effects (natural, expected and unavoidable drug actions)
> With excessive use: abnormally high blood potassium levels, abnormally low blood sodium levels, dehydration.
>
> Blue coloration of the urine (of no significance).

▷ **Possible Adverse Effects** (unusual, unexpected and infrequent reactions)
> **If any of the following develop, consult your physician promptly for guidance.**
>
> *Mild Adverse Effects*
> Allergic Reactions: Skin rash, itching.
> Headache, dizziness, unsteadiness, weakness, drowsiness, lethargy.
> Dry mouth, nausea, vomiting, diarrhea.
> *Serious Adverse Effects*
> Allergic Reaction: Anaphylactic reaction (see Glossary).
> Symptomatic potassium excess: confusion, numbness and tingling in lips and extremities, fatigue, weakness, shortness of breath, slow heart rate, low blood pressure.
> Rare blood cell disorders: megaloblastic anemia, causing weakness and fatigue; abnormally low white blood cell count, causing infection, fever or sore throat; abnormally low blood platelet count, causing abnormal bleeding or bruising.

▷ **Possible Effects on Sexual Function:**   None reported.

CAUTION
> 1. Do not take potassium supplements or increase your intake of potassium-rich foods while taking this drug.
> 2. Do not discontinue this drug abruptly unless abnormally high blood levels of potassium develop.
> 3. Avoid the liberal use of salt substitutes that contain potassium; these are a potential cause of potassium excess.

Precautions for Use
> *By Infants and Children:* This drug is not recommended for use in children.
> *By Those over 60 Years of Age:* The natural decline in kidney function may predispose to potassium retention in the body. Limit continual use of this drug to periods of 2 to 3 weeks. Observe for indications of potassium excess: slow heart rate, irregular heart rhythms, low blood pressure, confusion, drowsiness. The excessive use of diuretics can cause harmful loss of body water (dehydration), increased viscosity of the blood and an increased tendency of the blood to clot, predisposing to stroke, heart attack or thrombophlebitis.

▷ **Advisability of Use During Pregnancy**
> *Pregnancy Category:* B (tentative). See Pregnancy Code inside back cover.
> Animal studies: No birth defects due to this drug reported.
> Human studies: Information from adequate studies of pregnant women is not available.

This drug should not be used during pregnancy unless a very serious complication of pregnancy occurs for which this drug is significantly beneficial.

Advisability of Use if Breast-Feeding
Presence of this drug in breast milk: Yes.
Avoid drug or refrain from nursing.

Habit-Forming Potential: None.

Effects of Overdosage: Thirst, drowsiness, fatigue, weakness, nausea, vomiting, confusion, irregular heart rhythm, low blood pressure.

Possible Effects of Long-Term Use: Potassium accumulation to abnormally high blood levels.

Suggested Periodic Examinations While Taking This Drug (at physician's discretion)
Complete blood cell counts.
Measurements of blood sodium, potassium and chloride levels.
Kidney function tests.

▷ **While Taking This Drug, Observe the Following**
Foods: No restrictions. Avoid excessive restriction of salt.
Beverages: No restrictions. May be taken with milk.
▷ *Alcohol:* Use with caution until the combined effects have been determined. Alcohol may enhance the drowsiness and the blood-pressure-lowering effect of this drug.
Tobacco Smoking: No interactions expected.
▷ *Other Drugs*
Triamterene may *increase* the effects of
• amantadine (Symmetrel).
• digoxin (Lanoxin).
Triamterene *taken concurrently* with
• captopril (Capoten) may cause excessively high blood potassium levels.
• indomethacin (Indocin) may increase the risk of kidney damage.
• lithium may cause accumulation of lithium to toxic levels.
• potassium preparations may cause excessively high blood potassium levels.
▷ *Driving, Hazardous Activities:* This drug may cause dizziness and drowsiness. Restrict activities as necessary.
Aviation Note: The use of this drug *may be a disqualification* for piloting. Consult a designated Aviation Medical Examiner.
Exposure to Sun: Use caution until your sensitivity has been determined. This drug may cause photosensitivity (see Glossary).
Discontinuation: With high dosage or prolonged use, it is advisable to withdraw this drug gradually. Sudden discontinuation may cause rebound potassium excretion and resultant potassium deficiency. Ask your physician for guidance.

TRIAZOLAM
(tri AY zoh lam)

Introduced: 1974

Class: Hypnotic, benzodiazepines

Prescription: USA: Yes
Canada: Yes

Controlled Drug: USA: C-IV*
Canada: No

Available as Generic: USA: No
Canada: No

Brand Name: Halcion

BENEFITS versus RISKS

Possible Benefits	*Possible Risks*
EFFECTIVE HYPNOTIC with short duration of action	Habit-forming potential with long-term use
Wide margin of safety with therapeutic doses	Minor impairment of mental functions ("hangover" effect)

▷ **Principal Uses**

As a Single Drug Product: This member of the benzodiazepine class of "minor tranquilizers" is used exclusively as a bedtime sedative to induce sleep. It is useful in the short-term management of insomnia characterized by difficulty in falling asleep, frequent awakenings during the night and early morning awakening.

How This Drug Works: It is thought that this drug produces a calming effect by enhancing the action of the nerve transmitter gamma-aminobutyric acid (GABA), which in turn blocks the arousal of higher brain centers and helps to induce sleep.

Available Dosage Forms and Strengths
Tablets — 0.125 mg, 0.25 mg, 0.5 mg

▷ **Usual Adult Dosage Range:** 0.125 to 0.5 mg at bedtime. The total daily dosage should not exceed 0.5 mg. **Note: Actual dosage and administration schedule must be determined by the physician for each patient individually.**

▷ **Dosing Instructions:** Preferably taken on an empty stomach to hasten absorption and induce sleep rapidly. The tablet may be crushed for administration. Do not discontinue this drug abruptly if taken for more than 4 weeks.

Usual Duration of Use: Periods of 3 to 5 nights intermittently, repeated as needed with appropriate dosage adjustment. Avoid uninterrupted

---

*See Schedules of Controlled Drugs inside back cover.

and prolonged use. The duration of use should not exceed 2 weeks without reappraisal of continued need.

▷ **This Drug Should Not Be Taken If**
- you have had an allergic reaction to it previously.

▷ **Inform Your Physician Before Taking This Drug If**
- you are allergic to any benzodiazepine drug (see Drug Class, Section Four).
- you have a history of alcoholism or drug abuse.
- you are pregnant or planning pregnancy.
- you have impaired liver or kidney function.
- you have a history of serious depression or mental disorder.
- you are taking other drugs with sedative effects.
- you have any of the following: asthma, emphysema, epilepsy, myasthenia gravis.

Possible Side-Effects (natural, expected and unavoidable drug actions)
"Hangover" effects on arising: drowsiness (14%), lethargy and unsteadiness (4.6%).

▷ **Possible Adverse Effects** (unusual, unexpected and infrequent reactions)
If any of the following develop, consult your physician promptly for guidance.
Mild Adverse Effects
Allergic Reactions: Skin rash, itching.
Headache, dizziness, fatigue, blurred vision.
Nausea, indigestion, constipation, diarrhea.
Serious Adverse Effects
Idiosyncratic Reactions: Nervousness, talkativeness, irritability, apprehension, euphoria, excitement, hallucinations.
Confusion, mental depression.

▷ **Possible Effects on Sexual Function:**   None reported.

CAUTION
1. This drug should not be discontinued abruptly if it has been taken continually for more than 4 weeks.
2. The concurrent use of some over-the-counter drug products that contain antihistamines (allergy and cold preparations, sleep aids) can cause excessive sedation in sensitive individuals.
3. Regular nightly use of any hypnotic drug should be avoided.
4. If you experience a "hangover" effect, avoid hazardous activities (driving, etc.) and the use of alcohol.

Precautions for Use
By Infants and Children: Safety and effectiveness for use by those under 18 years of age have not been established.
By Those over 60 Years of Age: It is advisable to use smaller doses (0.125 mg) at first to determine your response. Observe for the possible de-

velopment of lethargy, indifference, fatigue, weakness, unsteadiness, disturbing dreams, nightmares and paradoxical reactions of excitement, agitation, anger, hostility and rage.

▷ **Advisability of Use During Pregnancy**
Pregnancy Category: X (tentative). See Pregnancy Code inside back cover.
Animal studies: Benzodiazepines cause significant birth defects in test animals.
Human studies: Information from adequate studies of pregnant women is not available.
Avoid use during entire pregnancy.

Advisability of Use if Breast-Feeding
Presence of this drug in breast milk: Probably yes.
Avoid drug or refrain from nursing.

Habit-Forming Potential: This drug can produce psychological and/or physical dependence (see Glossary) if used in large doses for an extended period of time. Avoid continual use.

Effects of Overdosage: Marked drowsiness, weakness, feeling of drunkenness, staggering gait, tremor, stupor progressing to deep sleep or coma.

Possible Effects of Long-Term Use: Psychological and/or physical dependence.

Suggested Periodic Examinations While Taking This Drug (at physician's discretion)
Complete blood cell counts during long-term use.

▷ **While Taking This Drug, Observe the Following**
Foods: No restrictions.
Beverages: Avoid excessive intake of caffeine-containing beverages (coffee, tea, cola) within 4 hours of taking this drug. May be taken with milk.
▷ *Alcohol:* Use with extreme caution until the combined effect has been determined. Alcohol may increase the absorption of this drug and add to its depressant effects on the brain. It is advisable to avoid alcohol completely throughout the day and night if it is necessary to drive or to engage in any hazardous activity.
Tobacco Smoking: Heavy smoking may reduce the hypnotic action of this drug.
Marijuana Smoking: Increased sedation and significant impairment of intellectual and physical performance.
▷ *Other Drugs*
Triazolam may ***increase*** the effects of
• digoxin (Lanoxin), and cause digoxin toxicity.
• phenytoin (Dilantin), and cause phenytoin toxicity.
Triazolam may ***decrease*** the effects of
• levodopa (Sinemet, etc.), and reduce its effectiveness in treating Parkinson's disease.

The following drugs may *increase* the effects of triazolam
- cimetidine (Tagamet).
- disulfiram (Antabuse).
- isoniazid (INH, Rifamate, etc.).
- oral contraceptives.
- valproic acid (Depakene).

The following drugs may *decrease* the effects of triazolam
- rifampin (Rimactane, etc.).
- theophylline (Aminophylline, Theo-Dur, etc.).

▷ *Driving, Hazardous Activities:* This drug can impair mental alertness, judgment, physical coordination and reaction time. Avoid hazardous activities accordingly.

Aviation Note: The use of this drug *is a disqualification* for piloting. Consult a designated Aviation Medical Examiner.

Exposure to Sun: No restrictions.

Exposure to Heat: Use caution until the effect of excessive perspiration is determined. Because of reduced urine volume, this drug may accumulate in the body and produce effects of overdosage.

Discontinuation: Avoid sudden discontinuation if this drug has been taken for over 4 weeks without interruption. Dosage should be tapered gradually to prevent a withdrawal syndrome that could include depression, confusion, hallucinations, tremor, seizures, muscle cramping, sweating and vomiting.

TRIFLUOPERAZINE
(tri floo oh PER a zeen)

Introduced: 1958

Class: Strong tranquilizer, phenothiazines

Prescription: USA: Yes
Canada: Yes

Controlled Drug: USA: No
Canada: No

Available as Generic: USA: Yes
Canada: No

Brand Names: ✦Apo-Trifluoperazine, ✦Novoflurazine, ✦Solazine, Stelazine, Suprazine, ✦Terfluzine

---

BENEFITS versus RISKS

Possible Benefits	*Possible Risks*
EFFECTIVE CONTROL OF ACUTE MENTAL DISORDERS in the majority of patients: beneficial effects on thinking, mood and behavior	SERIOUS TOXIC EFFECTS ON BRAIN with long-term use Liver damage with jaundice (infrequent) Rare blood cell disorders: abnormally low red and white blood cell and platelet counts

---

▷ **Principal Uses**

As a Single Drug Product: This antipsychotic drug is used primarily to treat psychotic thinking and behavior associated with acute psychoses of unknown nature, mania, paranoid states and acute schizophrenia. It is most effective in those who are withdrawn and apathetic and in those with agitation, delusions and hallucinations.

How This Drug Works: Not completely established. Present theory is that by inhibiting the action of dopamine, this drug acts to correct an imbalance of nerve impulse transmissions that is thought to be responsible for certain mental disorders.

Available Dosage Forms and Strengths
  Concentrate — 10 mg per ml
  Injection — 2 mg per ml
  Tablets — 1 mg, 2 mg, 5 mg, 10 mg

▷ **Usual Adult Dosage Range:**   Initially, 1 or 2 mg twice daily. The dose may be increased by 1 or 2 mg at 3- to 4-day intervals as needed and tolerated. Usual dosage range is 10 to 30 mg daily. The total daily dosage should not exceed 40 mg. **Note: Actual dosage and administration schedule must be determined by the physician for each patient individually.**

▷ **Dosing Instructions:**   May be taken with or following meals to reduce stomach irritation. The tablets may be crushed for administration.

Usual Duration of Use: Continual use on a regular schedule for several weeks is usually necessary to determine this drug's effectiveness in controlling psychotic disorders. If not significantly beneficial within 6 weeks, it should be discontinued. Long-term use (months to years) requires periodic evaluation of response, appropriate dosage adjustment and consideration of continued need. Consult your physician on a regular basis.

▷ **This Drug Should Not Be Taken If**
  • you are allergic to any of the drugs bearing the brand names listed above.
  • you have active liver disease.
  • you have cancer of the breast.
  • you have a current blood cell or bone marrow disorder.

▷ **Inform Your Physician Before Taking This Drug If**
  • you are allergic or abnormally sensitive to any phenothiazine drug (see Drug Class, Section Four).
  • you have impaired liver or kidney function.
  • you have any type of seizure disorder.
  • you have diabetes, glaucoma or heart disease.
  • you have a history of lupus erythematosus.
  • you are taking any drug with sedative effects.

- you plan to have surgery under general or spinal anesthesia in the near future.

Possible Side-Effects (natural, expected and unavoidable drug actions)
Drowsiness (usually during the first 2 weeks), orthostatic hypotension (see Glossary), blurred vision, dry mouth, nasal congestion, constipation, impaired urination.
Pink or purple coloration of urine, of no significance.

▷ **Possible Adverse Effects** (unusual, unexpected and infrequent reactions)
If any of the following develop, consult your physician promptly for guidance.

Mild Adverse Effects
Allergic Reactions: Skin rash, hives, low-grade fever.
Lowering of body temperature, especially in the elderly. (See Hypothermia in Glossary.)
Increased appetite and weight gain.
Dizziness, weakness, agitation, insomnia, impaired day and night vision.
Chronic constipation, fecal impaction.

Serious Adverse Effects
Allergic Reactions: Hepatitis with jaundice (see Glossary), severe skin reactions, anaphylactic reaction (see Glossary).
Depression, disorientation, seizures, loss of peripheral vision.
Rapid heart rate, heart rhythm disorders.
Blood cell disorders: significant reduction in all cellular elements of the blood (reduced counts of red cells, white cells and blood platelets).
Nervous system reactions: Parkinson-like disorders (see Glossary), severe restlessness, muscle spasms involving the face and neck, tardive dyskinesia (see Glossary) (10% to 20%).

▷ **Possible Effects on Sexual Function**
Altered timing and pattern of menstruation.
Male breast enlargement and tenderness.
Female breast enlargement with milk production.
Spontaneous male orgasm, paradoxical (1 case reported).
Inhibited ejaculation, painful ejaculation, priapism (see Glossary).
Delayed female orgasm.
False positive pregnancy test result.

▷ **Adverse Effects That May Mimic Natural Diseases or Disorders**
Nervous system reactions may suggest true Parkinson's disease.
Liver reactions may suggest viral hepatitis.
Reactions resembling systemic lupus erythematosus may occur.

Natural Diseases or Disorders That May Be Activated by This Drug
Latent epilepsy, glaucoma, diabetes mellitus, prostatism (see Glossary).

CAUTION
1. Many over-the-counter medications (see OTC Drugs in Glossary) for allergies, colds and coughs contain drugs that can interact unfa-

vorably with this drug. Ask your physician or pharmacist for guidance before using any such medications.

2. Antacids that contain aluminum and/or magnesium may prevent the absorption of this drug and reduce its effectiveness.

3. Obtain prompt evaluation of any change or disturbance of vision.

Precautions for Use

By Infants and Children: Use of this drug is not recommended in children under 6 years of age. Do not use this drug in the presence of symptoms suggestive of Reye syndrome (see Glossary). Children with acute infectious diseases ("flulike" infections, chicken pox, measles, etc.) are more prone to develop muscular spasms of the face, back and extremities when this drug is given.

By Those over 60 Years of Age: Small doses are advisable until individual response has been determined. You may be more susceptible to the development of drowsiness, lethargy, constipation, lowering of body temperature (hypothermia) and orthostatic hypotension (see Glossary). This drug may enhance existing prostatism (see Glossary). You may also be more susceptible to the development of Parkinson-like reactions and/or tardive dyskinesia (see discussion of these terms in Glossary). These reactions must be recognized early since they may become unresponsive to treatment and irreversible.

▷ Advisability of Use During Pregnancy

Pregnancy Category: C (tentative). See Pregnancy Code inside back cover.

Animal studies: Significant birth defects reported in mouse and rat studies.

Human studies: No increase in birth defects reported in 700 exposures. Information from adequate studies of pregnant women is not available.

Avoid drug during the first 3 months; avoid during the last month because of possible adverse effects on the newborn infant.

Advisability of Use if Breast-Feeding

Presence of this drug in breast milk: Yes, in minute amounts.

Monitor nursing infant closely and discontinue drug or nursing if adverse effects develop.

Habit-Forming Potential: None.

Effects of Overdosage: Marked drowsiness, weakness, tremor, agitation, unsteadiness, deep sleep, coma, convulsions.

Possible Effects of Long-Term Use: Tardive dyskinesia (see Glossary).

Suggested Periodic Examinations While Taking This Drug (at physician's discretion)

Complete blood cell counts, especially between the fourth and tenth weeks of treatment.

Liver function tests, electrocardiograms.

Complete eye examinations—eye structures and vision.

Careful inspection of the tongue for early evidence of fine, involuntary, wavelike movements that could indicate the beginning of tardive dyskinesia.

▷ **While Taking This Drug, Observe the Following**

Foods: No restrictions.

Nutritional Support: A riboflavin (vitamin B-2) supplement should be taken with long-term use.

Beverages: No restrictions. May be taken with milk.

▷ *Alcohol:* Avoid completely. Alcohol can increase the sedative action of phenothiazines and accentuate their depressant effects on brain function and blood pressure. Phenothiazines can increase the intoxicating effects of alcohol.

Tobacco Smoking: Possible reduction of drowsiness from drug.

Marijuana Smoking: Moderate increase in drowsiness; accentuation of orthostatic hypotension; increased risk of precipitating latent psychoses, confusing the interpretation of mental status and drug responses.

▷ *Other Drugs*

Trifluoperazine may ***increase*** the effects of
- all sedative drugs, especially narcotic analgesics, and cause excessive sedation.
- all atropinelike drugs, and cause nervous system toxicity.

Trifluoperazine may ***decrease*** the effects of
- guanethidine (Ismelin, Esimil), and reduce its effectiveness in lowering blood pressure.

Trifluoperazine ***taken concurrently*** with
- lithium (Lithobid, Lithotabs) may impair the effectiveness of lithium and cause nervous system toxicity.

The following drugs may ***decrease*** the effects of trifluoperazine
- antacids containing aluminum and/or magnesium.
- barbiturates (see Drug Class, Section Four).
- benztropine (Cogentin).
- disulfiram (Antabuse).
- trihexyphenidyl (Artane).

▷ *Driving, Hazardous Activities:* This drug can impair mental alertness, judgment and physical coordination. Avoid hazardous activities.

Aviation Note: The use of this drug ***is a disqualification*** for piloting. Consult a designated Aviation Medical Examiner.

Exposure to Sun: Use caution until sensitivity has been determined. Some phenothiazines can cause photosensitivity (see Glossary).

Exposure to Heat: Use caution and avoid excessive heat as much as possible. This drug may impair the regulation of body temperature and increase the risk of heat stroke.

Exposure to Cold: Use caution and dress warmly. This drug can increase the risk of hypothermia in the elderly.

Discontinuation: After a period of long-term use, do not discontinue this drug suddenly. Gradual withdrawal over 2 to 3 weeks under physician supervision is recommended. Do not discontinue this drug without your physician's knowledge and approval. The relapse rate of schizophrenia after discontinuation is 50% to 60%.

TRIMETHOBENZAMIDE
(tri meth oh BEN za mide)

Introduced: 1959

Class: Antiemetic

Prescription: USA: Yes

Controlled Drug: USA: No

Available as Generic: Yes

Brand Names: Arrestin, Hymetic, T-Gen, Tigan

BENEFITS versus RISKS

Possible Benefits	*Possible Risks*
Possibly effective prevention and control of nausea and vomiting in selected disorders	TOXIC EFFECTS ON BRAIN: disorientation, Parkinson-like tremors, muscle spasms and rigidity, seizures Rare liver damage Rare blood cell disorders: abnormally low white blood cell count

---

▷ **Principal Uses**

As a Single Drug Product: Used exclusively for the control of nausea and vomiting associated with motion sickness, inner ear infections, Meniere's syndrome, surgery and radiation therapy. It is not as effective as the phenothiazines in relieving nausea and preventing vomiting, but it is significantly safer to use for long-term therapy.

How This Drug Works: Not completely established. It is thought that this drug relieves nausea and prevents vomiting by suppressing the transmission of nerve impulses to the vomiting centers in the brain.

Available Dosage Forms and Strengths
Capsules — 100 mg, 250 mg
Injection — 100 mg per ml
Suppositories — 100 mg, 200 mg

▷ **Usual Adult Dosage Range:** 250 mg every 4 to 6 hours as needed. The total daily dosage should not exceed 1000 mg. **Note: Actual dosage and** administration schedule must be determined by the physician for each patient individually.

▷ **Dosing Instructions:**   May be taken without regard to food. The capsule may be opened for administration.

Usual Duration of Use: Continual use on a regular schedule for 24 to 48 hours is usually necessary to determine this drug's effectiveness in controlling nausea and vomiting. If this drug is not effective within 3 days, it should be discontinued. Long-term use requires supervision and periodic evaluation by your physician. Consult your physician on a regular basis.

▷ **This Drug Should Not Be Taken If**
  • you have had an allergic reaction to it previously.
  • you have any symptoms suggestive of Reye syndrome (see Glossary).
  • you have active liver disease.
  • you have any type of blood cell or bone marrow disorder.

▷ **Inform Your Physician Before Taking This Drug If**
  • you have had any unfavorable reactions to antihistamine drugs in the past.
  • you have impaired liver or kidney function.
  • you have a seizure disorder.
  • you have any type of parkinsonism.
  • you have a history of blood cell or bone marrow disorders, especially one induced by drugs.

Possible Side-Effects (natural, expected and unavoidable drug actions)
Drowsiness.
Temporary drop in blood pressure when given by injection.

▷ **Possible Adverse Effects** (unusual, unexpected and infrequent reactions)
  If any of the following develop, consult your physician promptly for guidance.
  Mild Adverse Effects
  Allergic Reaction: Skin rash.
  Headache, dizziness, blurred vision, muscle spasms.
  Diarrhea.
  Serious Adverse Effects
  Nervous system reactions: mental depression, disorientation, seizures, Parkinson-like syndrome (see Glossary).
  Liver damage with jaundice (see Glossary).
  Blood cell disorder: abnormally low white blood cell count, causing infections, fever, sore throat.

▷ **Possible Effects on Sexual Function:**   None reported.

▷ **Adverse Effects That May Mimic Natural Diseases or Disorders**
  Liver reaction may suggest viral hepatitis.

Natural Diseases or Disorders That May Be Activated by This Drug
Reye syndrome (see Glossary).

CAUTION
1. The suppository form of this drug contains 2% benzocaine; it should not be used by anyone who is allergic to benzocaine or related local anesthetics.
2. This drug has a toxicity pattern similar to the phenothiazines. It may lower the seizure threshold in epileptic individuals. Observe closely for any change in seizure patterns.

Precautions for Use
By Infants and Children: Do not use this drug in children of any age with symptoms suggestive of Reye syndrome or with illnesses that predispose to Reye syndrome (see Glossary). Children with "flulike" infections, measles, chicken pox, etc. are very susceptible to adverse effects when this drug is given to control nausea or vomiting.
By Those over 60 Years of Age: Observe closely for excessive sedation, weakness, unsteadiness or tendency to fall. Take precautions to prevent injury.

▷ **Advisability of Use During Pregnancy**
Pregnancy Category: B (tentative). See Pregnancy Code inside back cover.
Animal studies: No birth defects reported in rat and rabbit studies.
Human studies: No increase in birth defects reported in 700 exposures to this drug. Information from adequate studies of pregnant women is not available.
Avoid use of drug during the first 3 months if possible. Use it otherwise only if clearly needed. Ask your physician for guidance.

Advisability of Use if Breast-Feeding
Presence of this drug in breast milk: Unknown.
Avoid drug or refrain from nursing.

Habit-Forming Potential: None.

Effects of Overdosage: Drowsiness, weakness, incoordination, muscle spasms in neck and extremities, confusion, disorientation, seizures, coma.

Possible Effects of Long-Term Use: None reported.

Suggested Periodic Examinations While Taking This Drug (at physician's discretion)
Complete blood cell counts, liver function tests.

▷ **While Taking This Drug, Observe the Following**
Foods: No restrictions.
Beverages: No restrictions. May be taken with milk.
▷   *Alcohol:* Avoid completely. Alcohol may increase the depressant effects of this drug on brain function.

Tobacco Smoking: No interactions expected.
▷ *Other Drugs*
   Trimethobenzamide may **increase** the effects of
   • other drugs with sedative effects, and cause excessive sedation; con-
     current use may provoke other reactions of nervous system toxicity:
     severe spasms of neck and back muscles, seizures and coma.
▷ *Driving, Hazardous Activities:* This drug may cause dizziness and drow-
     siness. Restrict activities as necessary.
   Aviation Note: The use of this drug **is a disqualification** for piloting. Con-
     sult a designated Aviation Medical Examiner.
   Exposure to Sun: No restrictions.

TRIMETHOPRIM
(tri METH oh prim)

Introduced: 1966

Prescription: USA: Yes
   Canada: Yes

Available as Generic: USA: Yes
   Canada: No

Class: Anti-infective

Controlled Drug: USA: No
   Canada: No

Brand Names: ✦Apo-Sulfatrim [CD], ✦Apo-Sulfatrim DS [CD], Bactrim
   [CD], Bactrim DS [CD], Bethaprim [CD], Comoxol [CD], ✦Coptin
   [CD], Cotrim [CD], ✦Novotrimel [CD], ✦Novotrimel DS [CD], Prolo-
   prim, ✦Protrin [CD], ✦Protrin DF [CD], ✦Roubac [CD], Septra [CD],
   Septra DS [CD], Trimpex, Uroplus DS [CD], Uroplus SS [CD]

BENEFITS versus RISKS

Possible Benefits	*Possible Risks*
EFFECTIVE TREATMENT OF INFECTIONS due to susceptible microorganisms	Rare blood cell disorders: megaloblastic anemia, methemoglobinemia, abnormally low white blood cell and platelet counts

---

▷ **Principal Uses**
   As a Single Drug Product: Used primarily to treat the initial episode of
     certain infections of the urinary tract that are not complicated by the
     presence of kidney stones or obstructions to the normal flow of urine.
     It is sometimes used to prevent the recurrence of such infections.

As a Combination Drug Product [CD]: This drug is available in combination with sulfamethoxazole; the generic name co-trimoxazole is used in some countries to identify this combination. It is very effective in the treatment of certain urinary tract infections, middle ear infections, chronic bronchitis, acute enteritis and certain types of pneumonia.

How This Drug Works: This drug prevents the growth and multiplication of susceptible infecting organisms by inactivating the enzyme systems that are necessary for the formation of essential nuclear elements and cell proteins.

Available Dosage Forms and Strengths

    Tablets — 100 mg, 200 mg
    Tablets — 80 mg combined with 400 mg of
       sulfamethoxazole
    Tablets — 160 mg combined with 800 mg of
       sulfamethoxazole
  Oral suspension — 40 mg combined with 200 mg of
       sulfamethoxazole per 5-ml teaspoonful

▷ **Usual Adult Dosage Range:**   100 mg every 12 hours for 10 days. For certain pneumonias, the same dose is given every 6 hours. The total daily dosage should not exceed 640 mg. **Note: Actual dosage and administration schedule must be determined by the physician for each patient individually.**

▷ **Dosing Instructions:**   May be taken without regard to meals. However, it may also be taken with or following food if necessary to reduce stomach irritation. The tablet may be crushed for administration.

Usual Duration of Use: Continual use on a regular schedule for 7 to 14 days is usually necessary to determine this drug's effectiveness in controlling responsive infections. The actual duration of use will depend upon the nature of the infection.

Currently a "Drug of Choice" (when combined with sulfamethoxazole) for preventing pneumonia (due to pneumocystis carinii) in patients with AIDS.

▷ **This Drug Should Not Be Taken If**
- you have had an allergic reaction to it previously.
- you have an anemia due to folic acid deficiency.

▷ **Inform Your Physician Before Taking This Drug If**
- you have a history of folic acid deficiency.
- you have impaired liver or kidney function.
- you are pregnant or breast-feeding.

Possible Side-Effects (natural, expected and unavoidable drug actions)
 None with short-term use.

▷ **Possible Adverse Effects** (unusual, unexpected and infrequent reactions)
  If any of the following develop, consult your physician promptly for guidance.
  Mild Adverse Effects
  Allergic Reactions: Skin rash (2.9%), itching, drug fever.
  Headache, abnormal taste, sore mouth or tongue, loss of appetite, nausea, vomiting, abdominal cramping, diarrhea.
  Serious Adverse Effects
  Allergic Reactions: Severe dermatitis with peeling of skin.
  Blood cell disorders: megaloblastic anemia, methemoglobinemia, abnormally low white blood cell and platelet counts. (All are rare.)

▷ **Possible Effects on Sexual Function:** None reported.

CAUTION
  1. Certain strains of bacteria that cause urinary tract infections can develop resistance to this drug. If you do not show significant improvement within 10 days, consult your physician.
  2. Comply with your physician's request for periodic blood counts during long-term therapy.

Precautions for Use
  By Infants and Children: Safety and effectiveness for use by those under 2 months of age have not been established.
  By Those over 60 Years of Age: The natural decline in liver and kidney function may require smaller doses. If you develop itching reactions in the genital or anal areas, report this promptly.

▷ **Advisability of Use During Pregnancy**
  Pregnancy Category: C (tentative). See Pregnancy Code inside back cover.
  Animal studies: Birth defects due to this drug reported in rat and rabbit studies.
  Human studies: Information from adequate studies of pregnant women is not available.
  Avoid use of drug during the first 3 months and during the last 2 weeks of pregnancy. Use this drug otherwise only if clearly needed. Ask your physician for guidance.

Advisability of Use if Breast-Feeding
  Presence of this drug in breast milk: Yes.
  Avoid drug or refrain from nursing.

Habit-Forming Potential: None.

Effects of Overdosage: Headache, dizziness, confusion, depression, nausea, vomiting, bone marrow depression, possible liver toxicity with jaundice.

Possible Effects of Long-Term Use: Impaired production of red and white blood cells and blood platelets.

Suggested Periodic Examinations While Taking This Drug (at physician's discretion)
Complete blood cell counts.

▷ **While Taking This Drug, Observe the Following**
Foods: No restrictions.
Beverages: No restrictions. May be taken with milk.
▷ *Alcohol:* No interactions expected.
Tobacco Smoking: No interactions expected.
▷ *Other Drugs*
Trimethoprim may *increase* the effects of
• phenytoin (Dilantin), and cause phenytoin toxicity.
The following drugs may *decrease* the effects of trimethoprim
• rifampin (Rifadin, Rimactane).
▷ *Driving, Hazardous Activities:* No restrictions.
Aviation Note: The use of this drug is probably not a disqualification for piloting. Consult a designated Aviation Medical Examiner.
Exposure to Sun: No restrictions.

VALPROIC ACID
(val PROH ik)

Introduced: 1967

Class: Anticonvulsant

Prescription: USA: Yes
Canada: Yes

Controlled Drug: USA: No
Canada: No

Available as Generic: USA: Yes
Canada: No

Brand Names: Depa, Depakene, Depakote, Deproic

BENEFITS versus RISKS	
Possible Benefits	*Possible Risks*
EFFECTIVE CONTROL OF MULTIPLE SEIZURE TYPES: ABSENCE SEIZURES, TONIC-CLONIC SEIZURES, MYOCLONIC SEIZURES, PSYCHOMOTOR SEIZURES when used adjunctively with other antiseizure drugs	LIVER TOXICITY, infrequent but may be severe Rare reduction of blood platelets and impaired platelet function with risk of bleeding

▷ **Principal Uses**
As a Single Drug Product: Used effectively in the management of the following types of epilepsy: simple and complex absence seizures (petit

mal); tonic-clonic seizures (grand mal); myoclonic seizures; complex partial seizures (psychomotor, temporal lobe epilepsy). It is sometimes used adjunctively with other anticonvulsants as needed.

How This Drug Works: Not completely established. It is thought that by increasing the availability of the nerve impulse transmitter gamma-aminobutyric acid (GABA), this drug suppresses the spread of abnormal electrical discharges that cause seizures.

Available Dosage Forms and Strengths
Capsules — 250 mg
Syrup — 250 mg per 5-ml teaspoonful
Tablets, enteric-coated — 125 mg, 250 mg, 500 mg

▷ **Usual Adult Dosage Range:** Initially, 15 mg/kg/24 hours. The dose is increased cautiously by 5 to 10 mg/kg/24 hours every 7 days as needed and tolerated. *The usual daily dose is from 1000 mg to 1600 mg in divided doses.* The total daily dosage should not exceed 60 mg/kg. **Note: Actual dosage and administration schedule must be determined by the physician for each patient individually.**

▷ **Dosing Instructions:** Preferably taken 1 hour before meals. However, it may be taken with or following food if necessary to prevent stomach irritation. The capsule should not be opened and the tablet should not be crushed for administration. Do not administer the syrup in carbonated beverages. It may be diluted in water or milk.

Usual Duration of Use: Continual use on a regular schedule for 2 weeks is usually necessary to determine this drug's effectiveness in reducing the frequency and severity of seizures. Long-term use (months to years) requires supervision and periodic evaluation by your physician. Consult your physician on a regular basis.

▷ **This Drug Should Not Be Taken If**
- you have had an allergic reaction to it previously.
- you have active liver disease.
- you have an active bleeding disorder.

▷ **Inform Your Physician Before Taking This Drug If**
- you have a history of liver disease or impaired liver function.
- you have a history of any type of bleeding disorder.
- you are pregnant or planning pregnancy.
- you have myasthenia gravis.
- you are taking any of the following drugs: anticoagulants; other anticonvulsants; antidepressants, either the tricyclic type or monoamine oxidase (MAO) type A inhibitors (see Drug Classes, Section Four).
- you plan to have surgery or dental extraction in the near future.

Possible Side-Effects (natural, expected and unavoidable drug actions)
Drowsiness and lethargy (5%).

▷ **Possible Adverse Effects** (unusual, unexpected and infrequent reactions)
   If any of the following develop, consult your physician promptly for guidance.

Mild Adverse Effects

Allergic Reaction: Skin rash (rare).

Headache, dizziness, confusion, unsteadiness, slurred speech.

Nausea, indigestion, stomach cramps, diarrhea.

Temporary loss of scalp hair.

Serious Adverse Effects

Idiosyncratic Reactions: Bizarre behavior, hallucinations.

Drug-induced hepatitis with jaundice (see Glossary).

Drug-induced pancreatitis.

Possible Reye syndrome (see Glossary).

Reduced formation of blood platelets and impaired function of platelets, with increased risk of abnormal bleeding.

▷ **Possible Effects on Sexual Function**

Altered timing and pattern of menstruation.

Female breast enlargement with milk production.

Decreased libido.

Decreased effectiveness of oral contraceptives taken concurrently (6%).

▷ **Adverse Effects That May Mimic Natural Diseases or Disorders**

Liver reactions may suggest viral hepatitis.

CAUTION

1. The capsules and tablets should be swallowed whole without alteration to avoid irritation of the mouth and throat.
2. This drug can impair normal blood clotting mechanisms. In the event of injury, dental extraction, or need for surgery, inform your physician or dentist that you are taking this drug.
3. Because this drug can impair the normal function of blood platelets, it is advisable to avoid aspirin (which has the same effect).
4. Over-the-counter drug products that contain antihistamines (allergy and cold remedies, sleep aids) can enhance the sedative effects of this drug.

Precautions for Use

By Infants and Children: The concurrent use of aspirin with this drug can cause abnormal bleeding or bruising. Children with mental retardation, organic brain disease or severe seizure disorders may be at increased risk for severe liver toxicity while taking this drug. Observe closely for the development of fever that could indicate the onset of a drug-induced Reye syndrome (see Glossary). Avoid concurrent use of clonazepam (Clonopin); the combined use could result in continuous petit mal episodes.

By Those over 60 Years of Age: Start treatment with small doses and increase dosage cautiously. Observe closely for excessive sedation, confusion or unsteadiness that could predispose to falling and injury.

▷ **Advisability of Use During Pregnancy**

Pregnancy Category: D (tentative). See Pregnancy Code inside back cover.

Animal studies: Palate and skeletal birth defects reported in mouse, rat and rabbit studies.

Human studies: Information from adequate studies of pregnant women is not available. There have been several reports of birth defects attributed to the use of this drug during early pregnancy.

Consult your physician regarding the advantages and disadvantages of using this drug. If it is used, it is advisable to keep the dose as low as possible.

Advisability of Use if Breast-Feeding

Presence of this drug in breast milk: Yes, in small amounts.

Monitor nursing infant closely and discontinue drug or nursing if adverse effects develop.

Habit-Forming Potential: None.

Effects of Overdosage: Increased drowsiness, weakness, unsteadiness, confusion, stupor progressing to coma.

Possible Effects of Long-Term Use: None reported.

Suggested Periodic Examinations While Taking This Drug (at physician's discretion)

Complete blood cell counts and baseline liver function tests should be done before treatment is started. During treatment, blood counts should be repeated every month and liver function tests repeated every 2 months.

▷ **While Taking This Drug, Observe the Following**

Foods: No restrictions.

Beverages: Do not administer the syrup in carbonated beverages; this could liberate the valproic acid and irritate the mouth and throat. This drug may be taken with milk.

▷ *Alcohol:* Use extreme caution until the combined effects have been determined. Alcohol can increase the sedative effect of this drug. Also, this drug can increase the depressant effects of alcohol on brain function.

Tobacco Smoking: No interactions expected.

▷ *Other Drugs*

Valproic acid may *increase* the effects of
- anticoagulants (Coumadin, etc.), and increase the risk of bleeding.
- antidepressants, both monoamine oxidase (MAO) type A inhibitors and tricyclics, and cause toxicity.
- phenobarbital, and cause barbiturate intoxication.
- phenytoin (Dilantin), and cause phenytoin toxicity.

Valproic acid *taken concurrently* with
- antiplatelet drugs: aspirin, dipyridamole (Persantine), sulfinpyrazone (Anturane) may enhance the inhibition of platelet function and increase the risk of bleeding.

▷ *Driving, Hazardous Activities:* This drug may cause drowsiness, dizziness or confusion. Restrict activities as necessary.

Aviation Note: The use of this drug *is a disqualification* for piloting. Consult a designated Aviation Medical Examiner.

Exposure to Sun: No restrictions.

Discontinuation: **Do not discontinue this drug suddenly.** Abrupt withdrawal can cause repetitive seizures that are difficult to control.

VERAPAMIL
(ver AP a mil)

Introduced: 1967

Class: Antianginal, antiarrhythmic, antihypertensive, calcium channel blocker

Prescription: USA: Yes
Canada: Yes

Controlled Drug: USA: No
Canada: No

Available as Generic: USA: Yes
Canada: No

Brand Names: Calan, Calan SR, Isoptin, Isoptin SR

BENEFITS versus RISKS

Possible Benefits	*Possible Risks*
EFFECTIVE PREVENTION OF BOTH MAJOR TYPES OF ANGINA	Congestive heart failure
	Low blood pressure (2.9%)
	Heart rhythm disturbance
EFFECTIVE CONTROL OF HEART RATE IN CHRONIC ATRIAL FIBRILLATION AND FLUTTER	Fluid retention (1.7%)
	Liver damage without jaundice (very rare)
EFFECTIVE PREVENTION OF PAROXYSMAL ATRIAL TACHYCARDIA (PAT)	
EFFECTIVE TREATMENT OF HYPERTENSION	

▷ **Principal Uses**

As a Single Drug Product: Used primarily to treat (1) angina pectoris due to coronary artery spasm (Prinzmetal's variant angina) that occurs spontaneously and is not associated with exertion; (2) classical angina-of-effort (due to atherosclerotic disease of the coronary arteries) in individuals who have not responded to or cannot tolerate the nitrates and beta blocker drugs customarily used to treat this disorder; (3) abnormally rapid heart rate due to chronic atrial fibrillation or flutter; (4) recurrent paroxysmal atrial tachycardia; and (5) primary hypertension.

How This Drug Works: Not completely established. It is thought that by blocking the normal passage of calcium through certain cell walls (which is necessary for the function of nerve and muscle tissue), this drug slows the spread of electrical activity through the conduction system of the heart and inhibits the contraction of coronary arteries and peripheral arterioles. As a result of these combined effects, this drug

- prevents spontaneous spasm of the coronary arteries (Prinzmetal's type of angina).
- reduces the rate and contraction force of the heart during exertion, thus lowering the oxygen requirement of the heart muscle; this reduces the occurrence of effort-induced angina (classical angina pectoris).
- reduces the degree of contraction of peripheral arterial walls, resulting in their relaxation and consequent lowering of blood pressure. This further reduces the work load of the heart during exertion and contributes to the prevention of angina.
- slows the rate of electrical impulses through the conduction system of the heart and thereby prevents excessively rapid heart action (tachycardia).

Available Dosage Forms and Strengths
Injection — 5 mg per 2 ml
Tablets — 40 mg, 80 mg, 120 mg
Tablets, prolonged-action — 240 mg

▷ **Usual Adult Dosage Range:**   Initially, 80 mg 3 or 4 times daily. The dose may be increased gradually at 1- to 7-day intervals as needed and tolerated. The usual maintenance dose is from 240 mg to 480 mg daily in 3 or 4 divided doses. The total daily dosage should not exceed 480 mg. **Note: Actual dosage and administration schedule must be determined by the physician for each patient individually.**

▷ **Dosing Instructions:**   Preferably taken before meals and at bedtime. The tablet may be crushed for administration.

Usual Duration of Use: Continual use on a regular schedule for 2 to 4 weeks is usually necessary to determine this drug's effectiveness in reducing the frequency and severity of angina. Reduction of elevated blood pressure may be apparent within the first 1 to 2 weeks. For long-term use (months to years), determine the smallest effective dose; this requires supervision and periodic evaluation by your physician. Consult your physician on a regular basis.

Possible Advantages of This Drug
No adverse effects of blood levels of glucose, potassium or uric acid.
Does not increase blood cholesterol or triglyceride levels.
Does not impair capacity for exercise.

Currently a "Drug of Choice" for initiating treatment of hypertension with a single drug.

▷ **This Drug Should Not Be Taken If**
- you have had an allergic reaction to it previously.
- you have active liver disease.
- you have a "sick sinus" syndrome (and do not have an artificial pacemaker).
- you have been told that you have a second-degree or third-degree heart block.
- you have low blood pressure—systolic pressure below 90.

▷ **Inform Your Physician Before Taking This Drug If**
- you have had an unfavorable response to any calcium blocker drug in the past.
- you are currently taking any other drugs, especially digitalis or a beta blocker drug (see Drug Class, Section Four).
- you have had a recent stroke or heart attack.
- you have a history of congestive heart failure or heart rhythm disorders.
- you have impaired liver or kidney function.
- you have a history of drug-induced liver damage.

Possible Side-Effects (natural, expected and unavoidable drug actions)
Low blood pressure (2.9%), fluid retention (1.7%).

▷ **Possible Adverse Effects** (unusual, unexpected and infrequent reactions)
If any of the following develop, consult your physician promptly for guidance.
Mild Adverse Effects
Allergic Reactions: Skin rash, hives, itching, aching joints.
Headache (1.8%), dizziness (3.6%), fatigue (1.1%).
Nausea (1.6%), indigestion, constipation (6.3%).
Serious Adverse Effects
Serious disturbances of heart rate and/or rhythm, congestive heart failure (0.9%).
Drug-induced liver damage without jaundice (very rare).

▷ **Possible Effects on Sexual Function**
Altered timing and pattern of menstruation.
Male breast enlargement and tenderness.
Impotence (20%).

CAUTION
1. Be sure to inform all physicians and dentists you consult that you are taking this drug. Note the use of this drug on your card of personal identification.

2. You may use nitroglycerin and other nitrate drugs as needed to relieve acute episodes of angina pain. However, if you detect that your angina attacks are becoming more frequent or intense, notify your physician promptly.
3. If this drug is used concurrently with a beta blocker drug, you may develop excessively low blood pressure.
4. This drug may cause swelling of the feet and ankles. This may not be indicative of either heart or kidney dysfunction.

Precautions for Use

By Infants and Children: Safety and effectiveness for use by those under 12 years of age have not been established.

By Those over 60 Years of Age: You may be more susceptible to the development of weakness, dizziness, fainting and falling. Take necessary precautions to prevent injury. Report promptly any changes in your pattern of thirst and urination.

▷ Advisability of Use During Pregnancy

Pregnancy Category: C (tentative). See Pregnancy Code inside back cover.

Animal studies: Toxic effects on the embryo and retarded growth of the fetus (but no birth defects) reported in rat studies.

Human studies: Information from adequate studies of pregnant women is not available.

Avoid this drug during the first 3 months. Use during the last 6 months only if clearly needed. Ask your physician for guidance.

Advisability of Use if Breast-Feeding

Presence of this drug in breast milk: Possibly yes.

Avoid drug or refrain from nursing.

Habit-Forming Potential: None.

Effects of Overdosage: Flushed and warm skin, sweating, light-headedness, irritability, rapid heart rate, low blood pressure, loss of consciousness.

Possible Effects of Long-Term Use: None reported.

Suggested Periodic Examinations While Taking This Drug (at physician's discretion)

Evaluations of heart function, including electrocardiograms; liver and kidney function tests, with long-term use.

▷ While Taking This Drug, Observe the Following

Foods: No restrictions. Avoid excessive salt intake.

Beverages: No restrictions. May be taken with milk.

▷ *Alcohol:* Use with caution until combined effects have been determined. Alcohol may exaggerate the drop in blood pressure experienced by some individuals.

Tobacco Smoking: Nicotine can reduce the effectiveness of this drug. Avoid all forms of tobacco.

Marijuana Smoking: Possible reduced effectiveness of this drug; mild to moderate increase in angina; possible changes in electrocardiogram, confusing interpretation.

▷ *Other Drugs*

Verapamil may *increase* the effects of
- carbamazepine (Tegretol), and cause carbamazepine toxicity.
- digitoxin and digoxin, and cause digitalis toxicity.

Verapamil *taken concurrently* with
- beta blocker drugs (see Drug Class, Section Four) may affect heart rate and rhythm adversely. Careful monitoring by your physician is necessary if these drugs are taken concurrently.

The following drugs may *increase* the effects of verapamil
- cimetidine (Tagamet).

▷ *Driving, Hazardous Activities:* Usually no restrictions. This drug may cause dizziness. Restrict activities as necessary.

Aviation Note: Coronary artery disease *is a disqualification* for piloting. Consult a designated Aviation Medical Examiner.

Exposure to Sun: Use caution until sensitivity has been determined. This drug may cause photosensitivity (see Glossary).

Exposure to Heat: Caution advised. Hot environments can exaggerate the blood-pressure-lowering effects of this drug. Observe for light-headedness or weakness.

Heavy Exercise or Exertion: This drug may improve your ability to be more active without resulting angina pain. Use caution and avoid excessive exercise that could impair heart function in the absence of warning pain.

Discontinuation: Do not discontinue this drug abruptly. Consult your physician regarding gradual withdrawal to prevent the development of rebound angina.

WARFARIN
(WAR far in)

Introduced: 1941

Class: Anticoagulant, coumarins

Prescription: USA: Yes
Canada: Yes

Controlled Drug: USA: No
Canada: No

Available as Generic: USA: Yes
Canada: No

Brand Names: ✦Athrombin-K, Carfin, Coumadin, Panwarfin, Sofarin, ✦Warfilone

BENEFITS versus RISKS

Possible Benefits	Possible Risks
EFFECTIVE PREVENTION OF BOTH ARTERIAL AND VENOUS THROMBOSIS EFFECTIVE PREVENTION OF EMBOLIZATION IN THROMBOEMBOLIC DISORDERS	NARROW TREATMENT RANGE Dose-related bleeding (5% to 7%) Skin and soft tissue hemorrhage with tissue death (rare)

▷ **Principal Uses**

As a Single Drug Product: Used exclusively for its anticoagulant effect in treating the following conditions: (1) acute thrombosis (clot) or thrombophlebitis of the deep veins; (2) acute pulmonary embolism, resulting from blood clots that originate anywhere in the body; (3) atrial fibrillation, to prevent clotting of blood inside the heart that could result in embolization of small clots to any part of the body; (4) acute myocardial infarction (heart attack), to prevent clotting and embolization; (5) transient ischemic attack (TIA), a temporary reduction of blood flow to a part of the brain; used here to reduce the risk of repeated attacks or possible stroke. Other possible uses include the long-term prevention of recurrent heart attack, and prevention of embolization from the heart in those individuals with artificial heart valves.

How This Drug Works: The coumarin anticoagulants interfere with the production of four essential blood clotting factors by blocking the action of vitamin K. This leads to a deficiency of these clotting factors in circulating blood and inhibits blood clotting mechanisms.

Available Dosage Forms and Strengths
Injection — 50 mg/vial
Tablets — 2 mg, 2.5 mg, 5 mg, 7.5 mg, 10 mg

▷ **Usual Adult Dosage Range:** Initially, 10 to 15 mg daily for 2 to 3 days. A large loading dose is inappropriate and may be hazardous. For maintenance, 2 to 10 mg/day. The dosage is adjusted according to the prothrombin time. **Note: Actual dosage and administration schedule must be determined by the physician for each patient individually.**

▷ **Dosing Instructions:** Preferably taken when the stomach is empty, and at the same time each day to ensure uniform results. The tablet may be crushed for administration.

Usual Duration of Use: Continual use on a regular schedule for 3 to 5 days is usually necessary to determine this drug's effectiveness in providing significant anticoagulation. An additional 10 to 14 days is required to determine the optimal maintenance dose for each individual. Long-term use (months to years) requires supervision and periodic evaluation by your physician. Consult your physician on a regular basis.

▷ **This Drug Should Not Be Taken If**
- you have had an allergic reaction to it previously.
- you have an active peptic ulcer or active ulcerative colitis.
- you have had a recent stroke.

▷ **Inform Your Physician Before Taking This Drug If**
- you are now taking *any other drugs,* either prescription drugs or over-the-counter drug products.
- you are pregnant or planning pregnancy.
- you have a history of a bleeding disorder.
- you have high blood pressure.
- you have abnormally heavy or prolonged menstrual bleeding.
- you have diabetes.
- you are using an indwelling catheter.
- you have impaired liver or kidney function.
- you plan to have surgery or dental extraction in the near future.

Possible Side-Effects (natural, expected and unavoidable drug actions)
Minor episodes of bleeding may occur even though dosage and prothrombin times are well within the recommended range.

▷ **Possible Adverse Effects** (unusual, unexpected and infrequent reactions)
If any of the following develop, consult your physician promptly for guidance.
Mild Adverse Effects
Allergic Reactions: Skin rash, hives.
Loss of scalp hair.
Loss of appetite, nausea, vomiting, cramping, diarrhea.
Serious Adverse Effects
Allergic Reaction: Drug fever (see Glossary).
Idiosyncratic Reactions: Bleeding into skin and soft tissues causing gangrene of breast, toes and localized areas anywhere (rare).
Abnormal bleeding from nose, gastrointestinal tract, urinary tract or uterus.

▷ **Possible Effects on Sexual Function:**   None reported.

▷ **Adverse Effects That May Mimic Natural Diseases or Disorders**
Drug-induced fever may suggest infection.

Natural Diseases or Disorders That May Be Activated by This Drug
Bleeding from "silent" peptic ulcer, intestinal or bladder polyp or tumor.

CAUTION
1. Always carry with you a card of personal identification that includes a statement that *you are taking an anticoagulant drug.*

2. While taking this drug, always consult your physician *before* starting any new drug, changing the dosage schedule of any drug or
   discontinuing any drug.

Precautions for Use

By Those over 60 Years of Age: Small doses are mandatory until your individual sensitivity has been determined. Observe regularly for indications of excessive drug effects: prolonged bleeding from shaving
cuts, bleeding gums, bloody urine, rectal bleeding, excessive bruising.

▷ **Advisability of Use During Pregnancy**

Pregnancy Category: X. See Pregnancy Code inside back cover.
Animal studies: Fetal hemorrhage and death due to this drug reported
in mice.
Human studies: Information from studies of pregnant women indicates
fetal defects and fetal hemorrhage due to this drug.
The manufacturers state that this drug is contraindicated during entire
pregnancy.

Advisability of Use if Breast-Feeding

Presence of this drug in breast milk: Yes.
Avoid drug or refrain from nursing.

Habit-Forming Potential: None.

Effects of Overdosage: Episodes of bleeding from minor surface bleeding
(nose, gums, small lacerations) to major internal bleeding: vomiting
blood, bloody urine or stool.

Possible Effects of Long-Term Use: None reported.

Suggested Periodic Examinations While Taking This Drug (at physician's
discretion)

Regular determinations of prothrombin time are essential to safe dosage and proper control.
Urine analyses for blood.

▷ **While Taking This Drug, Observe the Following**

Foods: A larger intake than usual of foods rich in vitamin K may reduce
the effectiveness of this drug and make larger doses necessary. Foods
rich in vitamin K include: asparagus, bacon, beef liver, cabbage, cau-
liflower, fish, green leafy vegetables.

Beverages: No restrictions. May be taken with milk.

▷ *Alcohol:* Limit alcohol to one drink daily. Note: Heavy users of alcohol
with liver damage may be very sensitive to anticoagulants and require smaller than usual doses.

Tobacco Smoking: Heavy smokers may require relatively larger doses of
this drug.

▷ *Other Drugs*

Warfarin may *increase* the effects of
• phenytoin (Dilantin).

The following drugs may *increase* the effects of warfarin
- amiodarone.
- androgens.
- cephalosporins.
- chloral hydrate.
- cimetidine.
- clofibrate.
- dextrothyroxine.
- disulfiram.
- glucagon.
- metronidazole.
- phenylbutazone.
- quinidine.
- salicylates.
- sulfinpyrazone.
- sulfonamides.
- thyroid hormones.

The following drugs may *decrease* the effects of warfarin
- barbiturates.
- carbamazepine.
- cholestyramine.
- ethchlorvynol.
- glutethimide.
- griseofulvin.
- rifampin.
- vitamin K.

▷   *Driving, Hazardous Activities:* No restrictions.

Aviation Note: The use of this drug *is a disqualification* for piloting. Consult a designated Aviation Medical Examiner.

Exposure to Sun: No restrictions.

Discontinuation: Do not discontinue this drug abruptly unless abnormal bleeding occurs. Ask your physician for guidance regarding gradual reduction in dosage over a period of 3 to 4 weeks.

ZIDOVUDINE
(zi DOH vyoo deen)

Other Names: AZT, azidothymidine

Introduced: 1987   **Class:** Antiviral

Prescription: USA: Yes   **Controlled Drug:** USA: No
       Canada: Yes   Canada: No

Available as Generic: USA: No
       Canada: No

Brand Name: Retrovir

BENEFITS versus RISKS

Possible Benefits	*Possible Risks*
PROLONGATION OF LIFE AND REDUCED INCIDENCE OF INFECTIONS IN TREATING AIDS AND AIDS-RELATED COMPLEX	SERIOUS BONE MARROW DEPRESSION (see Glossary) Brain toxicity Lip, mouth and tongue sores

---

▷ **Principal Uses**

As a Single Drug Product: Used primarily to treat selected patients who have acquired immunodeficiency syndrome (AIDS) or acquired immunodeficiency syndrome-related complex (ARC) caused by human immunodeficiency virus (HIV); it is used specifically to treat those with interstitial plasma cell pneumonia or a marked deficiency of helper T-lymphocytes. This drug is not a cure for AIDS, and it does not reduce the risk of transmission of AIDS infection to others through sexual contact or contamination of blood.

How This Drug Works: By interfering with essential enzyme systems, this drug is thought to prevent the growth and reproduction of HIV particles within tissue cells, thus limiting the severity and extent of HIV infection.

Available Dosage Forms and Strengths

Capsules — 100 mg

▷ **Usual Adult Dosage Range:**   200 mg/4 hours throughout the day and night (no omission for activities or sleep). Smaller and larger doses may be used according to individual patient characteristics. **Note: Actual dosage and administration schedule must be determined by the physician for each patient individually.**

▷ **Dosing Instructions:**   Preferably taken on an empty stomach, but may be taken with or following food. Take exactly as prescribed. The capsule may be opened and the contents mixed with food just prior to administration.

Usual Duration of Use: Continual use on a regular schedule for 10 to 12 weeks is usually necessary to determine this drug's effectiveness in improving the course of symptomatic AIDS infection. Long-term use requires periodic evaluation of response and dosage adjustment. Consult your physician on a regular basis.

▷ **This Drug Should Not Be Taken If**
- you have had a serious allergic reaction to it previously.
- you have a serious degree of uncorrected bone marrow depression.

▷ **Inform Your Physician Before Taking This Drug If**
  • you have a history of either folic acid or vitamin B-12 deficiency.
  • you have impaired liver or kidney function.

Possible Side-Effects (natural, expected and unavoidable drug actions)
  None reported.

▷ **Possible Adverse Effects** (unusual, unexpected and infrequent reactions)
  If any of the following develop, consult your physician promptly for guidance.
  Mild Adverse Effects
  Allergic Reactions: Skin rash, hives, itching.
  Headache (50%), weakness (20%), drowsiness, dizziness, nervousness, insomnia.
  Nausea (50%), stomach pain (20%), diarrhea (12%), loss of appetite and vomiting (5% to 11%), altered taste, lip sores, swollen mouth or tongue.
  Muscle aches (8%), fever, sweating.
  Serious Adverse Effects
  Confusion, loss of speech, twitching, tremors, seizures (representing brain toxicity).
  Bone marrow depression (see Glossary): fatigue, weakness, fever, sore throat, abnormal bleeding or bruising. Anemia occurs most commonly after 4 to 6 weeks of treatment; abnormally low white blood cell counts occur after 6 to 8 weeks of treatment.

▷ **Possible Effects on Sexual Function:**   None reported.

  Possible Delayed Adverse Effects: Significant anemia and deficient white blood cell counts may develop after this drug has been discontinued.

▷ **Adverse Effects That May Mimic Natural Diseases or Disorders**
  Seizures may suggest the possibility of epilepsy.

  CAUTION
    1. This drug is not a cure for AIDS or AIDS-related complex. Nor does it protect completely against other infections or complications. Follow your physician's instructions and take all medications exactly as prescribed.
    2. This drug does not reduce the risk of transmitting AIDS to others through sexual contact or contamination of the blood. The use of an effective condom is mandatory. Needles for drug administration should not be shared.

  Precautions for Use
    By Infants and Children: Safety and effectiveness for use by those under 14 years of age have not been established.
    By Those over 60 Years of Age: Impaired kidney function will require dosage reduction.

▷ **Advisability of Use During Pregnancy**
  Pregnancy Category: C (tentative). See Pregnancy Code inside back cover.
  Animal studies: Rat studies reveal no birth defects.
  Human studies: Information from adequate studies of pregnant women
    is not available.
  Consult your physician for specific guidance.

Advisability of Use if Breast-Feeding
  Presence of this drug in breast milk: Unknown.
  Avoid drug or refrain from nursing.

Habit-Forming Potential: None.

Effects of Overdosage: Nausea, vomiting, diarrhea, bone marrow depression.

Possible Effects of Long-Term Use: Serious anemia and loss of white blood cells.

Suggested Periodic Examinations While Taking This Drug (at physician's discretion)
  Complete blood cell counts before starting treatment and weekly thereafter until tolerance is established. Continual monitoring for bone marrow depression is necessary during entire course of treatment.

▷ **While Taking This Drug, Observe the Following**
  Foods: No restrictions.
  Beverages: No restrictions. May be taken with milk.
▷ *Alcohol:* No interactions expected.
  Tobacco Smoking: No interactions expected.
▷ *Other Drugs*
  The following drugs may *increase* the effects of zidovudine and enhance
    its toxicity
  • acetaminophen.
  • acyclovir.
  • aspirin.
  • benzodiazepines (see Drug Class, Section Four).
  • cimetidine.
  • indomethacin.
  • morphine.
  • probenecid.
  • sulfonamides (see Drug Class, Section Four).
▷ *Driving, Hazardous Activities:* This drug may cause dizziness or fainting.
    Restrict activities as necessary.
  Aviation Note: The use of this drug *is a disqualification* for piloting. Consult a designated Aviation Medical Examiner.
  Exposure to Sun: No restrictions.
  Discontinuation: Do not discontinue this drug without your physician's knowledge and guidance.

DRUG CLASSES

Drug Classes

Throughout the Drug Profiles in Section Three reference is made to various drug classes. The reader may be advised to consult Section Four to become familiar with the drugs which belong to a particular class of drugs that share important characteristics in their chemical composition or in their actions within the body. Often it is important to know that *any* drug (or *all* drugs) within a given class can be expected to behave in a particular way. Such information may be useful in preventing interactions that could reduce the effectiveness of the drugs in use or result in unanticipated and sometimes hazardous adverse effects.

The presentation of each Drug Class is divided into two listings. The upper list contains the more widely recognized brand names of the drugs within the class; the lower list contains the generic names of the class members. In some instances the number of brand names in use is so large that a complete listing is not possible. In such cases, to be certain that you are consulting the correct drug class, determine the generic name of the drug that concerns you and consult the lower list to see if it is included there. The generic name listing is sufficiently complete to serve the scope of this book.

The following page lists the names of all the Drug Classes included in this section.

LIST OF DRUG CLASSES

Amphetaminelike Drugs
Analgesics, Mild
Analgesics, Strong (Narcotic Drugs)
Antiacne Drugs
Antiallergic Drugs
Antianginal Drugs
Antiarthritic/Anti-inflammatory
  Drugs (Aspirin Substitutes)
Antiasthmatic Drugs
  (Bronchodilators)
Antibiotics
Anticoagulants
Antidepressants
Antidiabetics, Oral (Sulfonylureas)
Antidiarrheal Drugs
Antiepileptic Drugs
  (Anticonvulsants)
Antiglaucoma Drugs
Antigout Drugs
Antihistamines
Antihypertensives
Anti-infective Drugs (Nonantibiotic-
  Antimicrobials)
Anti-itching Drugs (Antipruritics)
Anti-Motion Sickness/Antinausea
  Drugs (Antiemetics)
Antiparkinsonism Drugs
Antispasmodics, Synthetic
Appetite Suppressants
  (Anorexiants)
Atropinelike Drugs
Barbiturates
Benzodiazepines
Beta-Adrenergic-Blocking Drugs
  (Beta Blockers)
Calcium Channel-Blocking Drugs
  (Calcium Blockers)

Cephalosporins
Cholesterol-Reducing Drugs
Cortisonelike Drugs (Adrenocortical
  Steroids)
Cough Suppressants (Antitussives)
Decongestants
Digitalis Preparations
Diuretics
Female Sex Hormones
Fever-Reducing Drugs
  (Antipyretics)
Heart Rhythm Regulators
  (Antiarrhythmic Drugs)
Histamine (H-2)-Blocking Drugs
  (H-2 Blockers)
Male Sex Hormones (Androgens)
Monoamine Oxidase (MAO)
  Inhibitor Drugs
Muscle Relaxants
Nitrates
Penicillins
Phenothiazines
Salicylates
Sedatives/Sleep Inducers,
  Nonbarbiturate (Hypnotics)
Sulfonamides ("Sulfa" Drugs)
Sulfonylureas
Tetracyclines
Thiazide Diuretics
Tranquilizers, Mild (Antianxiety
  Drugs)
Tranquilizers, Strong
  (Antipsychotic Drugs)
Vasodilators
Xanthines

AMPHETAMINELIKE DRUGS

BRAND NAMES

Amodex
Benzedrine
Biphetamine
Desoxyn
Dexatrim
Dexedrine

Didrex
Fastin
Ionamin
Obalan
Plegine
Preludin

Ritalin
Tenuate
Tepanil
Tora
Wilpowr

GENERIC NAMES

amphetamine
benzphetamine
dextroamphetamine
diethylpropion
levamphetamine
methamphetamine

methylphenidate
phendimetrazine
phenmetrazine
phentermine
phenylpropanolamine

ANALGESICS, MILD

BRAND NAMES

Anaprox
A.S.A. Preparations
Darvocet
Darvon
Datril

Hycodan
Indocin
Motrin
Nebs
Percodan

Talwin
Taper
Tempra
Tylenol
Valadol

GENERIC NAMES

acetaminophen
aspirin
codeine
hydrocodone
ibuprofen
indomethacin

naproxen
oxycodone
paregoric
pentazocine
propoxyphene

ANALGESICS, STRONG

(Narcotic Drugs)

<u>BRAND NAMES</u>
Demerol
Dilaudid
Dolophine
Leritine

<u>GENERIC NAMES</u>

anileridine
hydromorphone
meperidine
methadone
morphine

ANTIACNE DRUGS

<u>BRAND NAMES</u>

Accutane
Achromycin V
Eryderm
Lucidol
Retin-A

<u>GENERIC NAMES</u>

benzoyl peroxide
erythromycin
isotretinoin
tetracycline
tretinoin

ANTIALLERGIC DRUGS

See: Antihistamines
Cortisonelike Drugs

ANTIANGINAL DRUGS

BRAND NAMES

Calan   Nitrostat
Cardene   Peritrate
Cardizem   Procardia
Corgard   Tenormin
Inderal
Isoptin
Isordil

GENERIC NAMES

beta blockers (see Class)   nifedipine
diltiazem   nitrates (see Class)
nicardipine   verapamil

ANTIARTHRITIC/ANTI-INFLAMMATORY DRUGS

(Aspirin Substitutes)

BRAND NAMES

Ansaid   Nalfon
Clinoral   Naprosyn
Dolobid   Orudis
Feldene   Suprol
Indocin   Tolectin
Meclomen   Voltaren
Motrin

GENERIC NAMES

diclofenac   meclofenamate
diflunisal   naproxen
fenoprofen   piroxicam
flurbiprofen   sulindac
ibuprofen   suprofen
indomethacin   tolmetin
ketoprofen

ANTIASTHMATIC DRUGS

(Bronchodilators)

BRAND NAMES

Aarane
Adrenalin
Alupent
Aminodur
Brethine
Bricanyl
Bronkodyl
Bronkometer
Bronkosol
Bronkotabs

Choledyl
Elixophyllin
Intal
Isuprel
Lufyllin
Medihaler-Epi
Medihaler-Iso
Metaprel
Neothylline
Norisodrine

Proternol
Proventil
Slo-Phyllin
Somophylline
Sus-Phrine
Theolair
Tornalate
Vaponefrin
Ventolin

GENERIC NAMES

albuterol
aminophylline
bitolterol
cromolyn
dyphylline
ephedrine
epinephrine

isoetharine
isoproterenol
metaproterenol
oxtriphylline
terbutaline
theophylline

ANTIBIOTICS

BRAND NAMES

See respective Classes listed under Generic Names.

GENERIC NAMES

cephalosporins
chloramphenicol
clindamycin
erythromycins

lincomycin
penicillins
rifampin
tetacyclines

ANTICOAGULANTS

Coumarin Class

BRAND NAMES

Coumadin
Dicumarol
Liquamar
Panwarfin
Sintrom
Tromexan

GENERIC NAMES

acenocoumarol
dicumarol
phenprocoumon
warfarin

Indandione Class

BRAND NAMES

Danilone
Dipaxin
Eridione
Hedulin
Miradon

GENERIC NAMES

anisindione
diphenadione
phenindione

ANTIDEPRESSANTS

Bicyclic Antidepressants

BRAND NAMES

Prozac

GENERIC NAMES

fluoxetine

Tricyclic Antidepressants

BRAND NAMES

Adapin	Pertofrane
Asendin	Presamine
Aventyl	Sinequan
Elavil	Surmontil
Endep	Tofranil
Norpramin	Vivactil
Pamelor	

GENERIC NAMES

amitriptyline	imipramine
amoxapine	nortriptyline
desipramine	protriptyline
doxepin	trimipramine

Tetracyclic Antidepressants

BRAND NAMES

Ludiomil

GENERIC NAMES

maprotiline

Other Antidepressants

BRAND NAMES
Desyrel

GENERIC NAMES

trazodone

ANTIDIABETICS, ORAL

Sulfonylurea Class

BRAND NAMES

Chloronase   Glucotrol
DiaBeta   Micronase
Diabinese   Mobenol
Dimelor   Orinase
Dymelor   Stabinol
Euglucon   Tolinase

GENERIC NAMES

acetohexamide
chlorpropamide
glipizide
glyburide
tolazamide
tolbutamide

ANTIDIARRHEAL DRUGS

BRAND NAMES

Donnagel
Imodium
Kaopectate
Lomotil
Parepectolin

GENERIC NAMES

atropine
diphenoxylate
kaolin
loperimide
paregoric
pectin

ANTIEPILEPTIC DRUGS

(Anticonvulsants)

BRAND NAMES

Clonopin	Mysoline
Depakene	Tegretol
Diamox	Valium
Dilantin	Zarontin
Luminal	

GENERIC NAMES

acetazolamide	phenobarbital
carbamazepine	phenytoin
clonazepam	primidone
diazepam	valproic acid
ethosuximide	

ANTIGLAUCOMA DRUGS

BRAND NAMES

Diamox
Glaucon
Isopto-carpine
Timoptic

GENERIC NAMES

acetazolamide
epinephrine
pilocarpine
timolol

ANTIGOUT DRUGS

BRAND NAMES

Anaprox
Anturane
Benemid
Clinoril
Naprosyn
Zyloprim

GENERIC NAMES

allopurinol
colchicine
naproxen
probenecid
sulfinpyrazone
sulindac

ANTIHISTAMINES

BRAND NAMES

Actidil	Dramamine	Optimine
Atarax	Hispril	Periactin
Benadryl	Histadyl	Phenergan
Bonine	Histalon	Pyribenzamine
Chlor-Trimeton	Inhiston	Seldane
Clistin	Marezine	Tavist
Decapryn	Neo-Antergan	Trimeton
Dimetane	Norflex	Vistaril

GENERIC NAMES

azatadine	dimenhydrinate	orphenadrine
brompheniramine	diphenhydramine	pheniramine
carbinoxamine	diphenylpyraline	promethazine
chlorpheniramine	doxylamine	pyrilamine
clemastine	hydroxyzine	terfenidine
cyclizine	meclizine	tripelennamine
cyproheptadine	methapyrilene	triprolidine

ANTIHYPERTENSIVES

BRAND NAMES

Aldomet	HydroDiuril	Normodyne
Anhydron	Hygroton	Prinivil
Apresoline	Hytrin	Renese
Blocadren	Inderal	Saluron
Capoten	Inversine	Sectral
Cardene	Ismelin	Serpasil
Catapres	Lasix	Tenex
Corgard	Levatol	Tenormin
Diuril	Loniten	Trandate
Enduron	Lopressor	Vasotec
Esbaloid	Lozol	Visken
Esidrix	Minipress	Zestril
Eutonyl	Naqua	
Exna	Naturetin	

GENERIC NAMES

bendroflumethiazide	enalapril	methyclothiazide
benzthiazide	furosemide	methyldopa
beta blockers (see Class)	guanethidine	minoxidil
	guanfacine	nicardipine
bethanidine	hydralazine	pargyline
captopril	hydrochlorothiazide	penbutolol
chlorothiazide	hydroflumethiazide	polythiazide
chlorthalidone	indapamide	prazosin
clonidine	lisinopril	reserpine
cyclothiazide	mecamylamine	terazosin
		trichlormethiazide

ANTI-INFECTIVE DRUGS

(Nonantibiotic-Antimicrobials)

BRAND NAMES

Bactrim	Macrodantin
Cipro	NegGram
Flagyl	Noroxin
Furadantin	Septra
Gantrisin	

GENERIC NAMES

ciprofloxacin
metronidazole
nalidixic acid
nitrofurantoin
norfloxacin
sulfonamides (see Class)
trimethoprim

ANTI-ITCHING DRUGS

(Antipruritics)

BRAND NAMES

Atarax
Cortaid
Dermolate
Periactin
Temaril
Vistaril

GENERIC NAMES

cortisonelike drugs (see Class)
cyproheptadine
hydroxyzine
trimeprazine

ANTI-MOTION SICKNESS/ANTINAUSEA DRUGS

(Antiemetics)

BRAND NAMES

Antivert	Compazine	Phenergan
Atarax	Dexedrine	Thorazine
Benadryl	Dramamine	Tigan
Bonine	Marezine	Vistaril

GENERIC NAMES

chlorpromazine	meclizine
cyclizine	prochlorperazine
dextroamphetamine	promethazine
dimenhydrinate	scopolamine
diphenhydramine	trimethobenzamide
hydroxyzine	

ANTIPARKINSONISM DRUGS

BRAND NAMES

Akineton	Eldepryl	Parsidol
Artane	Kemadrin	Permax
Bendopa	Larodopa	Phenoxene
Biodopa	Levodopa	Pipanol
Cogentin	Norflex	Sinemet
Disipal	Pagitane	Symmetrel
Dopar	Parda	Tremin
	Parlodel	

GENERIC NAMES

amantadine	levodopa
benztropine	orphenadrine
biperiden	pergolide
bromocriptine	procyclidine
chlorphenoxamine	selegiline
cycrimine	trihexyphenidyl
ethopropazine	

ANTISPASMODICS, SYNTHETIC

BRAND NAMES

Antrenyl	Nacton	Quarzan
Banthine	Pamine	Robinul
Bentyl	Pathilon	Tral
Cantil	Prantal	Trocinate
Darbid	Pro-Banthine	

GENERIC NAMES

clidinium	isopropamide	poldine
dicyclomine	mepenzolate	propantheline
diphemanil	methantheline	thiphenamil
glycopyrrolate	methscopolamine	tridihexethyl
hexocyclium	oxyphenonium	

APPETITE SUPPRESSANTS

(Anorexiants)

BRAND NAMES

Dexedrine	Preludin
Dietac	Pre-Sate
Fastin	Sanorex
Ionamin	Tenuate
Plegine	Tepanil
Pondimin	

GENERIC NAMES

chlorphentermine	phendimetrazine
dextroamphetamine	phenmetrazine
diethylpropion	phentermine
fenfluramine	phenylpropanolamine
mazindol	

ATROPINELIKE DRUGS

The drugs included in the following groups may exhibit atropinelike (anticholinergic) action. This can be important in the management of certain diseases and in potential interactions with other drugs used concurrently.

All drugs containing:

atropine	Antidepressants, tricyclic
belladonna	Antihistamines (some)
hyoscyamine	Antiparkinsonism Drugs
scopolamine	(some)
	Antispasmodics, Synthetic
	Muscle Relaxants (some)

BARBITURATES

BRAND NAMES

Alurate	Mebaral
Amytal	Nembutal
Butisol	Sandoptal
Lotusate	Seconal
Luminal	Sombulex

GENERIC NAMES

amobarbital	mephobarbital
aprobarbital	pentobarbital
butabarbital	phenobarbital
butalbital	secobarbital
hexobarbital	talbutal

BENZODIAZEPINES

BRAND NAMES

Ativan	Paxipam
Centrax	Restoril
Clonopin	Serax
Dalmane	Tranxene
Halcion	Valium
Libritabs	Verstran
Librium	Xanax

GENERIC NAMES

alprazolam	halazepam
chlordiazepoxide	lorazepam
clonazepam	oxazepam
clorazepate	prazepam
diazepam	temazepam
flurazepam	triazolam

BETA-ADRENERGIC-BLOCKING DRUGS

(Beta Blockers)

BRAND NAMES

Blocadren	Sectral
Corgard	Tenormin
Inderal	Trandate
Levatol	Visken
Lopressor	
Normodyne	

GENERIC NAMES

acebutolol	penbutolol
atenolol	pindolol
labetalol	propranolol
metoprolol	timolol
nadolol	

CALCIUM CHANNEL-BLOCKING DRUGS
(Calcium Blockers)

BRAND NAMES

Calan
Cardene
Cardizem
Isoptin
Procardia

GENERIC NAMES

diltiazem
nicardipine
nifedipine
verapamil

CEPHALOSPORINS

BRAND NAMES

Anspor   Keflex
Ceclor   Novolexin
Ceftin   Ultracef
Ceporex   Velosef
Duricef

GENERIC NAMES

cefaclor
cefadroxil
cefuroxime
cephalexin
cephradine

CHOLESTEROL-REDUCING DRUGS

BRAND NAMES

Atromid S   Lopid
Choloxin   Lorelco
Colestid   Mevacor
Cytellin   Nicobid
                 Questran

GENERIC NAMES

cholestyramine   gemfibrozil
clofibrate   lovastatin
colestipol   niacin
dextrothyroxine   probucol
                    sitosterols

CORTISONELIKE DRUGS

(Adrenocortical Steroids)

BRAND NAMES

Aristocort   Dexamethadrone   Meticorten
Colisone   Dexasone   Novadex
Cortef   Gammacorten   Novapred
Cortril   Hexadrol   Paracort
Decadron   Hydeltra   Prednis
Delta-Cortef   Hydrocortone   Servisone
Deltasone   Inflamase   Sterane
Deltra   Kenacort   Valisone
Deronil   Maxidex   Vanceril
Dexameth   Medrol   Wescopred

GENERIC NAMES

beclomethasone   methylprednisolone
betamethasone   prednisolone
cortisone   prednisone
dexamethasone   triamcinolone
hydrocortisone

COUGH SUPPRESSANTS

(Antitussives)

BRAND NAMES

Benylin   Phenergan
Benylin DM   Tessalon
Dilaudid   Tussionex
Hycodan

GENERIC NAMES

benzonatate   hydrocodone
codeine   hydromorphone
dextromethorphan   promethazine
diphenhydramine

DECONGESTANTS

BRAND NAMES

Afrin   Privine
Gluco-Fedrin   Propadrine
Neo-Synephrine   Sudafed
Novafed   Tyzine
Otrivin

GENERIC NAMES

ephedrine   pseudoephedrine
naphazoline   tetrahydrozoline
oxymetazoline   xylometazoline
phenylephrine
phenylpropanolamine

DIGITALIS PREPARATIONS

BRAND NAMES

Crystodigin	Lanoxicaps
Digifortis	Lanoxin
Digiglusin	Purodigin
Gitaligin	

GENERIC NAMES

digitalis	digoxin
digitoxin	gitalin

DIURETICS

BRAND NAMES

Aldactone	Hygroton
Bumex	Lasix
Diamox	Lozol
Diulo	Midamor
Diuril	Zaroxolyn
Dyrenium	(See Thiazide
Edecrin	Brand Names)

GENERIC NAMES

acetazolamide	indapamide
amiloride	metolazone
bumetanide	spironolactone
chlorthalidone	thiazides (see Class)
ethacrynic acid	triamterene
furosemide	

FEMALE SEX HORMONES

BRAND NAMES

Estrogens	*Progestogens*
Delestrogen	Amen
DES	Curretab
Estinyl	Megace
Estrace	Micronor
Estrovis	Morlutin
Evex	Ovrette
Feminone	Provera
Ogen	
Premarin	
TACE	

GENERIC NAMES

Estrogens	*Progestogens*
chlorotrianisene	medroxyprogesterone
diethylstilbestrol	megestrol
estradiol	norethindrone
estrogens, conjugated	norgestrel
estrogens, esterified	
estropipate	
ethinyl estradiol	
quinestrol	

FEVER-REDUCING DRUGS

(Antipyretics)

BRAND NAMES

Anaprox	Naprosyn
Clinoril	Ponstel
Indocin	Rufen
Motrin	Tolectin
Nalfon	Tylenol

GENERIC NAMES

acetaminophen	ibuprofen	naproxen
aspirin	indomethacin	sulindac
fenoprofen	mefenamic acid	tolmetin

HEART RHYTHM REGULATORS

(Antiarrhythmic Drugs)

BRAND NAMES

Calan	Pronestyl
Crystodigin	Purodigin
Inderal	Quinaglute
Isoptin	Quinidex
Lanoxin	Quinora
Mexitil	Tambocor
Norpace	Tonocard
Procan SR	

GENERIC NAMES

digitoxin	procainamide
digoxin	propranolol
disopyramide	quinidine
flecainide	tocainide
mexiletine	verapamil

HISTAMINE (H-2)-BLOCKING DRUGS

(H-2 Blockers)

BRAND NAMES

Axid
Pepcid
Tagamet
Zantac

GENERIC NAMES

cimetidine
famotidine
nizatidine
ranitidine

MALE SEX HORMONES

(Androgens)

<u>BRAND NAMES</u>

Android   Oratestin
Android F   Ora-Testryl
Depo-Testosterone   Oreton
Halotestin   Oreton Methyl
Metandren   Testred

<u>GENERIC NAMES</u>

fluoxymesterone
methyltestosterone
testosterone

MONOAMINE OXIDASE (MAO) INHIBITOR DRUGS

MAO Type A Inhibitors

(Food restrictions apply)

<u>BRAND NAMES</u>

Actomol   Marsilid
Catron   Nardil
Drazine   Niamid
Eutonyl   Parnate
Furoxone   Tersavid
Marplan

<u>GENERIC NAMES</u>

furazolidone   phenelzine
iproniazid   pheniprazine
isocarboxazid   phenoxypropazine
mebanazine   piohydrazine
nialamide   tranylcypromine
pargyline

MAO Type B Inhibitors
(Food restrictions do not apply)

BRAND NAMES

Eldepryl

GENERIC NAMES

selegiline

MUSCLE RELAXANTS

BRAND NAMES

Equanil	Rela
Flexeril	Robaxin
Lioresal	Skelaxin
Norflex	Soma
Paraflex	Valium
Parafon Forte	

GENERIC NAMES

baclofen	meprobamate
carisoprodol	metaxalone
chlorzoxazone	methocarbamol
cyclobenzaprine	orphenadrine
diazepam	

NITRATES

BRAND NAMES

Cardilate	Nitro-Bid	Peritrate
Isordil	Nitroglyn	SK-Petn
Laserdil	Nitrospan	Sorbide
Neo-Corovas	Nitrostat	Sorbitrate

GENERIC NAMES

erythrityl tetranitrate
isosorbide dinitrate
nitroglycerin
pentaerythritol tetranitrate

PENICILLINS

BRAND NAMES

Alpen	Omnipen	Principen
Amcill	Orbenin	Prostaphlin
Amoxil	Pathocil	Spectrobid
Bactocil	Penbritin	Tegopen
Dynapen	Pentids	Unipen
Geocillin	Pen-Vee K	V-Cillin K
Geopen	Polycillin	Veracillin
Larotid	Polymox	

GENERIC NAMES

amoxicillin	dicloxacillin
ampicillin	nafcillin
bacampicillin	oxacillin
carbenicillin	penicillin G
cloxacillin	penicillin V

PHENOTHIAZINES

BRAND NAMES

Chlor-PZ	Proketazine	Tacaryl
Compazine	Prolixin	Temaril
Largon	Promatar	Thorazine
Levoprome	Quide	Tindal
Mellaril	Repoise	Torecan
Parsidol	Serentil	Trilafon
Permitil	Sparine	Vesprin
Phenergan	Stelazine	

GENERIC NAMES

acetophenazine	methdilazine	propiomazine
butaperazine	methotrimeprazine	thiethylperazine
carphenazine	perphenazine	thioridazine
chlorpromazine	piperacetazine	trifluoperazine
ethopropazine	procholorperazine	triflupromazine
fluphenazine	promazine	trimeprazine
mesoridazine	promethazine	

SALICYLATES

BRAND NAMES

Arthropan	Empirin
Bufferin	Magan
Causalin	Neocylate
Ecotrin	Uracel

GENERIC NAMES

aspirin
choline salicylate
magnesium salicylate
potassium salicylate
sodium salicylate

SEDATIVES/SLEEP INDUCERS, NONBARBITURATE

(Hypnotics)

BRAND NAMES

Carbrital	Halcion	Restoril
Dalmane	Noctec	Somnafac
Doriden	Noludar	Sopor
Dorimide	Parest	Valmid
Felsules	Placidyl	

GENERIC NAMES

carbromal	glutethimide
chloral hydrate	methyprylon
ethchlorvynol	temazepam
ethinamate	triazolam
flurazepam	

SULFONAMIDES

("Sulfa" Drugs)

BRAND NAMES

Azulfidine	Gantanol	Sonilyn
Coco-Diazine	Gantrisin	Suladyne
Cosulfa	Kynex	Thiosulfil
Dagenan	Madribon	Triple Sulfas
Diamox	Midicel	Urobiotic
Elkosin	Neotrizine	

GENERIC NAMES

acetazolamide	sulfamethazine	sulfapyridine
sulfachlorpyridazine	sulfamethizole	sulfasalazine
sulfadiazine	sulfamethoxazole	sulfisomidine
sulfadimethoxine	sulfamethoxy-	sulfisoxazole
sulfamerazine	pyridazine	trisulfapyrimidines

SULFONYLUREAS

BRAND NAMES

Chloronase	Micronase
DiaBeta	Mobenol
Diabinese	Novobutamide
Dimelor	Orinase
Dymelor	Tolbutone
Euglucon	Tolinase
Glucotrol	

GENERIC NAMES

acetohexamide
chlorpropamide
glipizide
glyburide
tolazamide
tolbutamide

TETRACYCLINES

BRAND NAMES

Achromycin	Rondomycin	Tetracyn
Aureomycin	Steclin	Vectrin
Declomycin	Sumycin	Velacycline
Minocin	Terramycin	Vibramycin
Panmycin	Tetrachel	

GENERIC NAMES

chlortetracycline	minocycline
demeclocycline	oxytetracycline
doxycycline	rolitetracycline
methacycline	tetracycline

THIAZIDE DIURETICS

BRAND NAMES

Anhydron	Hydrazide	Naqua
Chemhydrazide	Hydrid	Naturetin
Diucardin	Hydrite	Neocodema
Diuchlor	Hydro-Aquil	Novohydrazide
Diuril	Hydrodiuretex	Oretic
Duretic	HydroDiuril	Renese
Edemol	Hydrosaluret	Saluron
Enduron	Hydrozide	Thiuretic
Esidrix	Metahydrin	Urozide
Exna		

GENERIC NAMES

bendroflumethiazide	hydroflumethiazide
benzthiazide	methyclothiazide
chlorothiazide	polythiazide
cyclothiazide	trichlormethiazide
hydrochlorothiazide	

TRANQUILIZERS, MILD

(Antianxiety Drugs)

Atarax	Miltown	Tybatran
Buspar	Paxipam	Ultran
Deprol	Serax	Valium
Equanil	Trancopal	Vistaril
Fenarol	Tranxene	Xanax
Librium		

alprazolam	halazepam
benactyzine	hydroxyzine
buspirone	meprobamate
chlordiazepoxide	oxazepam
chlormezanone	phenaglycodol
clorazepate	tybamate
diazepam	

TRANQUILIZERS, STRONG

(Antipsychotic Drugs)

Carbolith	Lithotabs	Serpasil
Eskalith	Loxitane	Taractan
Haldol	Moban	(See Phenothiazines,
Lithane	Navane	Brand Names)
Lithonate	Sandril	

chlorprothixene	phenothiazines (see Class)
haloperidol	reserpine
lithium	thiothixene
loxapine	
molindone	

VASODILATORS

BRAND NAMES

Arlidin

Cerespan

Cyclospasmol

Ethatab

Pavabid

Vasodilan

Vasospan

GENERIC NAMES

cyclandelate

ethaverine

isoxsuprine

nylidrin

papaverine

XANTHINES

BRAND NAMES

Aminodur

Bronkodyl

Choledyl

Droxine

Elixophylline

Quibron-T

Slo-Phyllin

Theo-Dur

Theolixir

Theovent

GENERIC NAMES

aminophylline

dyphylline

oxtriphylline

theophylline

A GLOSSARY
OF
DRUG-RELATED TERMS

Glossary

Addiction The traditional term used to identify the irresistible craving for and compulsive use of habit-forming drugs. The more recent preference for the term *dependence* has served to clarify the distinction between habituation and addiction. Drugs capable of producing addiction do so by interacting with the biochemistry of the brain in such a way that they assume a working role. This physical incorporation of the drug into the fundamental processes of brain tissue function is responsible for the agony of the "withdrawal syndrome"—the intense mental and physical pain experienced by the addict when intake of the drug is stopped abruptly. Thus addiction is a *physical dependence*. (See DEPENDENCE for a further account of physical and psychological dependence.)

Adverse Effect or Reaction An abnormal, unexpected, infrequent and usually unpredictable injurious response to a drug. Used in this restrictive sense, the term *adverse reaction* does *not* include effects of a drug which are normally a part of its pharmacological action, even though such effects may be undesirable and unintended. (See SIDE-EFFECT.) Adverse reactions are of three basic types: those due to drug *allergy*, those caused by individual *idiosyncrasy* and those representing *toxic* effects of drugs on tissue structure and function (see ALLERGY, IDIOSYNCRASY and TOXICITY).

Allergy (Drug) An abnormal mechanism of drug response that occurs in individuals who produce injurious antibodies* that react with foreign substances—in this instance, a drug. The person who is allergic by na-

*Antibodies are special tissue proteins that combine with substances foreign to the body. Protective antibodies destroy bacteria and neutralize toxins. Injurious antibodies, reacting with foreign substances, cause the release of histamine, the principal chemical responsible for allergic reactions.

ture and has a history of hay fever, asthma, hives or eczema is more likely to develop drug allergies. Allergic reactions to drugs take many forms: skin eruptions of various kinds, fever, swollen glands, painful joints, jaundice, interference with breathing, acute collapse of circulation, etc. Drug allergies can develop gradually over a long period of time, or they can appear with dramatic suddenness and require life-saving intervention.

Analgesic A drug that is used primarily to relieve pain. Analgesics are of three basic types: (1) Simple, nonnarcotic analgesics that relieve pain by suppressing the local production of prostaglandins and related substances; examples are acetaminophen, aspirin and the large group of nonsteroidal anti-inflammatory drugs known as aspirin substitutes (Motrin, Advil, Naprosyn, etc.). (2) Narcotic analgesics or opioids ("like opium" derivatives) that relieve pain by suppressing its perception in the brain; examples are morphine, codeine and hydrocodone (natural derivatives of opium), and meperidine or pentazocine (synthetic drug products). (3) Local anesthetics that prevent or relieve pain by rendering sensory nerve endings insensitive to painful stimulation; an example is the urinary tract analgesic phenazopyridine (Pyridium).

Anaphylactic (Anaphylactoid) Reaction A group of symptoms which represent (or resemble) a sometimes overwhelming and dangerous allergic reaction due to extreme hypersensitivity to a drug. Anaphylactic reactions, whether mild, moderate or severe, often involve several body systems. Mild symptoms consist of itching, hives, nasal congestion, nausea, abdominal cramping and/or diarrhea. Sometimes these precede more severe symptoms such as choking, shortness of breath and sudden loss of consciousness (usually referred to as anaphylactic shock).

Characteristic features of anaphylactic reaction must be kept in mind. It can result from a very small dose of drug; it develops suddenly, usually within a few minutes after taking the drug; it can be rapidly progressive and can lead to fatal collapse in a short time if not reversed by appropriate treatment. A developing anaphylactic reaction is a true medical emergency. Any adverse effect that appears within 20 minutes after taking a drug should be considered the early manifestation of a possible anaphylactic reaction. Obtain medical attention immediately! (See ALLERGY, DRUG and HYPERSENSITIVITY.)

Antihypertensive A drug used to lower excessively high blood pressure. The term *hypertension* denotes blood pressure above the normal range. It does not refer to excessive nervous or emotional tension. The term *antihypertensive* is sometimes used erroneously as if it had the same meaning as *antianxiety* (or tranquilizing) drug action.

Today there are more than 100 drug products in use for treating hypertension. Those most frequently prescribed for long-term use fall into three major groups:

drugs that increase urine production (the diuretics)
drugs that relax blood vessel walls
drugs that reduce the activity of the sympathetic nervous system

Regardless of their mode of action, all these drugs share an ability to lower the blood pressure. It is important to remember that many other drugs can interact with antihypertensive drugs: some add to their effect and cause excessive reduction in blood pressure; others interfere with their action and reduce their effectiveness. Anyone who is taking medications for hypertension should consult with his or her physician whenever drugs are prescribed for the treatment of other conditions as well.

Antipyretic A drug that is used to treat fever because of its ability to lower body temperature that is elevated above the normal. Antipyretics relieve fever through their effects on the temperature regulating center in the hypothalamus of the brain. Their actions cause dilation of the blood vessels (capillary beds) in the skin, bringing overheated blood to the surface for cooling; in addition, the sweat glands are stimulated to provide copious perspiration that cools the body further through evaporation. An antipyretic drug may also be analgesic (acetaminophen), or analgesic and anti-inflammatory (aspirin).

Aplastic Anemia A form of bone marrow failure in which the production of all 3 types of blood cells is seriously impaired (also known as pancytopenia). Aplastic anemia can occur spontaneously from unknown causes, but about one-half of reported cases are induced by certain drugs or chemicals. The symptoms reflect the consequences of inadequate supplies of all 3 blood cell types: deficiency of red blood cells (anemia) results in fatigue, weakness and pallor; deficiency of white blood cells (leukopenia) predisposes to infections; deficiency of blood platelets (thrombocytopenia) leads to spontaneous bruising and hemorrhage. Treatment is difficult and the outcome unpredictable. Even with the best of care, approximately 50% of cases end fatally.

These drugs and chemicals are known to be capable of inducing aplastic anemia:

acetazolamide
anticancer drugs
aspirin
benzene (solvent)
carbamazepine
carbon tetrachloride (solvent)
chlordane (insecticide)
chlordiazepoxide
chloromycetin
chlorothiazide
chlorpheniramine
chlorpromazine
chlorpropamide
colchicine
DDT (insecticide)
indomethacin
lithium
mephenytoin

meprobamate
methimazole
oxyphenbutazone
penicillin
phenacetin
phenylbutazone
phenytoin
primidone
promazine
quinacrine
sulfonamides
tetracyclines
thiouracil
tolbutamide
triflupromazine
trimethadione
tripelennamine

Although aplastic anemia is a rare consequence of drug treatment (3 in 100,000 users of quinacrine, for example), anyone taking a drug capable of inducing it should have complete blood cell counts periodically if the drug is to be used over an extended period of time.

Bioavailability The measurable characteristics of a drug product (usually a tablet or a capsule) that represent how rapidly the active drug ingredient is absorbed into the bloodstream and to what extent it is absorbed. Two types of measurements—(1) blood levels of the drug at certain time intervals after administration, and (2) the duration of the drug's presence in the blood—indicate how much of the drug is available for biological activity and for how long.

Another method of determining a drug product's bioavailability is to measure (1) the cumulative amount of the drug (or any breakdown product after transformation) that is excreted in the urine, and (2) the rate of drug accumulation in the urine.

The two major factors that govern a drug product's bioavailability are the chemical and physical characteristics (the formulation) of the dosage form given, and the functional state of the digestive system of the individual who takes it. A drug product that disintegrates rapidly in a normally functioning stomach and small intestine produces blood levels of the absorbed drug quite promptly. Such a drug product can be demonstrated to possess good bioavailability.

Specially designed laboratory tests are now available to evaluate a drug product's potential bioavailability when taken by the "average" individual.

Bioequivalence It is generally accepted that the ability of a drug product to produce its intended therapeutic effect is directly related to its bioavailability. When a particular drug is marketed by several manufacturers, often in a variety of dosage forms, it is critically important that the drug product selected for use be one that possesses the bioavailability necessary to be effective therapeutically. Substantial variations occur among manufacturers in the formulation of their drug products. Although the principal drug ingredient of products from different firms may be identical chemically, it cannot be assumed that these products possess equal bioavailability and are therefore equal therapeutically.

The bioavailability of any drug product is governed to a large extent by the physical characteristics of its formulation; these in turn determine how rapidly and how completely the drug product disintegrates and releases its active drug component(s) for absorption into the bloodstream. Drug products that contain the same principal drug ingredient but are combined with different inert additives, are coated with different substances or are enclosed in capsules of different composition may or may not possess the same bioavailability. Those that do are said to be bioequivalent, and can be relied upon to be equally effective in achieving therapeutic results.

If you consider having your prescription filled with the generic equivalent of a brand name drug product, ask your physician *and* pharmacist for guidance. This decision requires professional judgment in each case. In many treatment situations, reasonable differences in the bioavailability patterns among drug products are acceptable. In some situations, however, because of the serious nature of the illness, or because it is mandatory that blood levels of the drug be maintained within a narrowly defined range, it is essential to use the drug product that has been demonstrated to possess reliable bioavailability.

Blood Platelets The smallest of the three types of blood cells produced by the bone marrow. Platelets are normally present in very large numbers. Their primary function is to assist the process of normal blood clotting so as to prevent excessive bruising and bleeding in the event of injury. When present in proper numbers and functioning normally, platelets preserve the retaining power of the walls of the smaller blood vessels. By initiating appropriate clotting processes in the blood, platelets seal small points of leakage in the vessel walls, thereby preventing spontaneous bruising or bleeding (that which is unprovoked by trauma).

Certain drugs and chemicals may reduce the number of available blood platelets to abnormally low levels. Some of these drugs act by suppressing platelet formation; other drugs hasten their destruction. When the number of functioning platelets falls below a critical level, blood begins to leak through the thin walls of smaller vessels. The outward evidence of this leakage is the spontaneous appearance of scattered bruises in the skin of the thighs and legs. This is referred to as purpura. Bleeding may occur anywhere in the body, internally as well as superficially into the tissues immediately beneath the skin.

Bone Marrow Depression A serious reduction in the ability of the bone marrow to carry on its normal production of blood cells. This can occur as an adverse reaction to the toxic effect of certain drugs and chemicals on bone marrow components. When functioning normally, the bone marrow produces the majority of the body's blood cells. These consist of three types: the red blood cells (erythrocytes), the white blood cells (leukocytes) and the blood platelets (thrombocytes). Each type of cell performs one or more specific functions, all of which are indispensable to the maintenance of life and health.

Drugs that are capable of depressing bone marrow activity can impair the production of all types of blood cells simultaneously or of only one type selectively. Periodic examinations of the blood can reveal significant changes in the structure and number of the blood cells that indicate a possible drug effect on bone marrow activity.

Impairment of the production of red blood cells leads to anemia, a condition of abnormally low red cells and hemoglobin. This causes weakness, loss of energy and stamina, intolerance of cold environments and shortness of breath on physical exertion. A reduction in the formation of white blood cells can impair the body's immunity and lower its resistance to infection. These changes may result in the development of fever, sore throat or pneumonia. When the formation of blood platelets is suppressed to abnormally low levels, the blood loses its ability to quickly seal small points of leakage in blood vessel walls. This may lead to episodes of unusual and abnormal spontaneous bruising or to prolonged bleeding in the event of injury.

Any of these symptoms can occur in the presence of bone marrow depression. They should alert both patient and physician to the need for prompt studies of blood and bone marrow.

Brand Name The registered trade name given to a drug product by its manufacturer. Many drugs are marketed by more than one manufacturer or distributor. Each company adopts a distinctive trade name to distinguish its brand of the generic drug from that of its competitors. Thus a brand name designates a proprietary drug—one that is protected by patent or copyright. Generally brand names are shorter, easier to pronounce and more readily remembered than their generic counterparts.

Cause-and-Effect Relationship A possible causative association between a drug and an observed biologic event—most commonly a side-effect or an adverse effect. Knowledge of a drug's full spectrum of effects (wanted and unwanted) is highly desirable when weighing its benefits and risks in any treatment situation. However, it is often impossible to establish with certainty that a particular drug is the primary agent responsible for a suspected adverse effect. In the evaluation of every cause-and-effect relationship, therefore, meticulous consideration must be given to such factors as the time sequence of drug administration and possible reaction, the use of multiple drugs, possible interactions among these drugs, the effects of the disease under treatment, the physiological and psychological characteristics of the patient and the possible influence of unrecognized disorders and malfunctions.

The majority of adverse drug reactions occur sporadically, unpredictably and infrequently in the general population. A *definite* cause-and-effect relationship between drug and reaction is established when (1) the adverse effect immediately follows administration of the drug; or (2) the adverse effect disappears after the drug is discontinued (dechallenge) and promptly reappears when the drug is used again (rechallenge); or (3) the adverse effects are clearly the expected and predictable toxic consequences of drug overdosage.

In contrast to the obvious "causative" (definite) relationship, there exists a large gray area of "probable," "possible" and "coincidental" associations that are clouded by varying degrees of uncertainty. These classifications usually apply to alleged drug reactions that require a relatively long time to develop, are of low incidence and for which there are no clear-cut objective means of demonstrating a causal mechanism that links drug and reaction. Clarification of cause-and-effect relationships in these uncertain groups requires carefully designed observation over a long period of time, followed by sophisticated statistical analysis. Occasionally the public is alerted to a newly found "relationship" based upon suggestive but incomplete data. Though early warning is clearly in the public interest, such announcements should make clear whether the presumed relationship is based upon definitive criteria or is simply inferred because the use of a drug and an observed event were found to occur together within an appropriate time frame.

The most competent techniques for evaluating cause-and-effect relationships of adverse drug reactions have been devised by the Division of Tissue Reactions to Drugs, a research unit of the Armed Forces Institute of Pathology. Based upon a highly critical examination of all available evidence, the Division's study of 2800 drug-related deaths yielded the following levels of certainty regarding cause-and-effect relationship:

No association	5.0%
Coincidental	14.5%
Possible	33.0%
Probable	30.0%
Causative	17.5%

It is significant that expert evaluation of 2800 drug-related cases concluded that only 47.5% could be substantiated as definitely or probably causative.

Contraindication A condition or disease that precludes the use of a particular drug. Some cointraindications are *absolute*, meaning that the use of the drug would expose the patient to extreme hazard and therefore cannot be justified. Other contraindications are *relative*, meaning that the condition or disease does not entirely bar the use of the drug but requires that, before the decision to use the drug is made, special consideration be given to factors which could aggravate existing disease, interfere with current treatment or produce new injury.

Dependence The preferred term used to identify the drug-dependent states of *psychological dependence* (or *habituation*), and *physical dependence* (or *addiction*). In addition, a third kind of drug-dependence can be included under this term. This might be called *functional dependence*—the need to use a drug continuously in order to sustain a particular body function, the impairment of which causes annoying symptoms of varying degree and significance.

Psychological dependence is a form of neurotic behavior. Its principal characteristic is an obsession to satisfy a particular desire, be it one of self-gratification or one of escape from some real or imagined distress. Psychological dependence is a very human trait that is seen often in many socially acceptable patterns and practices such as entertainment, gambling, sports and collecting. A common form of this dependence in today's culture is the increasing reliance upon drugs to help in coping with the everyday problems of living: pills for frustration, disappointment, nervous stomach, tension headache and insomnia. The 20 million smokers of marijuana have found it to be a drug that eases their stress, one whose effectiveness fosters habit (psychological dependence) but not addiction.

Physical dependence, which is true addiction, includes two elements: habituation and tolerance. Addicting drugs provide relief from anguish and pain swiftly and effectively; they also induce a physiological tolerance that requires increasing dosage or repeated use if they are to remain effective. These two features foster the continued need for the drug and lead to its becoming a functioning component in the biochemistry of the brain. As this occurs, the drug assumes an "essential" role in ongoing chemical processes. (Thus some authorities prefer the term *chemical dependence.*) Sudden removal of the drug from the system causes a major upheaval in body chemistry and provokes a withdrawal syndrome—the intense mental and physical pain experienced by the addict when intake of the drug is stopped abruptly—that is the hallmark of addiction.

Functional dependence differs significantly from both psychological and physical dependence. It occurs when a drug effectively relieves an annoying or distressing condition and the particular body function involved becomes increasingly dependent upon the action of the drug to provide a sense of well-being. Drugs which are capable of inducing functional dependence are used primarily for the relief of symptoms. They do not act on the brain to produce alteration of mood or consciousness as do those drugs with potential for either psychological or physical dependence. The most familiar example of functional dependence is the "laxative habit." Some types of constipation are made worse by the wrong choice of laxative, and natural function gradually fades as the colon becomes more and more dependent upon the action of certain laxative drugs.

Disulfiramlike (Antabuselike) Reaction The symptoms that result from the interaction of alcohol and any drug that is capable of provoking the pattern of response typical of the "Antabuse effect." The interacting drug interrupts the normal decomposition of alcohol by the liver and thereby permits the accumulation of a toxic by-product that enters the bloodstream. When sufficient levels of both alcohol and drug are present in the blood the reaction occurs. It consists of intense flushing and warming of the face, a severe throbbing headache, shortness of breath, chest pains, nausea, repeated vomiting, sweating and weakness. If the amount of alcohol ingested has been large enough, the reaction may progress to blurred vision, vertigo, confusion, marked drop in blood pressure and loss of consciousness. Severe reactions may lead to convulsions and death. The reaction can last from 30 minutes to several hours, depending upon the amount of alcohol in the body. As the symptoms subside, the individual is exhausted and usually sleeps for several hours.

Diuretic A drug that alters kidney function to increase the volume of urine. Diuretics use several different mechanisms to increase urine volume, and these, in turn, have different effects on body chemistry. Diuretics are used primarily to (1) remove excess water from the body (as in congestive heart failure and some types of liver and kidney disease), and (2) treat hypertension by promoting the excretion of sodium from the body.

Dosage Forms and Strengths This information category in the individual

Drug Profiles (Section Three) uses several abbreviations to designate measurements of weight and volume. These are

mcg = microgram = 1,000,000th of a gram (weight)
mg = milligram = 1000th of a gram (weight)
ml = milliliter = 1000th of a liter (volume)
gm = gram = 1000 milligrams (weight)

There are approximately 65 mg in 1 grain.
There are approximately 5 ml in 1 teaspoonful.
There are approximately 15 ml in 1 tablespoonful.
There are approximately 30 ml in 1 ounce.
1 milliliter of water weighs 1 gram.
There are approximately 454 grams in 1 pound.

Drug, Drug Product Terms often used interchangeably to designate a medicine (in any of its dosage forms) used in medical practice. Strictly speaking, the term *drug* refers to the single chemical entity that provokes a specific response when placed within a biological system—the "active" ingredient. A *drug product* is the manufactured dosage form—tablet, capsule, elixir, etc.—that contains the active drug intermixed with inactive ingredients to provide for convenient administration.

Drug products which contain only one active ingredient are referred to as single entity drugs. Drug products with two or more active ingredients are called combination drugs (designed [CD] in the lists of brand names in the Drug Profiles, Section Three).

Drug Class A group of drugs that are similar in chemistry, method of action and use in treatment. Because of their common characteristics, many drugs within a class will produce the same side-effects and have similar potential for provoking related adverse reactions and interactions. However, significant variations among members within a drug class can occur. This sometimes allows the physician an important degree of selectivity in choosing a drug if certain beneficial actions are desired or particular side-effects are to be minimized.

Examples: Antihistamines, phentothiazines, tetracyclines (see Section Four).

Drug Fever The elevation of body temperature that occurs as an unwanted manifestation of drug action. Drugs can induce fever by several mechanisms; these include allergic reactions, drug-induced tissue damage, acceleration of tissue metabolism, constriction of blood vessels in the skin with resulting decrease in loss of body heat and direct action on the temperature-regulating center in the brain.

The most common form of drug fever is that associated with allergic reactions. It may be the only allergic manifestation apparent, or it may be part of a complex of allergic symptoms that can include skin rash, hives, joint swelling and pain, enlarged lymph glands, hemolytic anemia or hepatitis. The fever usually appears about 7 to 10 days after starting the drug and may vary from low-grade to alarmingly high levels. It may be sustained or intermittent, but it usually persists for as long as the drug is taken. In previously sensitized individuals drug fever may occur within 1 or 2 hours after taking the first dose of medication.

While many drugs are capable of producing fever, the following are more commonly responsible:

allopurinol
antihistamines
atropinelike drugs
barbiturates
coumarin anticoagulants
hydralazine
iodides
isoniazid
methyldopa
nadalol

novobiocin
para-aminosalicylic acid
penicillin
pentazocine
phenytoin
procainamide
propylthiouracil
quinidine
rifampin
sulfonamides

Extension Effect An unwanted but predictable drug response that is a logical consequence of mild to moderate overdosage. An extension effect is an exaggeration of the drug's normal pharmacological action; it can be thought of as a mild form of dose-related toxicity (see OVERDOSAGE and TOXICITY).

Example: The continued "hangover" of drowsiness and mental sluggishness that persists after arising in the morning is a common extension effect of a long-acting sleep-inducing drug (hypnotic) taken the night before.

Example: The persistent intestinal cramping and diarrhea that result from too generous a dose of laxative are extension effects of the drug's anticipated action.

Generic Name The official, common or public name used to designate an active drug entity, whether in pure form or in dosage form. Generic names are coined by committees of officially appointed drug experts and are approved by governmental agencies for national and international use. Thus they are nonproprietary. Many drug products are marketed under the generic name of the principal active ingredient and bear no brand name of the manufacturer.

While the total number of prescriptions written in the United States in 1986 increased by 0.6%, prescriptions specifying the *generic name* of the drug increased by 8.6%. Generically written prescriptions now account for 13.5% of all new prescriptions written in the United States. The drugs most commonly prescribed by generic name are listed below, ranked in descending order of the number of new prescriptions issued.

amoxicillin
penicillin VK
ampicillin
tetracycline
prednisone

erythromycin
hydrochlorothiazide
acetaminophen/codeine
doxycycline
phenobarbital

Habituation A form of drug dependence based upon strong psychological gratification rather than the physical (chemical) dependence of addiction. The habitual use of drugs that alter mood or relieve minor discomforts results from a compulsive need to feel pleasure and satisfaction or to escape the manifestations of emotional distress. The abrupt cessation of habituating drugs does not produce the withdrawal syndrome seen in addiction. Thus habituation is a *psychological dependence*. (See DEPENDENCE for a further account of psychological and physical dependence.)

Hemolytic Anemia A form of anemia (deficient red blood cells and hemoglobin) resulting from the premature destruction (hemolysis) of circulating red blood cells. Several mechanisms can be responsible for the development of hemolytic anemia; among these is the action of certain drugs and chemicals. Some individuals are susceptible to hemolytic anemia because of a genetic deficiency in the makeup of their red blood cells. If such people are given certain antimalarial drugs, sulfa drugs or numerous other drugs, some of their red cells will disintegrate on contact with the drug. (About 10% of American blacks have this genetic trait.)

Another type of drug-induced hemolytic anemia is a form of drug allergy. Many drugs in wide use (including quinidine, methyldopa, levodopa and chlorpromazine) are known to cause hemolytic destruction of red cells as a hypersensitivity (allergic) reaction.

Hemolytic anemia can occur abruptly (with evident symptoms) or silently. The acute form lasts about 7 days and is characterized by fever, pallor, weakness, dark-colored urine and varying degrees of jaundice (yellow coloration of eyes and skin). When drug-induced hemolytic anemia is mild, involving the destruction of only a small number of red blood cells, there may be no symptoms to indicate its presence. Such episodes are detected only by means of laboratory studies (see IDIOSYNCRASY and ALLERGY, DRUG).

Hepatitislike Reaction Changes in the liver, induced by certain drugs, which closely resemble those produced by viral hepatitis. The symptoms of drug-induced hepatitis and virus-induced hepatitis are often so similar that the correct cause cannot be established without precise laboratory studies.

Hepatitis due to drugs may be a form of drug allergy (as in reaction to many of the phenothiazines), or it may represent a toxic adverse effect (as in reaction to some of the monoamine oxidase inhibitor drugs). Liver reactions of significance usually result in jaundice and represent serious adverse effects (see JAUNDICE).

Hypersensitivity A term subject to varying usages for many years. One common use has been to identify the trait of overresponsiveness to drug action, that is, an intolerance to even small doses. Used in this sense, the term indicates that the nature of the response is appropriate but the degree of response is exaggerated.

The term is more widely used today to identify a state of allergy. To have a *hypersensitivity* to a drug is to be *allergic* to it (see ALLERGY, DRUG).

Some individuals develop cross-hypersensitivity. This means that once a person has developed an allergy to a certain drug, that person will experience an allergic reaction to other drugs which are closely related in chemical composition.

Example: The patient was known to be *hypersensitive* by nature, having a history of seasonal hay fever and asthma since childhood. His *allergy* to tetracycline developed after his third course of treatment. This drug *hypersensitivity* manifested itself as a diffuse, measleslike rash.

Hypnotic A drug that is used primarily to induce sleep. There are several classes of drugs that have hypnotic effects: antihistamines, barbiturates, benzodiazepines and several unrelated compounds. Within the past 15 years the benzodiazepines, because of their relative safety and lower potential for inducing dependence, have largely replaced the barbiturates as the most commonly used hypnotics. The body usually develops a tolerance to the hypnotic effect after several weeks of continual use. To maintain their effectiveness, hypnotics should be used intermittently for short periods of time.

Hypoglycemia A condition in which the amount of glucose (a sugar) in the blood is below the normal range. Since normal brain function is dependent upon an adequate supply of glucose, reducing the level of glucose in the blood below a critical point will cause serious impairment of brain activity. The resulting symptoms are characteristic of the hypoglycemic state. Early indications are headache, a sensation resembling mild drunkenness and an inability to think clearly. These may be accompanied by hunger. As the level of blood glucose continues to fall, nervousness and confusion develop. Varying degrees of weakness, numbness, trembling, sweating and rapid heart action follow. If sugar is not provided at this point and the blood glucose level drops further, impaired speech, incoordination and unconsciousness, with or without convulsions, will follow.

Hypoglycemia in any stage requires prompt recognition and treatment. Because of the potential for injury to the brain, the mechanisms and management of hypoglycemia should be understood by all who use drugs capable of producing it.

Hypothermia A state of the body characterized by an unexpected decline of internal body temperature to levels significantly below the norm of 98.6 degrees F or 37 degrees C. By definition, hypothermia means a body temperature of less than 95 degrees F or 35 degrees C. The elderly and debilitated are more prone to develop hypothermia if clothed inadequately and exposed to cool environments. Most episodes are initiated by room temperatures below 65 degrees F or 18.3 degrees C. The condition often develops suddenly, can mimic a stroke and has a mortality rate of 50%. Some drugs, such as phenothiazines, barbiturates and benzodiazepines, are conducive to the development of hypothermia in susceptible individuals.

Idiosyncrasy An abnormal mechanism of drug response that occurs in individuals who have a peculiar defect in their body chemistry (often hereditary) which produces an effect totally unrelated to the drug's normal pharmacological action. Idiosyncrasy is not a form of allergy. The actual chemical defects responsible for certain idiosyncratic drug reactions are well understood; others are not.

Example: Approximately 100 million people in the world (including 10% of American blacks) have a specific enzyme deficiency in their red blood cells that causes these cells to disintegrate when exposed to drugs such as sulfonamides (Gantrisin, Kynex), nitrofurantoin (Furadantin, Macrodantin), probenecid (Benemid), quinine and quinidine. As a result of this reaction, these drugs (and others) can cause a significant anemia in susceptible individuals.

Example: Approximately 5% of the population of the United States is susceptible to the development of glaucoma on prolonged use of cortisone-related drugs (see Cortisone Drug Class in Section Four).

Immunosuppressive A drug that significantly impairs (suppresses) the functions of the body's immune system. In some instances, immunosuppression is an intended drug effect as in the use of cyclosporine to prevent the immune system from rejecting a transplanted heart or kidney. In other instances, it is an unwanted side-effect as in the long-term use of cortisonelike drugs (to control chronic asthma) that suppresses the immune system sufficiently to permit reactivation of a dormant tuberculosis. Immunosuppressant drugs are being used to treat several chronic disorders that are thought to be autoimmune diseases, notably advanced rheumatoid arthritis, ulcerative colitis and systemic lupus erythematosus.

Interaction An unwanted change in the body's response to a drug that results when a second drug that is capable of altering the action of the first is administered at the same time. Some drug interactions can enhance the effect of either drug, producing an overresponse similar to overdosage. Other interactions may reduce drug effectiveness and cause inadequate response. A third type of interaction can produce a seemingly unrelated toxic response with no associated increase or decrease in the pharmacological actions of the interacting drugs.

Theoretically, many drugs can interact with one another, but in reality drug interactions are comparatively infrequent. Many interactions can be anticipated, and the physician can make appropriate adjustments in dosage to prevent or minimize unintended fluctuations in drug response.

Jaundice A yellow coloration of the skin (and the white portion of the eyes) that occurs when excessive bile pigments accumulate in the blood as a result of impaired liver function. Jaundice can be produced by several mechanisms. It may occur as a manifestation of a wide variety of diseases, or it may represent an adverse reaction to a particular drug. At times it is difficult to distinguish between disease-induced jaundice and drug-induced jaundice.

Jaundice due to a drug is always a serious adverse effect. Anyone taking a drug that is capable of causing jaundice should watch closely for any significant change in the color of urine or feces. Dark discoloration of the urine and paleness (lack of color) of the stool may be early indications of a developing jaundice. Should either of these symptoms occur, it is advisable to discontinue the drug and notify the prescribing physician promptly. Diagnostic tests are available to clarify the nature of the jaundice.

Lupus Erythematosus (LE) A serious disease of unknown cause that occurs in two forms, one limited to the skin (discoid LE) and the other involving several body systems (systemic LE). Both forms occur predominantly in young women. About 5% of cases of the discoid form convert to the systemic form. Basically, systemic LE is a disorder of the body's immune system which may result in chronic, progressive inflammation and destruction of the connective tissue framework of the skin, blood vessels, joints, brain, heart muscle, lungs and kidneys. Altered proteins in the blood lead to the formation of antibodies which react with certain organ tissues to produce the inflammation and destruction characteristic of the disease. A reduction in the number of white blood cells and blood platelets often occurs. The course of systemic LE is usually quite protracted and unpredictable. While no cure is known, satisfactory management may be achieved in some cases by the judicious use of cortisonelike drugs.

Several drugs in wide use are capable of initiating a form of systemic LE quite similar to that which occurs spontaneously. (More than 100 cases due to the use of procainamide have been reported.) Suggestive symptoms may appear as early as 2 weeks or as late as 8 years after starting the responsible drug. The initial symptoms usually consist of low-grade fever, skin rashes of various kinds, aching muscles and multiple joint pains. Chest pains (pleurisy) are fairly common. Enlargement of the lymph glands occurs less frequently. Symptoms usually subside following discontinuation of the responsible drug, but laboratory evidence of the reaction may persist for many months.

Drugs known to induce systemic LE include:

chlorpromazine	phenothiazines (some)
clofibrate	phenylbutazone
hydralazine	phenytoin
isoniazid	practolol
oral contraceptives	procainamide
penicillamine	thiouracil
phenolphthalein	

Orthostatic Hypotension A type of low blood pressure that is related to body position or posture (also called postural hypotension). The individual who is subject to orthostatic hypotension may have a normal blood pressure while lying down, but on sitting upright or standing he will experience sudden sensations of lightheadedness, dizziness and a feeling of impending faint that compel him to return quickly to a lying position. These symptoms are manifestations of inadequate blood flow (oxygen supply) to the brain due to an abnormal delay in the rise in blood pressure that always occurs as the body adjusts the circulation to the erect position.

Many drugs (especially the stronger antihypertensives) may cause orthostatic hypotension. Individuals who experience this drug effect should report it to their physician so that appropriate dosage adjustment can be made to minimize it. Failure to correct or to compensate for these sudden drops in blood pressure can lead to severe falls and injury.

The tendency to orthostatic hypotension can be reduced by avoiding sudden standing, prolonged standing, vigorous exercise and exposure to hot environments. Alcoholic beverages should be used cautiously until their combined effect with the drug in use has been determined.

Overdosage The meaning of this term should not be limited to the concept of doses that clearly exceed the normal dosage range recommended by the manufacturer. The optimal dose of many drugs (that amount which gives the greatest benefit with least distress) varies greatly from person to person. What may be an average dose for the majority of individuals will be an overdose for some and an underdose for others. Numerous factors, such as age, body size, nutritional status and liver and kidney function, have significant influence on dosage requirements. Drugs with narrow safety margins often produce indications of overdosage if something delays the regular elimination of the customary daily dose. In this instance, overdosage results from accumulation of prescribed daily doses. Massive overdosage—as occurs with accidental ingestion of drugs by children or with suicidal intention by adults—is referred to as poisoning.

Over-the-Counter (OTC) Drugs Drug products that can be purchased without prescription. Many are available in food stores, variety stores and newsstands as well as in conventional drug stores. Because of the unrestricted availability of these drugs, many people do not look upon OTC medicines as drugs. But drugs they are! And like the more potent drug products that are sold only on prescription, they are chemicals that are capable of a wide variety of actions on biological systems. Within the last 30 years, many OTC drugs have assumed greater importance because of their ability to interact unfavorably with some widely used prescription drugs. Serious problems in drug management can arise when (1) the patient fails to inform the physician of the OTC drug(s) he is taking ("because they really aren't drugs") and (2) the physician fails to specify that his question about what medicines are being taken currently *includes all OTC drugs*. During any course of treatment, whether medical or surgical, the patient should consult with the physician regarding any OTC drug that he wishes to take.

The major classes of OTC drugs for internal use include:

allergy medicines (antihistamines)	aspirin substitutes
antacids	asthma aids
antiworm medicines	cold medicines (decongestants)
aspirin and aspirin combinations	cough medicines

diarrhea remedies
digestion aids
diuretics
iron preparations
laxatives
menstrual aids
motion sickness remedies
pain relievers

reducing aids
salt substitutes
sedatives and tranquilizers
sleeping pills
stimulants (caffeine)
sugar substitutes (saccharin)
tonics
vitamins

Paradoxical Reaction An unexpected drug response that is not consistent with the known pharmacology of the drug and may in fact be the opposite of the intended and anticipated response. Such reactions are due to individual sensitivity or variability and can occur in any age group. They are seen more commonly, however, in children and the elderly.

Example: An 80-year-old man was admitted to a nursing home following the death of his wife. He had difficulty adjusting to his new environment and was restless, agitated and irritable. He was given a trial of the tranquilizer diazepam (Valium) to relax him, starting with small doses. On the second day of medication he became confused and erratic in behavior. The dose of diazepam was increased. On the third day he began to wander aimlessly, talked incessantly in a loud voice and displayed anger and hostility when attempts were made to help him. Suspecting the possibility of a paradoxical reaction, the diazepam was discontinued. All behavioral disturbances gradually subsided within 3 days.

Parkinson-like Disorders (Parkinsonism) A group of symptoms that resembles those caused by Parkinson's disease, a chronic disorder of the nervous system also known as shaking palsy. The characteristic features of parkinsonism include a fixed, emotionless facial expression (masklike in appearance), a prominent trembling of the hands, arms or legs and stiffness of the extremities that limits movement and produces a rigid posture and gait.

Parkinsonism is a fairly common adverse effect that occurs in about 15% of all patients who take large doses of strong tranquilizers (notably the phenothiazines) or use them over an extended period of time. If recognized early, the Parkinson-like features will lessen or disappear with reduced dosage or change in medication. In some instances, however, Parkinson-like changes may become permanent, requiring appropriate medication for their control.

Peripheral Neuritis (Peripheral Neuropathy) A group of symptoms that results from injury to nerve tissue in the extremities. A variety of drugs and chemicals are capable of inducing changes in nerve structure or function. The characteristic pattern consists of a sensation of numbness and tingling that usually begins in the fingers and toes and is accompanied by an altered sensation to touch and vague discomfort ranging from aching sensations to burning pain. Severe forms of peripheral neuritis may include loss of muscular strength and coordination.

A relatively common form of peripheral neuritis is that seen with the long-term use of isoniazid in the treatment of tuberculosis. If vitamin B-6 (pyridoxine) is not given concurrently with isoniazid, peripheral neuritis may occur in sensitive individuals. Vitamin B-6 can be both preventive and curative in this form of drug-induced peripheral neuritis.

Since peripheral neuritis can also occur as a late complication following many viral infections, care must be taken to avoid assigning a cause-and-effect relationship to a drug which is not responsible for the nerve injury (see CAUSE-AND-EFFECT RELATIONSHIP).

Peyronie's Disease A permanent deformity of the penis caused by the formation of dense fibrous (scarlike) tissue within the system of penile vessels that become engorged with blood during the process of erection. During sexual arousal, this inelastic fibrous tissue causes a painful downward bowing of the penis that hampers or precludes satisfactory intercourse. This condition has been associated with the use of phenytoin (Dilantin, etc.) and with most members of the beta blocker class of drugs (see Drug Class, Section Four).

Pharmacology The medical science that relates to the development and use of medicinal drugs, their composition and action in animals and man. Used in its broadest sense, pharmacology embraces the related sciences of medicinal chemistry, experimental therapeutics and toxicology.

Example: The widely used sulfonylurea drugs (Diabinese, Dymelor, Orinase, Tolinase) are effective in the treatment of some forms of diabetes because of the accidental discovery that some of their parent "sulfa" drugs produced hypoglycemia (low blood sugar) during their early therapeutic trials as anti-infectives. Subsequent investigation of the mechanisms of action (*pharmacology*) of these drugs revealed that they are capable of stimulating the pancreas to release more insulin.

Pharmacological studies on another group of "sulfa"-related drugs—the thiazide diuretics—revealed that they could induce the kidney to excrete more water and salt in the urine. This drug action is of great value in treating high blood pressure and heart failure.

Photosensitivity A drug-induced change in the skin that results in the development of a rash or exaggerated sunburn on exposure to the sun or ultraviolet lamps. The reaction is confined to uncovered areas of skin, providing a clue to the nature of its cause. (See Table 3 in Section Six.)

Porphyria The porphyrias are a group of hereditary disorders characterized by excessive production of prophyrins, essential respiratory pigments of the body. (One porphyrin is a component of hemoglobin, the pigment of red blood cells.) Two forms of porphyria—acute intermittent porphyria and cutaneous porphyria—can be activated by the use of certain drugs. Acute intermittent porphyria involves damage to the nervous system; an acute attack can include fever, rapid heart rate, vomiting, pain in the abdomen and legs, hallucinations, seizures, paralysis and coma. Twenty-three drugs (or drug classes) can induce an acute attack; among these are the barbiturates, "sulfa" drugs, chlordiazepoxide (Librium), chlorpropamide (Diabinese), methyldopa (Aldomet) and phenytoin (Dilantin). Cutaneous porphyria involves damage to the skin and liver. An episode can include reddening and blistering of the skin, followed by crust formation, scarring and excessive hair growth; repeated liver damage can lead to cirrhosis. This form of porphyria can be precipitated by chloroquine, estrogen, oral contraceptives and excessive iron.

Priapism The prolonged, painful erection of the penis usually unassociated with sexual arousal or stimulation. It is caused by obstruction to the outflow (drainage) of blood through the veins at the root of the penis. Erection may persist for 30 minutes to a few hours and then subside spontaneously; or it may persist for up to 30 hours and require surgical drainage of blood from the penis for relief. More than half of the episodes of priapism induced by drugs result in permanent impotence. Sickle cell anemia (or trait) may predispose to priapism; individuals with this disorder should avoid all drugs that may induce priapism.

Drugs reported to induce priapism include the following:

anabolic steroids (male hormone–like drugs: Anadrol, Anavar, Android, Halotestin, Metandren, Oreton, Testred, Winstrol)
chlorpromazine (Thorazine)
cocaine
guanethidine (Ismelin)
haloperidol (Haldol)
heparin
levodopa (Sinemet)
molindone (Moban)
prazosin (Minipress)
prochlorperazine (Compazine)
trazodone (Desyrel)
trifluoperazine (Stelazine)
warfarin (Coumadin)

Prostatism This term refers to the difficulties associated with an enlarged prostate gland. As the prostate enlarges (a natural development in aging men), it constricts the urethra (outflow passage) where it joins the urinary bladder and impedes urination. This causes a reduction in the size and force of the urinary stream, hesitancy in starting the flow of urine, interruption of urination and incomplete emptying of the bladder. Atropine and drugs with atropinelike effects can impair the bladder's ability to compensate for the obstructing prostate gland, thus intensifying all of the above symptoms.

Raynaud's Phenomenon This term refers to intermittent episodes of reduced blood flow into the fingers or toes, with resulting paleness, discomfort, numbness and tingling. It is due to an exaggerated constriction of the small arteries that supply blood to the digits. Characteristically an attack is precipitated either by emotional stress or exposure to cold. It can occur as part of a systemic disorder (lupus erythematosus, scleroderma), or it can occur without apparent cause (Raynaud's disease).

Some widely used drugs, notably beta-adrenergic blockers and products that contain ergotamine, are conducive to the development of Raynaud-like symptoms in predisposed individuals.

Reye (Reye's) Syndrome An acute, often fatal, childhood illness characterized by swelling of the brain and toxic degeneration of the liver. It usually develops during recovery from a flulike infection, measles or chickenpox. Symptoms include fever, headache, delirium, loss of consciousness and seizures. It is one of the 10 major causes of death in children aged 1 to 10 years. Evidence to date suggests that the syndrome may be due to the combined effects of viral infection and chemical toxins (possibly drugs) in a genetically predisposed child. Drugs that have been used just prior to the onset of symptoms include acetaminophen, aspirin, antibiotics and antiemetics (drugs to control nausea and vomiting). Although it has not been definitely established that drugs actually cause Reye syndrome, it is thought that they may contribute to its development or adversely affect its course. Current recommendations are to avoid the use of acetaminophen, aspirin and antiemetic drugs in children with flulike infections, chickenpox or measles.

Secondary Effect A by-product or complication of drug use which does not occur as part of the drug's primary pharmacological activity. Secondary effects are unwanted consequences and may therefore be classified as adverse effects.

Example: The reactivation of dormant tuberculosis can be a *secondary effect* of long-term cortisone administration for arthritis. Cortisone and related drugs (see Drug Class, Section Four) suppress natural immunity and lower resistance to infection.

Example: The cramping of leg muscles can be a *secondary effect* of diuretic (urine-producing) drug treatment for high blood pressure. Excessive loss of potassium through increased urination renders the muscle vulnerable to painful spasm during exercise.

Side-Effect A normal, expected and predictable response to a drug that accompanies the principal (intended) response sought in treatment. Side-effects are part of a drug's pharmacological activity and thus are unavoidable. Most side-effects are undesirable. The majority cause minor annoyance and inconvenience; some may cause serious problems in managing certain diseases; a few can be hazardous.

Example: The drug propantheline (Pro-Banthine) is used to treat peptic ulcer because one of the consequences of its pharmacological action is the reduction of acid formation in the stomach (an intended effect). Other consequences can include blurring of near vision, dryness of the mouth and constipation. These are *side-effects.*

Superinfection (Suprainfection) The development of a second infection that is superimposed upon an initial infection currently under treatment. The superinfection is caused by organisms that are not susceptible to the killing action of the drug(s) used to treat the original (primary) infection. Superinfections usually occur during or immediately following treatment with a broad spectrum antibiotic—one that is capable of altering the customary balance of bacterial populations in various parts of the body. The disturbance of this balance permits the overgrowth of organisms that normally exist in numbers too small to cause disease. The superinfection may also require treatment, using those drugs that are effective against the offending organism.

   Example: Recurrent infections of the kidney and bladder often require repeated courses of treatment with a variety of anti-infective drugs. When these are taken by mouth they can suppress the normally dominant types of bacteria present in the colon and rectum, encouraging the overgrowth of yeast organisms which are capable of causing *colitis.* When this occurs, colitis is a *superinfection.*

Tardive Dyskinesia A late-developing, drug-induced disorder of the nervous system characterized by involuntary bizarre movements of the jaws, lips and tongue. It occurs after long-term treatment with the more potent drugs used in the management of serious mental illness. While it may occur in any age group, it is more common in the middle-aged and the elderly. Older, chronically ill women are particularly susceptible to this adverse drug effect. Once developed, the pattern of uncontrollable chewing, lip puckering and repetitive tongue protruding (fly-catching movement) appears to be irreversible. No consistently satisfactory treatment or cure is available. To date, there is no way of identifying beforehand the individual who may develop this distressing reaction to drug treatment, and there is no known prevention. Fortunately, the persistent dyskinesia (abnormal movement) is not accompanied by further impairment of mental function or deterioration of intelligence. It is ironic, however, that the patient who shows significant improvement in his mental illness but is unfortunate enough to develop tardive dyskinesia may have to remain hospitalized because of a reaction to a drug that was given to make it possible for him to leave the hospital.

Tolerance An adaptation by the body that lessens responsiveness to a drug on continuous administration. Body tissues become accustomed to the drug's presence and react to it less vigorously. Tolerance can be beneficial or harmful in treatment.

   Examples: Beneficial tolerance occurs when the hay fever sufferer finds that the side-effect of drowsiness gradually disappears after 4 or 5 days of continuous use of antihistamines.

   Harmful tolerance occurs when the patient with "shingles" (herpes zoster) finds that the usual dose of codeine is no longer sufficient to relieve pain and that the need for increasing dosage creates a risk of physical dependence or addiction.

Toxicity The capacity of a drug to dangerously impair body functions or to damage body tissues. Most drug toxicity is related to total dosage: the larger the overdose, the greater the toxic effects. Some drugs, however, can produce toxic reactions when used in normal doses. Such adverse effects are not due to allergy or idiosyncrasy; in many instances their mechanisms are not fully understood. Toxic effects due to overdosage are generally a harmful extension of the drug's normal pharmacological actions and—to some extent—are predictable and preventable. Toxic reactions which occur with normal dosage are unrelated to the drug's known pharmacology and for the most part are unpredictable and unexplainable.

Tyramine A chemical present in many common foods and beverages that causes no difficulties to body functioning under normal circumstances. The main pharmacological action of tyramine is to raise the blood pressure. Normally, enzymes present in many body tissues neutralize this action of tyramine in the quantities in which it is consumed in the average diet. The principal enzyme responsible for neutralizing the blood-pressure-elevating action of tyramine (and chemicals related to it) is monoamine oxidase (MAO) type A. Monoamine oxidase type A serves an important regulatory function that helps to balance several of the chemical processes in the body that control certain activities of the nervous system. Stabilization of the blood pressure is one of these activities. If the action of monoamine oxidase type A is blocked, chemical substances like tyramine function unopposed, and relatively small amounts can cause alarming and dangerous elevations of blood pressure.

Several drugs in use today are capable of blocking the action of monoamine oxidase type A. These drugs are commonly referred to as monoamine oxidase (MAO) type A inhibitors (see Drug Class, Section Four). If an individual is taking one of these drugs and his diet includes foods or beverages that contain a significant amount of tyramine, he may experience a sudden increase in blood pressure. Before this interaction of food and drug was understood, several deaths due to brain hemorrhage occurred in persons taking MAO type A inhibitor drugs as a result of an extreme elevation of blood pressure following a meal of tyramine-rich foods.

It should be noted also that MAO inhibitor drugs can interact with many other drugs and cause serious adverse effects. Consult your physician before taking *any* drug concurrently with one that can inhibit the action of monoamine oxidase, type A or B.

Any protein-containing food that has undergone partial decomposition may present a hazard because of its increased tyramine content. The following foods and beverages have been reported to contain varying amounts of tyramine. Unless their tyramine content is known to be insignificant, they should be avoided altogether while taking a MAO type A inhibitor drug. Consult your physician about the advisability of using any of the foods or beverages on these lists if you are taking such drugs.

FOODS	BEVERAGES
Aged cheeses of all kinds*	Beer (unpasteurized)
Avocado	Chianti wine
Banana skins	Sherry wine

*Cottage cheese, cream cheese and processed cheese are safe to eat.

FOODS	BEVERAGES
Beef liver (unless fresh and used at once	Vermouth
"Bovril" extract	
Broad bean pods	
Chicken liver (unless fresh and used at once)	
Chocolate	
Figs, canned	
Fish, canned	
Fish, dried and salted	
Herring, pickled	
"Marmite" extract	
Meat extracts	
Meat tenderizers	
Raisins	
Raspberries	
Sour cream	
Soy sauce	
Yeast extracts	

NOTE: *Any* high-protein food that is aged or has undergone breakdown by putrefaction probably contains tyramine and could produce a hypertensive crisis in anyone taking MAO type A inhibiting drugs.

TABLES OF DRUG INFORMATION

TABLE 1

Your Drugs and Behavior

In addition to producing side-effects that can alter mood and disturb emotional stability, some drugs are capable of inducing unexpected and unpredictable patterns of abnormal thinking and behavior. Such responses are relatively infrequent, but the nature and degree of mental disturbance can, at times, be quite alarming and potentially dangerous for both patient and family. It is now well recognized that such paradoxical responses are often of an idiosyncratic nature, and that the individual with a history of a serious mental or emotional disorder is more likely to experience bizarre reactions involving disturbed behavior.

It is often difficult to judge whether a particular aberration of thought or behavior is primarily a feature of the disorder under treatment or an effect of one (or more) drugs the patient may be taking at the time. If in doubt, it is advisable to discontinue any drug with potential for such side-effects and observe for changes during a drug-free period.

Drugs reported to impair *concentration* and/or *memory*

antihistamines*	monoamine oxidase inhibitor
antiparkinsonism drugs*	drugs*
barbiturates*	phenytoin
benzodiazepines*	primidone
isoniazid	scopolamine

Drugs reported to cause *confusion, delirium* or *disorientation*

acetazolamide	digitoxin
aminophylline	digoxin
antidepressants*	disulfiram
antihistamines*	ethchlorvynol
atropinelike drugs*	ethinamate
barbiturates*	fenfluramine
benzodiazepines*	glutethimide
bromides	isoniazid
carbamazepine	levodopa
chloroquine	meprobamate
cimetidine	para-aminosalicylic acid
cortisonelike drugs*	phenelzine
cycloserine	phenothiazines*
digitalis	phenytoin

*See Drug Class, Section Four.

Drugs reported to cause *confusion, delirium* or *disorientation* (cont.)

piperazine
primidone
propranolol

reserpine
scopolamine

Drugs reported to cause *paranoid thinking*

bromides
cortisonelike drugs*
diphenhydramine

disulfiram
isoniazid
levodopa

Drugs reported to cause *schizophreniclike behavior*

amphetamines*
ephedrine
fenfluramine

phenmetrazine
phenylpropanolamine

Drugs reported to cause *maniclike behavior*

antidepressants*
cortisonelike drugs*

levodopa
monoamine oxidase inhibitor
    drugs*

Less apparent—but no less important—are the mood-altering *side-effects* of some drugs which are prescribed primarily for altogether unrelated conditions, with no intention of modifying emotional status. In keeping with the wide variation of individual response to the primary and intended effects of drugs, it is to be expected that the emotional and behavioral secondary effects will also be quite unpredictable and will vary enormously from person to person. However, the following experiences have been observed with sufficient frequency to establish recognizable patterns.

Drugs reported to cause *nervousness* (anxiety and irritability)

amamtadine
amphetaminelike drugs* (appetite
    suppressants)
antihistamines*
caffeine

chlorphenesin
cortisonelike drugs*
ephedrine
epinephrine
isoproterenol

*See Drug Class, Section Four.

Drugs reported to cause *nervousness* (cont.)

levodopa
liothyronine (in excessive dosage)
methylphenidate
methysergide
monoamine oxidase inhibitor
  drugs*

nylidrin
oral contraceptives
theophylline
thyroid (in excessive dosage)
thyroxine (in excessive dosage)

Drugs reported to cause *emotional depression*

amantadine
amphetamine* (on withdrawal)
benzodiazepines*
carbamazepine
chloramphenicol
cortisonelike drugs*
cycloserine
digitalis
digitoxin
digoxin
diphenoxylate
estrogens
ethionamide
fenfluramine (on withdrawal)
fluphenazine
guanethidine

haloperidol
indomethacin
isoniazid
levodopa
methsuximide
methyldopa
methysergide
metoprolol
oral contraceptives
phenylbutazone
procainamide
progesterones
propranolol
reserpine
sulfonamides*
vitamin D (in excessive dosage)

Drugs reported to cause *euphoria*

amantadine
aminophylline
amphetamines
antihistamines* (some)
antispasmodics, synthetic*
aspirin
barbiturates*
benzphetamine
chloral hydrate
clorazepate
codeine
cortisonelike drugs*

diethylpropion
diphenoxylate
ethosuximide
flurazepam
haloperidol
levodopa
meprobamate
methysergide
monoamine oxidase inhibitor
  drugs*
morphine
pargyline

*See Drug Class, Section Four.

Drugs reported to cause *euphoria* (cont.)

pentazocine
phenmetrazine
propoxyphene

scopalamine
tybamate

Drugs reported to cause *excitement*

acetazolamide
amantadine
amphetaminelike drugs*
antidepressants*
antihistamines*
atropinelike drugs*
barbiturates* (paradoxical
    response)
benzodiazepines* (paradoxical
    response)
cortisonelike drugs
cycloserine
diethylpropion
digitalis
ephedrine
epinephrine

ethinamate (paradoxical response)
ethionamide
glutethimide (paradoxical response)
isoniazid
isoproterenol
levodopa
meperidine and MAO inhibitor
    drugs*
methyldopa and MAO inhibitor
    drugs*
methyprylon (paradoxical response)
nalidixic acid
orphenadrine
quinine
scopolamine

*See Drug Class, Section Four.

TABLE 2

Your Drugs and Vision

Approximately 3.5% of all adverse drug effects involve impairment of vision or damage to structures of the eye. Some effects, such as blurring of vision or double vision, may occur shortly after starting a drug. These quickly disappear with adjustment of dosage. More subtle and serious effects, such as the development of cataracts or damage to the retina or optic nerve, may not occur until a drug has been in continuous use for an extended period of time. Some of these changes are irreversible. If you are taking a drug that can affect the eye in any way, you are urged to report promptly any eye discomfort or change in vision so that appropriate evaluation can be made and corrective action taken as soon as possible.

Drugs reported to cause *blurring of vision*

acetazolamide
antiarthritic/anti-inflammatory
  drugs
antidepressants*
antihistamines*
atropinelike drugs*
chlorthalidone
ciprofloxacin
cortisonelike drugs*

diethylstilbestrol
etretinate
fenfluramine
norfloxacin
oral contraceptives
phenytoin
sulfonamides*
tetracyclines*
thiazide diuretics*

Drugs reported to cause *double vision*

antidepressants*
antidiabetic drugs*
antihistamines*
aspirin
barbiturates*
benzodiazepines*
bromides
carbamazepine
carisoprodol
chloroquine
chlorprothixene
ciprofloxacin
clomiphene
colchicine

colistin
cortisonelike drugs*
digitalis
digitoxin
digoxin
ethionamide
ethosuximide
etretinate
guanethidine
hydroxychloroquine
indomethacin
isoniazid
levodopa
mephenesin

*See Drug Class, Section Four.

Drugs reported to cause *double vision* (cont.)

methocarbamol
methsuximide
morphine
nalidixic acid
nitrofurantoin
norfloxacin
oral contraceptives
orphenadrine
oxyphenbutazone
pentazocine

phenothiazines*
phensuximide
phenylbutazone
phenytoin
primidone
propranolol
quinidine
sedatives/sleep inducers*
thiothixene
tranquilizers*

Drugs reported to cause *farsightedness*

ergot
penicillamine

sulfonamides* (possibly)
tolbutamide (possibly)

Drugs reported to cause *nearsightedness*

acetazolamide
aspirin
carbachol
chlorthalidone
codeine
cortisonelike drugs*
ethosuximide
methsuximide
morphine

oral contraceptives
penicillamine
phenothiazines*
phensuximide
spironolactone
sulfonamides*
tetracyclines*
thiazide diuretics*

Drugs reported to *alter color vision*

acetaminophen
amodiaquine
amyl nitrite
aspirin
atropine
barbiturates*
belladonna
chloramphenicol

chloroquine
chlorpromazine
chlortetracycline
cortisonelike drugs*
digitalis
digitoxin
digoxin
disulfiram

*See Drug Class, Section Four.

Drugs reported to *alter color vision* (cont.)

epinephrine
ergotamine
erythromycin
ethchlorvynol
ethionamide
fluphenazine
furosemide
hydroxychloroquine
indomethacin
isocarboxazid
isoniazid
mephenamic acid
mesoridazine
methysergide
nalidixic acid
norfloxacin
oral contraceptives
oxyphenbutazone
paramethadione
pargyline
penicillamine

pentylenetetrazol
perphenazine
phenacetin
phenylbutazone
primidone
prochlorperazine
promazine
promethazine
quinacrine
quinidine
quinine
reserpine
sodium salicylate
streptomycin
sulfonamides*
thioridazine
tranylcypromine
trifluoperazine
triflupromazine
trimeprazine
trimethadione

Drugs reported to cause *sensitivity to light* (photophobia)

antidiabetic drugs*
atropinelike drugs*
bromides
chloraquine
clomiphene
digitoxin
doxepin
ethambutol
ethionamide
ethosuximide
etretinate
hydroxychloroquine
mephenytoin

methsuximide
monoamine oxidase inhibitor
   drugs*
nalidixic acid
norfloxacin
oral contraceptives
paramethadione
phenothiazines*
quinidine
quinine
tetracyclines*
trimethadione

*See Drug Class, Section Four.

Drugs reported to cause *halos around lights*

amyl nitrite
chloroquine
cortisonelike drugs*
digitalis
digitoxin
digoxin
hydrochloroquine

nitroglycerin
norfloxacin
oral contraceptives
paramethadione
phenothiazines*
quinacrine
trimethadione

Drugs reported to cause *visual hallucinations*

amantadine
amphetaminelike drugs*
amyl nitrite
antihistamines*
aspirin
atropinelike drugs*
barbiturates*
benzodiazepines*
bromides
carbamazepine
cephalexin
cephaloglycin
chloroquine
cycloserine
digitalis
digoxin
disulfiram
ephedrine
furosemide
griseofulvin

haloperidol
hydroxychloroquine
indomethacin
isosorbide
levodopa
nialamide
oxyphenbutazone
pargyline
pentazocine
phenothiazines*
phenylbutazone
phenytoin
primidone
propranolol
quinine
sedatives/sleep inducers*
sulfonamides*
tetracyclines*
tricyclic antidepressants*
tripelennamine

Drugs reported to impair the use of *contact lenses*

brompheniramine
carbinoxamine
chlorpheniramine
cyclizine
cyproheptadine
dexbrompheniramine
dexchlorpheniramine

dimethindene
diphenhydramine
diphenpyraline
furosemide
oral contraceptives
terfenadine
tripelennamine

*See Drug Class, Section Four.

Drugs reported to cause *cataracts* or *lens deposits*

allopurinol
busulfan
chlorpromazine
chlorprothixene
cortisonelike drugs*
fluphenazine
mesoridazine
methotrimeprazine
perphenazine
phenmetrazine

pilocarpine
prochlorperazine
promazine
promethazine
thioridazine
thiothixene
trifluoperazine
triflupromazine
trimeprazine

*See Drug Class, Section Four.

TABLE 3

Your Drugs and the Sun: Photosensitivity

Some drugs are capable of sensitizing the skin of some individuals to the action of ultraviolet light. This can cause uncovered areas of the skin to react with a rash or exaggerated burn on exposure to sun or ultraviolet lamps. If you are taking any of the following drugs, ask your physician for guidance and use caution with regard to sun exposure.

acetohexamide
amitriptyline
amoxapine
barbiturates
bendroflumethiazide
carbamazepine
chlordiazepoxide
chloroquine
chlorothiazide
chlorpromazine
chlorpropamide
chlortetracycline
chlorthalidone
clindamycin
cyproheptadine
demeclocycline
desipramine
diethylstilbestrol
diltiazem
diphenhydramine
doxepin
doxycycline
estrogen
fluphenazine
glyburide
gold preparations
griseofulvin
hydrochlorothiazide
hydroflumethiazide
imipramine
isotretinoin

lincomycin
maprotiline
mesoridazine
methacycline
methotrexate
nalidixic acid
nortriptyline
oral contraceptives
oxyphenbutazone
oxytetracycline
perphenazine
phenobarbital
phenylbutazone
phenytoin
prochlorperazine
promazine
promethazine
protriptyline
pyrazinamide
sulfonamides
tetracycline
thioridazine
tolazamide
tolbutamide
tranylcypromine
triamterene
trifluoperazine
trimeprazine
trimipramine
triprolidine

TABLE 4
Your Drugs and Sexuality

It is now well established that certain drugs have the potential for affecting sexual functions in a variety of unintended ways. Many commonly prescribed drugs can cause both obvious and subtle effects on one or more aspects of sexual expression. Patients are usually unaware that changes in sexual performance or response may be related to medications they are taking. If they should suspect it, they are often reluctant to discuss the possible association with their physician. In some situations, the sexual dysfunction may be a natural consequence of the disorder under treatment or of a concurrent and undetected disorder, possibilities often overlooked by both practitioner and patient. It is well known that disorders such as diabetes, kidney failure, hypertension, epression and alcoholism may reduce libido and cause failure of erection. In addition, many of the drugs commonly used to treat these conditions may have the ability to augment a subclinical sexual dysfunction through unavoidable pharmacological activity. Such situations require the closest cooperation between therapist and patient in order to correctly assess the possible cause-and-effect relationships and to modify the treatment program appropriately.

Possible Drug Effects on Male Sexuality

1. Increased libido
   androgens (replacement therapy in deficiency states)
   baclofen (Lioresal)
   chlordiazepoxide (Librium) (antianxiety effect)
   diazepam (Valium) (antianxiety effect)
   haloperidol (Haldol)
   levodopa (Larodopa, Sinemet) (may be an indirect effect due to improved sense of well-being)

2. Decreased libido
   antihistamines
   barbiturates
   chlordiazepoxide (Librium) (sedative effect)
   chlorpromazine (Thorazine) 10% to 20% of users
   cimetidine (Tagamet)
   clofibrate (Atromid-S)
   clonidine (Catapres) 10% to 20% of users
   danazol (Danocrine)
   diazepam (Valium) (sedative effect)
   disulfiram (Antabuse)
   estrogens (therapy for prostatic cancer)
   fenfluramine (Pondimin)
   heroin

licorice
medroxyprogesterone (Provera)
methyldopa (Aldomet) 10% to 15% of users
perhexilene (Pexid)
prazosin (Minipress) 15% of users
propranolol (Inderal) rarely
reserpine (Serpasil, Ser-Ap-Es)
spironolactone (Aldactone)
tricyclic antidepressants (TAD's)

3. Impaired erection (impotence)
anticholinergics
antihistamines
baclofen (Lioresal)
barbiturates (when abused)
beta blockers (see Drug Class, Section Four)
chlordiazepoxide (Librium) (in high dosage)
chlorpromazine (Thorazine)
cimetidine (Tagamet)
clofibrate (Atromid-S)
clonidine (Catapres) 10% to 20% of users
cocaine
diazepam (Valium) (in high dosage)
digitalis and its glycosides
disopyramide (Norpace)
disulfiram (Antabuse) (uncertain)
estrogens (therapy for prostatic cancer)
ethacrynic acid (Edecrin) 5% of users
ethionamide (Trecator-SC)
fenfluramine (Pondimin)
furosemide (Lasix) 5% of users
guanethidine (Ismelin)
haloperidol (Haldol) 10% to 20% of users
heroin
hydroxyprogesterone (therapy for prostatic cancer)
licorice
lithium (Lithonate)
marijuana
mesoridazine (Serentil)
methantheline (Banthine)
methyldopa (Aldomet) 10% to 15% of users
monoamine oxidase (MAO) type A inhibitors, 10% to 15% of users
perhexilene (Pexid)
prazosin (Minipres) infrequently
reserpine (Serpasil, Ser-Ap-Es)
spironolactone (Aldactone)
thiazide diuretics, 5% of users

thioridazine (Mellaril)
tricyclic antidepressants (TAD's)

4. Impaired ejaculation
anticholinergics
barbiturates (when abused)
chlorpromazine (Thorazine)
clonidine (Catapres)
estrogens (therapy for prostatic cancer)
guanethidine (Ismelin)
heroin
mesoridazine (Serentil)
methyldopa (Aldomet)
monoamine oxidase (MAO) type A inhibitors
phenoxybenzamine (Dibenzyline)
phentolamine (Regitine)
reserpine (Serpasil, Ser-Ap-Es)
thiazide diuretics
thioridazine (Mellaril)
tricyclic antidepressants (TAD's)

5. Decreased testosterone
adrenocorticotropic hormone (ACTH)
barbiturates
digoxin (Lanoxin)
haloperidol (Haldol)
   increased testosterone with low dosage
   decreased testosterone with high dosage
lithium (Lithonate)
marijuana
medroxyprogesterone (Provera)
monoamine oxidase (MAO) type A inhibitors
spironolactone (Aldactone)

6. Impaired spermatogenesis (reduced fertility)
adrenocorticosteroids (prednisone, etc.)
androgens (moderate to high dosage, extended use)
antimalarials
aspirin (abusive, chronic use)
chlorambucil (Leukeran)
cimetidine (Tagamet)
colchicine
co-trimoxazole (Bactrim, Septra)
cyclophosphamide (Cytoxan)
estrogens (therapy for prostatic cancer)
marijuana
medroxyprogesterone (Provera)
methotrexate
monoamine oxidase (MAO) type A inhibitors

niridazole (Ambilhar)
nitrofurantoin (Furadantin)
spironolactone (Aldactone)
sulfasalazine (Azulfidine)
testosterone (moderate to high dosage, extended use)
vitamin C (in doses of 1 gram or more)

7. Testicular disorders
    Swelling
        tricyclic antidepressants (TAD's)
    Inflammation
        oxyphenbutazone (Tandearil)
    Atrophy
        androgens (moderate to high dosage, extended use)
        chlorpromazine (Thorazine)
        cyclophosphamide (Cytoxan) (in prepubescent boys)
        spironolactone (Aldactone)

8. Penile disorders
    Priapism (see Glossary)
        anabolic steroids (male hormonelike drugs)
        chlorpromazine (Thorazine)
        cocaine
        guanethidine (Ismelin)
        haloperidol (Haldol)
        heparin
        levodopa (Sinemet)
        molindone (Moban)
        prazosin (Minipress)
        prochlorperazine (Compazine)
        trazodone (Desyrel)
        trifluoperazine (Stelazine)
        warfarin (Coumadin)
    Peyronie's disease (see Glossary)
        beta blocker drugs (see Drug Class, Section Four)
        phenytoin (Dilantin, etc.)

9. Gynecomastia (excessive development of the male breast)
    androgens (partial conversion to estrogen)
    BCNU
    busulfan (Myleran)
    chlormadinone
    chlorpromazine (Thorazine)
    chlortetracycline (Aureomycin)
    cimetidine (Tagamet)
    clonidine (Catapres) (infrequently)
    diethylstilbestrol (DES)
    digitalis and its glycosides
    estrogens (therapy for prostatic cancer)

    ethionamide (Trecator-SC)
    griseofulvin (Fulvicin, etc.)
    haloperidol (Haldol)
    heroin
    human chorionic gonadotropin
    isoniazid (INH, Nydrazid)
    marijuana
    mestranol
    methyldopa (Aldomet)
    phenelzine (Nardil)
    reserpine (Serpasil, Ser-Ap-Es)
    spironolactone (Aldactone)
    thioridazine (Mellaril)
    tricyclic antidepressants (TAD's)
    vincristine (Oncovin)

10. Feminization (loss of libido, impotence, gynecomastia, testicular atrophy)
    conjugated estrogens (Premarin, etc.)

11. Precocious puberty
    anabolic steroids
    androgens
    isoniazid (INH)

Possible Drug Effects on Female Sexuality

1. Increased libido
    androgens
    chlordiazepoxide (Librium) (antianxiety effect)
    diazepam (Valium) (antianxiety effect)
    mazindol (Sanorex)
    oral contraceptives (freedom from fear of pregnancy)

2. Decreased libido
    See list of drug effects on male sexuality. Some of these *may* have potential for reducing libido in the female. The literature is sparse on this subject.

3. Impaired arousal and orgasm
    anticholinergics
    clonidine (Catapres)
    methyldopa (Aldomet)
    monoamine oxidase inhibitors (MAOI's)
    tricyclic antidepressants (TAD's)

4. Breast enlargement
    penicillamine
    tricyclic antidepressants (TAD's)

5. Galactorrhea (spontaneous flow of milk)
   amphetamine
   chlorpromazine (Thorazine)
   cimetidine (Tagamet)
   haloperidol (Haldol)
   heroin
   methyldopa (Aldomet)
   metoclopramide (Reglan)
   oral contraceptives
   phenothiazines
   reserpine (Serpasil, Ser-Ap-Es)
   sulpiride (Equilid)
   tricyclic antidepressants (TAD's)

6. Ovarian failure (reduced fertility)
   anesthetic gases (operating room staff)
   cyclophosphamide (Cytoxan)
   cytostatic drugs
   danazol (Danacrine)
   medroxyprogesterone (Provera)

7. Altered menstruation (menstrual disorders)
   adrenocorticosteroids (prednisone, etc.)
   androgens
   barbiturates (when abused)
   chlorambucil (Leukeran)
   chlorpromazine (Thorazine)
   cyclophosphamide (Cytoxan)
   danazol (Danocrine)
   estrogens
   ethionamide (Trecator-SC)
   haloperidol (Haldol)
   heroin
   isoniazid (INH, Nydrazid)
   marijuana
   medroxprogesterone (Provera)
   oral contraceptives
   phenothiazines
   progestins
   radioisotopes
   rifampin (Rifadin, Rifamate, Rimactane)
   spironolactone (Aldactone)
   testosterone
   thioridazine (Mellaril)
   vitamin A (in excessive dosage)

8. Virilization (acne, hirsutism, lowering of voice, enlargement of clitoris)
   anabolic drugs
   androgens

haloperidol (Haldol)
oral contraceptives (lowering of voice)

9. Precocious puberty
   estrogens (in hair lotions)
   isoniazid (INH, Nydrazid)

TABLE 5
Your Drugs and Alcohol

Beverages containing alcohol may interact unfavorably with a wide variety of drugs. The most important (and most familiar) interaction occurs when the depressant action on the brain of sedatives, sleep-inducing drugs, tranquilizers and narcotic drugs is intensified by alcohol. Alcohol may also reduce the effectiveness of some drugs, and it can interact with certain other drugs to produce toxic effects. Some drugs may increase the intoxicating effects of alcohol, producing further impairment of mental alertness, judgment, physical coordination and reaction time.

While drug interactions with alcohol are generally predictable, the intensity and significance of these interactions can vary greatly from one individual to another and from one occasion to another. This is because many factors influence what happens when drugs and alcohol interact. These factors include individual variations in sensitivity to drugs (including alcohol), the chemistry and quantity of the drug, the type and amount of alcohol consumed and the sequence in which drug and alcohol are taken. If you need to use any of the drugs listed in the following tables, you should ask your physician for guidance concerning the use of alcohol.

Drugs with which it is advisable to avoid alcohol completely

Drug name or class	Possible interaction with alcohol
amphetamines	excessive rise in blood pressure with alcoholic beverages containing tyramine**
antidepressants*	excessive sedation, increased intoxication
barbiturates*	excessive sedation
bromides	confusion, delirium, increased intoxication
calcium carbamide	disulfiramlike reaction**
carbamazepine	excessive sedation
chlorprothixene	excessive sedation
chlorzoxazone	excessive sedation
disulfiram	disulfiram reaction**
ergotamine	reduced effectiveness of ergotamine
fenfluramine	excessive stimulation of nervous system with some beers and wines
furazolidone	disulfiramlike reaction**

*See Drug Class, Section Four.
**See Glossary.

Drug name or class	Possible interaction with alcohol
haloperidol	excessive sedation
MAO inhibitor drugs*	excessive rise in blood pressure with alcoholic beverages containing tyramine**
meperidine	excessive sedation
meprobamate	excessive sedation
methotrexate	increased liver toxicity and excessive sedation
metronidazole	disulfiramlike reaction**
narcotic drugs	excessive sedation
oxyphenbutazone	increased stomach irritation and/or bleeding
pentazocine	excessive sedation
pethidine	excessive sedation
phenothiazines*	excessive sedation
phenylbutazone	increased stomach irritation and/or bleeding
procarbazine	disulfiramlike reaction**
propoxyphene	excessive sedation
reserpine	excessive sedation, orthostatic hypotension**
sleep-inducing drugs (hypnotics)	excessive sedation
carbromal	
chloral hydrate	
ethchlorvynol	
ethinamate	
glutethimide	
flurazepam	
methaqualone	
methyprylon	
temazepam	
triazolam	
thiothixene	excessive sedation
tricyclic antidepressants*	excessive sedation, increased intoxication
trimethobenzamide	excessive sedation

Drugs with which alcohol should be used only in small amounts (use cautiously until combined effects have been determined)

acetaminophen (Tylenol, etc.)	increased liver toxicity
amantadine	excessive lowering of blood pressure

*See Drug Class, Section Four.
**See Glossary.

Drug name or class	Possible interaction with alcohol
antiarthritic/anti-inflammatory drugs	increased stomach irritation and/or bleeding
anticoagulants (coumarins)*	increased anticoagulant effect
antidiabetic drugs (sulfonylureas)*	increased antidiabetic effect, excessive hypoglycemia**
antihistamines*	excessive sedation
antihypertensives*	excessive orthostatic hypotension**
aspirin (large doses or continuous use)	increased stomach irritation and/or bleeding
benzodiazepines*	excessive sedation
carisoprodol	increased alcoholic intoxication
diethylpropion	excessive nervous system stimulation with alcoholic beverages containing tyramine**
dihydroergotoxine	excessive lowering of blood pressure
diphenoxylate	excessive sedation
dipyridamole	excessive lowering of blood pressure
diuretics*	excessive orthostatic hypotension**
ethionamide	confusion, delirium, psychotic behavior
fenoprofen	increased stomach irritation and/or bleeding
griseofulvin	flushing and rapid heart action
ibuprofen	increased stomach irritation and/or bleeding
indomethacin	increased stomach irritation and/or bleeding
insulin	excessive hypoglycemia**
iron	excessive absorption of iron
isoniazid	decreased effectiveness of isoniazid, increased incidence of hepatitis
lithium	increased confusion and delirium (avoid all alcohol if any indication of lithium overdosage)
methocarbamol	excessive sedation
methotrimeprazine	excessive sedation
methylphenidate	excessive nervous system stimulation with alcoholic beverages containing tyramine**
metoprolol	excessive orthostatic hypotension**
nalidixic acid	increased alcoholic intoxication

*See Drug Class, Section Four.
**See Glossary.

Drug name or class	Possible interaction with alcohol
naproxen	increased stomach irritation and/or bleeding
nicotinic acid	possible orthostatic hypotension**
nitrates* (vasodilators)	possible orthostatic hypotension**
nylidrin	increased stomach irritation
orphenadrine	excessive sedation
phenelzine	increased alcoholic intoxication
phenoxybenzamine	possible orthostatic hypotension**
phentermine	excessive nervous system stimulation with alcoholic beverages containing tyramine**
phenytoin	decreased effect of phenytoin
pilocarpine	prolongation of alcohol effect
prazosin	excessive lowering of blood pressure
primidone	excessive sedation
propranolol	excessive orthostatic hypotension**
sulfonamides*	increased alcoholic intoxication
sulindac	increased stomach irritation and/or bleeding
tolmetin	increased stomach irritation and/or bleeding
tranquilizers (mild) chlordiazepoxide clorazepate diazepam hydroxyzine meprobamate oxazepam phenaglycodol tybamate	excessive sedation
tranylcypromine	increased alcoholic intoxication

Drugs capable of producing a disulfiramlike reaction** when used concurrently with alcohol

antidiabetic drugs (sulfonylureas)*	nifuroxine
calcium carbamide	nitrofurantoin
chloral hydrate	procarbazine
chloramphenicol	quinacrine
disulfiram	sulfonamides*
furazolidone	tinidazole
metronidazole	tolazoline

*See Drug Class, Section Four.
**See Glossary.

TABLE 6
High-Potassium Foods

Diuretic drugs that cause loss of potassium from the body are often used to treat conditions that also require a reduced intake of sodium. The high-potassium foods listed below have been selected for their compatibility with a sodium restricted diet (500 to 1000 mg of sodium daily).

Beverages

orange juice
prune juice
skim milk

tea
tomato juice
whole milk

Breads and Cereals

brown rice
cornbread
griddle cakes
muffins

oatmeal
shredded wheat
waffles

Fruits

apricot
avocado
banana
fig
honeydew melon

mango
orange
papaya
prune

Meats

beef
chicken
codfish
flounder
haddock
halibut

liver
pork
rockfish
salmon
turkey
veal

Vegetables

baked beans
lima beans
mushrooms
navy beans
parsnips

radishes
squash
sweet potato
tomato
white potato

Sources

The following sources were consulted in the compilation and revision of this book:

Adverse Drug Reaction Bulletin. Edited by D. M. Davies. Newcastle upon Tyne, England: Regional Postgraduate Institute for Medicine and Dentistry, 1989.

AMA Department of Drugs, *AMA Drug Evaluations,* 6th ed. Chicago: American Medical Association, 1986.

Andreoli, T. E., Carpenter, C. C. J., Plum, F., Smith, L. H., eds., *Cecil Essentials of Medicine.* Philadelphia: W. B. Saunders Co., 1986.

Arndt, K. A., *Manual of Dermatologic Therapeutics,* 4th ed. Boston: Little, Brown and Co., 1989.

Atkinson, A. J., Ambre, J. J., *Kalman and Clark's Drug Assay, The Strategy of Therapeutic Drug Monitoring,* 2nd ed. New York: Masson Publishing USA, 1985.

Avery, G. S., ed., *Drug Treatment,* 2nd ed. Sydney, Australia: ADIS Press, 1980.

Berkow, R., ed., *The Merck Manual,* 15th ed. Rahway, New Jersey: Merck Sharp & Dohme Research Laboratories, 1987.

Bevan, J. A., ed., *Essentials of Pharmacology.* Hagerstown, Maryland: Harper & Row, 1976.

Billups, N. F., ed., *American Drug Index 1989.* Philadelphia: J. B. Lippincott Co., 1989.

Branch, W. T., *Office Practice of Medicine,* 2nd ed. Philadelphia: W. B. Saunders Co., 1987.

Briggs, G. G., Bodendorfer, T. W., Freeman, R. K., Yaffee, S. J., *Drugs in Pregnancy and Lactation.* Baltimore: Williams & Wilkins, 1983.

Brooke, M. H., *A Clinician's View of Neuromuscular Diseases,* 2nd ed. Baltimore: Williams & Wilkins, 1986.

Canadian Pharmaceutical Association, *Compendium of Pharmaceuticals and Specialties,* 24th ed. Ottawa: Canadian Pharmaceutical Association, 1989.

Cape, Ronald, *Aging: Its Complex Management.* Hagerstown, Maryland: Harper & Row, 1978.

Clin-Alert. Medford, New Jersey: Clin-Alert, Inc., 1988–1989.

Davies, D. M., ed., *Textbook of Adverse Drug Reactions*, 2nd ed. New York: Oxford University Press, 1981.

Diamond, S., Dalessio, D. J., eds., *The Practicing Physician's Approach to Headache*, 4th ed. Baltimore: Williams & Wilkins, 1986.

Drug Interaction Facts. Edited by R. J. Mangini. St. Louis: Facts and Comparisons Division, J. B. Lippincott Co., 1989.

Drug Interactions Newsletter. Edited by P. D. Hansten, J. R. Horn. Spokane, Washington: Applied Therapeutics, Inc., 1989.

Drug Newsletter. Edited by G. H. Schwach, B. R. Olin. St. Louis: Facts and Comparisons Division, J. B. Lippincott Co., 1989.

Drug Therapy, Clinical Therapeutics for Physicians. New York: Biomedical Information Corporation, 1989.

Dukes, M. N. G., ed., *Meyler's Side Effects of Drugs*, 9th ed. Amsterdam: Excerpta Medica, 1980.

Encyclopedia of Associations, 23rd ed., Vol. 1, Part 2. Detroit: Gale Research, Inc., 1989.

Facts and Comparisons. Edited by B. R. Olin. St. Louis: Facts and Comparisons Division, J. B. Lippincott Co., 1989.

F.D.A. Drug Bulletin. Rockville, Maryland: Department of Health and Human Services, Food and Drug Administration.

Fraunfelder, F. T., *Drug-Induced Ocular Side Effects and Drug Interactions*. Philadelphia: Lea & Febiger, 1976.

Goodman, L. S., Gilman, A., eds., *The Pharmacological Basis of Therapeutics*, 7th ed. New York: Macmillan, 1985.

Greenberger, N. J., Arvanitakis, C., Hurwitz, A., *Drug Treatment of Gastrointestinal Disorders*. New York: Churchill Livingstone, 1978.

Hansten, P. D., *Drug Interactions*, 6th ed. Philadelphia: Lea & Febiger, 1989.

Heinonen, O. P., Slone, D., Shapiro, S., *Birth Defects and Drugs in Pregnancy*. Littleton, Massachusetts: PSG Publishing Co., 1977.

Hollister, L. E., *Clinical Pharmacology of Psychotherapeutic Drugs*, 2nd ed. New York: Churchill Livingstone, 1983.

Huff, B. B., ed., *The Physicians' Desk Reference*, 43rd ed. Oradell, New Jersey: Medical Economics Company, 1989.

International Drug Therapy Newsletter. Edited by F. J. Ayd. Baltimore: Ayd Medical Communications, 1989.

Jefferson, J. W., Greist, J. H., *Primer of Lithium Therapy*. Baltimore: Williams & Wilkens, 1977.

Journal of the American Medical Association. Edited by G. D. Lundberg. Chicago: American Medical Association, 1989.

Koller, W. C., ed., *Handbook of Parkinson's Disease*. New York: Marcel Dekker, 1987.

Kolodny, R. C., Masters, W. H., Johnson, V. E., *Textbook of Sexual Medicine*. Boston: Little, Brown and Co., 1979.

Lawrence, R. A., *Breast-Feeding*. St. Louis: Mosby, 1980.

Lieberman, M. L., *The Sexual Pharmacy*. New York: New American Library, 1988.

Long, J. W., *Clinical Management of Prescription Drugs*. Philadelphia: Harper & Row, 1984.

McEvoy, G. K., ed., *American Hospital Formulary Service, Drug Information 89*. Bethesda, Maryland: American Society of Hospital Pharmacists, 1989.

Maddin, S., ed., *Current Dermatologic Therapy*. Philadelphia: W. B. Saunders Co., 1982.

The Medical Letter on Drugs and Therapeutics. Edited by H. Aaron. New Rochelle, New York: The Medical Letter, Inc., 1989.

Melmon, K. L., Morrelli, H. F., *Clinical Pharmacology*, 2nd ed. New York: Macmillan, 1978.

Messerli, F. H., ed., *Current Clinical Practice*. Philadelphia: W. B. Saunders Co., 1987.

Meyler, L., Herxheimer, A., eds., *Side-Effects of Drugs*, Vol. 8. Amsterdam: Excerpta Medica, 1975.

Mohler, S. R., *Medication and Flying: A Pilot's Guide*. Boston: Boston Publishing Co., 1982.

The New England Journal of Medicine. Edited by A. S. Relman. Boston: The Massachusetts Medical Society, 1989.

Pharmacotherapy, The Journal of Human Pharmacology and Drug Therapy. Edited by R. T. Scheife. Boston: Pharmacotherapy Publications, Inc., 1987.

Postgraduate Medicine, The Journal of Applied Medicine for the Primary Care Physician. Minneapolis: McGraw-Hill, Inc., 1989.

Raj, P. P., *Practical Management of Pain*. Chicago: Year Book Medical Publishers, Inc., 1986.

Rakel, R. E., ed., *Conn's Current Therapy 1989*. Philadelphia: W. B. Saunders Co., 1989.

Rational Drug Therapy, Pharmacology for Physicians. Bethesda, Maryland: American Society for Pharmacology and Experimental Therapeutics, 1989.

Reynolds, J. E. F., ed. *Martindale, The Extra Pharmacopoeia*, 28th ed. London: The Pharmaceutical Press, 1982.

Rodman, M. J., Smith, D. W., *Clinical Pharmacology in Nursing*. Philadelphia: J. B. Lippincott Co., 1984.

Rogers, C. S., McCue, J. D., eds., *Managing Chronic Disease*. Oradell, New Jersey: Medical Economics Books, 1987.

Sauer, G. C., *Manual of Skin Diseases*, 5th ed. Philadelphia: J. B. Lippincott Co., 1985.

Schardein, J. L., *Drugs As Teratogens*. Cleveland: CRC Press, 1976.

Shepard, T. H., *Catalog of Teratogenic Agents*, 3rd ed. Baltimore: Johns Hopkins University Press, 1980.

Smith, L. H., Thier, S. O., *Pathophysiology, The Biological Principles of Disease*, 2nd ed. Philadelphia: W. B. Saunders Co., 1985.

Speight, T. M., ed., *Avery's Drug Treatment*, 3rd ed. Auckland: ADIS Press, 1987.

Swash, M., Schwartz, M. S., *Neuromuscular Diseases*, 2nd ed. Berlin: Springer-Verlag, 1988.

Tuchmann-Duplessis, H., *Drug Effects on the Fetus*. Sydney, Australia: ADIS Press, 1975.

USAN 1989 and the USP Dictionary of Drug Names. Edited by M. C. Griffiths. Rockville, Maryland: United States Pharmacopeial Convention, Inc., 1988.

USP Dispensing Information 1989, 9th ed., Vol. 1, *Drug Information for the Health Care Provider*. Rockville, Maryland: United States Pharmacopeial Convention, 1989.

Utian, W. H., *Menopause in Modern Perspective*. New York: Appleton-Century-Crofts, 1980.

Wartak, J., *Drug Dosage and Administration*. Baltimore: University Park Press, 1983.

Worley, R. J., ed., *Clinical Obstetrics and Gynecology*, Vol. 24, No. 1: *Menopause*. Hagerstown, Maryland: Harper & Row, 1981.

Index

This index contains all the brand and generic drug names included in Section Three and the names and alternative names of the disorders and conditions for which drug management is described in Section Two.

Brand names of drugs appear in italic type and are capitalized.

Each brand name is followed by the generic name of its Drug Profile in Section Three.

The symbol [CD] indicates that the brand name represents a combination drug that contains the generic drug components listed below it. To be fully familiar with any combination drug [CD], it is necessary to read the Drug Profile of each of the components listed. The brand name of a combination drug *may* or *may not* appear in the brand name list of each Drug Profile that is cited in the index as a component of a particular combination drug. The index listing of component drugs for any combination drug product represents the manufacturer's formulation of that brand at the time this information was compiled for publication.

The symbol ✦ before the brand name of a combination drug indicates that the brand name is used in both the United States and Canada, but that the ingredients in the combination product in each country differ. The Canadian drug is marked with the symbol ✦ to distinguish it from the American drug which has the same name.

A generic name with no page designation indicates an active component of a combination drug for which there is no Profile in Section Three. It is included to alert you to its presence, should you wish to consult your physician regarding its significance.

*The symbol [CD] indicates that the brand name given is a combination drug consisting of generic drug components listed below it. If there is no page numbering following the name of the generic drug component, there is no Drug Profile for that ingredient in this book.

*The symbol [CD] indicates that the brand name given is a combination drug consisting of generic drug components listed below it. If there is no page numbering following the name of the generic drug component, there is no Drug Profile for that ingredient in this book.

*The symbol [CD] indicates that the brand name given is a combination drug consisting of generic drug components listed below it. If there is no page numbering following the name of the generic drug component, there is no Drug Profile for that ingredient in this book.

*The symbol [CD] indicates that the brand name given is a combination drug consisting of generic drug components listed below it. If there is no page numbering following the name of the generic drug component, there is no Drug Profile for that ingredient in this book.

*The symbol [CD] indicates that the brand name given is a combination drug consisting of generic drug components listed below it. If there is no page numbering following the name of the generic drug component, there is no Drug Profile for that ingredient in this book.

*The symbol [CD] indicates that the brand name given is a combination drug consisting of generic
drug components listed below it. If there is no page numbering following the name of the generic
drug component, there is no Drug Profile for that ingredient in this book.

*The symbol [CD] indicates that the brand name given is a combination drug consisting of generic drug components listed below it. If there is no page numbering following the name of the generic drug component, there is no Drug Profile for that ingredient in this book.

*The symbol [CD] indicates that the brand name given is a combination drug consisting of generic drug components listed below it. If there is no page numbering following the name of the generic drug component, there is no Drug Profile for that ingredient in this book.

---

*The symbol [CD] indicates that the brand name given is a combination drug consisting of generic drug components listed below it. If there is no page numbering following the name of the generic drug component, there is no Drug Profile for that ingredient in this book.

*The symbol [CD] indicates that the brand name given is a combination drug consisting of generic drug components listed below it. If there is no page numbering following the name of the generic drug component, there is no Drug Profile for that ingredient in this book.

*The symbol [CD] indicates that the brand name given is a combination drug consisting of generic drug components listed below it. If there is no page numbering following the name of the generic drug component, there is no Drug Profile for that ingredient in this book.

*The symbol [CD] indicates that the brand name given is a combination drug consisting of generic drug components listed below it. If there is no page numbering following the name of the generic drug component, there is no Drug Profile for that ingredient in this book.

About the Author

James W. Long, M.D., was born in Allentown, Pennsylvania. He received his premedical education from the University of Maryland and his medical degree from the George Washington University School of Medicine in Washington, D.C. For twenty years he was in the private practice of internal medicine in the Washington metropolitan area, and for over thirty-five years he was a member of the faculty of the George Washington University School of Medicine. He has served with the Food and Drug Administration, the National Library of Medicine, and the Bureau of Health Manpower of the National Institutes of Health. Prior to his retirement, Dr. Long was director of Health Services for the National Science Foundation in Washington. He lives in Oxford, Maryland.

Dr. Long's involvement in drug information activities includes service on the H.E.W. Task Force on Prescription Drugs, on the F.D.A. Task Force on Adverse Drug Reactions, as a delegate-at-large to the U.S. Pharmacopeial Convention, as editorial consultant for *Hospital Formulary*, as a director of the Drug Information Association, and as a member of the Toxicology Information Program Committee of the National Research Council/National Academy of Sciences. He was consultant to the Food and Drug Administration, serving as advisor to their staff on the development of patient package inserts. He is also the author of numerous articles in professional journals. *The Essential Guide to Prescription Drugs* is an outgrowth of his conviction that the general public needs and is entitled to practical drug information which is the equivalent of the professional "package insert." He believes the patient can be reasonably certain of using medications with the least risk and the greatest benefit only when the patient has all the relevant information about the drugs he or she is taking.

Schedules of Controlled Drugs*

Schedule I: Non-medicinal substances with high abuse potential and dependence liability. Used for research purposes only. Examples: heroin, marijuana, LSD. Not legally available for medicinal use by prescription.

Schedule II: Medicinal drugs in current use that have the highest abuse potential and dependence liability. Examples: opium derivatives (morphine, codeine, etc.), meperidine (Demerol), amphetamines (Dexedrine), short-acting barbiturates (Amytal, Nembutal, Seconal). A written prescription is required. Telephoned prescribing is prohibited. No refills are allowed.

Schedule III: Medicinal drugs with abuse potential and dependence liability less than Schedule II drugs but greater than Schedule IV or V drugs. Examples: codeine, hydrocodone and paregoric in combination with one or more non-narcotic drugs, some hypnotics (Doriden, Noludar), some appetite suppressants (Didrex, Tenuate, Sanorex). A telephoned prescription is permitted, to be converted to written form by the dispensing pharmacist. Prescriptions must be renewed every 6 months. Refills are limited to 5.

Schedule IV: Medicinal drugs with less abuse potential and dependence liability than Schedule III drugs. Examples: pentazocine (Talwin), propoxyphene (Darvon), all benzodiazepines (Librium, Valium, etc.), certain hypnotics (Placidyl, Noctec, Valmid, etc.). Prescription requirements are the same as for Schedule III.

Schedule V: Medicinal drugs with the lowest abuse potential and dependence liability. Examples: diphenoxylate (Lomotil), loperamide (Imodium). Drugs requiring a prescription are handled the same as any non-scheduled prescription drug. Some non-prescription drugs can be sold only with approval of the pharmacist; the buyer is required to sign a log of purchase at the time the drug is dispensed. Examples: codeine and hydrocodone in combination with other active, non-narcotic drugs, sold in preparations that contain limited quantities for control of cough and diarrhea.

*Under jurisdiction of the Controlled Substances Act of 1970.